Catheter Ablation of Cardiac Arrhythmias

Catheter Ablation of Cardiac Arrhythmias

SECOND EDITION

WITHDRAWN

Edited by

Shoei K. Stephen Huang, MD
Professor of Medicine
College of Medicine
Texas A&M University Health Science Center;
Section of Cardiac Electrophysiology and Pacing
Scott & White Heart and Vascular Institute
Scott & White Healthcare
Temple, Texas

Distinguished Chair, Professor of Medicine
College of Medicine
Tzu Chi University
Hualien, Taiwan

Mark A. Wood, MD
Professor of Medicine
Assistant Director
Cardiac Electrophysiology Laboratory
Virginia Commonwealth University Medical Center
Richmond, Virginia

ELSEVIER
SAUNDERS

ELSEVIER
SAUNDERS

1600 John F. Kennedy Blvd.
Ste 1800
Philadelphia, PA 19103-2899

CATHETER ABLATION OF CARDIAC ARRHYTHMIAS   ISBN: 978-1-4377-1368-8

Notices

Knowledge and best practice in this field are constantly changing. As new research and experience broaden our understanding, changes in research methods, professional practices, or medical treatment may become necessary.

Practitioners and researchers must always rely on their own experience and knowledge in evaluating and using any information, methods, compounds, or experiments described herein. In using such information or methods they should be mindful of their own safety and the safety of others, including parties for whom they have a professional responsibility.

With respect to any drug or pharmaceutical products identified, readers are advised to check the most current information provided (i) on procedures featured or (ii) by the manufacturer of each product to be administered, to verify the recommended dose or formula, the method and duration of administration, and contraindications. It is the responsibility of practitioners, relying on their own experience and knowledge of their patients, to make diagnoses, to determine dosages and the best treatment for each individual patient, and to take all appropriate safety precautions.

To the fullest extent of the law, neither the Publisher nor the authors, contributors, or editors assume any liability for any injury and/or damage to persons or property as a matter of products liability, negligence or otherwise, or from any use or operation of any methods, products, instructions, or ideas contained in the material herein.

Library of Congress Cataloging-in-Publication Data
Catheter ablation of cardiac arrhythmias / edited by Shoei K. Stephen Huang, Mark A. Wood. – 2nd ed.
   p. ; cm.
 Includes bibliographical references and index.
 ISBN 978-1-4377-1368-8 (hardcover)
 1. Catheter ablation. 2. Arrhythmia–Surgery. I. Huang, Shoei K. II. Wood, Mark A.
 [DNLM: 1. Tachycardia–therapy. 2. Arrhythmias, Cardiac–therapy. 3. Catheter Ablation–methods. WG 330]
 RD598.35.C39C36 2011
 617.4'12–dc22

                                           2010039806

Executive Publisher: Natasha Andjelkovic
Senior Developmental Editor: Mary Beth Murphy
Publishing Services Manager: Anne Altepeter
Team Manager: Radhika Pallamparthy
Senior Project Manager: Doug Turner
Project Manager: Preethi Kerala Varma
Designer: Steve Stave

Printed in Canada

Last digit is the print number: 9 8 7 6 5 4 3 2 1

To all the physicians, electrophysiology fellows, and friends who are interested in cardiac electrophysiology and catheter ablation as a means to treat patients with cardiac arrhythmias.

To my dearest wife, Su-Mei Kuo, for her love, support, and encouragement; my grown-up children, Priscilla, Melvin, and Jessica, for their love and inspiration; my late parents, Yu-Shih (father) and Hsing-Tzu (mother) for spiritual support.

To Pablo Denes, MD, Robert G. Hauser, MD, and Joseph S. Alpert, MD, who, as my respected mentors, have taught and inspired me.

Shoei K. Stephen Huang, MD

To my wife, Helen E. Wood, PhD, for all of her patience and love, and to our daughter, Lily Anne Fuyan Wood, who fills my life with joy.

Mark A. Wood, MD

Contributors

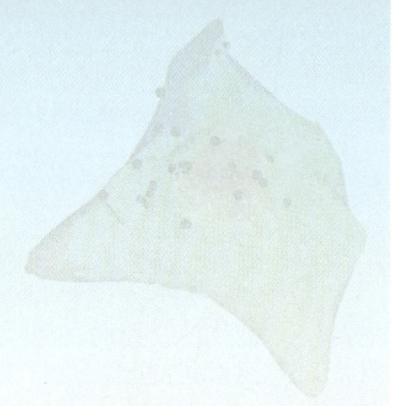

Amin Al-Ahmad, MD
Assistant Professor of Cardiovascular Medicine
Associate Director
Cardiac Arrhythmia Service;
Director
Cardiac Electrophysiology Laboratory
Stanford University Medical Center
Stanford, California

Robert H. Anderson, MD, PhD, FRCPath, FESC
Emeritus Professor of Paediatric Cardiac Morphology
London Great Ormond Street Hospital
University College
London, United Kingdom

Rishi Arora, MD
Assistant Professor of Medicine
Feinberg School of Medicine
Northwestern University
Chicago, Illinois

Nitish Badhwar, MD
Assistant Professor of Medicine
Division of Cardiology, Cardiac Electrophysiology
University of California, San Francisco
San Francisco, California

Javier E. Banchs, MD
Assistant Professor of Medicine
Penn State Hershey Heart & Vascular Institute
Penn State College of Medicine
Hershey, Pennsylvania

Juan Benezet-Mazuecos, MD
Arrhythmia Unit
Department of Cardiology
Fundación Jiménez Díaz-Capio
Universidad Autónoma de Madrid
Madrid, Spain

Deepak Bhakta, MD
Associate Professor of Clinical Medicine
Krannert Institute of Cardiology
School of Medicine
Indiana University
Indianapolis, Indiana

Eric Buch, MD
Assistant Professor of Medicine
Clinical Cardiac Electrophysiology;
Director
Specialized Program for Atrial Fibrillation
UCLA Cardiac Arrhythmia Center
David Geffen School of Medicine at UCLA
Los Angeles, California

José A. Cabrera, MD, PhD
Chief of Cardiology
Department of Cardiology
Hospital Quirón Pozuelo de Alarcón
Madrid, Spain

Hugh Calkins, MD
Professor of Medicine
Director of Electrophysiology
Johns Hopkins Medical Institutions
Johns Hopkins Hospital
Baltimore, Maryland

David J. Callans, AB, MD
Professor of Medicine
Department of Cardiology;
Director
Electrophysiology Laboratory
Department of Cardiology
Hospital of the University of Pennsylvania
Philadelphia, Pennsylvania

Shih-Lin Chang, MD
Division of Cardiology
Department of Medicine
National Yang-Ming University School of Medicine
Taipei Veterans General Hospital
Taipei, Taiwan

Henry Chen, MD
Stanford Hospital and Clinics
East Bay Cardiology Medical Group
San Pablo, California

Shih-Ann Chen, MD
Professor of Medicine
Division of Cardiology
Department of Medicine
National Yang-Ming University School of Medicine
Taipei Veterans General Hospital
Taipei, Taiwan

Thomas Crawford, MD
Lecturer
Division of Cardiovascular Medicine
University of Michigan
Ann Arbor, Michigan

Mithilesh K. Das, MBBS
Associate Professor of Clinical Medicine
Krannert Institute of Cardiology
School of Medicine
Indiana University
Indianapolis, Indiana

Sanjay Dixit, MD
Assistant Professor of Cardiovascular Division
Hospital of the University of Pennsylvania
Philadelphia, Pennsylvania

Shephal K. Doshi, MD
Director
Cardiac Electrophysiology
Pacific Heart Institute
St. Johns Health Center
Santa Monica, California

Marc Dubuc, MD, FRCPC, FACC
Staff Cardiologist and Clinical Electrophysiologist
Montreal Heart Institute;
Associate Professor of Medicine
Faculty of Medicine
University of Montreal
Montreal, Quebec, Canada

Srinivas Dukkipati, MD
Assistant Professor of Medicine
Mount Sinai School of Medicine
New York, New York

Sabine Ernst, MD, PhD
Consultant Cardiologist
Royal Brompton and Harefield NHS Foundation Trust;
Honorary Senior Lecturer
National Heart and Lung Institute
Imperial College
London, United Kingdom

Jerónimo Farré, MD, PhD, FESC
Professor of Cardiology and Chairman
Department of Cardiology
Fundación Jiménez Diaz-Capio
Universidad Autónoma de Madrid
Madrid, Spain

Gregory K. Feld, MD
Professor of Medicine
Department of Medicine;
Director
Electrophysiology Program
San Diego Medical Center
University of California, San Diego
San Diego, California

Westby G. Fisher, MD, FACC
Assistant Professor of Medicine
Feinberg School of Medicine;
Director
Cardiac Electrophysiology
Evanston Northwestern Healthcare
Northwestern University
Evanston, Illinois

Andrei Forclaz, MD
Physician
Hôpital Cardiologique du Haut Lévèque
Université Victor Segalen (Bordeaux II)
Bordeaux, France

Mario D. Gonzalez, MD, PhD
Professor of Medicine
Penn State Heart & Vascular Institute
Penn State University
Hershey, Pennsylvania

David E. Haines, MD
Professor
Oakland University-Beaumont Hospital
   School of Medicine;
Chairman
Department of Cardiovascular Medicine;
Director
Heart Rhythm Center
William Beaumont Hospital
Royal Oak, Michigan

Michel Haïssaguerre, MD
Professor of Cardiology
Hôpital Cardiologique du Haut Lévèque
Université Victor Segalen (Bordeaux II)
Bordeaux, France

Haris M. Haqqani, PhD, MBBS(Hons)
Senior Electrophysiology Fellow
Section of Electrophysiology
Division of Cardiology
University of Pennsylvania Health System
Philadelphia, Pennsylvania

Satoshi Higa, MD, PhD
Second Department of Internal Medicine
Faculty of Medicine
University of the Ryukyus
Okinawa, Japan

Mélèze Hocini, MD
Physician
Hôpital Cardiologique du Haut Lévèque
Université Victor Segalen (Bordeaux II)
Bordeaux, France

Bobbi Hoppe, MD
Cardiologist
Cardiovascular Consultants, Ltd
Minneapolis, Minnesota

Henry H. Hsia, MD
Associate Professor of Medicine
School of Medicine
Stanford University
Stanford, California

Lynne Hung, MD
Cardiac Electrophysiologist
Mission Internal Medical Group
Mission Viejo, California

Amir Jadidi, MD
Physician
Hôpital Cardiologique du Haut Lévèque
Université Victor Segalen (Bordeaux II)
Bordeaux, France

Pierre Jaïs, MD
Physician
Hôpital Cardiologique du Haut Lévèque
Université Victor Segalen (Bordeaux II)
Bordeaux, France

Alan Kadish, MD
Professor of Medicine
Northwestern University
Chicago, Illinois

Jonathan M. Kalman, MBBS, PhD
Professor of Medicine
Department of Cardiology
University of Melbourne;
Director of Cardiac Electrophysiology
The Royal Melbourne Hospital
Melbourne, Australia

David Keane, MD, PhD
Cardiac Electrophysiologist
Cardiac Arrhythmia Service
St. James's Hospital
Dublin, Ireland

Paul Khairy, MD, PhD
Research Director
Boston Adult Congenital Heart (BACH) Service
Harvard University
Boston, Massachusetts;
Associate Professor of Medicine
University of Montreal;
Director, Adult Congenital Heart Center
Canada Research Chair, Electrophysiology and Adult
    Congenital Heart Disease
Montreal Heart Institute Montreal, Quebec, Canada

George J. Klein, MD, FRCP(C)
Professor of Medicine
Division of Cardiology
Department of Medicine
University of Western Ontario and University Hospital
London, Ontario, Canada

Sebastien Knecht, MD
Physician
Hôpital Cardiologique du Haut Lévèque
Université Victor Segalen (Bordeaux II)
Bordeaux, France

Andrew D. Krahn, MD
Professor
Division of Cardiology
Department of Medicine
University of Western Ontario
London, Ontario, Canada

Ling-Ping Lai, MD
Professor of Medicine
College of Medicine
National Taiwan University
Taipei, Taiwan

Byron K. Lee, MD
Assistant Professor of Medicine
Division of Cardiology, Cardiac Electrophysiology
University of California Medical Center
University of California School of Medicine
San Francisco, California

Bruce B. Lerman, MD
H. Altshul Professor of Medicine
Division of Cardiology;
Chief, Division of Cardiology
Director of the Cardiac Electrophysiology Laboratory
Cornell University Medical Center
New York Presbyterian Hospital
New York, New York

David Lin, MD
Assistant Professor of Medicine
Department of Medicine
Attending Physician;
Medicine/Cardiac Electrophysiology
Hospital of the University of Pennsylvania
Philadelphia, Pennsylvania

Kuo-Hung Lin, MD
Instructor of Medicine
College of Medicine
China Medical University
Taichung, Taiwan

Yenn-Jiang Lin, MD
Division of Cardiology
Department of Medicine
National Yang-Ming University School of Medicine
Taipei Veterans General Hospital
Taipei, Taiwan

Nick Linton, MEng MRCP
Physician
Hôpital Cardiologique du Haut Lévèque
Université Victor Segalen (Bordeaux II)
Bordeaux, France

Li-Wei Lo, MD
Division of Cardiology
Department of Medicine
National Yang-Ming University School of Medicine
Taipei Veterans General Hospital
Taipei, Taiwan

Francis E. Marchlinski, MD
Professor of Medicine
School of Medicine
University of Pennsylvania;
Director of Electrophysiology
Hospital of the University of Pennsylvania
Philadelphia, Pennsylvania

Steven M. Markowitz, MD
Associate Professor of Medicine
Division of Cardiology
New York Presbyterian Hospital
Cornell University Medical Center
New York, New York

John M. Miller, MD
Professor of Medicine
Indiana University School of Medicine
Director, Clinical Cardiac Electrophysiology
Clarian Health Partners
Indianapolis, Indiana

Shinsuke Miyazaki, MD
Surgeon
Hôpital Cardiologique du Haut-Lévèque
Université Victor Segalen (Bordeaux II)
Bordeaux, France

Joseph B. Morton, PhD, MBBS, FRACP
Department of Cardiology
The Royal Melbourne Hospital
Melbourne, Australia

Isabelle Nault, MD
Cardiologist and Electrophysiologist
Hôpital Cardiologique du Haut Lévèque
Université Victor Segalen (Bordeaux II)
Bordeaux, France

Akihiko Nogami, MD, PhD
Clinical Professor
Department of Cardiology
Tokyo Medical and Dental University
Bunkyo, Tokyo;
Chief of Cardiac Electrophysiology Laboratory
Cardiology Division;
Director of Coronary Care Unit
Cardiology Division
Yokohama Rosai Hospital
Yokohama, Japan

Jeffrey E. Olgin, MD
Professor in Residence
Cardiac Electrophysiology
Division of Cardiology
Department of Medicine
Chief Cardiac Electrophysiology
University of California, San Francisco
San Francisco, California

Hakan Oral, MD
Associate Professor
Director, Cardiac Electrophysiology
University of Michigan
Ann Arbor, Michigan

Basilios Petrellis, MB, BS, FRACP
Consultant, Arrhythmia Service
University of Toronto
St. Michael's Hospital
Toronto, Ontario, Canada

Vivek Y. Reddy, MD
Professor of Medicine
Mount Sinai School of Medicine
New York, New York

Jaime Rivera, MD
Cardiac Electrophysiologist
Director of Cardiac Electrophysiology
Instituto Nacional de Ciencias Medicas y Nutricion
Hospital Médica Sur
Mexico City, Mexico

Alexander S. Ro, MD
Clinical Instructor, Electrophysiology
Northwestern University;
Director
Cardiac Device Therapies
Department of Electrophysiology
Evanston Northwestern Healthcare
Evanston, Illinois

Raphael Rosso, MD
Senior Electrophysiologist
Department of Cardiology
The Royal Melbourne Hospital
Melbourne, Australia

José M. Rubio, MD, PhD
Associate Professor of Cardiology
Director of the Arrhythmia Unit
Department of Cardiology
Fundación Jiménez Díaz-Capio
Universidad Autónoma de Madrid
Madrid, Spain

Damián Sánchez-Quintana, MD, PhD
Chair Professor of Anatomy
Department of Anatomy and Cell Biology
Universidad de Extremadura
Badajoz, Spain

Prashanthan Sanders, MD
Professor
Hôpital Cardiologique du Haut Lévèque
Université Victor Segalen (Bordeaux II)
Bordeaux, France

J. Philip Saul, MD, FACC
Professor of Pediatrics
Director, Pediatric Cardiology
Department of Pediatrics
Medical University of South Carolina
Charleston, South Carolina

Mauricio Scanavacca, MD, PhD
Assistant Professor
Department of Cardiology
Heart Institute (INCOR)
São Paulo Medical School
São Paulo, Brazil

Ashok Shah, MD
Physician
Hôpital Cardiologique du Haut Lévèque
Université Victor Segalen (Bordeaux II)
Bordeaux, France

Kalyanam Shivkumar, MD, PhD
Professor of Medicine & Radiology
Director, UCLA Cardiac Arrhythmia Center
 and EP Programs
David Geffen School of Medicine at UCLA
Los Angeles, California

Allan C. Skanes, MD
Associate Professor
Division of Cardiology
Department of Medicine
University of Western Ontario
London, Ontario, Canada

Kyoko Soejima, MD
Assistant Professor
Department of Cardiology
St. Marianna University School of Medicine
Kawasaki Municipal Hospital
Kawasaki, Japan

Eduardo Sosa, MD, PhD
Associate Professor
Director of Clinical Arrythmia and Pacemaker Units
Heart Institute (INCOR)
São Paulo Medical School
São Paulo, Brazil

Uma Srivatsa, MD
Assistant Professor of Medicine
Division of Cardiology
University of California Davis Medical Center
Sacramento, California

Ching-Tai Tai, MD
Professor of Medicine
Division of Cardiology
Department of Medicine
National Yang-Ming University School of Medicine
Taipei Veterans General Hospital
Taipei, Taiwan

Taresh Taneja, MD
Assistant Professor of Medicine
Cardiology
Scott & White Healthcare
Texas A&M Health Sciences Center
Temple, Texas

Mintu Turakhia, MD, MAS
Director of Cardiac Electrophysiology
Palo Alto VA Health Care System;
Investigator
Center for Health Care Evaluation;
Instructor of Medicine (Cardiovascular Medicine)
School of Medicine
Stanford University
Stanford, California

George F. Van Hare, MD
Professor of Pediatrics
School of Medicine
Washington University;
Director of Pediatric Cardiology
St. Louis Children's Hospital
St. Louis, Missouri

Edward P. Walsh, MD
Chief, Electrophysiology Division
Department of Cardiology
Children's Hospital Boston;
Professor of Pediatrics
Harvard Medical School
Boston, Massachusetts

Paul J. Wang, MD
School of Medicine
Stanford University
Stanford, California

Matthew Wright, PhD, MRCP
Cardiac Electrophysiology
Academic Clinical Lecturer
Rayne Institute
Department of Cardiology
St. Thomas' Hospital
London, United Kingdom;
EP Fellow
Hôpital Cardiologique du Haut Lévèque
Université Victor Segalen (Bordeaux II)
Bordeaux, France

Anil V. Yadav, MD
Associate Professor of Clinical Medicine
Krannert Institute of Cardiology
Indiana University School of Medicine
Indianapolis, Indiana

Raymond Yee, MD
Professor
Department of Medicine
University of Western Ontario;
Director
Department of Cardiology, Arrhythmias Services
London Health Sciences Center
London, Ontario, Canada

Paul C. Zei, MD, PhD
Clinical Associate Professor
Cardiac Electrophysiology Service
School of Medicine
Stanford University
Stanford, California

Preface

"Art is never finished, only abandoned."

Leonardo da Vinci

So it is with textbooks as well. Textbooks are inherently dated when they appear, especially in the era of electronic media. No sooner are the latest revisions for a chapter sent for typesetting than an important new article is published, a more illustrative figure appears, or a better phrasing for a passage is conceived. At some point and reluctantly, the revisions must be abandoned and the pages printed. Further amendments must await the next edition. Therefore, the nature of a textbook is based less on being the most current source than on being a permanent record. To be useful, the book's content should comprise enduring concepts and involatile knowledge. This principle underlies the philosophy for this book.

The first edition of this book was a fusion of purposes by the editors. Through his seminal work, Dr. Shoei K. Stephen Huang first demonstrated the vast scope of cardiac catheter ablation by publishing the original textbook on the subject in 1995. My own vision for the book began with a binder of handwritten notes, sketches, and copies of important publications that stayed "at bedside" within the electrophysiology laboratory. This rough collection served as a reference for critical values, algorithms, and information that always seemed beyond my memory. Conceived from these two necessities—the need to organize the vast literature on catheter ablation and the need for ready access to specific information—the publication of this book continues with the second edition.

To serve these purposes, we have placed a premium on organization and consistency throughout the book. The content is selected to facilitate catheter ablation before and during the procedure. The scope of the book is not intended to include the global management of arrhythmia patients.

We have retained the unique chapter format of the first edition. This includes the consistent organization and content among chapters. We have made liberal use of tables to summarize key points, diagnostic criteria, differential diagnosis, targets for ablation, and troubleshooting of difficult cases for each arrhythmia. In response to readers' feedback from the first edition, we have expanded the descriptions of catheter manipulation techniques for mapping and ablation of most arrhythmias and have paid particular attention to the completeness of the troubleshooting sections that have been widely acclaimed. In addition to the revisions and updates of each chapter, new chapters have been added to reflect the latest approaches to atrial fibrillation ablation. An emphasis has been placed on illustrative figures and their high quality reproduction.

We have striven to make the book useful to practitioners of ablation at all levels of experience. For those in training, the fundamentals of anatomy, pathophysiology, mapping, and catheter manipulation are presented. For more seasoned practitioners, the concepts of advanced mapping and troubleshooting are organized for easy access. We envision practitioners consulting the book in preparation for a procedure and keeping the book at bedside in the electrophysiology laboratory for reference. Finally, new to this second edition is online access to all the figures and tables in the book, as well as videos that supplement the text.

It is our sincerest hope that this book will be a valuable part of every electrophysiology laboratory. We have tried to build on the success of the first edition and always value reader comments, criticisms, and suggestions to improve future editions.

Mark A. Wood, MD
Shoei K. Stephen Huang, MD
August 31, 2010

Acknowledgments

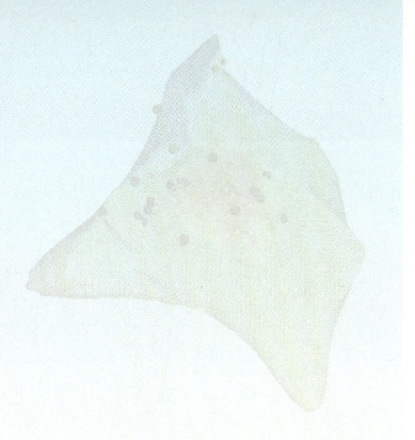

I offer my sincerest thanks to all the contributors to this textbook. Each is recognized as a leading expert in the field of catheter ablation. The vast time required to prepare each chapter is an act of dedication made by every author. Special thanks go to my department chairmen, Drs. George Vetrovec and Kenneth Ellenbogen, for providing the academic freedom to prepare the second edition of this textbook. I also thank Elsevier for their commitment to produce a book true to the editors' visions. Most importantly, I must recognize each of my colleagues at Virginia Commonwealth University Medical Center—Dr. Kenneth Ellenbogen, Dr. Richard Shepard, Dr. Gauthum Kalahasty, Dr. Jordana Kron, Dr. Jose Huizar, and Dr. Karoly Kaszala—for the support they have given me through this endeavor and all my absences. I can never repay their kindness.

Mark A. Wood, MD

I thank all the contributing authors for their efforts, allowing the second edition of this book to successfully publish on time. Many of them contributed to the first edition and kindly updated their chapters. I particularly thank those new authors for their incredible accomplishment. My special thanks go to Elsevier executive publisher, Natasha Andjelkovic; senior developmental editor, Mary Beth Murphy; senior project manager, Doug Turner; and the many other co-workers at Elsevier who devoted their efforts in such a professional manner to bring this book to completion. Finally, I need to give my sincerest thanks to my co-editor and dearest friend, Dr. Mark Wood, who devoted invaluable time and effort to this book.

Shoei K. Stephen Huang, MD

Contents

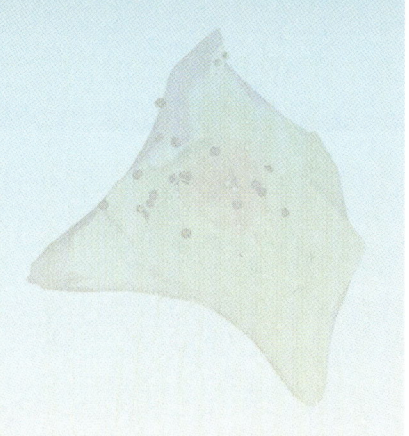

Fundamental Concepts
of Transcatheter Energy
Applications

1

Biophysics of Radiofrequency Lesion Formation

David E. Haines

Key Points

Radiofrequency (RF) energy induces thermal lesion formation through resistive heating of myocardial tissue. Tissue temperatures of 50°C or higher are necessary for irreversible injury.

Under controlled conditions, RF lesion size is directly proportional to delivered power, electrode-tissue interface temperature, electrode diameter, and contact pressure.

Power density declines with the square of distance from the source and tissue temperature declines inversely with distance from the heat source.

The ultimate RF lesion size is determined by the zone of acute necrosis as well as the region of microvascular injury.

Electrode cooling reduces the efficiency of tissue heating. For a fixed energy delivery, blood flow over the electrode-tissue interface reduces lesion size by convective tissue cooling. Cooled ablation increases lesion size by increasing the power that can be delivered before limiting electrode temperatures are achieved.

When Huang and colleagues first introduced radiofrequency (RF) catheter ablation in 1985[1] as a potentially useful modality for the management of cardiac arrhythmias,[2] few would have predicted its meteoric rise. In the past two decades, it has become one of the most useful and widely employed therapies in the field of cardiac electrophysiology. RF catheter ablation has enjoyed a high efficacy and safety profile, and indications for its use continue to expand. Improvements in catheter design have continued to enhance the operator's ability to target the arrhythmogenic substrate, and modifications in RF energy delivery and electrode design have resulted in more effective energy coupling to the tissue. It is likely that most operators view RF catheter ablation as a "black box" in that once the target is acquired, they need only push the button on the RF generator. However, gaining insight into the biophysics of RF energy delivery and the mechanisms of tissue injury in response to this intervention will help the clinician optimize catheter ablation and ultimately may enhance its efficacy and safety.

Biophysics of Tissue Heating

Resistive Heating

RF energy is a form of alternating electrical current that generates a lesion in the heart by electrical heating of the myocardium. A common form of RF ablation found in the medical environment is the electrocautery employed for tissue cutting and coagulation during surgical procedures. The goal of catheter ablation with RF energy is to effectively transform electromagnetic energy into thermal energy in the tissue and destroy the arrhythmogenic tissues by heating them to a lethal temperature. The mode of tissue heating by RF energy is resistive (electrical) heating. As electrical current passes through a resistive medium, the voltage drops, and heat is produced (similar to the heat that is created in an incandescent light bulb). The RF electrical current is typically delivered in a unipolar fashion with completion of the circuit through an indifferent electrode placed on the skin. Typically, an oscillation frequency of 500 kHz is selected. Lower frequencies are more likely to stimulate cardiac muscle and nerves, resulting in arrhythmia generation and pain sensation. Higher frequencies will result in tissue heating, but in the megahertz range the mode of energy transfer changes from electrical (resistive) heating to dielectric heating (as observed with microwave energy). With very high frequencies, conventional electrode catheters become less effective at transferring the electromagnetic energy to the tissue, and complex and expensive catheter "antenna" designs must be employed.[3]

Resistive heat production within the tissue is proportional to the RF power density and that, in turn, is proportional to the square of the current density (Table 1-1). When RF energy is delivered in a unipolar fashion, the current distributes radially from the source. The current density decreases in proportion to the square of the

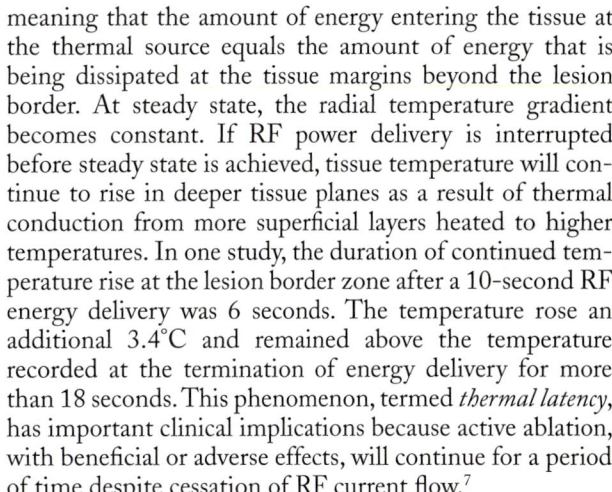

TABLE 1-1

EQUATIONS DESCRIBING BIOPHYSICS OF RADIOFREQUENCY ABLATION

$V = I\,R$	Ohm's law: V, voltage; I, current; R, resistance
Power $= V\,I\,(\cos \acute{\alpha})$	Cos $\acute{\alpha}$ represents the phase shift between voltage (V) and current (I) in alternating current
Current density $= I/4\,\pi\,r^2$	I, total electrode current; r, distance from electrode center
$H \approx p\,I^2/16\,\pi^2\,r^4$	H, heat production per unit volume of tissue; p, tissue resistivity; I, current; r, distance from the electrode center
$T\,(t) = T_{ss} + (T_{initial} - T_{ss})e^{-t/\tau}$	Monoexponential relationship between tissue temperature (T) and duration of radiofrequency energy delivery (t): $T_{initial}$, starting tissue temperature; T_{ss}, tissue temperature at steady state; τ, time constant
$r/r_i = (t_o - T)/(t - T)$	Relationship between tissue temperature and distance from heat source in ideal system: r, distance from center of heat source; r_i, radius of heat source; t_o, temperature at electrode tissue interface; T, basal tissue temperature; t, temperature at radius r

distance from the RF electrode source. Thus, direct resistive heating of the tissue decreases proportionally with the distance from the electrode to the fourth power (Fig. 1-1). As a result, only the narrow rim of tissue in close contact with the catheter electrode (2 to 3 mm) is heated directly. All heating of deeper tissue layers occurs passively through heat conduction.[4] If higher power levels are used, the depth of direct resistive heating will increase, and the volume and radius of the virtual heat source will increase as well.

Thermal Conduction

Most of the tissue heating resulting in lesion formation during RF catheter ablation occurs as a result of thermal conduction from the direct resistive heat source. Transfer of heat through tissue follows basic thermodynamic principles and is represented by the bioheat transfer equation.[5] The tissue temperature change with increasing distance from the heat source is called the *radial temperature gradient*. At onset of RF energy delivery, the temperature is very high at the source of heating and falls off rapidly over a short distance (Fig 1.1 and **Videos 1-1 and 1-2**). As time progresses, more thermal energy is transferred to deeper tissue layers by means of thermal conduction. The rise of tissue temperature at any given distance from the heat source increases in a monoexponential fashion over time. Sites close to the heat source have a rapid rise in temperature (a short half-time of temperature rise), whereas sites remote from the source heat up more slowly.[6] Eventually, the entire electrode-tissue system reaches steady state,

meaning that the amount of energy entering the tissue at the thermal source equals the amount of energy that is being dissipated at the tissue margins beyond the lesion border. At steady state, the radial temperature gradient becomes constant. If RF power delivery is interrupted before steady state is achieved, tissue temperature will continue to rise in deeper tissue planes as a result of thermal conduction from more superficial layers heated to higher temperatures. In one study, the duration of continued temperature rise at the lesion border zone after a 10-second RF energy delivery was 6 seconds. The temperature rose an additional 3.4°C and remained above the temperature recorded at the termination of energy delivery for more than 18 seconds. This phenomenon, termed *thermal latency*, has important clinical implications because active ablation, with beneficial or adverse effects, will continue for a period of time despite cessation of RF current flow.[7]

Because the mechanism of tissue injury in response to RF ablation is thermal, the final peak temperature at the border zone of the ablative lesion should be relatively constant. Experimental studies predict this temperature with hyperthermic ablation to be about 50°C.[3] This is called the *isotherm of irreversible tissue injury*. The point at which the radial temperature gradient crosses the 50°C isothermal line defines the lesion radius in that dimension. One may predict the three-dimensional temperature gradients with thermodynamic modeling and finite element analysis and by doing so can predict the anticipated lesion dimensions and geometry with the 50°C isotherm. In an idealized medium of uniform thermal conduction without convective heat loss, a number of relationships can be defined using boundary conditions when a steady-state radial temperature gradient is achieved. In this theoretical model, it is predicted that radial temperature gradient is inversely proportional to the distance from the heat source. The 50°C isotherm boundary (lesion radius) increases in distance from the source in direct proportion to the temperature at that source. It was predicted, then demonstrated experimentally, that in the absence of significant heat loss due to convective cooling, the lesion depth and diameter are best predicted by the electrode-tissue interface temperature.[4] In the clinical setting, however, the opposing effects of convective cooling by circulating blood flow diminish the value of electrode-tip temperature monitoring to assess lesion size.

The idealized thermodynamic model of catheter ablation by tissue heating predicted, then demonstrated, that the radius of the lesion is directly proportional to the radius of the heat source (Fig. 1-2).[8] When one considers the virtual heat source radius as the shell of direct resistive heating in tissue contiguous to the electrode, it is not surprising that larger electrode diameter, length, and contact area all result in a larger source radius and larger lesion size, and that this may result in enhanced procedural success. Higher power delivery not only increases the source temperature but also increases the radius of the heat source, thereby increasing lesion size in two ways. These theoretical means of increasing efficacy of RF catheter ablation have been realized in the clinical setting with large-tip catheters and cooled-tip catheters.[9–11]

The relationship of ablation catheter distance from the ablation target to the power requirements for clinical effect

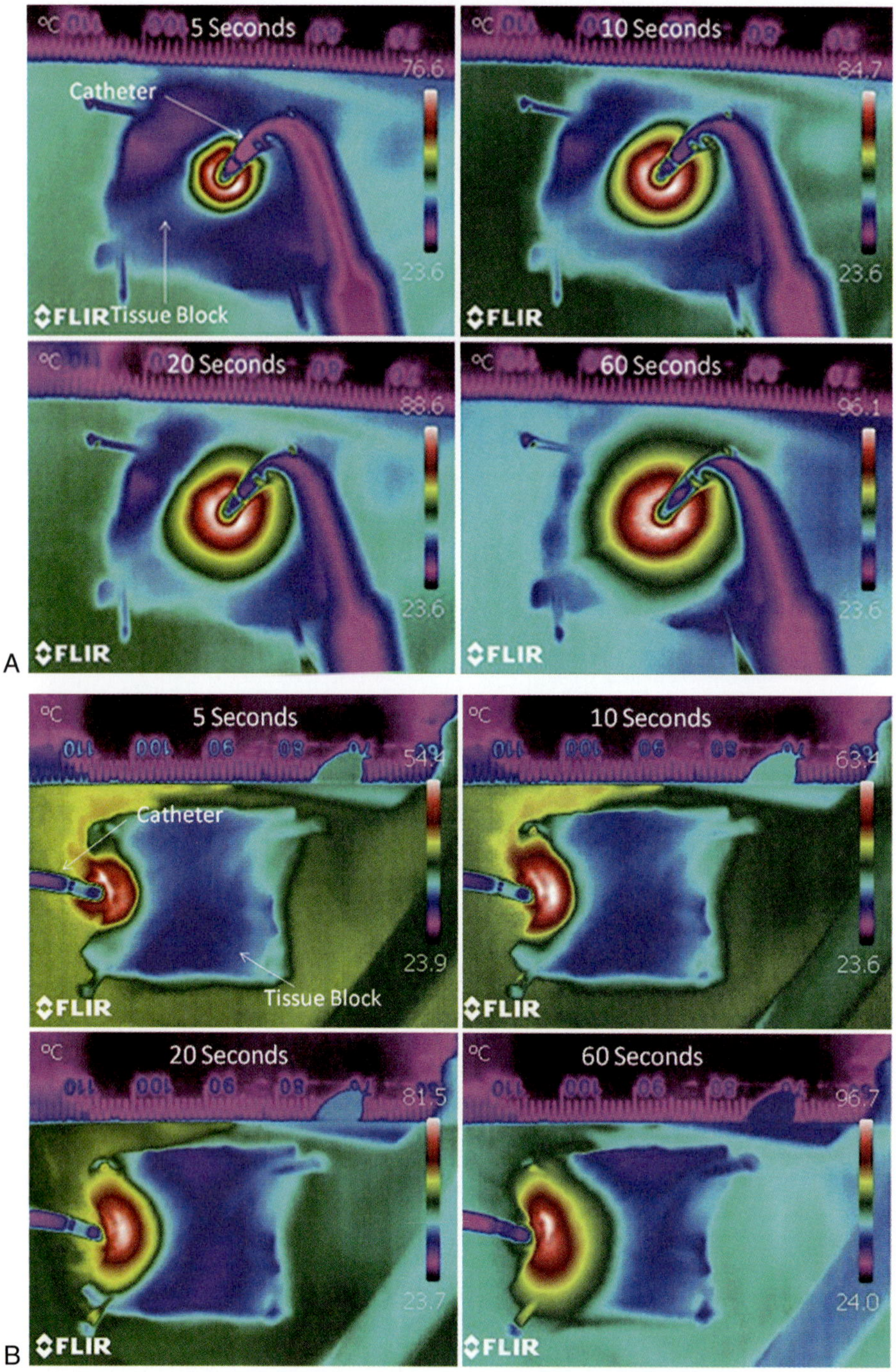

FIGURE 1-1. Infrared thermal imaging of tissue heating during radiofrequency ablation with a closed irrigation catheter. Power is delivered at 30 W to blocks of porcine myocardium in a tissue bath. The surface of the tissue is just above the fluid level to permit thermal imaging of tissue and not the fluid. Temperature scale (*right*) and a millimeter scale (*top*) are shown in each panel. **A,** Viewed from the surface, there is radial heating of the tissue from the electrode. **B,** Tissue heating visualized in cross section. The electrode is partially submerged in the fluid bath and perpendicular to the upper edge of the tissue. In both cases, very high tissue temperatures (>96°C) are achieved at 60 seconds because of the absence of fluid flow over the tissue surface.

were tested in a Langendorff-perfused canine heart preparation. Catheter ablation of the right bundle branch was attempted at varying distances, and while delivered, power was increased in a stepwise fashion. The RF power required to block right bundle branch conduction increased exponentially with increasing distance from the catheter. At a distance of 4 mm, most RF energy deliveries reached the threshold of impedance rise before block was achieved.

When pulsatile flow was streamed past the ablation electrode, the power requirements to cause block increased fourfold.[12] Thus, the efficiency of heating diminished with cooling from circulating blood, and small increases in distances from the ablation target corresponded with large increases in ablation power requirements, emphasizing the importance of optimal targeting for successful catheter ablation.

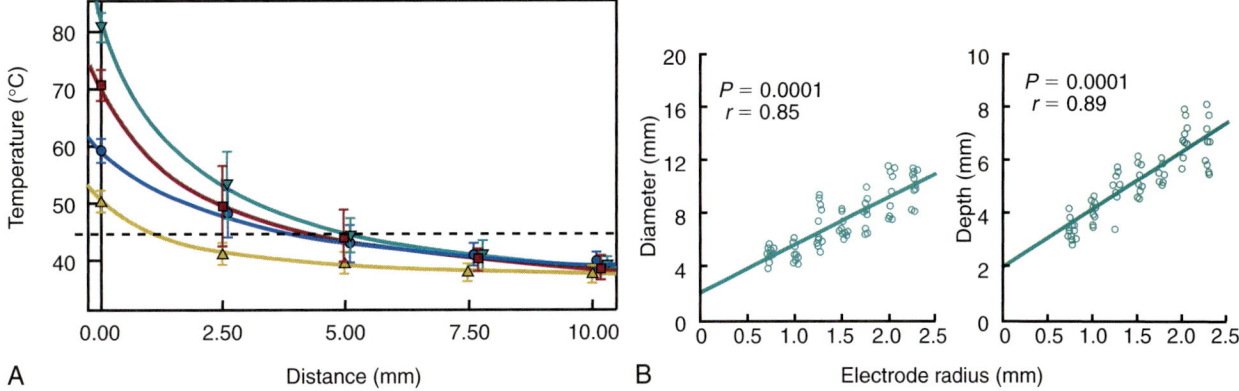

FIGURE 1-2. A, Radial temperature gradients measured during in vitro catheter ablation with source temperatures varying from 50° to 80°C. The tissue temperature falls in an inverse proportion to distance. The *dashed line* represents the 50°C isothermal line. The point at which the radial temperature gradient crosses the 50°C isotherm determines the boundary of the lesion. A higher source temperature results in a greater lesion depth. **B,** Lesion depth and diameter are compared to the electrode radius in temperature feedback power controlled radiofrequency ablation. A larger-diameter ablation electrode results in higher power delivery and a proportional increase in lesion dimension. *(From Haines DE, Watson DD, Verow AF. Electrode radius predicts lesion radius during radiofrequency energy heating: validation of a proposed thermodynamic model.* Circ Res. *1990;67:124–129. With permission.)*

Sudden Impedance Rise

In a uniform medium, the steady-state radial temperature gradient should continue to shift deeper into the medium as the source temperature increases. A very high source temperature, therefore, should theoretically yield a very deep 50°C isotherm temperature and, in turn, very large ablative lesions. Unfortunately, this process is limited in the biologic setting by the formation of coagulum and char at the electrode-tissue interface if temperatures exceed 100°C. At 100°C, blood literally begins to boil. This can be observed in the clinical setting with generation of showers of microbubbles if tissue heating is excessive.[13] As the blood and tissue in contact with the electrode catheter desiccate, the residue of denatured proteins adheres to the electrode surface. These substances are electrically insulating and result in a smaller electrode surface area available for electrical conduction. In turn, the same magnitude of power is concentrated over a smaller surface area, and the power density increases. With higher power density, the heat production increases, and more coagulum forms. Thus, in a positive-feedback fashion, the electrode becomes completely encased in coagulum within 1 to 2 seconds. In a study testing ablation with a 2-mm-tip electrode in vitro and in vivo, a measured temperature of at least 100°C correlated closely with a sudden rise in electrical impedance (Fig. 1-3).[14] Modern RF energy ablation systems all have an automatic energy cutoff if a rapid rise in electrical impedance is observed. Some experimenters have described soft thrombus that accumulates when temperatures exceed 80°C.[15] This is likely due to blood protein denaturation and accumulation, but fortunately appears to be more of a laboratory phenomenon than one observed in the clinical setting. When high temperatures and sudden rises in electrical impedance are observed, there is concern about the accumulation of char and coagulum, with the subsequent risk for char embolism. Anticoagulation and antiplatelet therapies have been proposed as preventative measures,[16] but avoidance of excessive heating at the electrode-tissue interface remains the best strategy to avoid this risk.

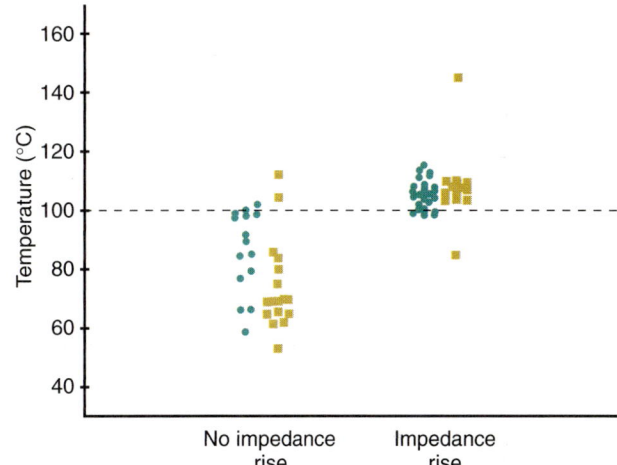

FIGURE 1-3. The association of measured electrode-tip temperature and sudden rise in electrical impedance is shown in this study of radiofrequency catheter ablation with a 2-mm-tip ablation electrode in vitro (*blue circles*) and in vivo (*yellow squares*). The peak temperature recorded at the electrode-tissue interface is shown. Almost all ablations without a sudden rise in electrical impedance had a peak temperature of 100°C or less, whereas all but one ablation manifesting a sudden rise in electrical impedance had peak temperatures of 100°C or more. *(From Haines DE, Verow AF. Observations on electrode-tissue interface temperature and effect on electrical impedance during radiofrequency ablation of ventricular myocardium.* Circulation. *1990;82:1034–1038. With permission.)*

Convective Cooling

The major thermodynamic factor opposing the transfer of thermal energy to deeper tissue layers is convective cooling. Convection is the process whereby heat is distributed through a medium rapidly by active mixing of that medium. With the case of RF catheter ablation, the heat is produced by resistive heating and transferred to deeper layers by thermal conduction. Simultaneously, the heat is conducted back into the circulating blood pool and metal electrode tip. Because the blood is moving rapidly past the electrode and over the endocardial surface, and because water (the main constituent of blood) has a high heat capacity, a large amount of the heat produced at the site of ablation can be carried away by the blood. Convective cooling is such an important factor that it dominates the thermodynamics of catheter ablation.[17] Efficiency of energy coupling to the tissue can be as low as 10%, depending on electrode size, catheter stability, and position relative to intracavitary blood flow.[18] Unstable, sliding catheter contact results in significant tip cooling and decreased efficiency of tissue heating.[19] This is most often observed with ablation along the tricuspid or mitral valve annuli.

Paradoxically, the convective cooling phenomenon has been used to increase lesion size. As noted earlier, maximal power delivery during RF ablation is limited by the occurrence of boiling and coagulum formation at the electrode tip. However, if the tip is cooled, a higher magnitude of power may be delivered without a sudden rise in electrical impedance. The higher magnitude of power increases the depth of direct resistive heating and, in turn, increases the radius of the effective heat source. In addition, higher temperatures are achieved 3 to 4 mm below the surface, and the entire radial temperature curve is shifted to a higher temperature over greater tissue depths. The result is a greater 50°C isotherm radius and a greater depth and diameter of the lesion. Nakagawa demonstrated this phenomenon in a blood-superfused exposed thigh muscle preparation. In this study, intramural tissue temperatures 3.5 mm from the surface averaged 95°C with an irrigated-tip catheter despite a mean electrode-tissue interface temperature of 69°C. Lesion depths were 9.9 mm compared with 6.1 mm in a comparison group of temperature-feedback power control delivery and no electrode irrigation (Fig. 1-4). An important finding of this study was that 6 of 75 lesions had a sudden rise in electrical impedance associated with an audible pop. In these cases, the intramural temperature

exceeded 100°C, resulting in sudden steam formation and a steam pop. The clinical concern about "pop lesions" is that sudden steam venting to the endocardial or epicardial surface (or both) can potentially cause perforation and tamponade.[20]

The observation of increasing lesion size with ablation-tip cooling holds true only so long as the ablation is not power limited. If a level of power is used that is insufficient to overcome the heat lost by convection, the resulting tissue heating may be inadequate. In this case, convective cooling will dissipate a greater proportion of energy, and less of the available RF energy will be converted into tissue heat. The resulting lesion may be smaller than it would be if there were no convective cooling. As power is increased to a higher level, more energy will be converted to tissue heat, and larger lesions will result. If power is unlimited and temperature feedback power control is employed, greater magnitudes of convective cooling will allow for higher power levels and very large lesions. Thus, paradoxically in this situation, lesion size may be inversely related to the electrode-tissue interface temperature if the ablation is not power limited.[21] However, if power level is fixed (most commercial RF generators limit power delivery to 50 W for use with these catheters), lesion size increases in proportion to electrode-tissue interface temperature even in the setting of significant convective cooling (Fig. 1-5).[22]

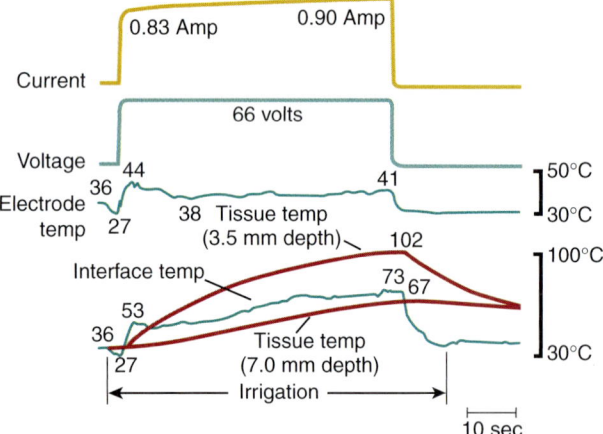

FIGURE 1-4. Current, voltage, and temperatures measured during radiofrequency catheter ablation with a perfused-tip electrode catheter in a canine exposed thigh muscle preparation are shown. Temperatures were recorded within the electrode, at the electrode-tissue interface, and within the muscle below the ablation catheter at depths of 3.5 and 7 mm. Because the electrode-tissue interface is actively cooled, high current and voltage levels can be employed. This results in an increased depth of direct resistive heating and superheating of the tissue below the surface of ablation. The peak temperature in this example at a depth of 3.5 mm was 102°C, and at 7 mm was 67°C, indicating that the 50°C isotherm defining the lesion border was significantly deeper than 7 mm. *(From Nakagawa H, Yamanashi WS, Pitha JV, et al. Comparison of in vivo tissue temperature profile and lesion geometry for radiofrequency ablation with a saline-irrigated electrode versus temperature control in a canine thigh muscle preparation.* Circulation. *1995;91:2264–2273. With permission.)*

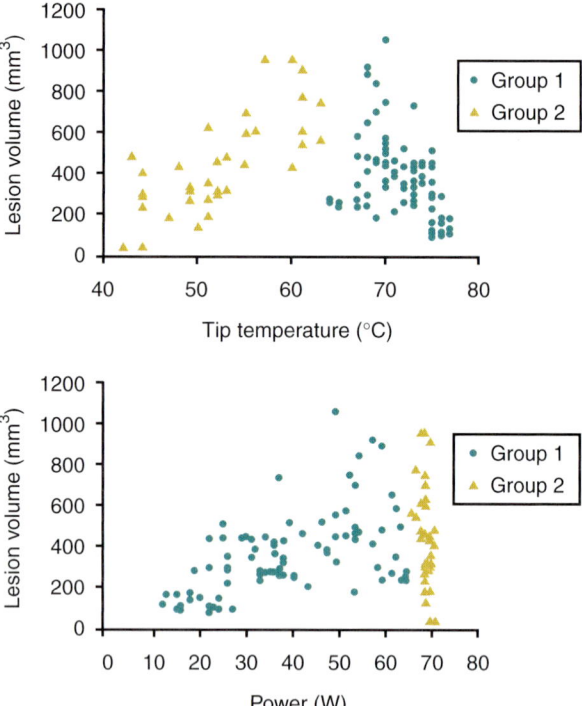

FIGURE 1-5. Temperatures measured at the tip of the electrode during experimental radiofrequency ablation and power are compared to the resulting lesion volume in this study. A maximal power of 70 W was employed. If lesion creation was not power limited (group 1), the lesion volume was a function of the delivered power. But if lesion production was limited by the 70-W available power maximum (group 2), the temperature measured at the electrode tip correlated with lesion size. *(From Petersen HH, Chen X, Pietersen A, et al. Lesion dimensions during temperature-controlled radiofrequency catheter ablation of left ventricular porcine myocardium: impact of ablation site, electrode size, and convective cooling.* Circulation. *1999;99:319–325. With permission.)*

Electrode-tip cooling can be achieved passively or actively. Passive tip cooling occurs when the circulating blood flow cools the mass of the ablation electrode and cools the electrode-tissue interface. This can be enhanced by use of a large ablation electrode.[23] Active tip cooling can be realized with a closed or open perfused-tip system. In each case, circulating saline from an infusion pump actively cools the electrode tip. One design recirculates the saline through a return port, and the opposing design infuses the saline through weep holes in the electrode into the bloodstream. Both designs are effective and result in larger lesions and greater procedure efficacy than standard RF catheter ablation. Theoretical advantages and disadvantages of open perfusion versus closed perfusion catheter designs are claimed by device manufacturers and their spokespeople, but the lesions produced and the clinical efficacy and safety profiles of these competing designs are very comparable.[24–27] The tip cooling or perfusion has the apparent advantage of reducing the prevalence of coagulum and char formation. However, because the peak tissue temperature is shifted from the endocardial surface to deeper intramyocardial layers, there is the risk for excessive intramural heating and pop lesions. The challenge for the clinician lies with the fact that with varying degrees of convective cooling, there is no reliable method for monitoring whether tissue heating is inadequate, optimal, or excessive. Cooling at the electrode-tissue interface limits the value of temperature monitoring to prevent excess power delivery and steam pops. With closed irrigation catheters, there is some value in the use of temperature feedback power control. In this case, target temperatures of 42° to 45°C have been empirically determined to optimize energy delivery.[27,28] If the ablation is power limited and the target temperature has not been reached, one may assume that the combination of passive cooling (from sliding or bouncing catheter-tissue contact) and active cooling is dissipating too much energy to allow for adequate tissue heating. In this situation, active electrode cooling can be held, and the operator can depend on passive cooling alone.

Catheter orientation will affect lesion size and geometry. Perpendicular catheter orientation results in less electrode surface area in contact with the tissue and more surface area in contact with the circulating blood pool. Parallel catheter orientation provides more electrode-tissue contact. With unrestricted power delivery, the parallel orientation should produce the larger lesion. In perfused-tip catheters, parallel orientation also results in more active tissue cooling and smaller lesion sizes than a perpendicular orientation.[29] The resultant interplay among active cooling, passive cooling, and power availability or limitation determines whether the lesions will be larger or smaller in these varying conditions. If perfused-tip catheters are positioned in a parallel orientation with greater tissue cooling, the lesions are smaller in vitro because of diminished efficiency of energy delivery. The effects of catheter orientation are less important with 4- or 5-mm-tip catheters but become more dominant when 8- or 10-mm tips are employed.

Since its inception, conventional RF ablation has been characterized by its excellent safety profile. This undoubtedly has been due to the relatively small size of the lesions. As new catheter technologies designed to increase the depth of the ablative lesion have been employed, it is not surprising

that complications due to collateral injury have increased. For example, left atrial ablation with cooled ablation catheters and high-intensity, focused ultrasound has resulted in cases of esophageal injury, perforation, and death. Despite the routine positioning of ablation catheters in close proximity to coronary arteries, there has been a dearth of coronary arterial complications with this procedure. The blood flow within the coronary artery is rapid, and the zone of tissue around the artery is convectively cooled by this blood flow. Fuller and Wood tested the effect of flow rate through a marginal artery of Langendorff perfused rabbit hearts.[30] RF ablation with an electrode-tissue interface temperature of 60° or 80°C was performed on the right ventricular free wall with two lesions straddling the artery, and conduction through this region was monitored. They observed that arterial flow rates as low as 1 mL/minute through these small (0.34 ± 0.1 mm diameter) arteries prevented complete transmural ablation and conduction block. This heat-sink effect is especially protective of the vascular endothelium. With higher power output of new ablation technologies, however, the convective cooling of the arterial flow may be overwhelmed, and there may be increased risk for vascular injury. With greater destructive power possible, operators need to be mindful to use only enough power to achieve complete ablation of the targeted tissue in order to safely accomplish the goal of arrhythmia ablation.

Electrical Current Distribution

Catheter ablation depends on the passage of RF electrical current through tissue. Tissue contact can be assessed by measuring baseline system impedance. In one clinical study, a very small (10 μA) current was passed through the ablation catheter, and the efficiency of heating was measured to assess tissue contact. A significant positive correlation between preablation impedance and heating efficiency was observed. As tissue is heated, there is a temperature-dependent fall in the electrical impedance.[31,32] A significant correlation is also observed between heating efficiency and the maximal drop in impedance during energy delivery. When electrode-tissue interface temperature monitoring is unreliable because of high-magnitude convective cooling, the slow impedance drop is a useful indicator that tissue heating is occurring. With the progressive fall in impedance during ablation, the delivered current increases along with tissue heating. If no impedance drop is observed, catheter repositioning is warranted.[33,34]

Because the magnitude of tissue heating is determined by the current density, the distribution of RF field around the electrodes in unipolar, bipolar, or phased RF energy delivery will determine the distribution of tissue heating. If energy is delivered in a unipolar fashion in a uniform medium from a spherical electrode to an indifferent electrode with infinite surface area, current density around the electrode should be entirely uniform. As geometries and tissue properties change, heating becomes nonuniform. Standard 4-mm electrode tips are small enough so that heating around the tip is fairly evenly distributed, even with varying tip contact angle to the tissue. One study showed that temperature monitoring with a thermistor located at the tip of a 4-mm electrode underestimated the peak electrode-tissue interface temperature recorded from multiple temperature sensors distributed around the electrode in only 4% of the applications. In RF applications where high power was employed and a sudden rise in electrical impedance occurred, the peak temperature recorded from the electrode tip was below 95°C in only one of 17 cases.[35] However, present-day electrode geometries vary considerably. The presence of fat will alter both electrical and thermal conductivity. Epicardial ablation over fat will result in minimal ablation of the underlying myocardium. Conversely, ablation of tissue insulated by fat outside of the ablation target will produce an "oven" effect, with higher temperatures for longer durations after cessation of energy delivery.[36] Also, tissue characteristics and placements of indifferent electrodes will affect tissue heating. Surface temperature recordings routinely underestimate peak subendocardial

tissue temperatures. For that reason, most operators limit ablation temperatures to 60° or 70°C during ablation with noncooled catheters.

Dispersive Electrode

The power dissipated in the complete circuit is proportional to the voltage drop and impedance for each part of the series circuit. The impedance of the ablation system and transmission lines is low, so there is little energy dissipation outside the body. The site of greatest impedance, voltage drop, and power dissipation is at the electrode-tissue interface (Fig. 1-6). However, most power is consumed with electrical conduction through the body and blood pool and into the dispersive electrode. In fact, only a fraction of the total delivered power actually is deposited in

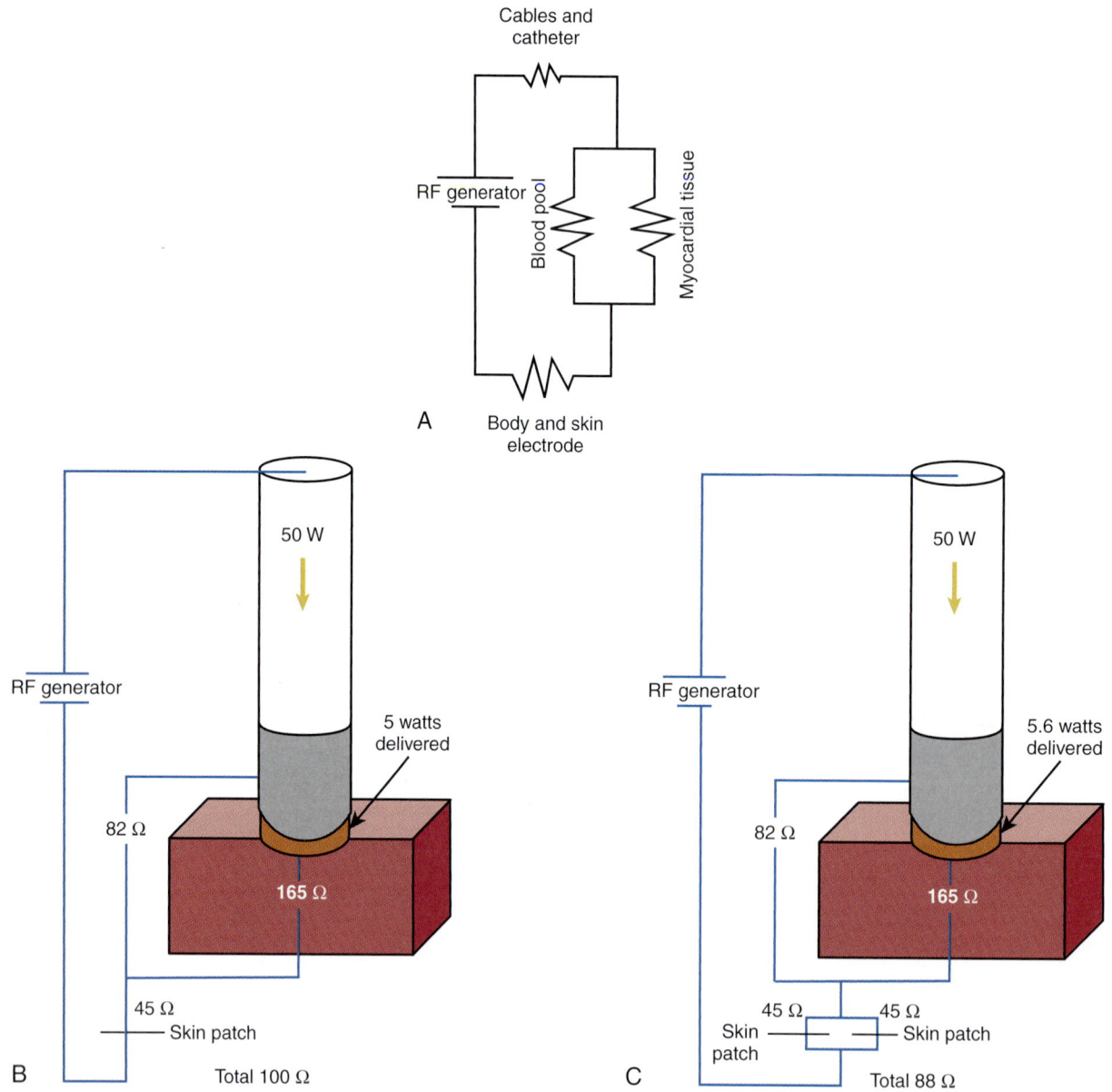

FIGURE 1-6. "Circuit diagrams" for radiofrequency (RF) ablation. **A,** From the RF generator, the cables and catheter present minimal resistance. The myocardial tissue and blood pool represent resistance circuits in parallel from the distal electrode. The return path from the ablation electrode to the generator comprises the patient's body and dispersive electrode in series. **B,** Hypothetical resistances for RF ablation circuit path. The resistance of the blood pool is about half that of the myocardial tissue. In this situation, for 50 W of energy delivered to the catheter, only 5 W is deposited in the myocardial tissue because of shunting of current through the lower resistance blood pool and power loss in the return path. **C,** Effect of adding a second dispersive skin electrode to the circuit. Assuming that the impedance of each dispersive electrode is 45 ohms and the generator voltage is constant, the total ablation circuit impedance is decreased by 12%. This allows for greater current delivery through the circuit and a proportional increase in power delivered to the tissue.

the myocardial tissue (Fig. 1-6). The return path of current to the indifferent electrode will certainly affect the current density close to that indifferent electrode, but its placement anterior versus posterior, and high versus low on the torso, has only a small effect on the distribution of RF current field lines within millimeters of the electrode. Therefore, lesion geometry should not be affected greatly by dispersive electrode placement. However, the proportion of RF energy contributing to lesion formation will be reduced if a greater proportion of that energy is dissipated in a long return pathway to the dispersive electrode. When the ablation is power limited, it is advantageous to minimize the proportion of energy that is dissipated along the current pathway at sites other than the electrode-tissue interface to achieve the greatest magnitude of tissue heating and the largest lesion. In an experiment that tested placement of the dispersive electrode directly opposite the ablation electrode versus at a more remote site, lesion depth was increased 26% with optimal placement.[37] Vigorous skin preparation to minimize impedance at the skin interface with the dispersive electrode, closer placement of the dispersive electrode to the heart, and use of multiple dispersive electrodes to increase skin contact area will all increase tissue heating in a power-limited energy delivery. Nath and associates reported that in the setting of a system impedance higher than 100 ohms, adding a second dispersive electrode increased the peak electrode-tip temperature during clinical catheter ablation (Fig. 1-7).[38]

Edge Effect

Electrical field lines are not entirely uniform around the tip of a unipolar ablation electrode. The distribution of field lines from an electrode source is affected by changes in electrode geometry. At points of geometric transition, the field lines become more concentrated. This so-called edge effect can result in significant nonuniformity of heating around

electrodes. The less symmetrical the electrode design (such as if found with long electrodes), the greater the degree of nonuniform heating. McRury and coworkers tested ablation with electrodes with 12.5-mm length.[39] They found that a centrally placed temperature sensor significantly underestimated the peak electrode-tissue interface temperature. Finite element analysis demonstrated a concentration of electrical current at the each of the electrode edges (Fig. 1-8). When dual thermocouples were placed on the edge of the electrode, the risk for coagulum formation and impedance rise was significantly reduced during ablation testing in vivo.

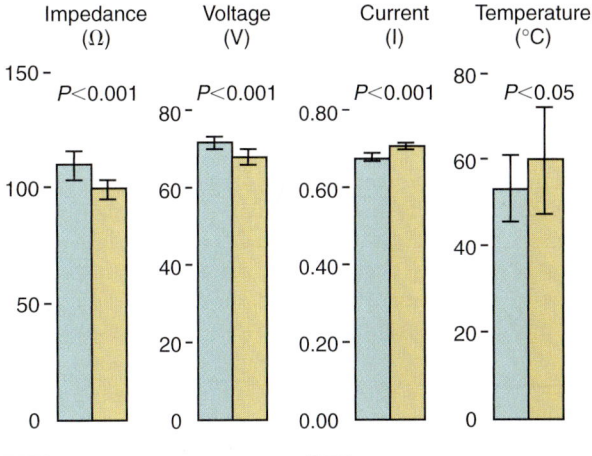

FIGURE 1-7. Impedance, voltage, current, and catheter-tip temperature readings during radiofrequency catheter ablation in a subset of patients with a baseline system impedance of more than 100 ohms. Ablations using a single dispersive electrode were compared with those using a double dispersive electrode. A lower system impedance was observed with addition of the second dispersive patch. This resulted in a greater current delivery and higher temperatures measured at the electrode-tissue interface. *(From Nath S, DiMarco JP, Gallop RG, et al. Effects of dispersive electrode position and surface area on electrical parameters and temperature during radiofrequency catheter ablation. Am J Cardiol. 1996;77:765–767. With permission.)*

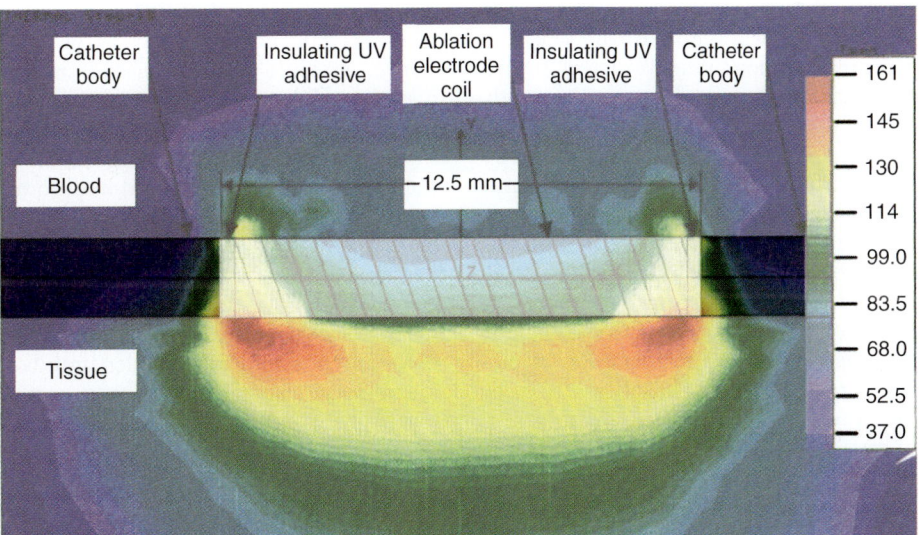

FIGURE 1-8. Steady-state temperature distribution derived from a finite element analysis of radiofrequency ablation with a 12-mm long coil electrode. In this analysis, the electrode temperature at the center of the electrode was maintained at 71°C. The legend of temperatures is shown at the right of the graph and ranges from the physiologic normal (violet = 37°C) to the maximal tissue temperature (red = 161°C) located below the electrode edges. There is a significant gradient of heating between the peak temperatures at the electrode edges and the center of the electrode. UV, ultraviolet. *(From McRury ID, Panescu D, Mitchell MA, Haines DE. Nonuniform heating during radiofrequency catheter ablation with long electrodes: monitoring the edge effect. Circulation. 1997;96:4057–4064. With permission.)*

Tissue Pathology and Pathophysiologic Response to Radiofrequency Ablation

Gross Pathology and Histopathology of the Ablative Lesion

The endocardial surface in contact with the ablation catheter shows pallor and sometimes a small depression due to volume loss of the acute lesion. If excessive power has been applied, there may be visible coagulum or char adherent to the ablation site. On sectioning the acute lesion produced by RF energy, a central zone of pallor and tissue desiccation characterizes its gross appearance. There is volume loss, and the lesion frequently has a teardrop shape with a narrower lesion width immediately subendocardially and a wider width 2 to 3 mm below the endocardial surface. This is because of surface convective cooling by the endocardial blood flow. Immediately outside the pale central zone is a band of hemorrhagic tissue. Beyond that border, the tissue appears relatively normal. The acute lesion border, as assessed by vital staining, correlates with the border between the hemorrhagic and normal tissue (Fig. 1-9). The histologic appearance of the lesion is consistent with coagulation necrosis. There are contraction bands in the sarcomeres, nuclear pyknosis, and basophilic stippling consistent with intracellular calcium overload.[40]

The temperature at the border zone of an acute hyperthermic lesion assessed by vital staining with nitro blue tetrazolium is 52° to 55°C.[3] However, it is likely that the actual isotherm of irreversible thermal injury occurs at a lower temperature boundary outside the lesion boundary, but that it cannot be identified acutely. Coagulation necrosis is a manifestation of thermal inactivation of the contractile and cytoskeletal proteins in the cell. Changes in the appearance of vital stains are due to loss of enzyme activity, as is the case with nitro blue tetrazolium staining and dehydrogenase activity.[41] Therefore, the acute assessment of the lesion border represents the border of thermal inactivation of various proteins, but the ultimate viability of the cell may depend on the integrity of more thermally sensitive organelles such as the plasma membrane (see later). In the clinical setting, recorded temperature does correlate with response to ablation. In patients with manifest Wolff-Parkinson-White syndrome, reversible accessory pathway conduction block was observed at a mean electrode temperature of 50° ± 8°C, whereas permanent block occurred at a temperature of 62° ± 15°C.[42] In a study of electrode-tip temperature monitoring during atrioventricular junctional ablation, an accelerated junctional rhythm was observed at a mean temperature of 51° ± 4°C. Permanent complete heart block was observed at ablation temperatures of 60° ± 7°C.[43] Because the targeted tissue was likely millimeters below the endocardial surface, the temperatures recorded by the catheter were likely higher than those achieved intramurally at the critical site of ablation.

The subacute pathology of the RF lesion is similar to what is observed with other types of injury. The appearance of typical coagulation necrosis persists, but the lesion border becomes more sharply demarcated with infiltration of mononuclear inflammatory cells. A layer of fibrin adheres to the lesion surface, coating the area of endothelial injury.

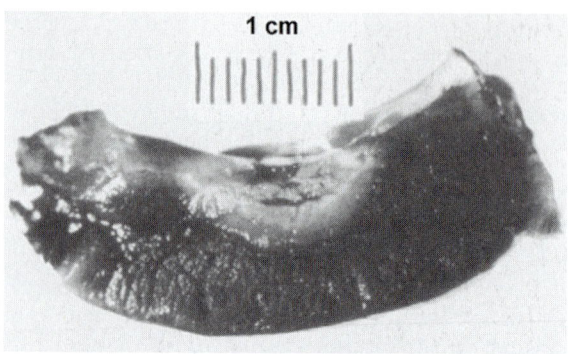

FIGURE 1-9. Typical appearance of radiofrequency catheter ablation lesion. There is a small central depression with volume loss, surrounded by an area of pallor, then a hemorrhagic border zone. The specimen has been stained with nitro blue tetrazolium to differentiate viable from nonviable tissue.

After 4 to 5 days, the transition zone at the lesion border is lost, and the border between the RF lesion and surrounding tissue becomes sharply demarcated. The changes in the transition zone within the first hours and days after ablation likely account for the phenomena of early arrhythmia recurrence (injury with recovery)[44] or delayed cure (progressive injury due to the secondary inflammatory response).[45] The coagulation necrosis in the body of the lesion shows early evidence of fatty infiltration. By 8 weeks after ablation, the necrotic zone is replaced with fatty tissue, cartilage, and fibrosis and can be surrounded by chronic inflammation.[46] The chronic RF ablative lesion evolves to uniform scar. The uniformity of the healed lesion accounts for the absence of any proarrhythmic effect of RF catheter ablation, unless multiple lesions with gaps are made. Like any fibrotic scar, there is significant contraction of the scar with healing. Relatively large and wide acute linear lesions have the final gross appearance of narrow lines of glistening scar when examined 6 months after the ablation procedure.[47]

Radiofrequency Lesion Ultrastructure

The ultrastructural appearance of the acute RF lesion offers some insight into the mechanism of tissue injury at the lesion border zone. In cases of experimental RF ablation in vivo, ventricular myocardium was examined in a band 3 mm from the edge of the acute pathologic lesion as defined by vital staining (Fig. 1-10). It showed marked disruption in cellular architecture characterized by dissolution of lipid membranes and inactivation of structural proteins. The plasma membranes were severely disrupted or missing. There was extravasation of erythrocytes and complete absence of basement membrane. The mitochondria showed marked distortion of architecture with swollen and discontinuous cristae membranes. The sarcomeres were extended with loss of myofilament structure or were severely contracted. The T-tubules and sarcoplasmic reticulum were absent or severely disrupted. Gap junctions were severely distorted or absent. Thus, despite the fact that the tissue examined was outside of the border of the acute pathologic lesion, the changes were profound enough to conclude that some progression of necrosis would occur within this border zone. The band of tissue 3 to 6 mm from the edge of the pathologic lesion was examined and manifested significant ultrastructural

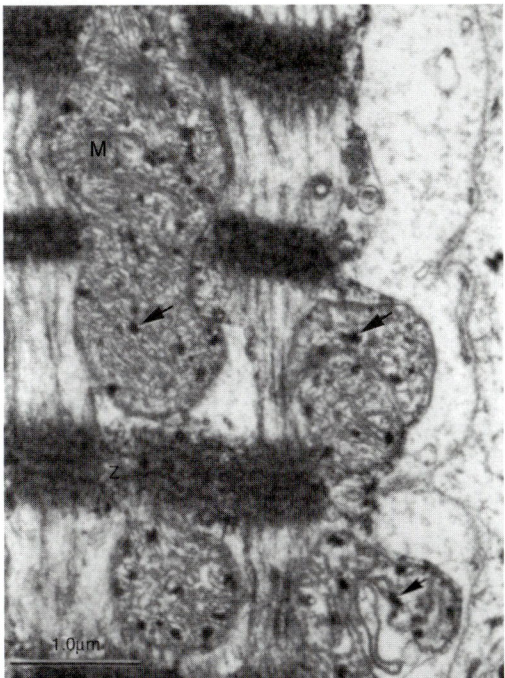

FIGURE 1-10. Electron micrograph of a myocardial sample 3 mm outside of the border zone of acute injury created by radiofrequency catheter ablation. There is severe disruption of the sarcomere with contracted Z bands, disorganized mitochondria, and basophilic stippling (*arrows*). Bar scale is 1.0 μm. *(From Nath S, Redick JA, Whayne JG, Haines DE. Ultrastructural observations in the myocardium beyond the region of acute coagulation necrosis following radiofrequency catheter ablation.* J Cardiovasc Electrophysiol. *1994;5:838–845. With permission.)*

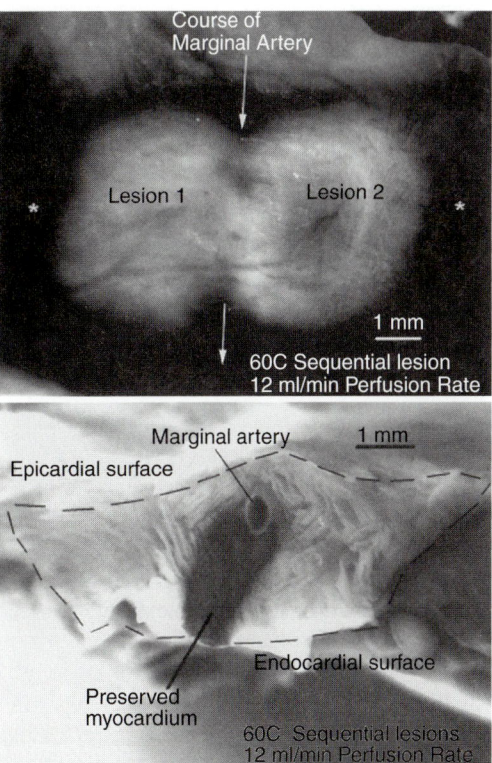

FIGURE 1-11. **Top,** Epicardial view of two radiofrequency lesions created during perfusion of a penetrating marginal artery in a rabbit heart. The lesions show central pallor that is apparent after vital staining. The course of the artery is marked. The *asterisks* mark the line used for perpendicular sectioning of the lesion. **Bottom,** Cross section through the middle of lesion perpendicular to marginal artery. The *broken lines* outline the lesion boundary. A region of myocardial sparing contiguous to the penetrating marginal artery (labeled) is apparent. Electrical conduction was present across this bridge of viable myocardium post ablation. *(From Fuller IA, Wood MA: Intramural coronary vasculature prevents transmural radiofrequency lesion formation: implications for linear ablation.* Circulation. *2003;107:1797–1803. With permission.)*

abnormalities, but not as severe as those described closer to the lesion core. Severe abnormalities of the plasma membrane were still present, but gap junctions and mitochondria were mainly intact. The sarcomeres were variable in appearance, with some relatively normal and some partially contracted. Although ultrastructural disarray was observed in the 3- to 6-mm zone, the myocytes appeared to be viable and would likely recover from the injury.[48]

Radiofrequency Ablation and Arterial Perfusion

In addition to direct injury to the myocytes, RF-induced hyperthermia has an effect on the myocardial vasculature and the myocardial perfusion. Impairment of the microcirculation could contribute to lesion formation by an ischemic mechanism. A study examined the effects of microvascular perfusion during acute RF lesion formation. In open chest canine preparations, the left ventricle was imaged with ultrasound from the epicardial surface, and a myocardial echocardiographic contrast agent was injected into the left anterior descending artery during endocardial RF catheter ablation. After ablation, the center of the lesion showed no echo contrast, consistent with severe vascular injury and absence of blood flow to that region. In the border zone of the lesion, a halo effect of retained myocardial contrast was observed. This suggested marked slowing of contrast transit rate through these tissues. The measured contrast transit rate at the boundary of the gross pathologic lesion was 25% ± 12% of the transit rate in normal tissue. In the 3-mm band of myocardium outside of the lesion edge, the contrast transit was 48% ± 27% of normal, and in the band of myocardium 3 to 6 mm outside of the lesion edge, the transit rate was 82% ± 28% of normal ($P < .05$ for all comparisons). The ultrastructural appearance of the arterioles demonstrated marked disruption of the plasma membrane and basement membrane and extravasation of red blood cells in these regions of impaired myocardial perfusion. The relative contribution of microvascular injury and myocardial ischemia to ultimate lesion formation is unknown but may play a role in lesion extension during the early phases after ablation.[49]

The effect of RF heating on larger arteries is a function of the size of the artery, the arterial flow rate, and the proximity to the RF source. In one study, flow rate through a marginal artery (or intramural perfusion cannula) in an in vitro rabbit heart preparation was varied between 0 and 10 mL/minute. A pair of epicardial ablations was produced with epicardial RF energy applications. Even at low flow rates, there was substantial sparing of the artery and the surrounding tissue owing to the heat-sink effect of the arterial flow (Fig. 1-11). However, if 45 W of power was applied along with RF electrode-tip cooling, complete ablation of the tissue contiguous to the intramural perfusion cannula was achieved.[30] Although this may be a desirable effect in the setting of small perfusing arteries through a region of conduction critical for arrhythmia propagation, it is not desirable if the artery is a large epicardial artery that happens to be contiguous to an ablation site, as is sometimes the case with accessory pathway or slow atrioventricular nodal pathway ablation, or ablation in the tricuspid-subeustachian isthmus for atrial flutter. Cases of arterial injury have been reported, particularly with the use of large-tip or tip-cooling technologies that allow for application of high RF powers.[50,51] In particular, when high-power ablation is required within the coronary sinus or great cardiac vein, it is prudent to define the course of the arterial anatomy to avoid unwanted arterial thermal injury.

Collateral Injury from Ablation

The injury to targeted myocardium is usually achieved if effort is made to optimize electrode-tissue contact. To ensure procedural success, particularly with ablation of more complex substrates like those found with atrial fibrillation, operators have employed a number of large-lesion RF technologies such as cooled-tip, perfused-tip, or large-tip catheters. With deep lesions sometimes comes unintended collateral injury to contiguous structures. An understanding of the anatomic relationships and careful titration of RF energy delivery can avoid adverse consequences of ablation in most cases. A rare but dangerous complication of ablation of the posterior left atrium is esophageal injury, often leading to atrioesophageal fistula or esophageal perforation.[52] The esophagus is located immediately contiguous to the atrium in most patients, with a distance from atrial endocardium to esophagus as small as 1.6 mm.[53] Hyperthermic injury leads to damage to structural proteins resulting in significant reduction in tensile strength of the esophageal musculature.[54] That, coupled with esophageal mucosal injury and ulcer formation, likely leads to ultimate perforation with a high case-fatality rate. Other structures that can be damaged with pulmonary vein isolation procedures are vagal and phrenic nerves.[55,56] Although these nerves usually regenerate after several months, permanent palsy can occur. Avoiding injury to these structures while achieving reliable transmural ablation of the myocardium can be challenging. Power should be limited, heating should be monitored carefully with multiple modalities (temperature, impedance drop, microbubbles on intracardiac echocardiogram imaging), and duration of energy delivery should be kept to a minimum. A complication of ablation of atrial fibrillation that was prevalent when ablation was being performed within the vein was pulmonary vein stenosis.[57] If the temperature rise of the venous wall is excessive, irreversible changes in the collagen and elastin of the vein wall will occur. In vitro heating of pulmonary vein rings showed a 53% reduction in circumference and a loss of compliance with hyperthermic exposure at or above 70°C. After exposure to those temperatures, the histologic examination showed loss of the typical collagen structure, presumably due to thermal denaturation of that protein.[58] For this reason, most pulmonary vein isolation is now performed outside the vein in the pulmonary vein antrum.

Cellular Mechanisms of Thermal Injury

The therapeutic effect of RF catheter ablation is due to electrical heating of tissue and thermal injury. The field of hyperthermia is broad, and the effects of long-duration exposures to mild and moderate hyperthermia have been well characterized in the oncology literature. Thermal injury is dependent upon both time and temperature. For example, when human bone marrow cells in culture are exposed to a temperature of 42°C, cell survival is 45% at 300 minutes. But when those cells are heated to 45.5°C, survival at 20 minutes is only 1%.[59] Data regarding the effects of brief exposure of myocardium to higher temperatures, as is the case during catheter ablation, is more limited and is reviewed in this section. The central zone of the ablation lesion reaches high temperatures and is simply coagulated. Lower temperatures are reached during the ablation in the border zones of the lesion. The responses of the various cellular components to low and moderate hyperthermia determine the pathophysiologic response to ablation. The thermally sensitive elements that contribute to overall thermal injury to the myocyte include the plasma membrane with its integrated channel proteins, the nucleus, and the cytoskeleton. Changes in these structures that occur during hyperthermic exposure all contribute to the ultimate demise of the cell.

Plasma Membrane

The plasma membrane is very thermally sensitive. A pure phospholipid bilayer will undergo phase transitions from a relatively solid form to a semiliquid form. Addition of integral proteins and the varying composition of the phospholipids with regard to the saturation of the hydrocarbon side chains affect the degree of membrane fluidity in eukaryotic cells. In one study, cultured mammalian cell membranes were found to have a phase transition at 8°C, and a second transition between 22° and 36°C. No phase changes were seen in the 37° to 45°C temperature range, but studies have not been performed examining this phenomenon in sarcomeres, or at temperatures above 45°C.[60] Regarding the function of integral plasma membrane proteins during exposure to heating, both inhibition and accentuation of protein activity have been observed. Stevenson and colleagues reported an increase in intracellular K^+ uptake in cultured Chinese hamster ovary (CHO) cells during heating to 42°C. This was blocked by ouabain, indicating an increased activity of the Na^+,K^+-ATPase pump.[61] Nath and colleagues examined action potentials in vitro in a superfused guinea pig papillary muscle preparation. In the low hyperthermic range between 38° and 45°C, there was an increase in the maximal dV/dt of the action potential, indicating enhanced sodium channel kinetics. In the moderate hyperthermia range from 45° to 50°C, the maximal dV/dt decreased below baseline values. The mechanism of this sodium channel inhibition was hypothesized to be either partial thermal inactivation of the sodium channel or, more likely, voltage-dependent sodium channel inactivation due to thermally mediated cellular depolarization[62] (see later).

Cytoskeleton

The cytoskeleton is composed of structural proteins that form microtubules, microfilaments, and intermediate filaments. The microfilaments coalesce into stress filaments. These include the proteins actin, actinin, and tropomyosin and form the framework to which the contractile elements of the myocyte attach. The cytoskeletal elements may have varying degrees of thermal sensitivity depending on the cell type. For example, in human erythrocytes, the cytoskeleton is composed predominantly of the protein spectrin. Spectrin is thermally inactivated at 50°C. When erythrocytes are exposed to temperatures above 50°C, the erythrocytes rapidly lose their biconcave shape.[63] There is no scientific literature reporting the inactivation temperature of the cytoskeletal proteins in myocytes. However, electron micrographs of the border zone of RF lesions show significant disruption in the cellular architecture with loss of the myofilament structure.[48] In the central portion of the RF lesion, thermal inactivation of the cytoskeleton contributes to the typical appearance of coagulation necrosis.

Nucleus

The eukaryote nucleus shows evidence of thermal sensitivity in both structure and function. Nuclear membrane vesiculation, condensation of cytoplasmic elements in the perinuclear region, and a decrease in heterochromatin content have been described.[64,65] The nucleolus appears to be the most heat-sensitive component of the nucleus. Whether or not hyperthermia induces DNA strand breaks is controversial. One reproducible finding after hyperthermic exposure is the elaboration of nuclear proteins called *heat shock proteins*. The function of heat shock proteins has not been entirely elucidated, but they appear to exert a protective effect on the cell. It is hypothesized that HSP 70 facilitates the effective production and folding of proteins and assists their transit among organelles.[66]

Cellular Electrophysiology

Hyperthermia leads to dramatic effects on the electrophysiology of myocardium. The thermal sensitivity of myocytes has been tested in a variety of experimental systems, and the mechanisms of the electrophysiologic responses to catheter ablation have been elucidated. In one series of in vitro experiments, isolated superfused guinea pig papillary muscles were subjected to 60 seconds of exposure to hyperthermic superfusate at temperatures varying from 38° to 55°C. Action potentials were recorded continuously during and after the hyperthermic pulse. If resting membrane potential was not restored after return to normothermia, the muscle was discarded, and testing proceeded with a new tissue sample. The resting membrane potential was assessed in unpaced preparations, and the action potential amplitude, duration, dV/dt, and excitability were tested during pacing. The preparations maintained a normal resting membrane potential in the low hyperthermic range (<45°C). In the intermediate hyperthermic range (45° to 50°C), the myocytes showed a temperature-dependent depolarization that was reversible on return to normothermic superfusion. Finally, experiments in the high hyperthermic range (>50°C) typically resulted in irreversible depolarization, contracture, and death

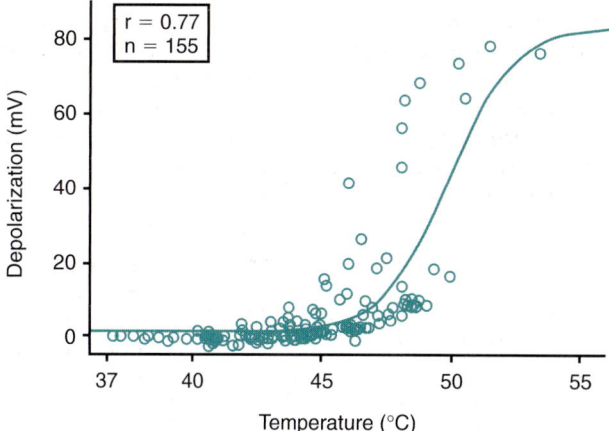

FIGURE 1-12. The magnitude of depolarization of guinea pig papillary muscle cells exposed to 1-minute pulses of hyperthermic perfusate versus perfusate temperature. At temperatures below 45°C, little depolarization is seen. The cells have progressive depolarization between 45° and 50°C. Above 50°C, few recordings are made because most cells have irreversible contracture and death. *(From Nath S, Lynch C III, Whayne JG, Haines DE. Cellular electrophysiological effects of hyperthermia on isolated guinea pig papillary muscle: implications for catheter ablation. Circulation. 1993;88:1826–1831. With permission.)*

(Fig. 1-12). There was a temperature-dependent decrease in action potential amplitude between 37° and 50°C as well as an inverse linear relationship between temperature and action potential duration. With increasing temperatures, the dV/dt increased, but above 46°C this measurement began to decrease in preparations that had a greater magnitude of resting membrane potential depolarization. Spontaneous automaticity was observed in both paced and unpaced preparations at a median temperature of 50°C, compared with a temperature of 44°C in preparations without automaticity. The occurrence of automaticity in unpaced preparations in the setting of hyperthermia-induced depolarization suggested abnormal automaticity as the mechanism. Beginning at temperatures higher than 42°C, loss of excitability to external-field stimulation was seen in some paced preparations and was dependent on the resting membrane potential. Mean resting membrane potential observed with loss of excitability was –44 mV, compared with –82 mV for normal excitability. The superfusate temperature measured during reversible loss of excitability was 43° to 51°C, but irreversible loss of excitability (cell death) occurred only at temperatures of 50°C or higher.[62] Thus, it appeared from these experiments that there was increased cationic entry into the hyperthermic cell and that the resultant depolarization led to loss of excitability and cell death.

Calcium Overload and Cellular Injury

In a preparation similar to that described previously, Everett and colleagues further elucidated the specific mechanisms for cellular depolarization and death in response to hyperthermia.[67] Isolated superfused guinea pig papillary muscles were attached to a force transducer to assess the pattern of contractility with varying hyperthermic exposure. Consistent with the observations of resting membrane potential changes during heating, there was a reversible increase in tonic resting muscle tension at temperatures between 45° and 50°C. Above 50°C, the preparations showed evidence of

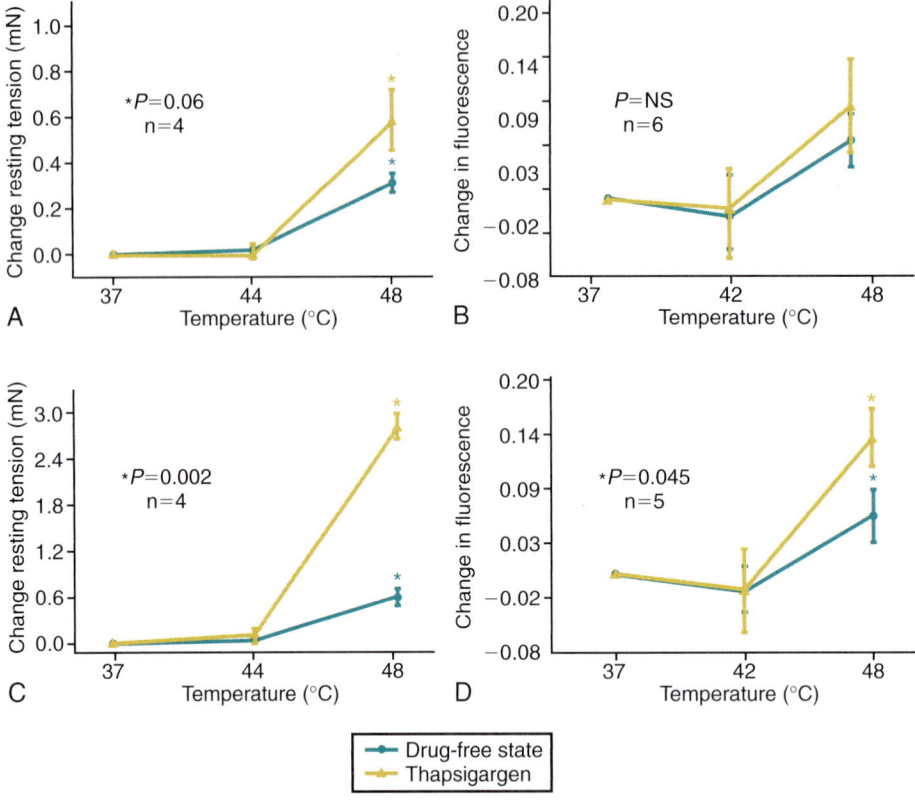

FIGURE 1-13. The effects of hyperthermic exposure on calcium entry into cells was tested in isolated perfused guinea pig papillary muscles. A change in resting tension was used as a surrogate measure for cytosolic calcium concentration (**A, C**), and a change in Fluo-3 AM fluorescence was used as a direct measure of free cytosolic calcium (**B, D**). With exposure to mild hyperthermia (42° to 44°C), little change in calcium levels was observed. With moderate hyperthermia (48°C), however, muscle tension and Fluo-3 AM fluorescence increased significantly. This increase was not channel specific because calcium channel blockade with cadmium or verapamil did not alter this response (**A, B**). The response was accentuated by thapsigargin (**C, D**), an agent that blocks calcium reuptake by the sarcoplasmic reticulum. *(From Everett TH, Nath S, Lynch C III, et al. Role of calcium in acute hyperthermic myocardial injury.* J Cardiovasc Electrophysiol. *2001;12:563–569. With permission.)*

irreversible contracture. This suggested that hyperthermia was causing calcium entry into the cell and ultimately calcium overload. This hypothesis was confirmed with calcium-sensitive Fluo-3 AM dye. Hyperthermic increases in papillary muscle tension correlated well with Fluo-3 AM luminescence. To elucidate the mechanism of calcium entry into the cell and its role in cellular injury, preparations were pretreated with either a calcium channel blocker (cadmium or verapamil) or an inhibitor of the sarcoplasmic reticulum calcium pump (thapsigargin). Preparations heated to 42° to 44°C showed no significant changes in tension at baseline or with drug treatment. With exposure to 48°C, treatment with calcium channel blockers did not reduce the increase in resting tension or Fluo-3 AM fluorescence, suggesting that the increase in cytosolic calcium was not the consequence of channel-specific calcium entry into the cell. In contrast, thapsigargin treatment led to irreversible papillary muscle contracture at lower temperatures (45% to 50°C) than observed without this agent. For preparations heated to 48°C, there was a greater increase in muscle tension and Fluo-3 AM fluorescence in the thapsigargin group compared with controls (Fig. 1-13). The authors concluded that hyperthermia results in significant increases in intracellular calcium, probably as a result of nonspecific transmembrane transit through thermally induced sarcolemmal pores. With increased intracellular calcium entry, the sarcoplasmic reticulum acts as a protective buffer against calcium overload,

unless this function is blocked with an agent like thapsigargin. In this case, cell contracture and death occur at lower temperatures than expected.[67]

Conduction Velocity

Simmers and coworkers have examined the effects of hyperthermia on impulse conduction in vitro in a preparation of superfused canine myocardium.[68] Average conduction velocity at baseline temperatures of 37°C was 0.35 m/second. When the superfusate temperature was raised, conduction velocity increased to supernormal values, reaching a maximum of 114% of baseline at 42.5°C. At temperatures above 45.4°C, conduction velocity slowed. Transient conduction block was observed between 49.5° and 51.5°C, and above 51.7°C permanent block was observed (Fig. 1-14).[68] These findings are exactly concordant with the temperature-related changes in cellular electrophysiology described previously. In a related experiment, the authors assessed myocardial conduction across a surgically created isthmus during heating with RF energy. The temperatures recorded during transient conduction block (50.7° ± 3.0°C) and permanent conduction block (58.0° ± 3.4°C) were nearly identical to those temperature ranges recorded in the experiments performed with hyperthermic perfusate. The authors concluded that the sole effects of RF ablation on the electrophysiologic properties of the myocardium were hyperthermic, and that there was no

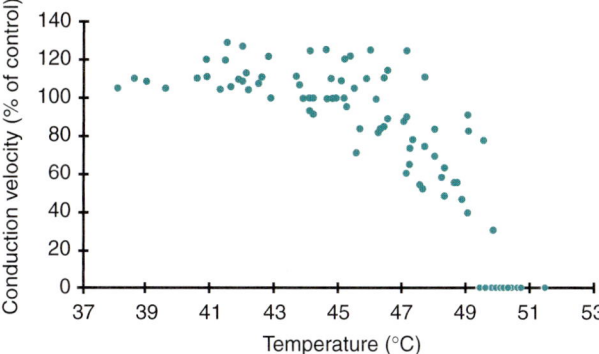

FIGURE 1-14. Conduction velocity of myocardium in superfused canine myocardium in vitro versus the temperature of the superfusate. A mild augmentation of conduction velocity due to an increase in dV/dt is observed at temperatures up to 45°C. Between 45° and 50°C, conduction velocity falls, and above 50°C, conduction is blocked. *(From Simmers TA, de Bakker JM, Wittkampf FH, Hauer RN. Effects of heating on impulse propagation in superfused canine myocardium.* J Am Coll Cardiol. *1995;25:1457–1464. With permission.)*

additional pathophysiologic response that could be attributed to direct effects of passage of electrical current through the tissue.[69] It is unknown whether these changes in conduction velocity are due solely to changes in intracellular ionic concentrations or whether thermal injury to gap junctions may also be implicated.

Determinants of Lesion Size

Targeting

The success of catheter ablation is dependent on a several factors. The first and foremost factor is optimizing targeting of the arrhythmogenic substrate. It is intuitive that increasing the size and depth of an ablative lesion will not improve the ablation success if the site selected for ablation is poor. To optimize site selection, it is necessary to understand the physiology and the anatomy of the arrhythmia in its entirety. The proximity of the electrode to the target will be the most important factor for ablation success.

Tissue Composition

Lesion sizes are decreased in areas of dense scar. In addition, an insulating layer of fat as thin as 2 mm overlying myocardial tissue (as in epicardial ablation) will prevent formation of a lesion with RF energy delivery.[70]

Power

Lesion size is proportional to power. Any method that will allow for greater power deposition into the tissue will result in more tissue heating and greater depth of thermal injury. In addition to power amplitude, efficiency of power coupling to the tissue (i.e., how much power is converted to tissue heat and how much is "wasted" with convective cooling) will affect ultimate lesion size.

Electrode Temperature

The electrode is passively heated by conduction of heat from the tissue during ablation. Lesion size increases

directly with electrode temperature up until the point of coagulum formation and impedance rise. The relationship between lesion size and electrode temperature is confounded by the effects of convective cooling and catheter motion in vitro.

Peak Tissue Temperature

Because of convective cooling, electrode temperature underestimates peak tissue temperature—the real determinant of lesion size. Future sensors such as infrared, microwave, or ultrasound elasticity monitors may allow the operator to monitor actual lesion growth.

Electrode Contact Pressure

Greater electrode-tissue contact pressure increases lesion size by improving electrical coupling with the tissue, increasing the electrode surface area in contact with the tissue, and reducing the shunting of current to the blood pool. In addition, greater contact pressure may prevent the electrode from sliding with cardiac motion. The optimal electrode contact pressure is believed to be 20 to 40 g.[6,71] Excessive contact that buries the electrode in the tissue, however, may prevent convective cooling of the electrode and reduce current delivery.

Convective Cooling

Ultimately, lesion size is a function of tissue heating, and tissue heating is a function of the magnitude of RF power that is converted into heat in the tissues. The greater magnitude of power delivered to the tissue, the greater the lesion size. Convective cooling at the electrode-tissue interface, either active or passive, will allow the operator to safely increase the power amplitude before impedance rises. However, if the ablation is power limited (i.e., the maximal available power is delivered throughout the ablation), greater degrees of convective cooling will draw heat from the tissue to create a smaller lesion size. The two factors that affect passive cooling at the electrode-tissue interface are the magnitude of regional blood flow and the stability of the electrode catheter on the tissue surface. Catheter motion over the tissue greatly increases the loss of heat to the blood pool. Intramyocardial blood flow draws heat from the tissue and not from the electrode and therefore decreases lesion size.

Electrode Size

When the goal is to maximize lesion size, larger electrodes will always be better than smaller electrodes. Larger electrodes increase the surface area and allow the operator to deliver higher total power without excessive current density at the electrode-tissue interface. Thus, coagulum formation with a sudden rise in electrical impedance can be avoided despite high total power delivery. The higher power delivery to the tissue increases the depth of direct volume heating and in turn increases the size of the virtual heat source. This translates directly into a larger lesion. As is the case with cooled electrodes, a large electrode will result in larger lesion formation only if it is accompanied by higher power

TABLE 1-2

FACTORS INFLUENCING RADIOFREQUENCY LESION SIZE

Factor	Effect on Lesion Size
Targeting	Close proximity to the target improves likelihood of success even with a small lesion size
Tissue composition	Smaller lesion sizes in scar and fat
Power	Directly proportional to lesion size
Ablation electrode temperature	Grossly proportional to lesion size but underestimates peak tissue temperature because of convective cooling effects
Peak tissue temperature	Directly proportional to lesion size
Electrode-tissue contact pressure	Directly proportional to lesion size
Convective cooling over electrode-tissue interface Active: perfused-tip catheter Passive: large tip, sliding contact Intramyocardial arterial flow	With fixed energy delivery, reduces lesion size; with unlimited energy, increases lesion size Reduces lesion size
Electrode size (radius and length)	Directly proportional to lesion size provided unrestricted power
Duration of energy delivery	Monoexponential relation to lesion size with half-time lesion formation of 5–10 seconds
Ablation circuit impedance	Lower body and dispersive (skin) patch resistance increases current delivery. Shunting current through blood decreases impedance but can reduced lesion size.
Electrode orientation	For nonirrigated electrode, parallel orientation increases lesion size. For irrigated electrode, perpendicular orientation increases lesion size.
Electrode geometry	Affects lesion size and shape by concentrating current density at electrode edges and asymmetries
Electrode material	Higher heat conductive materials increase lesion size by electrode cooling
Radiofrequency characteristics Pulsed Phased Frequency	May increase lesion size by allowing electrode cooling Increases continuity of linear lesions formed with multielectrode arrays Reduced heating efficiency at higher (MHz) frequencies

delivery. If a large electrode is employed with lower power, there may be a larger endocardial surface area ablated, but the lesion will not be as deep. RF energy delivery to multiple electrodes simultaneously may produce a large lesion as well, but other issues such as catheter and target geometry may limit energy coupling to the tissue if electrode-tissue contact is poor.

Duration of Energy Delivery

Tissue temperature follows a monoexponential rise during RF delivery (Table 1-2) until steady state is achieved. The half-time for lesion formation is 5 to 10 seconds. Therefore, lesion formation is assumed to be nearly complete after 45 to 60 seconds (five half-lives).

Ablation Circuit Impedance

By Ohm's law, lower resistance will allow for greater current delivery for the same applied voltage. For RF ablation, reducing resistance within the cables and dispersive electrode current path will increase current delivery to the tissue. The electrode-tissue interface represents two resistances in parallel, the tissue resistance and the blood pool resistance (Fig. 1-7). The resistance of the blood pool is about half that of the myocardial tissue.[72] Therefore, current preferentially flows through the blood pool from electrode surfaces not in contact with tissue. This becomes most apparent with the use of a large-tip electrode placed perpendicular to the tissue. Although

the system impedance is reduced, this results in current shunting through the blood and reduced current to the tissue unless high power outputs are applied.

Electrode Orientation

For nonirrigated electrodes with unrestricted power, an orientation parallel to the tissue generally results in larger lesions because of a larger electrode area in contact with the tissue and less current shunting to the blood pool. For irrigated electrodes delivering high power outputs, the parallel electrode orientation results in smaller lesion sizes because of a greater magnitude of tissue cooling.[29]

Electrode Geometry

Very long electrodes will provide greater surface area, allow higher power delivery, and usually yield larger lesions. If the electrode is too long, however, efficiency of electrode coupling to the tissue is lost, and lesion size is not increased.[22] Also, power is concentrated at points of geometric transitions (the edge effect), resulting in the possibility of excess heating at the electrode edges and less heating in the middle of the electrode.[39]

Electrode Material

Electrode materials with high heat transfer characteristics (such as gold) are more effectively cooled by passive blood flow and may allow for greater current deliveries.[73]

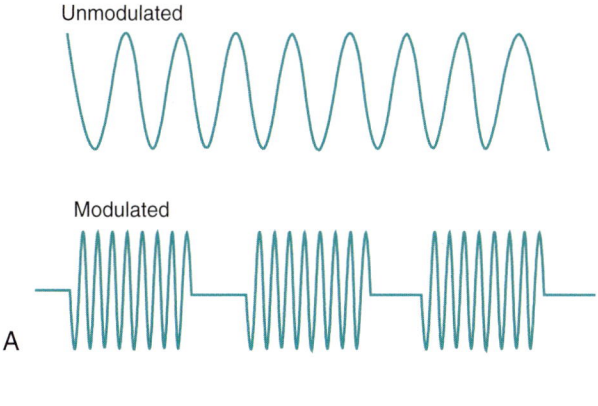

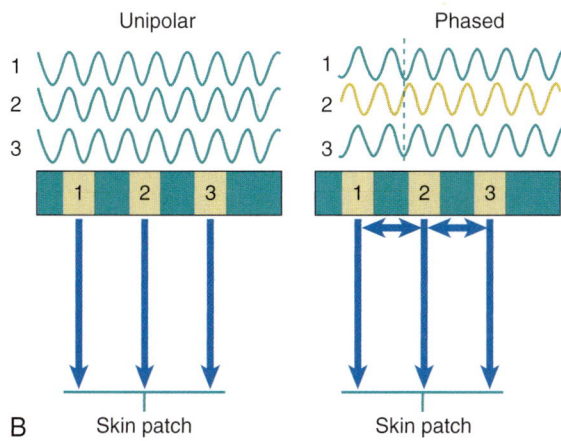

FIGURE 1-15. **A,** Unmodulated and modulated patterns of radiofrequency (RF) power. The modulated waveform is pulsed with periods of oscillating voltage separated by periods of quiescence. **B,** Unipolar and phased RF deliveries from a multielectrode array. With the unipolar delivery, the oscillating voltages among the electrodes are all in phase, and therefore there is no electrical potential for current flow between electrodes. With phased RF, the oscillations in voltage among contiguous electrodes are out of phase, creating an electrical potential for current to flow between electrodes as well as to the dispersive skin electrode.

Characteristics of Radiofrequency Energy

As noted, very high frequencies of alternating current lead to less efficient tissue heating, and lower frequencies may result in tissue stimulation. Pulsed RF current may allow for more electrode cooling than unmodulated RF and therefore increase power delivery (Fig. 1-15). With multielectrode ablation arrays, phased RF among the electrodes allows for more continuous linear lesions (Fig. 1-15).

Conclusion

RF catheter ablation remains the dominant modality for ablative therapy of arrhythmias. This technology is simple, has a high success rate, and has a low complication rate. Despite the fact that new ablation technologies such as ultrasound, laser, microwave, and cyrothermy are being tested and promoted as being easier, safer, or more efficacious, they are unlikely to supplant RF energy as the first choice for ablation of most arrhythmias. An appreciation of the biophysics and pathophysiology of RF energy heating

of myocardium during catheter ablation will help the operator to make the proper adjustments to optimize ablation safety and success. A tissue temperature of 50°C needs to be reached to achieve irreversible tissue injury. This likely occurs as a result of sarcolemmal membrane injury and intracellular calcium overload. The 50°C isotherm determines the boundary of the lesion. Greater lesion size is achieved with higher power delivery and higher intramural tissue temperatures. Monitoring surface temperature is useful to help prevent boiling of blood with coagulum formation and a sudden increase in electrical impedance. The selection of standard versus cooled tip; 4-mm versus 5-mm, 8-mm, or 10-mm electrode-tip size; maximal power delivered; and maximal electrode-tip temperature targeted will be achieved with a full understanding of the biophysics of catheter ablation. Finally, a complete understanding of the anatomy and physiology of the arrhythmogenic substrate will allow the operator to select the optimal ablation approach.

References

1. Huang SK, Jordan N, Graham A, et al. Closed-chest catheter desiccation of atrioventricular junction using radiofrequency energy: a new method of catheter ablation [abstract]. *Circulation*. 1985;72:III–1389 (abstract).
2. Huang SK, Bharati S, Graham AR, et al. Closed-chest catheter desiccation of the atrioventricular junction using radiofrequency energy: a new method of catheter ablation. *J Am Coll Cardiol*. 1987;9:349–358.
3. Whayne JG, Nath S, Haines DE. Microwave catheter ablation of myocardium in vitro: assessment of the characteristics of tissue heating and injury. *Circulation*. 1994;89:2390–2395.
4. Haines DE, Watson DD. Tissue heating during radiofrequency catheter ablation: a thermodynamic model and observations in isolated perfused and superfused canine right ventricular free wall. *Pacing Clin Electrophysiol*. 1989;12:962–976.
5. Erez A, Shitzer A. Controlled destruction and temperature distributions in biological tissues subjected to monoactive electrocoagulation. *J Biomech Eng*. 1980;102:42–49.
6. Haines DE. Determinants of lesion size during radiofrequency catheter ablation: the role of electrode-tissue contact pressure and duration of energy delivery. *J Cardiovasc Electrophysiol*. 1991;2:509–515.
7. Wittkampf FH, Nakagawa H, Yamanashi WS, et al. Thermal latency in radiofrequency ablation. *Circulation*. 1996;93:1083–1086.
8. Haines DE, Watson DD, Verow AF. Electrode radius predicts lesion radius during radiofrequency energy heating: validation of a proposed thermodynamic model. *Circ Res*. 1990;67:124–129.
9. Schreieck J, Zrenner B, Kumpmann J, et al. Prospective randomized comparison of closed cooled-tip versus 8-mm-tip catheters for radiofrequency ablation of typical atrial flutter. *J Cardiovasc Electrophysiol*. 2002;13:980–985.
10. Tsai CF, Tai CT, Yu WC, et al. Is 8-mm more effective than 4-mm tip electrode catheter for ablation of typical atrial flutter? *Circulation*. 1999;100:768–771.
11. Kasai A, Anselme F, Teo WS, et al. Comparison of effectiveness of an 8-mm versus a 4-mm tip electrode catheter for radiofrequency ablation of typical atrial flutter. *Am J Cardiol*. 2000;86:1029–1032 A10.
12. Simmers TA, de Bakker JM, Coronel R, et al. Effects of intracavitary blood flow and electrode-target distance on radiofrequency power required for transient conduction block in a Langendorff-perfused canine model. *J Am Coll Cardiol*. 1998;31:231–235.
13. Kilicaslan F, Verma A, Saad E, et al. Transcranial Doppler detection of microembolic signals during pulmonary vein antrum isolation: implications for titration of radiofrequency energy. *J Cardiovasc Electrophysiol*. 2006;17:495–501.
14. Haines DE, Verow AF. Observations on electrode-tissue interface temperature and effect on electrical impedance during radiofrequency ablation of ventricular myocardium. *Circulation*. 1990;82:1034–1038.
15. Demolin JM, Eick OJ, Munch K, et al. Soft thrombus formation in radiofrequency catheter ablation. *Pacing Clin Electrophysiol*. 2002;25:1219–1222.
16. Wang TL, Lin JL, Hwang JJ, et al. The evolution of platelet aggregability in patients undergoing catheter ablation for supraventricular tachycardia with radiofrequency energy: the role of antiplatelet therapy. *Pacing Clin Electrophysiol*. 1995;18:1980–1990.
17. Jain MK, Wolf PD. A three-dimensional finite element model of radiofrequency ablation with blood flow and its experimental validation. *Ann Biomed Eng*. 2000;28:1075–1084.
18. Strickberger SA, Hummel J, Gallagher M, et al. Effect of accessory pathway location on the efficiency of heating during radiofrequency catheter ablation. *Am Heart J*. 1995;129:54–58.
19. Kalman JM, Fitzpatrick AP, Olgin JE, et al. Biophysical characteristics of radiofrequency lesion formation in vivo: dynamics of catheter tip-tissue contact evaluated by intracardiac echocardiography. *Am Heart J*. 1997;133:8–18.

20. Nakagawa H, Yamanashi WS, Pitha JV, et al. Comparison of in vivo tissue temperature profile and lesion geometry for radiofrequency ablation with a saline-irrigated electrode versus temperature control in a canine thigh muscle preparation. *Circulation.* 1995;91:2264–2273.

21. Mukherjee R, Laohakunakorn P, Welzig MC, et al. Counter intuitive relations between in vivo RF lesion size, power, and tip temperature. *J Interv Cardiac Electrophysiol.* 2003;9:309–315.

22. Petersen HH, Chen X, Pietersen A, et al. Lesion dimensions during temperature-controlled radiofrequency catheter ablation of left ventricular porcine myocardium: impact of ablation site, electrode size, and convective cooling. *Circulation.* 1999;99:319–325.

23. Otomo K, Yamanashi WS, Tondo C, et al. Why a large tip electrode makes a deeper radiofrequency lesion: effects of increase in electrode cooling and electrode-tissue interface area. *J Cardiovasc Electrophysiol.* 1998;9:47–54.

24. Dorwarth U, Fiek M, Remp T, et al. Radiofrequency catheter ablation: different cooled and noncooled electrode systems induce specific lesion geometries and adverse effects profiles. *Pacing Clin Electrophysiol.* 2003;26:1438–1445.

25. Spitzer SG, Karolyi L, Rammler C, Otto T. Primary closed cooled tip ablation of typical atrial flutter in comparison to conventional radiofrequency ablation. *Europace.* 2002;4:265–271.

26. Atiga WL, Worley SJ, Hummel J, et al. Prospective randomized comparison of cooled radiofrequency versus standard radiofrequency energy for ablation of typical atrial flutter. *Pacing Clin Electrophysiol.* 2002;25:1172–1178.

27. Everett TH 4th, Lee KW, Wilson EE, et al. Safety profiles and lesion size of different radiofrequency ablation technologies: a comparison of large tip, open and closed irrigation catheters. *J Cardiovasc Electrophysiol.* 2009;20:325–335.

28. Watanabe I, Masaki R, Min N, et al. Cooled-tip ablation results in increased radiofrequency power delivery and lesion size in the canine heart: importance of catheter-tip temperature monitoring for prevention of popping and impedance rise. *J Interv Cardiac Electrophysiol.* 2002;6:9–16.

29. Wood MA, Goldberg SM, Parvez B, et al. Effect of electrode orientation on lesion sizes produced by irrigated radiofrequency ablation catheters. *J Cardiovasc Electrophysiol.* 2009;20:1262–1268.

30. Fuller IA, Wood MA. Intramural coronary vasculature prevents transmural radiofrequency lesion formation: implications for linear ablation. *Circulation.* 2003;107:1797–1803.

31. Ko WC, Huang SK, Lin JL, et al. New method for predicting efficiency of heating by measuring bioimpedance during radiofrequency catheter ablation in humans. *J Cardiovasc Electrophysiol.* 2001;12:819–823.

32. Thiagalingam A, D'Avila A, McPherson C, et al. Impedance and temperature monitoring improve the safety of closed-loop irrigated-tip radiofrequency ablation. *J Cardiovasc Electrophysiol.* 2007;18:318–325.

33. Seiler J, Roberts-Thomson KC, Raymond JM, et al. Steam pops during irrigated radiofrequency ablation: feasibility of impedance monitoring for prevention. *Heart Rhythm.* 2008;5:1411–1416.

34. Jain MK, Wolf PD. Temperature-controlled and constant-power radiofrequency ablation: what affects lesion growth? *Trans Biomed Eng.* 1999;46:1405–1412.

35. McRury ID, Whayne JG, Haines DE. Temperature measurement as a determinant of tissue heating during radiofrequency catheter ablation: an examination of electrode thermistor positioning for measurement accuracy. *J Cardiovasc Electrophysiol.* 1995;6:268–278.

36. Liu Z, Ahmed M, Weinstein Y, et al. Characterization of the RF ablation-induced "oven effect": the importance of background tissue thermal conductivity on tissue heating. *Int J Hypertherm.* 2006;22:327–342.

37. Jain MK, Tomassoni G, Riley RE, Wolf PD. Effect of skin electrode location on radiofrequency ablation lesions: an in vivo and a three-dimensional finite element study. *J Cardiovasc Electrophysiol.* 1998;9:1325–1335.

38. Nath S, DiMarco JP, Gallop RG, et al. Effects of dispersive electrode position and surface area on electrical parameters and temperature during radiofrequency catheter ablation. *Am J Cardiol.* 1996;77:765–767.

39. McRury ID, Panescu D, Mitchell MA, Haines DE. Nonuniform heating during radiofrequency catheter ablation with long electrodes: monitoring the edge effect. *Circulation.* 1997;96:4057–4064.

40. Huang SK, Bharati S, Graham AR, et al. Closed chest catheter desiccation of the atrioventricular junction using radiofrequency energy: a new method of catheter ablation. *J Am Coll Cardiol.* 1987;9:349–358.

41. Butcher RG. The measurement in tissue sections of the two formazans derived from nitroblue tetrazolium in dehydrogenase reactions. *Histochem J.* 1978;10:739–744.

42. Langberg JJ, Calkins H, el Atassi R, et al. Temperature monitoring during radiofrequency catheter ablation of accessory pathways [see comment]. *Circulation.* 1992;86:1469–1474.

43. Nath S, DiMarco JP, Mounsey JP, et al. Correlation of temperature and pathophysiological effect during radiofrequency catheter ablation of the AV junction. *Circulation.* 1995;92:1188–1192.

44. Langberg JJ, Calkins H, Kim YN, et al. Recurrence of conduction in accessory atrioventricular connections after initially successful radiofrequency catheter ablation. *J Am Coll Cardiol.* 1999;7:1588–1592.

45. DeLacey WA, Nath S, Haines DE, et al. Adenosine and verapamil-sensitive ventricular tachycardia originating from the left ventricle: radiofrequency catheter ablation [see comment]. *Pacing Clin Electrophysiol.* 1992;15:2240–2244.

46. Huang SK, Bharati S, Lev M, Marcus FI. Electrophysiologic and histologic observations of chronic atrioventricular block induced by closed-chest catheter desiccation with radiofrequency energy. *Pacing Clin Electrophysiol.* 1987;10:805–816.

47. Avitall B, Urbonas A, Urboniene D, et al. Time course of left atrial mechanical recovery after linear lesions: normal sinus rhythm versus a chronic atrial fibrillation dog model [see comment]. *J Cardiovasc Electrophysiol.* 2000;11:1397–1406.

48. Nath S, Redick JA, Whayne JG, Haines DE. Ultrastructural observations in the myocardium beyond the region of acute coagulation necrosis following radiofrequency catheter ablation. *J Cardiovasc Electrophysiol.* 1994;5:838–845.

49. Nath S, Whayne JG, Kaul S, et al. Effects of radiofrequency catheter ablation on regional myocardial blood flow: possible mechanism for late electrophysiological outcome. *Circulation.* 1994;89:2667–2672.

50. Duong T, Hui P, Mailhot J. Acute right coronary artery occlusion in an adult patient after radiofrequency catheter ablation of a posteroseptal accessory pathway. *J Invasive Cardiol.* 2004;16:657–659.

51. Sassone B, Leone O, Martinelli GN, Di Pasquale G. Acute myocardial infarction after radiofrequency catheter ablation of typical atrial flutter: histopathological findings and etiopathogenetic hypothesis. *Ital Heart J.* 2004;5:403–407.

52. Schmidt M, Nölker G, Marschang H, et al. Incidence of oesophageal wall injury post-pulmonary vein antrum isolation for treatment of patients with atrial fibrillation. *Europace.* 2008;10:205–209.

53. Helms A, West JJ, Patel A, et al. Real-time rotational ICE imaging of the relationship of the ablation catheter tip and the esophagus during atrial fibrillation ablation. *J Cardiovasc Electrophysiol.* 2009;20:130–137.

54. Evonich RF, Nori DM, Haines DE. A randomized trial comparing effects of radiofrequency and cryoablation on the structural integrity of esophageal tissue. *J Interv Card Electrophysiol.* 2007;19:77–83.

55. Sacher F, Monahan KH, Thomas SP, et al. Phrenic nerve injury after atrial fibrillation catheter ablation: characterization and outcome in a multicenter study. *J Am Coll Cardiol.* 2006;47:2498–2503.

56. Pisani CF, Hachul D, Sosa E, Scanavacca M. Gastric hypomotility following epicardial vagal denervation ablation to treat atrial fibrillation. *J Cardiovasc Electrophysiol.* 2008;19:211–213.

57. Saad EB, Marrouche NF, Saad CP, et al. Pulmonary vein stenosis after catheter ablation of atrial fibrillation: emergence of a new clinical syndrome [see comment] [summary for patients in *Ann Intern Med.* 2003;138:1; PMID: 12693916]. *Ann Intern Med.* 2003;138:634–638.

58. Kok LC, Everett TH, Akar JG, Haines DE. Effect of heating on pulmonary veins: how to avoid pulmonary vein stenosis. *J Cardiovasc Electrophysiol.* 2003;14:250–254.

59. Bromer RH, Mitchell JB, Soares N. Response of human hematopoietic precursor cells (CFUc) to hyperthermia and radiation. *Cancer Res.* 1982;42:1261–1265.

60. Lepock JR. Involvement of membranes in cellular responses to hyperthermia. *Radiat Res.* 1982;92:433–438.

61. Stevenson AP, Galey WR, Tobey RA, et al. Hyperthermia-induced increase in potassium transport in Chinese hamster cells. *J Cell Physiol.* 1983;115:75–86.

62. Nath S, Lynch III C, Whayne JG, Haines DE. Cellular electrophysiological effects of hyperthermia on isolated guinea pig papillary muscle: implications for catheter ablation. *Circulation.* 1993;88:1826–1831.

63. Coakley WT. Hyperthermia effects on the cytoskeleton and on cell morphology. *Symp Soc Exp Biol.* 1987;41:187–211.

64. Warters RL, Henle KJ. DNA degradation in Chinese hamster ovary cells after exposure to hyperthermia. *Cancer Res.* 1982;42:4427–4432.

65. Warters RL, Roti Roti JL. Hyperthermia and the cell nucleus. *Radiat Res.* 1982;92:458–462.

66. Warters RL, Brizgys LM, Sharma R, Roti Roti JL. Heat shock (45 degrees C) results in an increase of nuclear matrix protein mass in HeLa cells. *Int J Radiat Biol.* 1986;50:253–268.

67. Everett TH, Nath S, Lynch III C, et al. Role of calcium in acute hyperthermic myocardial injury. *J Cardiovasc Electrophysiol.* 2001;12:563–569.

68. Simmers TA, de Bakker JM, Wittkampf FH, Hauer RN. Effects of heating on impulse propagation in superfused canine myocardium. *J Am Coll Cardiol.* 1995;25:1457–1464.

69. Simmers TA, de Bakker JM, Wittkampf FH, Hauer RN. Effects of heating with radiofrequency power on myocardial impulse conduction: is radiofrequency ablation exclusively thermally mediated? *J Cardiovasc Electrophysiol.* 1996;7:243–247.

70. Hong KN, Russo MJ, Liberman EA, et al. Effect of epicardial fat on ablation performance: a three-energy source comparison. *J Card Surg.* 2007;22:521–524.

71. Yokoyama K, Nakagawa H, Shah D, et al. Novel contact force sensor incorporated in irrigated radiofrequency ablation catheter predicts lesion size and incidence of steam pop and thrombus. *Circ Arrhythm Electrophysiol.* 2008;1:354–362.

72. Wittkampf FHM, Nakagawa H. RF catheter ablation: lessons on lesions. *Pacing Clin Electrophysiol.* 2006;29:1285–1297.

73. Linhart M, Mollnau H, Bitzen A, et al. In vitro comparison of platinum-iridium and gold tip electrodes: lesion depth in 4 mm, 8 mm, and irrigated-tip radiofrequency ablation catheters. *Europace.* 2009;11:565–570.

Videos

Video 1-1. Infrared thermal imaging of tissue heating during radiofrequency ablation with a closed irrigation catheter as seen from the surface of the tissue. Power is delivered at 30 W to blocks of porcine myocardium in a tissue bath. The surface of the tissue is just above the fluid level to permit thermal imaging of tissue and not the fluid. Temperature scale (*right*) and a millimeter scale (*top*) are shown in each panel.

Video 1-2. Infrared thermal imaging of tissue heating during radiofrequency ablation with a closed irrigation catheter as seen in cross section. Power is delivered at 30 W to blocks of porcine myocardium in a tissue bath. The surface of the tissue is just above the fluid level to permit thermal imaging of tissue and not the fluid. Temperature scale (*right*) and a millimeter scale (*top*) are shown in each panel.

2

Guiding Lesion Formation during Radiofrequency Energy Catheter Ablation

Eric Buch and Kalyanam Shivkumar

Key Points

Radiofrequency (RF) energy is the most commonly used energy source in cardiac catheter ablation procedures. The goal of RF power titration is to maximize the safety and efficacy of energy application.

Stable catheter-tissue contact is important to achieve safe and effective RF ablation but is inadequately assessed by current methods, including fluoroscopy, tactile feedback, and electrogram characteristics.

Careful titration of energy delivery can avoid local complications, including coagulum formation, steam pop, and cardiac perforation. Collateral damage to surrounding structures, including the esophagus and phrenic nerves, can also be prevented.

Each method of RF energy titration has advantages and limitations. Common methods include ablation electrode temperature, changes in ablation circuit impedance, and electrogram amplitude reduction.

The discrepancy between catheter-tip temperature and myocardial tissue temperature is greater for large-tip and irrigated-tip catheters. Special precautions should be taken to avoid excessive myocardial and extracardiac heating.

RF ablation in nonendocardial sites, such as in the pericardial space or coronary sinus, requires modification to the general power titration approach.

General Principles of Power Titration

Catheter-based intervention has become the treatment of choice for many cardiac arrhythmias. Currently, the energy source used most often in these procedures is unipolar radiofrequency (RF) energy, typically 300 to 1000 KHz, which allows precise destruction of targeted tissue. The goal is to successfully ablate critical tissue within the tachycardia circuit or focus but avoid local complications and collateral damage to adjacent anatomic structures.

Several approaches are available to guide the operator in producing adequate, but not excessive, tissue heating and lesion size. Systematic methods of RF power titration using this information are discussed in detail. Alternative energy sources for ablation and the biophysics of RF lesion formation are reviewed in other chapters.

Assessment of Catheter-Tissue Contact

RF ablation is critically dependent on tissue contact because RF current is usually delivered in a unipolar mode from the ablation catheter tip electrode to a grounding patch (dispersive electrode) on the patient's skin. This results in resistive heating at the catheter-tissue interface because the surface area of the catheter tip is small compared with the area of the dispersive patch. In most cases, the zone of resistive heating extends only about 1 mm from the catheter electrode tip; heat production is inversely proportional to the fourth power of distance from the catheter tip. Without good contact, only intracavitary blood will be heated, with insufficient myocardial temperature to cause necrosis of targeted tissue.[1]

Parameters that can be used to assess degree of catheter-tissue contact include beat-to-beat variability in local electrograms, baseline electrode impedance, changes in electrode temperature and impedance during ablation, catheter movement on fluoroscopy, visual assessment by echocardiography, pacing capture threshold, and tactile feedback. Yet, even using all this information, substantial differences between estimated and actual contact force are common.[2] Experimental catheters that measure and report real-time contact force are in development but not yet commercially available.[3]

Power Titration for Ablation Efficacy

Catheter ablation should result in irreversible damage to targeted tissue and permanent loss of conduction. This is generally associated with coagulation necrosis, which results from sustained tissue temperature over 50°C.[4] The best predictor of lesion size is achieved tissue temperature because the ablation lesion closely corresponds to the zone of sufficiently heated tissue.[5] Key factors influencing the size and depth of an RF ablation lesion include current density at the electrode tip (in turn determined by delivered power and electrode surface area),[6] electrode-myocardium contact, orientation of catheter tip,[7] duration of energy delivery, achieved electrode tip temperature, and heat dissipation from intracavitary blood flow or nearby cardiac vessels. Because some of these factors are unknown during ablation, power is often increased to reach a prespecified goal (e.g., 40 to 50 W for ablation of the right atrial isthmus) or to a desired effect (e.g., loss of preexcitation or tachycardia termination). Power titration is also modulated by electrode impedance and temperature monitoring in the clinical setting.

Only tissue in direct contact with the electrode tip is significantly affected by resistive heating; most lesion volume results from conductive heating, which occurs much more slowly. The process can be modeled as nearly instantaneous production of a heated capsule at the catheter tip with slow subsequent conductive heating of adjacent tissue until thermal equilibrium is reached. In fact, ablation lesions continue to grow even after interruption of RF energy, a phenomenon called *thermal lag* or *thermal latency*.[8]

Power Titration for Ablation Safety

Although efficacy is important, it is also critical to avoid complications of excessive energy delivery. Careful titration of RF power can minimize the probability of coagulum formation, steam pops, cardiac perforation, and collateral damage to intracardiac and extracardiac structures.

Coagulum Formation

During the early use of RF energy in catheter ablation procedures, a sudden increase in impedance was often observed from boiling of blood at the electrode-tissue interface. This led to accumulation of gas (steam), an electrical insulator,

along the electrode surface and abrupt reduction in energy delivery due to high impedance. Usually coagulated blood adhered to the electrode tip, requiring removal before further ablation could be performed. Boiling at the tissue-electrode interface, called *interfacial boiling*, is necessary but not sufficient for this abrupt impedance rise. If gas is not trapped by intimate myocardial contact, but instead dissipated by brisk blood flow or open irrigation, overall circuit impedance may not change at all despite interfacial boiling.[9]

Coagulum on the electrode tip is another solid interface that can trap elaborated gas and increase ablation circuit impedance. Coagulum is caused by excessive heating of blood near the electrode-endocardial interface, denaturing proteins in blood cells and serum. This results in "soft thrombus" or char that initially anneals to the endocardium at the electrode-tissue interface, the site at the highest temperature (Fig. 2-1).[10] Eventually coagulum adheres to the electrode as well, often causing an increase in ablation circuit impedance because of its higher resistivity compared with blood. Coagulum is not formed by activation of clotting factors like typical thrombus and is not prevented by heparin or other anticoagulants. In temperature-controlled RF, the high temperature necessary for interfacial boiling is rarely reached, and therefore the dramatic impedance rise resulting from elaborated gas at the electrode is usually not seen. However, because proteins denature at temperatures well below boiling, probably at about 60°C, coagulum can form even in the absence of impedance rise.[11] Matsudaira and associates found that coagulum still formed in heparinized blood when

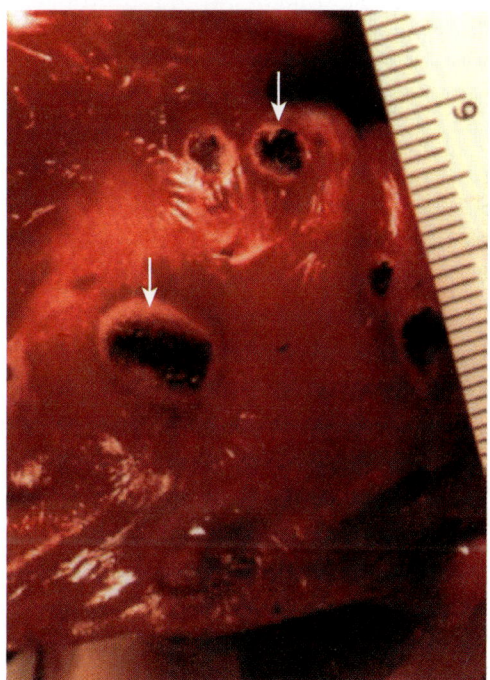

FIGURE 2-1. View of atrial endocardium after tetrazolium staining, demonstrating coagulum (*arrows*) overlying RF ablation lesions. (*From Schwartzman D, Michele JJ, Trankiem CT, Ren JF. Electrogram-guided radiofrequency catheter ablation of atrial tissue comparison with thermometry-guide ablation: comparison with thermometry-guide ablation. J Interv Card Electrophysiol. 2001;5:253-266. With permission.*)

electrode temperature was limited to 65°C with a 4-mm electrode, and 55°C with an 8-mm electrode.[12] Tissue interface temperatures remained well below 100°C, and coagulum did not always result in impedance rise. With large electrodes, it is possible to overheat portions of the electrode remote from the embedded thermistor or thermocouple.

Coagulum that anneals to tissue rather than the electrode tip may fail to affect electrode temperature or impedance, yet could detach from tissue and embolize. Embolic complications have been reported even in patients undergoing relatively short ablation procedures when few lesions were created and no abrupt increases in impedance were observed.[13] Even if embolism does not occur, coagulum formation requires removing the ablation catheter to clean the tip, increasing procedural and fluoroscopy time.

Myocardial Boiling (Steam Pop)

When tissue temperature exceeds 100°C, boiling of water in the myocardial tissue can cause a sudden buildup of steam in the myocardium, sometimes audible as a "steam pop " (**Video 2-1**).[14] This is often associated with a shower of microbubbles on intracardiac echocardiography, which have been shown to be composed of steam (**Video 2-2**).[15] The escaping gas can cause barotrauma with dissection of tissue planes. Damage ranging from superficial endocardial craters to full-thickness myocardial tears resulting in cardiac perforation and tamponade can occur (Fig. 2-2). The consequences of a steam pop vary widely depending on location, myocardial thickness, and proximity to vulnerable structures such as the atrioventricular (AV) node.

Temperature-controlled ablation with a conventional 4mm-tip catheter carries a low risk for steam pop because tissue and electrode temperature do not diverge widely, and temperature is limited to well below 100°C. However, this might not hold true in regions with very high rates of blood flow, in which convective cooling can permit significant discrepancy between tissue and electrode temperature. Steam pops are more likely with newer technologies aimed at creating larger lesions, such as large-electrode ablation catheters (8- to 12-mm tips) and cooled-tip ablation catheters with either internal or external irrigation. A common feature of these large-lesion catheters is that tissue temperature greatly exceeds electrode temperature, sometimes by as much as 40°C. Therefore, steam pops can occur even when electrode temperature is limited to ostensibly safe levels (Fig. 2-3).

Cardiac Perforation

RF energy delivery can cause perforation even in the absence of steam pop. This is more likely in a thin-walled chamber such as the left atrium, especially with high power and excessive contact force. Long deflectable sheaths allow extremely effective contact with myocardium. Unless caution is exercised (e.g., by limiting power), this may increase the chances of cardiac perforation during delivery of RF energy. Some structures are particularly prone to perforation, including the thin-walled left atrial appendage and the coronary sinus.

Left atrial ablation for atrial fibrillation is often performed with an irrigated catheter through a long sheath and carries a particularly high risk for cardiac perforation, effusion, and tamponade—more than 1.2% in two large series.[16,17] Considering that high power is delivered through intimate tissue contact in a thin-walled chamber, this is not unexpected. Titrating energy delivery down to the minimal level required to achieve the procedural end point reduces the risk for all local complications, including coagulum, steam pops, and perforation.

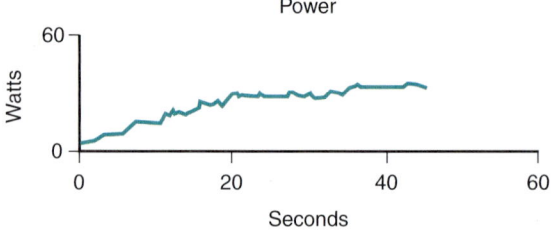

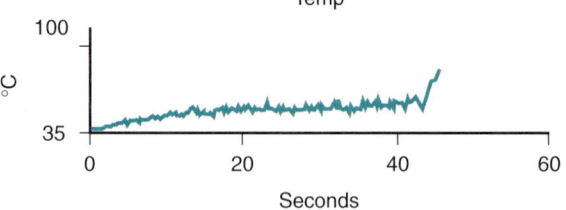

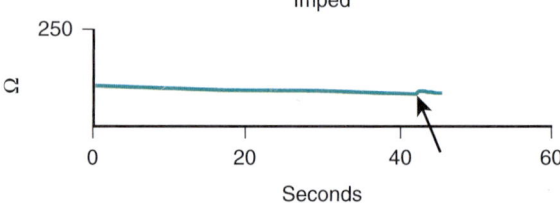

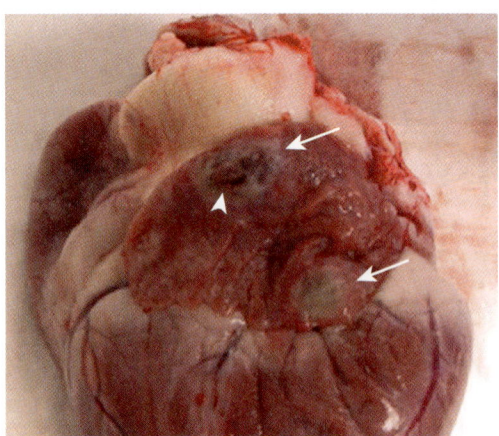

FIGURE 2-2. Lateral view of porcine heart following RF catheter ablation. Two transmural lesions in the left atrium appendage are shown (*arrows*). A steam pop occurred with the more superior lesion, and a surface tear is visible (*arrowhead*). (*From Cooper JM, Sapp JL, Tedrow U, et al. Ablation with an internally irrigated radiofrequency catheter: learning how to avoid steam pops.* Heart Rhythm. *2004;1:329–333. With permission.*)

FIGURE 2-3. Data recorded during lesion application that resulted in steam pop and transmural left atrial tear from barotrauma. At the moment of microbubble release on intracardiac echocardiography, a small, non-sustained rise in impedance was observed (*arrow*). A few seconds later, electrode temperature rose abruptly, as bubbles engulfed the ablation electrode.

Damage to Surrounding Structures

In addition to the local complications described previously, collateral damage to structures outside the heart can also result from excessive energy delivery. Depending on the arrhythmia being treated and location targeted, catheter ablation can result in damage to lung tissue,[18] coronary arteries,[19] phrenic nerves,[20,21] aorta, or esophagus.[22,23] Although many strategies have been developed to protect these structures during ablation,[24-26] one of the simplest and most effective is to reduce power to the minimum necessary level.

Methods of Titrating Energy Delivery with Conventional Radiofrequency Ablation Catheters

Multiple methods of titrating power have been used, alone and in combination. Although fixed power ablation is one option, most operators adjust power in response to real-time data. Commonly used parameters are electrode-tip temperature, ablation circuit impedance, local electrogram amplitude, and electrophysiologic end points.

Temperature-Titrated Energy Delivery

Power and duration of RF application alone do not accurately predict lesion size because unmeasured variables such as catheter orientation, cavitary blood flow, and catheter contact pressure significantly affect the volume of the resulting lesion. Early in the development of RF catheter ablation, investigators embedded a thermistor in the tip of an ablation catheter, showing that temperature monitoring of the tissue-electrode interface was useful in predicting lesion volume, both experimentally[4] and in clinical ablation procedures.[27] Closed-loop temperature-controlled ablation systems were devised, in which the RF generator decreases power automatically when temperature exceeds a prespecified cutoff. Usually the power, temperature, and impedance are continuously displayed to the operator as time plots during the energy application. In one large series, closed-loop temperature control reduced the rate of coagulum formation and RF shutdown due to sudden impedance rise by more than 80%.[28] Temperature control has proved useful in ablation of accessory pathways,[29] modification of the AV nodal slow pathway,[30] and treatment of many other arrhythmias. For most applications with a 4-mm electrode, temperatures of 50° to 65°C are sought. The electrode temperature must always be considered in the context of the delivered power and often impedance data. Controlling catheter-tip temperature reduces, but does not eliminate, the risk for coagulum formation and steam pops. As discussed earlier, coagulum can form at temperatures well below 100°C. The electrode temperature underestimates the tissue temperature, and the discrepency can be significant. Besides power and electrode temperature, other important determinants of tissue temperature include catheter orientation, electrode size, catheter contact, and convective cooling.[31,32] Not all these can be controlled, or even measured, in a clinical ablation procedure.

True tissue temperature control, as opposed to electrode-tip temperature control, has been tested in vitro. RF energy delivery has been titrated using a thermocouple needle extending 2 mm from the catheter tip into the myocardium.[33] This achieved adequate lesions without excessive intramyocardial temperature rise and prevented steam pops. In theory, tissue temperature–guided power titration would result in more predictable lesion size, reducing variability because of differences in catheter contact and convective blood flow cooling. However, significant engineering obstacles must be overcome, such as demonstrating the safety of inserting a needle into the beating human heart and reliably measuring tissue temperature regardless of catheter orientation.

Impedance-Titrated Energy Delivery

Because neither applied power nor electrode-tip temperature adequately reveals tissue temperature, investigators have sought other surrogate measures of tissue heating.[34] One such parameter is ablation circuit impedance, which reflects the resistance to current flow through the patient, from the tip of the ablation catheter to the skin grounding pad. At the high frequencies used for RF ablation, tissue impedance can be modeled as a simple resistor.[35] As the tissue is heated, ions in the tissue become more mobile, resulting in a fall in local resistivity,[36] measurable as a fall in ablation circuit impedance. Significant tissue heating is associated with a predictable fall in impedance, usually in the range of 5 to 10 ohms.[37] The absence of initial impedance fall may reflect inadequate energy delivery to the tissue, poor catheter-tissue contact, or catheter instability.

Impedance titration has been used successfully to guide ablation procedures. In one protocol used for accessory pathway ablation, power was adjusted manually to achieve a fall in impedance of 5 to 10 ohms, to a maximal power of 50 W.[38] A randomized comparison showed similar results for temperature and impedance power monitoring with 93% procedural success in each group, and no difference in the rate of coagulum formation. However, the same investigators found that impedance titration was not useful for AV nodal slow pathway modification, in which lower power and temperature are desirable to avoid AV block, with smaller resulting lesions.[39] Successful slow pathway sites showed a lower mean electrode temperature (48.5°C) and no significant change in impedance. This suggests that impedance drops are less dramatic (and impedance monitoring less useful) for ablations in which smaller lesions are indicated, such as slow pathway modification. Theoretically, a closed-loop system using impedance instead of electrode temperature to regulate power could be developed, but such systems are not commercially available.

Impedance monitoring can also be used to increase the safety of ablation procedures. Large drops in impedance, reflecting excessive tissue heating, predict subsequent impedance rises due to interfacial boiling. In one study, RF applications in which impedance fell by more than 10 ohms showed a high rate of coagulum formation (12%), but no coagulum was seen when impedance fell by less than 10 ohms.[40] Based on these results, the authors suggested reducing power during any application resulting in impedance drop of at least 10 ohms. Some investigators sought a correlation between the magnitude of impedance fall and electrode-tip temperature, before real-time monitoring of electrode temperature was widely available. Measuring only impedance, electrode-tip temperature could be predicted with reasonable accuracy, with an average difference of 5.2°C.[41] However, errors of more than 10°C were seen in 11% of applications. This is of largely historical interest because electrode-tip temperature is now routinely measured.

An important finding from these early studies was that impedance and electrode-tip temperature do not always correlate. For example, Strickberger and colleagues found a statistically significant inverse association between impedance and electrode-tip temperature, with each ohm corresponding to 2.63°C on average (Fig. 2-4).[40] However,

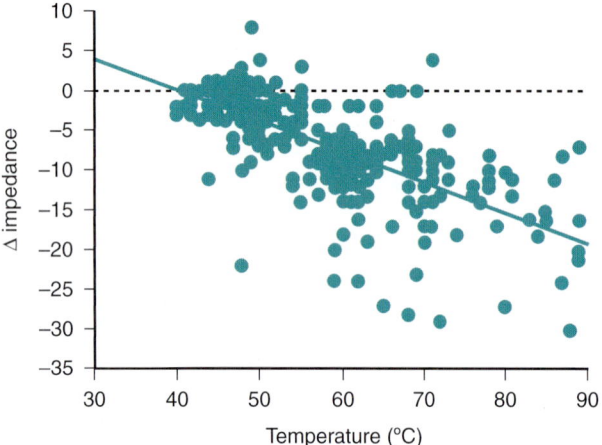

FIGURE 2-4. Correlation between final temperature and change in impedance during radiofrequency ablation. Temperature (°C) is represented on the *x* axis, and Δ impedance (ohms) is represented on the *y* axis ($y = 15.3 - 0.38x$; $p < .0001$; $R = 0.7$). *(Data from Strickberger SA, Ravi S, Daoud E, et al. Relation between impedance and temperature during radiofrequency ablation of accessory pathways. Am Heart J. 1995;130:1026–1030. With permission.)*

the data show significant scatter between the two variables with a correlation coefficient ($R = 0.7$, $R(2) = 0.49$), suggesting that only half the variability in impedance was associated with corresponding changes in electrode-tip temperature. Because impedance changes reflect changes in tissue characteristics, impedance drop can offer an independent means of assessing the true outcome of interest, tissue heating.

RF applications showing large impedance change relative to temperature increase are common in areas of brisk convective blood cooling, in which electrode temperature substantially underestimates tissue temperature (Fig. 2-5). Conversely, a large increase in electrode temperature without significant impedance drop may indicate intimate electrode-tissue contact without convective cooling; surface heating occurs without significant deep tissue heating. Power is limited by electrode-tip temperature, and a small lesion results.

In summary, both electrode-tip temperature and impedance offer indirect assessment of the true variable of interest, achieved tissue temperature, which cannot be measured directly with current technology. Taking both of these parameters into account allows the operator to titrate RF energy delivery to create large lesions safely, mitigating the inherent variability arising from differences in catheter contact and convective cooling.

Electrogram Amplitude-Titrated Energy Delivery

Even taken together, electrode-tip temperature and ablation circuit impedance are imperfect indicators of tissue destruction. Power can be titrated by using reduction in electrogram amplitude as a physiologic marker of effective ablation. During RF application, local electrogram amplitude typically falls as tissue heating causes necrosis and loss of excitability. However, the magnitude of this amplitude reduction varies, and the exact myocardial volume sensed by ablation catheter electrodes ("field of view") is

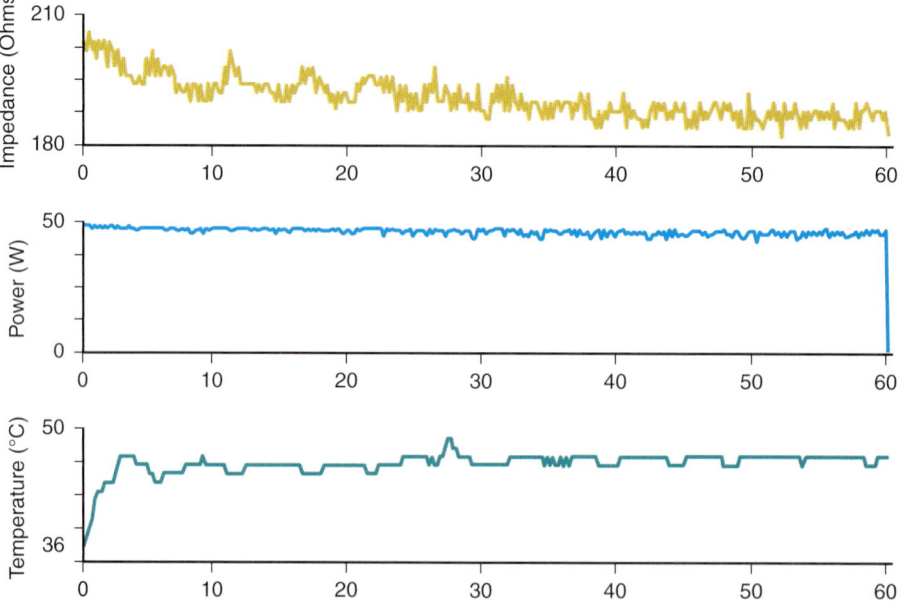

FIGURE 2-5. Plot of impedance, power, and temperature during catheter ablation of a left posteroseptal accessory pathway using a conventional 4-mm-tip catheter. Blood flow was brisk, and convective cooling kept the catheter-tip temperature below 50°C despite high power (50 W). However, even without a high temperature at the catheter tip, evidence of tissue damage was seen. Accessory pathway conduction was blocked in less than 3 seconds, and impedance fell by more than 15 ohms during energy application.

not known. A prospective evaluation was conducted using a 90% reduction in bipolar electrogram amplitude to titrate energy delivery.[42] Although the technique appeared to be safe, it often resulted in inadequate lesion size, and many lesions were not transmural.

In return for a potentially higher level of safety, electrogram amplitude reduction produces smaller lesions and would be expected to require a larger number of RF applications for a given procedure.[43] Concerns about procedural efficacy and procedure time have prevented this method of energy titration from being widely adopted. However, many operators increase power or duration, or repeat RF application at a given site, if no significant reduction in local electrogram amplitude is seen.

Titrating Energy Delivery by Electrophysiologic End Points

Some ablation procedures have clear electrophysiologic end points that can be used to titrate energy delivery.[44] One example is RF ablation of the cavotricuspid isthmus for typical atrial flutter. In this setting, relatively high power deliveries (50 W or higher) or irrigated catheters are often needed to permanently destroy the targeted myocardial tissue. Energy delivery can be modified to result in electrogram abatement or splitting of the electrogram into two components indicating local conduction block. Other examples may be delivery of RF current at progressively greater power until termination of scar-related ventricular tachycardia or focal atrial tachycardia.

Titrating Energy Delivery with Large-Tip Catheters

For many clinical applications of RF ablation, such as interruption of an accessory pathway, the goal is to produce a small, circumscribed lesion at a precisely targeted position. Standard 4-mm-tip ablation catheters are well suited to this purpose. However, for some ablation procedures, such as ventricular tachycardia ablation, small lesions are inadequate. Higher power cannot increase lesion size beyond a certain point because coagulum formation and impedance rise will occur. This can necessitate multiple RF applications at each site.

Early in the development of RF catheter ablation, investigators hypothesized that increasing the surface area of electrode-tissue contact would result in adequate current density over a larger area of myocardium, yielding a larger lesion.[4,45] This concept was systematically examined by Langberg and colleagues, who found that increasing electrode tip size from 2 to 4 mm doubled the resulting lesion volume, but larger electrodes (8 to 12 mm) resulted in smaller lesions.[46] However, the experimental design used a fixed power of only 13 W, insufficient to heat tissue with the largest electrodes because RF energy was dispersed over too wide an area (reducing current density) and shunted to the blood pool. Later studies showed that in temperature-controlled mode with higher maximal power (up to 100 W), larger lesions were indeed achieved with 8- and 10-mm-tip catheters.[47] Another mechanism of larger lesion formation is the increase in convective cooling seen across the large surface area of the 8-mm-tip

catheter.[48] Clinical results in ablation procedures have generally supported the concept that larger lesions are more effective. For typical atrial flutter, ablation using an 8-mm-tip instead of a 4-mm-tip catheter results in higher procedural success; bidirectional block can be achieved with fewer lesions and lower fluoroscopy time.[49,50] Large-tip catheters have also been used successfully in ablation of atrial fibrillation and ventricular tachycardia.

All other factors being equal, large-tip catheters require higher power for electrode tip heating and adequate lesion formation.[51] This is because of the need to compensate for the proportion of current shunted through the blood pool and to create a high current density around a larger electrode area that may be in contact with the tissue. Although initial impedance is lower for these catheters, a drop in impedance is still observed, and impedance titration can be used. However, the most common method in clinical practice is temperature guided. Because a greater volume of tissue is heated electrically and more convective cooling occurs, a lower target electrode temperature should be chosen, usually 50° to 55°C. Special caution is warranted, considering the large lesions produced by these catheters: heating of distant structures has been seen in an animal model, with lung injury from right atrial ablation occurring three times as often with a 10-mm-tip compared with a 4-mm-tip catheter.[47] Care should be exercised when ablating adjacent to the esophagus, phrenic nerves, or coronary arteries. In addition, there is a greater discrepancy between tip and tissue temperature with large-tip catheters,[52,53] which increases the chances of steam pop and perforation. Finally, the large surface area of these electrodes can obscure the usual signs of coagulum formation; impedance may not rise significantly if only a portion of the catheter tip is covered in coagulum. Table 2-1 lists some warning signs of impending complications that mandate discontinuation of RF application or reduction in RF power.

Titrating Energy Delivery with Irrigated Radiofrequency Ablation Catheters

Differences between Irrigated and Conventional Ablation Catheters

The observation that convective blood cooling allows delivery of higher power and creation of larger lesions led to the development of catheters that are cooled artificially by irrigating the catheter tip with saline, either internally[54] or externally[55] (Fig. 2-6). Cooling of the catheter tip also lowers the risk for coagulum formation by preventing interfacial boiling and possibly washing away denatured proteins.[56] However, it should be kept in mind that coagulum can still form on tissue because tip temperature may substantially underestimate maximal interfacial temperature. It is also possible that interfacial boiling does still occur and that irrigation simply prevents the usual rise in impedance to allow continued RF energy delivery.[9]

Irrigated catheters allow ablation at higher power, with a predictable increase in the surface area, depth, and volume of ablation lesions.[57] As expected, procedural efficacy is higher in arrhythmia substrates requiring large lesions,

TABLE 2-1

WARNING SIGNS OF IMPENDING COMPLICATIONS WITH CONVENTIONAL RADIOFREQUENCY ABLATION CATHETERS

Indicator	Cause	Notes
Excessive ablation catheter electrode temperature rise (>65°C for 4-mm electrode, 55°C for 8-mm electrode, 40° to 45°C for irrigated electrode)	Excellent catheter contact with little convective cooling, especially in fixed power mode	Risk for steam pop or coagulum; should not occur in temperature-controlled ablation mode
Impedance drop >10 ohms, especially if rapid	Excessive tissue heating	Increased risk for subsequent impedance rise
Increase in ablation circuit impedance	Formation of coagulum on electrode tip, trapping elaborated gas and insulating electrode	Formed by denatured blood proteins, not prevented by heparinization
Shower of microbubbles on intracardiac echocardiography	Boiling at electrode-tissue interface	Correlates with surface temperature, not tissue temperature[65]
Audible pop or sudden change in electrode temperature or impedance due to catheter movement	Boiling within myocardial tissue	Can result in myocardial tear, effusion, or tamponade, especially in thin-walled chambers
Esophageal temperature rise	Heating of esophagus during ablation of posterior left atrium	Risk for atrioesophageal fistula (usually fatal)
Loss of diaphragmatic capture with pacing from ablation distal electrode pair	Thermal injury to phrenic nerve	Seen especially with ablation at right-sided pulmonary veins and epicardial ablation
Physiologic end point, such as PR prolongation during AV node slow pathway modification	Slowed conduction in AV nodal fast pathway or compact AV node	Signifies impending AV block

AV, atrioventricular.

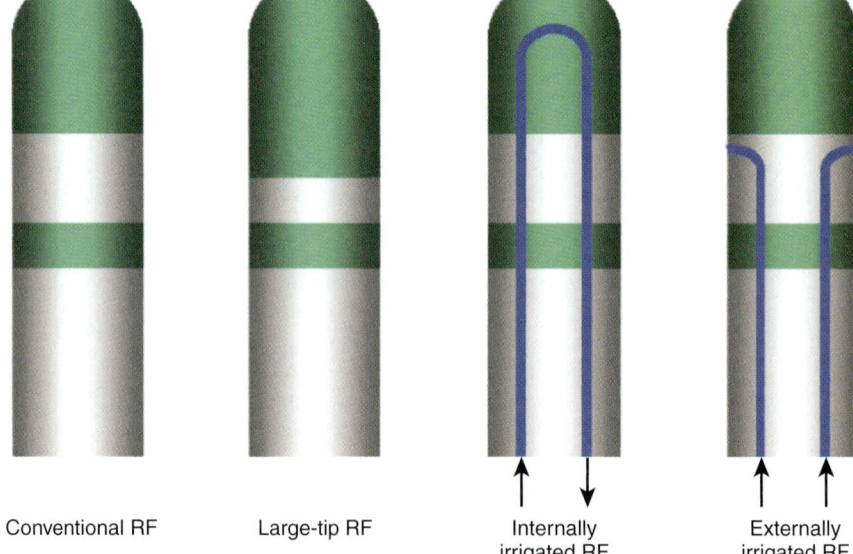

FIGURE 2-6. Currently available radiofrequency (RF) catheter designs. Lesion volume is larger with each of these technologies compared with conventional 4-mm-tip catheters. *(Adapted from Shivkumar K, Boyle NB, Cesario DA. Biophysics of radiofrequency ablation. In: Zipes DP, Jalife J, eds. Cardiac Electrophysiology: From Cell to Bedside. Philadelphia: Saunders, 2009.[85] With permission.)*

Conventional RF   Large-tip RF   Internally irrigated RF   Externally irrigated RF

including ablation of ventricular tachycardia[58] and atrial flutter.[59] Irrigated catheters also have been successful in the treatment of accessory pathways resistant to conventional ablation.[60]

A key difference between conventional and irrigated ablation catheters is the much higher discrepancy between catheter-tip and tissue temperature with irrigation. In fact, tip temperature is not a reliable indicator of tissue temperature at all, especially with higher irrigation flow rates. Tissue temperature may exceed tip temperature by 40°C or more, and the maximal tissue temperature typically occurs at least 2 mm away from the tip of the ablation catheter.[61] Therefore, steam pops can occur even with

normal tip temperature. Some investigators have argued that this divergence precludes controlling RF power by tip temperature.[33] However, the tip temperature still increases in response to adjacent tissue heating, especially at lower flow rates.[62] Therefore, a significant increase in catheter-tip temperature to more than 42° to 45°C during irrigated ablation signals the need to reduce power.

Factors Affecting Lesion Size during Irrigated Radiofrequency Ablation

Most irrigated-tip catheters use room-temperature saline (about 20°C) for cooling, but chilled saline can also be used

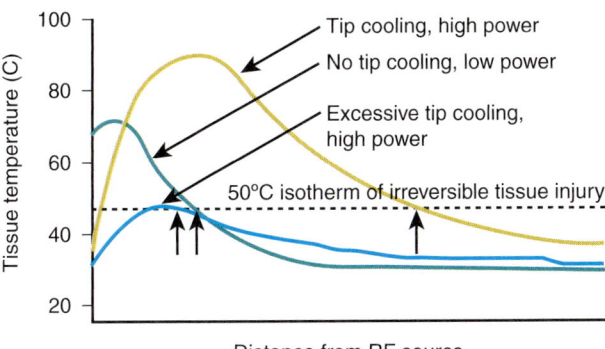

FIGURE 2-7. Tissue temperature gradients in three conditions. Tissue temperature higher than 50°C defines the border of the radiofrequency (RF) lesion (*vertical arrows*). During low-power ablation without tip cooling (*green plot*), electrode temperature only slightly underestimates peak tissue temperature, and the lesion is not deep. During ablation with tip cooling (*orange plot*), surface temperature remains low, allowing high-power delivery, and peak tissue temperature is reached below the endocardial surface, with a large resulting lesion. However, if flow rate is excessive (*blue plot*), a greater proportion of RF energy will be dissipated by convection, and the tissue will absorb less energy. The resulting lesion may be smaller than what would be created with standard, noncooled ablation.(*Adapted from Haines DE. Biophysics and pathophysiology of lesion formation by transcatheter radiofrequency ablation. In: Wilber DJ, Packer DL, Stevenson WG, eds. Catheter Ablation of Cardiac Arrhythmias: Basic Concepts and Clinical Applications. Malden, MA: Blackwell, 2008:20–34. With permission.*)

TABLE 2-2
EVIDENCE OF LESION FORMATION WITH IRRIGATED RADIOFREQUENCY ABLATION CATHETERS
Reduction in local electrogram amplitude (>50% to 90%)
Impedance drop (5-10 ohms)
Increase in local pacing threshold (>100%)
Emergence of double potentials, signifying local conduction block
Tachycardia termination during ablation (and noninducibility)

in either closed-loop or open-irrigated systems. In theory, this should allow delivery of greater power and create larger lesions, but in practice, the effect is minimal.[9] Irrigation flow rate can be important, especially when the catheter tip is located in an area with poor convective blood cooling, such as in a pouch or between tissue trabeculations. In such areas, increasing rate of irrigation flow may be necessary to permit desired power delivery without heating the electrode tip. At high flow rates, tip and tissue temperatures will diverge more widely. Excessive flow, beyond that needed to allow targeted power delivery, should be avoided because it will actually reduce tissue temperature and result in a smaller lesion (Fig. 2-7).[63] Electrode orientation also influences irrigated ablation lesion sizes. Electrode orientation perpendicular to the tissue produces larger lesions than a parallel orientation.

As with conventional ablation catheters, increasing the power and duration of RF application will also result in larger lesions. The time required to achieve thermal equilibrium, and therefore maximal lesion size, may be greater with irrigated-tip catheters.[62] The operator can also choose to allow a slightly larger rise in electrode tip temperature (e.g., 45° versus 40°C) if power delivery is limited despite irrigation.

Titrating Power during Irrigated Radiofrequency Ablation

The same principle applies with irrigated catheters: power should be set at the minimum required to achieve the desired outcome, in order to reduce risk for complications. With conventional catheters, electrode temperature is an important indicator of tissue heating, and a response to inadequate heating might be to increase RF power. With irrigated catheters, however, electrode temperature is not as useful, and other indicators of tissue damage must be

used instead. See Table 2-2 for a summary of factors suggesting adequate lesion formation with irrigated ablation catheters. None of these alone is a definite indicator of successful lesion formation, but taken together, they can help determine when targeted tissue has been ablated. In general, electrode temperatures of less than 40° to 45°C and impedance drops of 5 to 10 ohms are sought.

Warning signs of excessive energy delivery can be seen with irrigated-tip catheters. Although catheter cooling reduces the rate of interfacial boiling and coagulum formation, especially with external irrigation, steam pops may be more common.[56] Indicators of possible impending steam pop include temperature rise to above 42° to 45°C[14] and impedance drop of more than 18 ohms.[64] See Figure 2-8 for an example of excessive temperature rise during irrigated RF application. Microbubbles on intracardiac echocardiography have been investigated as another way to titrate energy delivery,[15] although they appear to be a better indicator of high interface temperature than of tissue temperature.[65] Table 2-3 presents practical recommendations on titrating RF energy during irrigated ablation.

Finally, monitoring for heating of extracardiac structures is important with irrigated ablation. During posterior left atrial ablation, temperature monitoring in the esophagus can be used to detect unwanted heating of esophageal tissue, allowing the operator to reduce power or reposition the catheter.[66] During ablation at the right-sided pulmonary vein ostia or in the epicardial space, phrenic nerve injury can occur, with symptoms ranging from mild to life-threatening.[67] To avoid this complication, many operators avoid RF application in sites with phrenic nerve capture on high-output pacing. Another option is to ablate at lower power during continuous pacing just above phrenic capture threshold, interrupting energy delivery if diaphragmatic stimulation is lost.[68] Several methods of phrenic nerve protection have been developed to allow safer ablation at a critical site in which phrenic nerve injury is otherwise likely.[25,69,70]

Titrating Energy Delivery in Unusual Anatomic Sites

The preceding sections described methods of RF power titration for endocardial ablation using conventional and irrigated ablation catheters. However, when catheter ablation is performed in other sites, it may be necessary to modify the approach to titrating RF energy delivery.

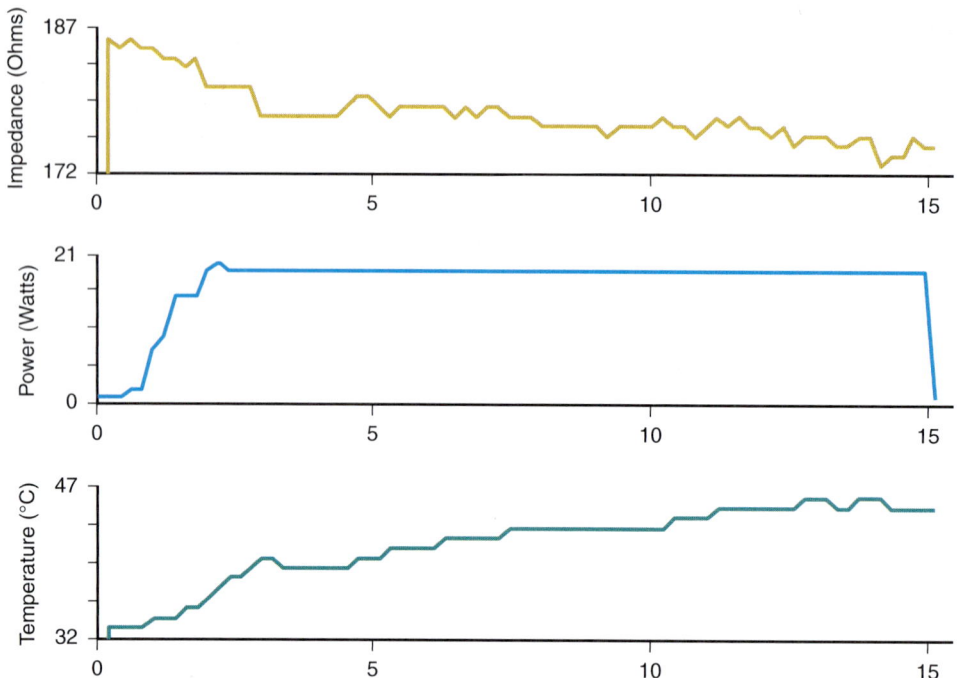

FIGURE 2-8. Excessive temperature rise during irrigated radiofrequency (RF) ablation. During ablation in the left atrium for atrial fibrillation, using an externally irrigated 4-mm-tip catheter with flow rate of 17 mL/min, the operator noticed a steadily rising temperature and discontinued RF when it reached 45°C. This probably resulted from intimate tissue contact that prevented adequate cooling of the electrode tip. Other possible responses would have been increasing the irrigation flow rate, reducing power, or repositioning the catheter.

TABLE 2-3

PRACTICAL RECOMMENDATIONS FOR RADIOFREQUENCY POWER TITRATION WITH EXTERNALLY IRRIGATED RADIOFREQUENCY ABLATION CATHETERS

Set irrigation flow rate to 17 mL/min for power under 30 W, otherwise 30 mL/min.[87]

Use power control instead of temperature control setting on radiofrequency (RF) generator, beginning at 15-30 W (depending on cardiac chamber and location).

Gradually increase RF power, watching for electrode-tip temperature to increase to 37° to 40°C. If tip temperature rises above 42°C, decrease power or reposition catheter to reduce risk for steam pop.

If temperature remains above 40°C despite power <20 W, the ablation catheter tip is likely wedged in tissue. Consider repositioning catheter or increasing irrigation flow rate. If problem persists, check integrity of the cooling system.

Impedance should fall by 5 to 10 ohms as tissue is ablated. If impedance does not change, catheter-tissue contact is likely inadequate, and repositioning may be needed.

If impedance falls by 18 ohms or more, titrate down power or pause energy delivery because this may signal impending steam pop.[64] If impedance rises, discontinue RF application, check cooling system, and inspect catheter tip for coagulum.

Power Titration during Epicardial Ablation

Nonsurgical epicardial catheter ablation, through a percutaneous subxiphoid approach, was first described by Sosa and colleagues.[71] Originally used to treat ventricular tachycardia in patients with Chagas disease, the technique has proved useful in the treatment of many arrhythmias, including ischemic ventricular tachycardia, accessory pathways, and other arrhythmias.[72]

One key difference compared with endocardial catheter ablation is the lack of blood flow in the pericardial space, resulting in minimal convective cooling. As a result, conventional noncooled ablation catheters reach high tip temperature at relatively low power (<10 W), limiting energy delivery and resulting in small lesions.[73] Intervening epicardial fat may also protect targeted myocardial tissue from effective ablation. However, internally or externally irrigated catheters allow higher RF power (25 to 50 W) without temperature rise; larger lesions are created, even when ablating over epicardial fat.[74] Most operators begin at 20 to 30 W and titrate up to a maximum of 50 W, maintaining adequate irrigation rate to keep tip temperature below 45°C.[73] Indicators of lesion formation are similar to those used in irrigated endocardial ablation, including fall in impedance and local electrogram amplitude.

Special precautions should be taken when ablating within the epicardial space. When using externally irrigated ablation, the epicardial sheath must be periodically aspirated to prevent accumulation of fluid, which could cause effusion and tamponade. Coronary arteries are epicardial structures, and care must be taken not to apply RF energy near them. Although in theory the coronary arteries are somewhat protected by the cooling effect of intraluminary blood flow, complications of RF ablation have been described, including coronary thrombosis, vessel wall damage, and vasospasm. Smaller vessels may be at particularly high risk.[75] Real-time coronary angiography is generally necessary to delineate the course of the arteries. RF application is usually avoided within 5 to 10 mm of a coronary artery, although no absolute safe distance has

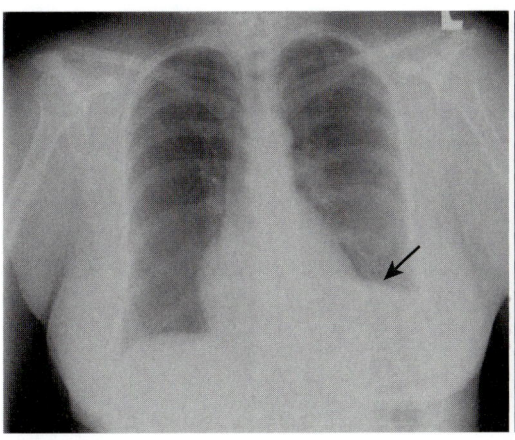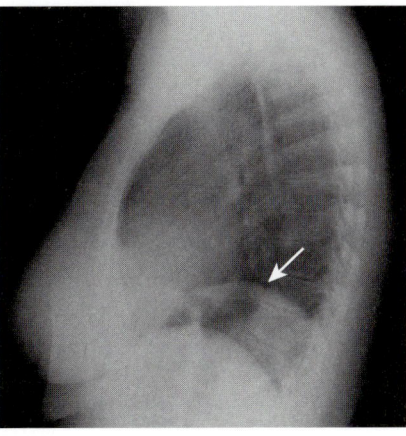

FIGURE 2-9. Phrenic nerve injury after ablation. Following epicardial ablation of ventricular tachycardia, this patient developed shortness of breath and was found to have an elevated left hemidiaphragm (*arrows*). This was managed conservatively and resolved completely within 3 months.

TABLE 2-4			
SUMMARY OF RADIOFREQUENCY ENERGY TITRATION TECHNIQUES			
Method	**Commonly Used Target Parameters**	**Advantages**	**Disadvantages**
Fixed power	No titration	Simple, no special equipment required	Increased risk for complications
Ablation electrode temperature	4-mm electrode: 55° to 60°C 8-mm electrode: <55°C Irrigated electrode: <42°C	Easy to apply, closed-loop systems regulate power automatically	Does not reliably predict lesion size or risk for complications, owing to difference between tip and tissue temperature
Change in ablation circuit impedance	5- to 10-ohm decrease	Can be used with any electrode, in some cases may correlate better with tissue temperature	Variable association with myocardial tissue temperature, insensitive for smaller lesions; less useful for irrigated catheters
Electrogram amplitude reduction	50% to 90% reduction in size of bipolar electrogram	Shows direct effects of ablation on targeted tissue	May result in small or nontransmural lesions, likely lower procedural efficacy

been defined.[73] Experimental evidence suggests that infusion of chilled saline into the coronary artery may help protect the endothelium, but this strategy is not yet widely used.[24,76] The phrenic nerves are also vulnerable to epicardial ablation (Fig. 2-9). Diaphragmatic capture with pacing identifies high risk for nerve injury, and ablation at these sites should be avoided. This diagnostic maneuver is possible only when procedural anesthesia does not include skeletal muscle relaxants.

Power Titration during Ablation within the Coronary Sinus

Occasionally, the optimal site for ablation is within the coronary venous system, accessed through the coronary sinus. Subepicardial accessory pathways,[77] premature ventricular complexes,[78] atypical atrial flutter,[7,79] and atrial fibrillation[80] have been successfully treated with RF ablation within the coronary sinus. One common reason for ablation in the coronary sinus is completing a mitral isthmus line as part of left atrial ablation for persistent atrial fibrillation. This is usually done with an irrigated ablation catheter: flow rate, 17 to 60 mL/minute; maximal temperature, 50°C; and power, 20 to 30 W.[81] However, despite the relatively high power used, successful creation of a mitral isthmus line remains technically challenging, even after combined endocardial and coronary sinus ablation. Some investigators hypothesize that this is due to coronary venous blood flow acting as a heat sink, carrying RF energy away and preventing adequate lesion formation.[82] In an animal study, D'Avila and colleagues tested a device that occluded the coronary sinus ostium to prevent blood flow during ablation.[83] They were able to achieve transmural lesions from endocardial ablation only when flow was prevented by balloon occlusion. Care must be taken during ablation in the coronary sinus, since the left circumflex coronary artery also runs within the AV groove. Occlusion of the circumflex artery has been described during ablation in the coronary sinus.[84]

Conclusion

Current methods of RF energy titration allow catheter ablation in the treatment of arrhythmias to be performed safely and effectively (Table 2-4). Most of these methods have a sound theoretical basis but have not been examined in rigorous prospective studies. In the future, technologies and techniques for titrating RF power and tissue response will continue to evolve, further improving the results of catheter ablation procedures.

References

1. Avitall B, Mughal K, Hare J, et al. The effects of electrode-tissue contact on radiofrequency lesion generation. *Pacing Clin Electrophysiol*. 1997;20:2899–2910.
2. Demazumder D, Schwartzman D. Titration of radiofrequency energy during endocardial catheter ablation. In: Huang SK, Wood MA, eds. *Catheter Ablation of Cardiac Arrhythmias*. Philadelphia: Saunders; 2006:691.

3. Yokoyama K, Nakagawa H, Shah DC, et al. Novel contact force sensor incorporated in irrigated radiofrequency ablation catheter predicts lesion size and incidence of steam pop and thrombus. *Circ Arrhythmia Electrophysiol.* 2008;1:354–362.

4. Haines DE, Watson DD. Tissue heating during radiofrequency catheter ablation: a thermodynamic model and observations in isolated perfused and superfused canine right ventricular free wall. *Pacing Clin Electrophysiol.* 1989;12:962–976.

5. Nath S, Lynch C, Whayne JG, Haines DE. Cellular electrophysiological effects of hyperthermia on isolated guinea pig papillary muscle: implications for catheter ablation. *Circulation.* 1993;88:1826–1831.

6. Wittkampf FH, Hauer RN, Robles de Medina EO. Control of radiofrequency lesion size by power regulation. *Circulation.* 1989;80:962–968.

7. Chugh SS, Chan RC, Johnson SB, Packer DL. Catheter tip orientation affects radiofrequency ablation lesion size in the canine left ventricle. *Pacing Clin Electrophysiol.* 1999;22:413–420.

8. Wittkampf FH, Nakagawa H, Yamanashi WS, et al. Thermal latency in radiofrequency ablation. *Circulation.* 1996;93:1083–1086.

9. Demazumder D, Mirotznik MS, Schwartzman D. Biophysics of radiofrequency ablation using an irrigated electrode. *J Interv Card Electrophysiol.* 2001;5:377–389.

10. Demolin JM, Eick OJ, Munch K, et al. Soft thrombus formation in radiofrequency catheter ablation. *Pacing Clin Electrophysiol.* 2002;25:1219–1222.

11. Wittkampf FH, Nakagawa H. RF catheter ablation: lessons on lesions. *Pacing Clin Electrophysiol.* 2006;29:1285–1297.

12. Matsudaira K, Nakagawa H, Wittkampf FH, et al. High incidence of thrombus formation without impedance rise during radiofrequency ablation using electrode temperature control. *Pacing Clin Electrophysiol.* 2003;26:1227–1237.

13. Thakur RK, Klein GJ, Yee R, Zardini M. Embolic complications after radiofrequency catheter ablation. *Am J Cardiol.* 1994;74:278–279.

14. Cooper JM, Sapp JL, Tedrow U, et al. Ablation with an internally irrigated radiofrequency catheter: learning how to avoid steam pops. *Heart Rhythm.* 2004;1:329–333.

15. Wood MA, Shaffer KM, Ellenbogen AL, Ownby ED. Microbubbles during radiofrequency catheter ablation: composition and formation. *Heart Rhythm.* 2005;2:397–403.

16. Spragg DD, Dalal D, Cheema A, et al. Complications of catheter ablation for atrial fibrillation: incidence and predictors. *J Cardiovasc Electrophysiol.* 2008;19:627–631.

17. Dagres N, Hindricks G, Kottkamp H, et al. Complications of atrial fibrillation ablation in a high-volume center in 1,000 procedures: still cause for concern? *J Cardiovasc Electrophysiol.* 2009;20:1014–1019.

18. Kongsgaard E, Foerster A, Aass H, et al. Power and temperature guided radiofrequency catheter ablation of the right atrium in pigs. *Pacing Clin Electrophysiol.* 1994;17:1610–1620.

19. Ouali S, Anselme F, Savoure A, Cribier A. Acute coronary occlusion during radiofrequency catheter ablation of typical atrial flutter. *J Cardiovasc Electrophysiol.* 2002;13:1047–1049.

20. Durante-Mangoni E, Del Vecchio D, Ruggiero G. Right diaphragm paralysis following cardiac radiofrequency catheter ablation for inappropriate sinus tachycardia. *Pacing Clin Electrophysiol.* 2003;26:783–784.

21. Lee BK, Choi KJ, Kim J, et al. Right phrenic nerve injury following electrical disconnection of the right superior pulmonary vein. *Pacing Clin Electrophysiol.* 2004;27:1444–1446.

22. Pappone C, Oral H, Santinelli V, et al. Atrio-esophageal fistula as a complication of percutaneous transcatheter ablation of atrial fibrillation. *Circulation.* 2004;109:2724–2726.

23. Scanavacca MI, D'Avila A, Parga J, Sosa E. Left atrial-esophageal fistula following radiofrequency catheter ablation of atrial fibrillation. *J Cardiovasc Electrophysiol.* 2004;15:960–962.

24. Thyer IA, Kovoor P, Barry MA, et al. Protection of the coronary arteries during epicardial radiofrequency ablation with intracoronary chilled saline irrigation: assessment in an in vitro model. *J Cardiovasc Electrophysiol.* 2006;17:544–549.

25. Buch E, Vaseghi M, Cesario DA, Shivkumar K. A novel method for preventing phrenic nerve injury during catheter ablation. *Heart Rhythm.* 2007;4:95–98.

26. Bahnson TD. Strategies to minimize the risk of esophageal injury during catheter ablation for atrial fibrillation. *Pacing Clin Electrophysiol.* 2009;32:248–260.

27. Langberg JJ, Calkins H, el-Atassi R, et al. Temperature monitoring during radiofrequency catheter ablation of accessory pathways. *Circulation.* 1992;86:1469–1474.

28. Calkins H, Prystowsky E, Carlson M, et al. Atakr Multicenter Investigators Group. Temperature monitoring during radiofrequency catheter ablation procedures using closed loop control. *Circulation.* 1994;90:1279–1286.

29. Willems S, Chen X, Kottkamp H, et al. Temperature-controlled radiofrequency catheter ablation of manifest accessory pathways. *Eur Heart J.* 1996;17:445–452.

30. Choi YS, Sohn KS, Sohn DW, et al. Temperature-guided radiofrequency catheter ablation of slow pathway in atrioventricular nodal reentrant tachycardia. *Am Heart J.* 1995;129:392–394.

31. Kongsgaard E, Steen T, Jensen O, et al. Temperature guided radiofrequency catheter ablation of myocardium: comparison of catheter tip and tissue temperatures in vitro. *Pacing Clin Electrophysiol.* 1997;20:1252–1260.

32. Haines DE, Verow AF. Observations on electrode-tissue interface temperature and effect on electrical impedance during radiofrequency ablation of ventricular myocardium. *Circulation.* 1990;82:1034–1038.

33. Eick OJ, Bierbaum D. Tissue temperature-controlled radiofrequency ablation. *Pacing Clin Electrophysiol.* 2003;26:725–730.

34. Nath S, DiMarco JP, Haines DE. Basic aspects of radiofrequency catheter ablation. *J Cardiovasc Electrophysiol.* 1994;5:863–876.

35. Zivin A, Strickberger SA. Temperature monitoring versus impedance monitoring during RF catheter ablation. In: Huang SK, Wilber DJ, eds. *Radiofrequency Catheter Ablation of Cardiac Arrhythmias: Basic Concepts and Clinical Applications.* Mount Kisco, NY: Futura; 1994.

36. Schwan HP, Foster KR. RF-field interactions with biological systems: electrical properties and biophysical mechanisms. *Proc IEEE.* 1980;68:104–113.

37. Haines DE. Determinants of lesion size during radiofrequency catheter ablation: the role of electrode-tissue contact pressure and duration of energy delivery. *J Cardiovasc Electrophysiol.* 1991;2:509–515.

38. Strickberger SA, Weiss R, Knight BP, et al. Randomized comparison of two techniques for titrating power during radiofrequency ablation of accessory pathways. *J Cardiovasc Electrophysiol.* 1996;7:795–801.

39. Strickberger SA, Zivin A, Daoud EG, et al. Temperature and impedance monitoring during slow pathway ablation in patients with AV nodal reentrant tachycardia. *J Cardiovasc Electrophysiol.* 1996;7:295–300.

40. Strickberger SA, Ravi S, Daoud E, et al. Relation between impedance and temperature during radiofrequency ablation of accessory pathways. *Am Heart J.* 1995;130:1026–1030.

41. Hartung WM, Burton ME, Deam AG, et al. Estimation of temperature during radiofrequency catheter ablation using impedance measurements. *Pacing Clin Electrophysiol.* 1995;18:2017–2021.

42. Schwartzman D, Michele JJ, Trankiem CT, Ren JF. Electrogram-guided radiofrequency catheter ablation of atrial tissue comparison with thermometry-guide ablation: comparison with thermometry-guide ablation. *J Interv Card Electrophysiol.* 2001;5:253–266.

43. Schwartzman D, Parizhskaya M, Devine WA. Linear ablation using an irrigated electrode electrophysiologic and histologic lesion evolution comparison with ablation utilizing a non-irrigated electrode. *J Interv Card Electrophysiol.* 2001;5:17–26.

44. Langberg JJ, Harvey M, Calkins H, et al. Titration of power output during radiofrequency catheter ablation of atrioventricular nodal reentrant tachycardia. *Pacing Clin Electrophysiol.* 1993;16:465–470.

45. Hoyt RH, Huang SK, Marcus FI. Factors influencing transcatheter radiofrequency ablation of the myocardium. *J Appl Cardiol.* 1986;1:469–486.

46. Langberg JJ, Lee MA, Chin MC, Rosenqvist M. Radiofrequency catheter ablation: the effect of electrode size on lesion volume in vivo. *Pacing Clin Electrophysiol.* 1990;13:1242–1248.

47. Anfinsen OG, Aass H, Kongsgaard E, et al. Temperature-controlled radiofrequency catheter ablation with a 10-mm tip electrode creates larger lesions without charring in the porcine heart. *J Interv Card Electrophysiol.* 1999;3:343–351.

48. Otomo K, Yamanashi WS, Tondo C, et al. Why a large tip electrode makes a deeper radiofrequency lesion: effects of increase in electrode cooling and electrode-tissue interface area. *J Cardiovasc Electrophysiol.* 1998;9:47–54.

49. Tsai CF, Tai CT, Yu WC, et al. Is 8-mm more effective than 4-mm tip electrode catheter for ablation of typical atrial flutter? *Circulation.* 1999;100:768–771.

50. Feld G, Wharton M, Plumb V, et al. Radiofrequency catheter ablation of type 1 atrial flutter using large-tip 8- or 10-mm electrode catheters and a high-output radiofrequency energy generator: results of a multicenter safety and efficacy study. *J Am Coll Cardiol.* 2004;43:1466–1472.

51. Dorwarth U, Fiek M, Remp T, et al. Radiofrequency catheter ablation: different cooled and noncooled electrode systems induce specific lesion geometries and adverse effects profiles. *Pacing Clin Electrophysiol.* 2003;26:1438–1445.

52. Bunch TJ, Bruce GK, Johnson SB, et al. Analysis of catheter-tip (8-mm) and actual tissue temperatures achieved during radiofrequency ablation at the orifice of the pulmonary vein. *Circulation.* 2004;110:2988–2995.

53. McRury ID, Panescu D, Mitchell MA, Haines DE. Nonuniform heating during radiofrequency catheter ablation with long electrodes: monitoring the edge effect. *Circulation.* 1997;96:4057–4064.

54. Ruffy R, Imran MA, Santel DJ, Wharton JM. Radiofrequency delivery through a cooled catheter tip allows the creation of larger endomyocardial lesions in the ovine heart. *J Cardiovasc Electrophysiol.* 1995;6:1089–1096.

55. Nakagawa H, Yamanashi WS, Pitha JV, et al. Comparison of in vivo tissue temperature profile and lesion geometry for radiofrequency ablation with a saline-irrigated electrode versus temperature control in a canine thigh muscle preparation. *Circulation.* 1995;91:2264–2273.

56. Yokoyama K, Nakagawa H, Wittkampf FH, et al. Comparison of electrode cooling between internal and open irrigation in radiofrequency ablation lesion depth and incidence of thrombus and steam pop. *Circulation.* 2006;113:11–19.

57. Skrumeda LL, Mehra R. Comparison of standard and irrigated radiofrequency ablation in the canine ventricle. *J Cardiovasc Electrophysiol.* 1998;9:1196–1205.

58. Soejima K, Delacretaz E, Suzuki M, et al. Saline-cooled versus standard radiofrequency catheter ablation for infarct-related ventricular tachycardias. *Circulation.* 2001;103:1858–1862.

59. Atiga WL, Worley SJ, Hummel J, et al. Prospective randomized comparison of cooled radiofrequency versus standard radiofrequency energy for ablation of typical atrial flutter. *Pacing Clin Electrophysiol.* 2002;25:1172–1178.

60. Yamane T, Jais P, Shah DC, et al. Efficacy and safety of an irrigated-tip catheter for the ablation of accessory pathways resistant to conventional radiofrequency ablation. *Circulation*. 2000;102:2565–2568.

61. Bruce GK, Bunch TJ, Milton MA, et al. Discrepancies between catheter tip and tissue temperature in cooled-tip ablation: relevance to guiding left atrial ablation. *Circulation*. 2005;112:954–960.

62. Petersen HH, Chen X, Pietersen A, et al. Tissue temperatures and lesion size during irrigated tip catheter radiofrequency ablation: an in vitro comparison of temperature-controlled irrigated tip ablation, power-controlled irrigated tip ablation, and standard temperature-controlled ablation. *Pacing Clin Electrophysiol*. 2000;23:8–17.

63. Weiss C, Antz M, Eick O, et al. Radiofrequency catheter ablation using cooled electrodes: impact of irrigation flow rate and catheter contact pressure on lesion dimensions. *Pacing Clin Electrophysiol*. 2002;25:463–469.

64. Seiler J, Roberts-Thomson KC, Raymond JM, et al. Steam pops during irrigated radiofrequency ablation: feasibility of impedance monitoring for prevention. *Heart Rhythm*. 2008;5:1411–1416.

65. Thompson N, Lustgarten D, Mason B, et al. The relationship between surface temperature, tissue temperature, microbubble formation, and steam pops. *Pacing Clin Electrophysiol*. 2009;32:833–841.

66. Perzanowski C, Teplitsky L, Hranitzky PM, Bahnson TD. Real-time monitoring of luminal esophageal temperature during left atrial radiofrequency catheter ablation for atrial fibrillation: observations about esophageal heating during ablation at the pulmonary vein ostia and posterior left atrium. *J Cardiovasc Electrophysiol*. 2006;17:166–170.

67. Bai R, Patel D, Di Biase L, et al. Phrenic nerve injury after catheter ablation: should we worry about this complication? *J Cardiovasc Electrophysiol*. 2006;17:944–948.

68. Bunch TJ, Bruce GK, Mahapatra S, et al. Mechanisms of phrenic nerve injury during radiofrequency ablation at the pulmonary vein orifice. *J Cardiovasc Electrophysiol*. 2005;16:1318–1325.

69. Matsuo S, Jais P, Knecht S, et al. Images in cardiovascular medicine: novel technique to prevent left phrenic nerve injury during epicardial catheter ablation. *Circulation*. 2008;117:e471.

70. Di Biase L, Burkhardt JD, Pelargonio G, et al. Prevention of phrenic nerve injury during epicardial ablation: comparison of methods for separating the phrenic nerve from the epicardial surface. *Heart Rhythm*. 2009;6:957–961.

71. Sosa E, Scanavacca M, d'Avila A, Pilleggi F. A new technique to perform epicardial mapping in the electrophysiology laboratory. *J Cardiovasc Electrophysiol*. 1996;7:531–536.

72. Schweikert RA, Saliba WI, Tomassoni G, et al. Percutaneous pericardial instrumentation for endo-epicardial mapping of previously failed ablations. *Circulation*. 2003;108:1329–1335.

73. Aliot EM, Stevenson WG, Almendral-Garrote JM, et al. EHRA/HRS Expert Consensus on Catheter Ablation of Ventricular Arrhythmias: developed in a partnership with the European Heart Rhythm Association (EHRA), a Registered Branch of the European Society of Cardiology (ESC), and the Heart Rhythm Society (HRS); in collaboration with the American College of Cardiology (ACC) and the American Heart Association (AHA). *Heart Rhythm*. 2009;6:886–933.

74. d'Avila A, Houghtaling C, Gutierrez P, et al. Catheter ablation of ventricular epicardial tissue: a comparison of standard and cooled-tip radiofrequency energy. *Circulation*. 2004;109:2363–2369.

75. D'Avila A, Gutierrez P, Scanavacca M, et al. Effects of radiofrequency pulses delivered in the vicinity of the coronary arteries: implications for nonsurgical transthoracic epicardial catheter ablation to treat ventricular tachycardia. *Pacing Clin Electrophysiol*. 2002;25:1488–1495.

76. Hammill SC. Epicardial ablation: reducing the risks. *J Cardiovasc Electrophysiol*. 2006;17:550–552.

77. Langberg JJ, Man KC, Vorperian VR, et al. Recognition and catheter ablation of subepicardial accessory pathways. *J Am Coll Cardiol*. 1993;22:1100–1104.

78. Yamauchi Y, Aonuma K, Sekiguchi Y, et al. Successful radiofrequency ablation of ventricular premature contractions within the coronary sinus. *Pacing Clin Electrophysiol*. 2005;28:1250–1252.

79. Tada H, Yamada M, Naito S, et al. Radiofrequency catheter ablation within the coronary sinus eliminates a macro-reentrant atrial tachycardia: importance of mapping in the coronary sinus. *J Interv Card Electrophysiol*. 2006;15:35–41.

80. Haissaguerre M, Hocini M, Takahashi Y, et al. Impact of catheter ablation of the coronary sinus on paroxysmal or persistent atrial fibrillation. *J Cardiovasc Electrophysiol*. 2007;18:378–386.

81. Jais P, Hocini M, Hsu LF, et al. Technique and results of linear ablation at the mitral isthmus. *Circulation*. 2004;110:2996–3002.

82. Fuller IA, Wood MA. Intramural coronary vasculature prevents transmural radiofrequency lesion formation: implications for linear ablation. *Circulation*. 2003;107:1797–1803.

83. D'Avila A, Thiagalingam A, Foley L, et al. Temporary occlusion of the great cardiac vein and coronary sinus to facilitate radiofrequency catheter ablation of the mitral isthmus. *J Cardiovasc Electrophysiol*. 2008;19:645–650.

84. Takahashi Y, Jais P, Hocini M, et al. Acute occlusion of the left circumflex coronary artery during mitral isthmus linear ablation. *J Cardiovasc Electrophysiol*. 2005;16:1104–1107.

85. Cesario DA, Boyle NB, Shivkumar K. Lesion-forming technologies for catheter ablation. In: Zipes DP, Jalife J, eds. *Cardiac Electrophysiology: From Cell to Bedside*. Philadelphia: Saunders; 2009:1051–1058.

86. Haines DE. Biophysics and pathophysiology of lesion formation by transcatheter radiofrequency ablation. In: Wilber DJ, Packer DL, Stevenson WG, eds. *Catheter Ablation of Cardiac Arrhythmias: Basic Concepts and Clinical Applications*. Malden, MA: Blackwell; 2008:20–34.

87. Stevenson WG, Cooper J, Sapp J. Optimizing RF output for cooled RF ablation. *J Cardiovasc Electrophysiol*. 2004;15:S24–S27.

Videos

Video 2-1. Microbubble formation in an isolated tissue preparation during ablation with an internally irrigated catheter. See figure for orientation. Note that there is steam formation and "boiling" within the block of tissue and profuse microbubble formation.

Video 2-2. Steam pop during pulmonary vein isolation procedure captured on echocardiography. An 8-mm-tip catheter was being used to deliver a lesion near the left superior pulmonary vein. Note the appearance of a few scattered microbubbles in the left atrial chamber before the explosion of microbubbles. Fortunately, the patient suffered no complication from the event.

3
Irrigated and Cooled-Tip Radiofrequency Catheter Ablation

Taresh Taneja, Kuo-Hung Lin, and Shoei K. Stephen Huang

Key Points

Irrigated or cooled ablation allows for larger lesion creation by allowing greater energy delivery.

Cooled ablation allows greater energy delivery to the tissue by preventing impedance rises, thus allowing higher powers, resulting in deeper and larger lesions.

In the clinical setting, efficacy of cooled-tip radiofrequency (RF) ablation is preferred over conventional RF ablation for the catheter-based treatment of atrial flutter, atrial fibrillation, and nonidiopathic ventricular tachycardias.

Temperature monitoring is less reliable for irrigated than nonirrigated ablation. Monitoring impedance changes during ablation is important.

The safety profile of cooled-tip RF ablation is comparable to conventional RF ablation.

Radiofrequency (RF) ablation has become a standard therapy for supraventricular tachycardias,[1–5] including atrial fibrillation (AF)[6] and ventricular tachycardias (VTs).[7] More recently, RF ablation has also been used increasingly for the treatment of more complicated arrhythmias, particularly VT associated with structural heart disease.[8,9] Although the results are promising, RF current delivered through a standard 7-French (7F), 4-mm-tip electrode catheter is limited to ablation of arrhythmogenic tissue located within a few millimeters of the ablation electrode. In 1% to 10% of patients with accessory pathways[3,10,11] and 30% to 50% of patients with nonidiopathic VT,[8,12–14] the arrhythmogenic tissue cannot be destroyed with a conventional ablation catheter. The overall success rate in these cases may be improved by using alternate technologies for RF application that increase lesion size and depth. In some situations, excessive ablation electrode temperatures may be reached with minimal power delivery, resulting in trivial lesion formation.

Temperature reduction at the tip of the ablation catheter has proved to be a solution for increasing the RF application duration and power, decreasing the impedance rise and coagulum formation, and thus developing a larger and deeper lesion.[15,16] The aim of this chapter is to review current understanding of the mechanism of irrigated and cooled-tip catheter ablation as well as the results of animal studies and clinical trials that have employed this technology.

Biophysics of Cooled Radiofrequency Ablation

During RF application, delivery of RF current through the catheter tip results in a shell of resistive heating that serves as a heat source conducting heat to the myocardium (Fig. 3-1). The shell of resistive heating is thin and 1 to 2 mm in thickness, only slightly greater than the diameter of the electrode tip. Conductive heat is responsible for thermal injury outside the zone of resistive heating.[17,18] For any given electrode size and tissue contact area, RF lesion size is a function of RF power level and exposure time.[19,20] At higher power, however, the exposure time is frequently limited by an impedance rise that occurs when the temperature at the electrode-tissue interface reaches 100 °C[17,20,21] because tissue desiccation, steam, and coagulum formation occur at this temperature. The impedance rise limits the duration of RF current delivery, the total amount of energy delivered, and the size of the lesion generated.

Although temperature-controlled[17,18,22,23] RF delivery systems are able to minimize the incidence of coagulum formation and impedance rise, this is achieved by limiting electrode temperature that may reach target values at very low power deliveries. During temperature-controlled RF ablation, the tip temperature, tissue temperature, and lesion size are affected by the electrode-tissue contact and by cooling effects resulting from blood flow. With good contact between catheter tip and tissue and low cooling of the catheter tip, the target temperature can be reached with little power, resulting in small lesions even though a high tip temperature is being measured. In contrast, a low tip temperature can be caused by a high level of convective cooling, which results in higher power delivery to reach the target temperature, yielding a larger lesion.

Two methods have been used to cool the catheter tip, prevent the impedance rise, and maximize power delivery. In one approach, larger ablation electrodes (8F, 8 to 10 mm in length) are used.[17,23,24] The larger electrode-tissue contact area results in a greater volume of direct resistive

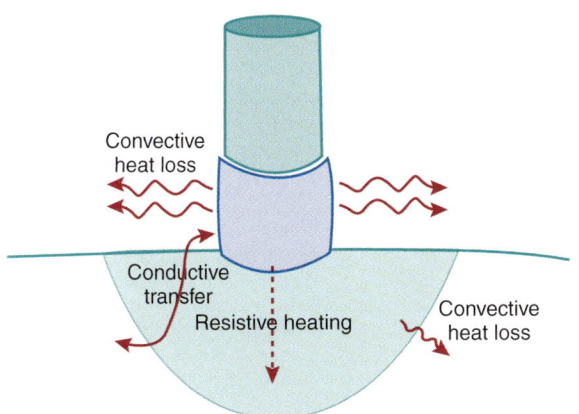

FIGURE 3-1. Schematic drawing of radiofrequency catheter ablation on the endocardium demonstrating zones of resistive and conductive heating and convective heat loss into the blood pool and coronary arteries. Superficial myocardium near the catheter is ablated by resistive heating, and deeper myocardium is heated by conductive heating. *(From EP Lab Digest. With permission.)*

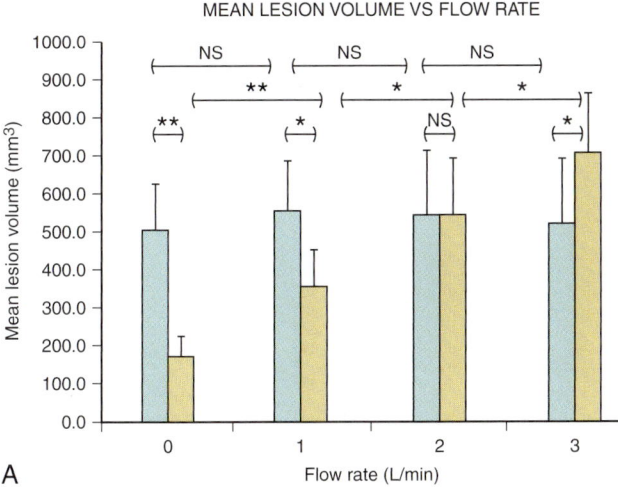

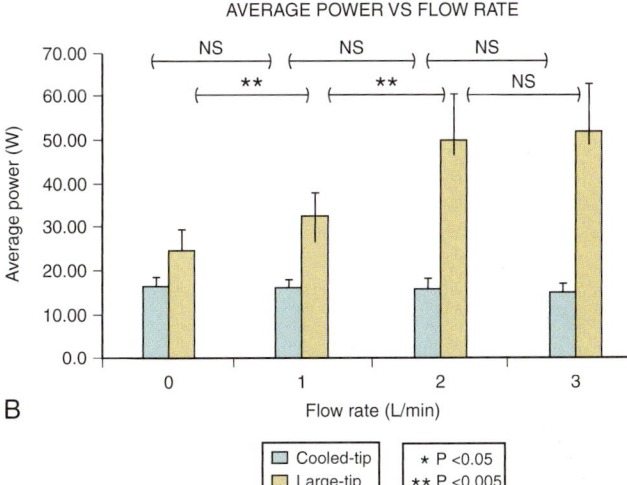

heating. In addition, the larger electrode surface area exposed to blood results in greater convective cooling of the electrode by the blood. This cooling effect helps to prevent an impedance rise, allowing longer application of RF current at higher power, which produces a larger and deeper lesion (Fig. 3-2).[17] As a caveat, however, a greater electrode area in contact with the blood pool increases the proportion of electrical current shunted away from the tissue. In this situation, greater power must be delivered to increase current flow through the tissue as well as to compensate for the current loss to the blood pool (Fig. 3-2C).

An alternative approach described by Wittkampf and associates[16] is to irrigate the ablation electrode with saline to reduce the electrode-tissue interface temperature and prevent an impedance rise.[15,16,25–29] This approach allows cooler saline to internally or externally bathe the ablation electrode, dissipating heat generated during RF application

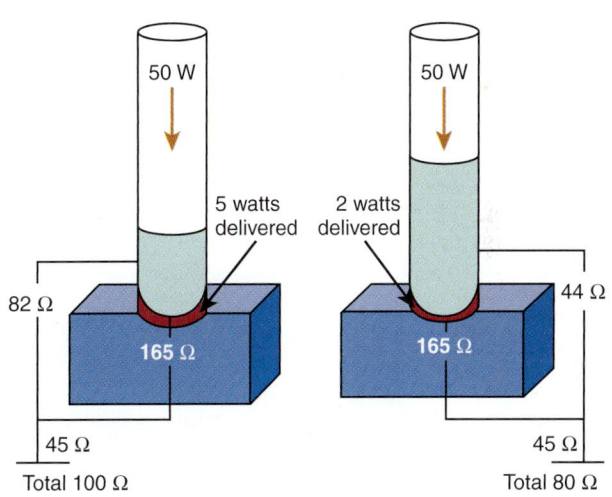

FIGURE 3-2. A, Relationship between lesion volume and superfusate flow rate over cooled-tip (irrigated) or large-tip (10 mm) electrodes in isolated porcine ventricular tissue. The flow rate of 3 L/min corresponded to a flow velocity of 15.5 cm/sec. Note that with increasing flow rate, larger lesions could be produced with the large-tip catheter in temperature control mode (65-70°C). The increased lesion size was based on the ability to deliver more power before reaching target electrode temperature (see panel **B**). For the irrigated electrode, no increase in lesion volume resulted. **B,** Average power delivered versus superfusate flow rate over the irrigated or large-tip electrodes. Note that no further power could be delivered to the irrigated electrode with increasing superfusate flow. For the large-tip electrode, increased flow rate provided incrementally more electrode cooling and allowed more power delivery. This resulted in larger lesion sizes for the large tip electrode. **C,** Current shunting with large-tip ablation catheter. Theoretical ablations with 4-mm (*left*) and 8-mm (*right*) catheters are shown. The current path for each electrode comprises the tissue resistance (165 ohms) and blood pool resistance (varies with electrode area) in parallel and the resistance to the skin electrode in series. Fifty watts of power is delivered to each electrode. Because the electrode diameter is the same for each catheter, in this orientation the tissue resistances to each electrode are the same. Because the 8-mm electrode places greater surface area in contact with the blood pool, the blood pool resistance is lower than for the 4-mm electrode. This shunts current away from the tissue (2 W versus 5 W delivered to tissue in this scenario) despite a lower total resistance (80 W versus 100 W). The result is a smaller lesion for the 8-mm electrode despite identical power deliveries to the catheters. *(**A** and **B**, Data from Pilcher TA, Sanford AL, Saul P, Dieter Haemmerich D. Convective cooling effect on cooled-tip catheter compared to large-tip catheter radiofrequency ablation. Pacing Clin Electrophysiol. 2006;29:1368–1374. With permission.)*

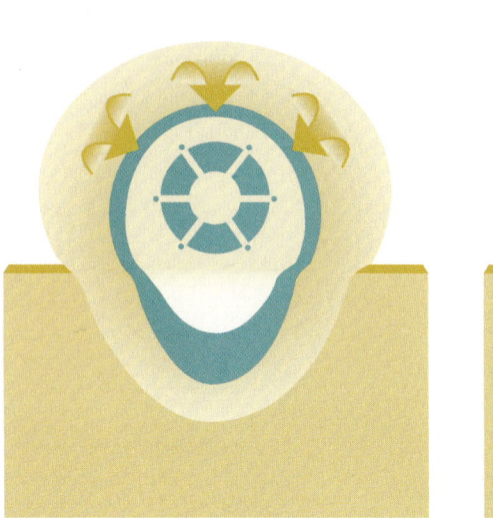

A **Cross section of cooled tip**   **B** **Cross section of standard RF tip**

FIGURE 3-3. Comparison between cooled-tip and standard radiofrequency (RF) ablation. **A,** Cross section of cooled-tip RF showing effect of saline envelope. **B,** Cross section of standard RF showing heat dissipation above ablation site. *(Courtesy of Boston Scientific Electrophysiology, San Jose, CA. With permission.)*

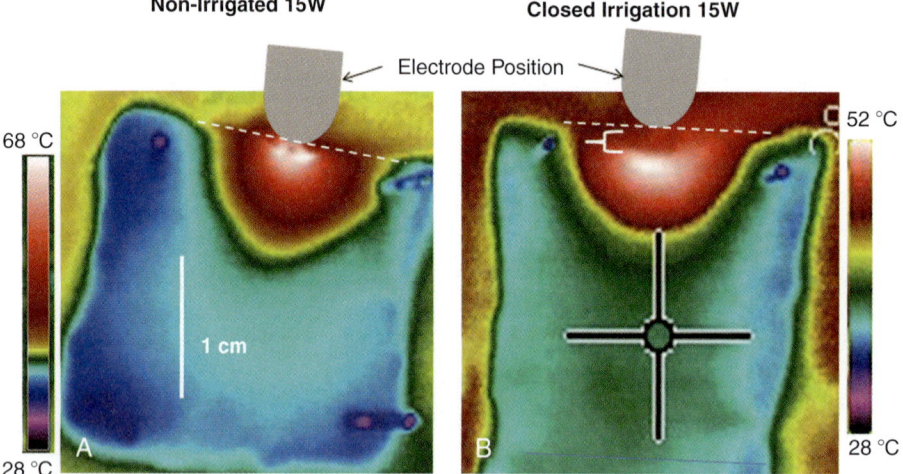

FIGURE 3-4. Infrared thermal images during radiofrequency ablation energy delivery to blocks of porcine left ventricular tissue in a saline bath. Nonirrigated 4-mm-tip (**A**) and closed-irrigation 4-mm-tip (**B**) catheters are used with the electrode positions shown. Energy delivered is at fixed 15 W power. The temperature scale for each figure is shown. The *dashed lines* indicate the edge of the tissue. For the nonirrigated catheter, the maximal tissue temperature is 68°C at the electrode-tissue interface and extending into the tissue (*white*). The electrode temperature measured 66°C. For the irrigated catheter, the maximal tissue temperature is 52°C and occurs remote from the electrode (*marker*) in the tissue because of the cooling of the tissue by the irrigation. The electrode temperature did not exceed 40°C. *(Courtesy of Mark Wood.)*

(Fig. 3-3).[30] Compared with conventional RF application, cooled ablation allows passage of both higher powers and longer durations of RF current with less likelihood of impedance rises. In addition, because convective cooling from the bloodstream is not required, an irrigated electrode may be capable of delivering higher RF power at sites of low blood flow, such as within ventricular trabecular crevasse.[31]

During cooled ablation, as the RF current is passed through the electrode to the myocardium, resistive heating still occurs around the electrode myocardial interface. However, unlike with standard RF application, the area of maximal temperature with cooled ablation is within the myocardium, rather than at the electrode-myocardium interface (Fig. 3-4). Nakagawa and colleagues[26] demonstrated that the maximal temperature generated by cooled RF application will be several millimeters away from the electrode-myocardium interface due to active electrode cooling. In a study by Dorwarth and coworkers,[32] the hottest point extended from the electrode surface to 3.2 to 3.6 mm within the myocardium from the electrode-tissue interface for cooled ablation modeled with a catheter cooled by internal perfusion of saline. Therefore, tissue temperature generated during cooled RF ablation increases from the electrode tip to a maximal temperature a couple of millimeters within the myocardium. The current density and the width of the shell of resistive heating are increased around the electrode-myocardium interface, resulting in a

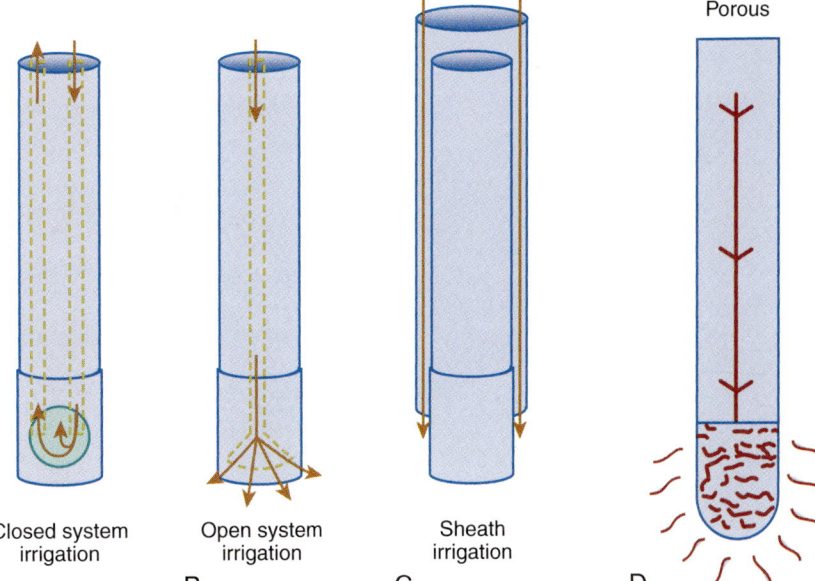

Porous

Closed system irrigation	Open system irrigation	Sheath irrigation	
A	B	C	D

FIGURE 3-5. Schematic drawings of four different methods of cooling; **A,** closed irrigation system; **B,** opened showerhead or sprinkler type; **C,** external sheath irrigation; and **D,** porous irrigated-tip catheter. *(From EP Lab Digest. With permission.)*

larger effective radiant surface diameter and larger lesion depth, width, and volume.

Because the catheter tip is cooled actively, the temperature at the tip-tissue interface during cooled RF application is unreliable as a marker for determining the duration of RF application. However, because the maximal tissue temperature is several millimeters away from the catheter tip during cooled ablation, the maximal tissue temperature may not be accurately monitored by a tip thermistor or thermocouple. Although RF current is increased with cooled RF application, intramyocardial tissues could be heated to 100°C, which would result in intramyocardial steam and crater formation, possibly associated with dissection, perforation, and thrombus formation.[32–38] Wharton and coworkers[36] demonstrated that impedance rises may be minimized to less than 6.3% if tip temperatures are maintained at less than 45°C.

Design of Irrigated Radiofrequency Catheters

Active cooling of the catheter tip during RF ablation is achieved by circulating saline through or around the tip of the ablation catheter while RF current is being delivered. In general, there are two types of irrigation catheters. The first type is the closed-loop irrigation catheter, which continuously circulates saline within the electrode tip, internally cooling the electrode tip. The second type is the open irrigation catheter, which has multiple irrigation holes located around the electrode, through which the saline is continuously flushed, providing both internal and external cooling. Four different cooled catheters have been designed as shown in Figure 3-5. The internally cooled catheter (Boston Scientific Electrophysiology, San Jose, CA) has an internally cooled tip electrode that is perfused with room-temperature saline (Fig. 3-6A). With this closed loop system, saline perfuses the tip of the catheter

through a conduit in the catheter shaft and returns back through a second conduit in the catheter. Saline is not infused into the body (Fig. 3-6A).

In clinical application, cooling is achieved by pumping 0.6 mL/second of saline to the tip of the catheter during RF application. RF energy is titrated to achieve an electrode temperature between 40° and 50 °C, to a maximum of 50 W.

The other cooled RF ablation systems that are available are the showerhead-type irrigated tip catheter (Biosense Webster and Medtronic CardioRhythm, San Jose, CA). The ThermoCool ablation catheter (Biosense Webster) (Fig. 3-6B) is also approved by U.S. Food and Drug Administration for AF ablation. Cooling is achieved with saline infused at a rate of 17 mL/minute or 30 mL/minute during RF application and 2 mL/minute during all other times at baseline. A new addition is the Therapy CoolPath Ablation catheter from St. Jude Medical (St. Paul, MN), which is a 4-mm externally irrigated ablation catheter with six equidistant ports with a nominal flow rate of 2 mL/minute or 13 mL/minute during ablation The maximal power setting is 50 W, and it has thermocouple temperature monitoring at the maximal set temperature of 50°C. Another Therapy CoolPath Duo (St. Jude Medical) irrigated-tip ablation catheter will be introduced soon with two sets of six ports evenly distributed on the distal and proximal portion of the tip electrode. Yokoyama and associates[39] found that open irrigation systems resulted in greater interface cooling with lower interface temperatures and lower incidences of both thrombus formation and steam pops than seen with closed-loop irrigated cooled-tip catheters.

Results of Animal Studies

Several authors have compared cooled RF catheter ablation to conventional ablation using animal models.[25,26,32,40] Nakagawa and coworkers[26] compared conventional RF current delivery without irrigation to saline irrigation through

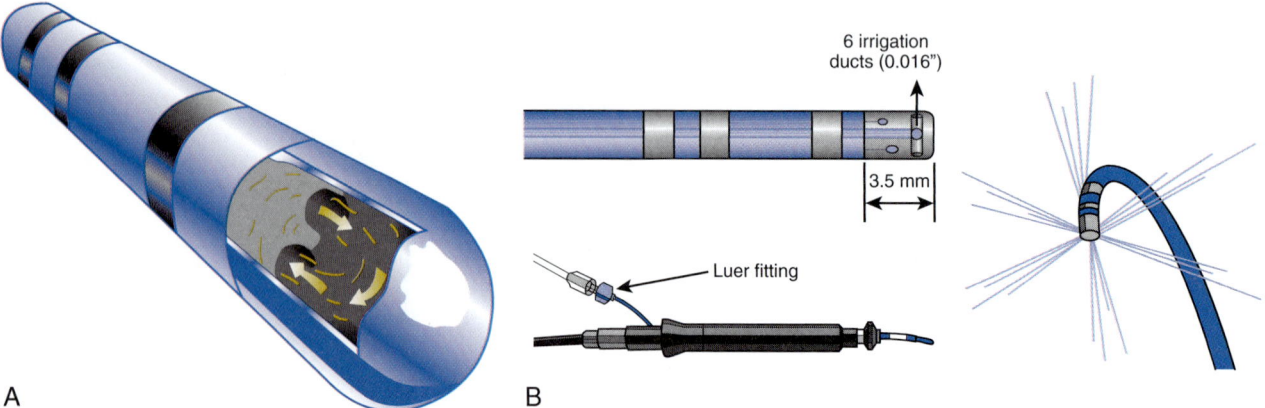

FIGURE 3-6. A, Schematic drawing of the Chilli internally cooled ablation catheter. **B,** Schematic drawing of the open-system irrigation ThermoCool ablation catheter showing location of irrigation ducts in the distal electrode. The pattern of irrigation fluid dispersion is shown at lower right. *(A, Courtesy of Boston Scientific Electrophysiology, San Jose, CA. B, Courtesy of Biosense-Webster, Diamond Bar, CA. With permission.)*

RF Lesion Dimensions

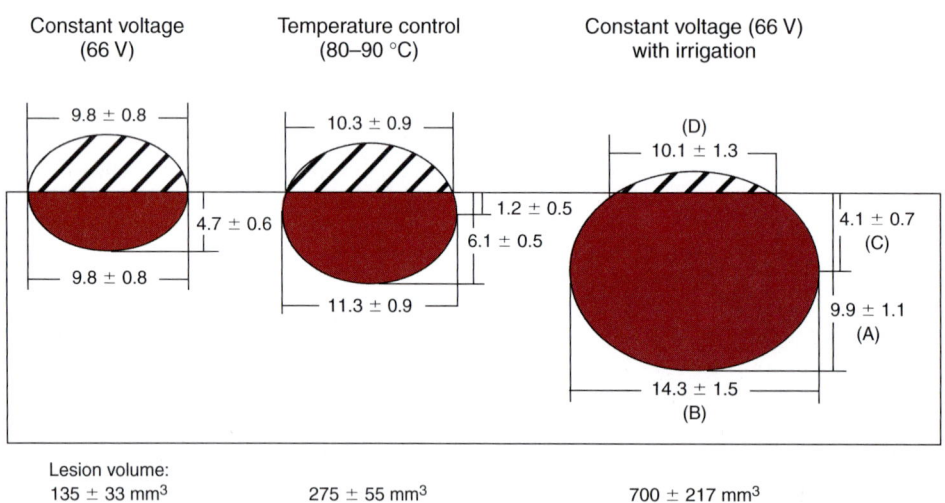

FIGURE 3-7. Diagram of radiofrequency (RF) lesion dimensions for the three groups of ablation conditions studied. Values are expressed in millimeters (mean ± standard deviation). A indicates maximal lesion depth; B, maximal lesion diameter; C, depth at maximal lesion diameter; and D, lesion surface diameter. Lesion volume was calculated by use of the formula for an oblate ellipsoid, by subtracting the volume of the "missing cap" *(hatched area)*. *(From Nakagawa H, Yamanashi SW, Pitha JV, et al. Comparison of in vivo tissue temperature profile and lesion geometry for radiofrequency ablation with a saline-irrigated electrode versus temperature control in a canine thigh muscle preparation. Circulation. 1995;91:2264–2273. With permission.)*

the catheter lumen and ablation electrode at 20 mL/minute. In the saline irrigation group, despite the tip-electrode temperature not exceeding 48°C and electrode tissue interface temperature not exceeding 80°C, the largest and deepest lesions (9.9 mm and 14.3 mm, respectively) were noted. They also demonstrated that the maximal tissue temperature of 94°C during cooled ablation occurred 3.5 mm from the tip of the electrode, as opposed to conventional ablation in which maximal temperatures were recorded at the electrode-tissue interface (Fig. 3-7). Mittleman et al.[25] also demonstrated that use of a saline irrigated luminal electrode with an end hole and two side holes (Bard Electrophysiology, Haverhill, MA) in the canine myocardium in vivo at 10 to 20 W produced significantly larger lesions than a standard catheter (Figs. 3-8 and 3-9). Dorwarth and coworkers[32] compared three different actively cooled systems (showerhead electrode tip, porous metal tip, and internally cooled system) to standard 4-mm and 8-mm ablation catheters in

isolated porcine myocardium. They found that the externally cooled systems had the largest lesion depth and diameter followed by the internally cooled system, which had a similar lesion depth with a slightly smaller diameter. The 8-mm tip had a similar lesion diameter with smaller depth. However, there were no differences in lesion volumes between the three cooled and the 8-mm ablation catheters. Maximal lesion volume was induced at a power setting of 30 W for the two open irrigated systems and 20 W for the internally cooled catheter.

Flow rates of saline infusion may also affect the size of a lesion created by cooled ablation.[41] A higher flow rate might cause a greater cooling effect to the catheter tip, which could potentially generate a larger lesion if more power could be delivered as a result. Overcooling the electrode and tissue by excessive irrigation rates may decrease lesion size, however. In contrast, a lower flow rate might result in a lesion size approaching that of conventional RF

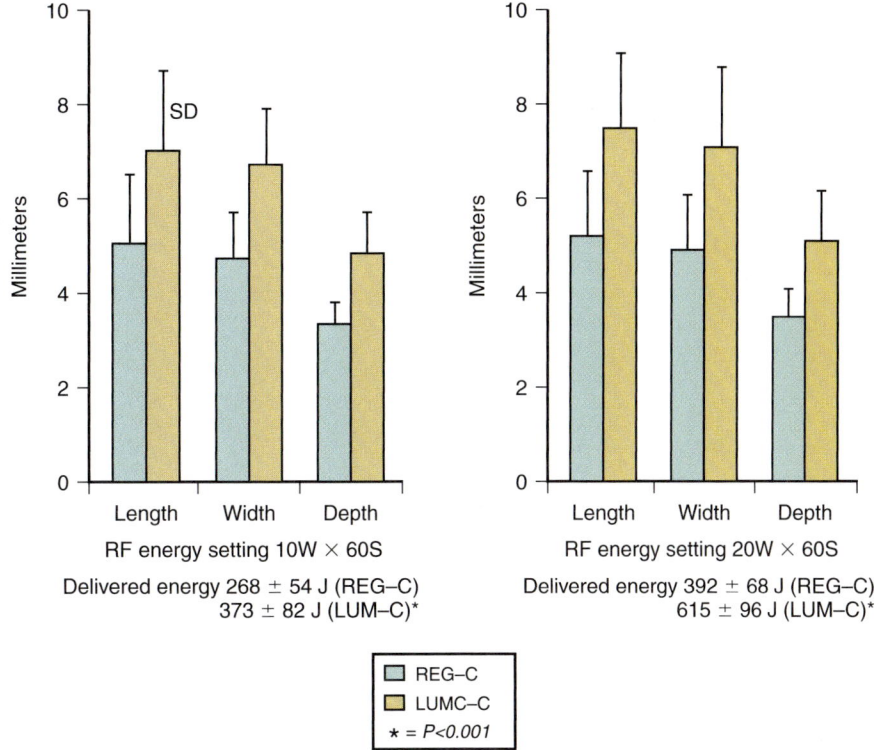

FIGURE 3-8. Dimensions of radiofrequency (RF) lesions (mean ± standard deviation) created at two set energy levels (10 W × 60 seconds and 20 W × 60 seconds). REG-C, standard electrode catheter; LUM-C, saline-infused electrode catheter; *, P < .001 versus standard catheter. *(Data from Mittleman RS, Huang SKS, De Guzman WT, et al. Use of the saline infusion electrode catheter for improved energy delivery and increased lesion size in radiofrequency catheter ablation.* Pacing Clin Electrophysiol. *1995;18:1022–1027. With permission.)*

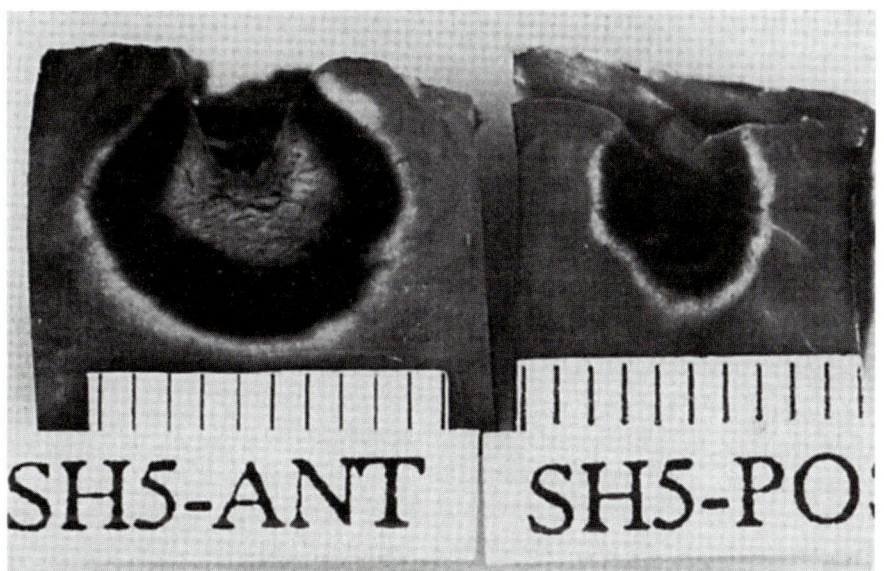

FIGURE 3-9. Examples of lesion created with either a saline-infused catheter (*left*) or a standard catheter (*right*), in the anterior and posterior wall of the left ventricle, respectively. The lesion on the left is bigger and exhibits a larger area of pitting and more extensive necrosis. The energy level for both lesions was 20 W for 60 seconds. Ruler divisions are at 1-mm intervals. *(From Mittleman RS, Huang SKS, De Guzman WT, et al. Use of the saline infusion electrode catheter for improved energy delivery and increased lesion size in radiofrequency catheter ablation.* Pacing Clin Electrophysiol. *1995;18:1022–1027. With permission.)*

ablation. Weiss and coworkers[42] compared three flow rates (5, 10, and 20 mL/minute) on sheep thigh muscle preparations (Table 3-1). There were no differences in tip temperature or thrombus formation or power delivery to deeper tissues. The higher flow rate (20 mL/minute), however, did result in a smaller surface diameter lesion.

Temperature monitoring during cooled RF application may be an unreliable marker because the actual surface temperature is underestimated. In the design of a longer catheter tip (6 to 10 mm) for increased convective cooling of the catheter tip, Petersen and colleagues[34] found a negative correlation between tip temperature reached and lesion

TABLE 3-1

TEMPERATURES DURING RADIOFREQUENCY APPLICATION WITH VARIOUS IRRIGATION FLOW RATES

Parameters of Radiofrequency Application	Irrigation Flow Rate (mL/min)		
	5 (n = 15)	10 (n = 14)	20 (n = 14)
Total power	929 ± 12	939 ± 12	935 ± 5
Maximum impedance (W)	133 ± 13	125 ± 12	113 ± 12
Maximum catheter tip temperature (°C)	43 ± 3	39 ± 3	37 ± 3
Maximum tissue temperature (°C)			
• At 3.5 mm	79 ± 8*	67 ± 5	57 ± 4
• At 7.0 mm	57 ± 4	67 ± 5	58 ± 6
Audible pops	0	0	0
Thrombus formation	0	0	0

*$P < .01$ versus 10 and 20 mL/min. All radiofrequency applications were achieved with a 30-W power output and a 30-second pulse duration.
From Weiss C, Antz M, Eick O, et al. Radiofrequency catheter ablation using cooled electrodes: impact of irrigation flow rate and catheter contact pressure on lesion dimensions. *Pacing Clinical Electrophysiol.* 2002;25:463–469.

volume for applications in which maximal generator output was not achieved, whereas delivered power and lesion volume correlated positively. They also directly examined the tissue temperature and lesion volumes formed by a showerhead-type cooled tip in the setting of either temperature control or power control. Power-controlled RF ablation at 40 W generated lesions that were similar to those achieved with temperature control at both 80° and 70°C, as opposed to 60°C, at which the lesions were significantly smaller. Importantly, positive correlations between lesion volume and real tissue temperature did not appear at the peak electrode-tip temperature. For this reason, it is important to monitor impedance drop with cooled electrode systems. Impedance drops of 5 to 10 ohms with RF delivery usually indicate tissue heating, but decreases of more than 10 ohms may herald steam formation and tissue pops.

Another potential application of RF ablation with active cooling might be used for epicardial ablation because of (1) the lack of convective cooling of the ablation catheter in the pericardial space (the conventional RF application would result in rapid rise in impedance and reduce the duration of RF energy delivery), and (2) the varying presence of epicardial adipose tissue interposed between the ablation electrode. D'Avila and associates[43] examined the dimensions and biophysical characteristics of RF lesions generated by either standard or cooled-tip ablation catheters delivered to normal and infarcted epicardial ventricular tissue in 10 normal goats and 7 pigs with healed anterior wall myocardial infarction. Cooled-tip RF delivery resulted in significantly deeper and wider lesions than conventional RF delivery. During cooled-tip RF application using a 4-mm tip with internal irrigation at 0.6 mL/second, 35.6 ± 7.1 W of power was required to achieve a temperature of $41.4° \pm 2.2°C$ (Fig. 3-10). Epicardial fat attenuated lesion formation.

Everett and colleagues[44] compared safety profiles and lesion sizes of 4-mm-tip, 10-mm-tip single thermistor and multitemperature sensor, 4-mm closed-loop and open-loop irrigated-tip ablation catheters in freshly excised canine thigh muscle placed in a chamber circulating with heparinized blood heated to 37°C and found for all catheters complications correlated to electrode-tip temperature and power setting with the cooled-tip catheters experiencing at least a sixfold greater odds of popping, bubbling, and impedance rises than with the conventional 4-mm-tip electrode, but most occurred at a power setting greater than 20 W.

Clinical Studies

Cooled Radiofrequency Ablation for Nonidiopathic Ventricular Tachycardia

Calkins and colleagues[45] enrolled 146 consecutive patients, most of whom had ischemic heart disease (82%) and an ejection fraction of 35% or less (73%). Using a Chilli cooled RF system (Boston Scientific Electrophysiology) and up-titration of power from 25 W (to 50 W) to reach a target temperature of 40° to 50°C, they were able to eliminate 75% of all mappable VTs, but only 41% of patients were completely noninducible, with a 1-year recurrence rate of 56%. Major complications occurred in 8%, with a mortality of 2.7%. Reddy and colleagues[46] evaluated the safety and acute procedural efficacy of the Navi-Star (Biosense Webster) 3.5-mm tip showerhead-type irrigated ablation catheter in 11 patients. The target VT was eliminated in 82% of patients, with elimination of all inducible monomorphic VT in 64% of patients. Soejima and associates[47] compared the efficacy of VT termination using standard versus cooled-tip RF application and showed that cooled-tip terminated VT more frequently at isthmus sites with or without an isolated potential and at inner loop sites. Termination rates were similarly low for bystander and outer-loop sites. The significantly higher termination rate at isthmus sites in the cooled RF group suggests that these reentry isthmuses exceed the width and depth of the standard RF lesion. Stevenson and coworkers[48] enrolled 231 patients with infarct-associated recurrent VTs in the Multicenter ThermoCool VT Ablation Trial and, using a 3.5-mm irrigated-tip ablation catheter, were successful in abolishing all inducible VTs in 49% of patients at 6 months with a procedure mortality rate of 3% and a 1-year mortality rate of 18% (72.5% of deaths attributable to ventricular arrhythmias). Deneke and colleagues[49]

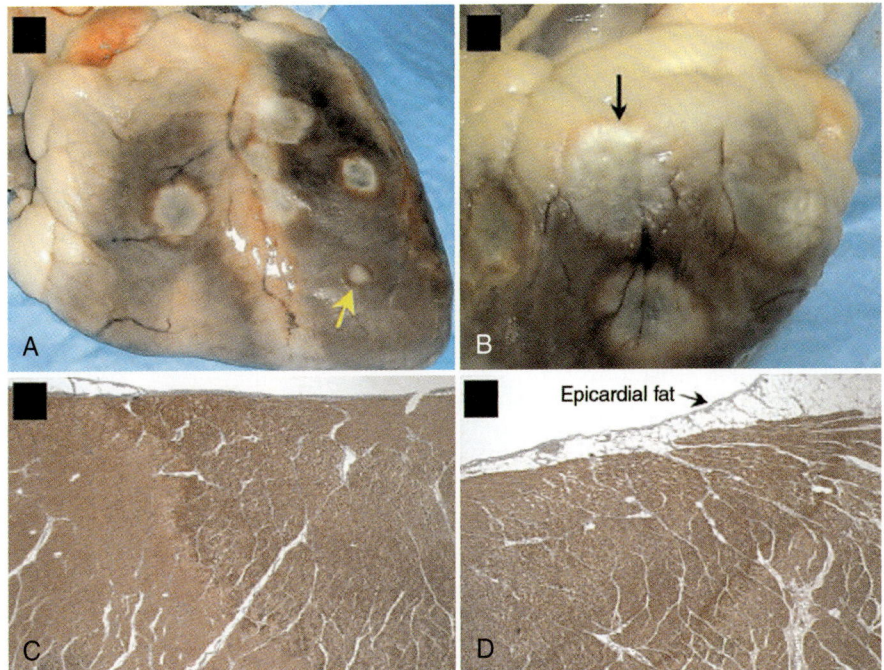

FIGURE 3-10. **A** and **B,** Cooled-tip and standard radiofrequency (RF) epicardial ablation lesions in an animal model. **A,** The smallest epicardial lesion was generated with standard RF energy (*yellow arrow*); the other five lesions on this heart were created with cooled-tip RF application. **B,** Contour of cooled-tip epicardial lesions on normal epicardial surface and on fat (*black arrow*). **C** and **D,** Histopathologic slides of epicardial lesions. Epicardial fat interposed between the tip of the ablation catheter and epicardium prejudiced creation of deep epicardial RF lesions. **C,** Lesion created with standard RF application shows a distinct border at the beginning of the epicardial fat layer. **D,** Significant attenuation toward the area covered by epicardial fat in a lesion created by cooled-tip RF application. *(From d'Avila A, Houghtaling C, Gutierrez P, et al. Catheter ablation of ventricular epicardial tissue: a comparison of standard and cooled-tip radiofrequency energy.* Circulation. *2004;109:2363–2369, 2004. With permission.)*

performed electroanatomic substrate mapping in a single patient with multiple VTs and coronary artery disease. After successful ablation with a cooled-tip radiofrequency ablation catheter in regions of "altered myocardium" (0.5 to 1.5 mV), the patient died 7 days later from worsening heart failure. On postmortem examination, they found that ablation with the cooled-tip system produced transmural coagulation necrosis of meshlike fibrotic tissue with interspersed remnants of myocardial cells up to a maximal depth of 7 mm.

Cooled Radiofrequency Ablation for Atrial Flutter

The most common type of atrial flutter is cavotricuspid isthmus dependent, in which the reentry is confined to the right atrium. Because of pouches, ridges, recesses, and trabeculations that may occur in the isthmus, it is often necessary to create lesions that are larger and deeper than those achieved using a 4-mm-tip ablation catheter by either using an 8-mm-tip or an irrigated-tip ablation catheter. Several studies have demonstrated that complete isthmus block is more easily achieved with a cooled-tip or irrigated-tip catheter than with a conventional ablation catheter.[50-55] However, Da Costa and associates[56,57] performed a meta-analysis of seven available randomized trials to compare the efficacy of cooled-tip and 8-mm tip-catheters for radiofrequency ablation of the cavotricuspid isthmus for isthmus-dependent atrial flutter. There were no significant differences in the achievement of bidirectional block, RF application time, and ablation procedure

time. Cooled ablation technology significantly reduces the recurrence rate of cavotricuspid isthmus dependent atrial flutter compared with noncooled catheters, however. Jais and colleagues[52] compared conventional and irrigated-tip (ThermoCool D curve system, Biosense Webster) catheter ablation of typical atrial flutter and showed that 100% of patients in the irrigated-tip group achieved successful creation of bidirectional isthmus block with significantly fewer RF applications and shorter procedure times, as opposed to 85% of patients in the conventional RF group achieving bidirectional block. Atiga and associates[50] compared standard RF ablation with cooled-tip ablation using the Chilli system in type I atrial flutter and showed that after 12 RF applications, 79% in the cooled-tip group achieved bidirectional cavotricuspid isthmus block, as opposed to 55% in the conventional RF group.

Bai and coworkers[58] performed a randomized comparison of open-system irrigated-tip (3.5 mm) and 8-mm-tip (without irrigation) ablation catheters in 70 patients with atypical atrial flutter after cardiac surgery or AF ablation and showed that both acute success and long-term success (10 months) were significantly higher in the open-system irrigated group despite shorter fluoroscopy and radiofrequency times. Blaufox and colleagues[59] analyzed the pediatric radiofrequency catheter ablation database of intra-atrial reentrant tachycardia (IART) in patients with structural heart disease and found 8 patients who had failed conventional ablation techniques with the 4-mm-tip catheter but had successful ablation performed in 11 of 13 IART using either passive cooling with an 8-mm tip or active cooling using the Chilli system.

Cooled Radiofrequency Ablation for Atrial Fibrillation

AF is the most common sustained cardiac rhythm disturbance increasing in prevalence with age. The observation that potentials arising in or near the ostia of the pulmonary veins (PVs) provoked AF and the demonstration that elimination of these foci abolished AF escalated enthusiasm for catheter-based ablation.[60] The technique of ablation has continued to evolve from early attempts to target individual ectopic foci within the PV to circumferential electrical isolation of the entire PV musculature using different ablation technologies. Marrouche and colleagues[61] performed ostial isolation of all PVs using 4-mm-tip (47 patients), 8-mm-tip (21 patients) or cooled-tip (122 patients) catheters and found at 6 months that the patients treated with the 8-mm-tip catheters had no recurrence of AF, whereas 21% and 15% of the 4-mm-tip and cooled-tip patients, respectively, had recurrence of AF. Dixit and colleagues[6] prospectively compared cooled-tip (40 patients) and 8-mm-tip (42 patients) ablation catheters in achieving electrical isolation of PVs for long-term AF control in 82 patients. Although electrical isolation of the PVs was achieved in a shorter time with the 8-mm ablation catheter, both ablation catheters had similar efficacy and safety. Matiello and coworkers,[62] in a series of 221 patients with symptomatic AF, performed circumferential PV ablation using an 8-mm-tip ablation catheter (55 W, 50°C) in 90 patients, a cooled-tip catheter (30 W, 45°C) in 42 patients, and a cooled-tip catheter (40 W, 45°C) in 89 patients. At 1-year follow-up, although there was no difference in complications, the probabilities of being arrhythmia free after a single procedure were 53%, 35%, and 55%, respectively, leading them to conclude that cooled-tip catheter ablation at 30 W led to a significantly higher recurrence rate.

Chang and colleagues[63] compared in 156 patients cooled-tip (54 patients) versus 4-mm-tip (102 patients) ablation catheters in the efficacy of acute ablative injury during circumferential PV isolation. The cooled-tip catheter caused more reduction in the electrical voltage in the PV antrum, lower incidence of acute (30 minutes) PV reconnection, inducibility of AF and gap-related atrial tachyarrhythmia despite the need for less ablation applications, and shorter procedure time. There were no significant differences in pain sensation or complications between the two groups with the 14-month recurrence rate being 13.5% in the cooled-tip group versus 33.7% in the 4-mm group.

Cooled Radiofrequency Ablation for Atrioventricular Reentrant Tachycardia

Between 5% and 17% of posteroseptal and left posterior accessory pathways have been reported to be epicardial and ablatable only within a branch of the coronary sinus (most commonly the middle cardiac vein), on the floor of the coronary sinus at the orifice of a venous branch, or within the coronary sinus diverticulum.[64] These pathways may consist of connections between the muscle coat of the coronary sinus and the ventricle. In the presence of a coronary sinus–ventricular accessory pathway, a conventional ablation catheter may completely occlude a branch of the coronary sinus, preventing cooling of the ablation electrode and

resulting in impedance rise when RF energy is delivered. This markedly reduced the amount of power that can be delivered and may result in adherence of the ablation electrode to the wall of the vein. An externally saline-irrigated ablation catheter allows more consistent delivery of RF energy with less heating at the electrode-tissue interface.

A small percentage of left free wall accessory pathways may also be epicardial, requiring ablation from within the coronary sinus. Other types of unusual accessory pathways that cannot be ablated with standard endocardial approach at the annulus have been described.[3,10,11] These include accessory pathways that connect the right atrial appendage to the right ventricle that were successfully ablated using a transcutaneous pericardial approach, and accessory pathways closely associated with the ligament of Marshall, ablated by targeting that ligament.[65–67] Several studies[68,69] have shown that RF application using an irrigated-tip catheter can be useful for the treatment of some right posteroseptal accessory pathways resistant to conventional catheter ablation. The optimum temperature suggested by the authors is no greater than 40° to 45°C, and the temperature setting should be even lower if cooled-tip RF ablation is applied to the cardiac veins.

Safety Profile of Cooled-Tip versus Noncooled-Tip Ablation Catheters

Several studies comparing irrigated-tip RF to conventional RF for ventricular tachycardia, atrial flutter, and AF have shown comparable safety profiles.[45,48,51,52,62,63] Zoppo and coworkers[70] looked at 991 consecutive patients who underwent AF ablation in an Italian multicenter registry, in which 86 patients had ablation performed by an 8-mm-tip catheter, and 905 patients were ablated with an open-system irrigated-tip ablation catheter. Even though the irrigated-tip ablation patients had a significantly longer clinical AF duration, larger left atrial size, and longer procedure time, the rates of cumulative complications were similar in the two groups. Kanj and coworkers[71] randomized 180 patients with AF to a 8-mm ablation catheter, open irrigation catheter 1 (OIC 1, peak power 50 W), and open irrigation catheter 2 (OIC 2, peak power 35 W), all of whom had a PV antral isolation performed. Although isolation of the PV antra was achieved in all patients with a significantly lower fluoroscopy and instrumentation time in the OIC 1 group with higher power titration, there was a significantly greater incidence of pops (1.3 pops/patient), pericardial effusion (20%), and gastrointestinal complaints (17% in OIC 1 versus 3% in the 8-mm versus 5% in OIC 2 groups) and focal areas of esophageal erythema (6.7% in OIC 1 versus none in the other two groups).

Conclusion

Research on cooled-tip ablation has been evolving over the past 10 years. The theoretical advantages of irrigated-tip catheters have been borne out in clinical trials. The efficacy

TABLE 3-2

COMPARISON OF STANDARD, IRRIGATED, AND LARGE-TIP ABLATION CATHETERS

	Standard Catheter	Irrigated Catheter	Large-Tip Catheter
Electrode length	4–5 mm	3.5–4 mm	6–10 mm
Power delivery	Up to 50 W	Up to 50 W	Up to 150 W
Power titration	Temperature control	Power control monitoring temperature and impedance	Usually temperature control monitoring impedance ± microbubble formation
Lesion size limited by:	Electrode temperature and impedance rise	Power setting	Electrode temperature, current shunting, impedance rise
Coagulum risk	Present	Low (especially open irrigation)	Present (possibly highest)
Steam pop risk	Low	Present	Present
Typical uses	Atrioventricular node reentry Accessory pathways Atrial tachycardias Ventricular tachycardia with normal heart Atrioventricular junctional ablation	Ventricular tachycardias with structural heart disease Atrial flutter Atrial fibrillation Coronary sinus ablation Epicardial ablation	Atrial flutter Possibly atrial fibrillation Possibly epicardial ablation

and safety of irrigated-tip ablation have been demonstrated in the treatment of several common arrhythmias, including recurrent accessory pathways after conventional RF ablation procedures, atrial flutter, ventricular tachycardia, and now AF. The inability to create transmural lesions by nonirrigation catheters could possibly be responsible for the arrhythmia recurrence after conventional RF ablation and also explain improved success with irrigated-tip catheters in scar-related arrhythmias. It appears that despite better outcomes with the irrigated-tip catheters, the overall complication rates are comparable to conventional RF ablation. There has been an increasing trend of using externally irrigated-tip catheters rather than the internally cooled-tip catheters because the former tend to increase the efficacy and decrease the complications of RF ablation (Table 3-2). Newer irrigated-tip electrode designs are expected to emerge to further increase the efficacy and safety of RF catheter ablation for difficult arrhythmias.

References

1. Calkins H, Yong P, Miller JM, et al. The Atakr Multicenter Investigators Group. Catheter ablation of accessory pathways, atrioventricular nodal reentrant tachycardia, and the atrioventricular junction: final results of a prospective, multicenter clinical trial [see comment]. *Circulation.* 1999;99:262–270.
2. Chen SA, Chiang CE, Yang CJ, et al. Sustained atrial tachycardia in adult patients: electrophysiological characteristics, pharmacological response, possible mechanisms, and effects of radiofrequency ablation [see comment]. *Circulation.* 1994;90:1262–1278.
3. Haissaguerre M, Gaita F, Fischer B, et al. Radiofrequency catheter ablation of left lateral accessory pathways via the coronary sinus. *Circulation.* 1992;86:1464–1468.
4. Jackman WM, Beckman KJ, McClelland JH, et al. Treatment of supraventricular tachycardia due to atrioventricular nodal reentry, by radiofrequency catheter ablation of slow-pathway conduction. *N Engl J Med.* 1992;327:313–318.
5. Kuck KH, Schluter M, Geiger M, et al. Radiofrequency current catheter ablation of accessory atrioventricular pathways. *Lancet.* 1991;337:1557–1561.
6. Dixit S, Gerstenfeld EP, Callans DJ, et al. Comparison of cool tip versus 8-mm tip catheter in achieving electrical isolation of pulmonary veins for long-term control of atrial fibrillation: a prospective randomized pilot study. *J Cardiovasc Electrophysiol.* 2006;17:1074–1079.
7. Nakagawa H, Beckman KJ, McClelland JH, et al. Radiofrequency catheter ablation of idiopathic left ventricular tachycardia guided by a Purkinje potential. *Circulation.* 1993;88:2607–2617.
8. Morady F, Harvey M, Kalbfleisch KG, et al. Radiofrequency catheter ablation of ventricular tachycardia in patients with coronary artery disease. *Circulation.* 1993;87:363–372.
9. Stevenson WG, Sager PT, Natterson PD, et al. Relation of pace mapping QRS configuration and conduction delay to ventricular tachycardia reentry circuits in human infarct scars. *J Am Coll Cardiol.* 1995;26:481–488.
10. Arruda MS, Beckman KJ, McClelland JH, et al. Coronary sinus anatomy and anomalies in patients with posteroseptal accessory pathway requiring ablation within a venous branch of the coronary sinus. *J Am Coll Cardiol.* 1994;17:224A.
11. Wang X, McClelland JH, Beckman KJ, et al. Left free-wall accessory pathways which require ablation from the coronary sinus: unique coronary sinus electrogram pattern. *Circulation.* 1992;86:I–581.
12. Downar E, Kimber S, Harris L, et al. Endocardial mapping of ventricular tachycardia in the intact human heart. II. Evidence for multiuse reentry in a functional sheet of surviving myocardium. *J Am Coll Cardiol.* 1992;20:869–878.
13. Kim YH, Sosa-Suarez G, Trouton TG, et al. Treatment of ventricular tachycardia by transcatheter radiofrequency ablation in patients with ischemic heart disease. *Circulation.* 1994;89:1094–1102.
14. Littmann L, Svenson RH, Gallagher JJ, et al. Functional role of the epicardium in postinfarction ventricular tachycardia: observations derived from computerized epicardial activation mapping, entrainment, and epicardial laser photoablation [see comment]. *Circulation.* 1991;83:1577–1591.
15. Huang SK, Cuenoud H, Tande Guzman W, et al. Increase in the lesion size and decrease in the impedance rise with saline infusion electrode catheter for radiofrequency catheter ablation. *Circulation.* 1989;80:II–324.
16. Wittkampf FH, Hauer RN, Robles De Medina EO. Radiofrequency ablation with a cooled porous electrode catheter. *J Am Coll Cardiol.* 1988;11:17A.
17. Pilcher TA, Sanford AL, Saul P, Dieter Haemmerich D. Convective cooling effect on cooled-tip catheter compared to large-tip catheter radiofrequency ablation. *Pacing Clin Electrophysiol.* 2006;29:1368–1374.
18. Haines DE, Watson DD. Tissue heating during radiofrequency catheter ablation: a thermodynamic model and observations in isolated perfused and superfused canine right ventricular free wall. *Pacing Clin Electrophysiol.* 1989;12:962–976.
19. Hoyt RH, Huang SK, Marcus FI, et al. Factors influencing trans-catheter radiofrequency ablation of the myocardium. *J Appl Cardiol.* 1986;1:469–486.
20. Wittkampf FH, Hauer RN, Robles de Medina EO. Control of radiofrequency lesion size by power regulation. *Circulation.* 1989;80:962–968.
21. Ring ME, Huang SK, Gorman G, Graham AR. Determinants of impedance rise during catheter ablation of bovine myocardium with radiofrequency energy. *Pacing Clin Electrophysiol.* 1989;12:1502–1513.
22. Haines DE. The biophysics of radiofrequency catheter ablation in the heart: the importance of temperature monitoring. *Pacing Clin Electrophysiol.* 1993;16:586–591.
23. Langberg JJ, Gallagher M, Strickberger SA, Amirana O. Temperature-guided radiofrequency catheter ablation with very large distal electrodes. *Circulation.* 1993;88:245–249.
24. Otomo K, Yamanashi WS, Tondo C, et al. Why a large tip electrode makes a deeper radiofrequency lesion: effects of increase in electrode cooling and electrode-tissue interface area. *J Cardiovasc Electrophysiol.* 1998;9:47–54.
25. Mittleman RS, Huang SK, de Guzman WT, et al. Use of the saline infusion electrode catheter for improved energy delivery and increased lesion size in radiofrequency catheter ablation. *Pacing Clin Electrophysiol.* 1995;18:1022–1027.
26. Nakagawa H, Yamanashi WS, Pitha JV, et al. Comparison of in vivo tissue temperature profile and lesion geometry for radiofrequency ablation with a saline-irrigated electrode versus temperature control in a canine thigh muscle preparation. *Circulation.* 1995;91:2264–2273.

27. Nibley C, Sykes CM, McLaughlin G, et al. Myocardial lesion size during radiofrequency current catheter ablation is increased by intra-electrode tip chilling. *J Am Coll Cardiol.* 1995;25:293A.

28. Ruffy R, Imran MA, Santel DJ, Wharton JM. Radiofrequency delivery through a cooled catheter tip allows the creation of larger endomyocardial lesions in the ovine heart. *J Cardiovasc Electrophysiol.* 1995;6:1089–1096.

29. Sykes C, Riley R, Pomeranz M, et al. Cooled tip ablation results in increased radiofrequency power delivery and lesion size. *Pacing Clin Electrophysiol.* 1994;88:782.

30. Eick OJ, Gerritse B, Schumacher B. Popping phenomena in temperature-controlled radiofrequency ablation: when and why do they occur? *Pacing Clin Electrophysiol.* 2000;23:253–258.

31. Petersen HH, Chen X, Pietersen A, et al. Lesion size in relation to ablation site during radiofrequency ablation. *Pacing Clin Electrophysiol.* 1990;21:322–326.

32. Dorwarth U, Fiek M, Remp T, et al. Radiofrequency catheter ablation: different cooled and noncooled electrode systems induce specific lesion geometries and adverse effects profiles. *Pacing Clin Electrophysiol.* 2003;26:1438–1445.

33. Petersen HH, Chen X, Pietersen A, et al. Lesion size in relation to ablation site during radiofrequency ablation. *Pacing Clin Electrophysiol.* 1998;21:322–326.

34. Petersen HH, Chen X, Pietersen A, et al. Tissue temperatures and lesion size during irrigated tip catheter radiofrequency ablation: an in vitro comparison of temperature-controlled irrigated tip ablation, power-controlled irrigated tip ablation, and standard temperature-controlled ablation. *Pacing Clin Electrophysiol.* 2000;23:8–17.

35. Skrumeda LL, Mehra R. Comparison of standard and irrigated radiofrequency ablation in the canine ventricle. *J Cardiovasc Electrophysiol.* 1998;9:1196–1205.

36. Wharton JM, Wilber DJ, Calkins H, et al. Utility of tip thermometry during radiofrequency ablation in humans using an internally perfused saline cooled catheter. *Circulation.* 1997;96:I–318.

37. Thiagalingam A, Campbell CR, Boyd A, et al. Catheter intramural needle radiofrequency ablation creates deeper lesions than irrigated tip catheter ablation. *Pacing Clin Electrophysiol.* 2003;26:2146–2150.

38. Weiss C, Stewart M, Franzen O, et al. Transmembranous irrigation of multipolar radiofrequency ablation catheters: induction of linear lesions encircling the pulmonary vein ostium without the risk of coagulum formation? *J Interv Cardiac Electrophysiol.* 2004;10:199–209.

39. Yokoyama K, Nakagawa H, Wittkampf FH, et al. Comparison of electrode cooling between internal and open irrigation in radiofrequency ablation lesion depth and incidence of thrombus and steam pop [see comment]. *Circulation.* 2006;113:11–19.

40. Nakagawa H, Wittkampf FH, Yamanashi WS, et al. Inverse relationship between electrode size and lesion size during radiofrequency ablation with active electrode cooling. *Circulation.* 1998;98:458–465.

41. Wong WS, VanderBrink BA, Riley RE, et al. Effect of saline irrigation flow rate on temperature profile during cooled radiofrequency ablation. *J Interv Cardiac Electrophysiol.* 2000;4:321–326.

42. Weiss C, Antz M, Eick O, et al. Radiofrequency catheter ablation using cooled electrodes: impact of irrigation flow rate and catheter contact pressure on lesion dimensions. *Pacing Clin Electrophysiol.* 2002;25:463–469.

43. D'Avila A, Houghtaling C, Gutierrez P, et al. Catheter ablation of ventricular epicardial tissue: a comparison of standard and cooled-tip radiofrequency energy. *Circulation.* 2004;109:2363–2369.

44. Everett TH, Lee KW, Wilson EE, et al. Safety profiles and lesion size of different radiofrequency ablation technologies: a comparison of large tip, open and closed irrigation catheters [see comment]. *J Cardiovasc Electrophysiol.* 2009;20:325–335.

45. Calkins H, Epstein A, Packer D, Cooled RF Multi Center Investigators Group. et al. Catheter ablation of ventricular tachycardia in patients with structural heart disease guided by cooled radiofrequency energy: results of a prospective multicenter study. *J Am Coll Cardiol.* 2000;35:1905–1914.

46. Reddy VY, Neuzil P, Taborsky M, et al. Short-term results of substrate mapping and radiofrequency ablation of ischemic ventricular tachycardia using a saline-irrigated catheter. *J Am Coll Cardiol.* 2003;41:2228–2236.

47. Soejima K, Delacretaz E, Suzuki M, et al. Saline-cooled versus standard radiofrequency catheter ablation for infarct-related ventricular tachycardias. *Circulation.* 2001;103:1858–1862.

48. Stevenson WG, Wilber DJ, Natale A, et al. Irrigated radiofrequency catheter ablation guided by electroanatomic mapping for recurrent ventricular tachycardia after myocardial infarction: the Multicenter ThermoCool Ventricular Tachycardia Ablation trial. *Circulation.* 2008;118:2773–2782.

49. Deneke T, Muller KM, Lemke B, et al. Human histopathology of electroanatomic mapping after cooled-tip radiofrequency ablation to treat ventricular tachycardia in remote myocardial infarction. *J Cardiovasc Electrophysiol.* 2005;16:1246–1251.

50. Atiga WL, Worley SJ, Hummel J, et al. Prospective randomized comparison of cooled radiofrequency versus standard radiofrequency energy for ablation of typical atrial flutter. *Pacing Clin Electrophysiol.* 2002;25:1172–1178.

51. Jais P, Haissaguerre M, Shah DC, et al. Successful irrigated-tip catheter ablation of atrial flutter resistant to conventional radiofrequency ablation. *Circulation.* 1998;98:835–838.

52. Jais P, Shah DC, Haissaguerre M, et al. Prospective randomized comparison of irrigated-tip versus conventional-tip catheters for ablation of common flutter. *Circulation.* 2000;101:772–776.

53. Scavee C, Jais P, Hsu LF, et al. Prospective randomised comparison of irrigated-tip and large-tip catheter ablation of cavotricuspid isthmus-dependent atrial flutter. *Eur Heart J.* 2004;25:963–969.

54. Schreieck J, Zrenner B, Kumpmann J, et al. Prospective randomized comparison of closed cooled-tip versus 8-mm-tip catheters for radiofrequency ablation of typical atrial flutter. *J Cardiovasc Electrophysiol.* 2002;13:980–985.

55. Spitzer SG, Karolyi L, Rammler C, et al. Primary closed cooled tip ablation of typical atrial flutter in comparison to conventional radiofrequency ablation. *Europace.* 2002;4:265–271.

56. Da Costa A, Cucherat M, Pichon N, et al. Comparison of the efficacy of cooled-tip and 8-mm-tip catheters for radiofrequency catheter ablation of the cavotricuspid isthmus: a meta-analysis. *Pacing Clin Electrophysiol.* 2005;28:1081–1087.

57. Da Costa A, Romeyer-Bouchard C, Jamon Y, et al. Radiofrequency catheter selection based on cavotricuspid angiography compared with a control group with an externally cooled-tip catheter: a randomized pilot study. *J Cardiovasc Electrophysiol.* 2009;20:492–498.

58. Bai R, Fahmy TS, Patel D, et al. Radiofrequency ablation of atypical atrial flutter after cardiac surgery or atrial fibrillation ablation: a randomized comparison of open-irrigation-tip and 8-mm-tip catheters. *Heart Rhythm.* 2007;4:1489–1496.

59. Blaufox AD, Numan MT, Laohakunakorn P, et al. Catheter tip cooling during radiofrequency ablation of intra-atrial reentry: effects on power, temperature, and impedance. *J Cardiovasc Electrophysiol.* 2002;13:783–787.

60. Haissaguerre M, Jais P, Shah DC, et al. Spontaneous initiation of atrial fibrillation by ectopic beats originating in the pulmonary veins. *N Engl J Med.* 1998;339:659–666.

61. Marrouche NF, Dresing T, Cole C, et al. Circular mapping and ablation of the pulmonary vein for treatment of atrial fibrillation: impact of different catheter technologies [see comment]. *J Am Coll Cardiol.* 2002;40:464–474.

62. Matiello M, Mont L, Tamborero D, et al. Cooled-tip vs. 8 mm-tip catheter for circumferential pulmonary vein isolation: comparison of efficacy, safety, and lesion extension. *Europace.* 2008;10:955–960.

63. Chang S, Tai C, Lin Y, et al. Comparison of cooled-tip versus 4-mm-tip catheter in the efficacy of acute ablative tissue injury during circumferential pulmonary vein isolation. *J Cardiovasc Electrophysiol.* 2009;20:1113–1118.

64. Sun Y, Arruda M, Otomo K, et al. Coronary sinus-ventricular accessory connections producing posteroseptal and left posterior accessory pathways: incidence and electrophysiological identification. *Circulation.* 2002;106:1362–1367.

65. Goya M, Takahashi A, Nakagawa H, Iesaka Y. A case of catheter ablation of accessory atrioventricular connection between the right atrial appendage and right ventricle guided by a three-dimensional electroanatomic mapping system [see comment]. *J Cardiovasc Electrophysiol.* 1999;10:1112–1118.

66. Hwang C, Peter CT, Chen PS, et al. Radiofrequency ablation of accessory pathways guided by the location of the ligament of Marshall. *J Cardiovasc Electrophysiol.* 2003;14:616–620.

67. Lam C, Schweikert R, Kanagaratnam L, Natale A. Radiofrequency ablation of a right atrial appendage-ventricular accessory pathway by transcutaneous epicardial instrumentation. *J Cardiovasc Electrophysiol.* 2000;11:1170–1173.

68. Garcia-Garcia J, Almendral J, Arenal A, et al. Irrigated tip catheter ablation in right posteroseptal accessory pathways resistant to conventional ablation. *Pacing Clin Electrophysiol.* 2002;25:799–803.

69. Yamane T, Jais P, Shah DC, et al. Efficacy and safety of an irrigated-tip catheter for the ablation of accessory pathways resistant to conventional radiofrequency ablation. *Circulation.* 2000;102:2565–2568.

70. Zoppo F, Bertaglia E, Tondo C, et al. High prevalence of cooled tip use as compared with 8-mm tip in a multicenter Italian registry on atrial fibrillation ablation: focus on procedural safety. *J Cardiovasc Med.* 2008;9:888–892.

71. Kanj MH, Wazni O, Fahmy T, et al. Pulmonary vein antral isolation using an open irrigation ablation catheter for the treatment of atrial fibrillation: a randomized pilot study. *J Am Coll Cardiol.* 2007;49:1634–1641.

4

Catheter Cryoablation: Biophysics and Applications

Paul Khairy and Marc Dubuc

Key Points

The biophysics and mechanisms of cryothermal injury comprise the following general phases: freeze-thaw, hemorrhage and inflammation, replacement fibrosis, and apoptosis.

Cryoablation lesion size is determined by refrigerant flow rate, electrode size, electrode contact pressure, electrode orientation, duration of energy delivery, and electrode temperature.

Advantages of cryoablation include the ability to titrate temperature and duration to produce reversible lesions before permanent tissue destruction (cryomapping), decreased risk for thromboembolism, superior catheter stability, and less risk for injury to vascular structures.

Cryoablation has been applied clinically to a variety of arrhythmic substrates, including atrioventricular (AV) nodal ablation, AV nodal reentrant tachycardia, mid-septal and paraseptal pathways, ventricular tachycardia, atrial flutter, and atrial fibrillation.

The introduction of percutaneous direct-current ablation more than 25 years ago launched an era of interventional cardiac electrophysiology that transformed the management of cardiac arrhythmias. Direct-current ablation was later supplanted by radiofrequency (RF) energy, which offered a more attractive efficacy and safety profile. Transcatheter RF ablation was broadly disseminated as the procedure of choice, with expanding indications that paralleled the growing global experience and knowledge base. Although benefits of RF ablation became widely appreciated, limitations were likewise increasingly recognized. These include thromboembolization, inadvertent collateral damage to surrounding vascular and electrical structures, and inability to assess electrophysiologic effects before permanent lesion creation.

The scientific community, therefore, persevered in its efforts to further improve patient safety and procedural outcomes by seeking alternative sources of energy and developing ablation systems capable of creating deeper, larger, and more contiguous lesions. It is within this context that cryothermal energy ablation emerged as an alternative treatment modality. With the first transcatheter procedure performed in humans at the Montreal Heart Institute in August 1998, the collective experience has increased exponentially during the past decade.[1] Potential advantages were recognized, including an impressive safety record with decreased thrombogenic potential, ability to produce reversible electrophysiologic effects before permanent lesion creation, improved catheter stability during cryoablation clinical applications, less propensity to damage vascular structures, and decreased levels of pain perceived by patients.

The purpose of this chapter is to provide the clinical electrophysiologist, trainee, and cardiologist with a solid understanding of the field of cryoablation, beginning with a brief historical overview, discussion of biophysics, and depiction of the components of a transvenous catheter cryoenergy delivery system. Advantages and limitations of cryoablation are reviewed, and current clinical applications are discussed.

History of Cryothermal Energy Use in Cardiovascular Medicine

The concept of hypothermic therapy dates back to the ancient Egyptian Edwin Smith Papyrus on surgical trauma, written between 3000 and 2500 BC, where it was introduced as a treatment for abscesses.[2,3] Cryosurgical devices cooled by liquid nitrogen were pioneered in the early 1960s.[4-8] Hass and colleagues first described predictable controlled myocardial lesions with cryoenergy in 1948 using carbon dioxide as a refrigerant.[5,6] Thus, although not novel as an energy modality, harnessing cryoenergy into a steerable transcatheter format represents a more recent landmark in the history of arrhythmia therapy. Table 4-1 summarizes key historical landmarks in the development of a transvenous cryoablation system for cardiac arrhythmias.[3–5,7–11]

It was in 1964 that Lister and associates[7] first described the application of cryoenergy to the cardiac conduction tissue by suturing a 4-mm U-shaped silver tube near the bundle of His. Progressive but reversible high-grade atrioventricular (AV) block was demonstrated. In 1977, Harrison and coworkers[8] introduced cryosurgery with hand-held bipolar electrode probes. Approaches not requiring extracorporeal bypass were later devised.[12–14]

Gallagher and coworkers[15] reported the first two cases of successful cryosurgical accessory pathway ablation in 1977. A different approach to ablation was later described with cryoprobes designed to enter the coronary sinus, thereby obviating the need for extracorporeal bypass.[16] Beginning with Gallagher's description of cryosurgical ablation for ventricular tachycardia in 1978,[17] cryosurgery became a recognized treatment for selected patients with refractory ventricular arrhythmias,[18–23] often as an adjunct to more extensive surgery.[24] Surgical cryoablation has also been described for less common arrhythmias, including nodoventricular tachycardia,[25] sinoatrial reentrant tachycardia,[26] disabling ventricular bigeminy,[27] bundle branch reentry tachycardia,[28] and fetal malignant tachyarrhythmias.[29] It has also been used for AV nodal reentrant tachycardia and other arrhythmias with rapid AV conduction with the objective of slowing but preserving nodal conduction.[30–32]

Gillette and colleagues reported the first animal study using a transvenous cryocatheter in 1991.[9] In five miniature swine, complete AV block was produced with an 11-French (11F) cryocatheter cooled by pressurized nitrous oxide. Although feasibility of transcatheter cryolesion formation was demonstrated, limited success was attributed to lack of steerability and recording electrodes. Cryocatheter placement required using a second catheter to record local signals. Transcatheter cryoablation was revived several years later, ultimately leading to clinical use. In 1998, we reported the first animal experiment using a steerable cryocatheter with integrated recording and pacing electrodes.[10] This 9F catheter system used Halocarbon 502 (Freon) as a refrigerant. Chronic histology was later characterized, with sharply demarcated ultrastructurally intact lesions devoid of thrombus. These and other preclinical studies contributed importantly to our understanding of the impact of cooling rate and catheter-tip temperature on tissue effects.[10,18,19,33,34]

Biophysics and Mechanisms of Cryothermal Energy Tissue Injury

The ultimate purpose of cryoablation is to freeze tissue in a discrete and focused fashion to destroy cells in a targeted area. The application of cryothermal energy results in the formation of an ice ball. Cooling first occurs at the distal catheter tip in contact with endocardial tissue. Freezing then extends radially into the tissue, establishing a temperature gradient. The lowest temperature and fastest freezing rate are generated at the point of contact, with slower tissue cooling rates more peripherally.[10,34–37] The mechanisms of tissue damage are complex and still debated but involve freezing and thawing, hemorrhage and inflammation, replacement fibrosis, and apoptosis (Fig. 4-1).[24]

Hypothermia causes cardiomyocytes to become less fluid as metabolism slows, ion pumps lose transport capabilities, and intracellular pH becomes more acidic.[33] These effects may be entirely transient, depending on the interplay between temperature and duration. The briefer the exposure to a hypothermic insult or the warmer the temperature, or both, the more rapidly cells recover. As a clinical correlate, this characteristic of cryoenergy permits functional assessment of putative ablation sites (i.e., cryomapping) without cellular destruction.

In contrast, the hallmark of permanent tissue injury induced by hypothermia is ice formation. As cells are rapidly cooled to freezing temperatures, ice crystals form within the extracellular matrix and then intracellularly.[38]

TABLE 4-1		
HISTORICAL LANDMARKS IN CARDIAC CRYOABLATION		
Year	**Study**	**Contribution**
1948	Hass[5]	Cryothermal myocardial lesions
1963	Cooper[4]	Cryosurgical apparatus development
1964	Lister et al.[7]	Cryothermal energy used to interrupt conduction with evidence of reversibility
1977	Harrison et al.[8]	Surgical application of cryothermal energy by handheld probe
1991	Gillette et al.[9]	Percutaneous application of cryothermal energy by transvenous catheter in animals
1998	Dubuc et al.[10]	Use of steerable cryocatheter system with pacing and recording electrodes
1999	Dubuc et al.[11]	Percutaneous transvenous catheter cryoablation in humans

From Khairy P, Dubuc M. Transcatheter cryoablation. In: Liem LB, Downar E, eds. *Progress in Catheter Ablation*. Dordrecht: Kluwer Academic; 2001:391.

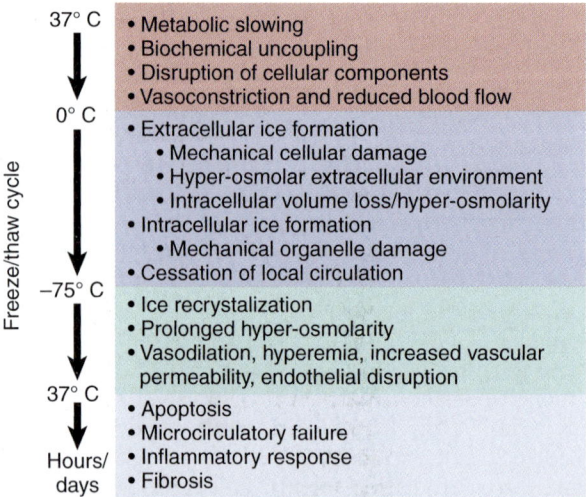

MECHANISMS OF CRYOTHERMAL INJURY

Freeze/thaw cycle

37° C
- Metabolic slowing
- Biochemical uncoupling
- Disruption of cellular components
- Vasoconstriction and reduced blood flow

0° C
- Extracellular ice formation
  - Mechanical cellular damage
  - Hyper-osmolar extracellular environment
  - Intracellular volume loss/hyper-osmolarity
- Intracellular ice formation
  - Mechanical organelle damage
- Cessation of local circulation

−75° C
- Ice recrystalization
- Prolonged hyper-osmolarity
- Vasodilation, hyperemia, increased vascular permeability, endothelial disruption

37° C
- Apoptosis
- Microcirculatory failure
- Inflammatory response
- Fibrosis

Hours/ days

FIGURE 4-1. Mechanisms of cryothermal injury during the freeze-thaw cycle of catheter cryoablation.

The size of ice crystals and their density are dependent on proximity to the cryoenergy source, the local tissue temperature achieved, and the rate of freezing. Ice crystals do not characteristically penetrate cellular membranes; rather, they cause compression and distortion of intracellular organelles, including nuclei and cytoplasmic components.[39,40] Mitochondria are particularly sensitive to ice crystals and are the first structures to suffer irreversible damage.[41–43] Extracellular ice crystal formation removes extracellular free water, resulting in intracellular desiccation. The remaining fluid becomes hyperosmotic, further contributing to cell death. Upon completion of freezing, the tissue passively returns to body temperature, resulting in a "thawing effect." This is an important component of cryoablation because rewarming causes intracellular crystals to enlarge and fuse into larger masses that extend cellular destruction.[33,38,44,45]

Within 48 hours after a freeze-thaw cycle, hemorrhage[35] and inflammation[6] characterize the second phase of cryoablation (coagulation necrosis) (Fig. 4-2A).[24] In what has been termed a "solution effect," water migrates out of myocardial cells to reestablish the osmotic equilibrium that was disturbed by ice crystals. In effect, the resulting increase in the intracellular solute concentration may damage cell membranes.[44] As the microcirculation is restored to previously frozen tissue, edema ensues. The fluid traverses damaged microvascular endothelial cells, resulting in ischemic necrosis. In the final phase of cryoinjury, replacement fibrosis and apoptosis of cells near the periphery of frozen tissue give rise to a mature lesion within weeks (Fig. 4-2B).[34]

Cryolesions produced by 4-, 6-, and 8-mm electrode-tip catheters are well circumscribed, with a sharply defined interface with normal myocardium, dense areas of fibrotic tissue, contraction band necrosis, and a conserved tissue matrix (Fig. 4-3A, *right panel*).[46,47] The endothelial cell layer is typically preserved, with no surface thrombosis (Fig. 4-3B, *right panel*). Lesion surface areas produced by 8-mm catheters are, on average, 92 mm² larger (177%) than with 4-mm catheters and 72 mm² greater (101%) than with 6-mm catheters.[47] Eight- and 6-mm catheters yield mean lesion volumes 253 mm³ (248%) and 116 mm³

(114%) larger than 4 mm catheters.[47] In contrast, RF lesions created by standard 4-mm electrode-tip catheters are less sharply demarcated, with less well-preserved architecture (Fig. 4-3A, *left panel*), endothelial disruption, and surface thrombosis (Fig. 4-3B, *left panel*).[46] Thermal profiles for cryoablation and radiofrequency ablation lesions obtained by infrared thermography are shown in Fig. 4-3D.

Cryoablation Technical Aspects

Console and Catheters

Principles such as the Joule-Thompson effect (cooling by expansion of a compressed gas after passage through a needle valve) and the Peltier effect (thermoelectric cooling) have been incorporated into the design of cryoablation systems.[18,45] A variety of devices were developed using several methods of refrigeration and numerous cryogens, including nitrogen, nitrous oxide, solid carbon dioxide, argon, and various fluorinated hydrocarbons.[33] Several systems for catheter cryoablation are in commercial use. Here, we describe the cryoablation system manufactured by Medtronic CryoCath LP (Montreal, Canada) (Fig. 4-4). Commonly used quadripolar steerable catheters come in 7F 4- and 6-mm-tip and 9F 8-mm-tip sizes. These catheters are equipped with a thermocouple (Fig. 4-5) at the distal electrode where cooling occurs and temperature is recorded. Three proximal electrodes serve to pace and record. In addition, an expandable cryoablation balloon catheter (Arctic Front), 18 to 28 mm in diameter, was specifically designed to isolate pulmonary veins in patients with atrial fibrillation.

Standard deflectable catheters are composed of two concentric lumens, with a hollow shaft, a distal cooling electrode tip, and three proximal ring electrodes for recording and pacing. A central console that contains the refrigerant fluid, currently nitrous oxide,[46] releases the cryogen under pressure. The cooling liquid travels through the inner delivery lumen to the distal electrode that is maintained under vacuum (Fig. 4-6). At the cryocatheter tip, the liquid cryogen boils. This accelerated liquid-to-gas phase change results in rapid cooling of the distal tip. The gas is then

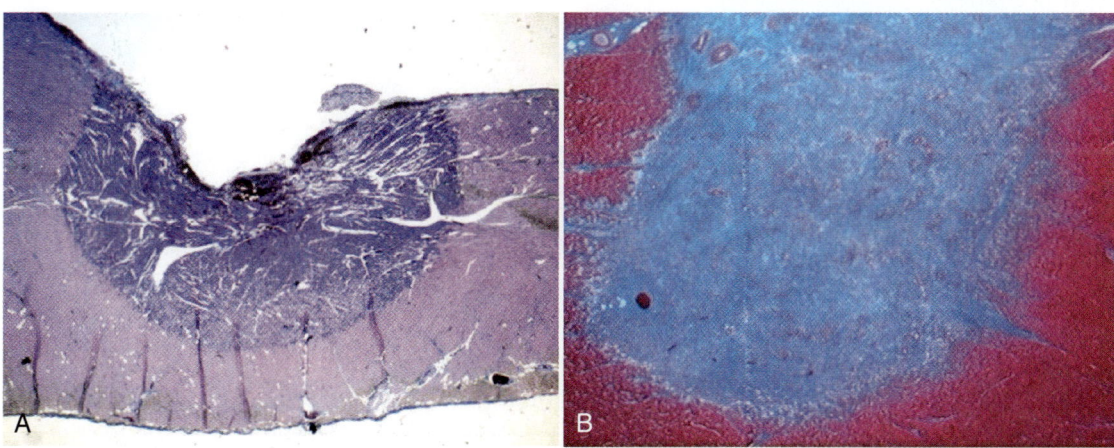

FIGURE 4-2. A, Low-power photomicrograph of a subacute cryothermal lesion; note the well-circumscribed borders of the lesion. **B,** Medium-power photomicrograph of a chronic cryothermal lesion with preserved tissue architecture. Both lesions were performed in mongrel dog left ventricular myocardium with a 4-minute cryoapplication at -55°C.

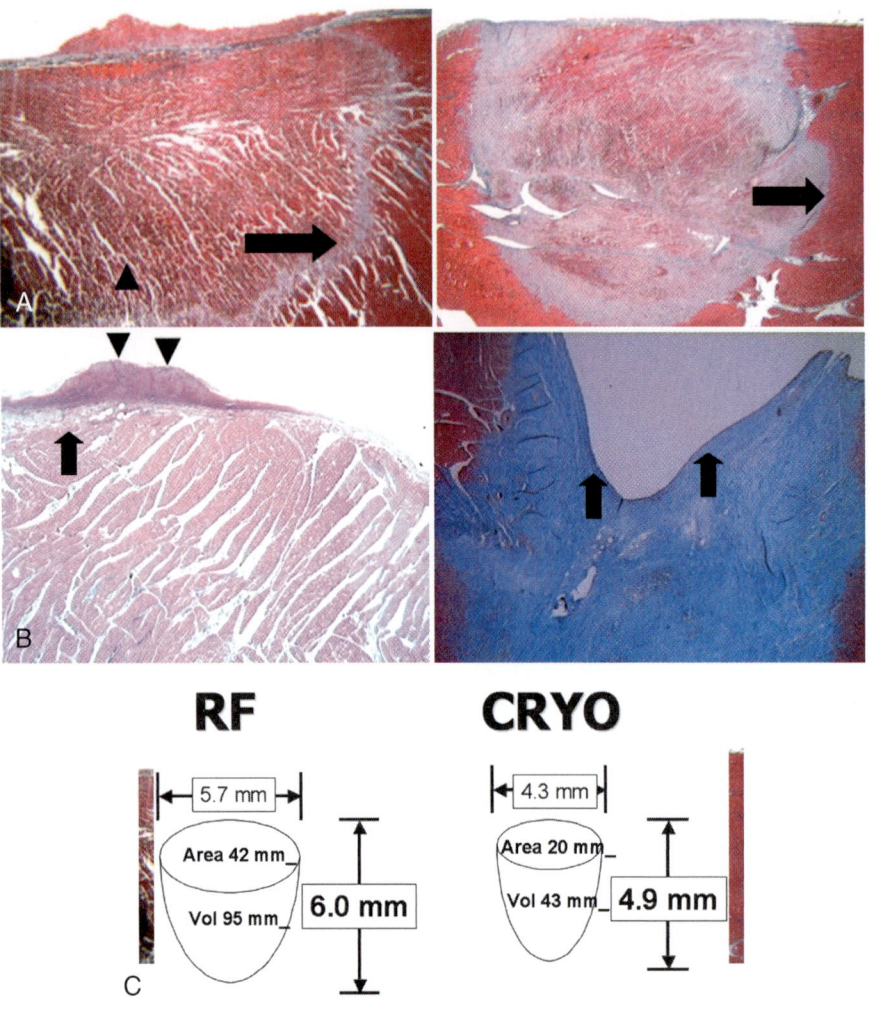

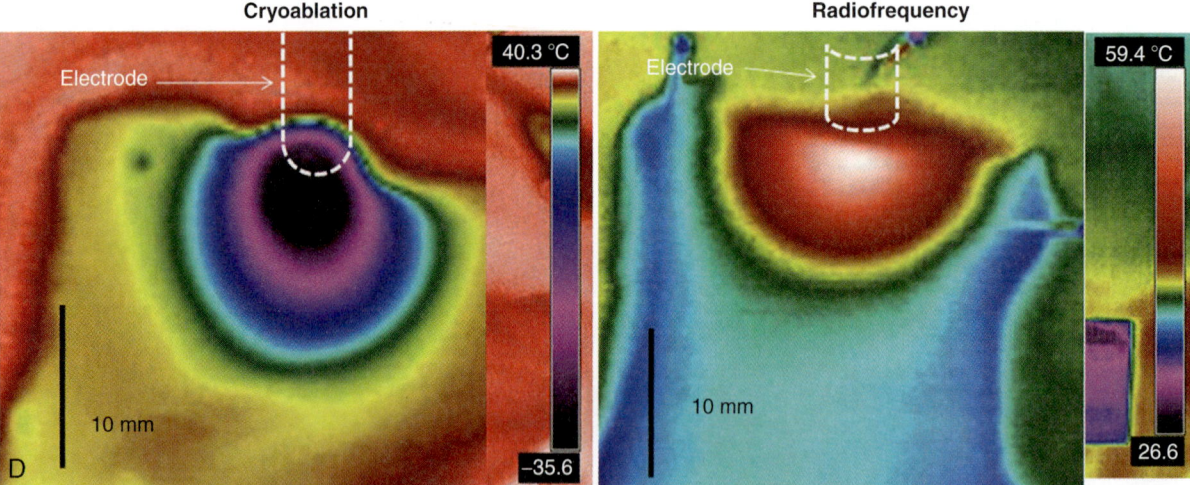

FIGURE 4-3. **A,** Photomicrographs of a chronic radiofrequency (RF) lesion (60 seconds at 70°C) *(left)* compared with a chronic cryothermal lesion (4 minutes at –75°C) *(right)*. Note the hemispherical necrosis of the cryothermal lesion as well as the discrete lesion demarcation *(right, arrow)* and preserved tissue architecture. In contrast, the RF lesion exhibits less discrete lesion demarcation *(left, arrow)* and less well-preserved architecture *(left, arrowhead)*. **B,** Photomicrographs of a chronic RF lesion (60 seconds at 70°C) *(left)* compared with a chronic cryothermal lesion (4 minutes at –75°C) *(right)*. Note the well-preserved endothelium free of thrombus in the cryothermal lesion *(right, arrows)* compared with the disrupted endothelium *(left, arrow)* and associated thrombus *(left, arrowheads)* of the RF lesion. **C,** Schematic diagram comparing lesion geometries between an RF lesion *(left)* and a cryoablation (CRYO) lesion *(right)*. The RF lesion has similar depth but larger lesion volume and area. **D,** Infrared thermal images of cryoablation lesion created with a 6-mm-tip electrode and RF lesion created with 4-mm internally irrigated electrode (25 W). The lesions are created in blocks of porcine ventricular myocardium in a warmed fluid bath with the tissue surface exposed just above the fluid level. The outlines of the submerged electrode locations are shown. *(A, left panel, Reproduced from, and C, created from data available in Khairy P, Chauvet P, Lehmann J, et al. Lower incidence of thrombus formation with cryoenergy versus radiofrequency catheter ablation. Circulation. 2003;107:2045–2050. With permission.)*

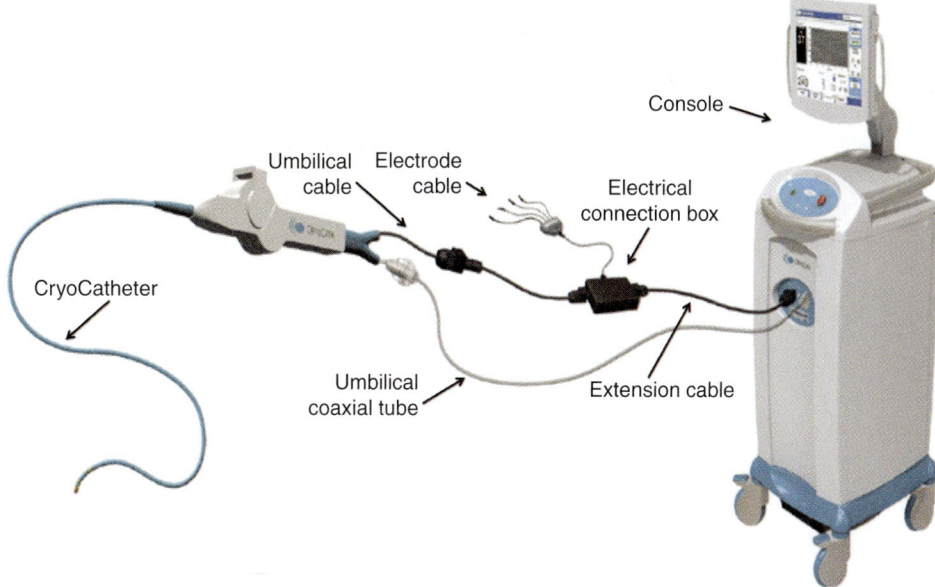

FIGURE 4-4. Cryoablation console and connectors. *(Courtesy of Medtronic CryoCath® LP, Montreal, Canada. With permission.)*

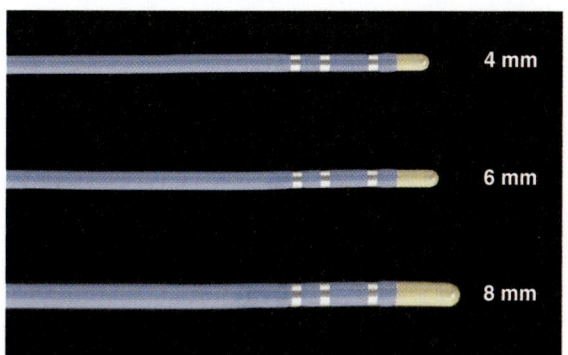

FIGURE 4-5. Cryoablation catheters with 4-, 6-, and 8-mm distal electrode tips. *(Courtesy of Medtronic CryoCath® LP, Montreal, Canada. With permission.)*

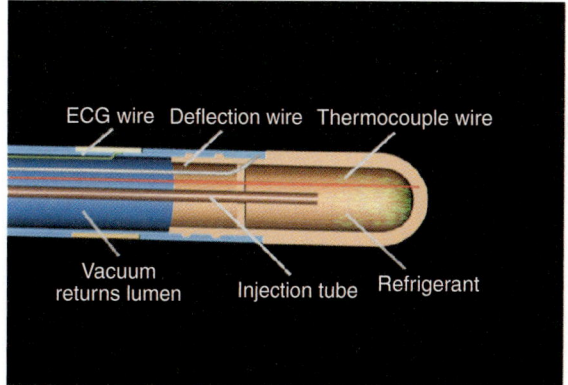

FIGURE 4-6. Schematic diagram demonstrating the CryoCath Freezor cryocatheter internal design and distal tip cooling by the Joule-Thompson effect. The electrocardiogram (ECG) wire, deflection wire, thermocouple wire, central injection tube, and vacuum return tip and lumen are shown. Refrigerant is injected from the central injection lumen into the distal tip, where it rapidly evaporates. The cooling of the tip causes ice ball formation around the external portion of the distal tip with freezing of adjacent tissue. *(Courtesy of Medtronic CryoCath® LP, Montreal, Canada. With permission.)*

conducted away from the catheter tip through a vacuum return lumen and back to the console, where it is collected and restored to its liquid state. Temperature is recorded at the distal tip by an integrated thermocouple device.

The console allows the operator two different modes of operation. The first is the cryomapping mode. In this mode, the tip is cooled to a temperature not lower than –30°C for a maximum of 80 seconds, to prevent irreversible tissue damage. Of note, this function is not available for 8-mm-tip catheters. The second mode is cryoablation, which results in cooling of the catheter tip to at least –75°C for a programmable period of time (nominally 4 minutes), producing the permanent lesion. The cryomapping mode may be used an indefinite number of times before cryoablation. Cryoablation may be initiated at any time during a cryomapping application or, from the onset, if the operator wishes to forgo the cryomapping function.

The design of the Arctic Front catheter consists of a bidirectional deflectable over-the-wire system with inner and outer balloons (Fig. 4-7).[48] Nitrous oxide is delivered to the inner balloon. To allow for some variation in venous ostial diameters, two balloon sizes are available: 23 and 28

mm in diameter. These catheters must be used in conjunction with a 12F transseptal sheath. The FlexCath transeptal sheath (Medtronic CryoCath LP) is deflectable, enhancing maneuverability in the left atrium.

Determinants of Cryoablation Lesion Size

During catheter cryoablation, tissue temperatures follow a monoexponential decline toward steady-state values around the ablation electrode (Fig. 4-8).[49] The size of catheter-based cryoablation lesions is dependent on many factors (Table 4-2).[49] Analogous to electrical current for RF ablation, the refrigerant is the mediator of thermal change in cryoablation systems. Higher flow rates of refrigerant are capable of extracting more heat from the tissue and, therefore, can result in increased lesion size. In addition,

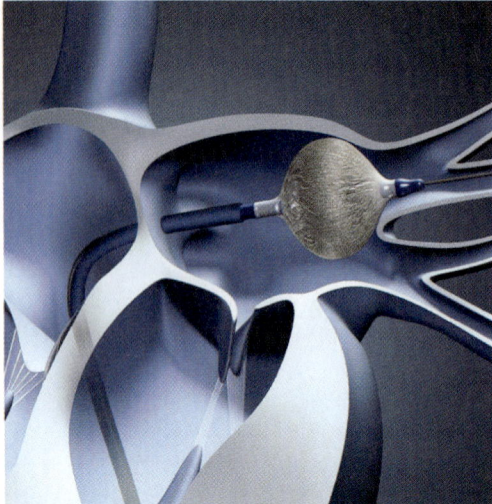

FIGURE 4-7. CryoCath Arctic Front cryoablation balloon. The procedure consists of deploying and inflating the balloon catheter in the left atrium before advance it toward the wired vein. The balloon comes in 23- and 28-mm sizes. *(Courtesy of Medtronic CryoCath LP, Montreal, Canada. With permission.)*

TABLE 4-2

DETERMINANTS OF LESION SIZE FOR CATHETER CRYOABLATION

Factor	Effect on Lesion Size
Refrigerant flow rate	Increased flow increases lesion size
Electrode size	Increased electrode size allows greater refrigerant flow rates
Tissue contact	Increased contact pressure increases lesion size
Electrode orientation	Larger lesion sizes with horizontal (parallel) electrode orientation to tissue
Convective warming	Blood flow over electrode/tissue reduces lesion size
Electrode temperature	Colder temperature creates larger lesion*
Duration of energy application	Longer delivery produces larger lesion

* See text. Heat extraction capacity of refrigerant is important. A refrigerant with greater heat extraction capacity may produce a larger lesion at a lower electrode temperature than a colder electrode using refrigerant with low heat extraction capacity.

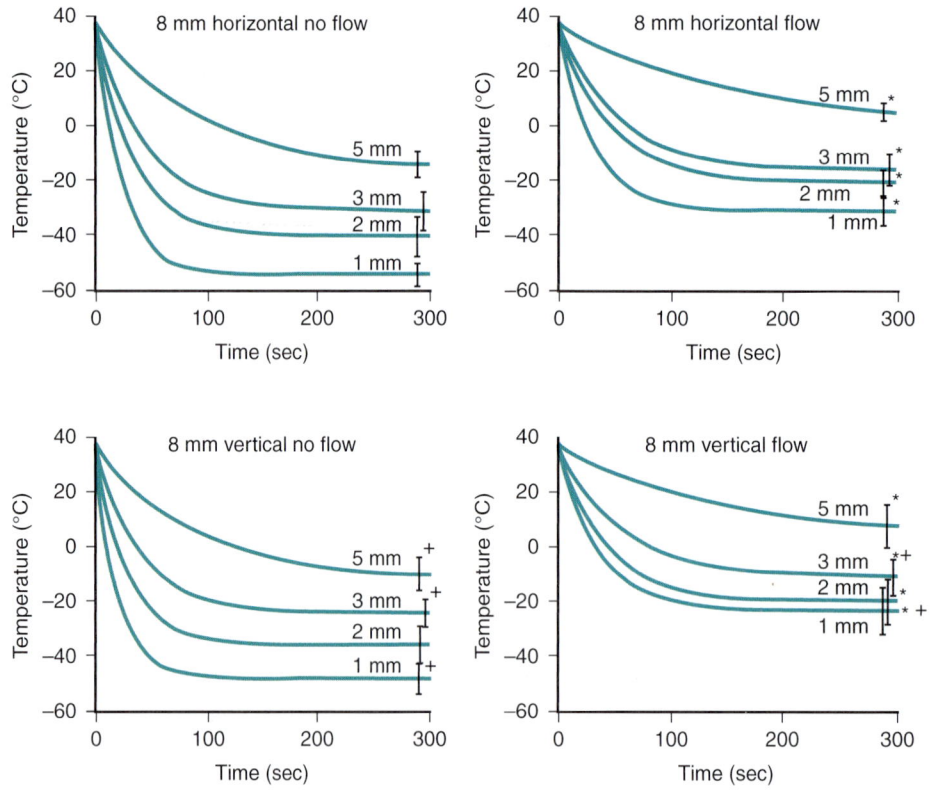

FIGURE 4-8. Graphs of average tissue temperature versus time in isolated myocardial tissue undergoing catheter cryoablation. Temperature recordings are made at 1-, 2-, 3-, and 5-mm depths from an 8-mm-tip cryoablation catheter. The individual temperature curves each follow a monoexponential decrease over time. The *vertical lines* represent 1 standard deviation above and below the average temperature just before energy termination. The four graphs represent differing conditions of vertical (perpendicular) or horizontal (parallel) electrode orientation to the tissue and either the presence or absence of simulated blood flow over the electrode-tissue interface. Note the marked effect of convective warming on tissue temperatures. *(Data from Wood MA, Parvez B, Ellenbogen AL, et al. Determinants of lesion sizes and tissue temperatures during catheter cryoablation. Pacing Clin Electrophysiol. 2007;30:644–654.)*

refrigerants differ in their capacity to extract heat based on their physical properties and physical phase delivered to the electrode tip. For example, a colder gas phase of refrigerant may well produce a smaller lesion than a liquid refrigerant undergoing a phase change within the electrode at a warmer temperature. Larger electrode sizes appear tied to larger lesions by way of allowing greater refrigerant flow rates.[49] Lesion sizes also increase with greater electrode contact pressure and with greater electrode surface area in contact with the tissue to allow greater heat extraction from the tissue and less from the local blood pool.[47,49] Electrode orientations that are parallel with the tissue therefore produce larger lesions than perpendicular orientations because of greater thermal coupling with the tissue.[47,49,50] Convective warming of electrode and tissue by local blood flow has a detrimental effect on lesion formation. In experimental preparations, simulated blood flow over cryoablation electrodes may reduce lesion volume by 75% compared with the absence of blood flow.[49] Even under strictly controlled experimental conditions, electrode temperature is an imperfect predictor of lesion size (Fig. 4-9). Because active cooling occurs within the electrode and near the embedded thermocouple, electrode temperature is insensitive to other factors critical to lesion formation such as convective warming, contact pressure, and electrode orientation.[49] In addition, maximal electrode cooling may occur in the absence of any tissue contact. This differs from RF ablation in which the electrode is passively heated from contact with the tissue. In isolated tissue experiments, lesion dimensions were increased by prolonging energy delivery or by repeating the freeze-thaw cycle when compared with single 2.5-minute applications.[50]

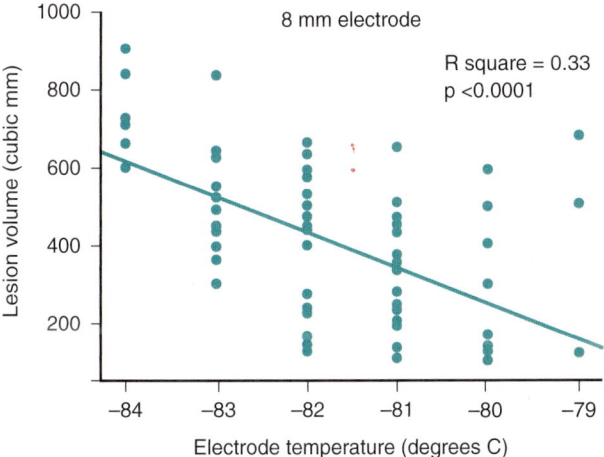

FIGURE 4-9. Lesion volumes versus cryoablation electrode temperature in isolated ventricular myocardial tissue under controlled conditions of vertical or horizontal electrode orientation, tissue contact pressure, and simulated blood flow over the electrode-tissue interface for an 8-mm-tip cryoablation catheter. Note the general trend toward larger lesions with colder electrode temperatures. However, for any given electrode temperature, the resulting lesion size may vary by threefold to fourfold depending on conditions such as electrode orientation and convective warming from blood flow. *(Data from Wood MA, Parvez B, Ellenbogen AL, et al. Determinants of lesion sizes and tissue temperatures during catheter cryoablation. Pacing Clin Electrophysiol. 2007;30:644–654. With permission.)*

Cryoablation versus Radiofrequency Ablation

Some factors influencing lesion size for catheter cryoablation are also critical to RF ablation, whereas others may have opposite effects for the two energy sources (Fig. 4-10).[51] Both modalities benefit from enhanced tissue contact pressure and larger electrode sizes if the larger electrode allows greater refrigerant flow or electrical current to be delivered. For RF ablation, convective cooling of the electrode by local blood flow can enhance power delivery. For cryoablation, local blood flow can be detrimental only by warming the electrode and tissue.[49,51] For cryoablation and noncooled RF ablation, an electrode orientation parallel to the tissue enhances lesion size. For irrigated RF catheters, a parallel electrode orientation reduces lesion size.[51] The superiority of cryoablation compared with RF ablation to increase lesion size depends on conditions such as convective thermal effects and electrode orientation.[51] Simultaneously applying standard RF and cryothermal energy through the same catheter may produce lesions of similar dimension to irrigated RF ablation.[52]

Cryomapping and Cryoablation Delivery

Standard ablation with the CryoCath system consists of advancing a steerable quadripolar catheter to the region of interest. The ablation target is identified with mapping techniques similar to RF ablation procedures. Once the target is identified, the operator may select either cryomapping (for 4- and 6-mm-tip catheters) or cryoablation mode. The cryomapping mode is typically performed before cryoablation when the arrhythmia substrate is in the vicinity of the AV node and His-Purkinje conduction system. The operator may choose to apply cryoablation directly if the region is deemed safe or at some distance from the conduction system. Importantly, dynamic cryomapping inherently occurs at the onset of cryoablation as the temperature gradient spreads centrifugally from the catheter-tissue contact. Cooling of cells (e.g., to a temperature of –30°C) with reversible electrophysiologic effects necessarily precedes irreversible tissue destruction (e.g., at temperatures of less than –50 to –60°C). Thus, vigilance is required throughout the cryoapplication as the temperature gradient spreads, despite an initially reassuring "cryomap."

When temperatures reach –20°C and colder, electrical noise appears on the distal electrode pair, with loss of the local electrogram signal due to ice ball formation. This electrical noise resolves once the temperature warms to more than –20°C. During the time that temperatures remain colder than –20°C, the catheter adheres to the cardiac endocardial tissue and, therefore, allows the operator to perform programmed stimulation to confirm safety and efficacy without concern for catheter dislodgment. In the event of an undesirable effect, prompt termination of the application usually results in complete recovery within seconds after rewarming, with no permanent effect. If desired effects are confirmed, cryoablation is typically maintained for 4 minutes because preclinical studies demonstrated that the lesion increases in size during the first 2 to 3 minutes and reaches a plateau thereafter. Thus, applications lasting less than 4 minutes may not provide histologic effects (Fig. 4-11A-C). Although one 4-minute application

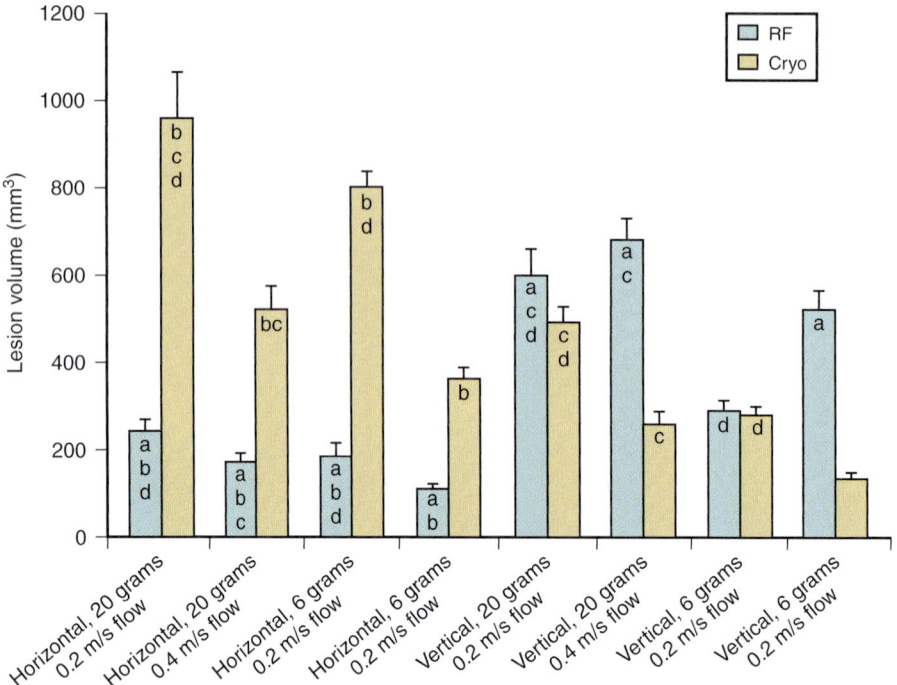

FIGURE 4-10. Lesion volumes for irrigated and radiofrequency (RF) ablation (*blue bars*) and cryoablation (*yellow bars*) under various conditions of electrode orientation (vertical or horizontal), contact pressure (6 or 20 g), and simulated blood flow over electrode-tissue interface (0.2 or 0.4 m/sec). a, $P < .05$ versus same conditions except cryoablation catheter; b, $P < .05$ versus same conditions except vertical orientation; c, $P < .05$ versus same conditions except 6 g pressure; d, $P < .05$ versus same conditions except 0.4 m/sec simulated blood flow. (*Data from Parvez B, Pathak V, Schubert CM, Wood M. Comparison of lesion sizes produced by cryoablation and open irrigated radiofrequency ablation catheters.* J Cardiovasc Electrophysiol. *2008;19:528–534. With permission.*)

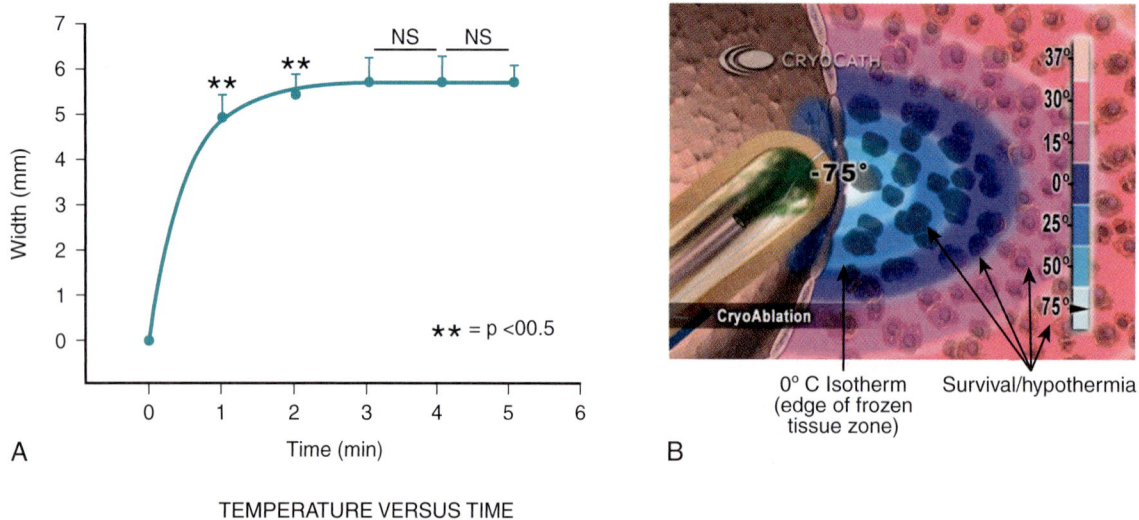

FIGURE 4-11. A, Plot of lesion width (mm) by time (min) of application demonstrating increase in lesion size during the first 3 minutes, with no substantial further increase thereafter. **, $P < .05$ versus previous time; NS, not significant. **B,** Schematic diagram demonstrating that, with freezing temperatures at the catheter tip, adjacent cardiac tissue is cooled, with ice ball formation and outward expansion in a concentric fashion. The longer the catheter is cooled, the larger the ice ball formation and the larger the lesion (until a plateau is reached). **C,** Schematic plot of cryothermal energy delivery demonstrating effect of temperature versus time. To create a permanent ablation lesion, the tissue adjacent to the catheter must reach a certain temperature, and this temperature must be applied for a given time. The colder the temperature, the shorter the duration of application required to achieve a permanent lesion. (*A, From Dubuc M, Roy D, Thibault B, et al. Transvenous catheter ice mapping and cryoablation of the atrioventricular node in dogs.* Pacing Clin Electrophysiol. *1999;22:1488–1498, 1999.* **B** *and* **C,** *Courtesy of Medtronic CryoCath LP, Montreal, Canada. With permission.*)

typically suffices to create permanent effects on conduction, double freeze-thaw cycles or multiple applications may be performed if desired or required.

The standard technique with the Arctic Front catheter consists of inserting a guidewire in a pulmonary vein, advancing the catheter over the wire to the desired location, inflating the balloon, assessing tissue contact by injecting contrast through the catheter's central lumen or demonstrating venous occlusion by intracardiac echo Doppler imaging, or both, and, in the absence of leaks, applying cryoablation for 4 minutes.

Clinical Advantages of Cryothermal Energy for Catheter Ablation

Theoretical advantages of cryothermal over RF ablation are summarized in Table 4-3,[3] and include reversibility, catheter stability, minimal risk for thromboembolism, safety near vascular structures, and decreased pain perception.

Reversible Effects

As previously discussed, one of the most exciting and truly remarkable characteristics of cryothermal energy is the ability to create reversible electrophysiologic effects before permanent tissue destruction by varying the temperature or time of application, or both (Fig. 4-12A-D). A functional effect may be obtained at sublethal temperatures, with complete recovery of all electrophysiologic properties and no histologically identifiable damage.[10,11] Not only is cryomapping theoretically possible, but also the broad temperature and time window between reversible and irreversible effects renders this feature readily clinically applicable. Thus, by identifying the desired substrate before definitive ablation, the appropriate catheter placement site may be confirmed to be efficacious (i.e., *efficacy* cryomapping) or safe (i.e., *safety* cryomapping), or both. Reversible cryomapping may be of particular importance when ablating arrhythmogenic substrates located near critical sites such as the AV node, where a missed target lesion may have major consequences. Reversibility observed with cryothermal energy contrasts starkly with RF energy.[53] With RF ablation, hyperthermal tissue injury leading to reversible loss of excitability occurs at a median tissue temperature of 48°C, whereas irreversible tissue destruction occurs at tissue temperatures greater than 50°C.[53,54] The RF "reversibility" window is, therefore, too narrow for safe clinical applications.

Catheter Stability

With hypothermia generated at the distal cooling electrode, the cryocatheter adheres to tissue affording greater catheter stability.[55] Metaphorically, this has been likened to a wet tongue sticking to a frozen pole. The operator may let go of the catheter once it has adhered onto the endocardial surface. Programmed electrical stimulation may be performed during cryoablation without concern for catheter dislodgment. Moreover, "brushing effects" that occur during beat-to-beat rocking

TABLE 4-3
POTENTIAL ADVANTAGES OF CRYOABLATION OVER RADIOFREQUENCY ABLATION

Advantages	Clinical Implications
Catheter adhesiveness	Greater catheter stability Programmed stimulation may be performed during ablation Avoidance of "brushing" effects
Homogeneous sharply demarcated lesion	Less arrhythmogenic More controllable titration of lesion size
Preservation of ultrastructural integrity	Decreased risk for thrombus formation Absence of aneurysmal dilation or rupture
Reversible suppression of conduction tissue	Prediction of successful site Avoidance of unwanted lesions Ablation of high-risk substrates
Lesion limited by warming blood flow	Safety to nearby epicardial coronary arteries
Visualization by ultrasound	Real-time monitoring Confirmation of endocardial contact Defining optimal freezing parameters
Pain-free ablation	Discomfort minimized under conscious sedation

heart motions and with respiratory variations are eliminated. This feature may be particularly advantageous if the arrhythmogenic substrate is located at a site where contact is difficult to maintain[10,11] or ablation of nearby tissue is deemed hazardous. It also permits ablation to be performed during tachycardia without the menace of catheter dislodgment on abrupt arrhythmia termination. In contrast, catheter stability may be an issue during RF ablation. The catheter must be held in place by the operator to ensure adequate delivery of power and subsequent tissue heating, which may prove difficult in the beating heart. Such effects may be magnified during tachycardia, on arrhythmia termination, and in patients with substantial valvular regurgitation. The lesser control and variable brushing effect may contribute to increasing the size, unpredictability, and imprecision of the lesion created.

Minimal Risk for Thromboembolism

To compare the propensity for RF and cryoenergy ablation to produce thrombus on the surface of the ablation lesion, we conducted a randomized preclinical study involving 197 ablation lesions in 22 dogs at right atrial, right ventricular, and left ventricular sites.[46] RF energy was more than five times more thrombogenic than cryoablation by histologic morphometric analyses 7 days after ablation. Moreover, thrombus volume was significantly greater with RF compared with cryoablation. Interestingly, the extent of hyperthermic tissue injury was positively correlated with thrombus bulk. This was unlike cryoenergy, in which lesion dimensions were not predictive of thrombus size. It was conjectured that this disparity likely reflected the fact that intact tissue

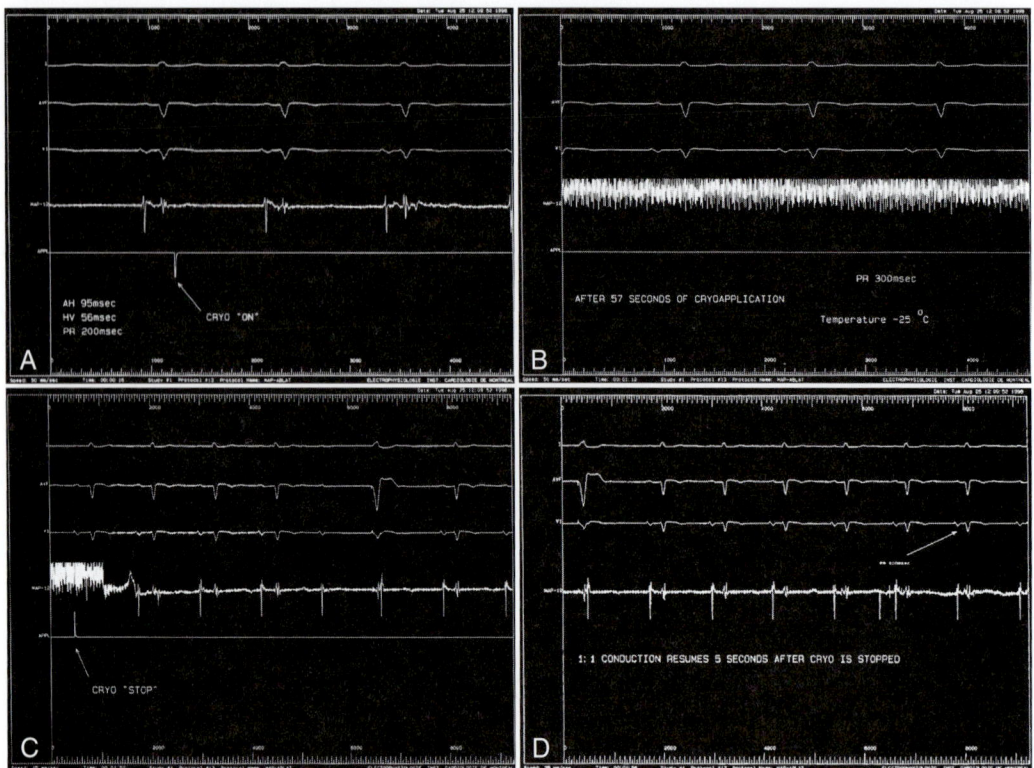

FIGURE 4-12. Electrograms demonstrating the reversible effect of cryomapping on the atrioventricular node. For all panels, I, AVF, and V1 are surface electrocardiographic (ECG) recordings; MAP 1–2 is the signal from the distal electrode pair of the cryocatheter; AH is the atrium-to-His activation time; HV is the His-to-ventricle activation time; and PR is the PR interval from the surface ECG. **A,** Normal baseline PR interval of 200 msec and AH interval of 95 msec before cryomapping application (paper speed = 50 mm/sec). **B,** After onset of cryomapping at a temperature of −25°C (evidenced by high-frequency signal on Map 1–2) for 57 seconds, the PR interval increased to 300 msec (paper speed = 50 mm/sec). **C,** At the end of the cryomapping application, a nonconducted atrial beat with a ventricular backup paced beat is shown. Upon rewarming, no further nonconducted atrial beats occurred (paper speed = 25 mm/sec). **D,** After 5 seconds of rewarming, normal 1:1 AV conduction resumed, and the PR interval returned to baseline (paper speed = 25 mm/sec). *(From Dubuc M, Khairy P, Rodriguez-Santiago A, et al. Catheter cryoablation of the atrioventricular node in patients with atrial fibrillation: a novel technology for ablation of cardiac arrhythmias.* J Cardiovasc Electrophysiol. *2001;12:439–444, 2001. With permission.)*

ultrastructure with endothelial cell preservation was maintained with cryoenergy. These results were later extended to larger-tip cryocatheters, further supporting the notion that the low risk for thrombosis is a feature of cryothermal energy, independent of lesion size.[47] Although the true incidence of thromboembolism associated with RF ablation is likely underreported, especially for right-sided interventions, clinically important thrombi have been reported to occur in 1.8% to 2.0% of procedures in systemic cardiac chambers.[56,57]

Minimal Risk to Vascular Structures

Concerns have been raised regarding RF ablation adjacent to or within the coronary sinus or pulmonary veins,[55] with damage to the vein, endoluminal thrombosis, fibrosis, and stenosis.[58] Perforation, tamponade, and coronary artery stenosis are potential complications. The circumflex or right coronary artery, or both, may course in close proximity to the arrhythmia substrate.[59–61] Moreover, the AV nodal artery passes near the mouth of the coronary sinus; ablation may conceivably damage this small vessel.[62] Preclinical studies suggest a lower incidence of coronary artery stenosis following cryoablation compared with RF ablation. In an experimental study in swine submitted to cryoablation within the mid and distal coronary sinus,

no angiographic coronary stenosis was observed, and coronary artery medial and intimal layers were preserved.[63] In a canine model, Aoyama and associates[64] demonstrated that cryoablation in the coronary sinus within 2 mm of the left circumflex artery produced transmural myocardial lesions similar to RF energy but with a lesser risk for coronary artery stenosis. Histologically, 50% of the animals randomized to RF energy had intimal coronary artery damage compared with none with cryoablation. There is also growing evidence that cryoablation in close proximity to pulmonary veins is associated with less risk for venous stenosis than RF energy.[65–67]

Painless

RF ablation may be painful to the patient under conscious sedation, particularly near thin-walled or venous structures, such as the inferior vena cava or the coronary sinus. Several studies have noted that pain perception, as assessed by standard Likert scales, is significantly less with cryoablation than RF ablation.[68]

Visualization by Ultrasound

In the 1990s, the ability to provide continuous real-time imaging of the freezing process was considered a major

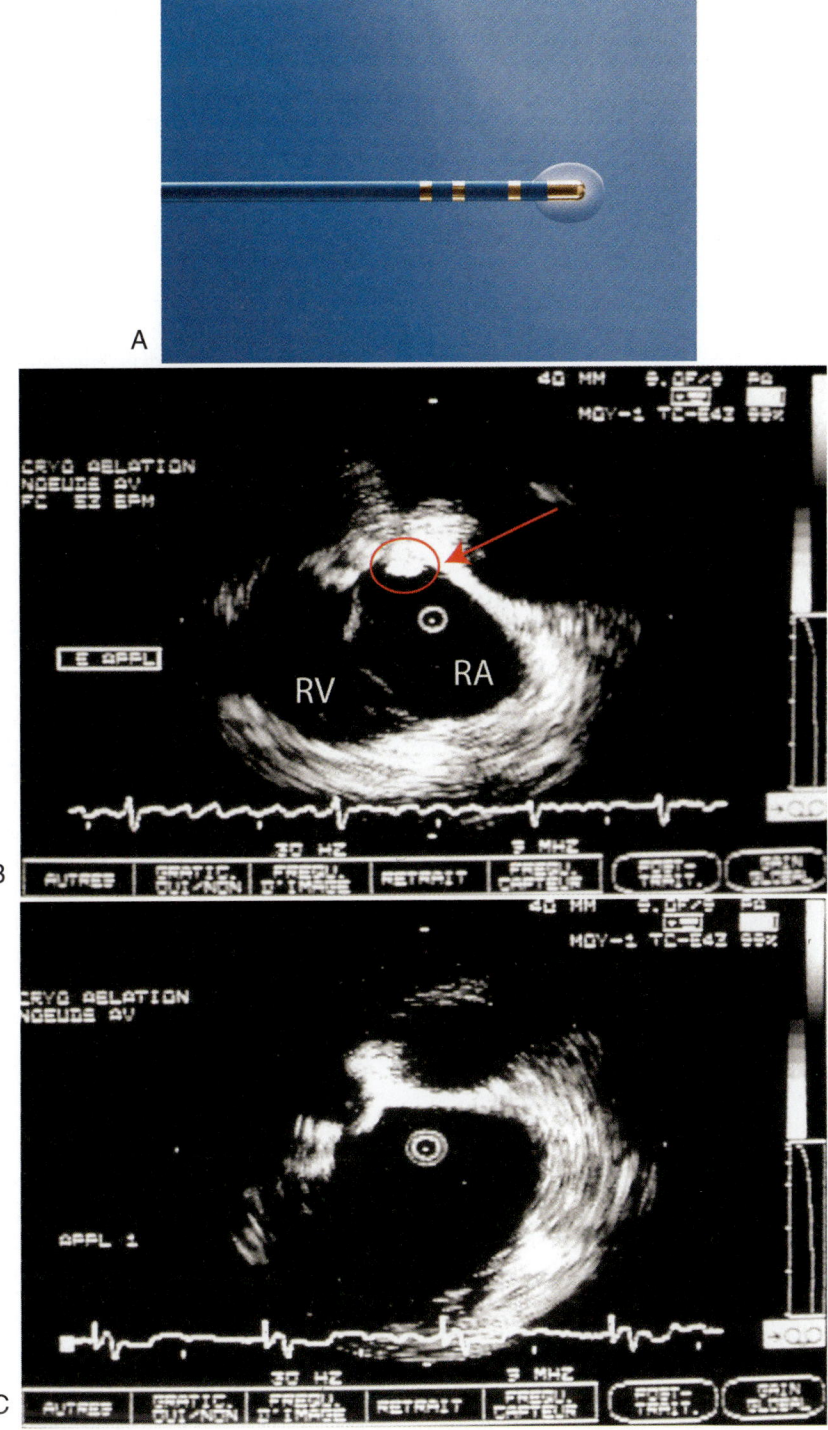

FIGURE 4-13. A, Ablation catheter adheres to adjacent cardiac tissue upon ice ball formation. **B,** The catheter situated in the right atrium (RA) is indicated by the arrow. RV denotes right ventricle. **C,** After application of cryoenergy, the presence of an ice ball is seen as a hypoechoic zone bordered by a hyperechoic rim with posterior shadowing. *(A, Courtesy of Medtronic CryoCath LP, Montreal, Canada. B and C, From Dubuc M, Khairy P, Rodriguez-Santiago A, et al. Catheter cryoablation of the atrioventricular node in patients with atrial fibrillation: a novel technology for ablation of cardiac arrhythmias. J Cardiovasc Electrophysiol. 12: 439–444, 2001. With permission.)*

technologic advancement that sparked renewed interest in visceral cryosurgery.[33] Indeed, ultrasonographic monitoring of the freeze-thaw cycle and frozen tissue volume contributed to rapid improvements in hepatic and prostatic surgery. The ability to visualize ice ball formation by ultrasonic means was likewise demonstrated in preclinical transcatheter cryoablation studies (Fig. 4-13A-C).[34] This feature of cryoablation has proved helpful in defining optimal freezing parameters.

Clinical Applications

Since its inception, transcatheter cryoablation technology has substantially improved. The refrigerant was modified to allow lower temperatures and faster freezing rates, larger electrode-tip sizes emerged, and innovative catheters of differing configurations were manufactured. Diverse clinical applications have since been explored as indications continue to be refined.[46,63,67,69–75]

Atrioventricular Nodal Ablation

Somewhat ironically, the first series of patients with transcatheter cryoablation had AV node ablation and pacemaker implantation as a rate-control strategy for atrial fibrillation.[11] Cryoablation is generally not advocated for this indication because of potentially lower long-term success rates. However, AV node ablation was deemed an appropriate substrate for initial safety and feasibility studies. Indeed, in the very first study with first-generation equipment (9F catheter; suboptimal handling characteristics; minimal achievable temperature of –55°C), AV node ablation was successful in 10 of 12 patients.[11]

Atrioventricular Nodal Reentrant Tachycardia

Atrioventricular nodal reentrant tachycardia (AVNRT) may be particularly well suited to cryomapping and cryoablation and is the arrhythmia substrate most extensively studied. Some centers, including our own, consider cryoablation first-line therapy for this indication.

In the first case series of 18 patients with cryoablation for AVNRT, cryomapping was demonstrated, 17 patients had successful ablation, and no recurrence was noted at 5 months of follow-up.[69] Important observations included the absence of an accelerated junctional rhythm during cryoablation, the ability to test for slow pathway conduction during the cryoapplication, and reversibility of AV block on rewarming. Other investigators subsequently confirmed these findings.[70,76,77] In a prospective multicenter cohort study (i.e., FROSTY), 103 patients with AVNRT had attempted cryoablation.[70] The acute procedural success rate was 91% using a 4-mm electrode-tip cryocatheter. At 6 months, arrhythmia-free survival in patients with acutely successful interventions was 94%. Although these figures appear somewhat lower than historically reported success rates with RF ablation, direct comparisons to RF were not made. Moreover, larger electrode-tip catheters (e.g., 6 mm) are more routinely employed today.

In a small pilot study directly comparing acute and long-term success with cryoablation versus RF ablation for AVNRT, no statistically significant difference in acute success was noted (97% versus 98%).[78] However, long-term success rates favored RF. A study of 63 patients randomized to RF or cryoablation for AVNRT also noted equivalent acute procedural success rates.[79] The median number of cryothermal applications was significantly lower than the number of RF applications (two versus seven). Fluoroscopy and procedural times were comparable. Long-term follow-up was later reported, suggesting no difference in outcomes.[80] It is important to note, however, that the lack of statistical significance is not synonymous with equivalency, which requires adequately powered studies.

We assessed whether recurrences could be predicted by the achieved procedural end point and found that persistent dual AV nodal physiology with or without echo beats was not associated with a higher recurrence rate than complete elimination of dual AV nodal physiology, if AVNRT remained noninducible on and off isoproterenol.[81] However,

the size of the electrode-tip catheter is an important determinant of arrhythmia-free survival. In a study of 289 patients with cryoablation using 4- or 6-mm electrode-tip catheters as a first-time procedure for AVNRT, a similar rate of acute procedural success was achieved.[82] However, recurrences were less common with 6-mm tips. Actuarial event-free survival rates at 1, 3, 6, and 12 months with 6-mm compared with 4-mm electrode-tip catheters were 97%, 93%, 92%, and 89% versus 90%, 87%, 84%, and 77%, respectively, with no recurrence thereafter. Indeed, ablation with a 4-mm-tip cryocatheter was associated with a 2.5-fold increased risk for recurrence.

Importantly, inadvertent permanent high-degree AV block has yet to be reported with cryoablation for AVNRT. Transient AV block occurs in up to 11% and typically resolves within seconds.[46,63,67,69–75,81] Some authors believe that the AV node is particularly resistant to cryothermal injury, offering an attractive safety margin for perinodal arrhythmia substrates.[83]

Septal and Parahisian Accessory Pathways

Most users of transcatheter cryoablation would probably agree that this technology permits them to tackle substrates that they would have otherwise refrained from ablating because of prohibitive risks. Mid-septal and parahisian pathways are classic examples.[70,76,77] For septal pathways, including parahisian locations, AV block with RF ablation has ranged from 12.5% to 20%.[84,85] In contrast, in a study that included 11 anteroseptal and 8 mid-septal accessory pathways undergoing cryoablation, transient AH (atrio-His) prolongation was noted in four of eight patients with mid-septal pathways and in none of the patients with anteroseptal pathways.[71] No permanent AV block occurred. Although the acute procedural success rate was 100%, 20% recurred at 15 months of follow-up. The series was later extended to include a total of 39 patients with perinodal accessory pathways, 15 mid-septal, and 24 parahisian.[86] An acute success rate of 95% was achieved. Other series have reported similar acute successes.[76,87] As for AVNRT, permanent inadvertent AV block has yet to be reported with ablation of perinodal pathways, although right bundle branch block has occurred on occasion.

Atrial Flutter

The treatment of cavotricuspid isthmus-dependent atrial flutter by RF ablation has been associated with high success rates and improvements in quality of life. Although reported success rates are in the range of 80% to 100%, cavotricuspid isthmus ablation with RF may be painful during lesion delivery and is rarely complicated by AV block or injury to the circumflex or right coronary artery. Several studies assessed cryoablation for atrial flutter and reported comparable success and recurrence rates, with lower pain perception.[68,77,88–90]

In an observational study of 95 patients with attempted cavotricuspid isthmus ablation using 9F 8-mm

(52 patients) or 7F 6-mm (43 patients) electrode-tip cryocatheters, a higher acute success rate was achieved with the larger catheters (100% versus 88%).[91] Despite comparable outcomes, modest advantages favored the larger-tip catheter with shorter fluoroscopy time and procedural duration and fewer applications. As an alternative technique, some investigators have advocated electrogram-guided "hot-spot" focal ablation.[92] The authors place an 8-mm electrode-tip cryocatheter at the isthmus, close to the mouth of the coronary sinus. The catheter is maneuvered laterally along the isthmus in search of electrograms with separated atrial and ventricular components and a local stimulus to onset time (70 milliseconds[93]). At these sites, cryoablation is performed at −75°C for 60 seconds. If conduction time across the cavotricuspid isthmus increases by 30 to 40 milliseconds, an 8-minute cryoapplication is delivered. Although this approach was acutely successful, by 3 months of follow-up 44% no longer had bidirectional block on repeat testing.[92]

Atrial Fibrillation

In general, there are two transcatheter cryoablation approaches to pulmonary vein isolation procedures for atrial fibrillation. The first technique, much like RF ablation, is point-by-point ablation to disconnect pulmonary veins or create linear lesions, or both. This has been shown to be feasible and safe, with successful pulmonary vein isolation in a high proportion of patients.[67,94] However, long procedural and fluoroscopy times render the procedure impractical. Concerns were also raised regarding nontransmurality of lesions, particularly for endocardial ablation of epicardial autonomic ganglia.[95]

The second approach use an expandable cryoablation balloon catheter, 18 to 28 mm in diameter, specifically designed for this purpose.[96,97] In a nonrandomized European study, 346 patients with paroxysmal or persistent atrial fibrillation had attempted pulmonary vein isolation with the cryoballoon.[96] Overall, 1360 of 1403 pulmonary veins were targeted with balloons or balloons in combination with point lesions. Cryoballoon ablation resulted in maintenance of sinus rhythm in 74% of patients with paroxysmal and 42% of patients with persistent atrial fibrillation. No pulmonary vein narrowing occurred. The most frequent complication was right phrenic nerve paralysis, particularly while ablating the right superior vein, with subsequent recovery.

Other investigators have recently expressed concern that drops in the luminal esophageal temperature may predispose to esophageal injury.[98] Postprocedural endoscopy showed esophageal ulcerations in 6 of 35 (17%) patients, with no atrial-esophageal fistulas. All ulcers had healed on follow-up endoscopy. The authors concluded that cryoballoon ablation can cause reversible esophageal ulcerations, particularly when targeting inferior pulmonary veins.

Currently, in North America, the Sustained Treatment of Paroxysmal Atrial Fibrillation (STOP AF) clinical trial is comparing cryoballoon ablation to antiarrhythmic therapy. The primary objective is to demonstrate equivalent safety to pharmacologic therapy, with superior efficacy. The study design includes a total of 243 patients recruited from 22 sites with 12 months of follow-up. Enrollment has been completed and follow-up is ongoing.

Ventricular Tachycardia

A few case series on cryoablation for ventricular tachycardia have been published.[99,100] Obel and colleagues reported three cases of left ventricular outflow tract tachycardia successfully ablated from the distal great cardiac vein.[101] In a larger series, cryoablation with an 8-mm-tip catheter was attempted in 14 patients with highly symptomatic frequent monomorphic ventricular premature beats or nonsustained ventricular tachycardia originating within the right ventricular outflow tract.[102] Cryoablation resulted in complete success in all but one patient. Three patients reported slight pain arising from local pressure of the catheter on the right ventricular outflow tract with no pain related to delivery of cryothermal energy. All patients with acutely successful procedures remained arrhythmia free at 3 months of follow-up.

Cryoablation in the Young

Due, in part, to smaller anatomic structures and distressing consequences of inadvertent AV block, cryoablation has emerged as an attractive treatment option for several arrhythmia substrates in children. Fortunately, persistent AV block has not been reported with cryoablation in the young. In children with AV nodal reentrant tachycardia, acute success rates are comparable to RF ablation. However, concerns persist over potentially higher recurrence rates.[103,104] Although these trends are not statistically significant and are influenced by learning curves, the concerns are valid, particularly with 4-mm-tip cryocatheters. Also, reported procedural times are longer with cryoenergy versus RF ablation (148 versus 112 minutes).[105]

Similar trends are noted with cryoablation of accessory pathways in children that are either close to the AV node or within the coronary venous system.[103,106] An acute success rate of 78% was noted in 35 young patients (mean age, 15.6 years).[106] Permanent PR prolongation occurred in one patient and right bundle branch block in another. At median follow-up of 207 days, recurrences were noted in 45%. Younger patient age and mid-septal pathways were associated with a higher likelihood of recurrence. Although acute success rates were comparable to RF ablation in a historical institutional control group, recurrences were significantly higher. The authors conjectured that safety benefits may nonetheless provide suitable compensation for higher recurrences.

Reports of other substrates in children successfully cryoablated include ectopic atrial trachycardia,[103] junctional ectopic tachycardia,[103,104] and permanent junctional reciprocating tachycardia.[105] In patients with congenital heart disease, particular indications may include presence of an intracardiac shunt to minimize thromboembolic risk[46] and anatomic displacement of the AV conduction system for cryomapping of the AV node or its inputs.[107]

References

1. Khairy P, Dubuc M. *Cryoablation for Cardiac Arrhythmias*. Montreal: Vision Communications; 2008.
2. Breasted JH. *The Edwin Smith Surgical Papyrus*. Chicago: University of Chicago Press; 1980.
3. Khairy P, Dubuc M. Transcatheter cryoablation. Part I: preclinical experience. *Pacing Clin Electrophysiol*. 2008;31:112–120.
4. Cooper IS. Cryogenic surgery: a new method of destruction or extirpation of benign or malignant tissues. *N Engl J Med*. 1963;268:743–749.
5. Hass GM. A quantitative hypothermal method for the production of local injury of tissue. *Arch Pathol*. 1948;45:563.
6. Taylor CB, Davis CB Jr, Vawter GF, Hass GM. Controlled myocardial injury produced by a hypothermal method. *Circulation*. 1951;3:239–253.
7. Lister JW, Hoffman BF, Kavaler F. Reversible cold block of the specialized cardiac tissues of the unanaesthetized dog. *Science*. 1964;145:723–725.
8. Harrison L, Gallagher JJ, Kasell J, et al. Cryosurgical ablation of the A-V node-His bundle: a new method for producing A-V block. *Circulation*. 1977;55:463–470.
9. Gillette PC, Swindle MM, Thompson RP, Case CL. Transvenous cryoablation of the bundle of His. *Pacing Clin Electrophysiol*. 1991;14:504–510.
10. Dubuc M, Talajic M, Roy D, et al. Feasibility of cardiac cryoablation using a transvenous steerable electrode catheter. *J Interv Card Electrophysiol*. 1998;2:285–292.
11. Dubuc M, Khairy P, Rodriguez-Santiago A, et al. Catheter cryoablation of the atrioventricular node in patients with atrial fibrillation: a novel technology for ablation of cardiac arrhythmias. *J Cardiovasc Electrophysiol*. 2001;12:439–444.
12. Bredikis J. Cryosurgical ablation of atrioventricular junction without extracorporeal circulation. *J Thorac Cardiovasc Surg*. 1985;90:61–67.
13. Bredikis JJ, Bredikis AJ. Surgery of tachyarrhythmia: intracardiac closed heart cryoablation. *Pacing Clin Electrophysiol*. 1990;13:1980–1984.
14. Louagie YA, Guiraudon GM, Klein GJ, Yee R. Closed heart cryoablation of the His bundle using an anterior septal approach. *Ann Thorac Surg*. 1991;51:616–619.
15. Gallagher JJ, Sealy WC, Anderson RW, et al. Cryosurgical ablation of accessory atrioventricular connections: a method for correction of the pre-excitation syndrome. *Circulation*. 1977;55:471–479.
16. Bredikis J, Bredikis A. Cryosurgical ablation of left parietal wall accessory atrioventricular connections through the coronary sinus without the use of extracorporeal circulation. *J Thorac Cardiovasc Surg*. 1985;90:199–205.
17. Gallagher JJ, Anderson RW, Kasell J, et al. Cryoablation of drug-resistant ventricular tachycardia in a patient with a variant of scleroderma. *Circulation*. 1978;57:190–197.
18. Ott DA, Garson A Jr, Cooley DA, et al. Cryoablative techniques in the treatment of cardiac tachyarrhythmias. *Ann Thorac Surg*. 1987;43:138–143.
19. Garratt C, Camm AJ. The role of cryosurgery in the management of cardiac arrhythmias. *Clin Cardiol*. 1991;14:153–159.
20. Krafchek J, Lawrie GM, Roberts R, et al. Surgical ablation of ventricular tachycardia: improved results with a map-directed regional approach. *Circulation*. 1986;73:1239–1247.
21. Page PL, Cardinal R, Shenasa M, et al. Surgical treatment of ventricular tachycardia: regional cryoablation guided by computerized epicardial and endocardial mapping. *Circulation*. 1989;80:I124–I134.
22. Ott DA, Garson A, Cooley DA, McNamara DG. Definitive operation for refractory cardiac tachyarrhythmias in children. *J Thorac Cardiovasc Surg*. 1985;90:681–689.
23. Guiraudon GM, Thakur RK, Klein GJ, et al. Encircling endocardial cryoablation for ventricular tachycardia after myocardial infarction: experience with 33 patients. *Am Heart J*. 1994;128:982–989.
24. Lustgarten DL, Keane D, Ruskin J. Cryothermal ablation: mechanism of tissue injury and current experience in the treatment of tachyarrhythmias. *Prog Cardiovasc Dis*. 1999;41:481–498.
25. Silka MJ, Kron J, Cutler JE, et al. Cryoablation of medically refractory nodoventricular tachycardia. *Pacing Clin Electrophysiol*. 1990;13:908–915.
26. Kerr CR, Klein GG, Guiraudon GM, Webb JG. Surgical therapy for sinoatrial reentrant tachycardia. *Pacing Clin Electrophysiol*. 1988;11:776–783.
27. Vermeulen FE, van Hemel NM, Guiraudon GM, et al. Cryosurgery for ventricular bigeminy using a transaortic closed ventricular approach. *Eur Heart J*. 1988;9:979–990.
28. Andress JD, Vander Salm TJ, Huang SK. Bidirectional bundle branch reentry tachycardia associated with Ebstein's anomaly: cured by extensive cryoablation of the right bundle branch. *Pacing Clin Electrophysiol*. 1991;14:1639–1647.
29. Assad RS, Aiello VD, Jatene MB, et al. Cryosurgical ablation of fetal atrioventricular node: new model to treat fetal malignant tachyarrhythmias. *Ann Thorac Surg*. 1995;60:S629–S632.
30. Nitta T, Ikeshita M, Asano T, et al. Perinodal cryomodification for supraventricular tachycardia. *Nippon Kyobu Geka Gakkai Zasshi*. 1995;43:344–349.
31. Szabo TS, Jones DL, Guiraudon GM, et al. Cryosurgical modification of the atrioventricular node: a closed heart approach in the dog. *J Am Coll Cardiol*. 1987;10:389–398.
32. Klein GJ, Guiraudon GM, Perkins DG, et al. Controlled cryothermal injury to the AV node: feasibility for AV nodal modification. *Pacing Clin Electrophysiol*. 1985;8:630–638.
33. Baust J, Gage AA, Ma H, Zhang CM. Minimally invasive cryosurgery: technological advances. *Cryobiology*. 1997;34:373–384.
34. Dubuc M, Roy D, Thibault B, et al. Transvenous catheter ice mapping and cryoablation of the atrioventricular node in dogs. *Pacing Clin Electrophysiol*. 1999;22:1488–1498.
35. Holman WL, Ikeshita M, Douglas JM Jr, et al. Cardiac cryosurgery: effects of myocardial temperature on cryolesion size. *Surgery*. 1983;93:268–272.
36. Peiffert B, Feldman L, Villemot JP, Verdier J. Cryosurgery in ventricular tachycardia: value of myocardial hypothermia in the extension of the depth of cryogenic lesions. *Chirurgie*. 1992;118:137–143.
37. Klein GJ, Harrison L, Ideker RF, et al. Reaction of the myocardium to cryosurgery: electrophysiology and arrhythmogenic potential. *Circulation*. 1979;59:364–372.
38. Budman H, Shitzer A, Dayan J. Analysis of the inverse problem of freezing and thawing of a binary solution during cryosurgical processes. *J Biomech Eng*. 1995;117:193–202.
39. Whittaker DK. Mechanisms of tissue destruction following cryosurgery. *Ann R Coll Surg Engl*. 1984;66:313–318.
40. Gill W, Fraser J, Carter DC. Repeated freeze-thaw cycles in cryosurgery. *Nature*. 1968;219:410–413.
41. Iida S, Misaki T, Iwa T. The histological effects of cryocoagulation on the myocardium and coronary arteries. *Jpn J Surg*. 1989;19:319–325.
42. Mikat EM, Hackel DB, Harrison L, et al. Reaction of the myocardium and coronary arteries to cryosurgery. *Lab Invest*. 1977;37:632–641.
43. Tsvetkov T, Tsonev L, Meranzov N, Minkov I. Functional changes in mitochondrial properties as a result of their membrane cryodestruction. II. Influence of freezing and thawing on ATP complex activity of intact liver mitochondria. *Cryobiology*. 1985;22:111–118.
44. Mazur P. Cryobiology: the freezing of biological systems. *Science*. 1970;168:939–949.
45. Markovitz LJ, Frame LH, Josephson ME, Hargrove WC 3rd. Cardiac cryolesions: factors affecting their size and a means of monitoring their formation. *Ann Thorac Surg*. 1988;46:531–535.
46. Khairy P, Chauvet P, Lehmann J, et al. Lower incidence of thrombus formation with cryoenergy versus radiofrequency catheter ablation. *Circulation*. 2003;107:2045–2050.
47. Khairy P, Rivard L, Guerra PG, et al. Morphometric ablation lesion characteristics comparing 4, 6, and 8 mm electrode-tip cryocatheters. *J Cardiovasc Electrophysiol*. 2008;19:1203–1207.
48. Guerra PG. Catheter cryoablation for the treatment of atrial fibrillation. In: Khairy P, Dubuc M, eds. *Cryoablation for Cardiac Arrhythmias*. Montreal: Vision Communications; 2008:83–92.
49. Wood MA, Parvez B, Ellenbogen AL, et al. Determinants of lesion sizes and tissue temperatures during catheter cryoablation. *Pacing Clin Electrophysiol*. 2007;30:644–654.
50. Tse HF, Ripley KL, Lee KL, et al. Effects of temporal application parameters on lesion dimensions during transvenous catheter cryoablation. *J Cardiovasc Electrophysiol*. 2005;16:201–204.
51. Parvez B, Pathak V, Schubert CM, Wood M. Comparison of lesion sizes produced by cryoablation and open irrigation radiofrequency ablation catheters. *J Cardiovasc Electrophysiol*. 2008;19:528–534.
52. Khairy P, Cartier C, Chauvet P, et al. A novel hybrid transcatheter ablation system that combines radiofrequency and cryoenergy. *J Cardiovasc Electrophysiol*. 2008;19:188–193.
53. Nath S, DiMarco JP, Haines DE. Basic aspects of radiofrequency catheter ablation. *J Cardiovasc Electrophysiol*. 1994;5:863–876.
54. Cote JM, Epstein MR, Triedman JK, et al. Low-temperature mapping predicts site of successful ablation while minimizing myocardial damage. *Circulation*. 1996;94:253–257.
55. Lemola K, Dubuc M, Khairy P. Transcatheter cryoablation part II: clinical utility. *Pacing Clin Electrophysiol*. 2008;31:235–244.
56. Hindricks G, The Multicentre European Radiofrequency Survey (MERFS) investigators of the Working Group on Arrhythmias of the European Society of Cardiology. The Multicentre European Radiofrequency Survey (MERFS): complications of radiofrequency catheter ablation of arrhythmias. *Eur Heart J*. 1993;14:1644–1653.
57. Zhou L, Keane D, Reed G, Ruskin J. Thromboembolic complications of cardiac radiofrequency catheter ablation: a review of the reported incidence, pathogenesis and current research directions. *J Cardiovasc Electrophysiol*. 1999;10:611–620.
58. Langberg J, Griffin JC, Herre JM, et al. Catheter ablation of accessory pathways using radiofrequency energy in the canine coronary sinus. *J Am Coll Cardiol*. 1989;13:491–496.
59. Lemola K, Mueller G, Desjardins B, et al. Topographic analysis of the coronary sinus and major cardiac veins by computed tomography. *Heart Rhythm*. 2005;2:694–699.
60. Becker AE. Left atrial isthmus: anatomic aspects relevant for linear catheter ablation procedures in humans. *J Cardiovasc Electrophysiol*. 2004;15:809–812.
61. Ho SY, Sanchez-Quintana D, Cabrera JA, Anderson RH. Anatomy of the left atrium: implications for radiofrequency ablation of atrial fibrillation. *J Cardiovasc Electrophysiol*. 1999;10:1525–1533.
62. Sanchez-Quintana D, Ho SY, Cabrera JA, et al. Topographic anatomy of the inferior pyramidal space: relevance to radiofrequency catheter ablation. *J Cardiovasc Electrophysiol*. 2001;12:210–217.
63. Skanes AC, Jones DL, Teefy P, et al. Safety and feasibility of cryothermal ablation within the mid- and distal coronary sinus. *J Cardiovasc Electrophysiol*. 2004;15:1319–1323.

64. Aoyama H, Nakagawa H, Pitha JV, et al. Comparison of cryothermia and radiofrequency current in safety and efficacy of catheter ablation within the canine coronary sinus close to the left circumflex coronary artery. *J Cardiovasc Electrophysiol.* 2005;16:1218–1226.

65. Saad EB, Rossillo A, Saad CP, et al. Pulmonary vein stenosis after radiofrequency ablation of atrial fibrillation: functional characterization, evolution, and influence of the ablation strategy. *Circulation.* 2003;108:3102–3107.

66. Wong T, Markides V, Peters NS, Davies DW. Percutaneous pulmonary vein cryoablation to treat atrial fibrillation. *J Interv Card Electrophysiol.* 2004;11:117–126.

67. Tse HF, Reek S, Timmermans C, et al. Pulmonary vein isolation using transvenous catheter cryoablation for treatment of atrial fibrillation without risk of pulmonary vein stenosis. *J Am Coll Cardiol.* 2003;42:752–758.

68. Timmermans C, Ayers GM, Crijns HJ, Rodriguez LM. Randomized study comparing radiofrequency ablation with cryoablation for the treatment of atrial flutter with emphasis on pain perception. *Circulation.* 2003;107:1250–1252.

69. Skanes AC, Dubuc M, Klein GJ, et al. Cryothermal ablation of the slow pathway for the elimination of atrioventricular nodal reentrant tachycardia. *Circulation.* 2000;102:2856–2860.

70. Friedman PL, Dubuc M, Green MS, et al. Catheter cryoablation of supraventricular tachycardia: results of the multicenter prospective "frosty" trial. *Heart Rhythm.* 2004;1:129–138.

71. Gaita F, Haissaguerre M, Giustetto C, et al. Safety and efficacy of cryoablation of accessory pathways adjacent to the normal conduction system. *J Cardiovasc Electrophysiol.* 2003;14:825–829.

72. Theuns DA, Kimman GP, Szili-Torok T, et al. Ice mapping during cryothermal ablation of accessory pathways in WPW: the role of the temperature time constant. *Europace.* 2004;6:116–122.

73. Wong T, Markides V, Peters NS, Davies DW. Clinical usefulness of cryomapping for ablation of tachycardias involving perinodal tissue. *J Interv Card Electrophysiol.* 2004;10:153–158.

74. Rodriguez LM, Leunissen J, Hoekstra A, et al. Transvenous cold mapping and cryoablation of the AV node in dogs: observations of chronic lesions and comparison to those obtained using radiofrequency ablation. *J Cardiovasc Electrophysiol.* 1998;9:1055–1061.

75. Gaita F, Paperini L, Riccardi R, Ferraro A. Cryothermic ablation within the coronary sinus of an epicardial posterolateral pathway. *J Cardiovasc Electrophysiol.* 2002;13:1160–1163.

76. Lowe MD, Meara M, Mason J, et al. Catheter cryoablation of supraventricular arrhythmias: a painless alternative to radiofrequency energy. *Pacing Clin Electrophysiol.* 2003;26:500–503.

77. Rodriguez LM, Geller JC, Tse HF, et al. Acute results of transvenous cryoablation of supraventricular tachycardia (atrial fibrillation, atrial flutter, Wolff-Parkinson-White syndrome, atrioventricular nodal reentry tachycardia). *J Cardiovasc Electrophysiol.* 2002;13:1082–1089.

78. Zrenner B, Dong J, Schreieck J, et al. Transvenous cryoablation versus radiofrequency ablation of the slow pathway for the treatment of atrioventricular nodal re-entrant tachycardia: a prospective randomized pilot study. *Eur Heart J.* 2004;25:2226–2231.

79. Kimman GP, Theuns DA, Szili-Torok T, et al. CRAVT: a prospective, randomized study comparing transvenous cryothermal and radiofrequency ablation in atrioventricular nodal re-entrant tachycardia. *Eur Heart J.* 2004;25:2232–2237.

80. Kimman GJ, Theuns DA, Janse PA, et al. One-year follow-up in a prospective, randomized study comparing radiofrequency and cryoablation of arrhythmias in Koch's triangle: clinical symptoms and event recording. *Europace.* 2006;8:592–595.

81. Khairy P, Novak PG, Guerra PG, et al. Cryothermal slow pathway modification for atrioventricular nodal reentrant tachycardia. *Europace.* 2007;9:909–914.

82. Rivard L, Dubuc M, Guerra PG, et al. Cryoablation outcomes for AV nodal reentrant tachycardia comparing 4-mm versus 6-mm electrode-tip catheters. *Heart Rhythm.* 2008;5:230–234.

83. Perez-Castellano N, Villacastin J, Moreno J, et al. High resistance of atrioventricular node to cryoablation: a great safety margin targeting perinodal arrhythmic substrates. *Heart Rhythm.* 2006;3:1189–1195.

84. Connors SP, Vora A, Green MS, Tang AS. Radiofrequency ablation of atrial tachycardia originating from the triangle of Koch. *Can J Cardiol.* 2000;16:39–43.

85. Yeh SJ, Wang CC, Wen MS, et al. Characteristics and radiofrequency ablation therapy of intermediate septal accessory pathway. *Am J Cardiol.* 1994;73:50–56.

86. Gaita F, Montefusco A, Riccardi R, et al. Acute and long-term outcome of transvenous cryothermal catheter ablation of supraventricular arrhythmias involving the perinodal region. *J Cardiovasc Med (Hagerstown).* 2006;7:785–792.

87. Atienza F, Arenal A, Torrecilla EG, et al. Acute and long-term outcome of transvenous cryoablation of midseptal and parahissian accessory pathways in patients at high risk of atrioventricular block during radiofrequency ablation. *Am J Cardiol.* 2004;93:1302–1305.

88. Collins NJ, Barlow M, Varghese P, Leitch J. Cryoablation versus radiofrequency ablation in the treatment of atrial flutter trial (CRAAFT). *J Interv Card Electrophysiol.* 2006;16:1–5.

89. Manusama R, Timmermans C, Limon F, et al. Catheter-based cryoablation permanently cures patients with common atrial flutter. *Circulation.* 2004;109:1636–1639.

90. Natale A, Newby KH, Pisano E, et al. Prospective randomized comparison of antiarrhythmic therapy versus first-line radiofrequency ablation in patients with atrial flutter. *J Am Coll Cardiol.* 2000;35:1898–1904.

91. Montenero AS, Bruno N, Antonelli A, et al. Comparison between a 7 French 6 mm tip cryothermal catheter and a 9 French 8 mm tip cryothermal catheter for cryoablation treatment of common atrial flutter. *J Interv Card Electrophysiol.* 2005;13:59–69.

92. Montenero AS, Bruno N, Antonelli A, et al. Low clinical recurrence and procedure benefits following treatment of common atrial flutter by electrogram-guided hot spot focal cryoablation. *J Interv Card Electrophysiol.* 2006;15:83–92.

93. Montenero AS, Bruno N, Zumbo F, et al. Cryothermal ablation treatment of atrial flutter: experience with a new 9 French 8 mm tip catheter. *J Interv Card Electrophysiol.* 2005;12:45–54.

94. Kettering K, Al-Ghobainy R, Wehrmann M, et al. Atrial linear lesions: feasibility using cryoablation. *Pacing Clin Electrophysiol.* 2006;29:283–289.

95. Gaita F, Riccardi R, Caponi D, et al. Linear cryoablation of the left atrium versus pulmonary vein cryoisolation in patients with permanent atrial fibrillation and valvular heart disease: correlation of electroanatomic mapping and long-term clinical results. *Circulation.* 2005;111:136–142.

96. Neumann T, Vogt J, Schumacher B, et al. Circumferential pulmonary vein isolation with the cryoballoon technique results from a prospective 3-center study. *J Am Coll Cardiol.* 2008;52:273–278.

97. Van Belle Y, Janse P, Theuns D, et al. One year follow-up after cryoballoon isolation of the pulmonary veins in patients with paroxysmal atrial fibrillation. *Europace.* 2008;10:1271–1276.

98. Ahmed H, Neuzil P, d'Avila A, et al. The esophageal effects of cryoenergy during cryoablation for atrial fibrillation. *Heart Rhythm.* 2009;6:962–969.

99. Reek S, Geller JC, Schildhaus HU, et al. Feasibility of catheter cryoablation in normal ventricular myocardium and healed myocardial infarction. *Pacing Clin Electrophysiol.* 2004;27:1530–1539.

100. Lustgarten DL, Bell S, Hardin N, et al. Safety and efficacy of epicardial cryoablation in a canine model. *Heart Rhythm.* 2005;2:82–90.

101. Obel OA, d'Avila A, Neuzil P, et al. Ablation of left ventricular epicardial outflow tract tachycardia from the distal great cardiac vein. *J Am Coll Cardiol.* 2006;48:1813–1817.

102. Kurzidim K, Schneider HJ, Kuniss M, et al. Cryocatheter ablation of right ventricular outflow tract tachycardia. *J Cardiovasc Electrophysiol.* 2005;16:366–369.

103. Papez AL, Al-Ahdab M, Dick M 2nd, Fischbach PS. Transcatheter cryotherapy for the treatment of supraventricular tachyarrhythmias in children: a single center experience. *J Interv Card Electrophysiol.* 2006;15:191–196.

104. Law IH, Von Bergen NH, Gingerich JC, et al. Transcatheter cryothermal ablation of junctional ectopic tachycardia in the normal heart. *Heart Rhythm.* 2006;3:903–907.

105. Gaita F, Montefusco A, Riccardi R, et al. Cryoenergy catheter ablation: a new technique for treatment of permanent junctional reciprocating tachycardia in children. *J Cardiovasc Electrophysiol.* 2004;15:263–268.

106. Bar-Cohen Y, Cecchin F, Alexander ME, et al. Cryoablation for accessory pathways located near normal conduction tissues or within the coronary venous system in children and young adults. *Heart Rhythm.* 2006;3:253–258.

107. Khairy P, Mercier LA, Dore A, Dubuc M. Partial atrioventricular canal defect with inverted atrioventricular nodal input into an inferiorly displaced atrioventricular node. *Heart Rhythm.* 2007;4:355–358.

5

Catheter Microwave, Laser, and Ultrasound: Biophysics and Applications

Shephal K. Doshi and David Keane

Key Points

Alternative energy sources have been explored to overcome the limitations in lesion size and need for tissue contact inherent to radiofrequency (RF) ablation. Microwave (MW), laser, and ultrasound (US) energies have been used in humans.

Problems with alternative energies have involved their incorporation into a catheter-based platform and titration of energy delivery. MW is particularly suited to penetrating scar tissue. Laser can create large, deep lesions by energy scatter within the tissue. US may be focused to create encircling lesions or focal lesions far from the transducer.

Since the initial descriptions of transcatheter ablation, optimal energy sources for creating myocardial lesions have been sought. Although direct current was initially used, radiofrequency (RF) energy has become the mainstay of transcatheter cardiac ablation.[1,2] RF has provided acceptable results for specific arrhythmias, with success rates in excess of 95% for the treatment of patients with atrioventricular nodal reentrant tachycardia (AVNRT), accessory pathway–mediated tachycardia, and atrioventricular (AV) junction ablation[2–4] with a relatively low complication rate (Fig. 5-1). However, as the targeted substrate for catheter ablation evolves from discrete focal ablation to linear ablation in tissue as thin as the posterior left atrial wall and as deep as the left ventricle, a need for more versatile and effective energy sources arises. This chapter reviews the mechanisms and data behind alternative energy sources for transcatheter ablation, including microwave (MW), laser, and ultrasound (US) energy.

As has been well described, thermal injury to myocardial tissue is a prerequisite for ablation by electromagnetic energy such as RF and MW. When RF voltage is applied, current is induced to flow between a pair of electrodes. RF tissue injury during catheter ablation is a result of resistive (ohmic) heating as electric currents (500 to 750 kHz) flow in radial paths from the ablation catheter electrode tip (high current density) into the tissue to a pad electrode applied to the body surface (low current density).[5,6] With RF, resistive heating decreases to the fourth power as the distance from the ablation electrode increases. Lesions are created beyond the electrode-tissue interface as a result of passive heat transfer. The point of maximal heating occurs below the surface in the subendocardium. Lesion volume is determined primarily by conductive heat transfer to adjacent tissue and convective heat loss. Tissue temperatures near 50°C are required to create irreversible injury.[7,8] Once temperatures approach 100°C, coagulum can form at the electrode tip. This desiccation and coagulation of tissue increases the resistance to the flow of current, which hinders tissue heating and limits lesion expansion.[8–10]

Attempts to reduce RF-mediated coagulum formation have focused on prevention of tissue overheating by reducing electrode temperature. RF electrode cooling has been achieved with internal irrigation and with saline infusion out of the electrode tip. Although this can create a larger lesion area by increasing the size and depth of injury, coagulation of tissue and desiccation can still occur.[11–16]

Microwave

Basic Principles

Like RF, MW injury is thermally mediated. In contrast to RF-mediated heating by electrical resistance, the mechanism of heating from a high-frequency MW energy source is dielectric.[17] Dielectric heating occurs when electromagnetic radiation stimulates oscillation of dipoles (e.g., water molecules) in the surrounding medium (Fig. 5-2). The electromagnetic energy is converted into kinetic energy (heat).[18] MW frequencies range from 30 to 3000 MHz.[19] These high-frequency electromagnetic waves can propagate in free space or in a conductive medium, through blood or desiccated tissue. Energy can be deposited directly into tissue at a distance regardless of the intervening medium, allowing for a greater amount of tissue being heated compared with that being heated directly by RF current.[20,21] It has been described that the propagation of MW in biologic tissue is regulated by tissue composition and dielectric permittivity, source frequency and power, and antenna radiation pattern and polarization.[17,22,23] With regard to biologic tissues of interest such as blood, muscle, and tissues with low water content (i.e., fat, bone, and desiccated tissue), there are differences in conductivity and dielectric constants as a function of frequency. These differences can be significant among the three types of tissues. As the MW field propagates in the tissue medium, energy is extracted

from the field and absorbed by the medium (converted to heat). This absorption results in a progressive reduction of MW power intensity as the field advances into the tissue.

Because of these differences in dielectric permittivity, tissues with low water content have a depth of penetration four times greater than that of tissues with high water content (e.g., muscle). Lin[22] quantified this reduction of MW power by the depth of penetration at 2450 MHz: 17, 19, and 79 mm for blood, muscle, and fat, respectively. In this way, an MW field can propagate through low-water (desiccated or fat) tissue to deliver energy to deeper tissue. The conductivities for blood and muscle are similar yet almost 300% lower than that of tissue with a low water content.[24] The basic properties of MW that render it favorable for ablation include the following[25]: (1) MW antennas radiate electromagnetic waves into the surrounding cardiac tissue; (2) power deposition follows a second-power law with distance, thereby heating tissue at a greater distance compared with RF; and (3) a dispersive electrode on the skin is not required. MW is contact forgiving; thus, for a linear antenna, direct contact with the endocardium throughout the length of the antenna may not be essential to obtain a transmural continuous lesion (Fig 5-3).

Microwave System Design

The first reported use of MW energy for ablation of cardiac arrhythmias in an experimental animal model was by Beckman and coworkers.[26] This report described the application of MW power using a probe applied directly to the His bundle during cardiopulmonary bypass. Langberg and colleagues[27] first described percutaneous catheter ablation of the AV junction using MW. Multiple reports have described variations in MW antenna design since these landmark studies, but the basic conceptual system design is consistent.

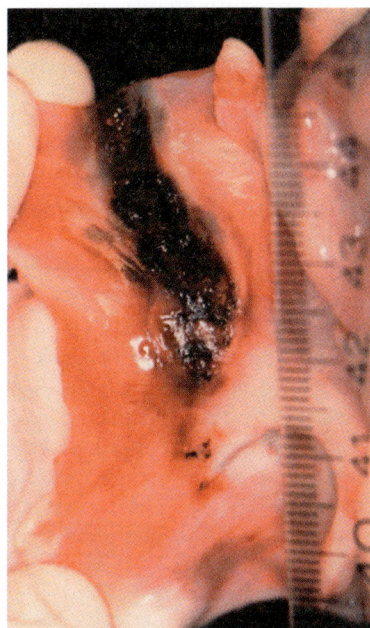

FIGURE 5-1. Gross pathology specimen of the posterior wall of a caprine right atrium. A radiofrequency (RF) 4-mm electrode catheter was deployed in vivo under electroanatomic guidance to create a linear lesion from the superior vena cava to the inferior cava. The resultant lesion demonstrates some of the limitations of conventional RF ablation, including extensive charring, as well as lack of lesion continuity at its inferior extension. For these reasons, the development of linear ablation approaches to the treatment of atrial fibrillation and ventricular tachycardia has stimulated interest in alternative energy sources for ablation.

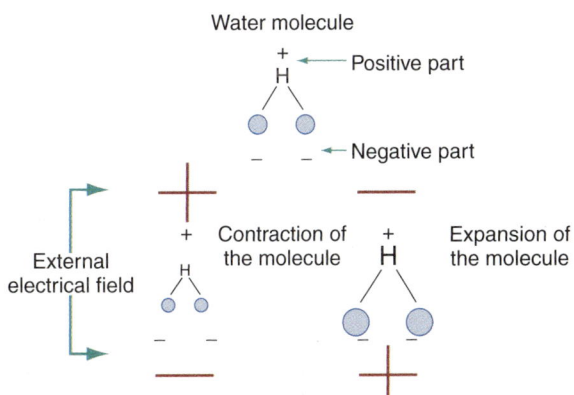

FIGURE 5-2. Microwave results in heating by causing contraction of expansion and rotation of dipole molecules such as water. The resulting physical motion causes thermal energy.

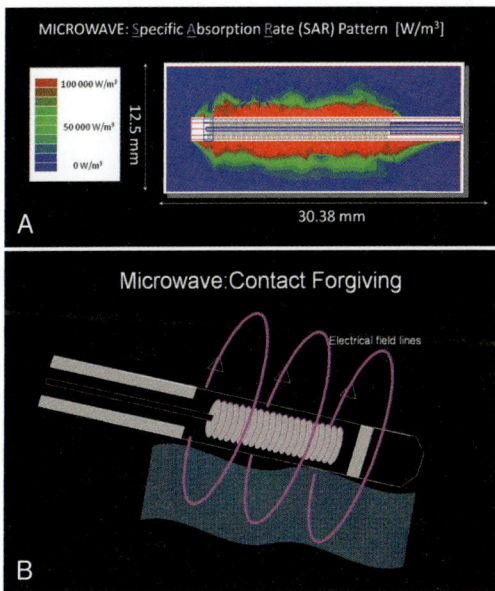

FIGURE 5-3. A, Microwave Specific Absorption Rate (SAR) pattern with a consistent pattern of absorption along antenna without edge effect. **B,** Microwave electrical fields permit contact forgiveness for lesion formation.

The MW system comprises four primary components: a MW power source, a switch assembly, power monitors, and control circuits.[24] The energy from the power source is transmitted through a coaxial cable to an antenna. MW catheter design is vital for efficient coupling of energy to the tissue. The impedance of the transmission line needs to be matched to the properties of the antenna, to prevent MW energy from being reflected back to its source, thereby minimizing heating of the catheter body (composed of a coaxial cable).[7] The vital element that determines the efficacy of the MW system is the antenna design. To characterize the MW antenna and its emission properties, the radiation efficiency, radiative field pattern, and power reflection coefficient are studied. The radiative field pattern—the change in temperature from instantaneous heating due to radiation from the MW field emitted from the antenna—is represented by the specific absorption rate (SAR) pattern.[28] The power reflection coefficient represents the amount of return loss of the forward power at a given frequency. This return loss (return of MW current up the transmission cable) should be at a minimum and has been reported to be 1% to 4% with certain antenna designs.[29,30] Multiple studies describing properties of various antenna designs have been published.[9,28,31–45]

To date, no one particular antenna design has been universally accepted. Most studies have used MW frequencies of 915 and 2450 MHz. The availability of MW frequencies for noncommunication medical applications is restricted by the U.S. Federal Communications Commission (FCC), which has limited exploration of other frequencies.[46] Because antenna dimensions are based on one-quarter wavelength, 2450 MHz allows use of a significantly smaller antenna, which is more favorable for percutaneous catheter-based systems.[7] In theory, lower frequencies are associated with deeper lesions and decreased cable heating; however, antenna characteristics are highly dependent on MW frequency.[47] The antenna requires a specific design for the selected MW frequency.[46] Large lesions have been reported with both frequencies.[35,37,48,49]

Data from in Vivo Experiments
Thigh Muscle Preparation
Because of the limited data regarding the optimal parameters for transcatheter delivery of microwave inside a vascular environment with blood flow (compared with conventional RF), Tse and associates[50] investigated the effect of the catheter-tip temperature, the duration of application, and the length of antenna on the lesion size, while holding contact pressure and local conditions constant, during transcatheter MW ablation in a swine thigh muscle preparation. The lesion size of MW ablation was compared with those of conventional RF ablation in the same experimental preparation. This study demonstrated that lesion size with transcatheter MW ablation can be controlled by adjusting targeted temperature, energy application duration, and antenna length. Lesion depth and width, but not length, were significantly increased by prolonging energy application duration from 120 to 240 seconds at a targeted temperature of 80°C. Compared with RF, microwave lesions were significantly longer but had comparable depth and width. A 20-mm microwave antenna produced longer

lesions than either a 10-mm antenna or RF ablation catheter. A targeted temperature of 80°C for more than 150 seconds provided optimal lesion dimensions and lower risk for surface desiccation or charring, which were significantly higher at targeted temperatures of 90°C.

Atrioventricular Nodal Ablation
MW ablation of the AV node has been studied in open-chest and closed-chest canine models using 2450 MHz of frequency and many different MW catheter designs.[27,35,37,38,51] These studies reliably resulted in discrete lesions without evidence of distant damage. Irreversible AV block strongly correlated with temperature rises greater than 55°C.[51] Yang and associates[35] demonstrated that the depth of the ablation lesions increases markedly with increasing power and duration of delivered energy, even beyond 100-second applications. Microscopically, the ablations produced hemorrhagic changes with coagulative necrosis and clearly demarcated borders.[37] There was no evidence of coagulum formation or charring at the catheter tip or antenna.[38]

Ablation of Ventricular Myocardium
Because lesion formation in ventricular myocardium, especially in the presence of scar, limits standard RF ablation, studies using MW have been performed to assess the efficacy of ablation in the ventricular myocardium.[35,49,53,54] These studies showed the feasibility of creating large lesions in the ventricular myocardium (Fig. 5-4). A dry epicardial study has shown that the acute, histologic lesions of microwave and radiofrequency energy appeared similar; however, the chronic lesions of microwave were deeper and wider than those created by RF.[52] MW ablation was found to lead to lesion volume expansion through 180 seconds.[35] Using a 4-mm split-tip antenna and 2450 MHz of MW energy, Huang and colleagues[53] performed closed-chest ablation in

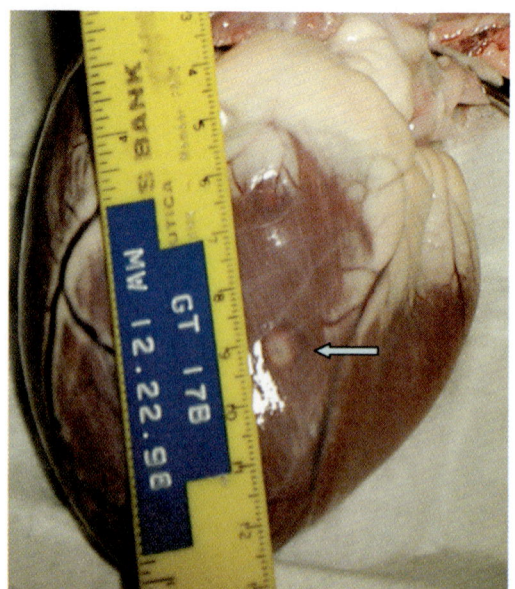

FIGURE 5-4. Microwave ablation. Caprine heart after percutaneous transvascular endocardial microwave ablation in vivo from an end-firing monopole antenna. The lesion (*arrow*) can be seen to be transmural, with a sharply defined circumferential appearance on the epicardial surface of the left ventricle.

mongrel dogs. Each animal received a single pulsed ablation of 30 W for 30 seconds. A total of 40 left ventricular and 18 right ventricular lesions were created. Mean lesion sizes were 10.4 × 9.1 × 7.0 mm (length × width × depth) or 379.0 mm^3 (volume) in the left ventricle and 10.4 × 8.4 × 5.2 mm or 249.3 mm^3 in the right ventricle. The lesions were discrete and hemielliptical or hemispherical in nature, consisting of a central crater with a thin layer of thrombus, along with a pale necrotic and hemorrhagic peripheral zone. These studies showed that MW energy should be efficacious even when ventricular tachycardia (VT) circuits involve the subepicardium. In vivo studies on goat models confirmed that the monopole antenna can produce a deep transmural lesion in the left ventricle without causing coagulation or charring on the endocardial surface.[55]

Ablation of the Cavotricuspid Isthmus

The efficacy of RF ablation of right atrial cavotricuspid isthmus-dependent flutter has been well documented.[56–58] Contiguous lesion formation with RF can be difficult because of variable contact and three dimensionally complex anatomy making contiguous ablation lines difficult. The complexity posed by the ridges and valleys of pectinate muscles and the eustachian ridge may favor the use of MW. A study based on MW energy field measurements was conducted to assess the feasibility of MW ablation without tissue contact at various catheter orientations.[59] Sixty-nine total lesions were created in vitro in bovine hearts with the MW antenna positioned parallel at 0, 1, 2, and 5 mm above the endocardium or perpendicular at 0 mm. Dimensions of lesions created at 0 and 1 mm were significantly greater than those made 2 and 5 mm above the endocardium. The authors concluded that MW lesions were feasible without tissue contact and at different orientations. MW ablation may provide utility, especially at sites where there is suboptimal tissue contact. Iwasa and colleagues[60] assessed the ability of a linear MW antenna capable of forming lesions up to 4 cm in length to ablate the isthmus from the inferior vena cava to the tricuspid annulus. A steerable 9-French (9F) catheter with a 4-cm MW antenna and a 900- to 930-MHz generator were used. Linear MW ablation of the tricuspid valve–inferior vena cava isthmus was successful in producing transmural isthmus ablation with bidirectional block as a treatment for atrial flutter in all 10 dogs studied. Few energy applications were required. The total ablation time ranged from 2 to 10 minutes, and no complications were reported in any of the animals. There was no evidence of charring, coagulum formation, or disruption of the atrial endocardium. Other authors have also concluded that single-application ablation can achieve isthmus block using MW energy delivered through an appropriately sized antenna.[61] Adragao and associates[62] published the first case of MW ablation of arrhythmia (atrial flutter) in humans. An 8F steerable MW ablation catheter with temperature sensing was used, and the flutter was terminated 50 seconds into the first application. The total application time was 60 seconds and resulted in bidirectional transisthmus conduction block. No coagulum was noted on the ablation catheter tip. No early or late complications occurred. The patient was reported to remain in sinus rhythm 3 months later. Other reports have since shown initial feasibility with right atrium–inferior vena cava isthmus ablation in human atrial flutter.[63,64] A total of eight patients have been reported using a steerable catheter with a distal 20-mm helical coil antenna and a generator delivering MW energy at 900 to 930 MHz. Each lesion was applied for 120 seconds at 21 W. Acute bidirectional cavotricuspid isthmus conduction block was demonstrated. The mean number of MW energy applications was 29 ± 14. One patient had documentation of atrial flutter 1 month after ablation. No complications were reported.

The principal advantages of MW ablation for percutaneous endocardial application include (1) contact forgiveness, (2) depth of penetration and lesion formation, and (3) avoidance of excessive endocardial temperatures to achieve adequate tissue temperature in deeper layers of the subepicardium. In addition to the percutaneous endocardial applications already described, MW energy has been used during the surgical maze procedure both on-pump in the arrested heart and off-pump in minimally invasive epicardial approaches.[65,66] The ability of MW energy to penetrate through epicardial fat and be absorbed by the atrial myocardium provides another distinct advantage for this latter application.

Laser

Basic Principles

Laser (**l**ight **a**mplification by **s**timulated **e**mission of **r**adiation) provides an additional energy source with which tissue ablation can be created. The generation of laser energy involves the basic principles of emission and absorption of electromagnetic radiation that occur when energy states are altered in atoms and molecules.[67] As described by Saksena and Gadhoke,[68] if a large number of identical atoms (or molecules) in a medium undergo a particular change in energy state at the same time, electromagnetic radiation with similar wavelengths, synchronized in time and space, will be emitted. Therefore, laser radiation is of a narrow frequency range (monochromatic), in phase (coherent), and in parallel (collimated). The ability of laser light to be highly focused permits a high power density to be administered to the target tissue. Laser systems have variable designs but generally consist of a lasing medium of solid, liquid, or gas contained in a chamber of reflecting surfaces. Typically, electricity is used to raise the energy state of the lasing medium, thereby causing a release of photons as the energy level of the medium falls back down to the baseline state. The difference between the two energy states determines the wavelength of the photon. These photons represent laser energy.[69] Numerous materials are used for laser action. Gaseous mediums used for excimer, and argon lasers emit light of wavelengths from 300 to 700 nm in the ultraviolet and visible light bands, respectively. Diode lasers involve the use of semiconductors and emit wavelengths between 700 and 1500 nm (near infrared). Solid lasers include neodymium-doped yttrium-aluminum-garnet (Nd-YAG) and holmium, which emit energy in the infrared spectrum of 1064 to 2000 nm.[47,70,71] Laser energy can be delivered in either a continuous or a pulsed mode. Laser energy is thermal in nature, and its effect is a function of laser power density on tissue. During tissue irradiation, light is scattered and absorbed to an extent that depends on beam diameter and the optical properties of the tissue. The laser energy is selectively absorbed by the tissues over a depth of several millimeters and produces heating of a volume of tissue.[72] Tissue heating produces focal myocardial tissue ablation through vaporization and coagulation necrosis. Myocardial tissue coagulation is produced by contraction and dehydration as light energy is absorbed. The volume of coagulated tissue can vary depending on laser energy absorption (transfer ratio) in the irradiated tissue.[73] Tissue temperatures in excess of 100°C typically cause tissue vaporization, whereas those in the range of 42° to 65°C can cause tissue damage from protein denaturation.[74,75] The laser beam power decreases within the tissue in an exponential manner. The rate of decay is multifactorial and involves laser beam absorption, scatter, and distance from the laser source.[19] Tissue injury may progress past the target site if the laser exposure time surpasses the thermal relaxation time of the target tissue. The distribution of spread follows a gaussian relationship and is expected to be focal.[76] In a study by Saksena and coworkers,[77] argon laser ablation in normal human ventricle was associated with an increase in mean lesion size and depth with increasing mean laser discharge energy dose, with tissue perforation at doses greater than 300 J. The diseased human ventricle had a higher safety margin with respect to perforation. Ultimately, lesion dimensions were determined by the total energy dose, medium used, and tissue characteristics. Isner and associates[78] demonstrated successful ablation of cardiovascular tissues with both infrared and ultraviolet laser radiation.

Argon Laser

Early work on argon laser radiation produced successful catheter ablation of the specialized AV conduction system in canines using fiberoptics.[79,80] The gross lesions were reported as circular, well-circumscribed areas of thermal injury at the site of discharge. Because the initial use of continuous argon laser discharges was associated with fiberoptic-tip damage, the efficacy of pulsed laser ablation was compared with that of continuous laser discharge in the diseased human ventricle.[81] Histologic examination showed crater formation due to tissue vaporization, with the crater lining consisting of charred tissue and a zone of coagulation necrosis. Lesion depth and diameter were comparable in the two approaches.

Evidence has accrued that the mechanical strength of tissue greatly influences the rate of ablation by pulsed lasers. A pulsed or high-energy continuous wave laser rapidly deposits energy and causes rapid heating of tissue. Because there may not be enough time for expansion of the heated water, there may be a significant pressure increase followed by an explosive abolition of tissue.[82] Argon lasers have been used intraoperatively in clinical settings for patients with refractory sustained VT and for atrial and accessory bypass tract ablation.[83,84]

Nd-YAG Laser

Initial studies involving the interaction of laser energy with the beating heart in vivo using an Nd-YAG laser created controlled endocardial lesions of 7.9 × 5.4 × 6.6 mm at 40 J.[85] The gross morphologic lesions consisted of a central vaporized crater surrounded by a rim of necrotic tissue. Lesion size increased as a function of total energy delivered. The duration of lasing was a more important determinant of lesion size than the absolute amount of energy delivered. This suggests that short but repetitive laser bursts could create shallow lesions with wider surface area, potentially decreasing the risk for cardiac perforation. Observations have also been made suggesting that, for Nd-YAG and argon lasers, blood enhances laser-induced tissue injury better than saline.[74] Ohtake and associates[73] confirmed that Nd-YAG laser energy was absorbed by blood due to hemoglobin absorption of light, causing more energy to be transferred into the myocardium.

When the Nd-YAG laser is compared with the argon laser, several differences are appreciated. The Nd-YAG laser has much greater forward scatter of energy than absorption at the surface.[73] This scattering effect of the beam on tissue causes coagulation to occur below rather than at the surface.[81] Continuous, percutaneous Nd-YAG laser coagulation was performed by Weber and colleagues[86,87] in the ventricular and atrial myocardium of canines, producing lesions as large as 7 mm in diameter and 11 mm in depth at 50 J in the ventricle and 5 mm in diameter in the atrium. Focal injuries of homogeneous coagulation or fibrosis were seen to be localized to the target area without vaporizing of tissue or crater formation in the ventricle. Chronic atrial lesions revealed sharply defined, oval-shaped areas of transmural fibrosis.

Initial clinical evaluation of epicardial laser use in patients without left ventriculotomy was performed by Pfeiffer and colleagues.[88] Nine patients with a history of myocardial infarction and monomorphic VT received epicardial laser ablation. The regions of interest where epicardial potentials during VT showed distinct mid-diastolic potentials received epicardial photocoagulation (50 to 80 W) with a continuous-wave Nd-YAG laser using a handheld probe. Seven patients remained free of clinical VT for a mean follow-up of 17 ± 11 months. This study elucidated the utility of deep tissue coagulation using the Nd-YAG laser with epicardial application for postinfarction VT caused by mid-myocardial or subepicardial reentrant circuits.

Clinical endocardial laser ablation, as described by Weber and coworkers,[89] involved 10 patients with common AVNRT. Using preshaped guiding catheters and a novel pin-electrode laser catheter, they applied Nd-YAG laser energy (one to five applications per patient) at 20 or 30 W for 10 to 45 seconds in the posteroinferior aspect of the tricuspid annulus. The tachycardia was rendered noninducible after ablation.

Diode Laser

A large hindrance to acceptance of laser technology has been concern about its size, expense, and complexity. Development of the diode laser, with size and costs analogous to those of an RF generator, has reduced these concerns. Ware and coworkers[90] used an intramyocardial diode laser operating at 805 nm and low power (2.0 to 4.5 W) in canines to create large, deep, well-circumscribed lesions up to 10 mm in width and depth without disrupting the endocardium or epicardium.

A slow rate of volumetric heating, provided by scattered photons, can enable the creation of deep, large-volume lesions by laser energy. This less intense but strictly intramural heating can permit maximal heat conduction that avoids the endocardium and epicardium.[91] The development of diode laser technology has also created the ability to customize wavelengths for optimal laser ablation because the optical properties of differing myocardial pathologies vary. An extensive study by d'Avila and associates[92] revealed experimental evidence of the efficacy of near-infrared endocardial and epicardial laser applications for catheter ablation of VT complicating Chagas' disease.

Applications for Linear Lesions

Interest in contiguous linear ablation lesions, particularly for arrhythmias such as atrial fibrillation (AF), has prompted the study of radial diffusing optical fibers that enable the laser energy to be distributed along the length of the active element. These optical fibers, with a gradient of titanium dioxide particles embedded in the flexible fiber tip, produce scattered radiation with near-uniform 360-degree radial delivery (Fig. 5-5), creating linear thermal lesions.[47] Fried and colleagues[93] demonstrated linear laser ablation using an Nd-YAG laser source in right ventricular myocardium without evidence of tissue charring and vaporization. Linear laser applications with a diode laser in the trabeculated anterior right atrial wall in a goat model produced transmural conduction block.[94] Use of optical fibers to deliver laser energy also provides a conduit

for light transmission and reflectance to provide real-time monitoring of lesion formation (Fig. 5-6A and B). It can also be used to provide endoscopic visualization for direct visual feedback, particularly when a balloon is used.

Laser Balloon Catheter Design

The efficacy of laser energy to create thermocoagulation is influenced by the irradiation angle, the distance between the laser tip and the target tissue, and the properties of the medium.[95] To this end, various catheter designs have been used for laser ablation.[89,90,95,96] The interest in transcatheter ablation of AF by pulmonary vein (PV) isolation and the inherent limitations of RF energy encouraged the design of a laser balloon system capable of projecting forward a circumferential ring of laser energy.[47,97–99] The balloon design has a collapsible profile and is filled with a 3-mL mixture of radiographic contrast agent and deuterium oxide (D_2O). D_2O is intended to eliminate self-heating of the balloon by shifting the absorption of wavelengths to greater than the 980 nm used. The light is transferred from the fiberoptic core with the use of a modified glass fiber tip, through an optically transparent shaft in the balloon, and projected as a ring onto the distal balloon surface (Fig. 5-7). The intensity of the emitted light delivered to the tissue around the ring is uniform and continuous without gaps.[47,98,99]

Laser energy is applied under endoscopic guidance in regions where balloon contact with tissue creates a bloodless environment, thereby preventing thrombus formation. This real-time visualization is achieved using a 500-μm

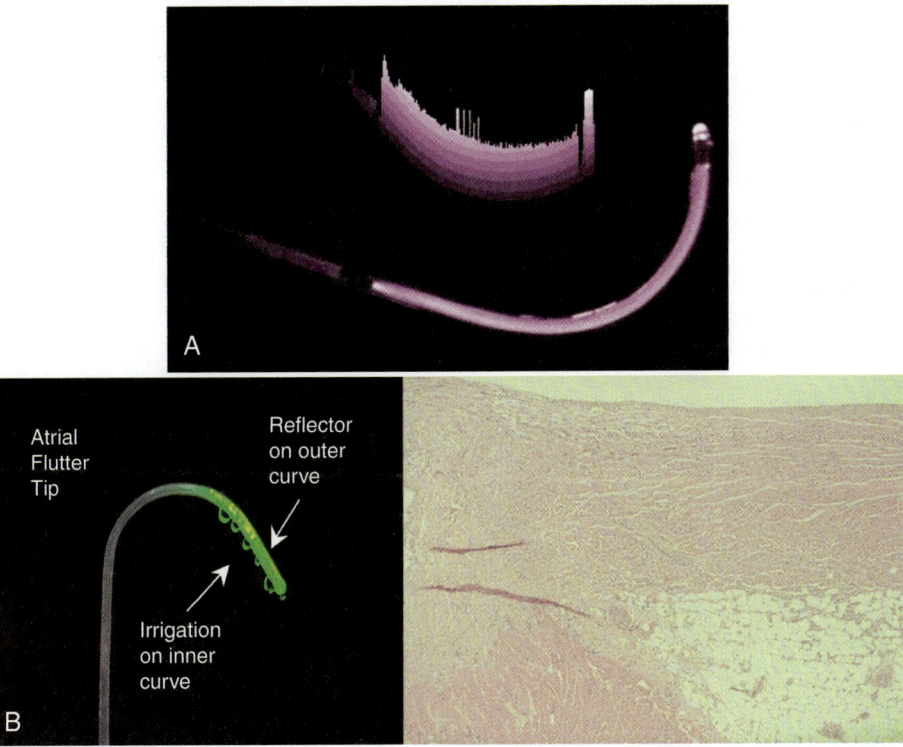

FIGURE 5-5. A, In vitro analysis of energy distribution of a curvilinear optical light diffuser used for linear lasing in the atrium. Despite the curvature, the uniformity of energy distribution is clear. **B,** Irrigated linear optical diffuser with gold reflector on the outer curve *(left)*. The curvilinear catheter was applied in vivo in the goat atrium and was shown on histology to produce transmural lesions across the isthmus from the inferior vena cava to the tricuspid annulus *(right)*.

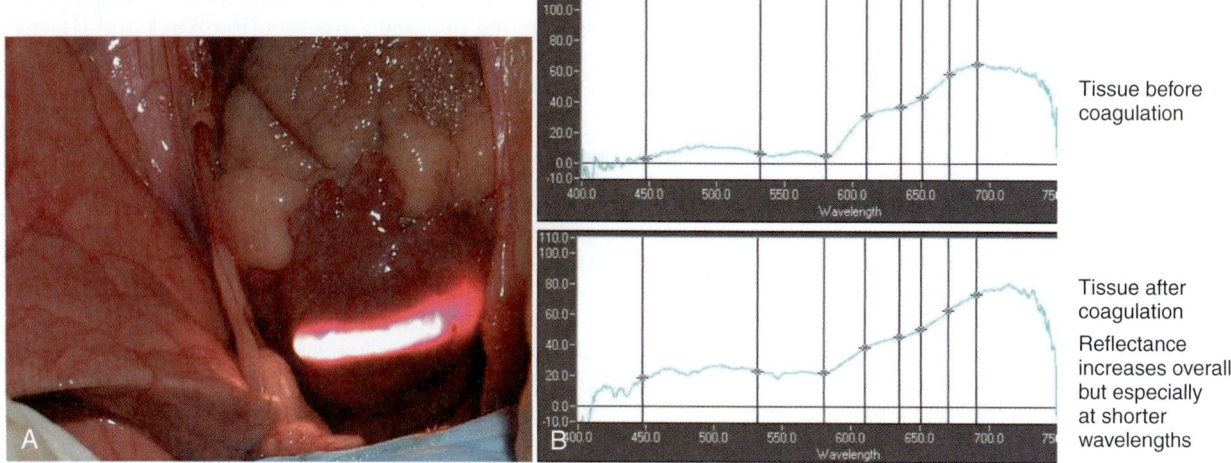

FIGURE 5-6. A, Epicardial appearance during endocardial light emission from a linear optical fiber (diffuser) before laser ablation. The reflected light is transmitted back through a second optical fiber and used for reflectance spectroscopy. The linear optical diffuser catheter has been introduced through the right femoral vein of a goat and is seen through an open thoracotomy to be in place for linear ablation of the right atrial free wall. **B,** Reflectance spectroscopy provides a potential means of monitoring lesion progression during ablation. The spectral display of light reflected back through an optical fiber during ablation of caprine atrium is shown. The ratio of green (shorter) to red (longer) wavelengths can provide a metric of lesion formation. If excessive ablation occurs, carbonization of the endocardium results in a reduction of reflected light.

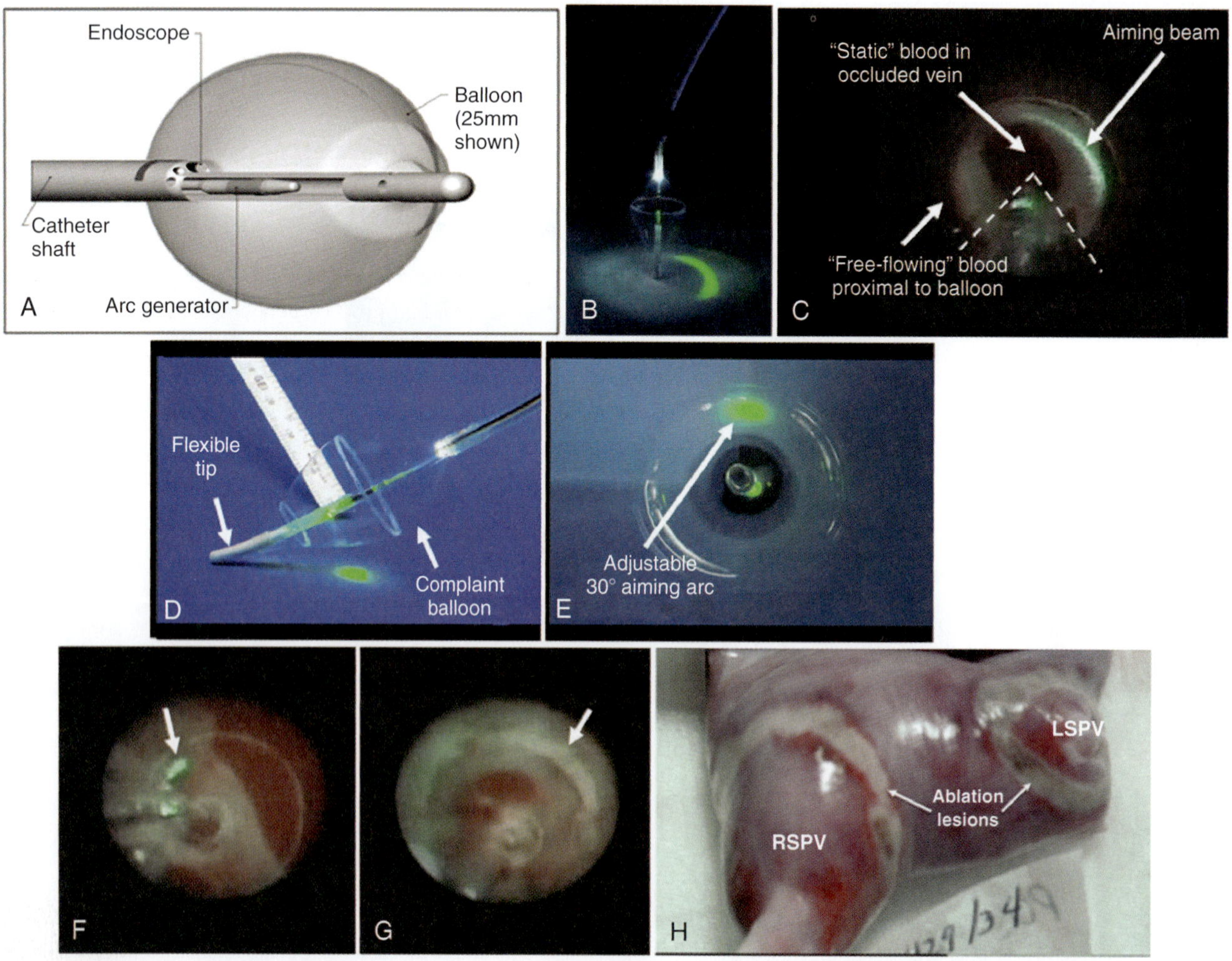

FIGURE 5-7. A, Forward-projecting endoscopic laser balloon components. **B** and **C,** Early-generation noncompliant laser balloon with 90-degree aiming beam and endoscopic visualization of the left superior pulmonary vein (LSPV) (see **Videos 5-1** through **5-3**). **D-H,** Current generation, compliant balloon catheter with 30-degree aiming beam and endoscopic visualization of lesion formation in a porcine model. RSPV, right superior pulmonary vein.

diameter endoscope, which is inserted into the balloon catheter. The most recent generation balloon catheter is compliant and with an adjustable diameter that permits greater circumferential contact and ablation. A 30-degree adjustable aiming arc is rotated to apply laser in regions of balloon-tissue contact.[100] A deflectable sheath permits improved navigation in the left atrium.

In first-generation systems, using an open-thoracotomy caprine model of endocardial access through a left atrial appendage sheath, Reddy and colleagues[98] demonstrated electrical isolation of 19 of 27 PVs after a single application of photonic energy. With the use of reflectance spectroscopy to ensure adequate orientation and contact of the laser balloon with the left atrial myocardium, complete PV isolation was achieved in 5 of 5 veins. Pathologic examination revealed no PV stenosis, no pericardial damage, minor lung lesions without pleural perforation, minimal endothelium disruption, and, in the presence of adequate heparinization, no endocardial charring or overlying thrombus. Using a percutaneous technique, Lemery and colleagues[99] delivered photonic energy successfully to 5 of 5 PVs, with gross inspection revealing endocardial lesions at the ostium in 4 of 5 veins. With the current generation balloon catheter, Dukkapati and colleagues performed an in vivo evaluation of visually guided ablation in acute and chronic porcine models to assess feasibility and reproducibility of achieving PV isolation.[101] PV isolation was assessed immediately and more than 30 minutes after ablation. Chronic lesions in survival animals were remapped at 4 weeks. All veins (30 of 30) were acutely isolated. Remapping at 4 weeks yielded 80% persistent PV isolation. Histologic examination of PV sections of the acute experiments identified 100% transmurality in 65% of acute veins and 97% of chronic veins. No esophageal or phrenic nerve injury was noted.[102] Laser balloon ablation also had a greater chronic isolation rate versus RF in a porcine model.[103] Clinical use was evaluated in a single-center open-labeled, nonrandomized trial for safety and efficacy of creating PV isolation in patients with refractory AF.[104] All PVs (total 65) were targeted in 18 patients. Pretreatment PV sizes ranged from 16 to 27 mm in diameter. PVs greater than 30 mm were excluded owing to limitations in balloon size. All PVs were successfully isolated, with 57 of 65 (88%) isolated after one circumferential lesion set. Mean fluoroscopy time was 21 minutes with a mean ablation time of 64 minutes per case. All PVs remained isolated after 30 minutes, At 8 weeks, 10 of 18 patients underwent remapping, and 36 of 38 (95%) of the PVs remained isolated.[105] The use of deflectable delivery systems has facilitated optimal balloon placement. The multicenter European experience is promising.[106] This generation laser balloon has now entered clinical trials in the United States.

Ultrasound

Basic Principles

US is yet another form of energy that can cause thermally mediated tissue injury. A form of vibration energy greater than 18,000 cycles per second (18 kHz), US is propagated as a mechanical wave by the motion of particles within the medium.[107] The motion causes alternating compression and decompression in the medium with the passage of sound waves. Thus, a pressure wave is propagated associated with the mechanical movement of particles. The particulate motion that a US field generates results in mechanical stress and strain. When applied to an absorbing medium, US energy is continuously absorbed and converted to heat within the medium. This thermal effect can cause substantial tissue injury if the temperature elevation is sufficient and is maintained for an adequate period.[108]

Early studies considered high-intensity focused ultrasound (HIFU) energy as a noninvasive technique capable of selectively injuring deep tissues within the body, particularly within the central nervous system.[109,110] Lesions were created in homogeneous tissue without damage to intervening tissue.[110–112] The ablation US transducer contains a piezoelectric element that vibrates at a fixed frequency when electricity is applied.[47] The lesion is formed within the focal region of the transducer and can be collimated to provide a greater depth of penetration.[113] Using frequencies of 500 kHz to 20 MHz, HIFU can create controlled, localized tissue injury through both mechanical energy (oscillation and collapse of gas bubbles, or microcavitation) and the primary mechanism, thermal energy (tissue absorption of acoustic energy).[114,115] As the incident energy is increased, boiling of tissue water may occur, leading to the formation of vapor cavities (bubbles).[116] The amount of energy transferred from the acoustic wave to the tissue is directly proportional to both the intensity of the wave and the absorption coefficient of the tissue.[117] If the US transducer transmits into a medium with low absorption (e.g., water, blood), the catheter tip will not need to be in direct contact with the myocardium.

Lessons from Experimental Studies

Zimmer and associates[118] studied the feasibility of using US for cardiac ablation. Frequencies from 10 to 15 MHz produced the deepest lesions at US intensities between 15 and 30 W/cm². The results showed the importance of tissue surface temperature monitoring to keep temperatures to less than the boiling threshold of 100°C. When temperatures reached these high levels, the lesions produced by sonication were typically wider and shallower than those created at a lower power level. This was thought to be a result of the scattering of sound by the gas bubbles formed from the boiling of water. Both in vitro and in vivo experiments verified the theoretical calculations that HIFU can ablate cardiac muscle within 60 seconds, creating lesions up to 9 mm deep with large areas up to 40 mm². Ohkubo and associates[113] studied the HIFU lesions created with transducers with frequencies in the range of 5 to 10 MHz on a beating heart in canine cardiac tissue and porcine heart specimens. HIFU was delivered through the ablation catheter at a preset temperature of 85°C for 180 seconds. The electrical power input was automatically adjusted to keep the temperature near the preset value, producing sharply demarcated endocardial lesions of varying size. In the in vitro study, when the temperature was maintained stable, lesion depth increased significantly with sonication of longer duration, and when the duration of sonication was kept constant, lesion depth increased significantly with higher temperatures of energy delivery.

Using a 10-MHz HIFU transducer mounted on a 7F catheter in canines, He and associates[108] obtained lesions with sonication for as little as 15 seconds. Myocardial lesions 11 mm in depth were produced with an acoustic power of 1.3 W applied for 60 seconds. Histologically, these lesions were well circumscribed, with a clear border zone between necrosis and intact cell layers. Hemorrhage, inflammation, and fibrin thrombi were consistently absent. Strickberger and colleagues[119] obtained similar histologic findings when performing extracardiac HIFU in an open-thoracotomy model to create AV block within the canine heart. Parallel two-dimensional US imaging was used to find the AV junction anatomically. Complete AV block was created in each of 10 animals with 30-second applications of HIFU gated to the cardiac cycle at a mean of 6.5 sites. Of interest, the myocardium immediately adjacent to the lesion, including the tissue between the lesion and the ablation US transducer (a distance of up to 6.3 cm), was histologically normal.

This study raises the possibility of noninvasive cardiac ablation.

Phased-Array High-Intensity Focused Ultrasound Systems

Phased-array HIFU systems composed of hundreds of US elements may be used to create lesions at specific target depths of up to 15 cm without significant heating of the intervening tissues.[120] Phased-array systems may be better suited to noninvasive cardiac ablation because of the ability to control the position of the target site by switching between different beam patterns at electronic speed, the ability to correct for aberrations that may be present due to complex inhomogeneous intervening tissue such as ribs and lungs, and the ability to change the effective aperture dimensions during treatment by adjusting the driving signals.[118] A novel "combo" catheter with real-time, three-dimensional imaging and a ring transducer for US ablation has been described.[121]

Ultrasound Balloon Catheters

Because US remains collimated or focused as it passes through an echo lucent fluid medium, it may be advantageous for application through a fluid-filled balloon.[47] US balloon delivery systems have been clinically investigated for ablation around the PVs. Two systems have been evaluated in humans. In the original concept, collimated US was delivered circumferentially around the equator of a balloon perpendicular to the axis of the catheter. Once it was realized that ablation inside the PV orifice may be less efficacious and safe than ablation in the PV antrum, a forward-projecting, focused US balloon was developed by incorporation of a parabolic acoustic reflector at the back of the balloon (Fig. 5-8 and **Video 5-4**). This HIFU balloon catheter consists of two attached noncompliant balloons. A distal balloon is filled with a mixture of water and contrast media (4:1 ratio) and an US crystal. A second proximal balloon, filled with carbon dioxide, forms a parabolic surface at the base of the balloon. This permits

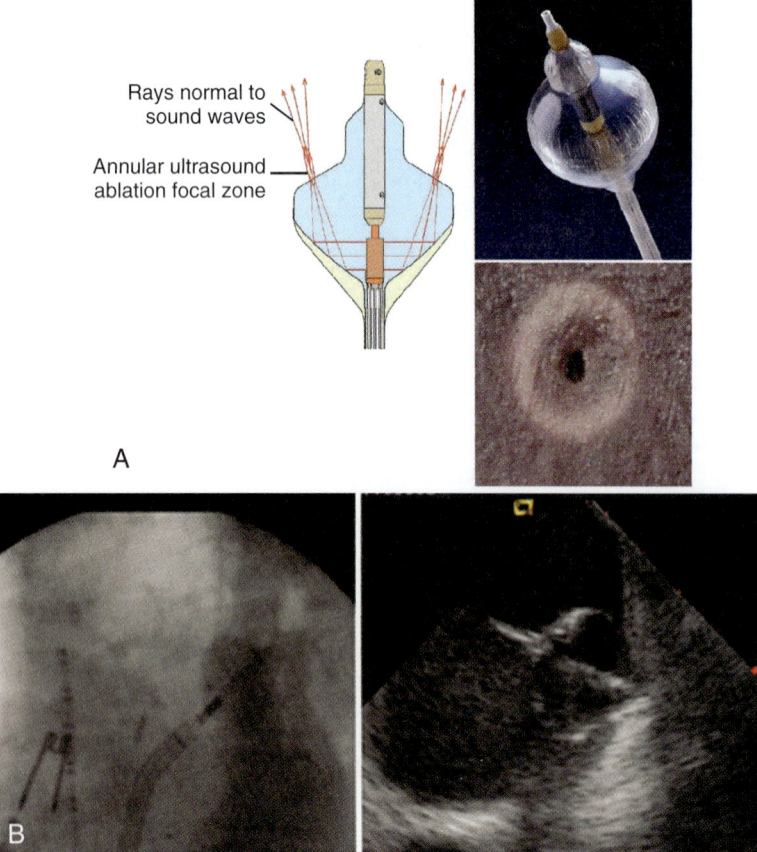

FIGURE 5-8. Forward-projecting high-intensity focused ultrasound balloon for pulmonary vein isolation. **A,** Radially emitted ultrasound is reflected from the back of the balloon, resulting in forward projection of ultrasound energy with a focal point at the balloon-endocardial interface. Application in vitro *(bottom right)* reveals the sharply demarcated edges and preserved inner core. **B,** Fluoroscopic and intracardiac echocardiographic images of clinical application of high-intensity focused ultrasound at the left superior pulmonary vein.

the US waves to reflect in a forward direction, focusing a 360-degree ring of ultrasound energy (sonicating ring) 2 to 6 mm distal to the balloon surface.[122] The US energy is delivered through a 9-MHz cylindrical transducer mounted on a catheter. The current passes through the transducer at its resonant frequency and causes it to vibrate. The emitted sound waves are absorbed by the cardiac tissue that is in contact with the balloon surface where the beam is incident with the tissue. This results in tissue heating, which, when applied for a sufficient duration, creates an irreversible thermal lesion of cardiac tissue.[123] Although unfocused collimated US energy has a decremental loss of energy as it emanates from the transducer, it may still penetrate significantly beyond the thin atrial or PV wall.

In animal studies of nonfocused US, Lesh and associates[124] reported the creation of uniformly heated lesions with a balloon catheter for anatomic isolation of the PVs. In a canine study,[125] a single US application targeted at 65°C was placed via a balloon catheter system in the right superior PV. PV stenosis with cartilaginous metaplasia was seen in two animals. All lesions were transmural, but PV branching and shorter applications accounted for incomplete circumferential lesions.

Natale and colleagues[126] first reported a single-center experience with the use of a through-the-balloon nonfocused circumferential US ablation system for patients with recurrent AF. Subsequently, these patients were included with patients from other centers who underwent circumferential US ablation.[127] This analysis consisted of 33 patients with a total of 85 veins ablated. The system used consisted of a 0.035-inch diameter luminal catheter with a distal balloon (maximal diameter, 2.2 cm) that contained a centrally located 8-MHz US transducer. The catheter was advanced over a sheath and guidewire to the ostium of the PV. The balloon was inflated at the ostium, causing total occlusion verified by contrast venography. Activated clotting times were maintained at greater than 250 seconds with heparin. During ablation, the energy was adjusted to maintain target temperatures of at least 60°C. A mean of 6.7 ablations per vein were applied. At 22-month follow-up, a total of 20 patients (60%) experienced recurrence of AF. Variable PV anatomy limiting proper balloon positioning and inability to reach temperatures greater than 60°C were technical limitations thought to be responsible for the high failure rate in this early-generation US balloon catheter. Procedural complications included cerebellar stroke (one patient), phrenic nerve palsy (two patients), severe PV stenosis (one patient), and hematoma (two patients).[127]

A forward-projecting, focused US ablation system (HIFU) for circumferential ablation outside the PV was developed to better direct the US energy.[128] Dispersion of the US energy beyond the highly focused target depth was thought to reduce the risk for deeper extracardiac damage compared with collimated US. In preclinical canine testing, Nakagawa and colleagues investigated PV isolation using an HIFU balloon catheter. This experiment yielded acute PV isolation in all animals, with persistent PV isolation in 88% 1 week to 3 months after ablation.[129] Lesions were present at sites without balloon-tissue contact, and no PV stenosis or thrombus formation was observed. Initial human experience consisted of 27 patients (19 paroxysmal and 8 persistent).[130]

PV antrum isolation was attempted in 78 of 104 PVs, but only 3 of 27 right inferior PVs were attempted because of limitations in catheter maneuverability. Successful isolation was achieved in 87% of the attempted PVs, with 1 to 26 (median, 3) HIFU applications. Complications included transient bleeding from guidewire manipulation and right phrenic nerve injury. No PV stenosis (>50% narrowing) or atrial-esophageal fistula occurred. At the 12-month follow-up, 16 (59%) of the 27 patients were free of symptomatic AF. A steerable HIFU balloon catheter was subsequently assessed in a consecutive study of 15 patients. Improved maneuverability increased the success rate for PV isolation to 89% (41 of 46) of PVs. Complications included 2 patients with right phrenic nerve injury.[131]

Okumura and associates studied the mechanism of tissue heating during HIFU and temperature effects on the phrenic nerve by recording tissue temperatures from epicardial thermocouples at the RSPV orifice and phrenic nerve in dogs.[132] This study demonstrated that HIFU energy delivery results in rapid direct heating at a limited area near the HIFU exit and conductive heating at a distance from HIFU exit with the ability to injure the phrenic nerve when it is located within 4 to 7 mm of the HIFU exit. This mandated careful monitoring of device positioning in relation to the vein geometry and adjacent structures and the use of oversized balloons to create more antral lesions near the right superior PV. It has also been previously described that HIFU applications close to the esophagus produced esophageal lacerations in an animal model.[133] This occurred when the balloon was positioned too close to the esophagus and HIFU was delivered unabsorbed in the PV (typically when the balloon was positioned too distally in the PV). It was recommended to maintain a balloon-to-esophagus distance of more than 5 mm with the concomitant monitoring of esophageal location and the exact sites of sonication using intracardiac ultrasound.[134] Despite careful monitoring, which included progression to esophageal temperature monitoring and postablation esophagogastroduodenoscopy, concerns regarding the potential for atrial-esophageal fistula creation resulted in suspension of clinical studies on the most recent HIFU balloon design with this fixed focal length.[135]

HIFU has also been applied successfully in patients with AF undergoing minimally invasive off-pump epicardial surgical maze procedures. The characteristics of transmission of energy through epicardial fat and contact forgiveness provided by US offer distinct advantages over RF applications (Fig. 5-9).

Alternative Ablative Techniques

Additional ablative energy sources that have been assessed in preclinical and clinical studies include direct heating (heated balloon for PV isolation), infrared radiation (epicardial maze), β radiation (atrial flutter and PV isolation), and pressure necrosis (PV stenting to produce conduction block). Each of these approaches carries a unique profile of relative merits, potential limitations, and technical challenges. The potential limitations include thermal conductivity properties and temperature monitoring of the heated balloon membrane, predisposition to char formation with infrared ablation, and delayed onset of the electrophysiologic end point (conduction block) for β radiation and pressure necrosis (PV stenting).

Conclusion

The limitations of RF ablation, including dependence on tissue contact, potential for coagulation at the catheter-tissue interface that limits power delivery, and difficulty in creating lesions in myocardial scar, have prompted the search for alternative sources of ablative energy (Table 5-1). MW energy has been shown in both in vitro and in vivo studies to be less dependent on tissue contact, to have the ability to transmit energy through desiccated and coagulated tissue, and to create larger lesions that expand with increased application time. The ability to create large, well-circumscribed lesions in myocardial scar is a characteristic favorable to laser energy. Focused ultrasound has the unique property of reaching specific target depths without injuring intervening tissues but has shown the propensity to injure other adjacent structures. These energy sources, when applied to new catheter designs and delivery techniques, may play an important role in the management of specific arrhythmias, including AF and VT, as the indication for ablation is broadened and the technical requirements shift from conventional focal ablation to circular and linear ablation.

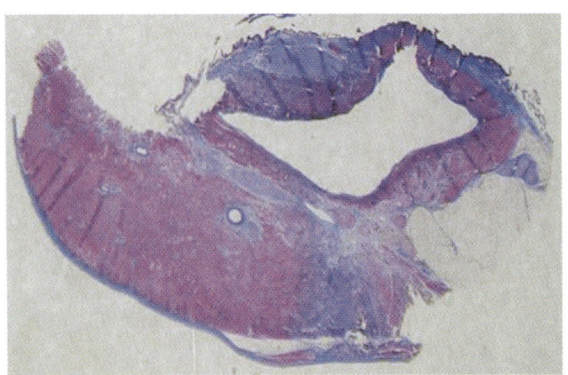

FIGURE 5-9. Epicardial high-intensity focused ultrasound (HIFU) ablation in a calf heart. Trichrome stain of posterior left atrial wall, including vein of Marshall *(top of image)*. HIFU was delivered in vivo from the epicardium in an open thoracotomy model to demonstrate the ability of HIFU to penetrate epicardial fat and venous tissue. The sharply defined, narrow transmural lesion *(blue)* can be seen to extend through to the endocardium *(bottom of section)*.

References

1. Scheinman MM, Morady F, Hess DS, et al. Catheter-induced ablation of the atrioventricular junction to control refractory supraventricular arrhythmias. *JAMA.* 1982;248:851–855.
2. Olgin JE, Scheinman MM. Comparison of high energy direct current and radiofrequency catheter ablation of the atrioventricular junction. *J Am Coll Cardiol.* 1993;21:557–584.
3. Jackman WM, Hunzhang W, Friday KJ, et al. Catheter ablation of accessory atrioventricular pathways (Wolff-Parkinson-White syndrome) by radiofrequency current. *N Engl J Med.* 1991;324:1605–1611.
4. Jackman WM, Beckman KJ, McClelland JH, et al. Treatment of supraventricular tachycardia due to atrioventricular nodal entry by radiofrequency catheter ablation of slow-pathway conduction. *N Engl J Med.* 1992;327:313–319.
5. Organ LW. Electrophysiologic principles of radiofrequency lesion making. *Appl Neurophysiol.* 1976;39:69–76.
6. Nath S, Lynch C, Whayne JG, et al. Cellular electrophysiological effects of hyperthermia on isolated guinea pig papillary muscle: implications for catheter ablation. *Circulation.* 1993;88:1826–1831.
7. Nath S, Haines DE. Biophysics and pathology of catheter energy delivery systems. *Prog Cardiovasc Dis.* 1995;37:185–204.
8. Haines DE, Watson DD. Tissue heating during radiofrequency catheter ablation: a thermodynamic model and observations in isolated perfused and superfused canine right ventricular free wall. *Pacing Clin Electrophysiol.* 1989;12:962–971.
9. Wonnell TL, Stauffer PR, Langberg JJ. Evaluation of microwave and radio frequency catheter ablation in a myocardium-equivalent phantom model. *IEEE Trans Biomed Eng.* 1992;39:1086–1095.
10. Jumrussirikul P, Chen JT, Jenkins M, et al. Prospective comparison of temperature guided microwave and radiofrequency catheter ablation in the swine heart. *Pacing Clin Electrophysiol.* 1998;21:1364–1374.
11. Ruffy R, Imran MA, Santel DJ, et al. Radiofrequency delivery through a cooled catheter tip allows the creation of larger endomyocardial lesions in the ovine heart. *J Cardiovasc Electrophysiol.* 1995;6:1089–1096.

TABLE 5-1

ENERGY SOURCES FOR CATHETER ABLATION

Energy Source	Frequency or Wavelength	Mechanism of Heating	Relation of Heating to Distance (r) from Source	Tissue Contact Needed	Advantages	Disadvantages
Radiofrequency	300-700 kHz	Resistive	$1/r^4$	Yes	Readily available, vast clinical experience	Limited lesion size, charring
Microwave	915-2450 MHz	Dielectric	$1/r^2$	No	Penetrates scar and fat, large lesions, linear catheters possible	Complex catheter design, energy titration
Laser	300-2000 nm	Photon absorption	Complex, exponential decline	No	Large lesions, can spare endocardium, linear and balloon catheters possible	Requires tissue contact to prevent char formation
Ultrasound	500 kHz to 20 MHz	Mechanical stress and strain	Varies with focal length	No	Can be focused for encircling lesions and focal lesions far from source	Difficulty controlling depth, highly directional, collateral damage

12. Petersen HH, Chen X, Pietersen A, et al. Temperature-controlled irrigated tip radiofrequency catheter ablation: comparison of in vivo and in vitro lesion dimensions for standard catheter and irrigated tip catheter with minimal infusion rate. *J Cardiovasc Electrophysiol*. 1998;9:409–414.

13. Petersen HH, Chen X, Pietersen A, et al. Tissue temperatures and lesion size during irrigated tip catheter radiofrequency ablation: an in vitro comparison of temperature-controlled irrigated tip ablation, power-controlled irrigated tip ablation, and standard temperature-controlled ablation. *Pacing Clin Electrophysiol*. 2000;23:8–17.

14. Dorwarth U, Fiek M, Remp T, et al. Radiofrequency catheter ablation: different cooled and noncooled electrode systems induce specific lesion geometries and adverse effects profiles. *Pacing Clin Electrophysiol*. 2003;26:1438–1445.

15. Cummings JE, Pacifico A, Drago JL, et al. Alternative energy sources for the ablation of arrhythmias. *Pacing Clin Electrophysiol*. 2005;28:434–443.

16. Wittkampf FH, Nakagawa H, Foresti S, et al. Saline-irrigated radiofrequency ablation electrode with external cooling. *J Cardiovasc Electrophysiol*. 2005;16:323–328.

17. Johnson CC, Guy AW. Nonionizing electromagnetic wave effects in biologic materials and systems. *Proc IEEE*. 1972;60:692–709.

18. Whayne JG, Nath S, Haines DE. Microwave catheter ablation of myocardium in vitro: assessment of the characteristics of tissue heating and injury. *Circulation*. 1994;89:2390–2395.

19. Avitall B, Khan M, Krum D, et al. Physics and engineering of transcatheter cardiac tissue ablation. *J Am Coll Cardiol*. 1993;22:921–932.

20. Gadhoke A, Aronovitz M, Zebede J, et al. Are tissue contact and catheter orientation important variables in microwave ablation? [abstract]. *Circulation*. 1992;86(suppl 1):I–191.

21. Erdogan A, Grumbrecht S, Neumann T, et al. Microwave, irrigated, pulsed, or conventional radiofrequency energy source: which energy source for which catheter ablation? *Pacing Clin Electrophysiol*. 2003;26:504–506.

22. Lin JC. Microwave propagation in biologic dielectrics with application cardiopulmonary interrogation. In: Larson LE, Jacobi JH, eds. *Medical Applications of Microwave Imaging*. New York: IEEE Press; 1986:47–58.

23. Lin JC. Engineering and biophysical aspects of microwave and radiofrequency radiation. In: Watmough DJ, Ross WM, eds. *Hyperthermia*. Glasgow, UK: Blackie and Sons; 1986:42–75.

24. Lin JC. Catheter microwave ablation therapy for cardiac arrhythmias. *Bioelectromagnetics*. 1999;4(suppl):120–132.

25. Lin JC. Studies on microwaves in medicine and biology: from snails to humans. *Bioelectromagnetics*. 2004;25:146–159.

26. Beckman KJ, Lin YC, Wang Y, et al. Production of reversible and irreversible atrioventricular block by microwave energy. *Circulation*. 1987;76:1612.

27. Langberg JJ, Wonnell T, Chin MC, et al. Catheter ablation of the atrioventricular junction using a helical microwave antenna: a novel means of coupling energy to the endocardium. *Pacing Clin Electrophysiol*. 1991;14:2105–2113.

28. Keane D, Ruskin J, Norris N, et al. In vitro and in vivo evaluation of the thermal patterns and lesions of catheter ablation with a microwave monopole antenna. *J Interv Card Electrophysiol*. 2004;10:111–119.

29. Lin JC, Wang YJ. A catheter antenna for percutaneous microwave therapy. *Microw Opt Technol Lett*. 1995;8:70–72.

30. Lin JC, Wang YJ. The cap-choke catheter antenna for microwave ablation treatment. *IEEE Trans Biomed Eng*. 1996;43:657–660.

31. Wang PJ, Schoen FJ, Aronovitz M, et al. Microwave catheter ablation under the mitral annulus: a new method of accessory pathway ablation? *Pacing Clin Electrophysiol*. 1993;16:866.

32. Huang SKS, Lin JC, Mazzola F, et al. Percutaneous microwave ablation of the ventricular myocardium using a 4-mm split-tip antenna electrode: a novel method for potential ablation of ventricular tachycardia [abstract]. *J Am Coll Cardiol*. 1994;351:24A.

33. Mazzola F, Huang SKS, Lin J, et al. Determinates of lesion size using a 4-mm split-tip antenna electrode for microwave catheter ablation. *Pacing Clin Electrophysiol*. 1994;17:814.

34. Ruder M, Mead RH, Baron K, et al. Microwave ablation: in vivo data. *Pacing Clin Electrophysiol*. 1994;17:781.

35. Yang X, Watanabe I, Kojima T, et al. Microwave ablation of the atrioventricular junction in vivo and ventricular myocardium in vitro and in vivo: effects of varying power and duration on lesion volume. *Jpn Heart J*. 1994;35:175–191.

36. Rho TH, Ito M, Pride HP, et al. Microwave ablation of canine atrial tachycardia induced by aconitine. *Am Heart J*. 1995;129:1021–1025.

37. Liem LB, Mead RH, Shenasa M, et al. In vitro and in vivo results of transcatheter microwave ablation using forward firing tip antenna design. *Pacing Clin Electrophysiol*. 1996;19:2004–2008.

38. Liem LB, Mead RH, Shenasa M, et al. Microwave catheter ablation using a clinical prototype system with a lateral firing antenna design. *Pacing Clin Electrophysiol*. 1998;21:714–721.

39. Nevels RD, Arndt GD, Raffoul GW, et al. Microwave catheter design. *IEEE Trans Biomed Eng*. 1998;45:885–890.

40. Gu Z, Rappaport CM, Wang PJ, et al. A 2 1/4-turn spiral antenna for catheter cardiac ablation. *IEEE Trans Biomed Eng*. 1999;46:1480–1482.

41. Thomas SP, Clout R, Deery C, et al. Microwave ablation of myocardial tissue: the effect of element design, tissue coupling, blood flow, power, and duration of exposure on lesion size. *J Cardiovasc Electrophysiol*. 1999;10:72–78.

42. Vanderbrink BA, Gu Z, Rodriguez V, et al. Microwave ablation using a spiral antenna design in a porcine thigh muscle preparation: in vivo assessment of temperature profile and lesion geometry. *J Cardiovasc Electrophysiol*. 2000;11:193–198.

43. Pisa S, Cavagnaro M, Bernardi P, et al. A 915-MHz antenna for microwave thermal ablation treatment: physical design, computer modeling and experimental measurement. *IEEE Trans Biomed Eng*. 2001;48:599–601.

44. Chiu HM, Mohan AS, Weily AR, et al. Analysis of a novel expanded tip wire (ETW) antenna for microwave ablation of cardiac arrhythmias. *IEEE Trans Biomed Eng*. 2003;50:890–899.

45. Rappaport C. Cardiac tissue ablation with catheter-based microwave heating. *Int J Hypertherm*. 2004;20:769–780.

46. Wang PJ, Estes NA. New technologies for catheter ablation. In: Saksena S, Luderitz B, eds. *Interventional Electrophysiology: A Textbook*. New York: Futura; 1996:557–560.

47. Keane D. New catheter ablation techniques for the treatment of cardiac arrhythmias. *Card Electrophysiol Rev*. 2002;6:341–348.

48. Iwasa A, Storey J, Yao B, et al. Efficacy of a microwave antenna for ablation of the tricuspid valve-inferior vena cava isthmus in dogs as a treatment for type 1 atrial flutter. *J Interv Card Electrophysiol*. 2004;10:191–198.

49. VanderBrink BA, Gilbride C, Aronovitz MJ, et al. Safety and efficacy of a steerable temperature monitoring microwave catheter system for ventricular myocardial ablation. *J Cardiovasc Electrophysiol*. 2000;11:305–310.

50. Tse HF, Songyan L, Chung-Wah S, et al. Determinants of lesion dimensions during transcatheter microwave ablation. *Pacing Clin Electrophysiol*. 2009;32:201–208.

51. Lin JC, Beckman KJ, Hariman RJ, et al. Microwave ablation of the atrioventricular junction in open-chest dogs. *Bioelectromagnetics*. 1995;16:97–105.

52. de Gouveia RH, Melo J, Santiago T, et al. Comparison of the healing mechanisms of myocardial lesions induced by dry radiofrequency and microwave epicardial ablation. *Pacing Clin Electrophysiol*. 2006;29:278–282.

53. Huang SKS, Lin JC, Mazzola F, et al. Percutaneous microwave ablation of the ventricular myocardium using a 4-mm split-tip antenna electrode: a novel method for potential ablation of ventricular tachycardia [abstract]. *J Am Coll Cardiol*. 1994;23:34A.

54. Pires LA, Huang SKS, Lin JC, et al. Comparison of radiofrequency (RF) versus microwave (MW) energy catheter ablation of the bovine ventricular myocardium. *Pacing Clin Electrophysiol*. 1994;17:782.

55. Keane D, Ruskin J, Norris N, et al. In vitro and in vivo evaluation of the thermal patterns and lesions of catheter ablation with a microwave monopole antenna. *J Interv Card Electrophysiol*. 2004;10:111–119.

56. Saoudi N, Atallah G, Kirkorian G, et al. Catheter ablation of the atrial myocardium in human type I atrial flutter. *Circulation*. 1990;81:762–771.

57. Feld GK, Fleck P, Chen PS, et al. Radiofrequency catheter ablation for the treatment of human type 1 atrial flutter: identification of a critical zone in the reentrant circuit by endocardial mapping techniques. *Circulation*. 1992;86:1233–1240.

58. Cosio FG, Lopez GM, Goicolea A, et al. Radiofrequency ablation of the inferior vena cava-tricuspid valve isthmus in common atrial flutter. *Am J Cardiol*. 1993;71:705–709.

59. Gadhoke A, Aronovitz M, Zebede J, et al. Are tissue contact and catheter orientation important variables in microwave ablation? [abstract]. *Circulation*. 1992;86(suppl 1):I–191.

60. Iwasa A, Storey J, Yao B, et al. Efficacy of a microwave antenna for ablation of the tricuspid valve-inferior vena cava isthmus in dogs as a treatment for type 1 atrial flutter. *J Interv Card Electrophysiol*. 2004;10:191–198.

61. Liem LB, Mead RH. Microwave linear ablation of the isthmus between the inferior vena cava and tricuspid annulus. *Pacing Clin Electrophysiol*. 1998;21:2079–2086.

62. Adragao P, Parreira L, Morgado F, et al. Microwave ablation of atrial flutter. *Pacing Clin Electrophysiol*. 1999;22:1692–1695.

63. Yiu KH, Siu CW, Lau CP, et al. Transvenous catheter based microwave ablation for atrial flutter. *Heart Rhythm*. 2007;4:221–223.

64. Chan JY, Fung JW, Yu CM, et al. Preliminary results with percutaneous transcatheter microwave ablation of typical atrial flutter. *J Cardiovasc Electrophysiol*. 2007;18:286–289.

65. Knaut M, Tugtekin SM, Matschke K. Pulmonary vein isolation by microwave energy ablation in patients with permanent atrial fibrillation. *J Card Surg*. 2004;19:211–215.

66. Wisser W, Khazen C, Deviatko E, et al. Microwave and radiofrequency ablation yield similar success rates for treatment of chronic atrial fibrillation. *Eur J Cardiothorac Surg*. 2004;25:1011–1017.

67. Einstein A. On the quantum theory of radiation. *Physikalische Zeitschrift*. 1917;18:121.

68. Saksena S, Gadhoke A. Laser therapy for tachyarrhythmias: a new frontier. *Pacing Clin Electrophysiol*. 1986;9:531–550.

69. Saksena S. Catheter ablation of tachycardias with laser energy: issues and answers. *Pacing Clin Electrophysiol*. 1989;12:196–203.

70. Zheng S, Kloner RA, Whittaker P. Ablation and coagulation of myocardial tissue by means of a pulsed holmium:YAG laser. *Am Heart J*. 1993;126:1474–1477.

71. Tomaru T, Geschwind HJ, Boussignac G, et al. Comparison of ablation efficacy of excimer, pulsed-dye, and holmium-YAG lasers relevant to shock waves. *Am Heart J*. 1992;123:886–895.

72. Verdaasdonk RM, Borst C, van Gemert MJC. Explosive onset of continuous wave laser tissue ablation. *Phys Med Biol*. 1990;35:1129–1144.

73. Ohtake H, Misaki T, Watanabe G, et al. Myocardial coagulation by intraoperative Nd:YAG laser ablation and its dependence on blood perfusion. *Pacing Clin Electrophysiol*. 1994;17:1627–1631.

74. Lee BI, Rodriguez ER, Notargiocomo A. Thermal effects of laser and electrical discharge on cardiovascular tissue: implications for coronary artery recanalization and endocardial ablation. *J Am Coll Cardiol*. 1986;8:193–200.

75. Splinter R, Semenov SY, Nanney GA, et al. Myocardial temperature distribution under cw Nd:YAG laser irradiation in "in vitro" and "in vivo" situations: theory and experiment. *Appl Optics*. 1995;34:391–399.

76. Levine JH, Merillat JC, Stern M, et al. The cellular electrophysiologic changes induced by ablation: comparison between argon laser photo ablation and high-energy electrical ablation. *Circulation*. 1987;76:217–225.

77. Saksena S, Ciccone JM, Chnadran P, et al. Laser ablation of normal and diseased human ventricle. *Am Heart J*. 1986;112:52–60.

78. Isner JM, DeJesus SR, Clarke RH, et al. Mechanism of laser ablation in an absorbing field. *Lasers Surg Med*. 1988;8:543–554.

79. Narula OS, Bharati S, Chan MC, et al. Laser microsection of the His bundle: a per-venous catheter technique. *J Am Coll Cardiol*. 1984;3:537.

80. Abele GS, Griffin JC, Hill JA, et al. Transvascular argon laser induced atrioventricular conduction ablation in dogs. *Circulation*. 1983;68:145.

81. Ciccone J, Saksena S, Pantopoulos D. Comparative efficacy of continuous and pulsed argon laser ablation of human diseased ventricle. *Pacing Clin Electrophysiol*. 1986;9:697–704.

82. Walsh JT, Deutsch TF. Pulsed CO₂ laser ablation of tissue: effect of mechanical properties. *IEEE Trans Biomed Eng*. 1989;36:1195–1201.

83. Saksena S, Hussain SM, Gielchinsky I, et al. Intraoperative mapping-guided argon laser ablation of malignant ventricular tachycardia. *Am J Cardiol*. 1987;59:78–83.

84. Saksena S, Hussain SM, Gielchinsky I, et al. Intraoperative mapping-guided argon laser ablation of supraventricular tachycardia in the Wolff-Parkinson-White syndrome. *Am J Cardiol*. 1987;60:196–199.

85. Lee BI, Gottdiener JS, Fletcher RD, et al. Transcatheter ablation: comparison between laser photoablation and electrode shock ablation in the dog. *Circulation*. 1985;71:579–586.

86. Weber HP, Enders HS, Keiditisch E. Percutaneous Nd:YAG laser coagulation of ventricular myocardium in dogs using a special electrode laser catheter. *Pacing Clin Electrophysiol*. 1989;12:899–910.

87. Weber HP, Enders HS, Ruprecht L, et al. Catheter-directed laser coagulation of atrial myocardium in dogs. *Eur Heart J*. 1994;15:971–980.

88. Pfeiffer D, Moosdorf R, Svenson RH, et al. Epicardial neodymium:YAG laser photocoagulation of ventricular tachycardia without ventriculotomy in patients after myocardial infarction. *Circulation*. 1996;94:3221–3225.

89. Weber HP, Kalternbrunner W, Heinze A, et al. Laser catheter coagulation of atrial myocardium for ablation of atrioventricular nodal reentrant tachycardia. *Eur Heart J*. 1997;18:487–495.

90. Ware DL, Boor P, Yang C, et al. Slow intramural heating with diffused laser light: a unique method for deep myocardial coagulation. *Circulation*. 1999;99:1630–1636.

91. Pierce J, Thomasen S. Rate process analysis of thermal damage. In: Welch AJ, van Gemert MJC, eds. *Optical-Thermal Responses of Laser-Irradiated Tissue*. New York: Plenum Press; 1995:561–606.

92. d'Avila A, Splinter R, Svenson RH. New perspectives on catheter-based ablation of ventricular tachycardia complicating Chagas' disease: experimental evidence of the efficacy of near infrared lasers for catheter ablation of Chagas' VT. *J Interv Card Electrophysiol*. 2002;7:23–38.

93. Fried NM, Lardo AC, Berger RD, et al. Linear lesions in myocardium created by Nd:YAG laser using diffusing optical fibers. *Lasers Surg Med*. 2000;27:295–304.

94. Keane D, Ruskin JN. Linear atrial ablation with a diode laser and fiberoptic catheter. *Circulation*. 1999;100:e59–e60.

95. Wagshall A, Abela GS, Maheshwari A, et al. A novel catheter design for laser photocoagulation of the myocardium to ablate ventricular tachycardia. *J Interv Card Electrophysiol*. 2002;7:13–22.

96. Littmann L, Svenson RH, Chuang CH, et al. Catheterization technique for laser photoablation of atrioventricular conduction from the aortic root in dogs. *Pacing Clin Electrophysiol*. 1993;16:401–406.

97. Johnson S, Su W, Da Salva LL, et al. Power dependence of laser energy in circumferential ablation of pulmonary veins [abstract]. *Pacing Clin Electrophysiol*. 2002;24:552.

98. Reddy VR, Houghtaling C, Fallon J, et al. Use of a diode laser balloon catheter to generate circumferential pulmonary venous lesions in an open-thoracotomy caprine model. *Pacing Clin Electrophysiol*. 2004;27:52–57.

99. Lemery R, Vienot JP, Tang ASL, et al. Fiberoptic balloon catheter ablation of pulmonary vein ostia in pigs using photonic energy delivery with diode laser. *Pacing Clin Electrophysiol*. 2002;25:32–36.

100. Ahmed H, Reddy VY. Technical advances in the ablation of atrial fibrillation. *Heart Rhythm*. 2009;6:S39–S44.

101. Dukkipati S, d'Avila A, Doshi SK, et al. Visually-guided isolation of the PV antrum using a compliant laser balloon catheter. *Heart Rhythm*. 2009;6:S7.

102. Dukkipati S, d'Avila A, Doshi SK, et al. Histological lesion characteristics following PV antral ablation using a visually guided compliant balloon catheter. *Heart Rhythm*. 2009;6:S342.

103. Dukkipati S, d'Avila A, Neuzil P, et al. Comparison of radiofrequency ablation vs. visually-guided laser balloon ablation in achieving chronic pulmonary vein isolation in a porcine model. *Circulation*. 2009;120:S706.

104. Doshi SK, Neuzil P, Reddy VY. First clinical experience with a novel, variable radius, endoscopic laser balloon for pulmonary vein isolation of atrial fibrillation. *Europace*. 2009;11:S1.

105. Reddy VY, Neuzil P, Doshi SK, et al. Does visually-guided placement of contiguous ablation lesions result in reliable and persistent pulmonary vein isolation? *Circulation*. 2009;120:S706.

106. Reddy VY, Neuzil P, Themistoclakis S, et al. Visually-guided balloon catheter ablation of atrial fibrillation: experimental feasibility and first-in-human multicenter clinical outcome. *Circulation*. 2009;120:20.

107. Stewart HF. Ultrasonic measurement techniques and equipment output levels. In: Repacholi MH, Benwell DA, eds. *Essentials of Medical Ultrasound*. Clifton, NJ: Humana; 1982:77–116.

108. He DS, Zimmer JE, Hynynen FI, et al. Application of ultrasound energy for intracardiac ablation of arrhythmias. *Eur Heart J*. 1995;16:961–966.

109. Lynn JG, Zwemer RL, Chick AJ, et al. A new method for the generation and use of focused ultrasound in experimental biology. *J Gen Physiol*. 1942;26:179–193.

110. Fry W, Mosberg W, Barnard J, et al. Production of focal destructive lesions in the central nervous system. *J Neurosurg*. 1954;11:471–478.

111. Ter Haar GR, Robertson D. Tissue destruction with focused ultrasound in vivo. *Eur Urol*. 1993;23:8–11.

112. Susani M, Madersbacher S, Kratzik C, et al. Morphology of tissue destruction induced by focused ultrasound. *Eur Urol*. 1993;23:34–38.

113. Ohkubo T, Okishige K, Goseki Y, et al. Experimental study of catheter ablation using ultrasound energy in canine and porcine hearts. *Jpn Heart J*. 1998;39:399–409.

114. Repacholi M, Grondolfo M, Rindi A. *Ultrasound: Medical Applications, Biological Effects and Hazard Potential*. New York: Plenum; 1987.

115. Lee LA, Simon C, Bove EL, et al. High intensity focused ultrasound effect on cardiac tissues: potential for clinical application. *Echocardiography*. 2000;17:563–566.

116. Malcolm AL, Ter Haar GR. Ablation of tissue volumes using high intensity focused ultrasound. *Ultrasound Med Biol*. 1996;22:659–669.

117. National Council on Radiation Protection. *Biological Effects of Ultrasound: Mechanisms and Clinical Implications*. NCRP Report No 74. Bethesda, MD: National Council on Radiation Protection; 1983.

118. Zimmer JE, Hynynen K, He DS, et al. The feasibility of using ultrasound for cardiac ablation. *IEEE Trans Biomed Eng*. 1995;42:891–897.

119. Strickberger SA, Tokano T, Kluiwstra JA, et al. Extracardiac ablation of the canine atrioventricular junction by use of high intensity focused ultrasound. *Circulation*. 1999;100:203–208.

120. Wan J, VanBaren P, Ebbini E, et al. Ultrasound surgery: comparison of strategies using phased array systems. *IEEE Trans UFFC*. 1996;43:1085–1098.

121. Gentry KL, Smith SW. Integrated catheter for 3-D intracardiac echocardiography and ultrasound ablation. *IEEE Trans UFFC*. 2004;51:799–807.

122. Schmidt B, Chun J, Kuck KH, et al. Pulmonary vein isolation using high intensity focused ultrasound. *Indian Pacing Electrophysiol*. 2006;7:126–133.

123. Hynynen K, Dennie J, Zimmer JE, et al. Cylindrical ultrasonic transducers for cardiac catheter ablation. *IEEE Trans Biomed Eng*. 1997;44:144–151.

124. Lesh MD, Diederich C, Guerra G, et al. An anatomic approach to prevention of atrial fibrillation: Pulmonary vein isolation with through-the-balloon ultrasound ablation (TTBUSA). *Thorac Cardiovasc Surg*. 1999;47:347–351.

125. Azegami K, Arruda MS, Anders R. Circumferential ultrasound ablation of pulmonary vein ostia: Relationship between ablation time and lesion formation [abstract]. *J Am Coll Cardiol*. 2002;39:106A.

126. Natale A, Pisano E, Shewchik J, et al. First human experience with pulmonary vein isolation using a through-the-balloon circumferential ultrasound ablation system for recurrent atrial fibrillation. *Circulation*. 2000;102:1879–1882.

127. Saliba W, Wilber D, Packer D, et al. Circumferential ultrasound ablation for pulmonary vein isolation: analysis of acute and chronic failures. *J Card Electrophysiol*. 2002;13:957–961.

128. Meininger GR, Calkins H, Lickfett L, et al. Initial experience with a novel focused ultrasound ablation system for ring ablation outside the pulmonary vein. *J Interv Card Electrophysiol*. 2003;8:141–148.

129. Nakagawa H, Aoyama H, Pitha JV, et al. Pre-clinical canine testing of a novel high intensity, forward-focused ultrasound balloon catheter for pulmonary vein isolation. *Pacing Clin Electrophysiol*. 2003;26:954A.

130. Nakagawa H, Natz M, Wong T, et al. Initial experience using a forward directed, high-intensity focused ultrasound balloon catheter for pulmonary vein antrum isolation in patients with atrial fibrillation. *J Card Electrophysiol*. 2007;18:136–144.

131. Schmidt B, Ernst S, Ouyang F, et al. Pulmonary vein isolation by high intensity focused ultrasound with the steerable balloon catheter: first in man study. *Heart Rhythm*. 2007;4:575–584.

132. Okumura Y, Kolasa M, Johnson S, et al. Mechanism of tissue heating during high intensity focused ultrasound pulmonary vein isolation: implications for atrial fibrillation efficacy and phrenic nerve protection. *J Card Electrophysiol*. 2008;19:945–951.

133. Yokoyama K, Nakagawa H, Pitha JV, et al. Can high intensity focused ultrasound applications very close to the esophagus produce left atrial-esophageal fistula? *Heart Rhythm*. 2006;3:S56.

134. Schmidt B, Chun J, Kuck KH, et al. Pulmonary vein isolation using high intensity focused ultrasound. *Indian Pacing Electrophysiol*. 2006;7:126–133.

135. Borchert B, Lawrenz T, Hansky B, et al. Lethal atrioesophageal fistula after pulmonary vein isolation using high-intensity focused ultrasound (HIFU). *Heart Rhythm*. 2008;5:145–148.

Video

Video 5-1. Sector ablation using steerable arc of laser energy applied at the antrum of the left superior pulmonary vein in a pig. The clear laser balloon displaces blood from the ablation site allowing visualization through the balloon.

Video 5-2. Steerable focused "spot" delivery of laser energy through the balloon ex vivo.

Video 5-3. Steerable focused "spot" delivery of laser energy through the balloon in vivo in the right superior pulmonary vein of a pig. Note the appearance of the light colored endocarial lesion at the sites of energy delivery.

Video 5-4. Application of high frequency focused ultrasound energy to a clear matrix phantom. Note the circumferential "ablation" of the matrix.

Cardiac Mapping and Imaging

PART II

6

Cardiac Anatomy for Catheter Mapping and Ablation of Arrhythmias

Jerónimo Farré, Robert H. Anderson, José A. Cabrera, Damián Sánchez-Quintana, José M. Rubio, and Juan Benezet-Mazuecos

Key Points

Catheter mapping and ablation require the understanding of the cardiac anatomy, a task that is facilitated by the use of *The Visible Human Slice and Surface Server,* an open access software that uses data sets of the *Visible Human Male and Female Project.*

Although new imaging techniques, such as intracardiac echocardiography, magnetic resonance, multislice computed tomography scans, and nonfluoroscopic navigational tools reconstructing computer-based surrogates of the endocardial surface of the cardiac chambers, are being used to perform arrhythmologic catheter interventions, simple fluoroscopy and angiography are the primary imaging modalities for ablation procedures.

Interventional arrhythmologists must become familiar with the principles of radiation protection.

For better planning and understanding of ablation procedures, it is crucial to obtain a perception of the macroscopic morphologic features, architecture, and anatomic relations of the triangle of Koch, the inferior right atrial or cavotricuspid isthmus, the pyramidal space, the right ventricular outflow tract, the atrioventricular grooves, the interatrial groove and oval fossa, and the right and left atria.

An attitudinally based nomenclature should be adopted to standardize anatomic descriptions.

Studies conducted during the past three decades have unravelled anatomic, architectural, and histologic details of the heart, enlightening the substrate of tachycardias and their ablation. In this chapter, we extend the scope of previous reviews focused on the fluoroscopic heart anatomy as observed during an electrophysiologic study and catheter ablation procedure.[1–3] We discuss not only the macroscopic morphologic features of the heart, but also some architectural information of interest for arrhythmologic interventions. When appropriate, we emphasize the relations of the heart chambers with extracardiac structures that are relevant in the appreciation of potential complications of ablation procedures. As a learning tool, we strongly recommend the use of *The Visible Human Slice and Surface Server,*[4] an open access software that uses data sets of the *Visible Human Male and Female Project* (Fig. 6-1).[5] Understanding the anatomy shown by fluoroscopy and angiography from the views obtained with magnetic resonance imaging (MRI) or transthoracic and transesophageal echocardiographic studies is more difficult than with the aforementioned software because the standard projections of the latter two imaging techniques are different from the planes presented to the eyes of the interventional arrhythmologist in the fluoroscopic screen. In this chapter, we use the fluoroscopically oriented nomenclature that takes into account the correct attitudinal position of the cardiac structures (Fig. 6-1).[6]

Sources of Cardiac Imaging Used in Mapping and Ablation Procedures

Mapping and ablation procedures have been traditionally performed under the guidance of simple fluoroscopy with the aid of angiographic techniques. With simple fluoroscopy, the only anatomic references are the cardiac shadow, the spine, the diaphragm or the thoracoabdominal boundary, the mediastinum, the "fat stripe" visible in the right anterior oblique (RAO) projection that is the landmark of both atrioventricular (AV) grooves,[7] and the moving catheter electrodes positioned at certain fixed locations such as the right atrial appendage, the right ventricular apex and outflow tract, the region of the His bundle, and the coronary sinus.

Right atrial angiography enables us to define the anatomic boundaries of the triangle of Koch and the inferior or cavotricuspid isthmus (Fig. 6-2).[8–12] The size and morphology of the inferior right atrial isthmus as depicted with right atrial angiography may play a role in the ease of ablation of isthmus-dependent atrial flutter.[10–14] Cardiac MRI has also been used to investigate the anatomic characteristics of the isthmus and their relation to the ease of ablation of atrial flutter.[15]

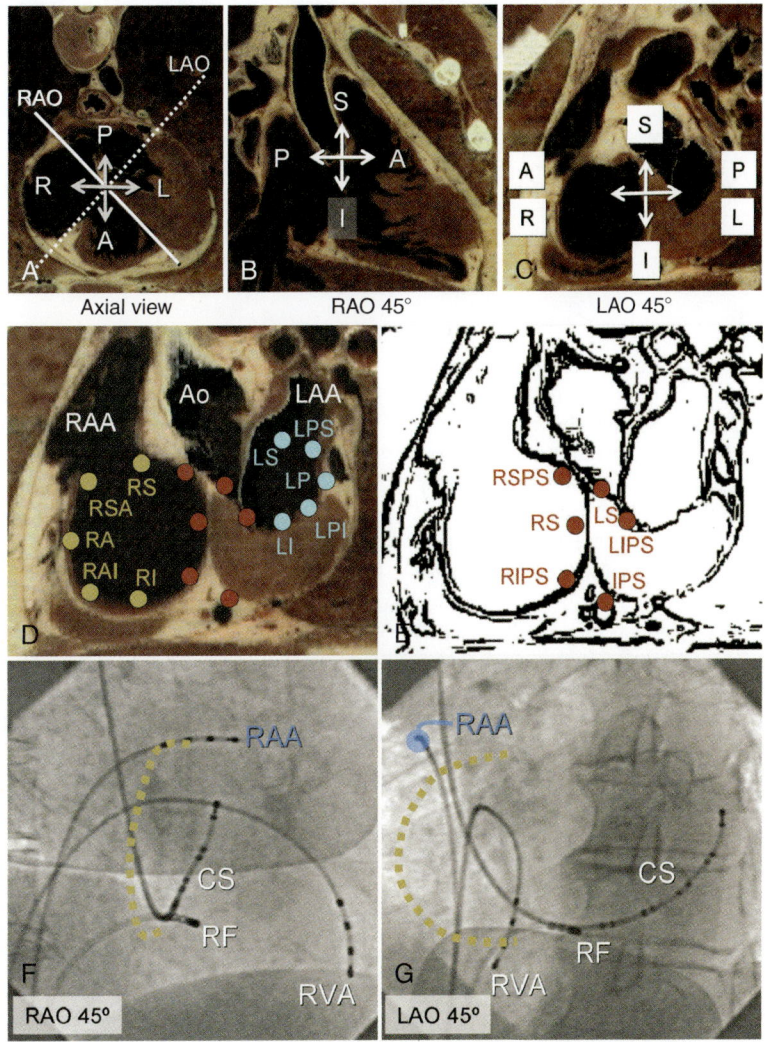

FIGURE 6-1. In this and in the rest of the figures, six slices of the heart have been obtained from *The Visible Human Slice and Surface Server*.[4] **A,** Axial slice of the heart of a male showing the four cardiac chambers. Two axes have been traced to indicate the planes of the 45-degree right and left anterior oblique projections (RAO and LAO). The right and left atrioventricular grooves are almost parallel to the fluoroscopic plane in the LAO view. The interatrial groove (interatrial septum) is almost perpendicular to the plane of the screen in the LAO projection. A frontal (antero-posterior) projection does not differentiate an anterior (A) from a posterior (P) position of the catheter. **B,** A 45-degree RAO slice obtained at the level indicated in panel **A.** This projection defines anterior (A) and posterior (P) locations, and superior (S) and inferior (I) sites. **C,** A 45-degree LAO slice that enables us to define what is right (R) and anterior (A), left (L) and posterior (P), as well as superior (S) and inferior (I). The plane of the triangle of Koch (panels **A** and **B**) is parallel to the fluoroscopic input in the RAO projection. **D** and **E,** Attitudinal nomenclature for positions in the right and left atrioventricular grooves as well as septal and paraseptal locations on an LAO slice of the heart. Ao, aorta; IPS, inferior paraseptal (in this case related to the middle cardiac vein); LI, left inferior; LIPS, left inferior paraseptal; LP, left posterior; LPI, left posteroinferior; LPS, left posterosuperior; LS, left superior (in **D**); LS, left septal (in **E**); RA, right anterior; RAI, right anteroinferior; RI, right inferior; RIPS, right inferior paraseptal; RS, right superior (in **D**); RS, right septal (in **E**), RSA, right superoanterior; RSPS, right superior paraseptal. Septal and paraseptal locations are represented by the *red circles*. There are septal accessory pathways at the right but also at the left side of the ventricular septum. **F,** A 45-degree fluorographic RAO projection showing catheter electrodes placed at the right atrial appendage (RAA), right ventricular apex (RVA), and coronary sinus (CS). A fourth catheter is used for the ablation of an accessory pathway (RF) at the ostium of the CS. **G,** A 45-degree fluorographic LAO projection. The tip of the RAA points toward the right of the screen in the RAO projection and to the left in the LAO view. In *yellow*, an imaginary line representing the theoretical location of the terminal crest in the RAO and LAO projections. The terminal crest is almost perpendicular to the imaging screen in the RAO view and forms a plane that is parallel to the image in the LAO projection. As shown in panels **F** and **G,** the RAO does not permit one to establish whether a catheter electrode is on the triangle of Koch or in the inferolateral aspect of the cavotricuspid isthmus. This can be determined using an LAO projection. *(Anatomic slices obtained from* The Visible Human Slice and Surface Server,[4] *courtesy of the Ecole Polytechnique Fédérale de Lausanne (EPFL), Professor R. D. Hersch, Peripheral Systems Laboratory,* http://visiblehuman.epfl.ch. *With permission.)*

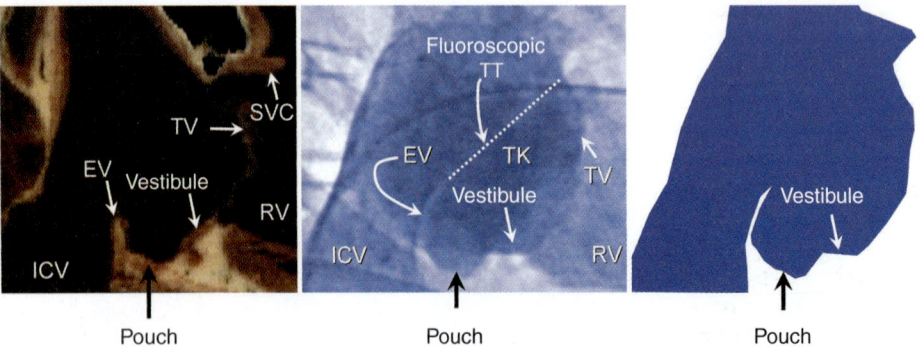

FIGURE 6-2. A, Anatomic cardiac slice in 45-degree right anterior oblique (RAO) projection.[4] **B,** Right atrial angiogram obtained by injecting contrast in the inferior caval vein, in a 45-degree RAO projection. **C,** Schematic representation of the angiogram of panel **B.** EV, eustachian valve; ICV, inferior caval vein; RV, right ventricle; TK, triangle of Koch; TT, tendon of Todaro; TV, tricuspid valve. The supraventricular crest (SVT) separates the right ventricular outflow and inflow tracts. The inferior isthmus is limited posteriorly by the eustachian valve and anteriorly by the tricuspid valve. The right atrial angiogram in the RAO projection depicts the pouch and the vestibule of the inferior right atrial isthmus. In the example of panel **B,** the tricuspid valve has a vertical orientation with a slight anterosuperior tilt. *(Anatomic slices obtained from* The Visible Human Slice and Surface Server,[4] *courtesy of the Ecole Polytechnique Fédérale de Lausanne (EPFL), Professor R. D. Hersch, Peripheral Systems Laboratory,* http://visiblehuman.epfl.ch. *With permission.)*

In addition, a coronary sinus venogram or the venous phase of a left coronary arteriogram may be obtained in patients with inferior paraseptal accessory pathways when the presence of a diverticulum is suspected (Fig. 6-3).[16–20] This malformation can also be diagnosed with multislice computed tomography (CT) and MRI studies,[21,22] but the latter investigations are rarely performed before the ablation procedure. Their additional cost is probably unjustified. Transthoracic echocardiography is useful in identifying a diverticulum of the coronary sinus, an examination that can be done at low cost before the ablation procedure in patients with inferior paraseptal, formerly known as posteroseptal, accessory pathways.[23]

Direct pulmonary venous angiography was used in the past in patients with atrial fibrillation undergoing catheter ablation procedures in and around the pulmonary veins.[24,25] These techniques were also employed to diagnose the development of pulmonary venous stenosis as a complication of applying radiofrequency (RF) pulses inside the pulmonary veins in patients with atrial fibrillation.[26,27] Direct pulmonary venous angiography is not routinely used today to depict the left atrial and pulmonary venous anatomy during ablation procedures in patients with atrial fibrillation. For this purpose, we currently use other imaging techniques, such as multislice CT scanning, MRI, or contrast-enhanced rotational radiographic angiography. Transesophageal echocardiography, multidetector CT, and MRI are also used to diagnose pulmonary venous stenosis after ablation procedures.[28–36]

Most interventional arrhythmologists currently employ nonfluoroscopic navigational tools able to reconstruct a computer-based surrogate of the endocardial surface of the heart chambers. CT and MRI studies of the cardiac chambers conducted before the ablation can be merged with these virtual reconstructions during the arrhythmologic intervention, thus combining the morphologic features of the cardiac cavities with a visually impressive degree of anatomic detail. Current systems produce a nonanimated display of the cardiac anatomy. As yet, they do not replicate the movements of the AV grooves during ventricular contraction, nor those of the diaphragm during respiration. This is why some investigators have found discrepancies between the location of an ablation spot and its representation on the electroanatomic map merged with the three-dimensional reconstructions of the

corresponding heart cavity prepared using CT or MRI techniques. Zhong and associates have assessed the accuracy of the CartoMerge software (Biosense Webster, Diamond Bar, CA) by comparing the location of the left atrial ablation points encircling the vestibules of the pulmonary veins, as determined with intracardiac echocardiography, with the corresponding locations saved on a CartoMerge image. They found an obvious inability of the CartoMerge image to localize the points of ablation in the right and left atrial vestibules.[37] This inaccuracy could be reduced by using CT and electroanatomic images obtained at the same point in the atrial mechanical cycle. This can be accomplished during a regular atrial rhythm but not during atrial fibrillation. Daccarett and associates have also found significant spatial discrepancies of up to 1 cm between locations of the catheter defined by the CartoMerge software and intracardiac echocardiography.[38] For an in-depth discussion of this topic, see Chapters 8, 9, and 10.

Despite these developments, simple fluoroscopy, with or without the aid of angiographic techniques, remains an essential guide for mapping and ablation procedures. Because of this, the integration of the perception of the cardiac anatomy with the abstract fluoroscopic landmarks is still crucial for the interventional electrophysiologist.

Radiation Protection Recommendations

Catheter ablation procedures may still require long fluoroscopic times in some instances, particularly during the learning curve of electrophysiologists in training. Radiography equipment based on an image intensifier is being replaced in many electrophysiology laboratories by flat-detector systems. These provide a better quality of image with a higher dynamic range, at a theoretically reduced dose of radiation. Without the appropriate tuning, nonetheless, the adoption of a flat detector does not necessarily imply an improvement in the quality of the image, nor does it produce a reduction in the radiation exposure for the patient and the staff, compared with the use of conventional image intensifier–based systems. The calibration of the equipment, the experience of the operator, and the methodology

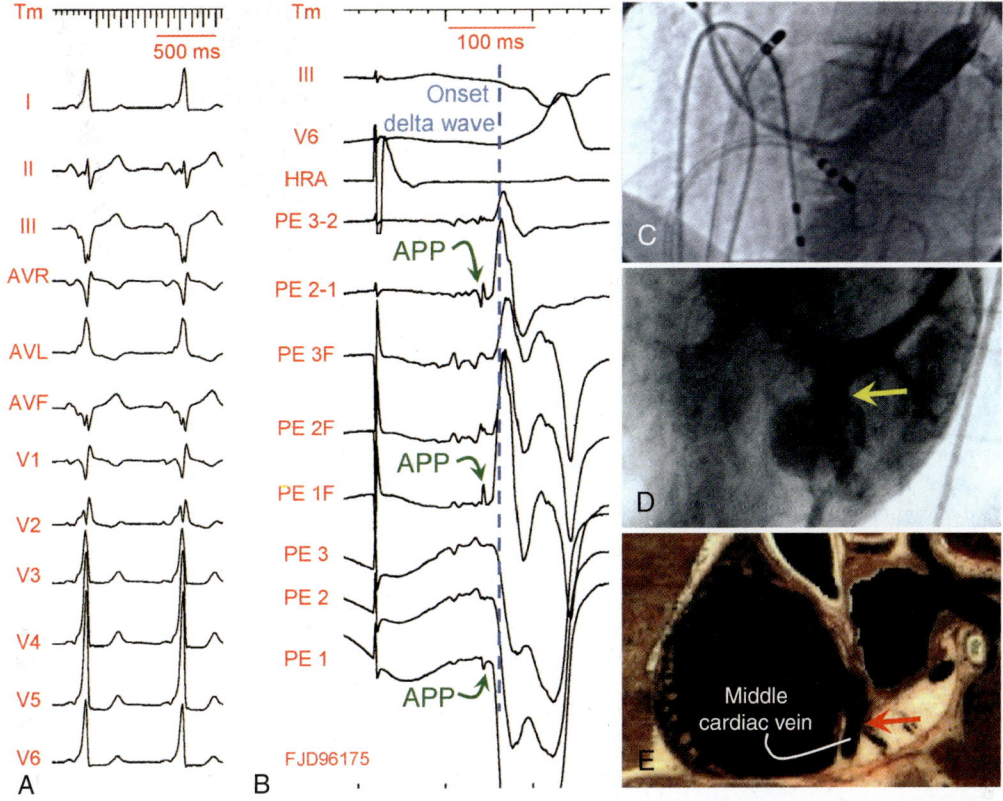

FIGURE 6-3. A, A 12-lead echocardiogram (ECG) from a patient with Wolff-Parkinson-White syndrome due to an inferior paraseptal accessory pathway. **B,** Leads III and V6 from the surface ECG are simultaneously displayed with bipolar intracardiac recording from the high right atrium (HRA), and bipolar and unipolar recordings from the probing electrode (PE) at the site of ablation of the accessory pathway. In the filtered bipolar recording from the distal pair of electrodes of the ablation catheter (PE 2-1), a fast deflection preceding the onset of the delta wave was registered that most likely represents the so-called accessory pathway potential (APP). This potential was also present at the near-DC (0.1 to 500 Hz) unfiltered unipolar recording from the distal ablating electrode (PE 1) and the filtered (30 to 500 Hz) distal unipolar recording (PE 1F). **C,** Left anterior oblique (LAO) fluorographic projection showing the ablation catheter at the site of block of the accessory pathway during the application of the radiofrequency current. A coronary sinus venogram has also been obtained, which retrogradely fills a diverticular formation in the middle cardiac vein. **D,** Venous phase of a left coronary artery angiography depicting the coronary sinus diverticulum and an inferior left ventricular venous branch ending at the neck of the diverticulum. This was the site of ablation of the accessory pathway. **E,** Anatomic slice in an LAO projection showing the entry into the coronary sinus and the middle cardiac vein as well as the ending of an inferior left ventricular venous affluent (*red arrow*). *(Anatomic slices obtained from* The Visible Human Slice and Surface Server,[4] *courtesy of the Ecole Polytechnique Fédérale de Lausanne (EPFL), Professor R. D. Hersch, Peripheral Systems Laboratory,* http://visiblehuman.epfl.ch. *With permission.)*

used at every individual laboratory play a crucial role in terms of image quality and radiation protection. In Europe, interventional cardiologists must follow accreditation training courses to be certified to use radiologic equipment. The observation of certain principles with flat-panel–or image intensifier–based systems results in a lower radiation dose for patients and staff and in improved image quality. These principles include the following[39–54]:

- Use x-ray beam systems entering the posterior and not the anterior side of the patient, thus attenuating radiation to thyroid, breasts, and eyes of the patient, and keep the radiation source far from the staff.
- Position the image intensifier or the flat detector as close as possible to the chest of the patient.
- Use collimation to limit the size of the explored field and to reduce scattered radiation (flat detectors in this regard have the advantage of collimating the x-ray beam to the size of the detector).
- Use the largest possible field of the image intensifier or flat panel because magnification increases the dose (for electrophysiologic studies and ablation procedures, the largest field is the most appropriate one); when using large fields, collimation is usually necessary even with flat panels.

- Use the semitransparent wedge filters to overcome blooming of the lung image when the automatic gain control is centered over the heart shadow, particularly in the RAO and left anterior oblique (LAO) projections with more than a 30-degree tilt, and to reduce excessive radiation at the corresponding skin areas of the patient.
- Use pulsed, not continuous, fluoroscopy at the lowest possible frame rate and the lowest possible dose per second that results in an acceptable appreciation of the fluoroscopic details; for transseptal puncture, it may be needed to allow a higher level of radiation dose for better fluoroscopic detail; once the left atrium has been reached, a lower radiation dose for the fluoroscopy regimen must be selected.
- Use digital fluorography at the lowest possible frame rate and for the shortest possible duration rather than 35-mm filming to store positions of catheters or angiographic information; 35-mm cine-films are seldom obtained today in cardiovascular interventional laboratories; documentation of the relevant catheter positions can be done from fluoroscopy or with single-shot fluorography, thus reducing the radiation exposure of the patient and personnel.

- Keep fluoroscopy time as low as possible (use an intermittent rather than a continuous view of catheters during RF application).
- Maintain the personnel as far as possible from the radiation source and the patient because scatter radiation decreases with the square of the distance from the radiation source, which is the patient in this case.
- Use all possible protections, such as a leaded acrylic glass between patient and operator, leaded aprons, neck collars and glasses, and filtration of the primary x-ray beam.
- Manipulate catheters as little as possible from a subclavian or jugular approach and use preferably the femoral approach that results in less scattered radiation for the exploring physician.
- When possible, use the RAO or anteroposterior (AP) projection rather than the LAO projection because the latter is the worst in terms of secondary radiation for the exploring physician.
- Lateral projections are rarely needed in ablation procedures; some interventional cardiologists use the lateral projection for transseptal puncture; if that is the case, the right lateral rather than the left lateral projection is used to avoid having the radiation source close to the interventional cardiologist; lateral projections demand higher

radiation outputs and result in more scatter radiation for the personnel close to the patient.

Potential problems associated with radiation during catheter ablation procedures are the development of various forms of malignant tumors, genetic abnormalities, and skin injuries. Failed procedures are associated with significantly longer fluoroscopy times than successful interventions.[54] The dose needed to cause radiation skin injury is exceeded in about one fifth of the procedures, at least with image intensifier systems.[54]

Cardiac Fluoroscopic Projections and Nomenclature

The understanding of the attitudinally oriented nomenclature of cardiac anatomy endorsed by the European Society of Cardiology and the North American Society of Pacing and Electrophysiology[6] is facilitated by *The Visible Human Slice and Surface Server*, a software program developed by Hersch and coworkers from the Geneva Hospitals and WDS Technologies SA[4] from data sets of the *Visible Human Male and Female Project* of the National Library of Medicine, United States.[5] The right atrium is indeed positioned on the right, but the left atrium is mainly a posterior structure (Fig. 6-4; see also Fig. 6-1A). Only the tip

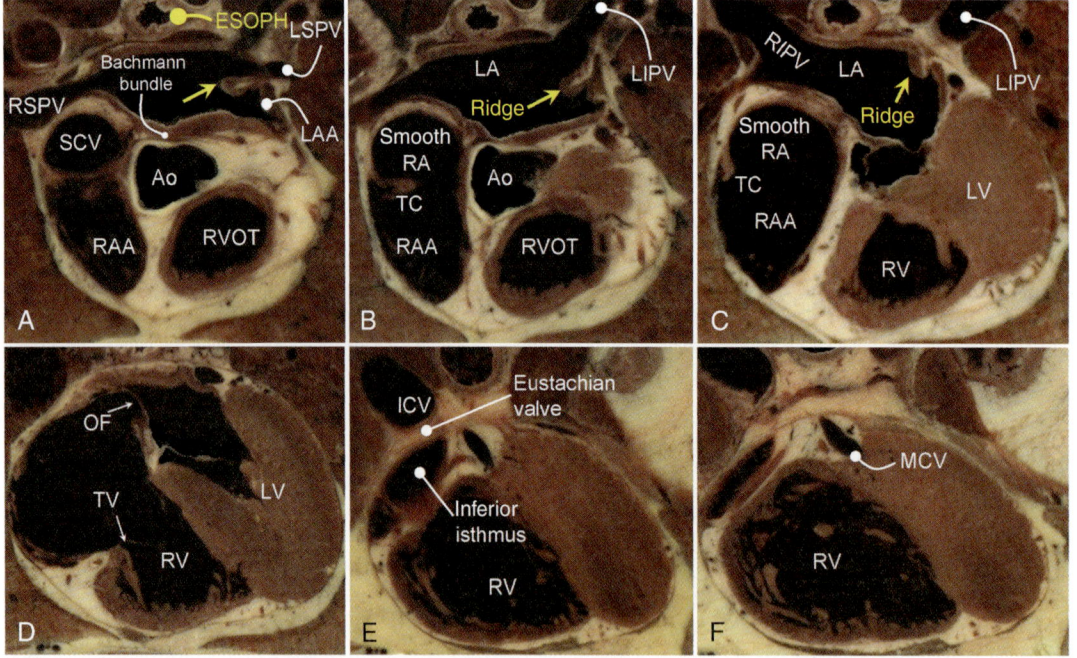

FIGURE 6-4. Right and left atrial anatomy as depicted with axial slices from a male heart.[4] Panels **A** to **F** are succeeding slides obtained in a cranial-to-caudal sequence. The slice in **A** has been obtained at the junction between the superior caval vein (SCV) and the right atrium. Anterior to the SCV can be seen the trabeculated right atrium forming the right atrial appendage (RAA). At this level, the terminal crest originates from the interatrial groove where the atrial myocytes are confluent with the beginning of the Bachmann bundle that extends itself into the left atrium. The superior apex of the RAA (**A** and **B**) is close to the myocardium of the right ventricular outflow tract (RVOT). Within the left atrium (LA), we observe that the left atrial appendage (LAA) is anterior to the left superior pulmonary vein (LSPV). The slice in **B** shows the terminal crest (TC) separating the posterior smooth right atrium and the trabeculated RAA. The right superior pulmonary vein (RSPV) is behind the smooth right atrium at this level. The *yellow arrow* (**A** to **C**) signals the lateral ridge of the left lateral atrial wall. In this case, the ridge extends beyond the origin of the left inferior pulmonary vein. The esophagus (ESOPH) is in close relation to the posterior left atrial wall (**A** to **C**). The right and left atrial myocardia (**C**) form a sandwich that contains fibrofatty tissue. Anatomically speaking, this is an interatrial groove more than an interatrial septum. The right inferior pulmonary vein (RIPV) drains into the left atrium at a more caudal level than the left inferior pulmonary vein (LIPV). More caudally (**D**) is seen the oval fossa (OF), a fibrous tissue that is a true interatrial septum. At a more caudal location (**E** and **F**) is the inferior isthmus between the inferior caval vein (ICV) and the tricuspid valve (TV). The eustachian valve separates the ICV from the inferior right atrial isthmus. The inferolateral components of the isthmus are shown in **F**. MCV, mid-cardiac vein. Note that the more caudal region of the posterior left atrial wall (**D**) is thicker than the more superior segments, particularly at the level of the areas where the pulmonary veins originate (**A** to **C**). (*Anatomic slices obtained from* The Visible Human Slice and Surface Server[4], *courtesy of the Ecole Polytechnique Fédérale de Lausanne (EPFL), Professor R. D. Hersch, Peripheral Systems Laboratory,* http://visiblehuman.epfl.ch. *With permission.*)

of the left atrial appendage contributes to the left cardiac silhouette in a frontal fluoroscopic view of the body. For the same reasons, the right ventricle is not a right-sided, but an anterior, cavity. In this chapter, we use the attitudinal nomenclature, albeit retaining traditional names such as right and left atria and right and left ventricles, for the sake of clarity.

The fluoroscopic examination during catheter-electrode mapping and ablation procedures is performed using the frontal and oblique projections. The frontal view is used to introduce and position catheters in the apex and outflow tract of the right ventricle, in the right atrial appendage or in the lateral aspect of the right atrium, and in the region of the His bundle. We also use the frontal projection to enter into the left ventricle from a retrograde aortic approach. Although positioning of the so-called halo catheter is usually accomplished using an LAO projection, the RAO serves to

finally ensure that the distal electrodes are at the right inferior cavotricuspid isthmus (Fig. 6-5A and C). The His bundle catheter can usually be placed at the right spot using a frontal projection, but occasionally an LAO view may help in obtaining a good recording of the His bundle potential. The LAO projection is generally used to catheterize the coronary sinus independently of the venous approach.

Although different laboratories may have their own preferences regarding the degree of rotation to obtain the oblique projections, we usually prefer a 45-degree tilt for both of them. From an attitudinal point of view, the RAO projection defines what is anterior, posterior, superior, and inferior (Fig. 6-1). The LAO projection defines superior, inferior, anterior, and posterior locations for both the right and left AV grooves, which are almost parallel to the plane of the fluoroscopic image in this view (Fig. 6-1).

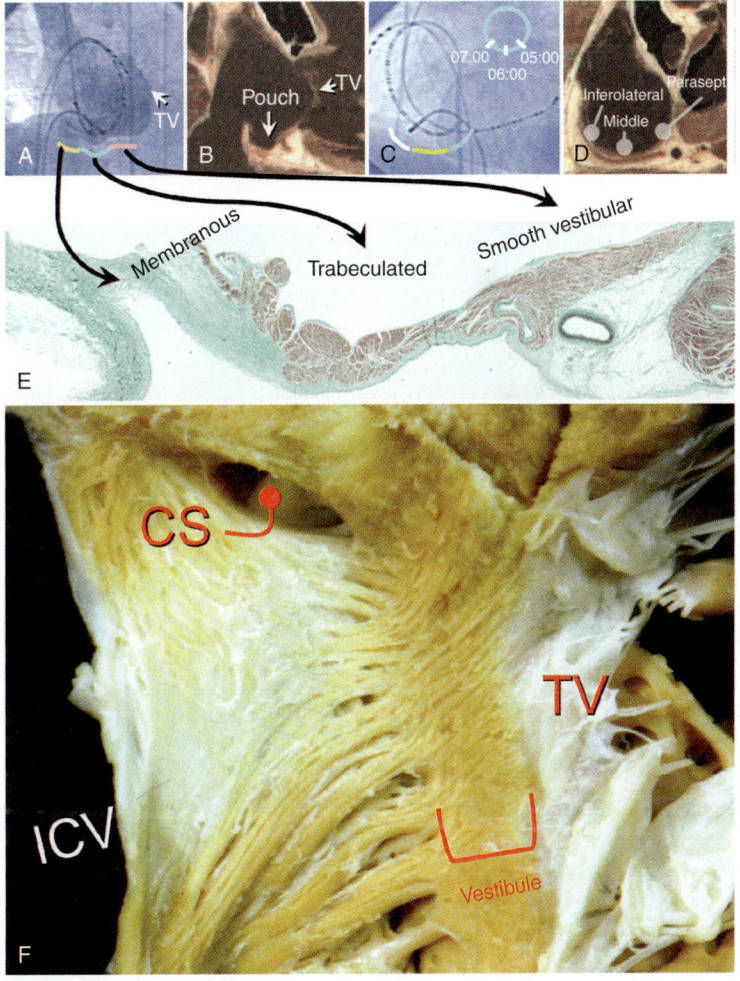

FIGURE 6-5. A, Right atrial angiogram in a right anterior oblique (RAO) projection showing three regions in the inferior isthmus (see text). **B,** Cardiac slice in RAO projection.[4] **C,** Fluoroscopic view of the catheters in left anterior oblique (LAO) projection. The ablation catheter is located in the inferolateral region of the inferior isthmus. The three regions that must be identified in this projection (inferolateral, middle, and paraseptal) are also shown in white, yellow, and cyan. **D,** Anatomic slice in LAO projection illustrating the aforementioned three regions of the inferior isthmus in this projection. **E,** Histologic section of the isthmus obtained between the middle and the paraseptal regions and depicting the architecture of the posterior membranous sector, the intermediate trabeculated muscular area, and the smooth anterior vestibular area, which also contains atrial myocardium (see text). **F,** Dissection of the inferior isthmus showing the pectinate muscles inserting at the vestibule. The endocardium has been peeled out to visualize the myocardial content of the vestibule. Note the parallel distribution of the vestibular myocardial bundles running almost perpendicular to the hinge of the tricuspid valve. ICV, inferior caval vein; CS, coronary sinus; TV, tricuspid valve. *(Anatomic slices obtained from* The Visible Human Slice and Surface Server,[4] *courtesy of the Ecole Polytechnique Fédérale de Lausanne (EPFL), Professor R. D. Hersch, Peripheral Systems Laboratory,* http://visiblehuman.epfl.ch. *With permission.)*

Right Atrium

Terminal Crest and Smooth-Walled Right Atrium

The right atrium consists of a flat-walled posterior venous portion, along with a trabeculated anterolateral sector, which is the pectinated right atrial appendage. These two right atrial compartments are separated by the terminal crest (Fig. 6-4). Although it is often thought that the right atrial appendage is only the tip of the trabeculated anterolateral sector, the correct concept is to consider the entirety of the pectinated anterolateral compartment of the right atrium as the appendage. When considering the location of the terminal crest, this prominent muscular bundle extends from its origin at the interatrial groove anteriorly to the mouth of the superior caval vein and runs laterally and inferiorly to terminate in the region of the vestibule of the tricuspid valve adjacent to the mouth of the coronary sinus (Fig. 6-6; see also Fig. 6-4). In the RAO projection, the terminal crest is almost perpendicular to the fluoroscopic screen (see Fig. 6-1F). In the LAO projection, the C-shaped structure of the crest is more or less parallel to the plane of the image intensifier (Fig. 6-1G). At its origin, the crest is confluent with the beginning of the Bachmann bundle, which extends into the left atrium (Fig. 6-7; see also Fig. 6-4). The aggregation of the myocytes within the pectinate muscles varies from heart to heart, and usually there are abundant crossovers, with small interlacing trabeculations interconnecting the individual pectinate muscles. Within the muscles themselves, nonetheless, the myocytes are aligned parallel to the long axis of the pectinate muscles.[55] In between the edges of the pectinate muscles, the right atrial wall is very thin, almost parchment-like. The pectinate muscles do not reach the orifice of the tricuspid valve. On the contrary, there is always a smooth muscular rim surrounding the insertions of the leaflets of the tricuspid valve. This is called the *right atrial vestibule* (Figs. 6-5 and 6-6). The terminal crest is important in interventional arrhythmology for at least three reasons. First, it is a barrier to conduction, probably more functional than anatomic, in isthmus-dependent atrial flutter.[56,57] Second, it is the origin of many focal right atrial tachycardias in patients without structural heart disease.[58] Third, ablation of the terminal crest has been used in patients with inappropriate sinus tachycardia.[59]

Region of the Sinus Node

The human sinus node is a crescent-like formation just over 1 cm in length located in the superior part of the terminal groove, close to the junction between the superior caval vein and the right atrial appendage.[60] It extends laterally along the terminal groove, gradually penetrating through the thickness of the terminal crest to terminate in a tail that is buried deep in the myocardium of the terminal crest. The margins of the sinus node are irregular, with multiple short radiations extending toward the superior caval vein, to the subepicardium, and intramurally into the ordinary myocardium of the terminal crest or intercaval area (Fig. 6-8A). These radiations, together with the noncompact arrangement of the nodal tail in many cases, may account for the absence of a single discrete site of exit of the normal sinus node activation front into the right atrium.[60,61] The radiations from the sinus node may also explain why, during sinus nodal reentry tachycardia, it is possible to ablate the earliest site of atrial activation, only to find thereafter that the tachycardia is still inducible but with a usually more caudal right atrial exit point.

The myocytes of the sinus node are supported by a dense matrix of connective tissue, but there are no sheaths of fibrous tissue insulating it from the neighboring working myocardium. Nevertheless, the sinus node is relatively protected against RF catheter ablation for different reasons. First, most of the sinus node is a subepicardial structure, relatively distant from the right atrial endocardium. Second, the almost constantly present central artery exerts a cooling effect on the cells of the node. Third, a significant mass of the node is separated from the right atrial endocardium by the thick terminal crest. Fourth, it is an extensive structure not amenable to a focal complete injury. Fifth, as already emphasized, the nodal cells are packed in a dense matrix of connective tissue.[60] These factors probably explain why endocardial catheter ablation of the node is difficult (Fig. 6-8). In patients with inappropriate sinus tachycardia, the results of RF catheter ablation have been poorer than those of other atrial tachycardias, even with three-dimensional electroanatomic mapping or endoepicardial approaches.[59,62–65] Improved outcomes have been obtained using intracardiac ultrasound to achieve transmural lesions.[66] Even better results have been reported with a complex methodology involving noncontact mapping, saline-cooled catheter ablation, complete autonomic blockade with atropine and

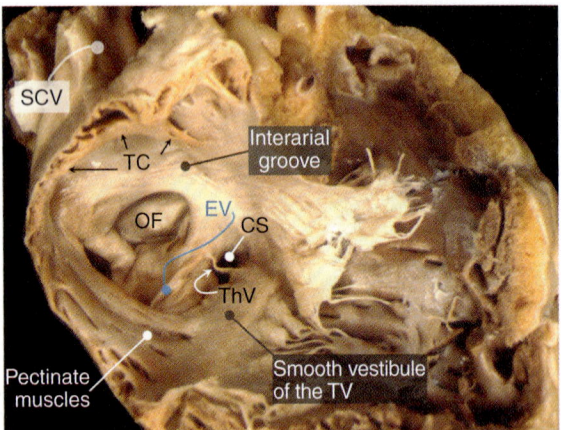

FIGURE 6-6. Gross human necropsy specimen showing the right atrium and its most important anatomic landmarks as viewed in an attitudinal right anterior oblique projection. The so-called muscular interatrial septum is in fact an interatrial groove formed by the apposition of the right and left atrial myocardia that are separated by fibrofatty tissue. Anterior to the oval fossa (OF) there is a prominent muscular rim known as the *anterior limbus*. The terminal crest (TC) is a C-shaped thick muscular bundle that distally ramifies to form the pectinate muscles. The eustachian valve (EV) separates the inferior caval vein from the inferior right atrial isthmus. At this level and toward the tricuspid valve insertion, the right atrium forms a smooth vestibule. The thebesian valve (ThV) guards the entry into the coronary sinus (CS).

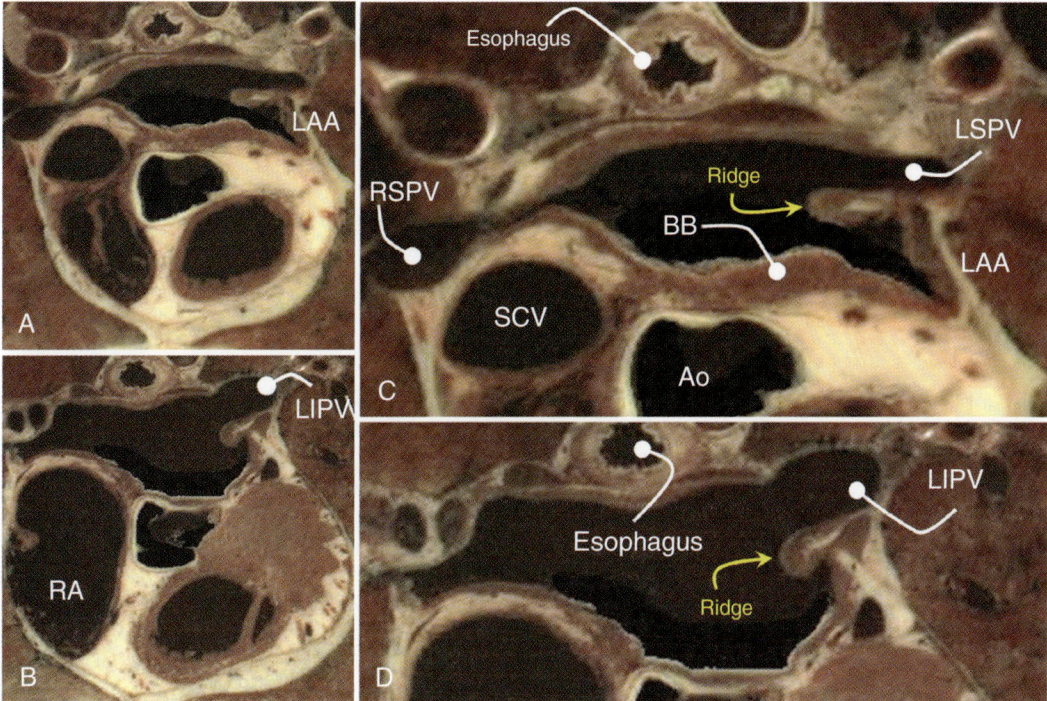

FIGURE 6-7. A and **B,** Two axial slices of a male human heart.[4] **A,** This slice has been obtained at the level of the left atrial appendage (LAA) and the junction between the right atrium (RA) and the superior caval vein (SCV). **B,** A more caudal slice (note the origin of the left inferior pulmonary vein [LIPV] from the left atrium). **C** and **D,** Enlargements of **A** and **B,** respectively. Medially, the myocardium of the terminal crest is confluent with the beginning of the Bachmann bundle (BB) (**A** and **C**). **A** and **C** also depict the thick anterior left atrial wall at the level of the BB. The anterior left atrial wall becomes thinner caudally, close to the mitral valve (**B** and **D**). The left superior and inferior pulmonary veins (LSPV, LIPV) are a little more cranially located than the right pulmonary veins. Note (in **C** and **D**) the close relation of the esophagus with the left atrial posterior wall. Finally, the left atrial lateral ridge is a fold of the left atrial wall behind the left atrial appendage (LAA), which in this case extends from the left superior pulmonary vein to the orifice of the left inferior pulmonary vein. Ao, aorta; RSPV, right superior pulmonary vein. *(Anatomic slices obtained from* The Visible Human Slice and Surface Server,[4] *courtesy of the Ecole Polytechnique Fédérale de Lausanne (EPFL), Professor R. D. Hersch, Peripheral Systems Laboratory,* http://visiblehuman.epfl.ch. *With permission.)*

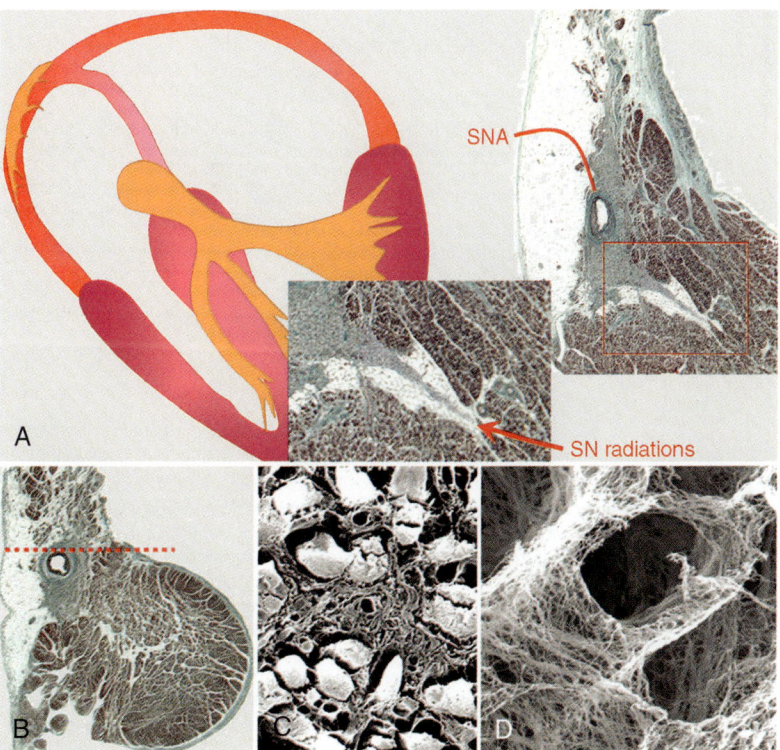

FIGURE 6-8. A, Schematic representation of the heart and its electrical installation where the sinus node (SN) has been represented as a long structure at the junction between the superior caval vein and the right atrium, with various radiations along its course. On the right, a histologic section of the right atrial wall at the level of the sinus node shows the nodal tissue around the sinus node artery (SNA). Note the radiation of sinus node tissue extending in between the working right atrial myocardial bundles (*insert and red arrow*). The sinus node, despite lacking a sheath of connective tissue, is relatively protected against radiofrequency catheter ablation for different reasons: (1) its subepicardial rather than subendocardial location (**A** and **B**), (2) the protection provided by the thick terminal crest over a significant mass of the node, usually the area below the upper limit of the sinus node artery (**B,** *red dotted line*), (3) the packing of the nodal cells in a dense matrix of connective tissue (**C** and **D** displaying the structure of the sinus node as observed with scanning electronic microscopy), (4) the cooling effect of the central sinus node artery (**A** and **B**), (5) its length, which prevents a focal complete injury (**A**).

propranolol, and the infusion of isoproterenol to ablate all P-wave morphologies.[67]

Recently, morphologic and immunocytochemical studies, combined with analysis of ion channels, have revealed the presence of a previously unidentified extensive paranodal area, close to but not continuous with the sinus node and composed of a loosely packed combination of nodal and atrial myocytes. The role of this area in the normal sinoatrial conduction, in the genesis of tachycardias originating from the terminal crest, and in atrial fibrillation is still unclear.[68]

Right Atrial Appendage

As we have emphasized, the entirety of the trabeculated wall of the right atrium anterior to the terminal crest is the right atrial appendage, not only its triangular tip. This pectinated component extends all around the smooth vestibule of the tricuspid valve (Fig. 6-6). To position a catheter electrode in the triangular tip of the right atrial appendage, we prefer to use the frontal or AP projection. In this fluoroscopic view, the catheter tip, when at the apex of the appendage, moves from left to right, and from right to left, the so-called negation movement. The tip of the appendage is superior and anterior, overlying the anterosuperior aspect of the right AV groove (Fig. 6-4A and B). When a catheter is placed at the apex of the right atrial appendage,

its tip points to the right of the screen in the RAO projection and to the left in the LAO view (Fig. 6-9; see also Fig. 6-1F and G). The arrhythmologic interest of the right atrial appendage is the existence of accessory pathways connecting this structure with the right ventricular myocardium (Fig. 6-9)[69] and of some focal atrial tachycardias arising at this area.[70] The injection of contrast from the junction between the inferior caval vein and the right atrium in the LAO projection facilitates the identification of the ablating catheter within the apex of the right atrial appendage (Fig. 6-9).

Junction between the Superior Caval Vein and Right Atrium

As shown in Figure 6-4A, the right superior pulmonary vein passes posterior to the superior caval vein at its junction with the right atrium. There are extensions of the right atrial myocardium toward the superior caval vein in the normal heart as well as in patients with atrial fibrillation and less frequently over the inferior caval vein.[71] These myocardial sleeves over the caval veins have been identified in three fourths of human hearts and may be an arrhythmogenic trigger of atrial fibrillation in some individuals. Ablative interventions approaching these caval extensions have been reported in patients with atrial fibrillation.[72–75]

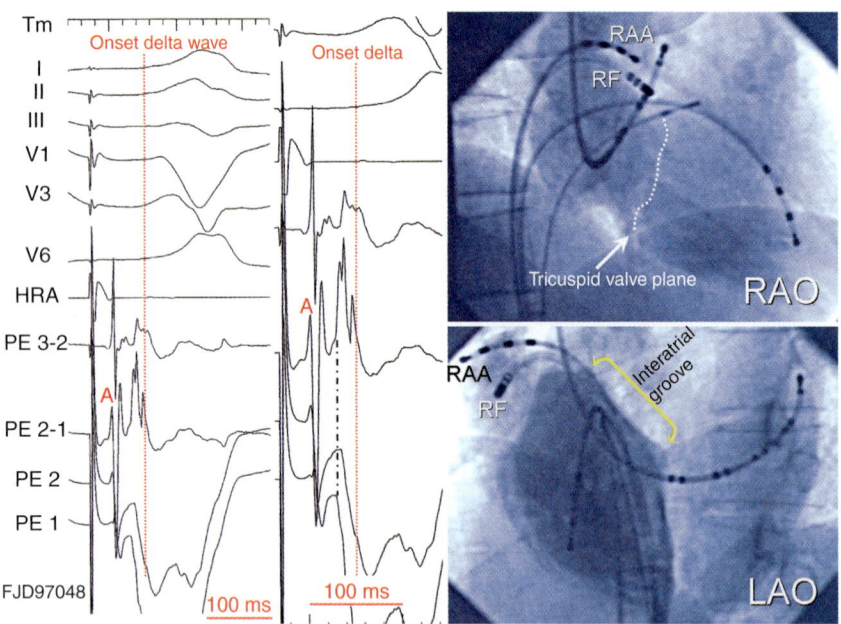

FIGURE 6-9. Accessory pathway connecting the right atrial appendage with the right ventricle. The *left panel* shows the simultaneous display of six surface electrocardiogram (ECG) leads and several intracardiac bipolar and unipolar recordings. HRA, high right atrium; PE, probing electrode. In the bipolar recording from the two distal electrodes of the ablation catheter (PE 2-1), there is an electrogram between the local atrial activation (**A**) and the onset of the delta wave in the surface ECG leads. This predelta local activation is coincidental with the onset of a QS potential in the unfiltered unipolar lead (PE 1), as shown in detail in the magnified recording of the *middle panel*. The *right panel* shows the fluorographic right anterior oblique (RAO) and left anterior oblique (LAO) views of the catheters with the probing electrode at the site of successful ablation of the accessory pathway (RF). Both fluorographic frames have been obtained during the injection of radiographic contrast in the right atrium. Note that the position of the tip of the ablation catheter is far from the level of the tricuspid valve plane. Also note that the terminal portion of the ablation catheter appears to be outside the boundaries of the right atrium as outlined by the radiographic contrast. This is because the manual injection of contrast did not fill the tip of the right atrial appendage, which is where the catheter was located, to ablate this very rare type of accessory pathway. Note that the interatrial groove is perpendicular to the plane of the image intensifier in the LAO projection. The tricuspid valve in the RAO projection has a vertical orientation with a slight anterosuperior tilt.

Eustachian Valve, Eustachian Ridge, and Tendon of Todaro

In the adult, the eustachian valve separates the inferior caval vein from the smooth vestibular inferior right atrium (Figs. 6-4E and 6-6). The eustachian valve can be fluoroscopically visualized in the RAO projection only after injecting contrast into the inferior caval vein close to its right atrial junction (Fig. 6-10; see also Fig. 6-2). In some instances, the eustachian valve is very well developed, with a fibromuscular content. Under those circumstances, it may pose an obstacle when catheterizing the coronary sinus from the femoral venous approach. Occasionally, the eustachian valve is perforated, or takes the form of a mesh or thick spiderweb, the so-called Chiari network. A catheter electrode may be entrapped during its manipulation in the Chiari network, a situation that can be worrisome, but one that can be solved when a continuous traction is applied on the catheter during a certain period of time.

The eustachian ridge is a rim between the oval foramen and the coronary sinus in continuation with the

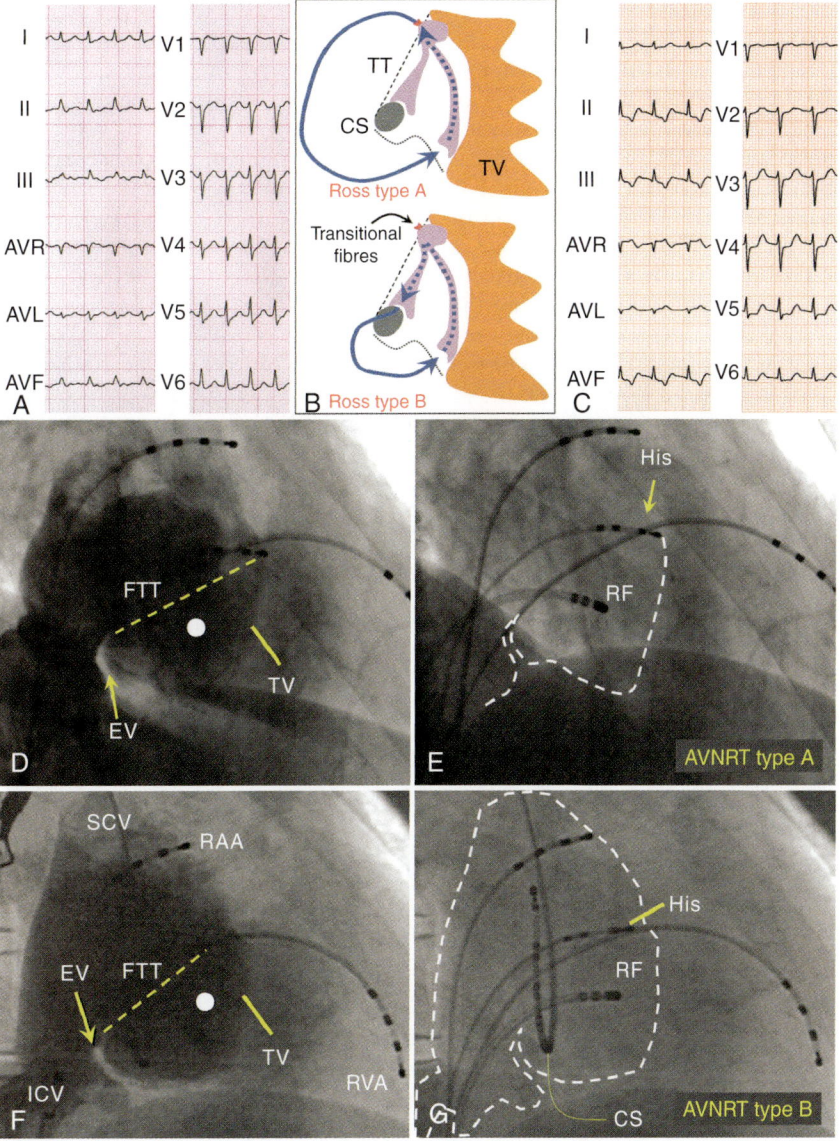

FIGURE 6-10. Two examples of atrioventricular nodal reentry tachycardia (AVNRT) of the so-called slow-fast type (**A**) and slow-slow type (**C**), also known as *types A and B of Ross*, respectively. **B,** The possible mechanisms of these two types of AVNRT and the role of the inferior extensions of the atrioventricular (AV) node as the potential substrate for the slow-type pathway of the circus movement mechanism. The triangle of Koch is schematically represented with the compact AV node at its superior angle, which has two inferior nodal extensions, one directed toward the coronary sinus and the other traveling along the border of the hinge of the septal leaflet of the tricuspid valve. **D** and **E,** Fluorographic frames in right anterior oblique projection showing a right atrial angiogram depicting the eustachian valve (EV), the fluoroscopic tendon of Todaro (FTT), and the tricuspid valve (TV). **E,** The site of ablation of the slow pathway in this patient who had a common slow-fast AV nodal reentry tachycardia (shown in **A**). The *interrupted white line* reproduces the limits of the eustachian and tricuspid valves as defined with the right atrial angiogram. The ablation site is represented in **D** as a *white circle.* **F** and **G,** Fluorographic frames in the right anterior oblique projection of the right atrial angiogram and the site of ablation of the slow pathway in a patient with a slow-slow AVNRT (**C**). The right atrial boundaries, as depicted during angiography, have been superimposed on the frame showing the ablation site. The *white circle* in **F** represents the approximate ablation site. Note that the margins of the tricuspid valve have a vertical orientation (**F**) or a slight anterosuperior tilt (**D**). CS, coronary sinus; ICV, inferior caval vein; RAA, right atrial appendage; RF, radiofrequency; RVA, right ventricular apex; SCV, superior caval vein.

insertion of the eustachian valve. It contains the tendon of Todaro, a fibrous structure not constantly present in the adult human heart.[76, 77] When the tendon of Todaro is fully developed, it has a superior course under the eustachian ridge toward the central fibrous body, ending at the junction between the AV node and the His bundle, or directly above the bundle.[77] The fluoroscopic equivalent of the tendon of Todaro—or better, of the eustachian ridge—is an imaginary line traced between the upper border of the orifice of the coronary sinus or the uppermost extreme of the eustachian valve, the latter being depicted only with right atrial angiography and the anterosuperior limit of the septal leaflet of the tricuspid valve (Fig. 6-2) or, better, the distal electrode of the catheter obtaining the largest His bundle potential (Fig. 6-10). Although this fluoroscopic representation of the tendon of Todaro is an imaginary concept, its best estimation is the line between the uppermost extreme of the eustachian valve and distal electrode of the His bundle catheter because the latter is related to the central fibrous body where the tendon of Todaro should insert. Conversely, when the reference is the anterosuperior limit of the septal leaflet of the tricuspid valve, as shown in Figure 6-2, we might be taking the supraventricular crest rather than the location of the central fibrous body, and our estimation of the course of the tendon would be not very accurate.

Inferior (Cavotricuspid) Right Atrial Isthmus

The inferior right atrial isthmus is the zone of slow conduction of the macro-reentrant circuit responsible for isthmus-dependent atrial flutters, namely the common counter-clockwise flutter, the uncommon clockwise form, and the more exceptional lower-loop reentry atrial flutter.[78–82] The right atrial inferior isthmus is limited posteriorly by the eustachian valve and anteriorly by the annular insertion of the septal leaflet of the tricuspid valve (Figs. 6-2, 6-4E, 6-5, and 6-6).

Anterior and inferior to the eustachian valve, there is a pouchlike formation, or recess, that continues more anteriorly with the smooth-walled vestibule of the tricuspid valve (Figs. 6-2, 6-5, and 6-10). This pouch and the vestibule of the tricuspid valve are clearly depicted in the RAO projection by injecting contrast into the inferior caval vein (Figs. 6-2, 6-5, and 6-10). The degree of development of the pouch and its angiographic demarcation in relation to the tricuspid vestibule vary from patient to patient.[9–15] The vestibule of the tricuspid valve, under its smooth endocardial aspect (Fig. 6-6), contains bundles of myocytes that become apparent upon peeling out the endocardium or with histologic sections (Fig. 6-5). These vestibular myocardial bundles are usually aligned in a parallel fashion, packed almost perpendicularly to the hinge of the tricuspid valve (Fig. 6-5). The myocardial architecture of the isthmus explains why the propagation of the activation wavefront along this area during isthmian atrial flutter has to be necessarily slow.

In patients with isthmus-dependent atrial flutter, the relations of the ablation catheter with the inferior isthmus must be explored using both RAO and LAO projections. This cavotricuspid isthmus is the inferior border of the right atrium in both the RAO and LAO projections (Figs. 6-2, 6-5, and 6-10). In the right atrial angiogram obtained in the RAO view, the isthmus consists of three areas. The posterior region is mainly membranous, the intermediate pouch is muscular and trabeculated, and the anterior smooth region, also muscular, is the vestibule of the tricuspid valve (Figs. 6-2, 6-4E, 6-5, and 6-6).[79,83] Fluoroscopically, these three regions of the inferior isthmus cannot be visualized without angiographic techniques. The myocardial content of the posterior (membranous) and middle (pouch) sectors, as viewed in the RAO projection, is scanty.[83] The LAO projection also reveals three zones. The medial or paraseptal region is seen at 5 o'clock, with the mid-inferior area seen at 6 o'clock, and the lateral portion, which attitudinally speaking is inferolateral, at 7 o'clock (Fig. 6-5). These three regions can readily be identified with simple fluoroscopy. In terms of myocardial content, the central or inferior isthmus is thinnest. The paraseptal isthmus has the thickest wall, being relatively close to the AV nodal artery and the inferior extensions of the AV node. The endocardial aspect of the inferolateral isthmus was shown to be within 0.5 cm of the right coronary artery in half of the hearts examined at autopsy.[83] These findings may be of some interest in selecting the ablation target, looking for areas with less myocardial content and far from vascular or electrophysiologically important structures at potential risk during RF application, particularly when the latter is performed with 8-mm-tip or cooled-tip electrodes.[83] The pretricuspid subendocardial bundles of atrial vestibular myocardium are a frequent target for the ablation of isthmian atrial flutters, particularly when the ablation is performed at the paraseptal area of the inferior isthmus (Fig. 6-11).

Angiographically, the dimensions of the right atrium and the inferior isthmus are larger in patients with isthmus-dependent atrial flutter than in normal controls.[9] This enlarged right atrium, including the inferior isthmus, may provide the pathophysiologic basis for sustaining atrial flutter within an otherwise universally existing anatomic substrate. It remains controversial, however, whether the variable angiographic expression of the inferior isthmus may influence the ease of creation of a complete bidirectional block across this anatomic landmark.[10–15] In a recent study using preablation multislice CT, the only predictor for the ease of creation of bidirectional isthmus block in patients with atrial flutter was the distance between the cavotricuspid isthmus and the right coronary artery.[82] This dimension was taken as a surrogate for the thickness of the isthmus and was measured as the shortest distance between the right coronary artery wall in the AV groove and the endocardial interface of the inferior isthmus. Others, using right atrial angiography at the time of the ablation procedure, have found that the shape and dimensions of the isthmus may serve to select the most appropriate catheter for ablation. It was suggested that an 8-mm-tip catheter electrode is effective and cheaper for ablating an isthmian atrial flutter when the inferior isthmus has a straight angiographic morphology, whereas externally cooled-tip catheters are a better choice for an angiographically concave isthmus.[12] In a subsequent controlled study from the same group, the angiographic evaluation enabled them to select the most appropriate catheter for ablation with an advantage over the empirical use of an

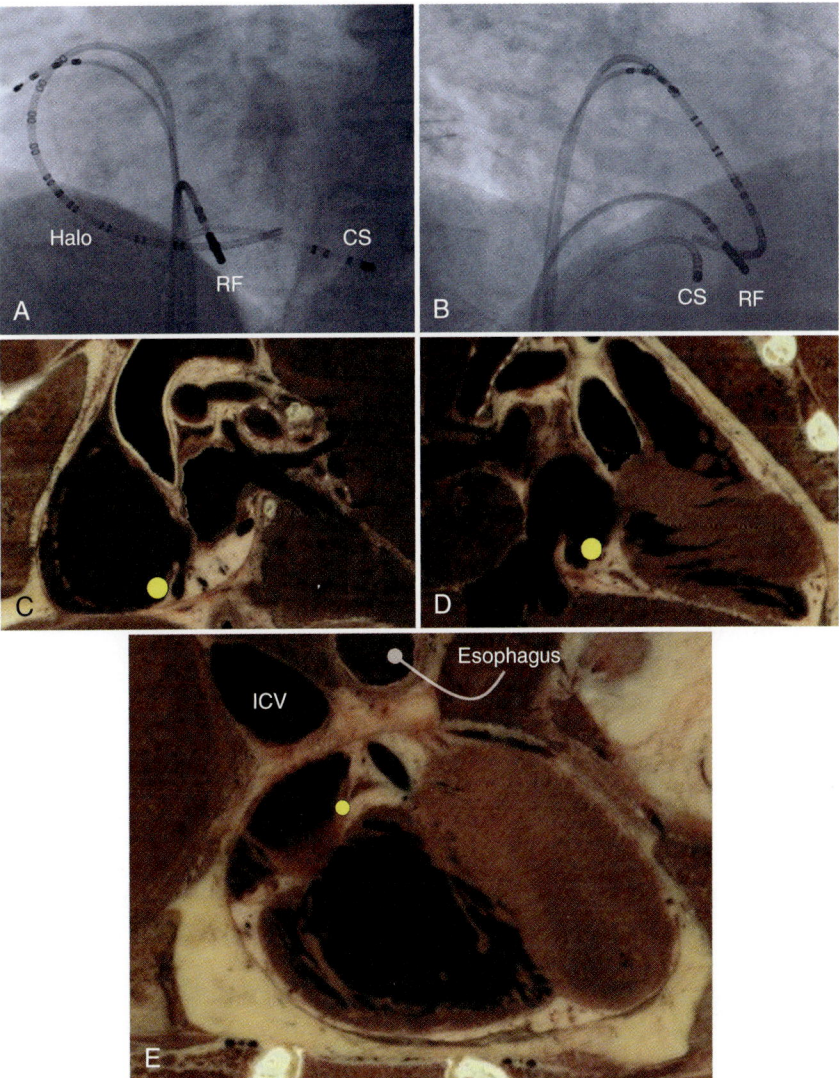

FIGURE 6-11. Ablation of the inferior right atrial isthmus at its paraseptal area in a patient with a common, isthmus-dependent, atrial flutter. **A** and **B,** Location of the ablation catheter at the site of creation of bidirectional isthmus block as observed in left anterior oblique (LAO) and right anterior oblique (RAO) fluorographic projections. Note that the inferior part of the halo catheter is placed at the cavotricuspid isthmus with its distal tip entering into the coronary sinus (CS). RF, radiofrequency. **C** to **E,** LAO, RAO, and axial sections of the heart at the level of the isthmus.[4] The *yellow circle* represents the approximate location of the tip of the ablating electrode, which was on the paraseptal vestibular pretricuspideal region. ICV, inferior caval vein. *(Anatomic slices obtained from* The Visible Human Slice and Surface Server,[4] *courtesy of the Ecole Polytechnique Fédérale de Lausanne (EPFL), Professor R. D. Hersch, Peripheral Systems Laboratory,* http://visiblehuman.epfl.ch. *With permission.)*

externally cooled-tip catheter in terms of radiation exposure, number of RF applications, and catheter crossovers. These investigators selected an 8-mm-tip catheter if the isthmus had a straight anatomy and an externally cooled-tip catheter when the isthmus had a concave or pouchlike morphology.[14]

Cardiac MRI studies of the isthmus performed before the ablation procedure in patients with atrial flutter can identify some anatomic characteristics, such as a long cavotricuspid isthmus, which predict a difficult intervention.[15] It has been claimed that right atrial angiographic studies may overestimate the length of the isthmus compared with cardiac MRI evaluation, but this assertion is not based on a head-to-head comparison of both imaging methods.[15] The justification of the added costs of an MRI study before the ablation in atrial flutter patients is questionable.

Triangle of Koch

The triangle of Koch is the inferior paraseptal right atrial region containing the AV node, its inferior extensions, and the transitional myocytes approaching the compact AV nodal area.[84,85] In addition, the triangle of Koch is the seat of the atrial insertion of many AV accessory pathways usually described as being septal and paraseptal.[6,86–95] The AV component of the membranous septum forms the anterosuperior apex of the triangle. The eustachian ridge, containing the tendon of Todaro, and the attachment of the septal leaflet of the tricuspid valve are its lateral margins. The base of the triangle is the orifice of the coronary sinus and the vestibular region, from the coronary sinus to the tricuspid valve (Figs. 6-2 and 6-10). The orifice of the coronary sinus is usually guarded by a small crescent-like flap of fibrous tissue known as the *thebesian valve.* This may be fenestrated and, in the occasional patient, may interfere with the catheterization of the coronary sinus (Fig. 6-6). The eponym for the triangle is widely used by morphologists, surgeons, and arrhythmologists despite the fact that Walter Koch did not describe as such the landmarks of this area. He did, nonetheless, in his description of the sinus node, provide an illustration clearly displaying this anatomic region.[77]

In the 45-degree RAO projection, the plane of the triangle is parallel to that of the fluoroscopic screen (Figs. 6-1B, 6-2, and 6-10). To establish that an electrode catheter is on the triangle of Koch, we must combine the RAO and LAO views (Figs. 6-1F, 6-1G, and 6-5). The LAO projection differentiates paraseptal locations from inferior ones, formerly described as posterior, along with anteroinferior and inferolateral sites, formerly said to be posterolateral, and anterior, which were termed in the past right lateral positions of the probing electrode (Figs. 6-1 and 6-5). The region of the His bundle is superior, whereas the orifice of the coronary sinus is inferior (Fig. 6-1).

Right atrial angiography obtained in a 45-degree RAO projection allows us to define the size and orientation of the triangle of Koch as well as the relation between the site of recording of the largest His bundle potential and the plane of the tricuspid valve. The triangle of Koch may have different sizes and configurations. In some patients, it is more vertically oriented, whereas in others, it has a more horizontal display. The pre-eustachian pouch, as well as the tricuspid vestibule, may also vary in size (Fig. 6-12; see also Figs. 6-2 and 6-10). The position of the node within the triangle of Koch is variable, a fact that we have established in our studies of human heart specimens as well as by means of right atrial angiograms.[85] Thus, the site of recording of the largest His bundle deflection does not always coincide with the anterosuperior vertex of the triangle as judged angiographically (Fig. 6-12). This has implications regarding the position of the compact node, which is just proximal to the His bundle.

The compact AV node is an unprotected structure, very sensitive to the application of RF current. The reason for this is the lack of any protective shield of connective tissue interposed between the node and the overlying atrial transitional cells and the right atrial endocardium. In our study of unselected necropsy human hearts, the distance between the right atrial endocardium and the compact node ranged from 0.3 to 1.2 mm, illustrating the ease of damaging this structure with direct RF current application.[85] This fact also explains why catheter mapping in the vicinity of the compact node can induce mechanical AV block. Unless we want to produce AV block voluntarily, delivery of RF current near the compact part of the node must be avoided. The length, thickness, and width of the compact node vary from heart to heart.[85]

As already stated, the triangle of Koch contains not only the compact AV node but also its inferior extensions and the transitional myocytes that at its anterosuperior apex may form the fast AV nodal pathway. In nearly 95% of the hearts, the compact node is in continuity with rightward and leftward inferior extensions that pass to either side of the AV nodal artery. There is no relation among the width and length of these inferior extensions, the size of the compact node, and the dimensions of the triangle of Koch.[85]

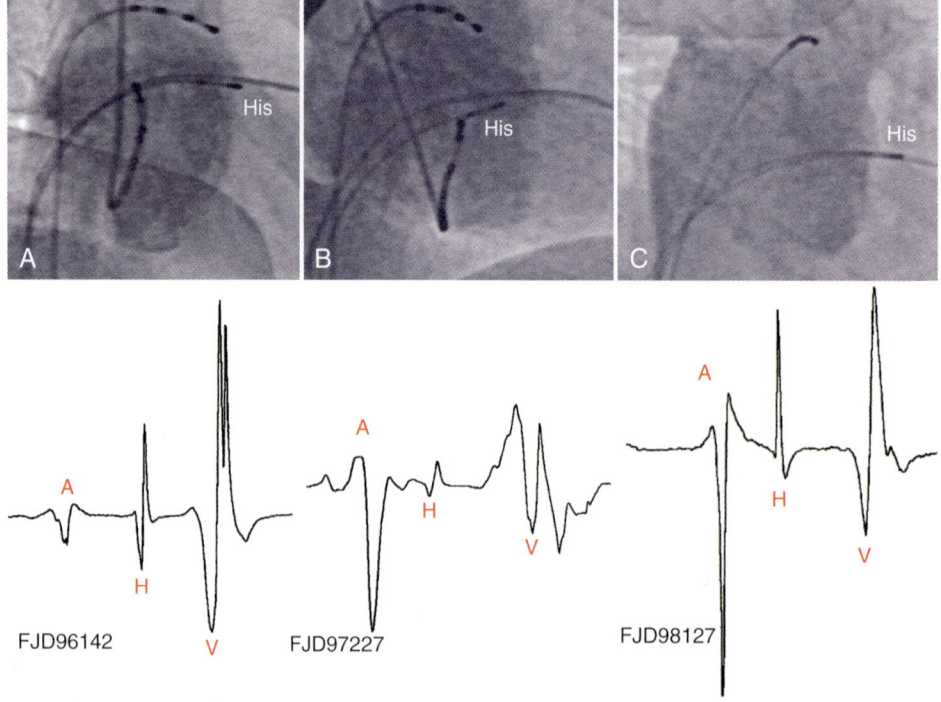

FIGURE 6-12. Relations between the site of recording of the His bundle potential and the triangle of Koch as outlined during right atrial angiography. Note the different shapes of the triangle of Koch. **A,** The His bundle potential was recorded at the level of the tricuspid valve. **B,** The His bundle potential was recorded at a pretricuspideal site. **C,** The His bundle potential is recorded beyond the tricuspid valve. Note that despite being at a right ventricular location in the right atrioventricular groove, the recording displays not only local His and ventricular deflections (H and V) of a good voltage, but also a large atrial electrogram (A). The tricuspid valve margins have a vertical orientation (**B** and **C**) or a slight anterosuperior tilt (**A**).

The leftward extension is superior relative to the rightward extension, and it is directed toward the coronary sinus. The rightward extension has a course parallel and adjacent to the hinge of the tricuspid valve. The maximal width of the rightward extension was 5 mm in our studies, whereas that of the leftward one was 4 mm.[85] These inferior extensions are also close to the endocardial surface of the triangle of Koch. Like the compact AV node, they lack any fibrous protective shield isolating them from the remaining myocardium. A schematic representation of the compact AV node and its inferior extensions is given in Figure 6-10.

Tawara, in his monograph published in 1906, had already described the posteroinferior extensions of the AV node in the human heart.[96] Inoue and Becker in 1999 reemphasized the existence of these nodal extensions, suggesting that there were two groups of myocytes, one along the tricuspid line of the triangle of Koch and the other directed toward the coronary sinus, both of them histologically identical in composition to the myocytes making up the compact AV node.[97] These inferior extensions may represent the slow AV nodal pathway participating in AV nodal reentry tachycardia and most likely are the target of our ablation procedures to cure the latter type of arrhythmia in its most common variety, the slow-fast or Ross type A, and also the slow-slow or type B (Fig. 6-10).[98,99]

The node becomes the His bundle as the AV conduction axis enters the central fibrous body, becoming enclosed by fibrous tissue. The bundle of His, therefore, is better protected than the compact node against RF current. The cellular components of the penetrating bundle of His can have a parallel, but also an interweaving, array.[85] Perihisian accessory AV pathways are superficial to the collagenous cup of the His bundle and have a subendocardial course. This is why they are very sensitive to mechanical block during catheter mapping. Also because of this superficial location, their ablation is possible without inducing His bundle block despite recording a His bundle potential at the site of the successful interruption of the bypass tract.

Right atrial angiography in the RAO projection not only displays the limits and variable dimensions of the triangle of Koch but also identifies the exact position of the catheter used for ablation in relation to the anterosuperior and posteroinferior limits of the tricuspid valve (Figs. 6-2, 6-5, 6-10, and 6-12). This applies to ablative procedures in patients with AV nodal reentry tachycardia, with inferior paraseptal, septal, and superior paraseptal (including perihisian) accessory pathways, with certain forms of atrial tachycardia arising from the triangle of Koch, and with isthmus dependent atrial flutter. The angiographic dimensions of the triangle of Koch may warn the interventional electrophysiologist of the potential dangers of inducing unwanted damage over the compact node.

In ablative procedures aimed at approaching the slow nodal pathway where the electrogram markers for ablation are relatively nonspecific, the LAO oblique fluoroscopic projection enables us to determine that the probing electrode is pointing toward the triangle of Koch, rather than to the inferior isthmus.

Having said that accessory pathways ablated in the region of the triangle of Koch are currently termed septal, this area, in the strictest sense, is not a septal structure if, by such, we understand those cardiac walls that can be excised

without exiting from the cavities of the heart.[100] The triangle of Koch is an overlap of the atrial and ventricular musculature, previously incorrectly called the muscular AV septum. In reality, the atrial and ventricular musculatures at this level are like a sandwich, containing an extension of the fibrofatty tissues of the inferior AV groove.[85]

Interatrial Groove (Septum) and Oval Fossa

The so-called muscular interatrial septum is formed for the most part by the apposition of the right and left atrial myocardia, which are separated by fibrofatty tissues that extend from the extracardiac fat. This is why we prefer to use the term *interatrial groove* rather than muscular interatrial septum. The interatrial groove has an oblique course, running from a left anterior to a right posterior position (Fig. 6-2C and D). The angle in relation to the sagittal plane varies with the size of the atrial chambers and the body build of the thorax. In the LAO projection, the interatrial groove is almost perpendicular to the plane of the screen (Figs. 6-1A and 6-9). The right atrial angiogram obtained in the LAO enables us to identify the interatrial groove (Fig. 6-9).

The oval fossa is a depression in the right atrial aspect of the area traditionally considered to be the interatrial septum (Fig. 6-13; see also Figs. 6-1A and 6-4D). The floor of the fossa is a fibromembranous structure that overlaps the infolded rims and, when complete, seals the passage of blood from one atrium to the other. Along with the anteroinferior buttress, the flap represents the true interatrial septum in the sense that it can be crossed without exiting the heart.[100] The anteroinferior part of the fossa anchoring the flap valve, also known as the *anterior limbus*, is also a true septal structure (Figs. 6-6 and 6-13).

The oval fossa is an interesting anatomic landmark in the electrophysiology laboratory because of the increased need to perform transseptal punctures, particularly for ablative procedures in patients with atrial fibrillation and left-sided atrial tachyarrhythmias. In 1958, John Ross, Jr., in Bethesda, developed the concept of transseptal catheterization of the heart.[101-104] The technique relied on using fluoroscopic landmarks to identify anatomic boundaries. The interventional cardiologist notices the "jump" of the Brockenbrough needle on entering the oval fossa. Electrophysiologists currently perform more transseptal punctures than any other interventional cardiologist. Perhaps because of this they have suggested modifications of the traditional technique for transseptal catheterization.[105-108] Fluoroscopic angulations used for transseptal punctures must be individualized because of the variability in the position of the heart in the thorax. Experienced operators may perform very efficiently the puncture of the oval fossa in the posteroanterior projection. Others prefer very angulated (>45 degrees) LAO or lateral projections. In the RAO projection, the oval fossa is posterior to the site of recording of the His bundle potential. In both the RAO and LAO projections, the oval fossa is posterior and superior relative to the entry into the coronary sinus (Figs. 6-6 and 6-13).[105,106] Right atrial angiography may help to identify the site of the oval fossa, particularly in the LAO projection, but this issue demands a more systematic study.[108] The use of a transthoracic or transesophageal

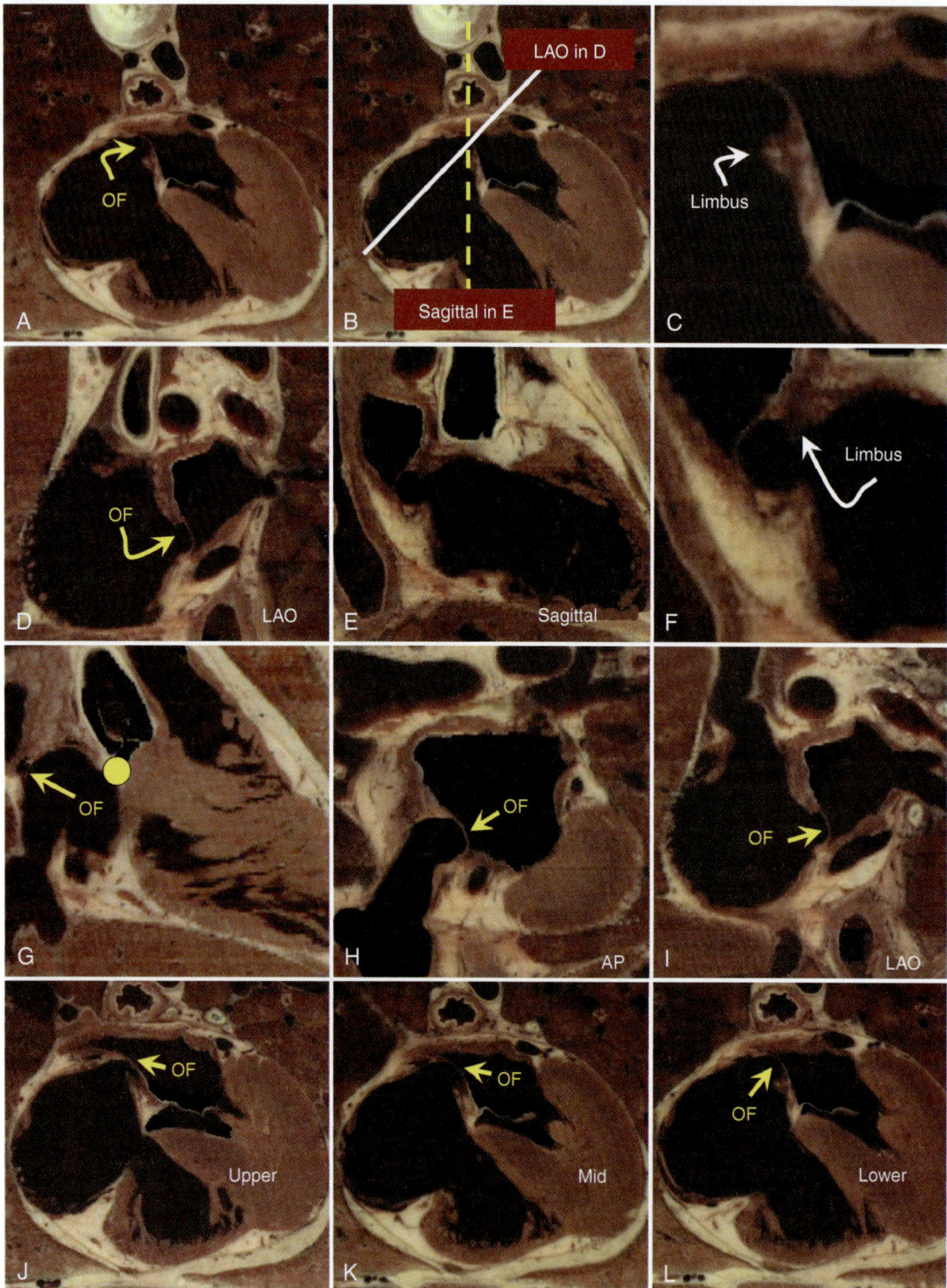

FIGURE 6-13. The oval fossa is an inferior and posterior depression of the interatrial groove. **A,** Axial slice at the level of the oval fossa (OF). **B,** The same slice showing two axes, with the *white line* showing the plane at which the section in left anterior oblique (LAO) projection has been taken and depicted in **D,** and with the *yellow line* showing the sagittal plane whose section is shown in **E. C** and **F,** Enlarged views of the oval fossa in the axial and sagittal planes. Anteriorly and superiorly, the oval fossa is limited by the thick muscular rim of the limbus. Puncture of the interatrial groove above the oval fossa enters into the left atrium through the apposition of the right and left atrial myocardia and the vascularized fibrofatty tissue sandwiched between them (see text). **G** and **H,** Slices in a right anterior oblique (RAO) and frontal plane projection at the level of the oval fossa. Note how, in the RAO (**G**), the oval fossa is at the same level or slightly superior in relation to the site of the recording of the His bundle potential (*yellow circle*) and posterior to it. **I,** A more anteriorly obtained LAO slice showing the oval fossa. **J** to **L,** Axial slices at the upper, middle, and lower regions of the fossa. Note the posterior and caudal location of the oval fossa. AP, anteroposterior. *(Anatomic slices obtained from* The Visible Human Slice and Surface Server,[4] *courtesy of the Ecole Polytechnique Fédérale de Lausanne (EPFL), Professor R. D. Hersch, Peripheral Systems Laboratory,* http://visiblehuman.epfl.ch. *With permission.)*

echocardiographic guide is not recommended for various logistic reasons. Intracardiac ultrasound is being used in several laboratories to guide transseptal puncture. This approach is expensive, and its routine use is unjustified in experienced hands.[109-111]

It is important to perform the transseptal puncture through the oval fossa. A puncture throughout the interatrial groove may result in hemopericardium in a highly anticoagulated patient because blood will dissect the vascular fibrofatty tissue that is sandwiched between the right and left atrial myocardium at this level (Fig. 6-13).

Coronary Sinus and Pyramidal Space

We discuss the coronary sinus and the pyramidal space within the right atrial section because we approach this region from a right atrial entry. The pyramidal space is an area of the heart in which the superior vertex is the central fibrous body, the lateral sides the right and left atria, and the floor the muscular ventricular septum and left ventricle. The coronary sinus limits with the base of this area, which has a trihedral pyramidal configuration. Tissues that are continuous with the inferior epicardial AV groove occupy the pyramidal space. The anatomy of the pyramidal space was first emphasized by Sealy and Gallagher during the days of surgical ablation of septal accessory pathways.[90]

The coronary sinus collects the venous blood from the ventricular septum and the left heart and drains into the right atrium. The continuation of the great cardiac vein, it is an epicardial structure that is situated at a plane that is more superior than the left AV groove (Fig. 6-14). Apart from the great cardiac or anterior interventricular vein, the

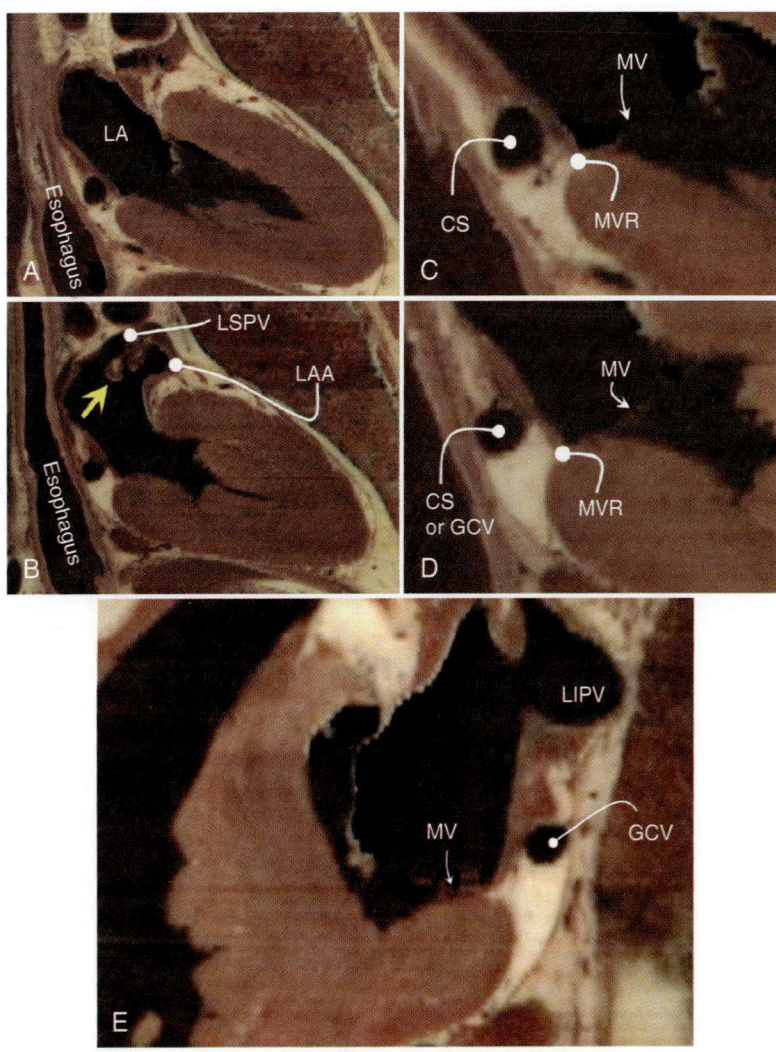

FIGURE 6-14. Relations among the coronary sinus (CS), and great cardiac vein (GCV), and the mitral valve annulus. **A** and **B,** Anatomic slices in the right anterior oblique projection. The slice in **B** has been obtained in a more posterolateral plane than that shown in **A**. The left atrial appendage (LAA) is anterior to the left superior pulmonary vein (LSPV) in **B**. The *yellow arrow* points to the lateral ridge (see text). **C** and **D,** Enlargements of the former two slices to depict the relations of the coronary sinus and the mitral valve ring (MVR). The vein within the epicardial fat is, at least for the slice shown in **A**, the coronary sinus. In the slice in **B** and **D**, the vein within the epicardial fat pad can be the coronary sinus or already the great cardiac vein. Neither the coronary sinus nor the great cardiac vein is a good marker to establish the level of the mitral valve ring. Also note the relations of the esophagus with the upper posterior left atrial wall. **E,** An almost sagittal section of the heart at the level of the mitral isthmus between the left inferior pulmonary vein (LIPV) and the mitral valve (MV). At this level, the coronary sinus tributary within the epicardial fat is the great cardiac vein. The myocardial content of the posterior left atrial wall decreases from the level of the orifice or the left inferior pulmonary vein towards the mitral valve (see text). *(Anatomic slices obtained from The Visible Human Slice and Surface Server,*[4] *courtesy of the Ecole Polytechnique Fédérale de Lausanne (EPFL), Professor R. D. Hersch, Peripheral Systems Laboratory,* http://visiblehuman.epfl.ch. *With permission.)*

other major tributaries of the coronary sinus are the middle cardiac vein (Fig. 6-3), the veins draining the inferior left ventricular wall, the left marginal vein, and the oblique vein of the left atrium (or the vein of Marshall). The middle cardiac vein, attitudinally, is an inferior interventricular vein. It can be the seat of accessory pathways that are included in the broad concept of inferior paraseptal but that should be specifically identified for a correct ablation (Fig. 6-15). The so-called diverticulum of the coronary sinus usually develops in relation to the middle cardiac vein (Fig. 6-3).

Accessory AV pathways in the pyramidal space are referred to as *septal* and *paraseptal*. This terminology is too broad and simplistic to help the ablationist. Accessory pathways that are specifically ablated from the right side of the heart outside or inside the coronary sinus, in the middle cardiac vein, or from the left side of the heart, in the immediate subaortic region, will be referred to as *inferior paraseptal* when dealing with spots that are several centimeters apart (Figs. 6-1, 6-3, and 6-15). The middle cardiac vein ends up in the proximal coronary sinus and initially runs an inferior course as seen in both the LAO and RAO projections (Figs. 6-3 and 6-15) before bending anteriorly along the inferior epicardial surface of the muscular interventricular septum.

Mid-septal accessory pathways, a term introduced by Jackman and colleagues,[87] are those located between the His bundle region and the orifice of the coronary sinus.

These accessory pathways are ablated from the triangle of Koch and were termed *septal* in the new nomenclature despite the fact that the triangle of Koch is not a true septal region. As repeatedly stated, to be certain that our ablation catheter is on the triangle of Koch, we must combine the two oblique projections (Fig. 6-16). Figure 6-16 illustrates an example of an accessory pathway whose categorization as septal (mid-septal) or right inferior paraseptal (right posteroseptal) could be debatable. In our opinion, the important issue is that this accessory pathway be ablated on the triangle of Koch, anterior to and outside the coronary sinus, well below the His bundle, in an inferior position of the triangle at the vicinity of the tricuspid valve insertion.

Right Atrioventricular Groove

The right AV groove is oriented either vertically or with a slight anterosuperior tilt (Figs. 6-2, 6-9, 6-10, 6-12, and 6-16). Accessory pathways may connect the atrial and ventricular myocardium across the right AV groove. Most ablative procedures in patients with right-sided accessory pathways approach the atrial rather than the ventricular insertion of the bypass tract. Figure 6-17 shows the ablation of a right anterior accessory pathway. Note the presence of atrial and ventricular electrograms at the ablation site. Special sheaths may be used to attain catheter stability during ablation procedures in the right AV groove.

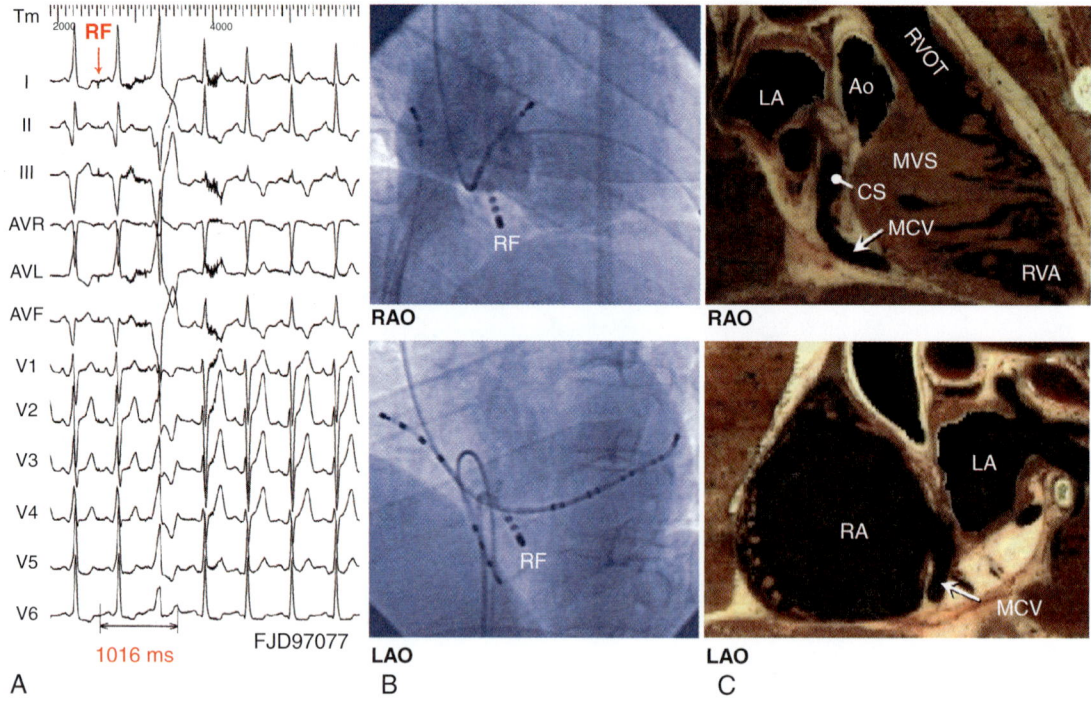

FIGURE 6-15. Ablation of an inferior paraseptal accessory pathway within the mid-cardiac vein (MCV). **A,** The accessory pathway is blocked 1016 msec after the onset of the application of radiofrequency current (RF). **B,** Right anterior oblique (RAO) and left anterior oblique (LAO) fluorographic images displaying the position of the ablation catheter (RF). The injection of contrast in the RAO projection enables one to determine that the ablation catheter is outside the outlines of the right atrium as defined by the angiographic contrast. This is indeed true because the catheter is inside the mid-cardiac vein. **C,** RAO and LAO slice of the heart. The MCV drains in the proximal coronary sinus (CS) running an inferior course before bending anteriorly along the epicardial surface of the muscular ventricular septum (MVS). Ao, aorta; LA, left atrium; RA, right atrium; RVA, right ventricular apex; RVOT, right ventricular outflow tract. *(Anatomic slices obtained from* The Visible Human Slice and Surface Server,[4] *courtesy of the Ecole Polytechnique Fédérale de Lausanne (EPFL), Professor R. D. Hersch, Peripheral Systems Laboratory,* http://visiblehuman.epfl.ch. *With permission.)*

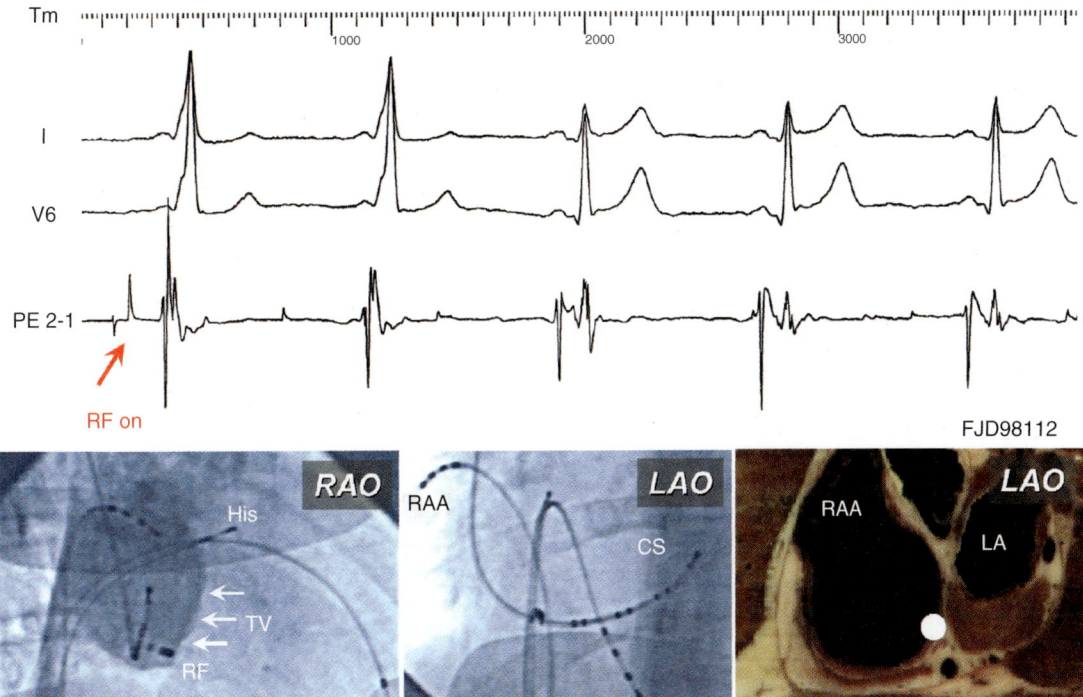

FIGURE 6-16. Ablation of a septal accessory atrioventricular pathway (mid-septal in the traditional nomenclature). The *upper panel* shows the simultaneous display of two surface electrocardiogram leads (I and V6) and the filtered bipolar distal recording from the ablation electrode. The *arrow* signals the onset of the application of radiofrequency current (RF). Preexcitation disappears in less than 2 seconds after the initiation of the delivery of RF. The position of the ablation catheter at the site of application of RF is shown in the 45-degree right anterior oblique (RAO) and 45-degree left anterior oblique (LAO) fluorographic frames. In the lower *right panel*, we represent the site of RF application on a 45-degree LAO section of the heart.[4] The right atrial angiogram (*left lower panel*) shows that the site of ablation was close to the tricuspid valve (*horizontal arrows*, TV). The LAO projection serves to demonstrate that the ablation catheter has a septal location (*middle lower panel*). The tricuspid valve in the RAO right atrial angiogram has a vertical orientation with a slight anterosuperior tilt. CS, coronary sinus; LA, left atrium; RAA, right atrial appendage. (*Anatomic slices obtained from* The Visible Human Slice and Surface Server,[4] *courtesy of the Ecole Polytechnique Fédérale de Lausanne (EPFL), Professor R. D. Hersch, Peripheral Systems Laboratory,* http://visiblehuman.epfl.ch. *With permission.*)

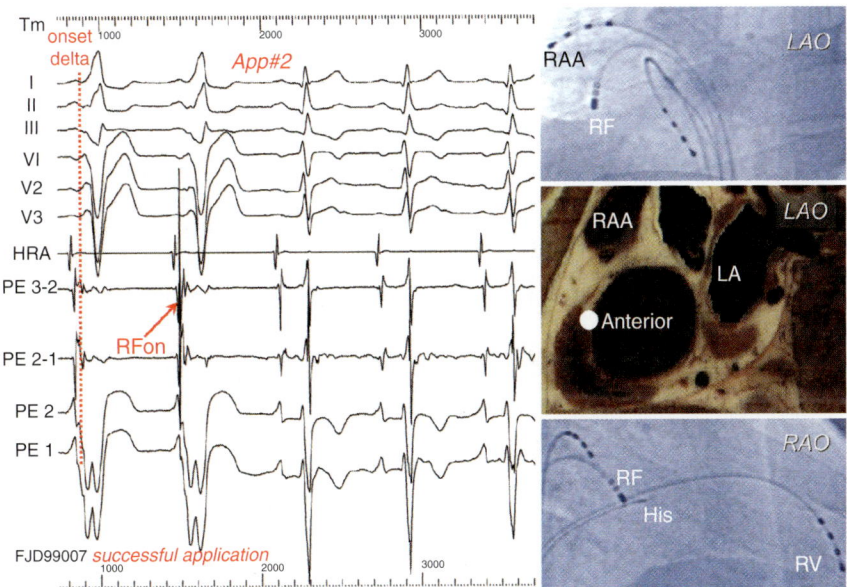

FIGURE 6-17. Ablation of a right anterior accessory atrioventricular pathway. The *left panel* shows the simultaneous display of six surface electrocardiogram leads and several intracardiac bipolar and unipolar recordings. The *arrow* signals the artifact at the onset of the application of radiofrequency current (RF). Preexcitation disappears in the first beat after the initiation of the delivery of RF. The position of the ablation catheter at the site of application of RF is shown in the 45-degree left anterior oblique (LAO) and 45-degree right anterior oblique (RAO) projections. In the *middle panel of the right*, we represent the site of RF application on a 45-degree LAO section of the heart.[4] LA, left atrium; RAA, right atrial appendage; RV, right ventricle. (*Anatomic slices obtained from* The Visible Human Slice and Surface Server,[4] *courtesy of the Ecole Polytechnique Fédérale de Lausanne (EPFL), Professor R. D. Hersch, Peripheral Systems Laboratory,* http://visiblehuman.epfl.ch. *With permission.*)

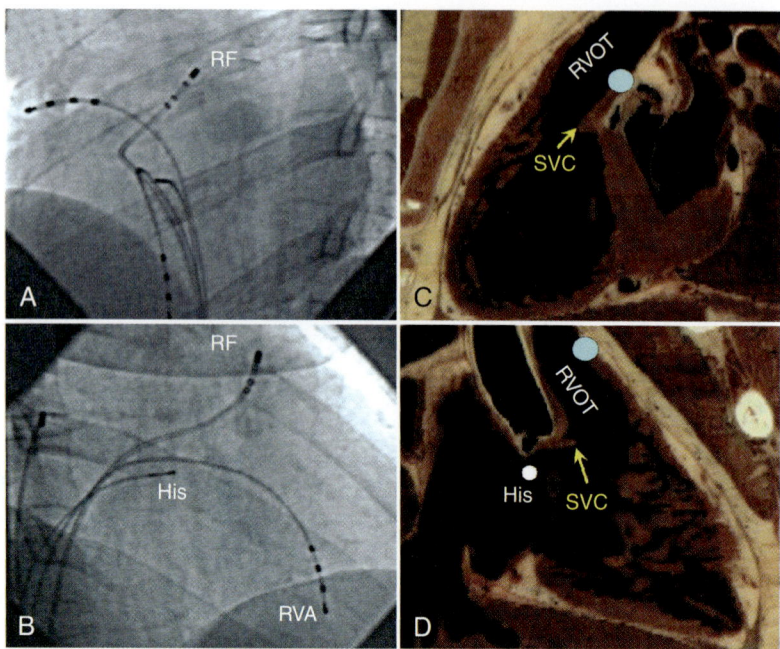

FIGURE 6-18. **A** and **B,** The ablation catheter (RF) in the right ventricular outflow tract at the site of ablation of an idiopathic ventricular tachycardia arising from this area (fluoroscopic projections are left anterior oblique [LAO] projections in **A** and right anterior oblique [RAO] projections in **B**). Note the position of the His bundle catheter, posterior and inferior in relation to the right ventricular outflow tract. The *light blue circles* in **C** and **D** represent the approximate location of the site of origin of this form of ventricular tachycardia on anatomic slices from *The Visible Human Slice and Surface Server*[4] in LAO (**C**) and RAO (**D**) projections. The *white circle* in panel **D** represents the approximate site of recording of the His bundle potential. RVA, right ventricular apex; RVOT, right ventricular outflow tract; SVC, superior vena cava. *(Anatomic slices obtained from* The Visible Human Slice and Surface Server,[4] *courtesy of the Ecole Polytechnique Fédérale de Lausanne (EPFL), Professor R. D. Hersch, Peripheral Systems Laboratory,* http://visiblehuman.epfl.ch. *With permission.)*

Right Ventricle

The right ventricle is almost systematically catheterized during an electrophysiologic study, and very frequently during an ablation procedure. In some stimulation studies, both the right ventricular apex and its outflow tract are catheterized simultaneously or sequentially. The frontal fluoroscopic projection is usually used to position an electrode catheter at the right ventricular apex. The right ventricular outflow tract can also be reached using a frontal fluoroscopy view, but it is safer, particularly with the relatively rigid catheters used for ablation, to use an LAO projection that enables us to avoid entering and forcing by mistake the coronary sinus (Fig. 6-18). Electrogram monitoring can also assist in preventing this error by demonstrating that an atrial and ventricular electrogram is being recorded (typical of the proximal coronary sinus) where we thought we had entered the right ventricle under the supraventricular crest. The right ventricle is anterior in relation to the left. As seen in Figure 6-4, this relation is true for the right versus the left ventricular cavities, but not for the right and left ventricular myocardial masses.

The right ventricular outflow tract is separated from the inflow tract of the right ventricle by the supraventricular crest (Fig. 6-18). The supraventricular crest is a prominent muscular band with a parietal part formed by the superior right ventricular free wall and a medial part merging with the ventricular septum (Fig. 6-19; see also Fig. 6-18).

Some accessory pathways with a superior paraseptal location (formerly considered anteroseptal) can have an insertion at the supraventricular crest. The fluoroscopic RAO projection cannot differentiate a ventricular ending at the crest from a perihisian insertion. When the ventricular insertion of such an accessory pathway is in the supraventricular crest, the catheter in the LAO projection separates from the area of the membranous septum fluoroscopically marked by the site of recording of the His bundle potential. Although the crest is a safe site at which to apply RF current, a slight displacement of the catheter can damage the normal AV conduction axis, which is very close.

The right bundle branch runs an anterior course. In patients with bundle branch reentry tachycardia, the right bundle branch is the preferred target to apply RF current. Sites for ablation should be selected to be as distant as possible from the His. The RAO fluoroscopic projection enables us to estimate the distance between the His bundle and the selected target site of the right bundle branch. The LAO projection is helpful in these instances to direct the probing electrode to the superior paraseptal aspect of the right ventricle where the trunk of the right bundle branch is located before dividing itself into several fascicles.

Right Ventricular Outflow Tract and Its Relation to the Aortic Leaflets and the Epicardial Superior Left Ventricle

The right ventricular outflow tract or infundibulum is a muscular tube that provides support to the pulmonary valve. The infundibulum is thickest at its origin, and its walls are progressively thinner toward the pulmonary valve. The right ventricular outflow tract is anterior and superior in relation to the supraventricular crest and, therefore, to the bundle of His (Figs. 6-4 and 6-18). As shown in Figure 6-4, the right ventricular outflow tract is anterior and to the left of

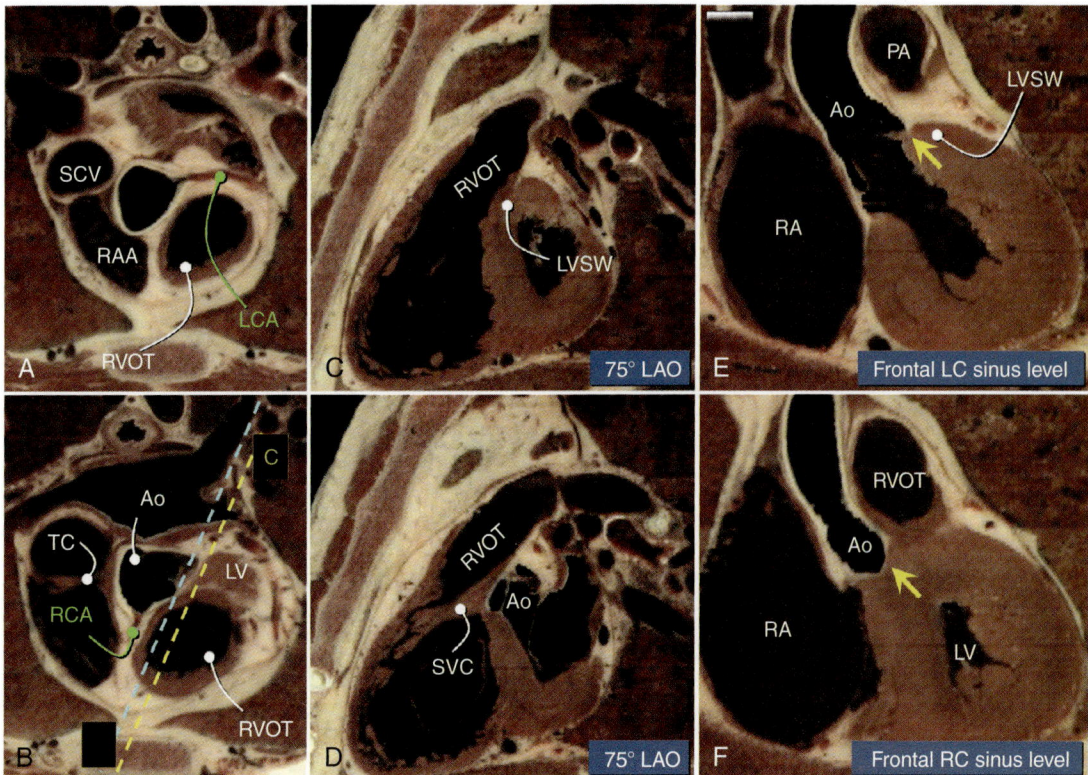

FIGURE 6-19. A and **B,** Axial slices obtained at the levels where the right and left coronary arteries (RCA and LCA) originate from the aortic sinus of Valsalva. The LCA has a more cranial origin than the RCA. The right ventricular outflow tract (RVOT) is related at the right with the right atrial appendage (RAA), and more posteriorly and above all inferiorly with the aortic root at the level or the origin of the RCA, and with the epicardial superior left ventricle (LV). Ventricular tachycardias arising from this epicardial superior LV need to be ablated from the right or left coronary aortic sinuses of Valsalva. The noncoronary, posterior, aortic sinus of Valsalva is unrelated to either the right or left ventricular myocardia. The lines marked as C and D in panel **B** represent the planes at which two slices have been obtained in a 75-degree left anterior oblique (LAO) projection. These two slices (**C** and **D**) illustrate the relations of the RVOT with the superior wall of the left ventricle (LVSW) and with the supraventricular crest (SVC). **E** and **F,** The relations of the aorta with areas close to the RVOT but belonging to the superior subaortic ventricular septum. The frontal slice in **E** has been obtained at the level of the left coronary (LC) sinus of Valsalva, and that of **F,** at the level of the right coronary (RC) aortic sinus. Slice **E** is more posterior than slice **F.** The left sinus is related to the superior left ventricular wall, not to the septum. The right aortic sinus is related to the epicardial superior paraseptal left ventricular wall. Ventricular tachycardias arising at sites such as those pointed by the *yellow arrows* cannot be ablated from the RVOT and are approached from the aorta or the immediately subaortic left ventricle (those illustrated in **E**). Ao, aorta; LV, left ventricle; RA, right atrium; RAA, right atrial appendage; PA, pulmonary artery; TC, terminal crest. *(All cardiac slices are obtained from* The Visible Human Slice and Surface Server,[4] *courtesy of the Ecole Polytechnique Fédérale de Lausanne (EPFL), Professor R. D. Hersch, Peripheral Systems Laboratory,* http://visiblehuman.epfl.ch. *With permission.)*

the aorta, and to the left of the right atrial appendage. The infundibulum of the right ventricle can be perforated with a catheter at several places. Its more superior part (Fig. 6-4A) may be perforated in almost its entire circumference. More caudally, the posterior aspect of the right ventricular outflow tract is in continuity with the superior segments of the left ventricle (Figs. 6-4B and 6-18).

Mapping of the right ventricular outflow tract becomes important in patients with idiopathic ventricular tachycardias that originate from this region, in certain forms of arrhythmogenic right ventricular cardiomyopathy, in some scar-related ventricular tachycardias developing after a complete correction of a tetralogy of Fallot, and in a rare form of atriofascicular accessory pathway with a Mahaim physiology that instead of having its distal insertion in the apical arborization of the right bundle branch, as it is usually the case in this variety of preexcitation, terminates at the junction between the septal right ventricle and the right ventricular outflow tract (Fig. 6-20).

There is some confusion regarding the anatomic basis of ventricular tachycardias that electrocardiographically resemble those originating from the right ventricular out-

flow tract but that can only be ablated from the aortic root or from the immediately subaortic left ventricle. The left coronary sinus of Valsalva is related to the superior left ventricular wall, whereas the right sinus of Valsalva is close to the epicardial aspect of the ventricular septum or, probably more correctly, of the paraseptal superior left ventricular wall (Fig. 6-19). Attitudinally, the left sinus of Valsalva is more cranially located than the right sinus. The right ventricular outflow tract, at the level of the origin of the right sinus of Valsalva, is related posteriorly and, above all, inferiorly to the aortic root and to the epicardial superior left ventricle. Whether some of the ventricular tachycardias thought to arise in the right ventricular outflow tract do in fact originate at the superior, more epicardially located left ventricular myocardial bundles, with which the right ventricular infundibulum is closely related, is unknown.

These anatomic relations explain why tachycardias ablated from the right coronary sinus of Valsalva have an earlier than V3 transition in the precordial leads—because they come from the epicardial superior paraseptal left ventricle. Conversely, those ventricular tachycardias ablated from the

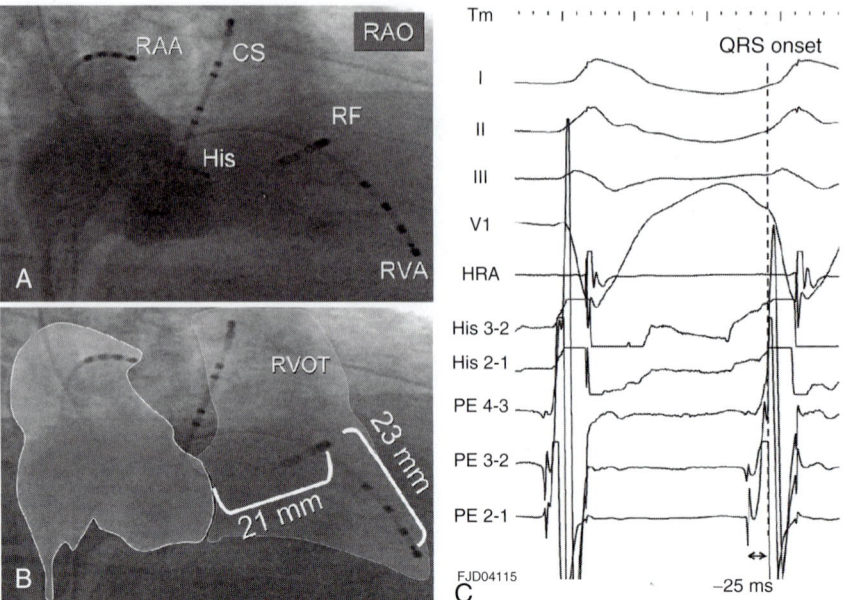

FIGURE 6-20. Ablation of an atrioventricular accessory pathway with long conduction times (Mahaim physiology) having a ventricular insertion high in the right ventricular septum, close to the right ventricular outflow tract (RVOT). **A,** The position of the ablation catheter (RF) in the right anterior oblique (RAO) projection during the injection of contrast into the right atrium. Note that the ablation catheter is far from the plane of the tricuspid valve. **B,** Superimposed outlines of the right atrium and right ventricle. The tip of the ablation catheter is at 21 mm from the tricuspid plane and at 23 mm from the tip of the right ventricular apex. **C,** Recordings obtained at the site of ablation during pacing from the right atrial appendage. Note the long atrioventricular conduction times during atrial pacing. Also note the presence of a Purkinje-like potential 25 msec before the onset of the maximally preexcited ventricular complexes. CS, coronary sinus; RAA, right atrial appendage; RVA, right ventricular apex.

left coronary aortic sinus may lead to positive QRS complexes in V1 or V2 because they come from the epicardial superior left ventricular wall.[112] Also of interest is that the noncoronary, posterior aortic sinus of Valsalva is unrelated to either the right or left ventricular myocardia but is related to the Bachmann bundle and the interatrial groove from which the terminal crest originates. This explains why pacing from the noncoronary aortic sinus results in atrial, not ventricular, capture.[112]

Accessory Pathways with a Mahaim Physiology

In 1971, Wellens, in his doctoral thesis, described an 8-year-old boy with a PR interval of 0.12 second, minor "type B" preexcitation during sinus rhythm, and wide QRS complex tachycardias with left bundle branch block configuration.[113] Although Wellens initially postulated that a nodoventricular Mahaim tract was involved in this form of preexcitation, it was subsequently demonstrated that the bypass tract in most of these patients consists of a right free-wall anomalous node that continues with an accessory His-Purkinje system distally inserting at the normal right bundle branch, or directly at the right ventricular myocardium. The term *Mahaim physiology* has been used for this kind of accessory pathway. Such a name is a misnomer because Mahaim described connections between the AV node or the left bundle branch and the ventricular myocardium. These are now known as *nodoventricular* or *fasciculoventricular connections.*[114]

Several approaches have been suggested for the ablation of these so-called Mahaim accessory pathways, including catheter-induced mechanical block of the

anomalous pathway, identification of the accessory pathway potential, either the proximal anomalous His or a more distant Purkinje-like potential of the anomalous AV bundle.[115–117] We perform the ablation at sites where a Purkinje-like potential precedes the onset of a maximally preexcited QRS complex by 20 to 40 milliseconds. More proximal sites may be encased by a shield of connective tissue, making them less susceptible to RF ablation. Approaching the atrial insertion by frequently provoking long-lasting mechanical block makes the ablation procedure more difficult. Distal segments close to the ventricular exit probably branch and are inappropriate targets for radiofrequency catheter ablation with only temporary success.[117] As already stated, most of these accessory pathways have a distal insertion that tends to be close to the right ventricular apex, but exceptionally, some of them may end in the neighborhood of the right ventricular outflow tract (Fig. 6-20).

Left Atrium and Pulmonary Veins

The left atrial anatomy is more complex than usually conceived.[118] The chamber is separated from the right atrium by the valve of the oval foramen. In up to one third of the adult population, the valve of the oval foramen is not mechanically joined to the rims of the fossa so that a catheter can be passed to the left atrium from the atrial cavity without requiring puncture of the valve covering the oval foramen.[118] The introduction of ablation procedures over left atrial structures in patients with atrial fibrillation and various forms of atrial tachycardia has increased the interest on

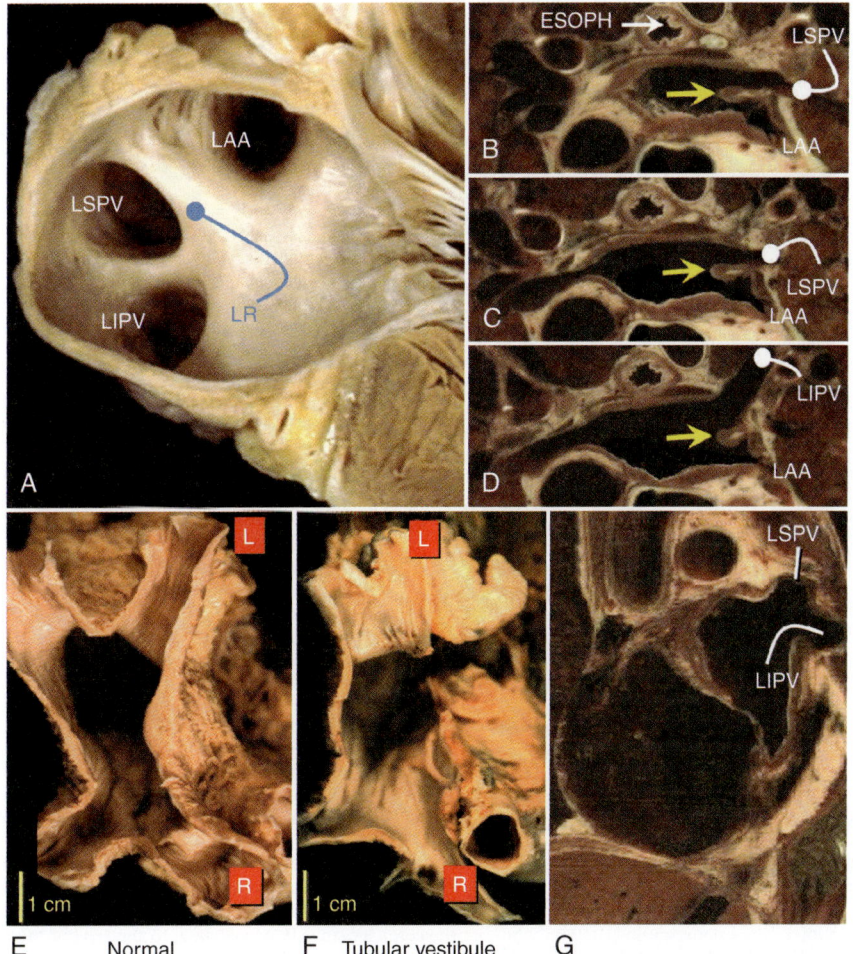

FIGURE 6-21. Endocardial visualization of a postmortem human left atrial specimen (**A**) and three axial cardiac slices obtained in a craniocaudal sequence from panels **B** to **D**. The left atrial appendage (LAA) is separated from the left superior and inferior pulmonary veins (LSPV, LIPV) by the lateral ridge (LR). This ridge (*yellow arrow* in **B**, **C** and **D**) is an infold of the lateral left atrial wall behind the left atrial appendage. Note the close relation between the esophagus (ESOPH) and the left atrial posterior wall (**B** to **D**). **E,** A postmortem human heart in which the left atrium has been opened to show the four pulmonary veins draining through four individual orifices into the left atrial cavity. **F,** Both left-sided pulmonary veins flow into the left atrium through a common tube or vestibule. **G,** Left anterior oblique slice from a female cadaver obtained with *The Visible Human Slice and Surface Server*[4] in which the left superior and left inferior pulmonary veins enter into the left atrium through a common vestibule. (*Anatomic slices obtained from* The Visible Human Slice and Surface Server,[4] *courtesy of the Ecole Polytechnique Fédérale de Lausanne (EPFL), Professor R. D. Hersch, Peripheral Systems Laboratory,* http://visiblehuman.epfl.ch. *With permission.*)

the macroscopic and architectural features of this cardiac chamber. In this section, we consider the venous part of the left atrium that receives the pulmonary veins, the left atrial appendage and the lateral left atrial ridge, the Bachmann bundle and the left atrial walls, the left atrial vestibule that conducts to the mitral ring and valve, also called the *left atrial isthmus*, and the relations of left atrial structures with the esophagus and phrenic nerves. The interatrial septum has already been considered.

Pulmonary Veins and Venoatrial Junctions

Defining the junction between the pulmonary veins and the left atrium is difficult in the electrophysiology laboratory, even when using angiographic techniques and merging multislice CT or MRI three-dimensional reconstructions of the left atrium with electroanatomic computer-generated casts. A common error is to consider that we are in the pulmonary veins only when the mapping catheter is outside

the contour of the heart silhouette in the AP projection when using fluoroscopic studies. We can be inside any of the four pulmonary veins without having crossed the projection of the heart on the AP fluoroscopic view. In fact, the initial portion of the right superior pulmonary vein is behind the smooth-walled right atrium at its junction with the posterior side of the superior caval vein (Fig. 6-21; see also Figs. 6-4 and 6-7). The best fluoroscopic projection to explore the left-sided pulmonary veins is the LAO (Fig. 6-22). The right-sided pulmonary veins are best explored in the AP and RAO projections (Fig. 6-22). Although the orifice of the left superior pulmonary vein is posterior to that of the left atrial appendage, the right superior pulmonary vein originates from the interatrial groove behind the junction of the superior caval vein with the posterior smooth right atrium (Figs. 6-4, 6-7, 6-14, 6-21, and 6-22). The right inferior pulmonary vein is the one that has a more caudal origin from the posterior left atrial wall and a posterior course that is very patent in the RAO projection (Fig. 6-22).

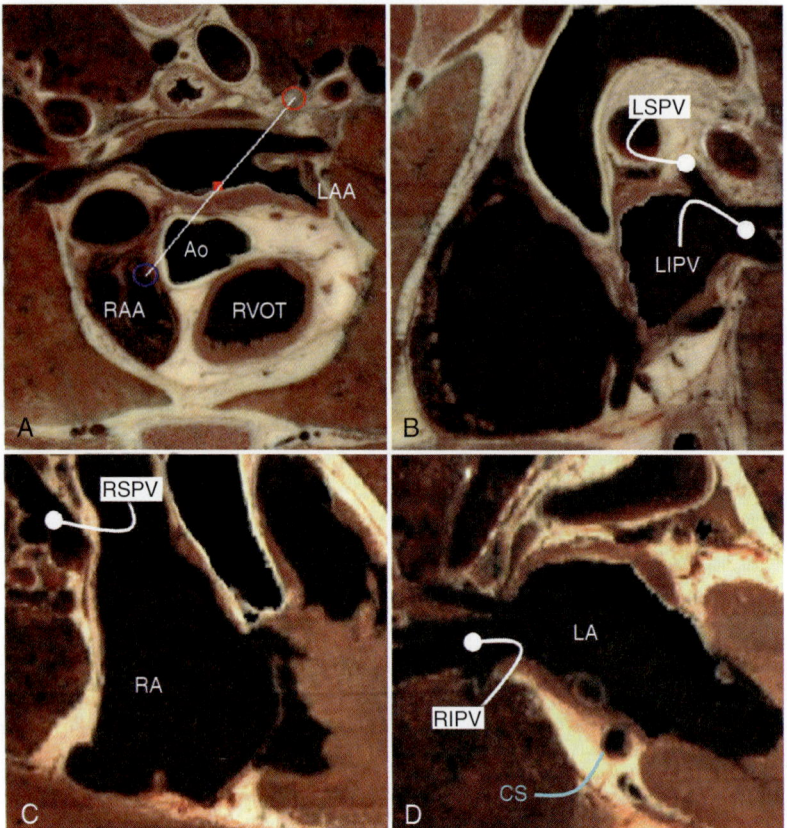

FIGURE 6-22. A, Axial slice showing the axis used to obtain the left anterior oblique (LAO) section shown in **B**. The slice avoided the left atrial appendage (LAA) to demonstrate that the LAO projection enables us to view the left pulmonary veins. Ao, aorta; LIPV, left inferior pulmonary vein; LSPV, left superior pulmonary vein; RAA, right atrial appendage. **C** and **D,** Right anterior oblique (RAO) slices depicting the right superior pulmonary vein (RSPV) and the right inferior pulmonary vein (RIPV). Note that the coronary sinus (CS) is cranial to the level of the mitral ring (see text). LA, left atrium; RA, right atrium. *(Anatomic slices obtained from* The Visible Human Slice and Surface Server,[4] *courtesy of the Ecole Polytechnique Fédérale de Lausanne (EPFL), Professor R. D. Hersch, Peripheral Systems Laboratory,* http://visiblehuman.epfl.ch. *With permission.)*

Multislice CT, MRI, and postmortem necropsy studies have established that the traditional picture of four pulmonary veins ending in individual orifices into the left atrium is not always the case in the individual patient.[119–122] Dual venous orifices at each side are present in about three fourths of the human hearts we studied at autopsy, but among these, in about one third of cases, the two veins from one side joined into a common short tube or vestibule before opening, through a common orifice, into the left atrium. This situation is usually observed at the left side and rarely in the right pulmonary veins (Fig. 6-21). This common vestibule should not be confused with another possible situation known as a *single pulmonary vein*. A single pulmonary vein is defined as one branching at the level of the pulmonary hilum, found in one tenth of the human hearts we studied. In one sixth of our specimens, we found more than four pulmonary veins, usually five, typically with three orifices at the right side and two at the left. The extra orifice at the right side corresponds to a middle-lobe right pulmonary vein, a finding also observed in CT studies.[121,122]

The left atrial myocardium extends beyond the venoatrial junctions, clothing the terminations of the veins as they join the left atrial cavity. These myocardial sleeves extend over longer distances in the superior than in the inferior pulmonary veins, and the superior extensions are usually thicker than the inferior ones. The myocardial sleeves are up to 3 mm in thickness at the venoatrial junctions, and they become progressively thinner when traced distally. In addition, the thickness is not uniform when assessed circumferentially. In the superior veins, the myocardial walls are thicker in their inferior than in their superior halves, whereas the opposite is true for the inferior veins. This difference likely reflects the fact that the aggregated left atrial myocytes surround the pulmonary veins by extending from the intervenous saddle, the breakthroughs of activation from the left atrium to the veins most usually being found at the inferior halves of the openings of the superior pulmonary veins, but on the superior poles of the inferior veins.[123] Study of autopsied human hearts shows that myocardial bundles cross from the superior to the inferior veins in two fifths of cases on the left side and in one fourth of hearts on the right side.[120]

Left Atrial Appendage and Lateral Ridge

Most of the left endocardial surface of the left atrial wall is smooth apart for the left atrial appendage, in which the left-sided pectinate muscles are confined in some three fourths of our autopsy specimens. In the remaining fourth, the pectinate muscles spill over to the anterosuperior part

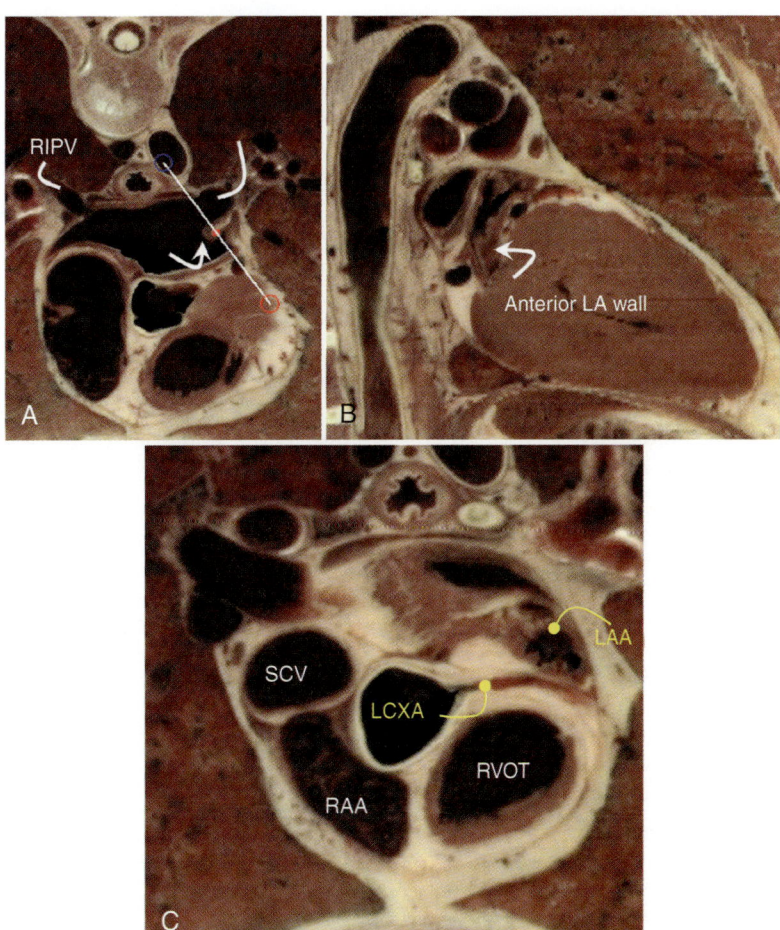

FIGURE 6-23. A, Axial section of the heart showing the ridge separating the left atrial appendage (LAA) from the left-sided pulmonary veins (in this slice, the left inferior pulmonary vein [LIPV]). The ridge in this case extends until the origin of the LIPV. The right inferior pulmonary vein (RIPV) is the one with a more caudal origin from the posterior left atrial (LA) wall. Also shown is the axis to obtain the right atrial oblique section (**B**) demonstrating how close the anterior left atrial wall (in this case the anterior wall of the left atrial appendage) is to the basal superoposterior left ventricular myocardium. At this level, accessory atrioventricular pathways can exist, and their ablation can be obtained from an endocardial approach. **C,** The relation of the left circumflex artery (LCXA) with the left atrial appendage (see text). RAA, right atrial appendage; RVOT, right ventricular outflow tract; SCV, superior caval vein. *(Anatomic slices obtained from The Visible Human Slice and Surface Server,[4] courtesy of the Ecole Polytechnique Fédérale de Lausanne (EPFL), Professor R. D. Hersch, Peripheral Systems Laboratory,* http://visiblehuman.epfl.ch. *With permission.)*

of the vestibule of the mitral valve but never extend to involve the inferior component of the vestibule.[120]

The left atrial appendage is anterior in relation to the orifice of the left superior pulmonary vein (Figs. 6-4, 6-7, 6-14, 6-21, and 6-22). There is a lateral ridge between the orifice of the left atrial appendage and the ostium of the left superior pulmonary vein (Fig. 6-23; see also Figs. 6-4, 6-7, 6-14, 6-21, and 6-22), which frequently extends inferiorly toward the left inferior pulmonary vein and beyond (Figs. 6-4B and C, 6-7B, and 6-21D). This ridge is no more than a fold of the lateral wall of the left atrium, producing a protrusion on the endocardial surface. The ridge should not be interpreted as being equivalent to the terminal crest as seen in the right atrium. Although the terminal crest is formed by a thick aggregation of myocytes, the lateral ridge is no more than an infolding of the atrial walls (Fig. 6-21). The lateral ridge incorporates myocytes from the leftward extension of the Bachmann bundle together with inferior branches of the septopulmonary bundle and the septoatrial bundle. The vein of Marshall and elements of the autonomic nervous system are located on the epicardial aspect of the ridge. The ridge contains more autonomic nerves close to the left superior pulmonary vein than more inferiorly.[124] The ridge, furthermore, has been shown to be no different in patients with and without atrial fibrillation during multislice CT studies.[119] The lateral ridge can vary in extent, terminating inferiorly either at the limit of the left inferior pulmonary vein or extending to the level of the isthmus between the orifices of the two left-sided pulmonary veins.[119] The relations also vary between the left atrial appendage and the left superior pulmonary vein, with the options of the orifice of the appendage being superior, at the same level, or inferior in relation to the orifice of the left superior pulmonary vein.[119]

The left atrial appendage is an extension of the left atrial cavity that in four fifths of hearts has a multilobulated appearance.[125] Its orifice is asymmetrical and oval shaped when viewed with multislice CT.[119] In patients with atrial fibrillation, the orifice and neck of the left atrial appendage are significantly larger than in controls without this arrhythmia.[119] Accessory pathways can connect the left atrial appendage with the left ventricle, usually from the neck of the appendage, a site that is accessible to endocardial catheter ablation (Fig. 6-23). The left circumflex coronary artery is closely related to the left atrial appendage (Fig. 6-23), being within 1 or 2 mm in nearly three fourths of the cases.[119]

Bachmann Bundle and Walls of the Left Atrium

Anteriorly, the Bachmann bundle connects the right and left atria (Figs. 6-4A and 6-7). It originates from the terminal crest, at the junction between the right atrium and the superior caval vein (Fig. 6-7B). It is not equally developed in all hearts and is not the only interatrial myocardial bridge.[7] The Bachmann bundle is located superior to the area of the His bundle and the oval fossa, but posterior to the apex of the right atrial appendage (Figs. 6-4 and 6-7). Axially, it is more or less at the level of the orifice of the superior pulmonary veins (Figs. 6-4 and 6-7). In the frontal fluoroscopic view, the bundle is at the level of the cranial portions of the right atrial appendage. If we intend to map the bundle endocardially, in addition to taking note of these fluoroscopic landmarks, we must confirm that the probing catheter is pointing anteriorly using the RAO projection. In the RAO projection, a catheter exploring the bundle needs to be behind an electrode catheter positioned inside the apex of the right atrial appendage (Figs. 6-4 and 6-7). Relatively rapid activation along the bundle is the consequence of the regular and parallel alignment of the myocytes within the muscular walls.

The anterior left atrial wall is behind the proximal ascending aorta (Figs. 6-4 and 6-7). It can be up to 0.5 cm in thickness but decreases markedly when traced caudally, and near the vestibule of the mitral valve, it is rarely more than 2 mm thick (Fig. 6-7). As we move caudally, the anterior wall becomes contiguous medially with the interatrial groove (Fig. 6-4) and even more inferiorly with the left atrial aspect of the oval fossa (Fig. 6-13J to L).

The thickness of the left atrial roof varies from 4 to 7 mm, whereas the lateral wall can extend up to 5 mm in thickness.[120] The posterior left atrial wall extends cranially at both sides of the midline (Fig. 6-4A to C), but when traced caudally, it becomes a left-sided structure (Figs. 6-4D and 6-13J to L). This wall of the left atrium is related to the esophagus and the vagal nerves (Figs. 6-4 and 6-7). As with the rest of the left atrium, the thickness of its posterior wall is far from uniform, being thickest immediately above the site of the coronary sinus where it has a myocardial component of up to 5 mm and a variable fibrofatty tissue component of about 2 mm.[126] It is the posterior wall at the level of the origin of the pulmonary veins that is the thinnest part of the left atrium in terms of myocardial content, less than 2.5 mm (Fig. 6-4).

Mitral Isthmus or Vestibule of the Left Atrium

The mitral isthmus is that part of the left atrial wall between the inferior border of the orifice of the left inferior pulmonary vein and the hinge of the mural leaflet of the mitral valve, this being the target of linear ablation during catheter interventions for atrial fibrillation to prevent tachyarrhythmia recurrences.[127] At this level, the left atrial myocardium is covered by an epicardial fat pad containing the great cardiac vein, not the coronary sinus taking the origin of the oblique vein of Marshall, or the location of the valve of Vieussens, as the marker for transition between the coronary sinus and the great cardiac vein (Fig. 6-14).[127] The dimensions of the isthmus ranged from 2 to 5 cm, but the distance from the great cardiac vein to the hinge of the mitral valve was no more than 15 mm.[127] The great cardiac vein and the coronary sinus are not good indicators for determining the level of the hinge of the mural leaflet of the mitral valve. It is also relevant for the ablationist to know that the wall thickness of the left atrium at the level of the orifice of the left inferior pulmonary vein ranges from 2 to 8 mm, decreasing toward the hinge of the mitral valve.[127] Others, however, have found that the thickest part of the isthmus was midway between the orifice of the left inferior pulmonary vein and the hinge of the mitral valve, with tapering at either side of this point.[127] These discrepancies may in part be due to different orientations of the slices obtained in the various studies.[128,129]

Relations of the Left Atrium with the Esophagus and Phrenic Nerves

The current techniques for catheter ablation used in patients with atrial fibrillation employ tools capable of creating deeper and larger lesions. Because of this, ablation lines created at the roof and along the left atrial posterior wall may produce important complications, such as atrioesophageal fistula or injury to the vagal and phrenic nerves.

Our studies in cadaveric specimens showed that the esophagus follows a variable course along the posterior aspect of the left atrium, but that in at least two fifths of the examined hearts, the esophageal wall was less than 5 mm from the left atrial endocardium. We have already emphasized the variability in thickness of the posterior left atrial wall, which is thickest adjacent to the coronary sinus and the great cardiac vein and thinnest more superiorly. Also variable is the thickness of the fibrofatty tissue behind the wall, which contains blood vessels and the vagus neural plexus. Esophageal arteries and the vagal plexus on the anterior surface of the esophagus, therefore, may be affected by ablative procedures. Because of this, current recommendations are to reduce the power, temperature, and duration of the RF applications, as well as creating the ablation line between both superior pulmonary veins over the left atrial roof rather than on its posterior wall.[120,126]

The right phrenic nerve can be damaged on approaching the right superior pulmonary vein—its anterior wall was within 2 mm of the nerve in about one third of our autopsy specimens.[130] The left phrenic nerve could also be damaged during implantations of leads into the great cardiac and left obtuse marginal veins or during ablation procedures on the left atrial appendage or its neighborhood.[126]

Left Ventricle

The left ventricle differs from the right ventricle in four major anatomic details. First, the left ventricular walls are much thicker than those of the right ventricle (Figs. 6-1, 6-4, 6-13, and 6-17). Second, in the left ventricle, there is no muscular separation between the inflow and outflow valves, and there is a mitroaortic continuity (Fig. 6-24). Third, the hinge of the leaflets of the mitral valve are positioned cranially relative to those of the tricuspid valve, with the AV sandwich occupying the space between the insertions. Fourth, the orifices of the right and left AV junctions diverge when viewed in the RAO projection, merging anterosuperiorly but separating inferoposteriorly. The latter two features explain why the triangle of Koch possesses a supratricuspid right atrial myocardial component separated by the inferior AV groove from the inframitral ventricular myocardium. The relations between the epicardial superior paraseptal and free wall left ventricular areas with the aortic sinuses of Valsalva and the right ventricular outflow tract have already been described.

The left ventricle is usually catheterized to ablate the ventricular insertion of left-sided accessory pathways and ventricular tachycardias. Generally, the cavity is approached by retrograde aortic access (Fig. 6-24). A transseptal approach can also be used. The septal area of the left ventricle is best examined using an LAO fluoroscopic projection. A combination of LAO and RAO projections is usually necessary to locate the site of successful ablation in the three orthogonal planes of the left ventricle. Although many ablationists prefer to have a catheter inside the coronary sinus to guide ablations, in patients with left-sided accessory pathways, with sufficient fluoroscopic experience, it is possible to map the left AV groove without the catheter in the coronary sinus.[131] The so-called single-catheter technique in practice requires two catheters: the ablation electrode and a right-sided catheter used for subsequent atrial and ventricular pacing after the ablation. In patients with left-sided accessory pathways with minor degrees of preexcitation during sinus rhythm, this second catheter is needed to pace the atrium to increase the contribution of the bypass tract to ventricular activation (Fig. 6-24).

Accessory pathways connecting the left atrial appendage with the ventricle must be approached using transseptal catheterization. In our experience, when using a retrograde aortic approach, the latter type of accessory

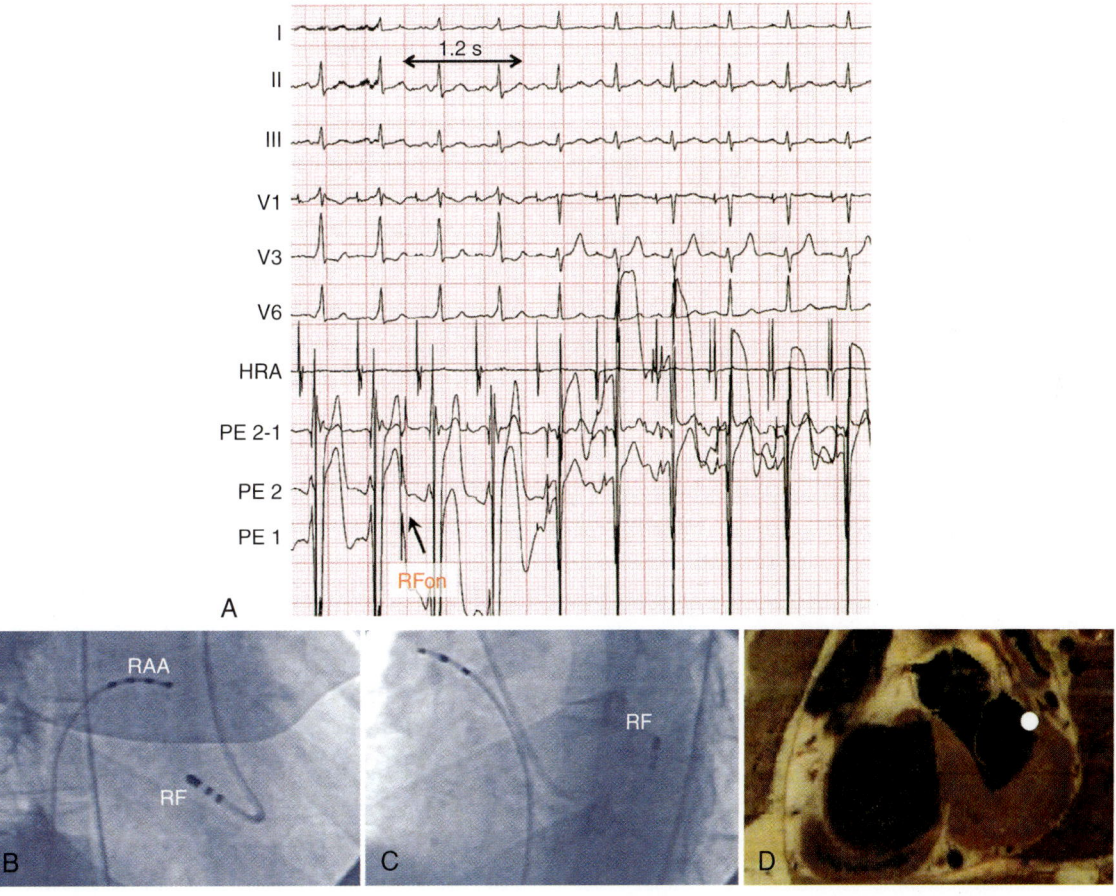

FIGURE 6-24. Ablation of a posterior left-sided accessory pathway with the so-called single catheter technique. **A,** Disappearance of preexcitation 1.2 seconds after the onset of the radiofrequency pulse application. **B** and **C,** Left and right anterior oblique (LAO and RAO) fluorographic views of the catheters used during this intervention. Note that apart from the ablation catheter (RF), a second catheter was placed at the right atrial appendage (RAA). This catheter was used during the procedure for right atrial pacing to increase the degree of preexcitation that was not well evident during sinus rhythm. **D,** LAO slice of the heart showing the mitroaortic continuity and the approximate ablation spot (*white circle*). *(Anatomic slice obtained from The Visible Human Slice and Surface Server,[4] courtesy of the Ecole Polytechnique Fédérale de Lausanne (EPFL), Professor R. D. Hersch, Peripheral Systems Laboratory,* http://visiblehuman.epfl.ch. *With permission.)*

pathway cannot be reached because the accessory pathways frequently connect the left atrial myocardium just at or below the mouth of the left atrial appendage with the opposite ventricular myocardium through the epicardial fat (Fig. 6-23). Because the ventricular insertion is rather epicardial, we must approach the atrial insertion of these accessory pathways.

Acknowledgments

This chapter is extensively illustrated with anatomic slices obtained from *The Visible Human Slice and Surface Server,*[4] courtesy of the Ecole Polytechnique Fédérale de Lausanne (EPFL), Professor R. D. Hersch, Peripheral Systems Laboratory, http://visiblehuman.epfl.ch.

References

1. Farre J, Rubio JM, Cabrera JA. Fluoroscopic heart anatomy. In: Farre J, Moro C, eds. *Ten Years of Radiofrequency Catheter Ablation.* Armonk, NY: Futura; 1998:3–19.
2. Farre J, Anderson RH, Cabrera JA, et al. Fluoroscopic cardiac anatomy for catheter ablation of tachycardia. *Pacing Clin Electrophysiol.* 2002;25:76–94.
3. Farre J, Cabrera JA, Sánchez-Quintana D, et al. Fluoroscopic and angiographic heart anatomy for catheter mapping and ablation of arrhythmias. In: Huang SKS, Wood MA, eds. *Catheter Ablation of Cardiac Arrhythmias.* Philadelphia: Saunders; 2006:85–106.
4. *Visible Human Slice and Surface Server.* Available at http://visiblehuman.epfl.ch.
5. *Visible Human Male and Female Project.* Available at http://www.nlm.nih.gov/research/visible/visible_human.html.
6. Cosio FG, Anderson RH, Kuck KH, et al. Living anatomy of the atrioventricular junctions: a guide to electrophysiologic mapping. A Consensus Statement from the Cardiac Nomenclature Study Group, Working Group of Arrhythmias, European Society of Cardiology, and the Task Force on Cardiac Nomenclature from NASPE. *Circulation.* 1999;100:e31–e37.
7. Moulton KP. The annular fat stripe as a fluoroscopic guide to anatomic sites during diagnostic and interventional electrophysiology studies. *Pacing Clin Electrophysiol.* 2003;26:2151–2156.
8. Cabrera JA, Medina A, Suárez-de-Lezo J, et al. Angiographic anatomy of Koch's triangle, atrioventricular nodal artery, and proximal coronary sinus in patients with and without atrioventricular nodal reentrant tachycardia. In: Farre J, Moro C, eds. *Ten Years of Radiofrequency Catheter Ablation.* Armonk, NY: Futura; 1998:91–102.
9. Cabrera JA, Sanchez-Quintana D, Ho SY, et al. Angiographic anatomy of the inferior right atrial isthmus in patients with and without history of common atrial flutter. *Circulation.* 1999;99:3017–3023.
10. Heidbuchel H, Willems R, van Rensburg H, et al. Right atrial angiographic evaluation of the posterior isthmus: relevance for ablation of typical atrial flutter. *Circulation.* 2000;101:2178–2184.
11. Da Costa A, Faure E, Thevenin J, et al. Effect of isthmus anatomy and ablation catheter on radiofrequency catheter ablation of the cavotricuspid isthmus. *Circulation.* 2004;110:1030–1035.
12. Da Costa A, Romeyer-Bouchard C, Dauphinot V, et al. Cavotricuspid isthmus angiography predicts atrial flutter ablation efficacy in 281 patients randomized between 8 mm- and externally irrigated-tip catheter. *Eur Heart J.* 2006;27:1833–1840.
13. Da Costa A, Jamon Y, Romeyer-Bouchard C, et al. Catheter selection for ablation of the cavotricuspid isthmus for treatment of typical atrial flutter. *J Interv Card Electrophysiol.* 2006;17:93–101.
14. Da Costa A, Romeyer-Bouchard C, Jamon Y, et al. Radiofrequency catheter selection based on cavotricuspid angiography compared with a control group with an externally cooled-tip catheter: a randomized pilot study. *J Cardiovasc Electrophysiol.* 2009;20:492–498.
15. Kirchhof P, Özgün M, Zellerhoff S, et al. Diastolic isthmus length and "vertical" angulation identify patients with difficult catheter ablation of typical atrial flutter—a pre-procedural MRI study. *Europace.* 2009;11:42–47.
16. Stamato N, Goodwin M, Foy B. Diagnosis of coronary sinus diverticulum in Wolff-Parkinson-White syndrome using coronary angiography. *Pacing Clin Electrophysiol.* 1989;12:1589–1591.
17. Lesh MD, Van Hare G, Kao AK, Scheinman MM. Radiofrequency catheter ablation for Wolff-Parkinson-White syndrome associated with a coronary sinus diverticulum. *Pacing Clin Electrophysiol.* 1991;14:1479–1484.
18. Tebbenjohanns J, Pfeiffer D, Schumacher B, et al. Direct angiography of the coronary sinus: impact on left posteroseptal accessory pathway ablation. *Pacing Clin Electrophysiol.* 1996;19:1075–1081.
19. Weiss C, Cappato R, Willems S, et al. Prospective evaluation of the coronary sinus anatomy in patients undergoing electrophysiologic study. *Clin Cardiol.* 1999;22:537–543.
20. Binder TM, Rosenhek R, Frank H, et al. Congenital malformations of the right atrium and the coronary sinus: an analysis based on 103 cases reported in the literature and two additional cases. *Chest.* 2000;117:1740–1748.
21. Funabashi N, Asano M, Komuro I. Giant coronary sinus diverticulum with persistent left superior vena cava demonstrated by multislice computed tomography. *Int J Cardiol.* 2006;111:468–469.
22. Tham EB, Ross DB, Giuffre M, et al. Images in cardiovascular medicine: cardiac magnetic resonance imaging of a coronary sinus diverticulum associated with congenital heart disease. *Circulation.* 2007;116:e541–e544.
23. Omran H, Pfeiffer D, Tebbenjohanns J, et al. Echocardiographic imaging of coronary sinus diverticula and middle cardiac veins in patients with preexcitation syndrome: impact on radiofrequency catheter ablation of posteroseptal accessory pathways. *Pacing Clin Electrophysiol.* 1995;18:1236–1243.
24. Haissaguerre M, Jais P, Shah DC, et al. Spontaneous initiation of atrial fibrillation by ectopic beats originating in the pulmonary veins. *N Engl J Med.* 1998;339:659–666.
25. Lin WS, Prakash VS, Tai CT, et al. Pulmonary vein morphology in patients with paroxysmal atrial fibrillation initiated by ectopic beats originating from the pulmonary veins: implications for catheter ablation. *Circulation.* 2000;101:1274–1281.
26. Robbins IM, Colvin EV, Doyle TP, et al. Pulmonary vein stenosis after catheter ablation of atrial fibrillation. *Circulation.* 1998;98:1769–1775.
27. Scanavacca MI, Kajita LJ, Vieira M, Sosa EA. Pulmonary vein stenosis complicating catheter ablation of focal atrial fibrillation. *J Cardiovasc Electrophysiol.* 2000;11:677–681.
28. Saad EB, Marrouche NF, Saad CP, et al. Pulmonary vein stenosis after catheter ablation of atrial fibrillation: emergence of a new clinical syndrome. *Ann Intern Med.* 2003;138:634–638.
29. Fink C, Schmaehl A, Bock M, et al. Images in cardiovascular medicine: pulmonary vein stenosis after radiofrequency ablation for atrial fibrillation: image findings with multiphasic pulmonary magnetic resonance angiography. *Circulation.* 2003;107:e129–e130.
30. Saad EB, Rossillo A, Saad CP, et al. Pulmonary vein stenosis after radiofrequency ablation of atrial fibrillation: functional characterization, evolution, and influence of the ablation strategy. *Circulation.* 2003;108:3102–3107.
31. Packer DL, Keelan P, Munger TM, et al. Clinical presentation, investigation, and management of pulmonary vein stenosis complicating ablation for atrial fibrillation. *Circulation.* 2005;111:546–554.
32. Dong J, Vasamreddy CR, Jayam V, et al. Incidence and predictors of pulmonary vein stenosis following catheter ablation of atrial fibrillation using the anatomic pulmonary vein ablation approach: results from paired magnetic resonance imaging. *J Cardiovasc Electrophysiol.* 2005;16:845–852.
33. Di Biase L, Fahmy TS, Wazni OM, et al. Pulmonary vein total occlusion following catheter ablation for atrial fibrillation: clinical implications after long-term follow-up. *J Am Coll Cardiol.* 2006;48:2493–2499.
34. Schneider C, Ernst S, Malisius R, et al. Transesophageal echocardiography: a follow-up tool after catheter ablation of atrial fibrillation and interventional therapy of pulmonary vein stenosis and occlusion. *J Interv Card Electrophysiol.* 2007;18:195–205.
35. Sigurdsson G, Troughton RW, Xu XF, et al. Detection of pulmonary vein stenosis by transesophageal echocardiography: comparison with multidetector computed tomography. *Am Heart J.* 2007;153:800–806.
36. Barrett CD, Di Biase L, Natale A. How to identify and treat patient with pulmonary vein stenosis post atrial fibrillation ablation. *Curr Opin Cardiol.* 2009;24:42–49.
37. Zhong H, Lacomis JM, Schwartzman D. On the accuracy of CartoMerge for guiding posterior left atrial ablation in man. *Heart Rhythm.* 2007;4:595–602.
38. Daccarett M, Segerson NM, Günther J, et al. Blinded correlation study of three-dimensional electro-anatomical image integration and phased array intra-cardiac echocardiography for left atrial mapping. *Europace.* 2007;9:923–926.
39. Calkins H, Niklason L, Sousa J, et al. Radiation exposure during radiofrequency catheter ablation of accessory atrioventricular connections. *Circulation.* 1991;84:2376–2382.
40. Lindsay BD, Eichling JO, Ambos HD, Cain ME. Radiation exposure to patients and medical personnel during radiofrequency catheter ablation for supraventricular tachycardia. *Am J Cardiol.* 1992;70:218–223.
41. Scanavacca M, d'Avila A, Velarde JL, et al. Reduction of radiation exposure time during catheter ablation with the use of pulsed fluoroscopy. *Int J Cardiol.* 1998;63:71–74.
42. Wittkampf FH, Wever EF, Vos K, et al. Reduction of radiation exposure in the cardiac electrophysiology laboratory. *Pacing Clin Electrophysiol.* 2000;23:1638–1644.
43. Perisinakis K, Damilakis J, Theocharopoulos N, et al. Accurate assessment of patient effective radiation dose and associated detriment risk from radiofrequency catheter ablation procedures. *Circulation.* 2001;104:58–62.
44. McFadden SL, Mooney RB, Shepherd PH. X-ray dose and associated risks from radiofrequency catheter ablation procedures. *Br J Radiol.* 2002;75:253–265.
45. Macle L, Weerasooriya R, Jais P, et al. Radiation exposure during radiofrequency catheter ablation for atrial fibrillation. *Pacing Clin Electrophysiol.* 2003;26:288–291.
46. Tsapaki V, Kottou S, Kollaros N, et al. Dose performance evaluation of a charge coupled device and a flat-panel digital fluoroscopy system recently installed in an interventional cardiology laboratory. *Radiat Prot Dosimetry.* 2004;111:297–304.

47. Vano E, Geiger B, Schreiner A, et al. Dynamic flat panel detector versus image intensifier in cardiac imaging: dose and image quality. *Phys Med Biol.* 2005;50:5731–5742.

48. Efstathopoulos EP, Katritsis DG, Kottou S, et al. Patient and staff radiation dosimetry during cardiac electrophysiology studies and catheter ablation procedures: a comprehensive analysis. *Europace.* 2006;8:443–448.

49. Ector J, Dragusin O, Adriaenssens B, et al. Obesity is a major determinant of radiation dose in patients undergoing pulmonary vein isolation for atrial fibrillation. *J Am Coll Cardiol.* 2007;50:234–242.

50. Dragusin O, Weerasooriya R, Jaïs P, et al. Evaluation of a radiation protection cabin for invasive electrophysiological procedures. *Eur Heart J.* 2007;28:183–189.

51. Mesbahi A, Mehnati P, Keshtkar A, Aslanabadi N. Comparison of radiation dose to patient and staff for two interventional cardiology units: a phantom study. *Radiat Prot Dosimetry.* 2008;131:399–403.

52. Lin PJ. Technical advances of interventional fluoroscopy and flat panel image receptor. *Health Phys.* 2008;95:650–657.

53. Lakkireddy D, Nadzam G, Verma A, et al. Impact of a comprehensive safety program on radiation exposure during catheter ablation of atrial fibrillation: a prospective study. *J Interv Card Electrophysiol.* 2009;24:105–112.

54. Rosenthal LS, Mahesh M, Beck TJ, et al. Predictors of fluoroscopy time and estimated radiation exposure during radiofrequency catheter ablation procedures. *Am J Cardiol.* 1998;82:451–458.

55. Sanchez-Quintana D, Anderson RH, Cabrera JA, et al. The terminal crest: morphological features relevant to electrophysiology. *Heart.* 2002;88:406–411.

56. Olgin JE, Kalman JM, Fitzpatrick AP, Lesh MD. Role of right atrial endocardial structures as barriers to conduction during human type I atrial flutter: activation and entrainment mapping guided by intracardiac echocardiography. *Circulation.* 1995;92:1839–1848.

57. Friedman PA, Luria D, Fenton AM, et al. Global right atrial mapping of human atrial flutter: the presence of posteromedial (sinus venosa region) functional block and double potentials. A study in biplane fluoroscopy and intracardiac echocardiography. *Circulation.* 2000;101:1568–1577.

58. Kalman JM, Olgin JE, Karch MR, et al. "Cristal tachycardias": origin of right atrial tachycardias from the crista terminalis identified by intracardiac echocardiography. *J Am Coll Cardiol.* 1998;31:451–459.

59. Lee RJ, Kalman JM, Fitzpatrick AP, et al. Radiofrequency catheter modification of the sinus node for "inappropriate" sinus tachycardia. *Circulation.* 1995;92:2919–2928.

60. Sánchez-Quintana D, Cabrera JA, Farré J, et al. Sinus node revisited in the era of electroanatomical mapping and catheter ablation. *Heart.* 2005;91:189–194.

61. Boineau JP, Canavan TE, Schuessler RB, et al. Demonstration of a widely distributed atrial pacemaker complex in the human heart. *Circulation.* 1988;77:1221–1237.

62. Man KC, Knight B, Tse HF, et al. Radiofrequency catheter ablation of inappropriate sinus tachycardia guided by activation mapping. *J Am Coll Cardiol.* 2000;35:451–457.

63. Koplan BA, Parkash R, Couper G, Stevenson WG. Combined epicardial-endocardial approach to ablation of inappropriate sinus tachycardia. *J Cardiovasc Electrophysiol.* 2004;15:237–240.

64. Marrouche NF, Beheiry S, Tomassoni G, et al. Three-dimensional nonfluoroscopic mapping and ablation of inappropriate sinus tachycardia. *J Am Coll Cardiol.* 2002;39:1045–1054.

65. Schweikert RA, Saliba WI, Tomassoni G, et al. Percutaneous pericardial instrumentation for endo-epicardial mapping of previously failed ablations. *Circulation.* 2003;108:1329–1335.

66. Ren JF, Marchlinski FE, Callans DJ, Zado ES. Echocardiographic lesion characteristic associated with successful ablation of inappropriate sinus tachycardia. *J Cardiovasc Electrophysiol.* 2001;12:814–818.

67. Lin D, Garcia F, Jacobson J, et al. Use of noncontact mapping and saline-cooled ablation catheter for sinus node modification in medically refractory inappropriate sinus tachycardia. *Pacing Clin Electrophysiol.* 2007;30:236–242.

68. Chandler NJ, Greener ID, Tellez JO, et al. Molecular architecture of the human sinus node: insights into the function of the cardiac pacemaker. *Circulation.* 2009;119:1562–1575.

69. Ho SY. Accessory atrioventricular pathways: getting to the origins. *Circulation.* 2008;117:1502–1504.

70. Roberts-Thomson KC, Kistler PM, Haqqani HM, et al. Focal atrial tachycardias arising from the right atrial appendage: electrocardiographic and electrophysiologic characteristics and radiofrequency ablation. *J Cardiovasc Electrophysiol.* 2007;18:367–372.

71. Kholová I, Kautzner J. Morphology of atrial myocardial extensions into human caval veins: a postmortem study in patients with and without atrial fibrillation. *Circulation.* 2004;110:483–488.

72. Ooie T, Tsuchiya T, Ashikaga K, Takahashi N. Electrical connection between the right atrium and the superior vena cava, and the extent of myocardial sleeve in a patient with atrial fibrillation originating from the superior vena cava. *J Cardiovasc Electrophysiol.* 2002;13:482–485.

73. Huang BH, Wu MH, Tsao HM, et al. Morphology of the thoracic veins and left atrium in paroxysmal atrial fibrillation initiated by superior caval vein ectopy. *J Cardiovasc Electrophysiol.* 2005;16:411–417.

74. Liu H, Lim KT, Murray C, Weerasooriya R. Electrogram-guided isolation of the left superior vena cava for treatment of atrial fibrillation. *Europace.* 2007;9:775–780.

75. Wang XH, Liu X, Sun YM, et al. Pulmonary vein isolation combined with superior vena cava isolation for atrial fibrillation ablation: a prospective randomized study. *Europace.* 2008;10:600–605.

76. Ho SY, Anderson RH. How constant anatomically is the tendon of Todaro as a marker for the triangle of Koch? *J Cardiovasc Electrophysiol.* 2000;11:83–89.

77. James TN. The tendons of Todaro and the "triangle of Koch": lessons from eponymous hagiolatry. *J Cardiovasc Electrophysiol.* 1999;10:1478–1496.

78. Nakagawa H, Lazzara R, Khastgir T, et al. Role of the tricuspid annulus and the eustachian valve/ridge on atrial flutter: relevance to catheter ablation of the septal isthmus and a new technique for rapid identification of ablation success. *Circulation.* 1996;94:407–424.

79. Cabrera JA, Sanchez-Quintana D, Ho SY, et al. The architecture of the atrial musculature between the orifice of the inferior caval vein and the tricuspid valve: the anatomy of the isthmus. *J Cardiovasc Electrophysiol.* 1998;9:1186–1195.

80. Shah DC, Jais P, Haissaguerre M, et al. Three-dimensional mapping of the common atrial flutter circuit in the right atrium. *Circulation.* 1997;96:3904–3912.

81. Cheng J, Cabeen WR, Scheinman M. Right atrial flutter due to lower loop reentry: mechanism and anatomic substrate. *Circulation.* 1999;99:1700–1705.

82. Knecht S, Castro-Rodriguez J, Verbeet T, et al. Multidetector 16-slice CT scan evaluation of cavotricuspid isthmus anatomy before radiofrequency ablation. *J Interv Card Electrophysiol.* 2007;20:29–35.

83. Cabrera JA, Sánchez-Quintana D, Farré J, et al. The inferior right atrial isthmus: further architectural insights for current and coming ablation technologies. *J Cardiovasc Electrophysiol.* 2005;16:402–408.

84. Sanchez-Quintana D, Davies DW, Ho SY, et al. Architecture of the atrial musculature in and around the triangle of Koch: its potential relevance to atrioventricular nodal reentry. *J Cardiovasc Electrophysiol.* 1997;8:1396–1407.

85. Sanchez-Quintana D, Ho SY, Cabrera JA, et al. Topographic anatomy of the inferior pyramidal space: relevance to radiofrequency catheter ablation. *J Cardiovasc Electrophysiol.* 2001;12:210–217.

86. Becker AE, Anderson RH, Durrer D, Wellens HJ. The anatomical substrates of Wolff-Parkinson-White syndrome: a clinicopathologic correlation in seven patients. *Circulation.* 1978;57:870–879.

87. Jackman WM, Friday KJ, Fitzgerald DM, et al. Localization of left free-wall and posteroseptal accessory atrioventricular pathways by direct recording of accessory pathway activation. *Pacing Clin Electrophysiol.* 1989;12:204–214.

88. Scheinman MM, Wang YS, Van Hare GF, Lesh MD. Electrocardiographic and electrophysiologic characteristics of anterior, midseptal and right anterior free wall accessory pathways. *J Am Coll Cardiol.* 1992;20:1220–1229.

89. Kuck KH, Schluter M, Gursoy S. Preservation of atrioventricular nodal conduction during radiofrequency current catheter ablation of midseptal accessory pathways. *Circulation.* 1992;86:1743–1752.

90. Sealy WC, Gallagher JJ. The surgical approach to the septal area of the heart based on experiences with 45 patients with Kent bundles. *J Thorac Cardiovasc Surg.* 1980;79:542–551.

91. Takahashi A, Shah DC, Jais P, et al. Specific electrocardiographic features of manifest coronary posteroseptal accessory pathways. *J Cardiovasc Electrophysiol.* 1998;9:1015–1025.

92. Davis LM, Byth K, Ellis P, et al. Dimensions of the human posterior septal space and coronary sinus. *Am J Cardiol.* 1991;68:621–625.

93. Sousa J, el-Atassi R, Rosenheck S, et al. Radiofrequency catheter ablation of the atrioventricular junction from the left ventricle. *Circulation.* 1991;84:567–571.

94. Schluter M, Kuck KH. Catheter ablation from right atrium of anteroseptal accessory pathways using radiofrequency current. *J Am Coll Cardiol.* 1992;19:663–670.

95. Haissaguerre M, Marcus F, Poquet F, et al. Electrocardiographic characteristics and catheter ablation of parahissian accessory pathways. *Circulation.* 1994;90:1124–1128.

96. Tawara S. Das Reitzleitungssystem des Saugetierherzens: Eine anatomischhistologische Studie über das Atrioventrikularbundel und die Purkinjeschen Faden. Jena, Germany: Gustav Fischer; 1906.

97. Inoue S, Becker AE. Posterior extensions of the human compact atrioventricular node: a neglected anatomic feature of potential clinical significance. *Circulation.* 1998;97:188–193.

98. Medkour D, Becker AE, Khalife K, Billette J. Anatomic and functional characteristics of a slow posterior AV nodal pathway: role in dual-pathway physiology and reentry. *Circulation.* 1998;98:164–174.

99. Katritsis DG, Becker AE, Ellenbogen KA, et al. Right and left inferior extensions of the atrioventricular node may represent the anatomic substrate of the slow pathway in humans. *Heart Rhythm.* 2004;1:582–586.

100. Anderson RH, Webb S, Brown NA. Clinical anatomy of the atrial septum with reference to its developmental components. *Clin Anat.* 1999;12:362–374.

101. Ross J Jr. Trans-septal catheterization: a new method of left atrial puncture. *Ann Surg.* 1959;149:395–401.

102. Ross J Jr, Braunwald E, Morrow AG. Trans-septal left atrial puncture: a new method for the measurement of left atrial pressure in man. *Am J Cardiol.* 1959;3:653–655.

103. Ross J Jr. Transseptal left heart catheterization a 50-year odyssey. *J Am Coll Cardiol.* 2008;51:2107–2115.

104. Brockenbrough E, Braunwald E. A new technique for left ventricular angiography and transseptal left heart catheterization. *Am J Cardiol.* 1960;6:219–231.

105. De Ponti R, Zardini M, Storti C, et al. Trans-septal catheterization for radiofrequency catheter ablation of cardiac arrhythmias: results and safety of a simplified method. *Eur Heart J.* 1998;19:943–950.

106. Gonzalez MD, Otomo K, Shah N, et al. Transseptal left heart catheterization for cardiac ablation procedures. *J Interv Card Electrophysiol.* 2001;5:89–95.

107. de Asmundis C, Chierchia GB, Sarkozy A, et al. Novel trans-septal approach using a Safe Sept J-shaped guidewire in difficult left atrial access during atrial fibrillation ablation. *Europace.* 2009;11:657–659.

108. Rogers DP, Lambiase PD, Dhinoja M, et al. Right atrial angiography facilitates transseptal puncture for complex ablation in patients with unusual anatomy. *J Interv Card Electrophysiol.* 2006;17:29–34.

109. Kim SS, Hijazi ZM, Lang RM, Knight BP. The use of intracardiac echocardiography and other intracardiac imaging tools to guide noncoronary cardiac interventions. *J Am Coll Cardiol.* 2009;53:2117–2128.

110. Dravid SG, Hope B, McKinnie JJ. Intracardiac echocardiography in electrophysiology: a review of current applications in practice. *Echocardiography.* 2008;25:1172–1175.

111. Saliba W, Thomas J. Intracardiac echocardiography during catheter ablation of atrial fibrillation. *Europace.* 2008;10(suppl 3):42–47.

112. Lin D, Ilkhanoff L, Gerstenfeld E, et al. Twelve-lead electrocardiographic characteristics of the aortic cusp region guided by intracardiac echocardiography and electroanatomic mapping. *Heart Rhythm.* 2008;5:663–669.

113. Wellens HJJ. In: *Electrical Stimulation of the Heart in the Study and Treatment of Tachycardias.* Leiden: Stenfert Kroese; 1971:97–109.

114. Mahaim I. Kent's fibers and the AV paraspecific conduction through the upper connections of the bundle of His-Tawara. *Am Heart J.* 1947;33:651–659.

115. McClelland JH, Wang X, Beckman KJ, et al. Radiofrequency catheter ablation of right atriofascicular (Mahaim) accessory pathways guided by accessory pathway activation potentials. *Circulation.* 1994;89:2655–2666.

116. Cappato R, Schluter M, Weiss C, et al. Catheter-induced mechanical conduction block of right-sided accessory fibers with Mahaim-type preexcitation to guide radiofrequency ablation. *Circulation.* 1994;90:282–290.

117. Haissaguerre M, Cauchemez B, Marcus F, et al. Characteristics of the ventricular insertion sites of accessory pathways with anterograde decremental conduction properties. *Circulation.* 1995;91:1077–1085.

118. Ho SY, Sanchez-Quintana D, Cabrera JA, Anderson RH. Anatomy of the left atrium: implications for radiofrequency ablation of atrial fibrillation. *J Cardiovasc Electrophysiol.* 1999;10:1525–1533.

119. Wongcharoen W, Tsao HM, Wu MH, et al. Morphologic characteristics of the left atrial appendage, roof, and septum: implications for the ablation of atrial fibrillation. *J Cardiovasc Electrophysiol.* 2006;17:951–956.

120. Cabrera JA, Farré J, Ho SY, Sánchez-Quintana D. Anatomy of the left atrium relevant to atrial fibrillation ablation. In: Aliot E, Haïssaguerre M, Jackman WM, eds. *Catheter Ablation of Atrial Fibrillation.* Oxford, UK: Blackwell-Futura; 2008:3–31.

121. Cronin P, Sneider MB, Kazerooni EA, et al. MDCT of the left atrium and pulmonary veins in planning radiofrequency ablation for atrial fibrillation: a how-to guide. *AJR Am J Roentgenol.* 2004;183:767–778.

122. Scharf C, Sneider M, Case I, et al. Anatomy of the pulmonary veins in patients with atrial fibrillation and effects of segmental ostial ablation analyzed by computed tomography. *J Cardiovasc Electrophysiol.* 2003;14:150–155.

123. Yamane T, Shah DC, Jaïs P, et al. Electrogram polarity reversal as an additional indicator of breakthroughs from the left atrium to the pulmonary veins. *J Am Coll Cardiol.* 2002;39:1337–1344.

124. Sharma S, Devine W, Anderson RH, Zuberbuhler JR. The determination of atrial arrangement by examination of appendage morphology in 1842 heart specimens. *Br Heart J.* 1988;60:227–231.

125. Cabrera JA, Ho SY, Climent V, Sánchez-Quintana D. The architecture of the left lateral atrial wall: a particular anatomic region with implications for ablation of atrial fibrillation. *Eur Heart J.* 2008;29:356–362.

126. Sánchez-Quintana D, Cabrera JA, Climent V, et al. Anatomic relations between the esophagus and left atrium and relevance for ablation of atrial fibrillation. *Circulation.* 2005;112:1400–1405.

127. Becker AE. Left atrial isthmus: anatomic aspects relevant for linear catheter ablation procedures in humans. *J Cardiovasc Electrophysiol.* 2004;15:809–812.

128. Wittkampf FH, van Oosterhout MF, Loh P, et al. Where to draw the mitral isthmus line in catheter ablation of atrial fibrillation: histological analysis. *Eur Heart J.* 2005;26:689–695.

129. Sánchez-Quintana D, Cabrera JA, Climent V, et al. How close are the phrenic nerves to cardiac structures? Implications for cardiac interventionalists. *J Cardiovasc Electrophysiol.* 2005;16:309–313.

130. Sánchez-Quintana D, Ho SY, Climent V, et al. Anatomic evaluation of the left phrenic nerve relevant to epicardial and endocardial catheter ablation: implications for phrenic nerve injury. *Heart Rhythm.* 2009;6:764–768.

131. Kuck KH, Schluter M. Single-catheter approach to radiofrequency current ablation of left-sided accessory pathways in patients with Wolff-Parkinson-White syndrome. *Circulation.* 1991;84:2366–2375.

7

Fundamentals of Intracardiac Mapping

Rishi Arora and Alan Kadish

Key Points

Intracardiac electrograms provide timing and morphologic information.

Local tissue activation is best identified by the point of maximal downslope of unipolar electrograms and maximal amplitude of bipolar electrograms.

Cardiac mapping techniques include activation mapping, pace mapping, entrainment mapping, and computerized mapping.

This chapter discusses the fundamentals of intracardiac mapping as it relates to the mapping and ablation of cardiac arrhythmias. The initial sections are dedicated to the basis and methodology of intracardiac, extracellular recording techniques; this is followed by a description of intracardiac electrograms as recorded in the normal myocardium, and subsequently by a description of intracardiac signals in the abnormal heart. The remainder of the chapter is dedicated to the application of various endocardial mapping techniques, including activation, pace, and entrainment mapping, in the diagnosis and ablation of atrial and ventricular arrhythmias in both normal and diseased hearts. Computerized mapping is discussed in Chapter 8.

Underlying Basis for the Extracellular Electrogram

Cardiac electrical activity originates from ion channel movement across cell membranes. The cardiac action potential is generated within individual cells and reflects cardiac electrical activation. Although some net charge flow occurs in the extracellular space, most cardiac electrical activity is generated within individual myocardial cells. Extracellular electrodes record potentials generated in the extracellular space and therefore differ markedly from action potentials recorded intracellularly. The differences are due not only to differences in recording location (extracellular versus intracellular) but also to the inherent summation of electrical activity from multiple cells that occurs when an extracellular potential is generated.

The "field of view" of extracellularly recorded electrograms reflects the relative contribution of individual cells both near to and far from recording electrodes that generate extracellular potentials. Computer modeling studies have created simulated extracellular potentials using various assumptions regarding intracellular action potentials.[1] Factors that affect the field of view of recording electrodes include whether the recordings are unipolar or bipolar, interelectrode distance (for bipolar recordings), electrode size and composition, and inherent myocardial properties such as tissue resistivity and space constant. In view of the summation of intracellular potentials that occurs to generate extracellular potentials, some fundamental questions regarding cardiac mapping require further investigation. For example, when one asks what is the "activation time" determined from extracellular potentials, there may not be a single answer to this question because different cells within the field of view of an extracellular recording electrode may be activated at different times. Thus, uniform rules regarding interpretation of extracellular electrograms need to account for differences in underlying physiology, and different "rules" may be appropriate in different circumstances. For example, it has generally been accepted that the HV interval should be measured from the onset of the His bundle electrogram. The basis for this approach is that regardless of the location of the recording electrode, one wishes to determine the onset of activation within the His bundle to best evaluate conduction time within the His-Purkinje system. In contrast, mapping of tachycardia origin uses techniques such as the baseline crossing in a bipolar electrogram that seek to determine not the onset of activation but the occurrence of activation at a specific location, in most cases to predict the effects of ablation at that site. Thus, understanding the physiology that generates extracellular potentials and the purpose of a particular mapping technique is required to determine the best theoretical as well as practical techniques to use for intracardiac mapping.

Electrogram Recording: Amplification, Filtering, and Digitization of Signals

Physiologic signals acquired through intracardiac electrodes are typically less than 10 mV in amplitude and therefore require considerable amplification before they can be digitized, displayed, and stored. In most modern electrophysiology laboratories, the signal processor (filters and amplifiers), visualization screen, and recording apparatus are often incorporated as a computerized laboratory recording system. The amplifiers used for recording intracardiac electrograms must have the ability to have gain modification as well as to alter both high-bandpass and low-bandpass filters to permit appropriate attenuation of the incoming signals.[2]

After amplification, signals are digitized and filtered by a computerized data acquisition system and are written to a hard disk or optical drive, while at the same time displaying signals in real time on a monitor. Digitization is a form of data reduction, whereby an analog waveform is "sampled" at a constant rate (sampling rate) by an analog-to-digital converter. The amplitude of the analog waveform is translated into a binary number (e.g., 8-, 10-, or 12-bit conversion resolution of the A/D converter), which represents the full dynamic input range of the A/D converter (typically ± 2.5 or ± 10 V). Sampling rates of 600 Hz or more allow for the recording of most of the data contained in the intracardiac electrogram waveforms, with most modern mapping systems sampling at or about 1000 Hz. The ideal system should be able to provide a variety of display configurations with a wide range of sweep speeds (most modern systems can display up to 400 mm/second) and should allow adjustment of the size and gain and other characteristics of the amplified electrogram.

Filtering is an important aspect of electrogram processing (Table 7-1). High-pass filters eliminate components below a given frequency. In the surface electrocardiogram (ECG), components such as the T wave are of relatively low frequency, and high-pass filtering of 0.05 to 0.1 Hz is used to preserve these components while eliminating baseline drift. When examining bipolar intracardiac electrograms, high-frequency components are of the most interest, and high-pass filtering of 30 to 50 Hz is used to eliminate the low-frequency components. Unipolar electrograms usually go through a high-pass filter of 0.05 Hz, however, because the polarity of the signal (which reflects the direction of myocardial activation) and the signal morphology (and

therefore low-frequency components) must be preserved. To eliminate noise at higher frequencies, low-pass filters are generally set to about 500 Hz for intracardiac signals (because there are essentially no intracardiac signals of interest much above 300 Hz).[3] Notch filters remove specific frequencies such as 60-Hz noise from power supplies. Figure 7-1 shows the effect of different filter settings on intracardiac atrial, ventricular, and His-Purkinje signals.

Unipolar and Bipolar Signals

The morphology and amplitude of the recorded electrograms depend on (1) the type of normal or abnormal depolarization responsible for the electrical potential and on local myocardial characteristics such as ischemia or infarction; (2) the orientation of the activation wavefront in relation to myocardial fiber orientation[4]; (3) the distance between the source of the potential and the recording electrode; (4) the size, configuration, and interpolar distance of the recording electrode[5]; (5) the orientation of the wavefront in relation to the poles of a bipolar electrode; (6) the conducting medium in which electrograms are recorded[6]; and (7) other factors.

The unipolar electrogram is recorded as the potential difference between a single electrode in direct contact with the heart ("exploring" electrode) and an "indifferent" electrode, which is placed at a distance from the heart[7] (such as in the inferior vena cava) or at the Wilson central terminal.[8] The recording is therefore not truly unipolar because all recordings depend on voltage differences between two poles; the "unipolar" designation signifies that one of the poles is distant from the heart. During cardiac activation, the approach of this dipole toward an exploring electrode gives a small positive deflection, and its passage gives a rapid deflection in the negative direction, with a final return to baseline.[9] The amplitude of the unipolar electrogram is proportional to the area of the dipole layer and the reciprocal value of the square of the distance between the dipole layer and the recording site.[10] Thus, the unipolar electrogram records a combination of local and distant electrical events, with the contribution of distant electrical events decreasing in proportion to the square of the distance from the exploring electrode.[11] As mentioned earlier, extracellular recordings are not synonymous with intracellular microelectrode recordings. Nonetheless, in normal myocardium with relatively homogeneous conduction and repolarization, several studies (as well as theoretical models) have shown conformity of activation times between intracellular microelectrode and extracellular recordings (Fig. 7-2), with the maximal downslope of the unipolar electrogram coinciding with the upstroke of the transmembrane potential.[12,13] Therefore, at least in normal hearts, there is agreement on using the maximal downslope of the unipolar electrogram for activation detection; there is significant controversy about the optimal value of the slope threshold, however, with recommended thresholds from different studies ranging from –0.2 to –2.5 mV/millisecond; the large range can be at least partially attributed to the fact that these studies were performed under a variety of different baseline conditions in normal, acutely ischemic as well as chronically infarcted hearts (animal and human).

TABLE 7-1		
TYPICAL FILTER SETTINGS FOR ELECTROPHYSIOLOGY LABORATORY RECORDINGS		
Recording	**High Pass**	**Low Pass**
Surface electrocardiogram	0.05-0.1 Hz	100 Hz
Bipolar intracardiac	30-50 Hz	300-500 Hz
Unipolar intracardiac	DC-0.05 Hz	>500 Hz

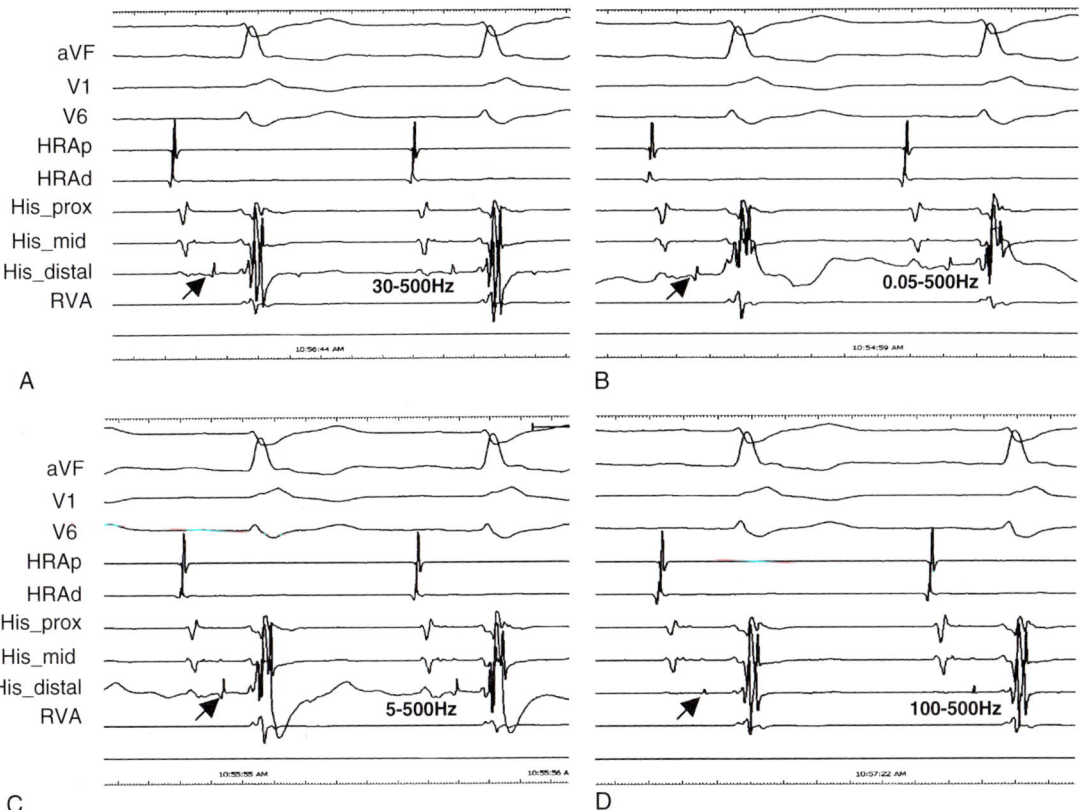

FIGURE 7-1. Effects of various filtering frequencies on the morphologic appearance of intracardiac electrograms. **A** to **D**, The tracings from *top* to *bottom* are electrocardiographic leads aVF, V1, V6, right atrial (HRAp, HRAd), three His bundle (His-prox, His-mid, His-distal) electrograms, and right ventricle (RVA). In each panel, both beats are of sinus origin. The top two His tracings (prox and mid), RA, and right ventricular (RV) tracings are filtered at 30 to 500 Hz (i.e., the usual filtering frequencies). The bottom His distal tracing shows the effect of various filtering frequencies on the appearance. The low-frequency signals are mostly eliminated at high-bandpass filter frequency settings greater than 10 Hz. Note that the high-bandpass setting reduces the overall magnitude of the electrogram, necessitating an increase in amplification. At all frequencies depicted, the His bundle deflection can be clearly identified. *(From Akhtar M. Invasive cardiac electrophysiologic studies: an introduction. In Parmley WW, Chatterjee K (eds): Cardiology. Vol. 1. Physiology, Pharmacology, Diagnosis. Philadelphia: Lippincott; 1991:1. With permission.)*

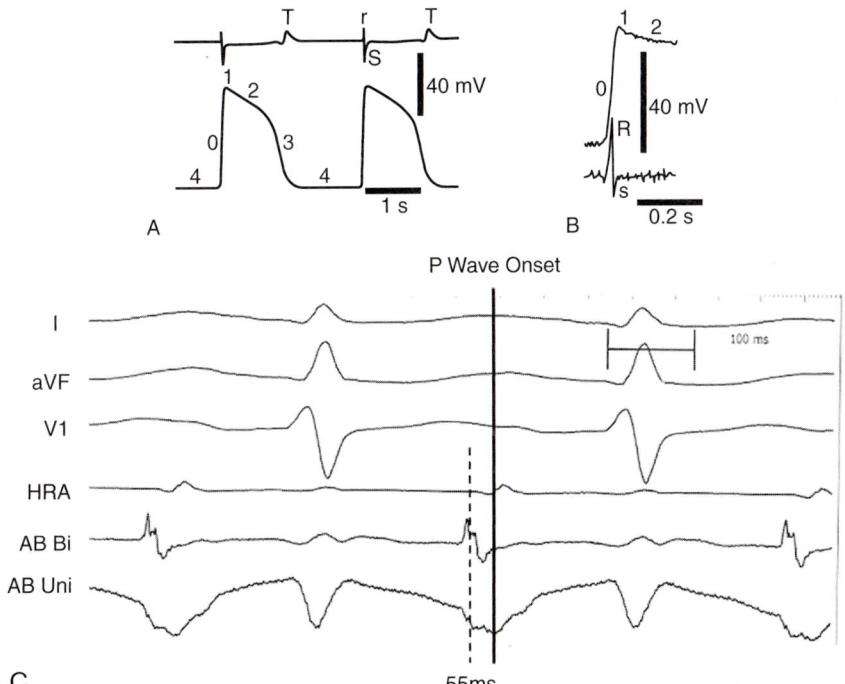

FIGURE 7-2. Concordance between extracellular electrogram and intracellular action potential recordings. **A,** Relationship between unipolar electrogram *(top trace)* and the transmembrane potential *(bottom trace)* recorded simultaneously from bullfrog ventricle. **B,** Display of the initial part of the simultaneously recorded transmembrane action potential *(top trace)* and unipolar electrogram from a different frog *(bottom trace)*, showing concordance between the upstrokes of the two potentials. **C,** Surface and intracardiac electrograms recorded during mapping of a right atrial tachycardia. The peak of the bipolar ablation electrogram (AB Bi) coincides with the maximal negative downslope of the distal ablation unipolar recording (AB Uni). These points reflect local activation time at the recording electrodes, and both precede P-wave onset by 55 msec. HRA, high right atrium. *(A and B, Modified from Yoshida S. Simple techniques suitable for student use to record action potentials from the frog heart. Adv Physiol Educ. 2001;25:176-186, 2001. With permission.)*

The bipolar electrogram is recorded as the potential difference between two closely spaced electrodes in direct contact with the heart; it can be calculated as the difference between two unipolar electrograms at each of the two electrode sites[14] (Fig. 7-3). In the electrophysiology laboratory, this is typically done with analog amplifiers rather than with digital subtraction between unipolar signals. The amplitude of the bipolar electrogram is inversely proportional to the third power of the distance between recording site and dipole.[15]

The major advantage of bipolar recordings lies in the distinction between local and distant activity. A limitation of bipolar electrograms is their directional sensitivity; as a result, if the activation wavefront is parallel in relation to the electrode pair, the bipolar spike will be of maximal amplitude, whereas if it is perpendicular, both electrodes will record the same waveform at the same time, and no spike will result.[16] In addition, activation at the two poles of the bipolar electrogram is not simultaneous, making activation detection more difficult in bipolar electrograms. The following criteria have been suggested for activation detection in bipolar electrograms: (1) the maximal absolute value of the bipolar electrogram; (2) the first elevation of the electrogram of more than 45 degrees from the baseline; (3) the baseline crossing with the steepest slope; and (4) morphologic algorithms that search for symmetry in the bipolar waveform. Of these, the maximal amplitude of the bipo-

lar electrogram is the most easily measured and has been shown to closely coincide with the maximal downslope of the unipolar electrogram (and the maximal upstroke of the monophasic action potential).[17]

Recording Artifacts

The identification of artifactual electrograms is of crucial importance in any system of cardiac mapping and may have major influence on the final interpretation of an activation sequence, such as whether a fractionated electrogram represents a motion artifact or local activation in an assumed zone of slow conduction[18] (Table 7-2). Typical recording artifacts induced at the myocardium-electrode interface include (1) polarization of electrodes, which can cause slow shifts of the baseline of the signals; (2) local myocardial injury resulting from inappropriate pressure by recording electrodes[12]; (3) motion artifacts, which are often rhythmic and linked to cardiac events, therefore simulating fractionated electrograms, or which can be sudden shifts of potential that may be misinterpreted as activations by computer algorithms; (4) poor contact between electrode and myocardium, leading to heavier weighing of far-field effects and increased 50- or 60-Hz noise; (5) potentials produced by two electrodes from different catheters touching each other; and (6) repolarization signals masquerading as a mid-diastolic potential. Ensuring good contact between the recording electrode and the underlying myocardium (to remove far-field effects), eliminating all possible sources of noise, including adequate grounding for 50 to 60 Hz (and if necessary the use of notch filters), and locating preamplifiers and amplifiers as close as possible to the mapped heart all may help eliminate most of the artifacts that are seen in the clinical electrophysiology laboratory. Undue pressure by the recording catheter on the underlying myocardium can be reflected by the appearance of ST-segment elevation on the unipolar electrogram; slight catheter repositioning usually results in resolution of the ST segment to baseline. Motion artifact (from the patient or the surrounding environment) can be minimized by preventing contact of perfusion pumps and other equipment capable of generating cyclical noise with the patient table and mapping equipment.

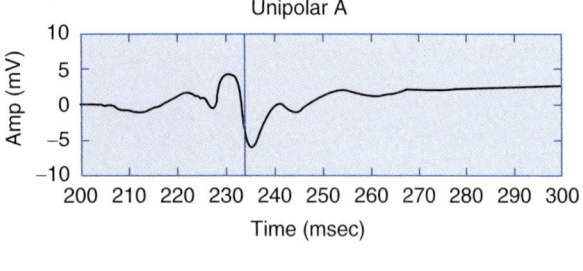

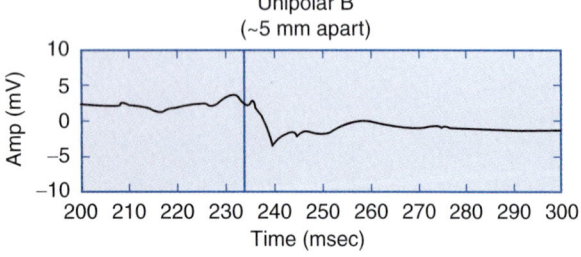

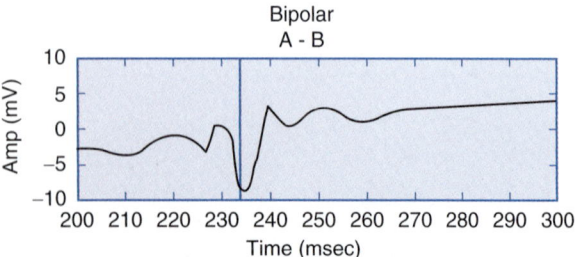

FIGURE 7-3. Relationship between unipolar and bipolar electrograms. The bipolar electrogram represents the difference between two closely spaced unipolar electrodes that have the same reference. The result is that the far-field effects and noise that are present in both unipolar electrograms get canceled out. Amp, amplitude.

TABLE 7-2	
SOURCES OF INTRACARDIAC RECORDING ARTIFACTS	
Cause	**Manifestation**
Electrode polarization	Electrogram drift
Excessive contact pressure	ST elevation
Catheter motion	Fractionation
Poor contact	Low amplitude
Contact with other catheters	High-frequency signals
Repolarization	Late or mid-diastolic potentials
Electromagnetic interference	High-frequency noise
Poor grounding	High-frequency noise

Characteristics of Intracardiac Signals: Normal Heart

Unipolar endocardial electrograms obtained from experiments in normal canine hearts and from the human atrium and ventricle are characterized by a QS morphology with a rapid downstroke in the first part of the QRS complex (intrinsic deflection).[10,19] Bipolar endocardial electrograms in the normal human left ventricle from catheters with 10-mm interelectrode distance have amplitudes of greater than 3 mV and durations of less than 70 milliseconds, and no split, fractionated electrograms are found.[17] Unipolar and bipolar electrograms in diseased myocardium are typically characterized by slower upstrokes and fragmentation (see later discussion).

Although slow conduction and fractionated, low-amplitude signals are not as widespread in the normal heart compared with the diseased atrium or ventricle, low-amplitude, high-frequency electrograms have been well described at the thoracic vein–atrium junction, within both the pulmonary veins and the vena cava,[20–22] as well as at other sites in the normal heart, such as the crista terminalis and coronary sinus.[23]

Electrical Abnormalities in the Absence of Structural Heart Disease

Electrograms need not be entirely "normal" even in the absence of overt fibrosis or fatty replacement. For example, low-amplitude, fractionated bipolar electrograms may be seen at the earliest activation sites of focal tachycardias, even in the presence of a normal-looking unipolar electrogram. Figure 7-4 shows the bipolar electrogram at the successful ablation site of two different focal tachycardias

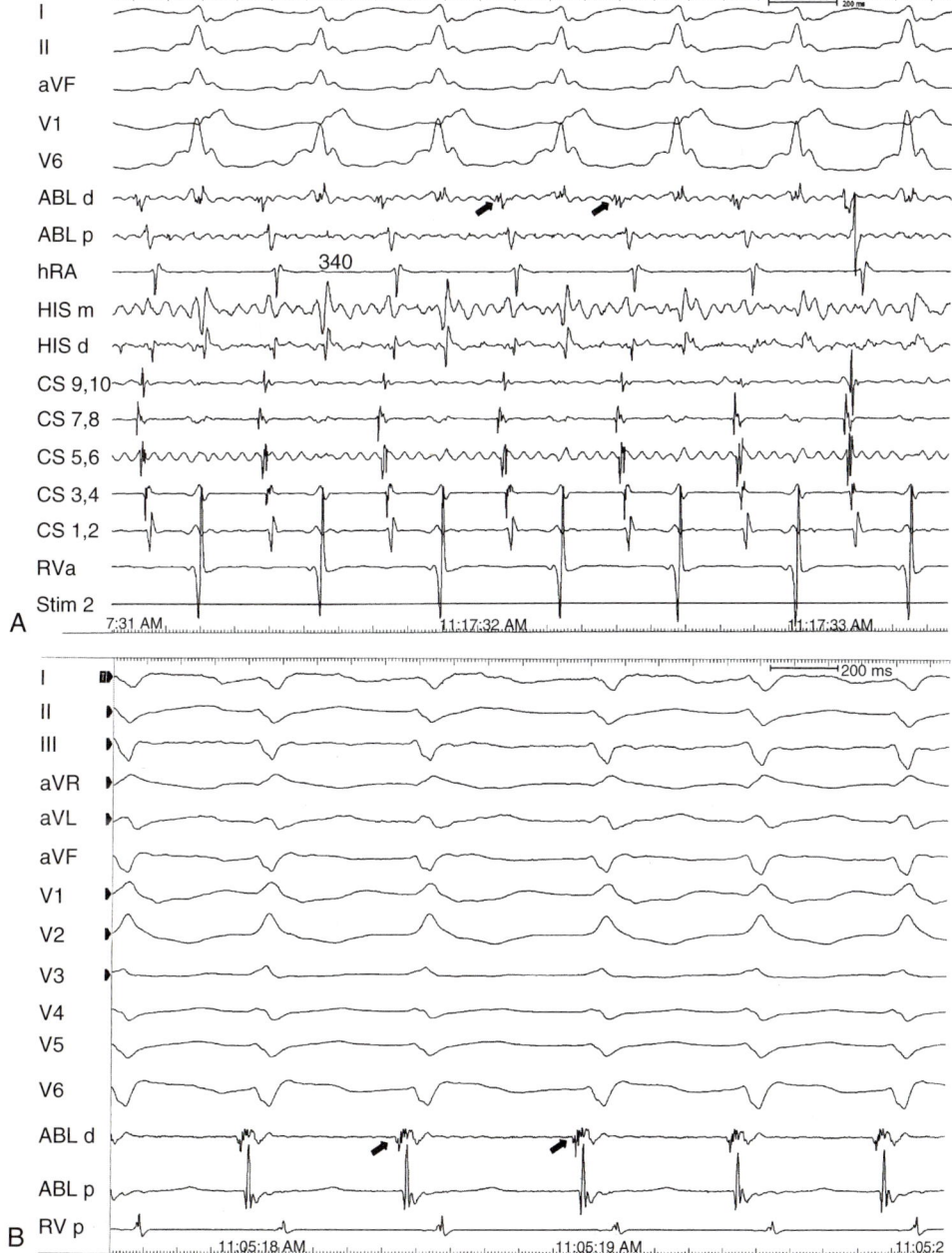

FIGURE 7-4. Low-amplitude bipolar electrogram at successful ablation site of two focal tachycardias: a focal tachycardia originating from the ostium of the coronary sinus (**A**) and a focal ventricular tachycardia arising from the inferolateral left ventricle (**B**). In both instances, notice the lower amplitude and prolonged duration of the electrogram at the site of earliest activation (i.e., the ablation site) *(arrows)*. ABL, ablation; CS, coronary sinus; d, distal; HRA, high right atrium; m, mid; p, proximal; RV, right ventricle.

in the absence of any overt structural heart disease: a focal tachycardia originating from the coronary sinus os and a focal ventricular tachycardia (VT) arising from the inferolateral left ventricle. We have also noted late potentials during sinus rhythm in hearts that are otherwise morphologically normal; Figure 7-5 shows late potentials in the right ventricle of a patient who had exercise-induced

left bundle superior axis VT, but no evidence of scar or any other abnormality on ECG or cardiac magnetic resonance imaging (MRI).

The basis for these potentials is not entirely clear. In the absence of overt scar on sensitive imaging modalities such as MRI, it is tempting to speculate that at least some of the delay seen in these electrograms may be functional in nature. In fact, "functional" anisotropic conduction is well described in the normal heart (e.g., at the crista terminalis)[23] and may be responsible for the creation of macroreentrant circuits, such as isthmus-dependent atrial flutter. More recently, anisotropic conduction has also been demonstrated within the pulmonary veins[24] and the superior vena cava. Figure 7-6 shows that the conduction times into and out of the pulmonary vein can be very different, which is an example of anisotropic conduction.[25]

It is conceivable, therefore, that at least some of the focal tachycardias described in the normal heart may be microreentrant in origin. Other factors that have been postulated include poor intercellular coupling, such as that due to decreased gap junctions at sites of origin of focal tachycardias, leading to decreased electrotonic inhibition of the focus by surrounding tissue.[26] In general, electrograms at successful ablation sites for focal tachycardias are less than 50 milliseconds presystolic. However, pulmonary vein tachycardias may be more than 50 seconds presystolic, at least partially on account of the slow conduction noted in this area.

Fractionated, bipolar electrograms (both during tachycardia and during sinus rhythm) have also been well

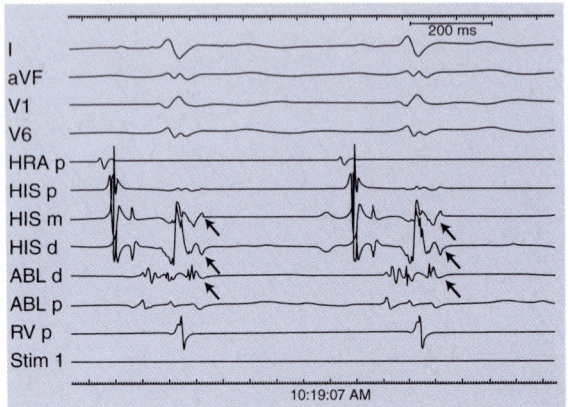

FIGURE 7-5. Late systolic potentials in a heart with no known myocardial disease. The figure demonstrates late potentials that extend beyond the end of the QRS *(arrows)* at the septal right ventricle (base of the right ventricular outflow tract) of a patient who had exercise-induced left bundle superior axis ventricular tachycardia but no evidence of scar or any other abnormality on echocardiography or cardiac magnetic resonance imaging. ABL, ablation; d, distal; HRA, high right atrium; m, mid; p, proximal; RV, right ventricle; Stim, stimulus.

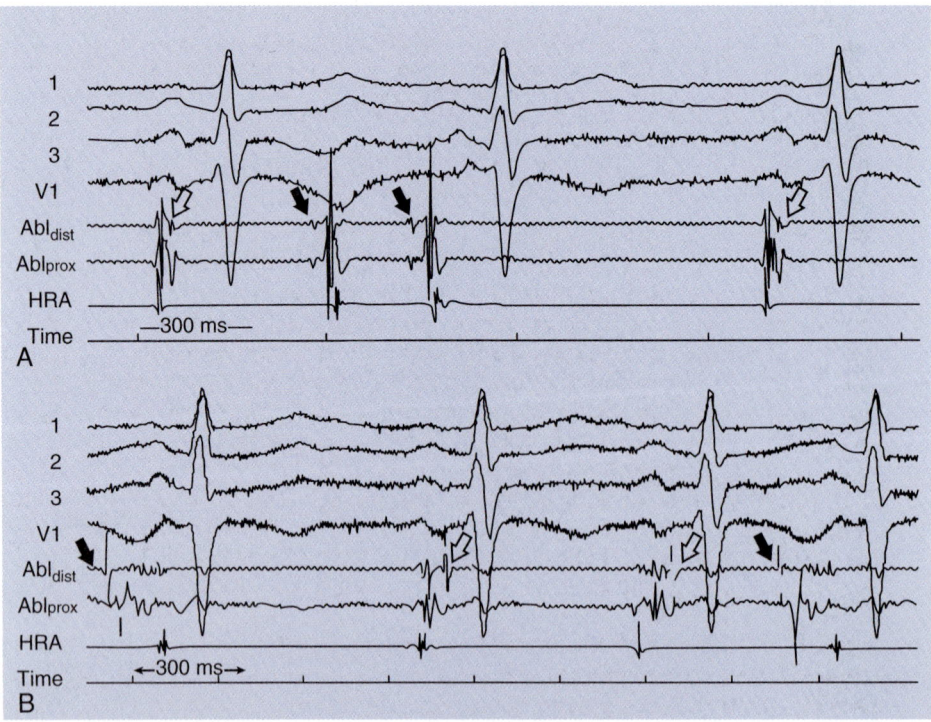

FIGURE 7-6. Anisotropic conduction in the superior vena cava (SVC) and pulmonary vein. In both **A** and **B**, *open arrows* indicate atrial electrograms, and *solid arrows* indicate pulmonary vein potentials. **A,** Sinus rhythm with conduction into the posterosuperior right atrium (close to its junction with the SVC). **B,** The right superior pulmonary vein. In both **A** and **B**, the bipolar ablation electrogram shows an atrial signal followed by an SVC or a pulmonary vein myocardial signal. Atrial premature contractions (APCs) coming from the SVC or from pulmonary veins show the venous myocardial potential first, followed by the atrial myocardial signal. Note that conduction out of the SVC or pulmonary vein (APCs) is longer than conduction into the SVC or pulmonary vein during sinus rhythm. *(From Miller JM, Olgin JE, Das MK. Atrial fibrillation: what are the targets for intervention? J Interv Card Electrophysiol. 2003;9:249-257. With permission.)*

described in idiopathic VT arising from the left ventricular septum. In fact, it is the presence of these Purkinje-like potentials some distance away from the septum that has led some to postulate a reentrant circuit of considerable size as the basis for this VT.[27] Split electrograms may sometimes be recorded in the normal heart, such as in the right posteroseptal area from conduction block across the eustachian ridge.

Electrogram Abnormalities in the Presence of Structural Heart Disease

The signature of scar in the atrium or ventricle is a low-amplitude, high-frequency electrogram (during sinus rhythm or during tachycardia), with the duration and amplitude of the electrogram showing some correlation with the degree of slow conduction in and around the area of fibrosis.[28] Low-amplitude, fractionated electrograms may be recorded during or after the QRS complex and are typically less than 1 mV in amplitude; these can be recorded during sinus rhythm and VT. The characteristic unipolar electrogram in the setting of chronic myocardial scar, such as myocardial infarction, may show a single, rapid biphasic deflection of Rs morphology following a wide QS potential, a double Rs deflection, or fragmentation with multiple deflections.[29] Continuous, low-amplitude electrical activity, such as a fractionated electrogram spanning the entire tachycardia cycle length, can also be seen in the setting of myocardial scar or disease. Figure 7-7 shows an example of low-amplitude continuous activity at a successful ablation site for a reentrant atrial tachycardia and flutter in a patient who had undergone Mustard repair for D-transposition of the great arteries.

Animal studies performed in the setting of chronic experimental myocardial infarction have examined the intracellular basis of the previously mentioned changes on the extracellularly recorded electrograms and have demonstrated that action potential amplitude and upstroke are similar to those of normal myocardium.[30,31] Despite the presence of normal action potentials, slow and discontinuous conduction is present, which may provide an electrophysiologic and anatomic basis for arrhythmias. One explanation of the low amplitude, prolonged duration, and notched extracellular potentials in the infarcted areas is that the slow conduction represents activation of normal cells separated by areas of fibrous tissue producing discontinuities in conduction. Kadish and colleagues used vector mapping, a technique based on summing orthogonally bipolar electrograms, to determine the direction of activation in cardiac tissue and showed that although vector loops recorded from normal myocardial tissue were found to be smooth and pointing in a single direction, those recorded from areas of healed myocardial infarction were notched, irregular, and occasionally pointing in more than one direction.[32] Using the vector technique, the authors demonstrated complex activation patterns in areas where abnormal extracellular electrograms are recorded in which discrete activation times may be difficult to identify, such as in areas of fractionated electrograms where multiple peaks are present.[33]

Ischemic heart disease is by far the most common cause of scar in the ventricle, although less common conditions such as arrhythmogenic right ventricular dysplasia and cardiomyopathy may demonstrate similar electrophysiologic characteristics because of fibrofatty replacement in the right (and occasionally left) ventricle. Fibrosis has also been described in dilated cardiomyopathy but is seen far less commonly than in ischemic heart disease. In the atrium, scar is commonly the result of surgery for congenital

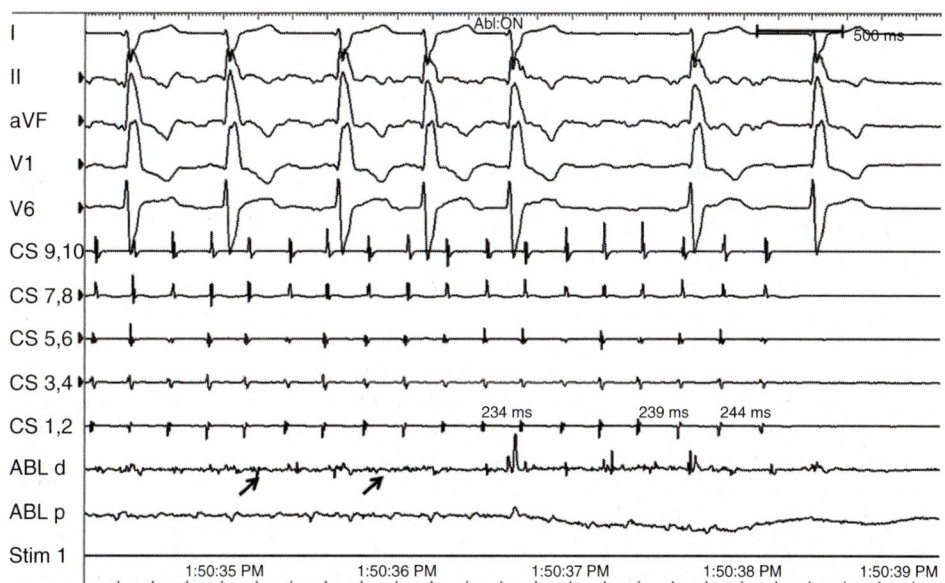

FIGURE 7-7. Continuous, low-amplitude activity at the site of ablation in atrial flutter in the setting of D-transposition of the great artery repair. In this patient, the atrial flutter was mapped to the subeustachian isthmus. The isthmus was first approached and ablated from the systemic or subaortic ventricle. However, the entire isthmus could not be ablated from the subaortic side (because of baffle and suture lines). Additional mapping and ablation were therefore performed through the baffle on the subpulmonic or left side. From the subpulmonic side, it was possible to reach a portion of the subeustachian isthmus that had previously not been reached with a subaortic approach. Mapping along this portion of the subeustachian isthmus (i.e., along the same line where ablation was performed from the right ventricle) revealed the continuous, low-amplitude activity shown by the *arrows*. Ablation here resulted in slowing and termination of the flutter.

heart disease, and atrial septal defect repair, tricuspid atresia (Fontan repair), tetralogy of Fallot repair, and transposition of great arteries (Mustard-Senning repair) are the most common reasons for scar in the right atrium.[34] Left atrial surgery can create substrate for left or right atrial reentry,[35] the latter likely on account of cannulation sites during bypass.

As mentioned earlier, the low-amplitude electrograms during sinus rhythm are often noted late in systole; Figure 7-8 shows an example of late systolic potentials in the right ventricle of a patient with arrhythmogenic right ventricular dysplasia. Such low-amplitude, high-frequency electrograms are thought to underlie the late potentials that are seen on a positive signal-average ECG.[36] Significantly, even though late potentials are typically seen in and around an area of scar or infarction, late potentials have not been shown to be a clear predictor of ablation success.[37] Although late potentials are frequently noted at or close to sites of successful ablation (of reentrant tachycardias), they lack specificity in that they may also be found at sites that are remote from a successful ablation site (indicating diseased myocardium in other areas). A list of abnormal electrogram morphologies and the possible interpretations is given in Table 7-3.

Endocardial Mapping Techniques

"Contact" endocardial mapping can be performed during sinus rhythm as well as during tachycardia. Mapping techniques can be broadly categorized as follows: (1) activation sequence mapping, (2) fractionated local electrogram and voltage mapping, (3) pace mapping, (4) entrainment mapping, and (5) miscellaneous pacing maneuvers (performed during sinus rhythm or tachycardia). Although these techniques are usually used in combination, the relative utility of each depends on arrhythmia inducibility, stability of the induced arrhythmia, underlying substrate (i.e., normal versus diseased heart), and arrhythmia mechanisms, among other factors. For example, entrainment can be used only in the setting of a sustained, reentrant arrhythmia.

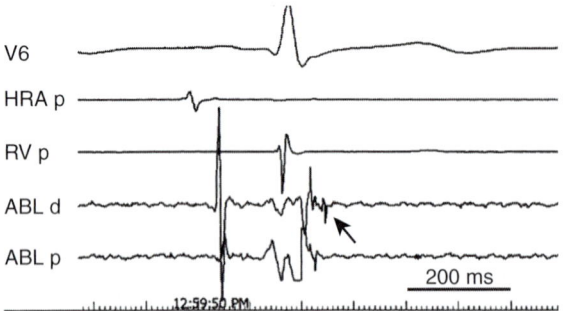

FIGURE 7-8. Late potential mapping in the right ventricle. In a patient with arrhythmogenic right ventricular (RV) dysplasia, many of the electrograms were abnormal, especially at the RV inflow, the RV apex, and the RV outflow tract. The figure shows late potentials during sinus rhythm in the region of the RV apex on the ablation (ABL) catheter *(arrows)*. HRA, high right atrium.

The previous two sections have described the electrogram and voltage characteristics in normal and diseased hearts. The following paragraphs describe the underlying basis for the remainder of the techniques and highlight their use (singly or in combination) in the diagnosis and ablation of atrial and ventricular arrhythmias.

Activation Sequence Mapping

The most commonly used method of identifying the site of origin of a tachyarrhythmia is activation mapping to locate the site of earliest endocardial activation or to determine the activation sequence during the tachycardia. Focal arrhythmias are typically characterized by presystolic timings less than 50 millisecond. Reentrant arrhythmias on the other hand, both in the normal and in diseased hearts, typically demonstrate diastolic activity that is significantly earlier than 50 milliseconds. In fact, for reentrant arrhythmias, intracardiac activity should be present at some point in the heart throughout the cardiac cycle. Electrograms are typically recorded through at least 70% of the tachycardia cycle length in macro-reentrant arrhythmias. In the normal heart, such as in the setting of subeustachian isthmus–dependent typical atrial flutter, the macro-reentrant circuit is of considerable size—bound by the two anatomic barriers of the

TABLE 7-3		
ABNORMAL ELECTROGRAM MORPHOLOGIES		
Morphology	**Definition**	**Interpretations**
Low amplitude	<0.5 mV atrium <1.5 mV ventricle	Myocardial infarction, fibrosis, infiltrative process, poor contact, far-field
Fractionated	Prolonged (>70 msec), low-amplitude potential with multiple peaks or multiple baseline crossings	Peri-infarction, slow conduction, catheter motion, arborized myocardial connection
Split	>70 msec duration with two components separated by isoelectric interval	Local conduction block, surgical scar, slow conduction
Late component	Potential occurs after end of surface QRS or P wave	Delayed activation, line of block, slow conduction
Continuous	Absence of isoelectric interval throughout diastole	Slow conduction, electromagnetic interference artifact
Mid-diastolic	Potential occurs in mid-diastole bounded by isoelectric intervals	Protected isthmus, bystander connection, repolarization, or motion artifact
Low frequency	Low dV/dt	Far-field, artifact
Monophasic action potential	Injury current pattern	Excessive contact pressure, local tissue injury (unipolar)

crista terminalis and the tricuspid annulus—and need not demonstrate the low-amplitude, high-frequency electrograms that are typical of scar-related reentrant arrhythmias. In a reentrant arrhythmia in the setting of myocardial scar, a zone of slow conduction over a pathway of possibly quite complex geometry (e.g., nonlinear, nonhomogeneously anisotropic) provides the diastolic limb of the reentrant circuit. After emerging from the zone of slow conduction, the wavefront propagates rapidly throughout the ventricles to generate the QRS complex. Thus, early or presystolic activation occurs in close proximity to the exit region from the zone of slow conduction.

What is considered to be early activation and a suitable ablation site in a focal arrhythmia (30 to 50 milliseconds presystolic) may not necessarily be early activation in a reentrant arrhythmia. Reentrant atrial tachycardias

or VTs are typically characterized by earlier electrogram timing in diastole, with mid-diastolic (or even earlier) potentials (discussed later) having been correlated with successful ablation sites for these arrhythmias. Figure 7-9 shows an example of atrial tachycardia that was induced in a patient with no known atrial disease; mapping with the ablation catheter revealed electrograms in and around the tricuspid annulus that were significantly more than 50 milliseconds presystolic, thereby raising suspicion for a macro-reentrant tachycardia; a halo duodecapolar catheter was subsequently inserted into the right atrium and showed an activation sequence consistent with counterclockwise reentry around the tricuspid annulus (Fig. 7-9B). Entrainment maneuvers confirmed the diagnosis and led to successful ablation of the arrhythmia at the cavotricuspid isthmus.

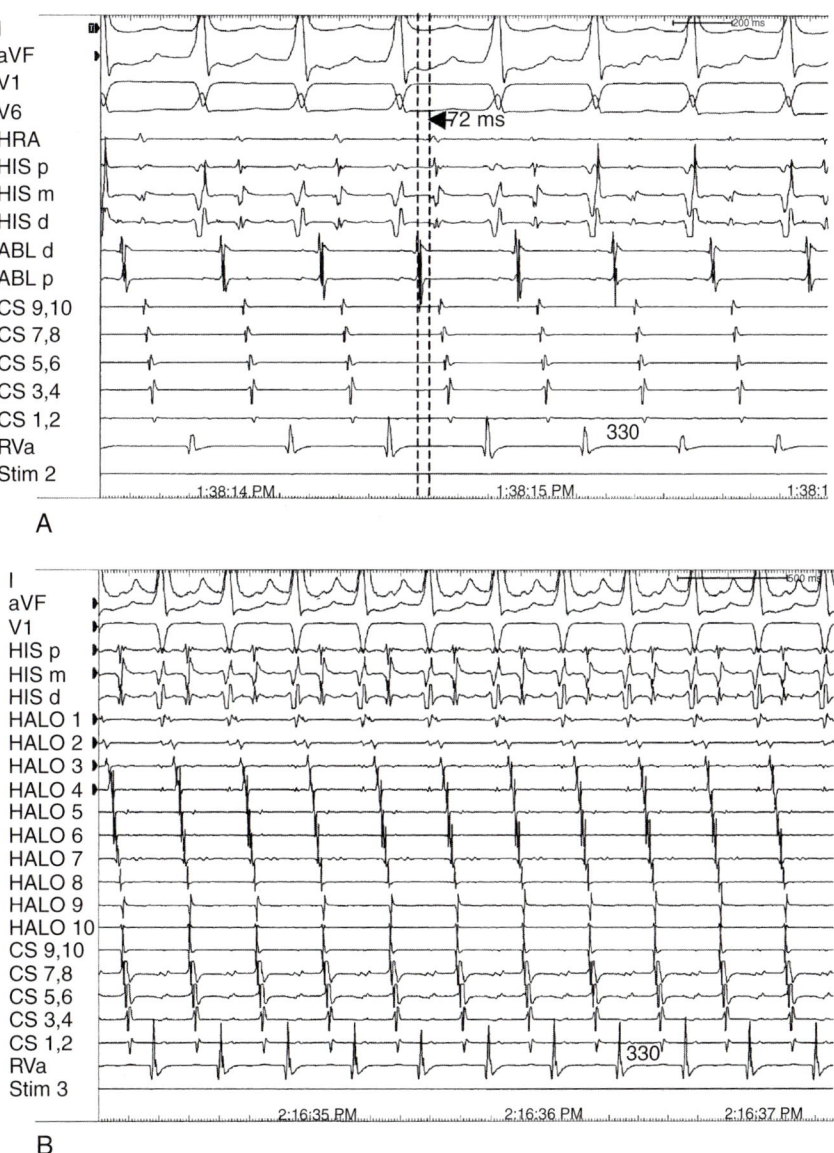

FIGURE 7-9. Apparent atrial tachycardia with sites that had greater than 50 msec presystolic activation times in a patient with no known atrial disease. The P-wave morphology and cycle length suggested that atrial tachycardia rather than atrial flutter was present. However, the mid-diastolic activation times suggested reentry rather than focal tachycardia. **A,** Mapping with the ablation catheter revealed electrograms in and around the tricuspid annulus that were more than 50 msec presystolic, thereby raising suspicion for a reentrant tachycardia. **B,** A halo catheter inserted subsequently showed an activation sequence consistent with clockwise, isthmus-dependent atrial tachycardia and flutter. Entrainment maneuvers confirmed the diagnosis and led to successful ablation of the arrhythmia.

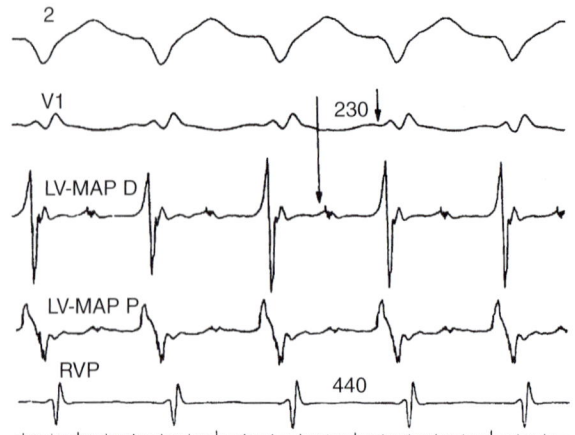

FIGURE 7-10. Activation mapping in a diseased heart. The figure shows mid-diastolic potentials in the setting of infracted-related ventricular tachycardia (VT). Leads 2 and V1 are shown with distal (D) and proximal (P) bipolar signals recorded from a presumed protected isthmus of the VT circuit. An isolated mid-diastolic potential (*long arrow*) is recorded 230 msec before the QRS during VT (*short arrow*), with a cycle length of 440 msec. *(From Josephson ME. Clinical Cardiac Electrophysiology: Techniques and Interpretation, 3rd ed. Philadelphia: Lippincott Williams & Wilkins; 2002. With permission.)*

Mid-diastolic Potentials

If an intervening isoelectric segment exists, the prepotentials are called *mid-diastolic potentials* (Fig. 7-10); it has been suggested that they identify the region of slow conduction. These prepotentials may precede the major ventricular deflection by tens to hundreds of milliseconds.

It is important to demonstrate that during initiation and resetting of an arrhythmia, loss of the mid-diastolic potential is associated with termination of the arrhythmia.[27] Although there are some recent data to support the specificity of diastolic potentials during sinus rhythm as the potentially successful ablation sites (i.e., critical isthmus sites during VT),[38] most studies have looked at diastolic potentials during sustained tachycardia as markers of a protected isthmus.

Mid-diastolic potentials that do not dynamically precede the QRS complex of the VT may represent blind-end alleys of late activation or motion artifact.[27,28] In one study, almost continuous electrical activity spanning the diastolic segment was frequently seen in patients with VT due to ischemic heart disease or arrhythmogenic right ventricular dysplasia. However, in 85% of patients, the episodes of continuous electrical activity could be dissociated from the VT.[23] Such behavior presumably is due to slow and fractionated conduction into nonessential areas of diseased myocardium.

Unipolar Potential Mapping

Unipolar electrograms provide useful adjunctive mapping information to bipolar electrograms during mapping for focal atrial and VTs. Amerendral and associates noted that the presence of a QS complex was highly sensitive in identifying successful ablation sites.[39] However, nearly 70% of unsuccessful sites also manifested a QS unipolar complex, with QS complexes being recorded more than 1 cm away in 65% of patients.[40] The unipolar electrogram morphology with standard ablation electrodes is therefore a highly

sensitive but nonspecific marker for target sites in patients with idiopathic right ventricular and other ventricular tachycardias as well as atrial tachycardias. Unipolar electrograms are of limited utility, however, in the setting of myocardial scar or fibrosis because the criteria established for unipolar activation (i.e., peak dV/dt) cannot be relied on in the presence of slow, disordered conduction, with the initial deflection in unipolar recordings in this setting frequently showing a delayed initial deflection.

Much has been written about the utility of the unipolar electrogram in localizing insertion and successful ablation sites for accessory pathways.[41] Note that most of these data are for anterograde mapping in the setting of overt preexcitation, although some investigators have demonstrated the utility of unipolar mapping for retrogradely conducting accessory pathways.[42] Electrograms characteristic of the insertion sites of accessory pathways have been described in detail elsewhere in this book (see Chapters 21, 22, and 23).

Pace Mapping

Pace mapping involves manipulation of the mapping catheter to the region of origin of the tachycardia. Pacing at this site, using the same cycle length as the tachycardia, should generate P waves or QRS complexes resembling those during tachycardia. The greater the degree of concordance between the P wave or QRS morphology during pacing and tachycardia, the closer the catheter is to the exit site of the tachycardia. In addition, the stimulus to QRS interval of more than 40 to 70 milliseconds is an indication of slow conduction.

Pace mapping has advantages over activation mapping in that induction of arrhythmia is not required; as a result, it allows identification of the site of origin when the induced arrhythmia is poorly tolerated or when VT is not inducible by electrophysiologic techniques but when P-wave or QRS morphology from a 12-lead ECG is available. However, others have argued that pace mapping is not as sensitive or precise as activation mapping and may be more time-consuming. Pace mapping has generally been more useful as a means of localizing sites, with a combination of activation and pace mapping used to best identify the optimal target site of ablation. For generalized localization of an arrhythmia exit site, such as with substrate mapping of unstable ventricular arrhythmias, matching 10/12 leads may be sufficient. For precise arrhythmia localization, 12/12 leads should match the clinical tachycardia.

Most investigators report successful ablation at sites with identical or nearly identical matches in all 12 surface leads.[43,44] Differences in QRS configuration between pacing and spontaneous tachycardia in a single lead may be critical. An example is shown in Figure 7-11, in which ablation success was achieved (in the left coronary cusp) only at the site of a 12/12 or perfect pace map. Figure 7-12 shows an example of premature ventricular contractions (PVCs) arising from the right coronary cusp. Unlike in Figure 7-11A, in which there is a small R wave in the unipolar electrogram, the distal unipolar electrogram in Figure 7-12A has a QS complex; pace mapping at this site also resulted in a nearly perfect pace map (see Fig. 7-12B). Ablation at this site resulted in termination of all PVCs.

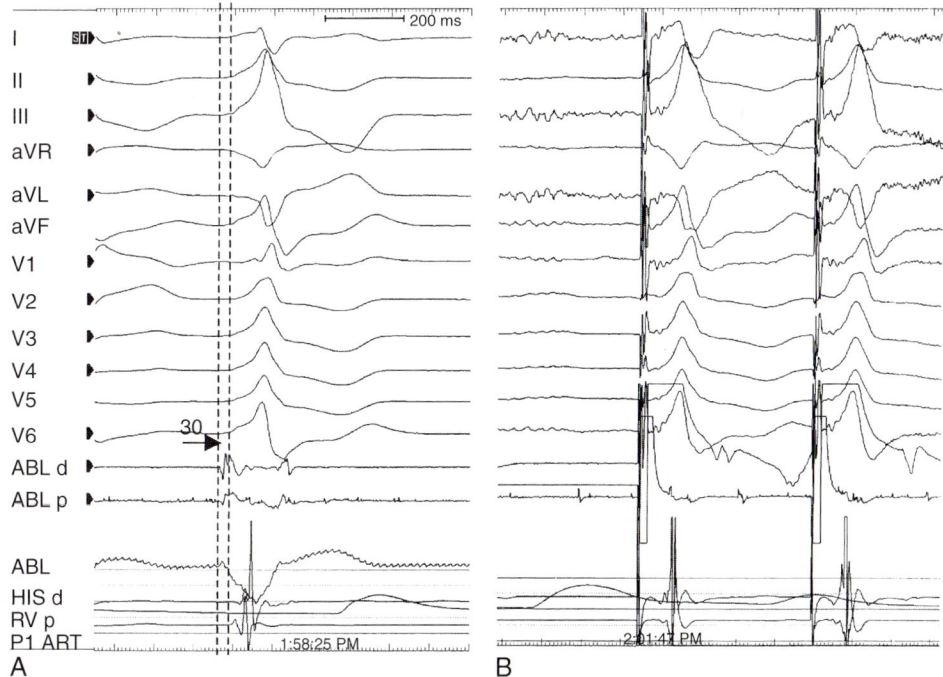

FIGURE 7-11. Excellent pace map in a patient with right bundle inferior axis premature ventricular contractions (PVCs). **A,** Right bundle PVCs mapped to the left coronary cusp. The ablation catheter shows an activation time that was 30 msec presystolic. The distal unipolar electrogram coincides with the earliest bipolar electrogram. Note that the unipolar electrogram (ABL) has a small r wave before the inscription of the QS. **B,** Pace mapping performed at the site shown in **A** revealed a 12/12 match with the PVC in **A.** It was decided to ablate at this site because activation sites with a QS pattern on the unipolar electrogram (i.e., no r wave) were less than 0.5 cm from the left main artery. Ablation resulted in termination of PVCs.

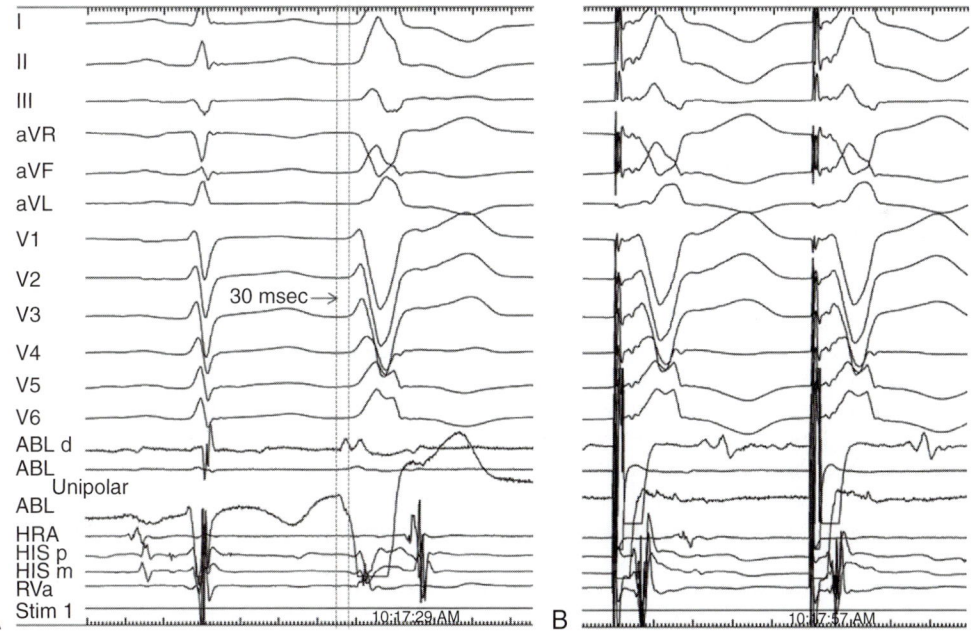

FIGURE 7-12. Excellent pace map in a patient with right coronary cusp premature ventricular contractions (PVCs). **A,** Right bundle PVCs mapped to the right coronary cusp. The ablation catheter shows an activation time that was 30 msec presystolic. The distal unipolar electrogram coincides with the earliest bipolar electrogram and has a QS complex. **B,** Pace mapping performed at the site shown in **A** revealed a 12/12 match with the PVC in **A.** Ablation at this site resulted in termination of PVC.

The use of single ECG leads or body surface mapping may improve the precision of pace mapping.[45] Kadish and colleagues examined the spatial resolution of unipolar pacing with respect to the degree of pace map matching and found that under optimal conditions—that is, when minor differences in configuration (notching, new small component,

change in amplitude of individual component, or overall change in QRS shape) in at least one lead were accounted for—the spatial resolution of an exact pace map match may be less than 5 mm.[46] Bipolar pacing may introduce additional variability in the ventricular paced electrocardiogram, but these changes may be minimized by low pacing outputs

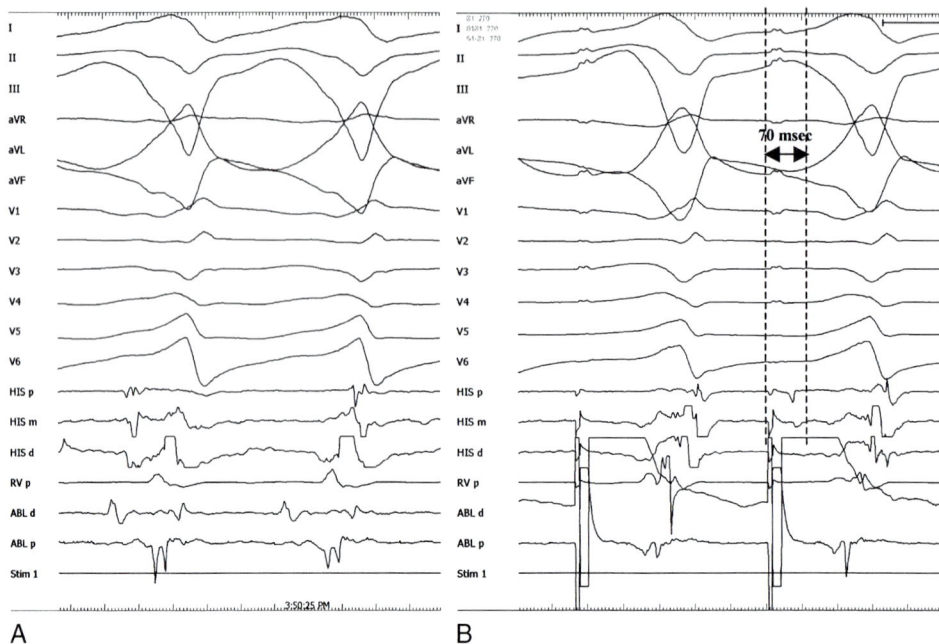

FIGURE 7-13. Pace mapping in the setting of myocardial scar. **A,** Ventricular tachycardia (cycle length, 260 msec). **B,** Pace mapping in a region of scar (low-amplitude potentials) in the right ventricle of a patient with arrhythmogenic right ventricular dysplasia. Note the 12/12 leads pace map and the long, mid-diastolic stimulus-to-QRS interval (70 msec); the stimulus-to-QRS interval was suggestive of a location in the middle of a protected isthmus. Ablation in this region rendered the ventricular tachycardia noninducible.

and small interelectrode distances (≤5 mm) or by unipolar pacing. Pace mapping should be performed as close as possible to the cycle length of the spontaneous tachycardia to minimize rate-dependent aberration in paced P-wave or QRS configuration (owing to increasing degrees of incomplete repolarization and fusion with the preceding T wave during shorter cycle lengths).[47]

Pace mapping during sinus rhythm has been shown to be less sensitive in the setting of scarred myocardium, even when pacing is performed close to the tachycardia circuit. The activation wavefront may take the "path of least resistance" and, instead of mimicking the tachycardia wavefront (through the protected tachycardia isthmus), may activate normal myocardium first, thereby creating a very different pace map. In addition, the boundaries of a protected isthmus may be functional in nature and therefore difficult to replicate with pacing during sinus rhythm. More recently, several investigators have shown that pace mapping may be performed at the infarct border[48] with good sensitivity and specificity and can provide successful target sites for ablation based on the closeness of the pace map to the tachycardia and the stimulus-to-QRS interval (helping outline the critical isthmus from entrance to exit) (Fig. 7-13).

Entrainment Mapping

Entrainment is one of the most powerful tools in the electrophysiologist's arsenal that serves the following purposes: (1) allows confirmation of reentry as the underlying mechanism of a sustained arrhythmia, (2) allows localization of an underlying reentrant circuit (e.g., to the right or left atrium in the setting of a reentrant atrial tachycardia), and (3) allows identification of myocardium that is critical to the reentrant circuit (i.e. critical isthmus). The critical isthmus may be narrow enough to be amenable to ablation, with resulting interruption of the tachycardia.[49] A full discussion of resetting curves, entrainment criteria, and the pitfalls of entrainment is beyond the scope of this chapter; the reader is referred to other authoritative texts for a more in-depth study of the principles of entrainment.[49-53]

Entrainment is continuous resetting of a reentrant circuit with an excitable gap by a series of stimuli. The presence of entrainment is established when pacing at a rate slightly faster than the tachycardia cycle length accelerates all P waves or QRS complexes (or intracardiac electrograms) to the pacing rate and termination of pacing is followed by resumption of the same tachycardia with the presence of constant surface or intracardiac fusion during pacing (or progressive fusion during pacing at progressively faster cycle lengths). The four criteria for manifest entrainment are (1) constant fusion during overdrive pacing, except for the last captured beat, which is entrained but not fused; (2) progressive fusion during overdrive pacing; (3) localized conduction block to a site for one paced beat associated with interruption of the tachycardia, followed by activation of that site by the next paced beat from a different direction and with a shorter conduction time; and (4) a change in conduction time to and electrogram morphology at an electrode recording site when pacing at two different rates during a tachycardia (this is the intracardiac equivalent of criterion 2 because surface criteria may be difficult to visualize on occasion, such as for atrial tachycardia).

Figure 7-14 shows an example of manifest entrainment (based on intracardiac electrograms); activation around the tricuspid annulus is shown during overdrive pacing of what appeared to be typical, counterclockwise atrial flutter in a

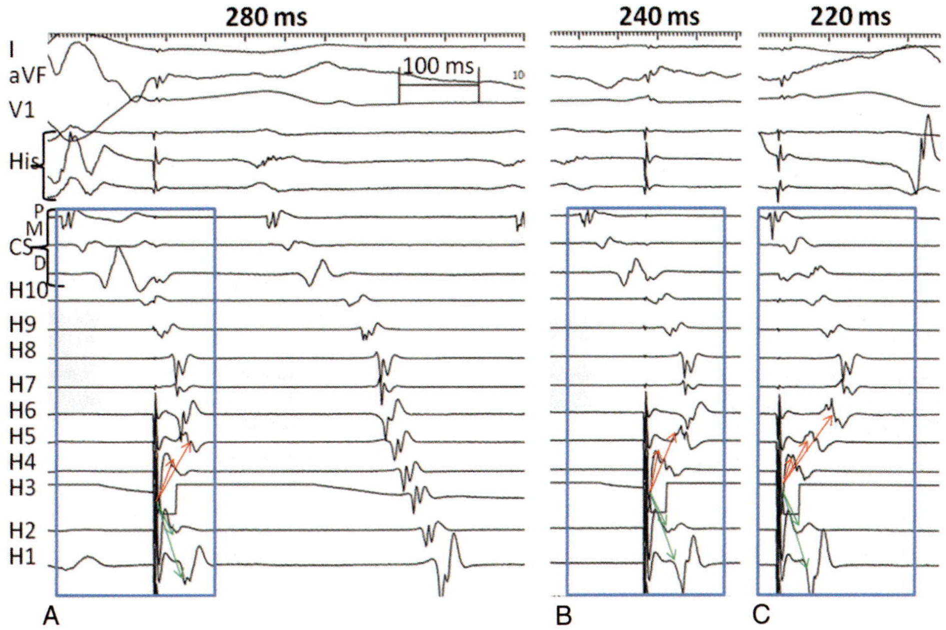

FIGURE 7-14. Progressive fusion with demonstration of (manifest) entrainment. The figure shows activation around the tricuspid annulus during attempted entrainment of what appeared to be typical, counterclockwise atrial flutter in a patient with a normal heart. **A,** Pacing from halo (H) 3 that is slightly faster than the tachycardia (entrainment) reveals fusion along the halo catheter; halo 5 is captured antidromically, but the rest of the halo is captured orthodromically (no change in activation sequence or polarity along the halo except in halo 7). **B,** Pacing at 240 ms demonstrates progressive fusion: now halo 5 and halo 6 are captured antidromically (*red arrows* show clear change in timing and morphology of halo 6 in **B** compared with **A**), thereby confirming entrainment (based on intracardiac fusion, the fourth entrainment criterion). **C,** Pacing at 220 msec results in antidromic activation of halo 6 and halo 7.

patient with a normal heart. Pacing at progressively faster rates demonstrates progressive fusion—one of the diagnostic criteria for entrainment and therefore reentry—which is best demonstrated by a change in activation (as well as timing) of the bipolar electrograms in the distal halo electrodes. In fact, even when changes in timing are subtle, electrogram morphology may provide important clues to a diagnosis.

After entrainment has been demonstrated (i.e., "manifest" entrainment), it can be used for mapping. Entrainment mapping is centered on obtaining a match between the entrained surface P wave or QRS complex or intracardiac electrograms and tachycardia morphology ("concealed" entrainment; discussed later) and on obtaining a postpacing interval (PPI; described later) that is equal to the tachycardia cycle length. Although the demonstration of resetting with fusion (or manifest entrainment) confirms reentry, the presence of concealed entrainment allows the ablationist to "home in" on a protected isthmus—a frequent site of ablation success. Concealed entrainment is characterized by a failure to demonstrate fusion (i.e., criteria 1, 2, and 4) during pacing from a protected isthmus within a tachycardia circuit (Fig. 7-15) and is associated with a PPI that is equal to the tachycardia cycle length. The PPI is the time between the last pacing stimulus that entrained the tachycardia and the next recorded electrogram at the pacing site. The PPI should be equal to the tachycardia cycle length (within 20 to 30 milliseconds) if the pacing site is within a critical part of the reentrant circuit. If the pacing site is outside of the circuit, the PPI should be equal to the tachycardia cycle length plus the time required for the stimulus to propagate from the pacing site to the tachycardia circuit and back. Problems

arise when the electrogram at the pacing site is distorted immediately after pacing. To overcome this shortcoming, alternative methods of estimating the PPI have been developed.[53] The first method is used when the electrogram on the pacing or mapping electrode is obscured in the first cycle after the termination of pacing and is given by the following equation:

$$ER(N+1 DIFFE_{Eg}) = [S - Eg_{(N+1)}] - [L_{(N+2)} - Eg_{(N+3)}]$$

where:

- $ER(N + 1 DIFFE_{Eg})$ is the entrainment response (estimated PPI – TCL) by the N + 1 method
- $S - Eg_{(N+1)}$ is the interval from the last stimulus (S) that entrains the tachycardia to the reference electrogram (Eg) during the first beat of tachycardia after $S[Eg_{(N+1)}]$
- $L_{(N + 2)} - Eg_{(N + 3)}$ is the interval from the local activation (L) at the pacing site during the second beat of tachycardia after $S[L_{(N+2)}]$ to Eg during the third beat of tachycardia after $S[Eg_{(N+3)}]$

The second method is given by the following equation:

$$ERPPIR = (PD - TD) + (PPIR - TCL)$$

where:

- ERPPIR is entrainment response (estimated PPI – TCL) by the PPI remote electrogram method
- PD (pacing delay) is the interval from the last stimulus that entrains the tachycardia (S) to the Eg during the last entrained beat of tachycardia [PD = S –$Eg_{(N)}$] interval

- TD (tachycardia delay) is the interval from the local activation at the pacing site during the second beat of tachycardia after S to the Eg during the second beat after S [TD = $L_{(N+2)}$ – $Eg_{(N+2)}$] interval
- PPIR is the postpacing interval recorded at the remote electrode [PPIR = $Eg_{(N)}$ – $Eg_{(N+1)}$] interval
- TCL is the tachycardia cycle length

Both of these methods have been shown to be equivalent and comparable to the standard PPI (Fig. 7-15D).[53]

Miscellaneous Pacing Maneuvers

Atrial or ventricular pacing during sinus rhythm or during tachycardia is a useful maneuver for determining the mechanism of a tachycardia and may also help in mapping a tachycardia.

Response to Atrial or Ventricular Pacing

In our laboratory, we perform overdrive ventricular pacing in an attempt to demonstrate entrainment in resetting a

narrow-complex supraventricular tachycardia with a concentric retrograde activation sequence, where we perform ventricular pacing (entrainment) as a diagnostic maneuver to differentiate between atrioventricular nodal reentrant tachycardia (AVNRT), atrioventricular reentrant tachycardia (AVRT), and atrial tachycardia. We pace 10 to 30 milliseconds faster than the tachycardia cycle length for at least 8 to 10 beats to allow continuous resetting of the atrial rate to occur; the atrial activation sequence of the tachycardia must remain unchanged during orthodromic capture of an AVRT or reentrant atrial tachycardia circuit as well as during AVNRT (the latter is a microreentrant circuit in which fusion cannot be seen during pacing)—only the third entrainment criterion (outlined previously) has been used to demonstrate entrainment during AVNRT. If the tachycardia resumes after pacing, we look for a V-A-V versus a V-A-A-V response on the return cycle length,[54] with the latter indicating an atrial tachycardia. If a V-A-V response is noted, we proceed to compare the stimulus-to-A (and HA, if a retrograde His is visible) interval during pacing with the VA (and HA)

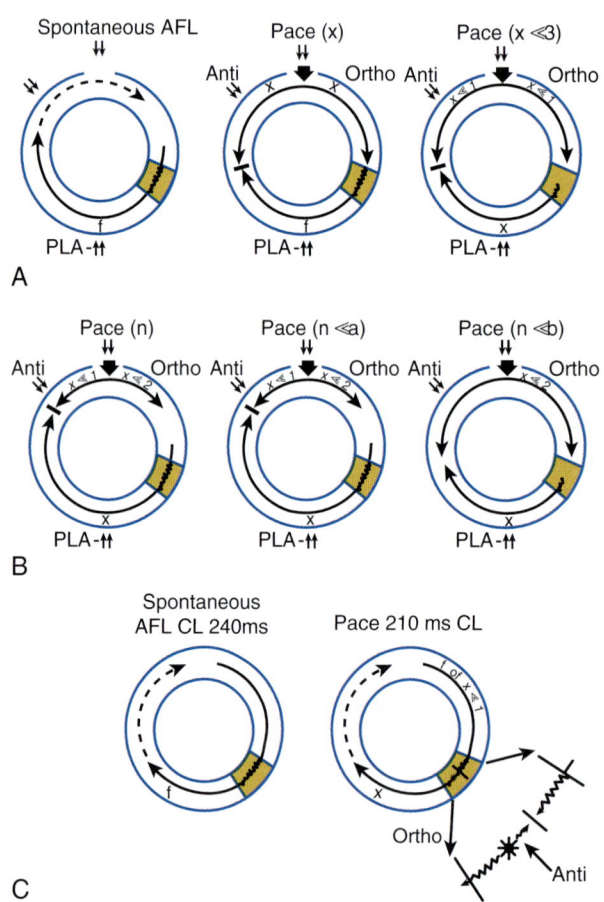

FIGURE 7-15. Manifest and concealed entrainment of atrial flutter. The figure shows schematic diagrams of manifest and concealed entrainment respectively. **A** and **B** demonstrate fixed and progressive fusion, respectively, with overdrive pacing during tachycardia; the contribution of the antidromic wavefront to the tachycardia morphology progressively increases. **C** represents concealed fusion; that is, progressively faster pacing from a protected isthmus does not lead to manifest fusion because the antidromic wavefront does not contribute significantly to the morphology of the tachycardia beat. *Shaded areas* indicate protected isthmus. AFL, atrial flutter; CL, cycle length; x, pacing stimulus in a sequence of stimuli; n, pacing cycle lengths with n > n + a > n + b; anti, antidromic; ortho, orthodromic; PLA, posteroinferior left atrium.

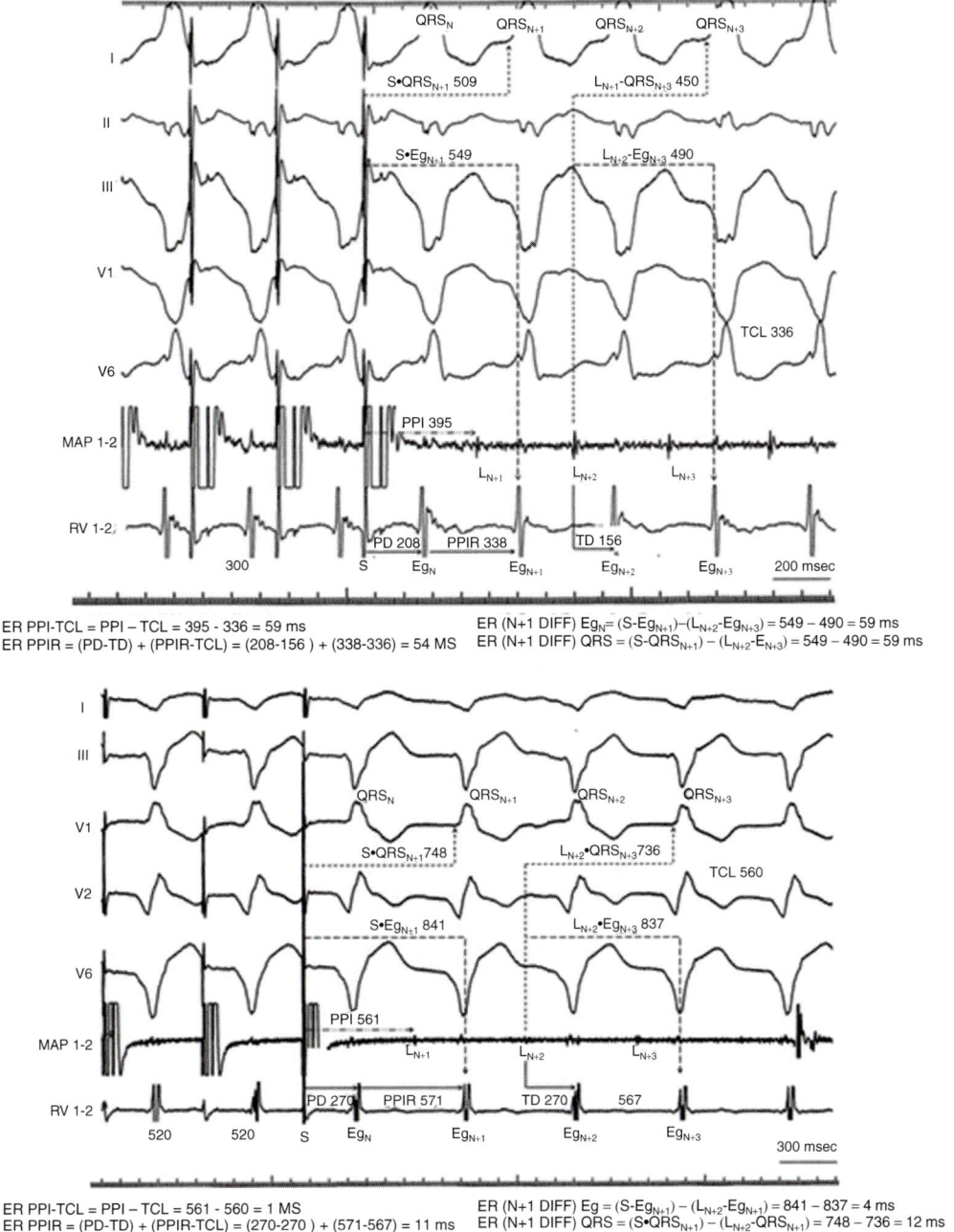

ER PPI-TCL = PPI − TCL = 395 − 336 = 59 ms
ER PPIR = (PD−TD) + (PPIR−TCL) = (208−156) + (338−336) = 54 MS

ER (N+1 DIFF) Eg$_N$= (S−Eg$_{N+1}$)−(L$_{N+2}$-Eg$_{N+3}$) = 549 − 490 = 59 ms
ER (N+1 DIFF) QRS = (S−QRS$_{N+1}$) − (L$_{N+2}$−E$_{N+3}$) = 549 − 490 = 59 ms

ER PPI-TCL = PPI − TCL = 561 − 560 = 1 MS
ER PPIR = (PD−TD) + (PPIR−TCL) = (270−270) + (571−567) = 11 ms

ER (N+1 DIFF) Eg = (S−Eg$_{N+1}$) − (L$_{N+2}$−Eg$_{N+1}$) = 841 − 837 = 4 ms
ER (N+1 DIFF) QRS = (S•QRS$_{N+1}$) − (L$_{N+2}$−QRS$_{N+1}$) = 748 − 736 = 12 ms

D

FIGURE 7-15, cont'd. D, Alternative methods for estimating postpacing interval when the pacing electrogram is obscured. Comparison of conventional method and alternative methods for assessing entrainment response in ventricular tachycardia (VT) circuits. Surface electrocardiogram leads and intracardiac bipolar electrograms recorded from the mapping catheter (MAP 1-2) and from the reference catheter (RV 1-2) are shown. *Top panel:* Overdrive pacing from a bystander dead-end pathway entrains VT with concealed fusion. PPI is 395 msec, and TCL is 336 msec. PPI − TCL is 395 − 336 = 59 msec. Measurements for ER (N + 1 DIFF) using QRS complex as the reference point are as follows: S − QRSN + 1 interval is 509 msec and LN + 2 − QRSN + 3 interval is 450 msec. ER (N + 1 DIFFQRS) = (S − QRSN + 1) − (LN + 2 − QRSN + 3) = 509 − 450 = 59 msec, and matches exactly measured PPI − TCL. Measurements using remote electrogram (RV 1-2) as the reference point are also presented: S − EgN +1 interval is 549 msec and LN + 2 − EgN + 3 interval is 490 msec and calculated ER (N + 1 DIFFEg) = (S − EgN + 1) − (LN + 2 − EgN + 3) = 549 − 490 = 59 msec. Computations for the PPIR method are also: PD interval is 208 msec, TD interval is 156 msec, PPIR interval is 338 msec and almost matches TCL, which is 336 msec. Thus, ER PPIR = (PD − TD) + (PPIR − TCL) = (208 − 156) + (338 − 336) = 52 + 2 = 54 msec. *Bottom panel,* VT entrained with concealed fusion during pacing from the isthmus of the VT circuit. PPI is 561 msec and TCL is 560 msec. PPI − TCL difference is 561 − 560 = 1 msec. Measurements for ER (N + 1 DIFF) using QRS complex as the reference point are as follows: S − QRSN + 1 interval is 748 msec and LN + 2 − QRS interval is 736 msec. Thus, ER (N + 1 DIFFQRS) = (S − QRSN + 1) − (LN + 2 − QRSN + 3) = 748 − 736 = 12 msec. Measurements using remote electrogram (RV 1-2) as the reference point are also presented. Eg − QRSN + 1 interval is 841 msec and LN + 2 − QRS interval is 837 msec and calculated. *(A to C, Modified from Waldo AL. Atrial flutter: entrainment characteristics.* J Cardiovasc Electrophysiol. *1997;8:337-352, 1997.* **D** *from Derejko P, Szumowski LJ, Sanders P, et al. Clinical validation and comparison of alternative methods for evaluation of entrainment mapping.* J Cardiovasc Electrophysiol. *2009;20:741-748. With permission.)*

interval during tachycardia.[54-56] We also measure the PPI and compare it with the tachycardia cycle length[54] to differentiate between AVRT and AVNRT.[54] Figure 7-16 shows an example each of AVNRT and AVRT in response to ventricular entrainment.

Ventricular pacing can also be performed at the tachycardia cycle length during sinus rhythm, and the diagnostic criteria mentioned earlier (i.e., comparison of VA and HA times during tachycardia and pacing) are used to differentiate between AVNRT and AVRT.

Another maneuver that may be helpful in deciphering the mechanism of long R-P supraventricular tachycardias is atrial pacing at the tachycardia cycle length; a comparison of AH times may allow differentiation among atrial tachycardia, AV nodal reentry, and AVRT; AH intervals that occur during pacing are expected to be similar to those that occur during tachycardia (≤ 20 milliseconds) for atrial tachycardia but are longer during AVRT (delta-AH between 20 and 40 milliseconds) and AVNRT (delta-AH ≥ 40 milliseconds).[57]

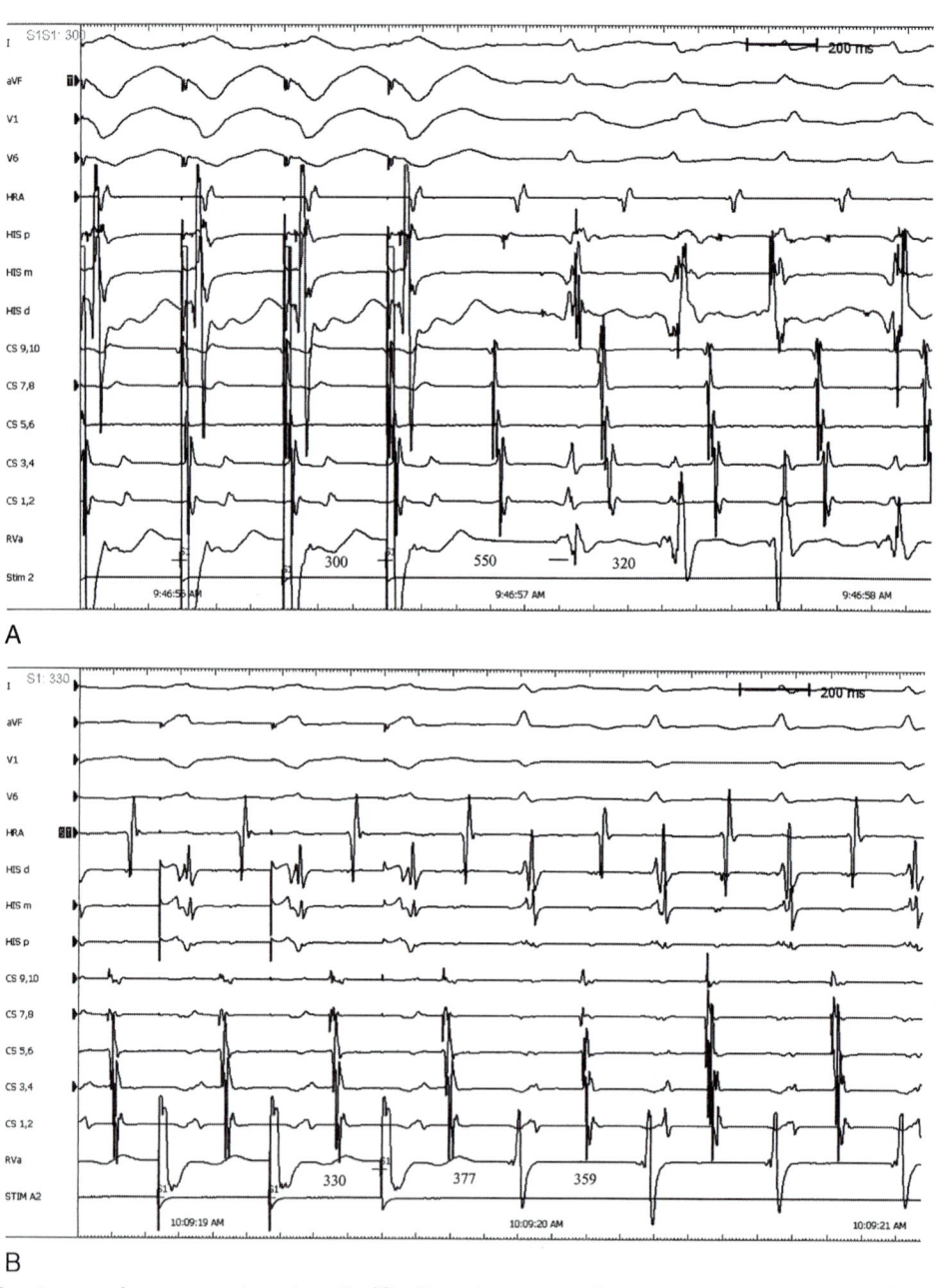

FIGURE 7-16. Entrainment of supraventricular tachycardia. The figure demonstrates the response of atrioventricular nodal reentrant tachycardia (AVNRT) and atrioventricular reentrant tachycardia (AVRT) (with concentric activation sequences) to entrainment from the ventricle. **A,** Entrainment is consistent with AVNRT: the stimulus-to-A interval during ventricular pacing exceeds the VA interval during tachycardia by more than 85 msec. The postpacing interval (PPI) exceeds the tachycardia cycle length by more than 115 msec, also consistent with AVNRT. **B,** Entrainment here is consistent with AVRT, with the difference between the stimulus-to-A interval (during pacing) and the VA interval (during tachycardia) being less than 85 msec and the PPI being about equal to the tachycardia cycle length.

Premature Ventricular Contractions during Narrow-Complex Tachycardia

It is almost standard practice in most laboratories to deliver premature ventricular stimuli at the onset of a sustained, hemodynamically stable, and regular (i.e., no variability in cycle length) supraventricular tachycardia. Exceptions to this rule include a regular tachycardia with changing VA times (indicating probable atrial tachycardia) and tachycardias lacking a 1:1 AV association (excluding AV reentry and making AVNRT unlikely). Single PVCs delivered during His refractoriness are of diagnostic utility if they advance, retard, or terminate the tachycardia. Each of these phenomena indicates the presence of a retrogradely conducting accessory pathway, with the latter two, if reproducible, confirming the participation of the pathway as the retrograde limb of the tachycardia. Although a PVC on His advancing the atrium with the same retrograde activation sequence as the tachycardia is highly suggestive of a participating bypass tract, it is by no means diagnostic, with an atrial tachycardia arising from close to the insertion of a bypass tract being a remote possibility. Figure 7-17 shows a PVC delivered during His refractoriness; although no His depolarization is seen, the presence of ECG fusion during the PVC confirms anterograde His depolarization, thereby indicating His refractoriness. More premature PVCs (more than 30 milliseconds before the next expected His bundle depolarization) delivered close to the site of earliest atrial activation can be considered diagnostic of the absence of an accessory pathway, if the atrium is not affected.[58] PVCs that reset the A can also help indicate the presence of an accessory pathway if they significantly change the VA, such as during supraventricular tachycardia with an eccentric retrograde atrial activation. A left bundle PVC (from the right ventricular apex) that advances the A, along with an increase in the VA interval, is diagnostic of a left-sided accessory pathway.

Termination of Tachycardia during Pacing Maneuvers

If a narrow-complex tachycardia terminates during ventricular pacing without any change in the atrial cycle length (indicating no depolarization of the atrium by the ventricular stimuli), atrial tachycardia is excluded as a possible diagnosis. (See also "Premature Ventricular Contractions during Narrow-Complex Tachycardia," earlier.)

On occasion, the mode of termination may provide valuable information about the location of a protected isthmus in the setting of a scar-related tachycardia. Figure 7-18 shows left ventricle mapping during VT, with mid-diastolic recordings from a site on the anterior wall; pacing at this site showed that it was integral to the VT circuit. A single extrastimulus delivered at this site reproducibly terminated VT without local propagation or depolarization.[59] Moreover, a single extrastimulus delivered at this site during sinus rhythm initiated VT. Radiofrequency energy delivered at this site terminated VT after one beat. This suggests that the ablation catheter tip was positioned in a critical portion of the circuit before tissues in the circuit immediately distal to this site had recovered excitability. The inference is that because the stimulus did not elicit a QRS complex, it affected cells that were in a protected area, such that (1) a single extrastimulus delivered at that site during sinus rhythm might have only one possible direction of propagation and could initiate VT and (2) this site would be an excellent ablation target site.

Electrogram Morphology in Response to Pacing

Close observation of electrogram morphology and polarity can also help differentiate between disparate activation pathways during electrophysiologic maneuvers performed in the absence of tachycardia. Bipolar electrogram morphology and polarity during atrial pacing,

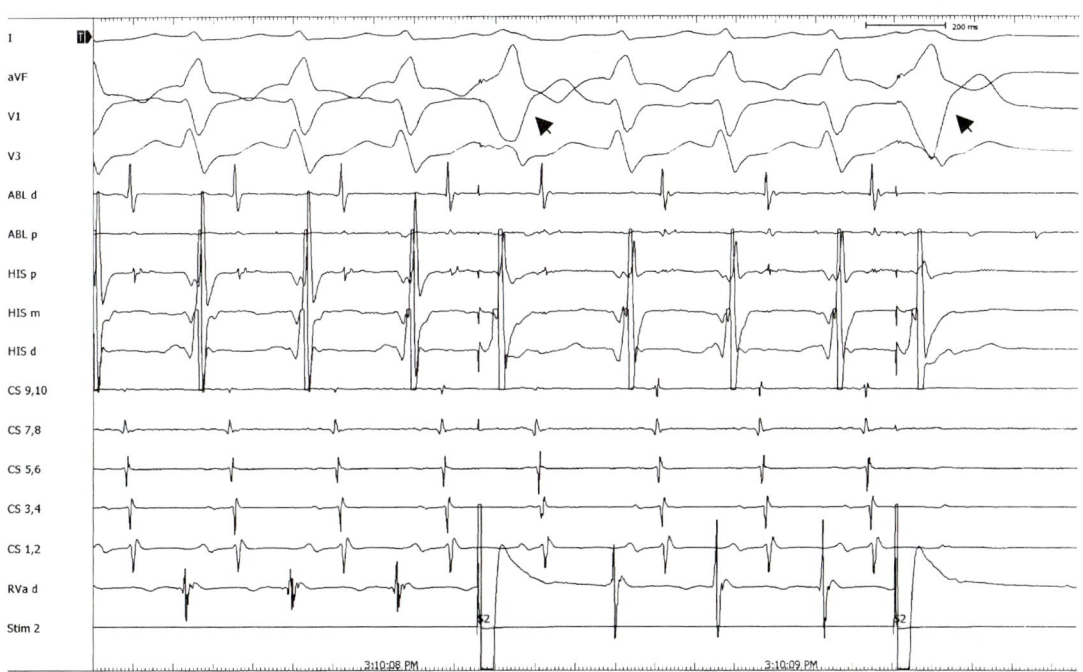

FIGURE 7-17. Premature ventricular stimuli (PVCs) delivered during His refractoriness (during supraventricular tachycardia). Although no His depolarization is seen, the presence of electrocardiographic fusion during the first PVC, compared with the second PVC, which closely resembles a fully paced beat during sinus rhythm (not shown here), confirms anterograde His depolarization, thereby indicating His refractoriness during the first PVC.

for example, can be helpful in targeting successful ablation sites in an otherwise normal, healthy heart in the setting of a reentrant tachycardia (e.g., during typical, isthmus-dependent atrial flutter). Figure 7-19 shows the local bipolar electrogram at a site where radiofrequency was applied with success; ablation had previously been performed along the isthmus but with-

out conduction block. The isthmus ablation line was further explored for areas where conduction through the isthmus remained. At one site along the line of block, the electrogram shown in Figure 7-19 was noted; although split, the electrograms were not as far apart as others along the ablation line. A single radiofrequency application at this site (applied during coronary sinus

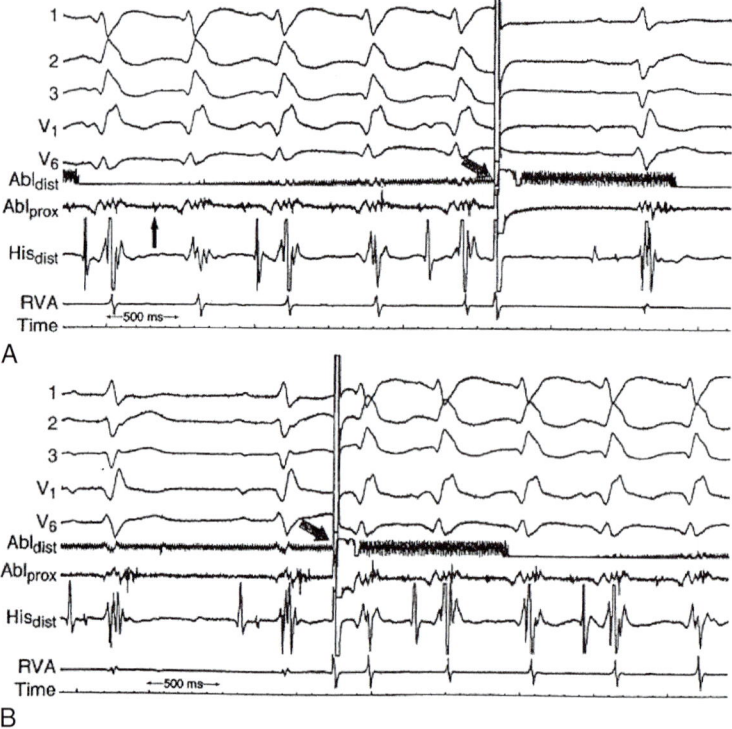

FIGURE 7-18. Termination of ventricular tachycardia (VT) by a nonpropagated extrastimulus. **A,** A single extrastimulus *(arrow)* terminated VT without local propagation. **B,** A single extrastimulus delivered at this site during sinus rhythm initiated VT. See text for discussion. *(From Altemose GT, Miller JM. Termination of ventricular tachycardia by a nonpropagated extrastimulus.* J Cardiovasc Electrophysiol. *2000;11:125, 2000. With permission.)*

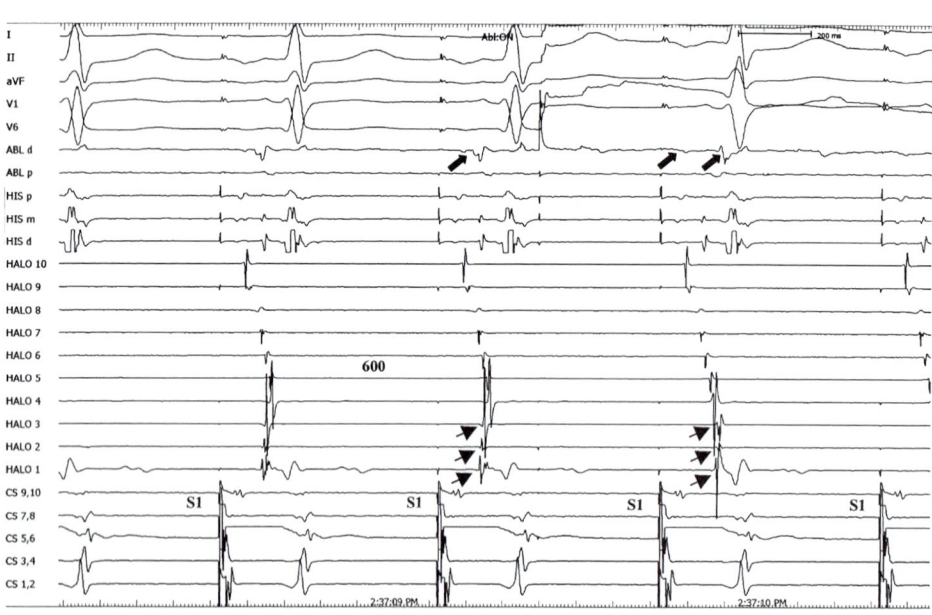

FIGURE 7-19. Reversal of bipolar electrogram polarity with ablation. The figure shows right atrial electrograms from a patient undergoing ablation for typical, isthmus-dependent atrial flutter. Ablation had been performed along the isthmus but without resulting in conduction block. When the isthmus ablation line was further explored for nonablated areas, the electrograms shown here were recorded. The *first arrow* highlights the local bipolar electrogram at a 6-oclock position along the subeustachian isthmus, close to where radiofrequency had been applied previously. Although split, the electrograms were not as far apart here as at other sites along the ablation line. A single radiofrequency application at this site resulted in further separation of the electrograms *(double arrows)*, with a change in electrogram polarity for the second component of the split electrogram, indicating activation from the opposite direction, and evidence of conduction block on the halo catheter.

pacing) resulted in further separation of the electro-grams (with a change in electrogram polarity for the second component of the split electrogram, indicating activation from the opposite direction) and evidence of conduction block on the halo catheter.

More recently, bipolar electrograms have been found to have utility in mapping the pulmonary veins for ablation of atrial fibrillation. Sites where the bipolar electrogram changes direction or polarity—thought to indicate break-throughs from the left atrium into the pulmonary vein—have been found to be predictive for ablation success of a

myocardial sleeve (with resulting pulmonary vein isolation from the rest of the atrial myocardium) (Fig. 7-20).[60]

Activation Sequence during Pacing Maneuvers

Close attention to atrial activation sequence and electro-gram polarity during ventricular pacing (in sinus rhythm) can also provide important diagnostic clues to underly-ing accessory pathway and AV nodal physiology—clues that may be helpful to individualizing ablation strategies. Figure 7-21 shows an example in which subtle changes

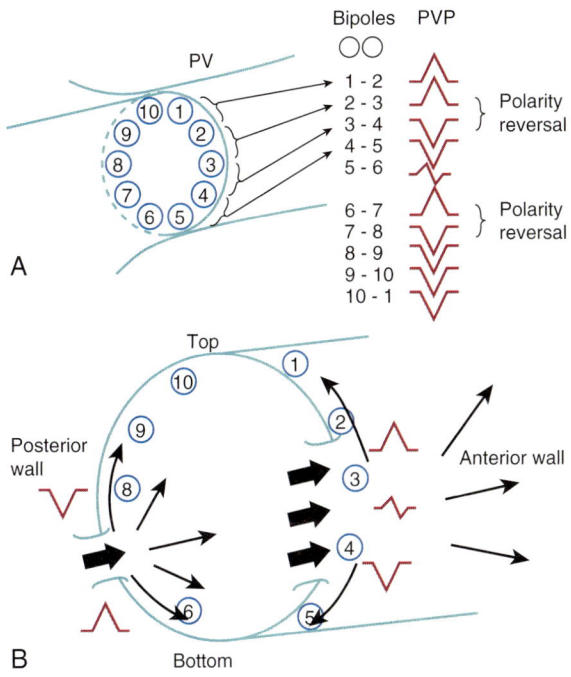

FIGURE 7-20. Bipolar electrogram polarity reversal as an additional indica-tor of breakthroughs from the left atrium to the pulmonary veins. **A,** Schematic representation of the circular mapping catheter with 10 electrodes. Pulmonary vein (PV) muscle potentials were recorded at the proximal PV in bipolar mode from 10 bipoles. Polarity reversal was defined as a sudden change of the main deflection of pulmonary vein potential (PVP) from positive to negative when analyzing adjacent bipoles in ascending order. **B,** Schematic diagram of radial propagation of activation fronts from two different breakthroughs in the left superior PV. The numbers positioned at the ostium of the vein represent the 10 electrodes of the circular mapping catheter. There are two distinct break-throughs, at both the anterior and posterior aspects of the vein. Radial propaga-tion of the activation front through one breakthrough (posterior wall) is reflected by an electrogram polarity reversal across the adjacent two bipoles (6 to 7 and 7 to 8). In the case of wider breakthrough (anterior wall), an electrogram polarity reversal is observed across three consecutive bipoles (2 to 3, 3 to 4, and 4 to 5), with the intervening bipole (3 to 4) showing relatively isoelectric initial deflec-tion. *(From Yamane T, Shah DC, Jais P, et al. Electrogram polarity reversal as an additional indicator of breakthroughs from the left atrium to the pulmonary veins. J Am Coll Cardiol. 2002;39:1337-1344. With permission.)*

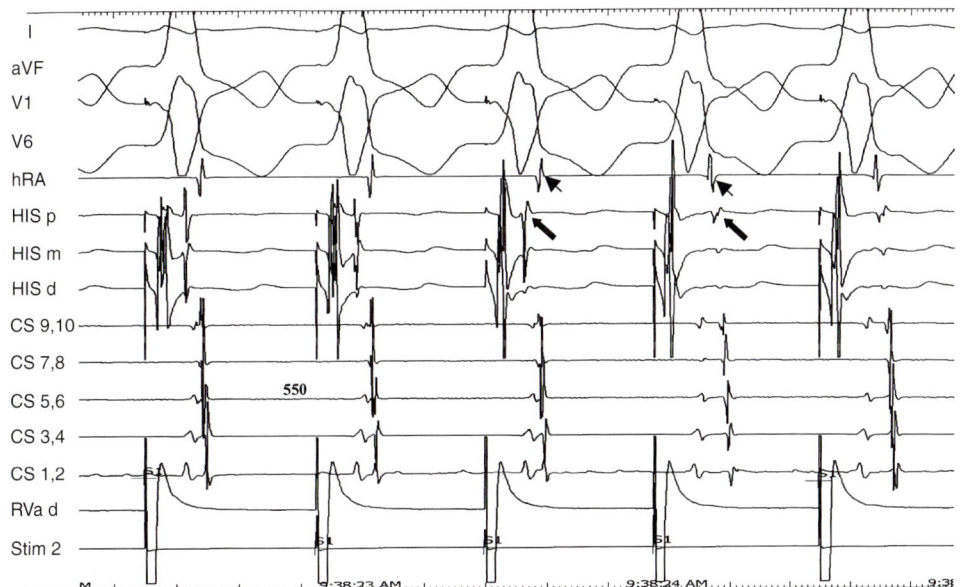

FIGURE 7-21. Reversal of polarity in high right atrial (HRA) bipolar electrogram with a change in retrograde activation sequence during ventricular pacing. Subtle changes in electrogram morphology are noted during ventricular pacing (at 550 msec) in the presence of a right lateral accessory pathway. The first three beats suggest that activation is up the atrioventricular (AV) node, whereas the fourth and later beats show a change in activation sequence, with the HRA now being earliest, suggesting retrograde activation up a right-sided accessory pathway. Although the stimulus-to-atrium time in the HRA is about the same for both activation sequences, suggesting that fusion up the AV node and accessory pathway may be occurring during the first three beats, the polarity of the HRA electrogram changes with the second activation sequence. This suggests that retrograde activation for the first three beats is entirely up the AV node, whereas activation for the fourth and subsequent beats is entirely up the accessory pathway.

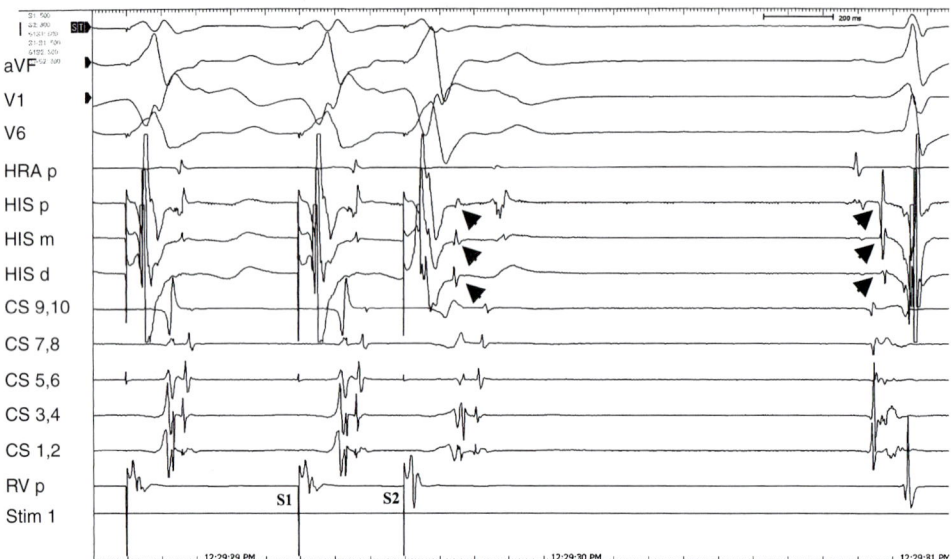

FIGURE 7-22. Anterograde versus retrograde His bundle activation. An example of retrograde His bundle activation, as shown by the distal (d)–to–proximal (p) activation of the His bundle potential *(first set of arrows)* with a ventricular extrastimulus (seen clearly due to retrograde right bundle branch block with a prolonged VH time), as opposed to proximal-to-distal or anterograde activation during sinus rhythm *(second set of arrows)*.

in electrogram morphology are noted during ventricular pacing in the presence of a right lateral accessory pathway. Although a cursory look at the activation sequence suggests that fusion may be present in the first three beats (i.e., retrograde activation may progress up the accessory pathway and the AV node), because there is no significant change in timing of the high right atrial electrogram (i.e., the VA time between the first three beats, which have a "concentric" retrograde activation sequence and the subsequent beats, which have an "eccentric" retrograde sequence), the near reversal of polarity of the distal high right atrial electrogram in the fourth and fifth beats (compared with the first three beats) suggests that retrograde activation for the first three beats is solely up the AV node and solely up the accessory pathway for the fourth and fifth beats. In fact, detailed assessment of atrial and AV accessory pathway activation direction using bipolar mapping has been performed by Damle and coworkers, who showed that vector mapping (performed by summing three orthogonally oriented bipolar electrograms) can help accurately localize accessory pathways insertion sites.[61]

Even if direct information is not present on a single bipolar electrogram (e.g., a high-frequency recording such as the His bundle electrogram), analysis of the electrogram when performed in the presence of its neighboring electrograms may indicate direction of activation. Figure 7-22 shows an example of retrograde His bundle activation, as shown by the distal-to-proximal activation of the His bundle potential with a ventricular extrastimulus (seen clearly owing to retrograde right bundle branch block with a prolonged VH time), as opposed to proximal-to-distal or antegrade activation during sinus rhythm (Fig. 7-23).

Parahisian Pacing

Parahisian pacing is of utility in differentiating between a retrogradely conducting septal pathway and the AV node. When direct His bundle capture is obtained, retrograde conduction can occur rapidly over the AV node if retrograde septal conduction is present.[62] In contrast, if conduction is proceeding only up an accessory pathway, His bundle capture will not alter the VA interval. Thus, the presence of a retrogradely conducting septal pathway can be identified by a fixed VA interval regardless of capture. Retrograde fusion complicates this finding. Shortening of the VA interval may occur if retrograde conduction is proceeding up both the AV node and an accessory pathway. In such a case, examination for closely spaced atrial recording sites can help identify a change in activation sequence that occurs when His bundle capture shortens the VA interval. An example of this is shown in Figure 7-24; the activation sequence is different between parahisian capture (narrow beat indicated by a single, heavy arrow in lead II) and ventricular capture (wider beat indicated by two heavy arrows in lead II). Closer inspection reveals that VA time is unchanged in $CS_{1,2}$ to $CS_{7,8}$, indicating that atrial activation in these electrodes is through an accessory pathway. However, VA time during ventricular capture is longer in Abl (close to high right atrium), His, and $CS_{9,10}$ compared with during parahisian capture, indicating that activation in these electrodes is up the AV node. Figure 7-25 shows a schematic outlining the use of parahisian pacing.

Figure 7-26 shows an instance in which parahisian pacing may be fraught with error, with retrograde activation being different with ventricular compared with combined (ventricular and His bundle) capture; ventricular pacing alone causes a longer VA interval because conduction is over a posteroseptal pathway (although some AV nodal conduction, i.e., fusion, cannot be ruled out in the His bundle recording) that conducts more slowly than the AV node. Combined His bundle and ventricular capture causes conduction to proceed up the AV node, but with a shorter VA time (and a different activation sequence than when retrograde conduction is over the accessory pathway).

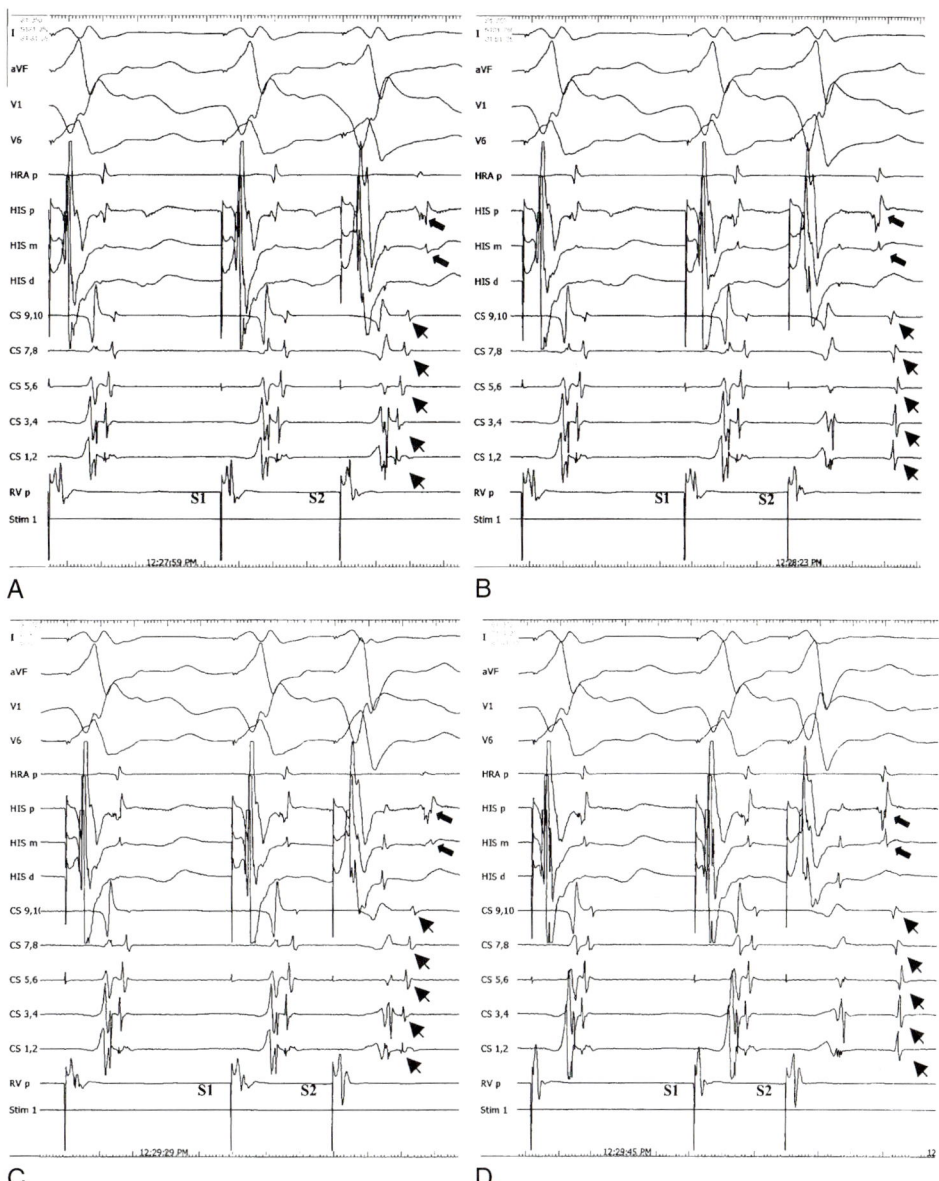

FIGURE 7-23. Changes in retrograde activation sequence with ventricular pacing in a patient with a left lateral accessory pathway. Retrograde activation from the ventricular drive train appears to be fusion up the atrioventricular (AV) node and the accessory pathway. The VA time in the His bundle is shorter because the His is probably within the early portion of the QRS. Multiple activation sequences are detected by ventricular extrastimulus testing. In the same patient as in Figure 7-14, disparate pathways of activation with single ventricular extrastimulus testing are shown. **A,** Change in atrial activation in the His channel and in coronary sinus (CS) 9, 10 (with a change in polarity in the latter) with the ventricular extrastimulus, with retrograde atrial activation appearing to go entirely up a left-sided accessory pathway. Note that a His deflection can be seen after the ventricular depolarization, suggesting retrograde right bundle branch block (due to the premature extrastimulus) with activation up the left bundle branch. **B,** With a more premature extrastimulus, the VH prolongs further; this is accompanied by a further increase in the VA time in the His recording channels, although the HA time remains unchanged. The atrial activation in the CS has now changed and is more concentric, suggesting activation up the AV node (i.e., block in the accessory pathway). **C,** With a still more premature extrastimulus, there is conduction up the accessory pathway again (with a change in polarity in the CS electrograms); the timing and polarity of the His and HRA electrograms remains unchanged again, with the HA being constant. The retrograde activation represents fusion up the accessory pathway and the AV node. **D,** A further increase in prematurity of the extrastimulus results in block in the accessory pathway once again. There is a further increase in the VH time, with the VA time increasing accordingly (i.e., constant HA), indicating activation up the AV node.

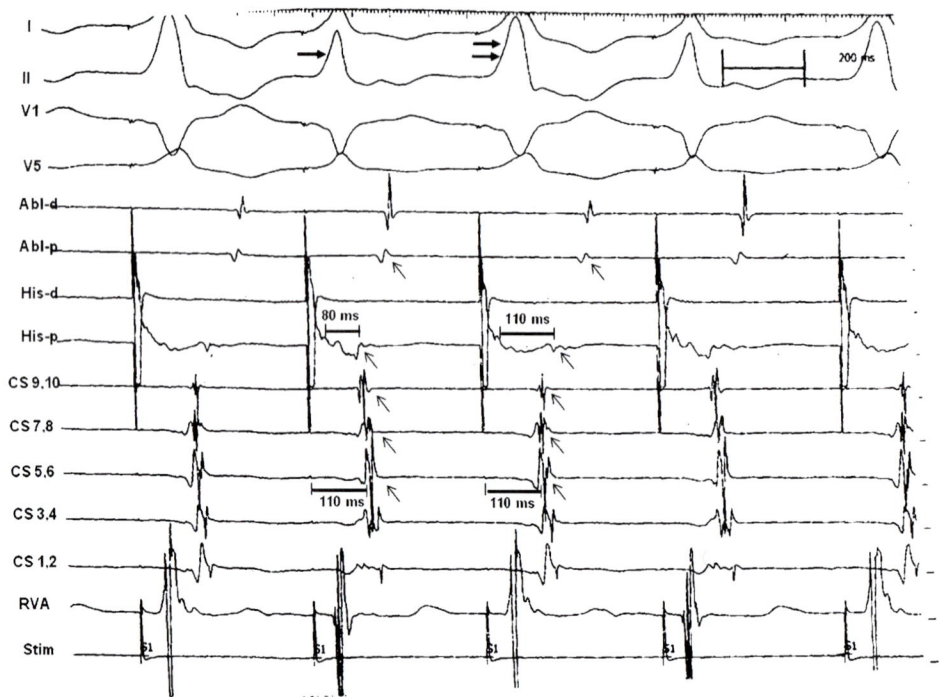

FIGURE 7-24. Fusion up the AV node and an accessory pathway during parahisian pacing. Activation sequence is different between combined His and ventricular capture (narrow beat indicated by a *single, heavy arrow* in lead II) and ventricular capture (wider beat indicated by *two heavy arrows* in lead II). Closer inspection reveals that VA time is unchanged in $CS_{1,2}$ to $CS_{7,8}$ (110 msec in $CS_{5,6}$), indicating that atrial activation in these electrodes is through an accessory pathway. However, VA time during ventricular capture is longer in Abl (close to high right atrium), His-p (VA increases from 80 to 110 msec), and $CS_{9,10}$ compared with during parahisian capture, indicating that activation in these electrodes is up the AV node.

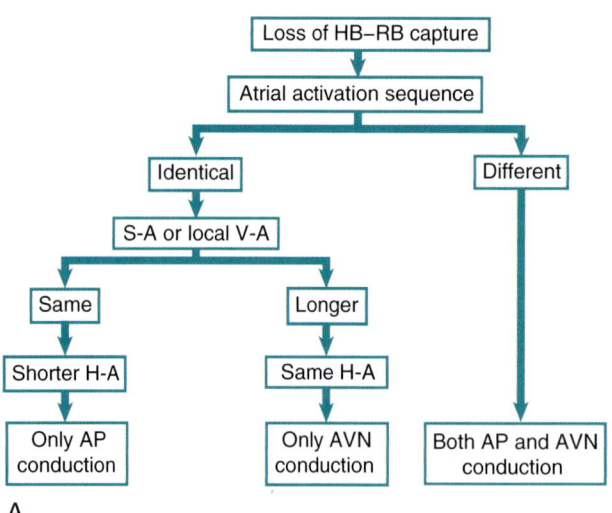

A

FIGURE 7-25. A, Abbreviated schematic for use in parahisian pacing to differentiate retrograde conduction over an accessory pathway from retrograde conduction over the atrioventricular (AV) node. AP, accessory pathway; AVN, atrioventricular node; H-A, interval from His bundle to atrial signal; HB, His bundle; RB, right bundle; S-A, interval from stimulus to atrial signal; V-A, interval from ventricular to atrial signal.

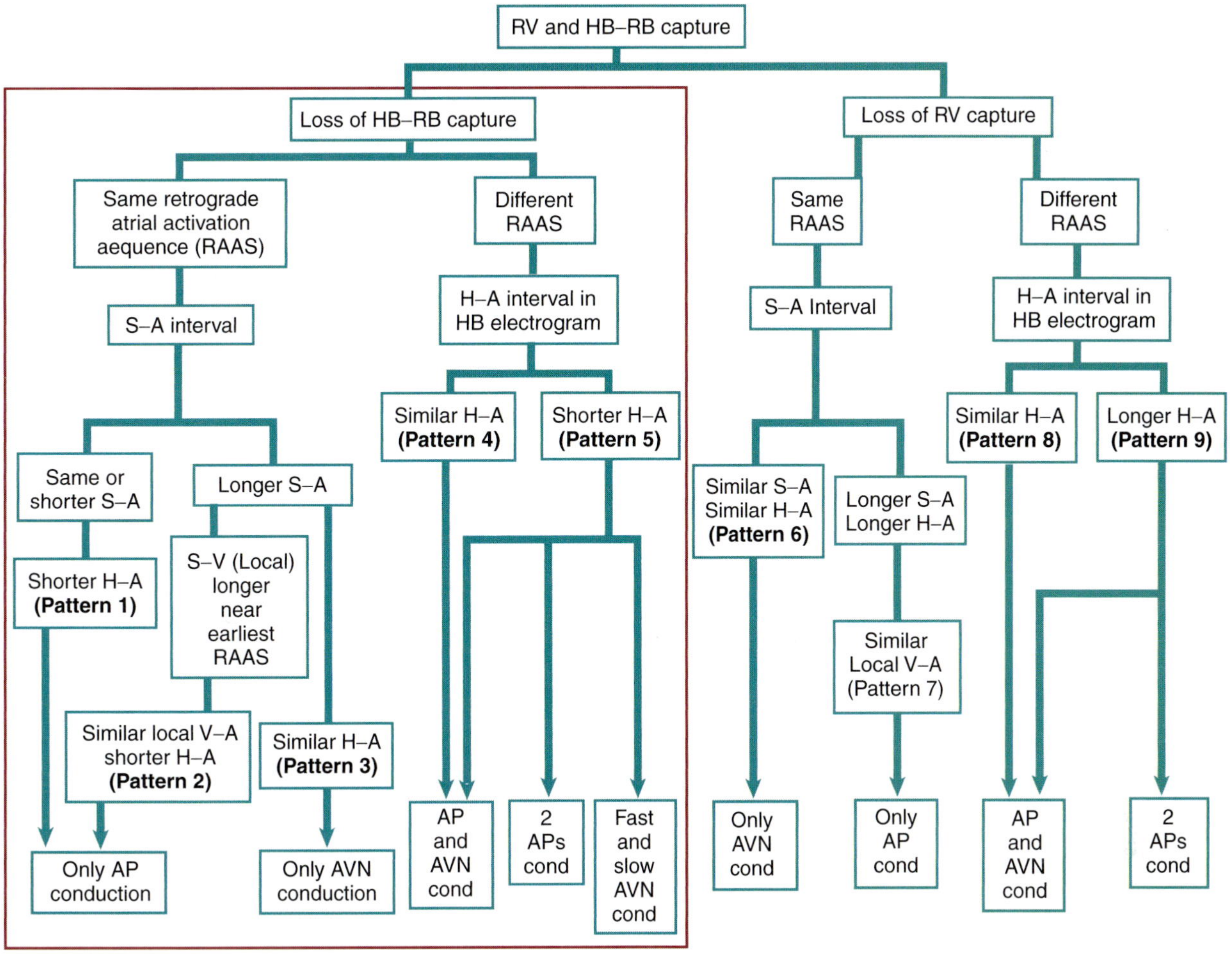

RV and HB–RB capture
Loss of HB–RB capture
Loss of RV capture
Same retrograde atrial activation aequence (RAAS)
Different RAAS
Same RAAS
Different RAAS
S–A interval
H–A interval in HB electrogram
S–A Interval
H–A interval in HB electrogram
Similar H–A (Pattern 4)
Shorter H–A (Pattern 5)
Similar H–A (Pattern 8)
Longer H–A (Pattern 9)
Same or shorter S–A
Longer S–A
Similar S–A Similar H–A (Pattern 6)
Longer S–A Longer H–A
Shorter H–A (Pattern 1)
S–V (Local) longer near earliest RAAS
Similar Local V–A (Pattern 7)
Similar local V–A shorter H–A (Pattern 2)
Similar H–A (Pattern 3)
AP and AVN cond
2 APs cond
Fast and slow AVN cond
Only AVN cond
Only AP cond
AP and AVN cond
2 APs cond
Only AP conduction
Only AVN conduction

B

FIGURE 7-25, cont'd. B, Complete schematic for parahisian pacing responses. The enclosed area corresponds to the three responses shown in panel **A**. RAAS, retrograde atrial activation sequence. *(**A,** From Hirao K, Otomo K, Wang X, et al. Para-hisian pacing: a new method for differentiating retrograde conduction over an accessory AV pathway from conduction over the AV node.* Circulation. *1996;94:1027-1035. **B,** Nakagawa H, Jackman WM. Parahisian pacing. A useful clinical technique to differentiate retrograde conduction between accessory atrioventricular pathways and atrioventricular nodal pathways.* Heart Rhythm. *2005; 2:667-672. With permission.)*

I
500 ms
aVF
V1
V6
HRA
HIS d
HIS p
CS 9,10
CS 7,8
CS 5,6
CS 3,4
CS 1,2
RVa
STIM A1
S1
10:17:47 AM
10:17:48 AM
10:17:49 AM
10:17:50 AM

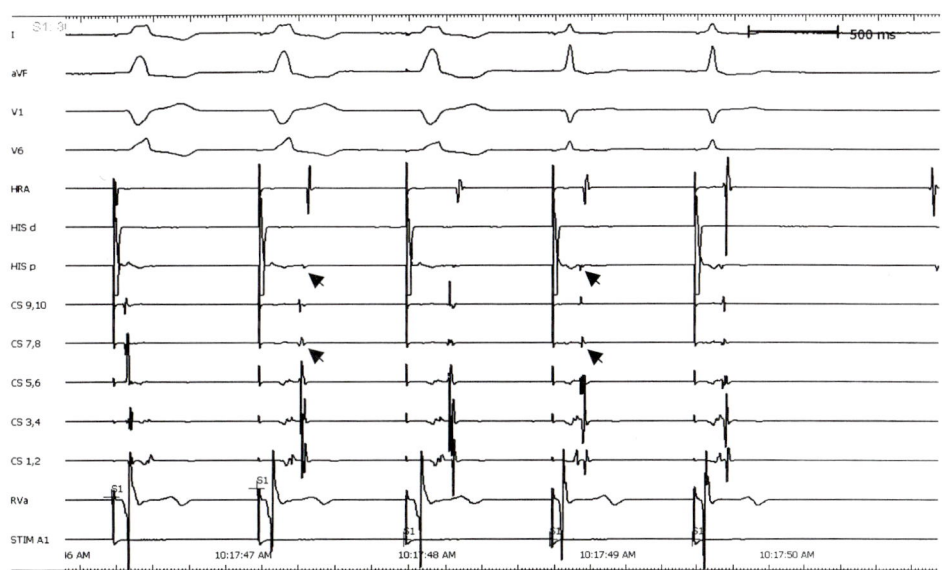

FIGURE 7-26. Parahisian pacing is performed in a patient with a known posteroseptal pathway, with retrograde activation being different with ventricular compared with combined (i.e., ventricular and His bundle capture) pacing. The *first arrow* shows ventricular pacing (wider QRS) with a longer VA time, whereas the *second arrow* shows His bundle as well as ventricular capture (narrower QRS) with a shorter VA time. Note, however, that the retrograde activation sequence with the first beat is earliest in the proximal coronary sinus (CS), and with the second beat it is earliest at the AV junction. Conduction in the former instance is up a slowly conducting posteroseptal pathway, although some AV nodal conduction (i.e., fusion) cannot be ruled out in the His bundle recording; in the latter instance, conduction is up the AV node alone. See text for discussion.

References

1. Rudy Y, Luo CH. A dynamic model of the cardiac ventricular action potential. I. Simulations of ionic currents and concentration changes. *Circ Res.* 1994;74:1097–1113.

2. Josephson ME. *Clinical Cardiac Electrophysiology: Techniques and Interpretation.* 3rd ed. Philadelphia: Lippincott Williams & Wilkins; 2002.

3. Murgatroyd FD, Krahn A. *Handbook of Cardiac Electrophysiology: A Practical Guide to Invasive EP Studies and Catheter Ablation.* London, UK: ReMedica; 2002.

4. Roberts DE, Hersh LT, Scher AM. Influence of cardiac fiber orientation on wavefront voltage, conduction velocity, and tissue resistivity in the dog. *Circ Res.* 1979;44:701–712.

5. Breirimann M, Shenasa M, Borgreffe M, et al. The interpretation of cardiac electrograms. In: Shenasa M, Borgreffe M, Breithardt G, eds. *Cardiac Mapping.* Elmsford, New York: Futura; 2003:15–39.

6. Green LS, Taccardi B, Ershler PR, Lux RL. Epicardial potential mapping: effects of conducting media on isopotential and isochrone distributions. *Circulation.* 1991;84:2513–2521.

7. Lewis T, Rothschild MA. The excitatory process in the dog's heart. II. The ventricles. *Philos Trans R Soc Lond (Biol).* 1915;206B:181–226.

8. Wilson FN, Johnston FE, Macleod AG, Barker PS. Electrocardiograms that represent the potential variations of a single electrode. *Am Heart J.* 1934;9:447–458.

9. Gallagher JJ, Kasell J, Sealy WC, et al. Epicardial mapping in the Wolff-Parkinson-White syndrome. *Circulation.* 1978;57:854–866.

10. Scher AM, Young AC. Ventricular depolarization and the genesis of the QRS. *Ann NY Acad Sci.* 1957;65:768–778.

11. Kupersmith J. Electrophysiologic mapping during open heart surgery. *Prog Cardiovasc Dis.* 1976;19:167–202.

12. Durrer D, Van der Tweel LH. Excitation of the left ventricular wall of the dog and goat. *Ann NY Acad Sci.* 1957;65:779–803.

13. Spach MS, Barr RC, Serwer GA, et al. Extracellular potentials related to intracellular action potentials in the dog Purkinje system. *Circ Res.* 1972;30:505–519.

14. Gallagher JJ, Kasell JH, Cox JL, et al. Techniques of intraoperative electrophysiologic mapping. *Am J Cardiol.* 1982;49:221–240.

15. Durrer D, Van der Tweel LH. The spread of the activation in the left ventricular wall of the dog. *Am Heart J.* 1953;46:683–691.

16. Ideker RE, Smith WM, Blanchard SM, et al. The assumptions of isochronal cardiac mapping. *Pacing Clin Electrophysiol.* 1989;12:456–478.

17. Cassidy DM, Vassallo JA, Marchlinski FE, et al. Endocardial mapping in humans in sinus rhythm with normal left ventricles: activation patterns and characteristics of electrograms. *Circulation.* 1984;70:37–42.

18. Biermann M. Precision and reproducibility of cardiac mapping. In: Shenasa M, Borggrefe M, Breithardt G, eds. *Cardiac Mapping.* 2nd ed. Elmsford, NY: Futura/Blackwell; 2003:157–186.

19. Scher AM, Young AC, Malmgren AL, et al. Spread of electrical activity through the wall of ventricle. *Circ Res.* 1953;1:539–547.

20. Yasuda T, Tojo H, Noguchi H, et al. Pulmonary vein electrogram characteristics in patients with focal sources of paroxysmal atrial fibrillation. *Pacing Clin Electrophysiol.* 2000;23:1823–1827.

21. Kumaji K, Yasuda T, Tojo H, et al. Role of rapid focal activation in the maintenance of atrial fibrillation originating from the pulmonary veins. *Pacing Clin Electrophysiol.* 2000;23:1823–1827.

22. Chen PS, Wu TJ, Hwang C, et al. Thoracic veins and the mechanisms of nonparoxysmal atrial fibrillation. *Cardiovasc Res.* 2002;54:295–301.

23. Kalman JM, Olgin JE, Karch MR, et al. "Cristal tachycardias": origin of right atrial tachycardias from the crista terminalis identified by intracardiac echocardiography. *J Am Coll Cardiol.* 1998;31:451–459.

24. Arora R, Verheule S, Navarrete A, et al. Effects of autonomic stimulation on the electrophysiology of the pulmonary vein and venoatrial junction. *Pacing Clin Electrophysiol.* 2001;24:550.

25. Miller JM, Olgin JE, Das MK. Atrial fibrillation: what are the targets for intervention? *J Interv Cardiac Electrophysiol.* 2003;9:249–257.

26. Arora R, Verheule S, Scott L, et al. Arrhythmogenic substrate of the pulmonary veins assessed by high-resolution optical mapping. *Circulation.* 2003;107:1816–1821.

27. Wen MS, Yeh SJ, Wang CC, et al. Successful radiofrequency ablation of idiopathic left ventricular tachycardia at a site away from the tachycardia exit. *J Am Coll Cardiol.* 1997;30:1024–1031.

28. Stevenson WG, Wiss JN, Wiener I, et al. Fractionated endocardial electrograms are associated with slow conduction in humans: evidence from pace-mapping. *J Am Coll Cardiol.* 1989;13:369–376.

29. Lacroix D, Savard P, Shenasa M, et al. Spatial domain analysis of late ventricular potentials: intraoperative and thoracic correlations. *Circ Res.* 1990;66:55–68.

30. Ursell PC, Gardner PI, Albala A, et al. Structural and electrophysiological changes in the epicardial border zone of canine myocardial infarcts during infarct healing. *Circ Res.* 1985;56:436–451.

31. Spear JF, Michelson EL, Moore EN. Cellular electrophysiologic characteristics of chronically infarcted myocardium in dogs susceptible to sustained ventricular tachyarrhythmias. *J Am Coll Cardiol.* 1983;1:1099–1110.

32. Kadish AH, Spear JF, Levine JH, et al. Vector mapping of myocardial activation. *Circulation.* 1986;74:603–615.

33. Balke CW, Lesh MD, Spear JF, et al. Activation patterns in healed experimental myocardial infarction. *Circ Res.* 1990;66:202–217.

34. Van Hare GF, Lesh MD, Ross BA, et al. Mapping and radiofrequency ablation of intraatrial reentrant tachycardia after the Senning or Mustard procedure for transposition of the great arteries. *Am J Cardiol.* 1996;77:985–991.

35. Markowitz SM, Brodman RF, Stein KM, et al. Lesional tachycardias related to mitral valve surgery. *J Am Coll Cardiol.* 2002;39:1973–1983.

36. Kinoshita O, Fontaine G, Rosas F, et al. Time- and frequency-domain analyses of the signal-averaged ECG in patients with arrhythmogenic right ventricular dysplasia. *Circulation.* 1995;91:715–721.

37. Cassidy DM, Vassallo JA, Buxton AE, et al. The value of catheter mapping during sinus rhythm to localize site of origin of ventricular tachycardia. *Circulation.* 1984;69:1103–1110.

38. Bogun F, Hohnloser S, Groenefeld G, et al. Characteristics of critical reentry sites of postinfarct hemodynamically stable ventricular tachycardia during sinus rhythm. *Pacing Clin Electrophysiol.* 2001;24:726.

39. Amerandral J, Peinado R. Radiofrequency catheter ablation of idiopathic right ventricular outflow tract tachycardia. In: Farre J, Moro C, eds. *Ten Years of Radiofrequency Catheter Ablation.* Armonk, NY: Futura; 1998:249–262.

40. Man KC, Daoud EG, Knight BP, et al. Accuracy of the unipolar electrogram for identification of the site of origin of ventricular activation. *J Cardiovasc Electrophysiol.* 1997;8:974–979.

41. Barlow MA, Klein GJ, Simpson CS, et al. Unipolar electrogram characteristics predictive of successful radiofrequency catheter ablation of accessory pathways. *J Cardiovasc Electrophysiol.* 2000;11:146–154.

42. Farre J, Grande A, Martinell J, et al. Atrial unipolar waveform analysis during retrograde conduction over left-sided accessory atrioventricular pathways. In: Brugada P, Wellens HS, eds. *Cardiac Arrhythmias: Where Do We Go from Here?* Mount Kisco, NY: Futura; 1987:243.

43. Klein LS, Shih HT, Hackett FK, et al. Radiofrequency catheter ablation of ventricular tachycardia in patients without structural heart disease. *Circulation.* 1992;85:1666–1674.

44. Calkins H, Kalbfleisch SJ, el-Atassi R, et al. Relation between efficacy of radiofrequency catheter ablation and site of origin of idiopathic ventricular tachycardia. *Am J Cardiol.* 1993;71:827–833.

45. Wilber D. Ablation of idiopathic right ventricular tachycardia. In: Huang SKS, Wilber DJ, eds. *Radiofrequency Catheter Ablation of Cardiac Arrhythmias: Basic Concepts and Clinical Applications.* 2nd ed. Armonk, NY: Futura/Blackwell; 2000:621–651.

46. Kadish AH, Childs K, Schmaltz S, Morady F. Differences in QRS configuration during unipolar pacing from adjacent sites: implications for the spatial resolution of pace-mapping. *J Am Coll Cardiol.* 1991;17:143–151.

47. Goyal R, Harvey M, Daoud EG, et al. Effect of coupling interval and pacing cycle length on morphology of paced ventricular complexes: implications for pace mapping. *Circulation.* 1996;94:2843–2849.

48. Brunckhorst CB, Stevenson WG, Soejima K, et al. Relationship of slow conduction detected by pace-mapping to ventricular tachycardia re-entry circuit sites after infarction. *J Am Coll Cardiol.* 2003;41:802–809.

49. Stevenson WG, Khan H, Sager P, et al. Identification of reentry circuit sites during catheter mapping and radiofrequency ablation of ventricular tachycardia late after myocardial infarction. *Circulation.* 1993;88:1647–1670.

50. Waldo AL. Atrial flutter: entrainment characteristics. *J Cardiovasc Electrophysiol.* 1997;8:337–352.

51. Henthorn RW, Okumura K, Olshansky B, et al. A fourth criterion for transient entrainment: the electrogram equivalent of progressive fusion. *Circulation.* 1988;77:1003–1012.

52. Waldo AL, Henthorn RW. Use of transient entrainment during ventricular tachycardia to localize a critical area in the reentry circuit for ablation. *Pacing Clin Electrophysiol.* 1989;12:231–244.

53. Derejko P, Szumowski LJ, Sanders P, et al. Clinical validation and comparison of alternative methods for evaluation of entrainment mapping. *J Cardiovasc Electrophysiol.* 2009;20:741–748.

54. Knight BP, Ebinger M, Oral H, et al. Diagnostic value of tachycardia features and pacing maneuvers during paroxysmal supraventricular tachycardia. *J Am Coll Cardiol.* 2000;36:574–582.

55. Michaud GF, Tada H, Chough S, et al. Differentiation of atypical atrioventricular node re-entrant tachycardia from orthodromic reciprocating tachycardia using a septal accessory pathway by the response to ventricular pacing. *J Am Coll Cardiol.* 2001;38:1163–1167.

56. Miller JM, Rosenthal ME, Gottlieb CD, et al. Usefulness of the delta HA interval to accurately distinguish atrioventricular nodal reentry from orthodromic septal bypass tract tachycardias. *Am J Cardiol.* 1991;68:1037–1044.

57. Man KC, Niebauer M, Daoud E, et al. Comparison of atrial-His intervals during tachycardia and atrial pacing in patients with long RP tachycardia. *J Cardiovasc Electrophysiol.* 1995;6:700–710.

58. Otomo K, Wang Z, Lazzara R, et al. Atrioventricular nodal reentrant tachycardia: electrophysiological characteristics of fours forms and implications for the reentrant circuit. In: Zipes JJ, eds. *Cardiac Electrophysiology: From Cell to Bedside.* Philadelphia: Saunders; 2000:504–521.

59. Altemose GT, Miller JM. Termination of ventricular tachycardia by a nonpropagated extrastimulus. *J Cardiovasc Electrophysiol.* 2000;11:125.

60. Yamane T, Shah DC, Jais P, et al. Electrogram polarity reversal as an additional indicator of breakthroughs from the left atrium to the pulmonary veins. *J Am Coll Cardiol.* 2002;39:1337–1344.

61. Damle RS, Choe W, Kanaan NM, et al. Atrial and accessory pathway activation direction in patients with orthodromic supraventricular tachycardia: insights from vector mapping. *J Am Coll Cardiol.* 1994;23:684–692.

62. Nakagawa H, Jackman WM. Para-hisian pacing: a useful clinical technique to differentiate retrograde conduction between accessory atrioventricular pathways and atrioventricular nodal pathways. *Heart Rhythm.* 2005;2:667–672.

8

Advanced Catheter Three-Dimensional Mapping Systems

Kyoko Soejima

Key Points

Different advanced catheter mapping systems are available, each with specific strengths and weaknesses. Each system requires familiarity with its principles of operation and serves as an adjunct to basic mapping and diagnostic techniques.

Common features of advanced mapping systems are the ability to display activation and voltage maps and to tag sites of previous ablation catheter positions. Systems now allow integration of catheter-derived electrical information with imported radiographic or ultrasonic cardiac images.

The optimal mapping system for any patient depends on the characteristics of the arrhythmia to be mapped and operator familiarity with the system.

Misinterpretation of the mapping data and improper data acquisition or processing are potential pitfalls associated with advanced mapping systems.

Catheter ablation has become a first-line therapy for a variety of arrhythmias and is progressively being used for more complex arrhythmias, such as scar-related ventricular tachycardia (VT) and atrial tachycardia and fibrillation. Technologic advances in electroanatomic mapping systems, ablation catheters, and other energy source ablations have greatly contributed to the improvement of ablations for such arrhythmias. In particular, the "advanced" mapping systems have been critical for ablation of complex arrhythmias while reducing radiation exposure. Modern mapping systems have the ability to localize at least one catheter in three-dimensional (3D) space and create a 3D map of the cardiac chambers of interest. In addition, preacquired or simultaneously acquired imaging, such as computed tomography (CT), magnetic resonance imaging (MRI), or intracardiac ultrasound, can be superimposed on the acquired 3D map, which will provide more detailed anatomic information. Currently, several advanced mapping systems are available, and each has both advantages and disadvantages. Understanding the characteristics of the system maximizes it use.

When to Use Electroanatomic Mapping Systems

For most supraventricular tachycardias (atrioventricular [AV] nodal reentry, AV reciprocating tachycardia), electroanatomic mapping systems are not necessary. Although they can decrease fluoroscopic time, the procedure time can be extended. The ability to tag catheter sites of interest in virtual space can be useful, however. With more complex arrhythmias and substrate-based ablation, electroanatomic mapping systems provide numerous advantages, including (1) identification of the abnormal scar area and slow conduction area, which may contribute to the formation of the reentry circuit in conjunction with anatomical landmarks; (2) tagging of sites with important information, such as excellent pace match sites and sites with delayed isolated potential, fragmentation, and delayed conduction; and (3) use of preacquired image information. Advanced mapping systems are therefore necessary to perform substrate-based atrial or ventricular ablation. The systems are also useful for efficiently mapping focal arrhythmias such as atrial tachycardias and for mapping and tracking the progress of linear ablation such as atrial flutters. There are several types of mapping systems available. Common features of advanced mapping systems are listed in Table 8-1.

Carto Advanced Mapping System

The Carto advanced mapping system (Biosense Webster, Diamond Bar, CA) is one of the most extensively used 3D mapping systems. The system uses ultralow-intensity

TABLE 8-1

COMMON FEATURES OF ADVANCED CATHETER THREE-DIMENSIONAL MAPPING SYSTEMS

Feature	Description	Uses
Virtual anatomy	Rendering of three- dimensional cardiac chamber anatomy by point-to-point acquisition of spatial coordinates with mapping catheter	Enables fluoroscopy-free catheter navigation framework to display electrophysiologic information
Activation map	Displays local activation times for a cardiac chamber in relation (earlier or later) to timing of a reference electrogram	Determines tachycardia mechanism as focal or macroreentrant Identifies ablation target sites
Location tagging	Marks catheter positions in virtual space	Designates location critical structures Catalogues ablation sites Allows return to sites of interest
Voltage map	Displays electrogram amplitude (in mV) throughout cardiac chamber	Substrate-based ablation Identifies areas of scar to be excluded from activation maps or as boundaries for reentry
Propagation map	Animated form of activation map showing spread of activation wavefront throughout cardiac cycle	Visualize spread of wavefront as adjunct to activation map
Isochronal map	Depicts all points with an activation time within a certain range with the same color	Assist in visualizing direction wavefront propagation Indicates local conduction velocities (e.g., crowded lines suggest slow conduction)
Image merge	Importation of radiographic anatomy (computed tomography, magnetic resonance imaging, fluoroscopy) for use in nonfluoroscopic catheter navigation	Facilitates extensive ablation about anatomic structures (pulmonary veins, left atrium, ventricular scar)

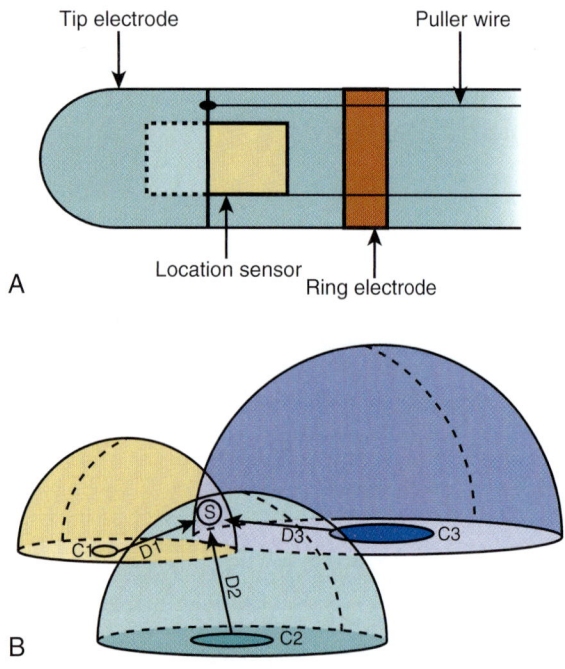

FIGURE 8-1. Carto mapping catheter (**A**) and the process of location determination (**B**). **A,** The mapping catheter is composed of tip and ring electrodes and a location sensor totally embedded within the catheter. **B,** A location pad is composed of three coils (C1, C2, C3) that generate a magnetic field that decays as a function of distance from that coil. The sensor (S) measures the strength of the field, and the distance from each coil (D1, D2, D3) can be measured. The location of the sensor is determined from the intersection of the theoretical spheres whose radii are the distances measured by the sensor.

proximally to the tip of a specialized mapping catheter. The strength of each coil's magnetic field decays as a function of distance from the coil, and by integrating each coil's field strength and converting this measurement into a distance, the catheter-tip position can be triangulated in space. The patient is positioned so that the heart is in the middle of the electromagnetic field. An anatomic reference patch adherent to the patient's back is used to monitor changes in the patient's position within the magnetic field. The anatomic reference can also be used in the form of an intracardiac catheter, which reduces the motion artifact created by cardiac movement in relation to the fixed external reference. The proprietary mapping and ablation catheter is then moved into the chamber of interest, and mapping points are acquired at the sites with contact. The special information is used to generate 3D chamber geometry. The geometry is in turn used to display electrical information, such as activation sequence or local electrogram amplitude, which is simultaneously recorded at each catheter position. In addition to the catheter location, the orientation (roll, pitch, and yaw) of the catheter is determined. The accuracy of the system is less than 1 mm. The activation and voltage information are displayed in rainbow colors. The ability to display real-time positions of multiple mapping catheters should be available by 2010 with the introduction of a new system (Carto 3).

How to Begin Mapping

The pad is placed beneath the operating table. The location patch (REF-STAR) is placed on the patient's back, roughly overlying the cardiac chamber of interest. Significant respiratory positional change of the heart (1 to 2 cm) may occur and must be taken into consideration. Acquiring mapping

magnetic fields (5×10^{-6} to 5×10^{-5} Tesla) emitted from nine coils in a locator pad beneath the laboratory table (Fig. 8-1).[1] The magnetic field strength from each coil is different and is detected by a location sensor embedded

points during expiration is recommended. The system allows tracking of the mapping catheter position and accurate reconstruction of chamber geometry. The activation timing reference should then be chosen. For supraventricular tachycardia activation mapping, a stable location, such as the coronary sinus or the right atrial appendage, is chosen for the atrial electrogram as a reference or fiduciary point to compare the timing of electrical signals from the mapping catheter. For VT, surface electrocardiography (ECG) is used because it is more stable; a right ventricular recording is an alternative.

Based on the local bipolar electrogram characteristics, the triggering criterion is selected (reference annotation): maximal deflection, minimal deflection, maximal upslope (dV/dt), maximal downslope. After the selection of the activation reference, it should be ensured that the reference is triggered at the same point in each beat. The activation reference can be adjusted after each point is taken; however, it will add a significant amount of time (Fig. 8-2). It is important that the window of interest for analyzing activation times be properly adjusted. If this window is too large,

incorporating data from two cardiac cycles, an ambiguous map will result for macro-reentrant circuits. Tagging anatomically and clinically important sites, such as the His bundle, sites with fractionated or delayed potentials, or good pace-match sites is also useful for successful ablation. Tagging the position of ablation lesions greatly facilitates the creation of linear lesions to treat macro-reentrant arrhythmias.

Activation Map

The activation map is constructed using a stable timing reference electrogram as a fiduciary point. The window of interest for mapping should be set at a slightly shorter interval than the tachycardia cycle length (typically, 90% of the cycle length). The timing reference can be adjusted after the mapping, but this is extremely time-consuming. Selection of a stable and reliable timing reference is critical for efficient and successful mapping. The activation map for reentry circuit shows the "early meets late" pattern (Fig. 8-3), and for focal arrhythmias, the earliest

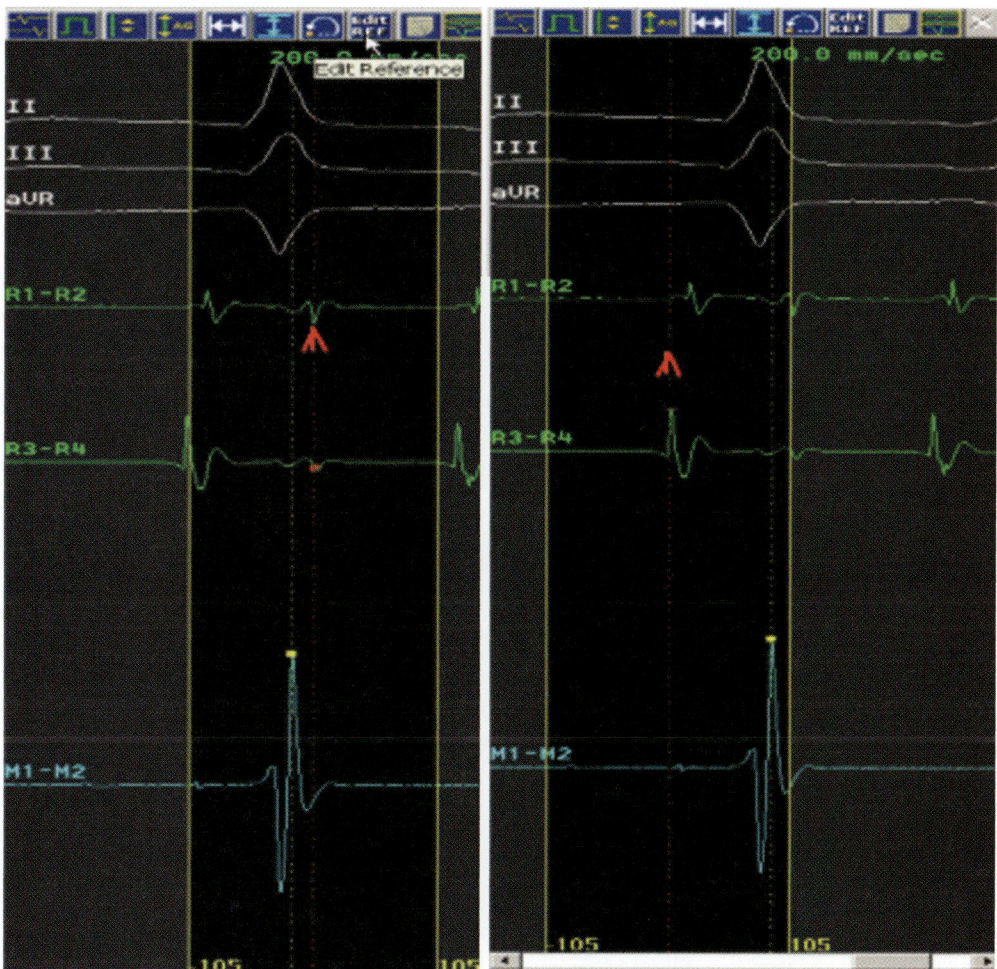

FIGURE 8-2. Window of interest display for Carto system during atrial activation mapping. The timing reference for atrial activation needs to be adjusted in the *left panel*. If the timing reference is set for minimal value reference catheter bipole 1 and 2 (R1-R2), it can pick up the ventricular activation as in *left panel*. To avoid this situation, the timing reference should be reference electrodes 3 and 4 (R3-R4) because the amplitude of the atrial signal is significantly larger than the ventricular signal. In the *right panel*, the timing reference is moved to the correct electrogram. Similarly, the mapping catheter (M1-M2) is recording only a ventricular electrogram but is annotated as the signal of interest by the algorithm.

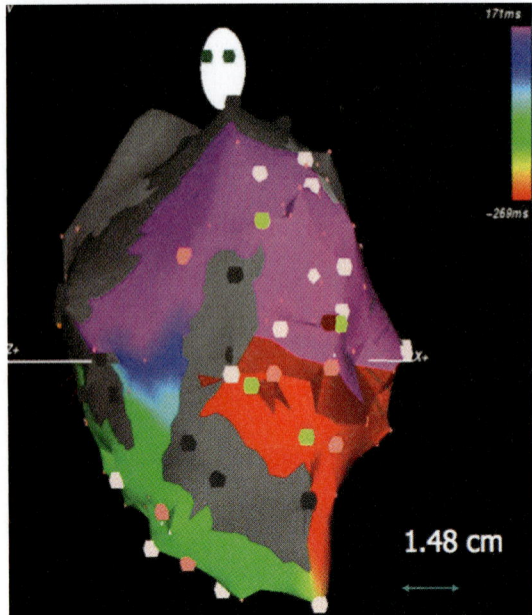

FIGURE 8-3. Carto left ventricular activation map during reentrant ventricular tachycardia (VT) (CL 440 msec) is shown. The patient had a large anterior myocardial infarction. The activation map shows "early *(red)* meets late *(purple)*" and covers the entire tachycardia cycle length (440 msec).

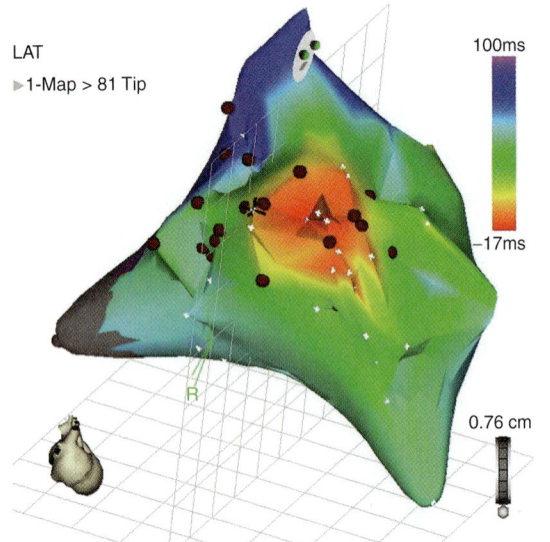

FIGURE 8-4. Carto activation map of focal ventricular tachycardia is shown. The earliest activation site (shown in *red*) is surrounded by the later activation.

activation is surrounded concentrically by the later activation (Fig. 8-4). Also, unipolar electrograms are recorded by the system, and their morphology, such as a QS pattern, is useful for focal arrhythmias. It is important to determine annotation of the local electrogram if there are multiple components recorded at the mapping site. Using entrainment mapping during tachycardia, the captured, local electrogram can be identified, and the activation timing should be adjusted to that local electrogram[2] (Fig. 8-5). It is important to acquire a sufficient number of points

around the chamber of interest to limit the interpolation performed by the system to fill gaps between data points. Isochronal maps and animated propagation maps may also be displayed using the activation data.

One of the weaknesses of the current system is the slow point-by-point acquisition of information. As such, it is not well suited for mapping hemodynamically unstable arrhythmias or nonsustained arrhythmias. Patients with these disorders can be treated by the use of substrate mapping during sinus rhythm or pacing. Recently, the ability to map simultaneously from multiple electrodes on a dedicated multipolar catheter has been introduced to expedite the mapping process.

Voltage Map

The amplitude of the local electrogram is displayed using the color-display function. Based on a prior study, bipolar amplitudes of 1.5 mV or greater suggest that the site is normal ventricular tissue, and lower voltage sites are considered abnormal.[3] Therefore, the maximal voltage of 1.5 mV is frequently used for the voltage map, and these areas, displayed as *purple,* are considered to be normal tissue (Fig. 8-6). Some use the minimal voltage of 0.5 mV to define a dense ventricular scar.[3] This system has been critical to the development of substrate-based catheter ablation for VT.[3–6] Pace mapping along the border of the low voltage area can identify the exit site for VT and sites with long stimulus to the QRS,[7] as well as sites with isolated delayed components that can be tagged on the map.[8] Clustering of these sites with slow conduction or a conduction block has been closely associated with the isthmus of the VT. Substrate mapping is also being used for multiple atrial tachycardias.

Complex Fractionated Atrial Electrogram Mapping

This algorithm analyzes several seconds of continuous electrograms from each catheter position for fractionation and short complex intervals. Bipolar or unipolar signals can be acquired. Within a 2.5-second sampling window, the algorithm determines the shortest complex interval, average complex interval, and an interval confidence level. Each of these measures can be displayed on the chamber geometry in color-coded scales.

Image Merge

The 3D electroanatomic mapping system (Carto XP) comes equipped with image integration software (CartoMerge Image Integration Module) that allows superimposing previously segmented CT or MRI and real-time anatomic information acquired through catheter mapping. Preacquired CT or MRI may not reflect the physiologic condition at the time of procedure. CT scans provide more precise insight into the left atrial and pulmonary vein (PV) morphology than MRI scans, especially in patients with atrial fibrillation.

Usually used for the left atrial registration, the mapping catheter is deployed into the PV and pulled back to the

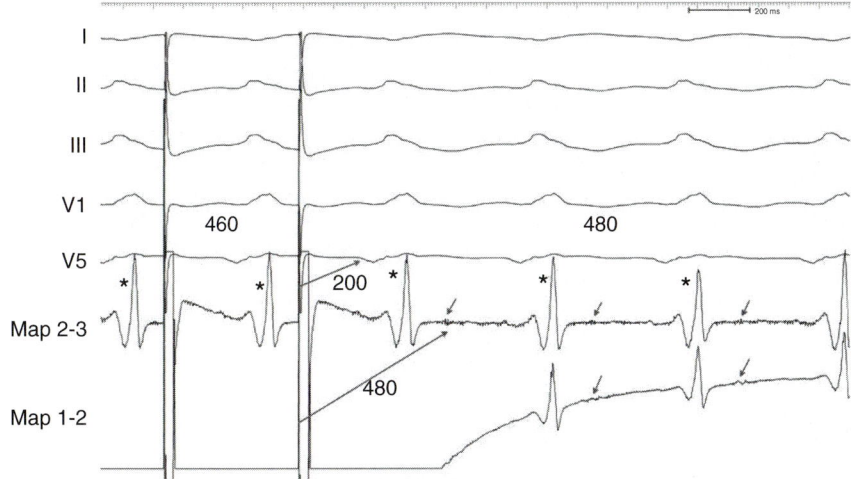

FIGURE 8-5. Local component of complex electrogram (EGM) can be differentiated from far-field signals by the entrainment. The mapping catheter records multiple components, including a blunt, larger potential and a sharp smaller potential. Entrainment mapping showed that the captured EGM is the sharp smaller signal, not the larger signal (*asterisk*) because one can see the larger potential during pacing. Therefore, for the activation mapping, the local activation time should be measured to the sharp EGM. Such subtlety demonstrates the need to over-read computer-generated annotations and measures.

focused endocardial surface registration had better alignment compared with the landmark registration. The ablation's point-to-CT image distance was significantly shorter in the group that underwent ICE-guided focused endocardial surface registration (1.73 ± 0.29 mm versus 3 ± 0.99 mm; $P < .001$).[10]

CartoSound

A 3D ultrasound image is acquired by a three-coil, electroanatomic mapping sensor and locator within the tip of the ICE catheter (SoundStar 3D catheter) and displayed with CartoSound software (Biosense Webster). The location and the direction of the phased-array image fan, with characteristic pitch, yaw, and roll components of catheter-tip motion, are displayed within the x-, y-, and z-axes. Three-second segments of two-dimensional (2D) ICE images are acquired during ECG gating. A single gated image is displayed on the ultrasound viewer, and the endocardial contour is manually or automatically drawn. By repeating this process, a series of contours in the chamber is acquired and is collated into a complete volume depicting point-to-point component interpolation and displayed.

The merit of the system is real-time acquisition of the anatomic information during the procedure. An ICE can be used for the transseptal puncture, location of the esophagus, location of PV–left atrium junction, view of the lasso (or spiral) catheter position in the veins, and monitoring for possible pericardial effusion development during the procedure. The validation study in animals using CartoSound showed that the actual anatomy and 3D ultrasound sites were only divergent by 2.1 ± 1.1 mm for atrial and 2.4 ± 1.2 mm for ventricular sites.[11] Using the CartoSound system, potential errors for CartoMerge approach can be corrected (Fig. 8-7).

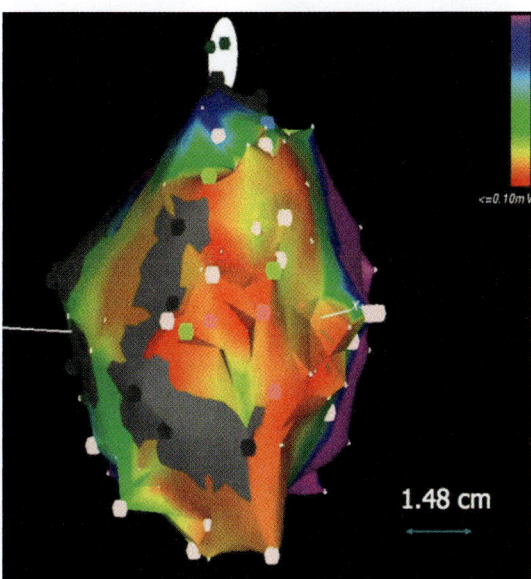

FIGURE 8-6. Carto voltage map of the left ventricle is shown. Activation map of the same patient during the ventricular tachycardia is shown in Figure 8-3. Maximal voltage is set up for 1.5 mV; *purple* is the normal voltage. This patient has large anterior myocardial infarct (*red*). Gray area indicates dense scar.

left atrium.[9] During this process, multiple PV points are sampled. The roof and floor of the vein are then identified using intracardiac echo or PV angiograms. The estimated corresponding locations of these left atrial–PV junctions are annotated on the imported 3D left atrial CT surface reconstruction. Usually, three or four landmark pairs are created by the user. A software algorithm called *landmark registration* is performed to approximate the left atrial CT surface reconstruction to the real-time catheter mapping space by matching the landmark pairs. Multiple left atrial endocardial locations are then sampled to reconstruct the left atrium. On completion of the reconstruction of the left atrial electroanatomic map, a software algorithm called *surface registration* is performed to fit the surface of the left atrial CT reconstruction to the surface of the left atrial electroanatomic map by rendering the smallest average distance between the two image data sets. Recent reports have shown that the intracardiac echocardiogram (ICE)–guided

Endocardial Solutions Advanced Mapping System

EnSite NavX Mapping System

The Ensite NavX mapping system (Endocardial Solutions, St. Jude Medical, St. Paul, MN) displays multiple catheter positions in real time and has the ability to reconstruct

CARTO SOUND

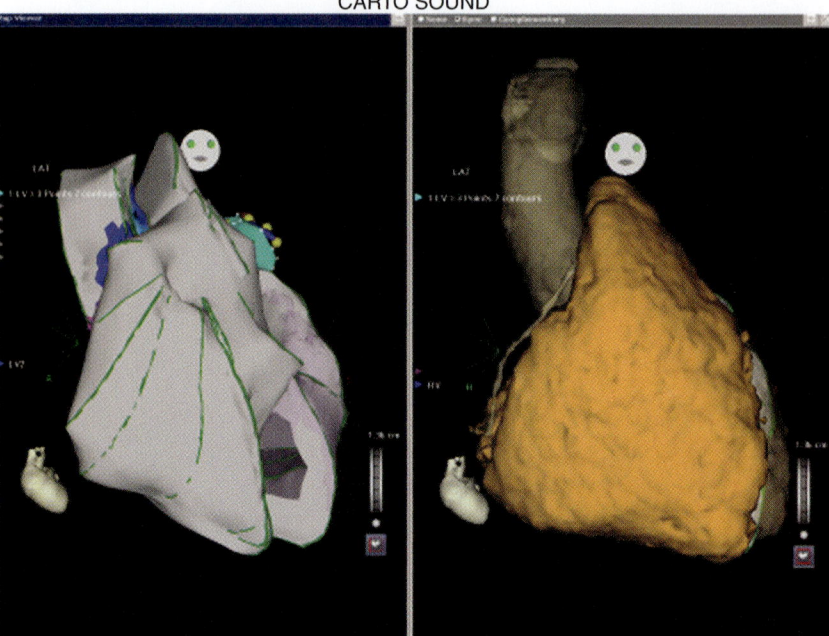

FIGURE 8-7. *Left panel* shows a CartoSound image of the right and left ventricles. *Right panel* shows the merged image of computed tomography using CartoSound.

virtual anatomy and point-by-point electroanatomic mapping. It is compatible with all diagnostic and ablation catheters. This system uses three pairs of patches placed in orthogonal planes (*x*, *y*, *z*); both sides of the patient's thorax (*x*-axis), chest and back (*y*-axis), and back of the neck and inner left thigh (*z*-axis). A 5.68-kHz electrical signal is delivered alternately across each pair of patches, creating a voltage gradient along the axis between them (Fig. 8-8). Using the sensed voltages compared with the voltage gradient on all three axes, the system calculates the 3D position of each catheter electrode and allows simultaneous localization of up to 64 electrodes on 12 conventional catheters more than 90 times per second. A respiration compensation algorithm, based on identification of gradual changes in transthoracic impedance, can be applied to help reduce artifact induced by respiration. A stable intracardiac positional reference catheter, such as one placed at the noncoronary cusp or coronary sinus, can significantly improve stability of catheter localization.

By moving any type of catheter to trace the endocardial contours of the chamber of interest, a 3D model of the geometry can be reconstructed at a reasonable speed. This poses a major advantage with the ability to accommodate multielectrode catheters, which allows quick mapping of the chamber. For example, penta-array catheters (PentaRay, Biosense Webster), with 20-pole steerable mapping catheter with five soft radiating spines (1-mm electrodes separated by 4-mm interelectrode spacing) or Reflection HD high-density mapping diagnostic catheter (St. Jude Medical) can be used to create the geometry and also to create the activation map quickly and efficiently[12] (Fig. 8-9). Having entered known catheter parameters such as electrode length and interelectrode spacing, the system can accurately reconstruct and display the shape of the electrode-containing part of the catheter and its 3D position and proximity to the geometric model. Ablation sites can be marked either as projections on the reconstructed endocardium or as independent 3D spheres.

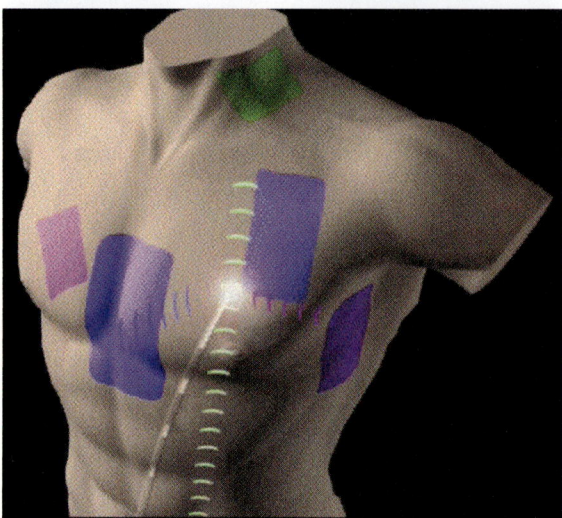

FIGURE 8-8. Orthogonal surface patches are placed on the patient for the NavX system. A 5.68-kHz electrical signal is delivered alternately across each pair of patches, creating a voltage gradient along the axis between them. Once the gradient is established, any mapping, ablation, or diagnostic catheter can be placed in the field and can act as a second receiver. The composite measurements represent the electrode positions of the catheters in three-dimensional virtual space.

Diagnostic Landmark Mapping Tool

This is the EnSite version of contact mapping. Data from the conventional catheters are organized and displayed on the 3D map. Samples are taken from various locations in the heart while the patient is in a stable rhythm using EnGuide-visualized conventional catheters. The 3D locations of these sampled points are saved along with voltage and activation data, which can be displayed on the geometry surface as color.

Basically, there are five steps for the mapping: (1) decide on the type of map, (2) set low voltage identification, (3) select reference, (4) select the roving catheter that will collect data, and (5) begin collecting the data.

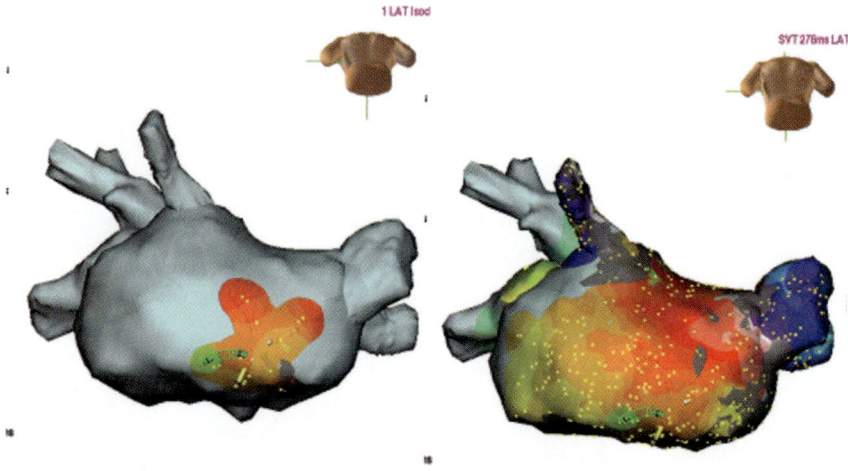

FIGURE 8-9. NavX three-dimensional mapping system. *Left panel*, using a multielectrode catheter, such as PentaRay, activation map can be obtained quickly by simultaneously recording data from the multiple electrodes. In this patient, atrial tachycardia exiting a gap from the left superior pulmonary vein was found (*right panel*), and radiofrequency ablation at the gap successfully abolished atrial tachycardia.

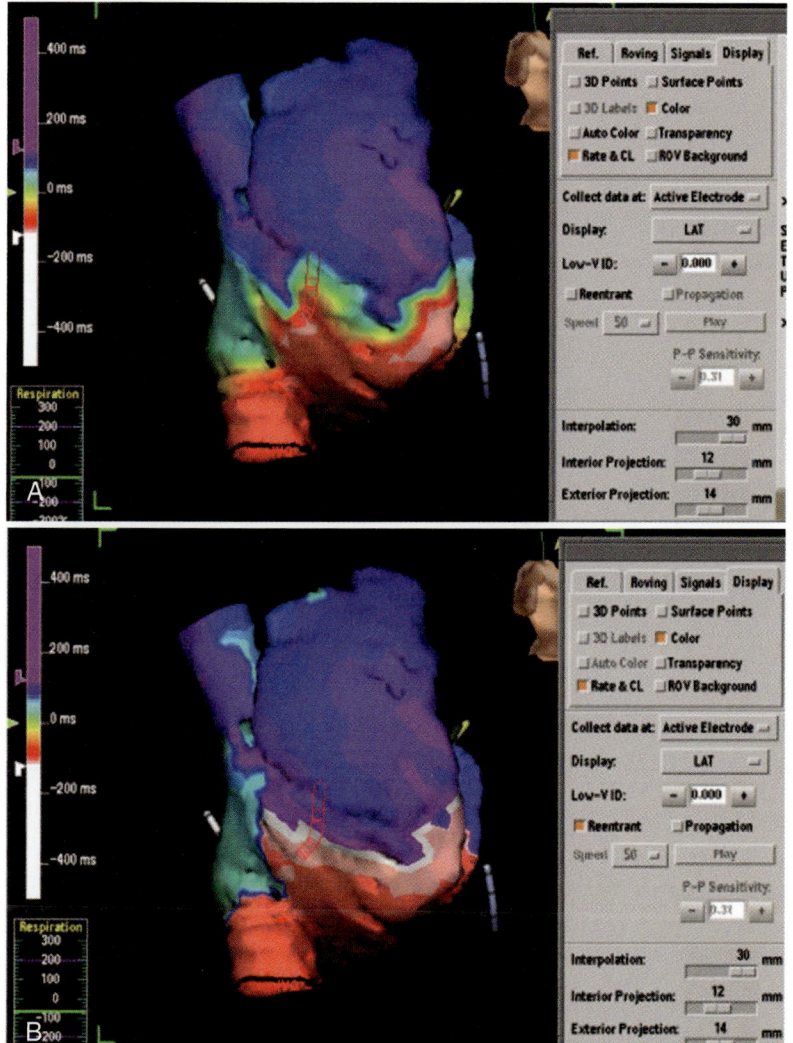

FIGURE 8-10. NavX System. **A,** Standard local activation time display; the transition from "early to late" spans the entire color range. In some situations, this may make identification of the transition zone difficult to visualize. **B,** The same map is displayed with reentrant function. The reentrant function is designed to emphasize the early-to-late activation. When applied, reentrant adjusts the color scale so that *purple* (late) is next to *white* (early) and eliminates the colors in between. This process makes it easy to visualize the transition zone and verify that the rhythm is reentrant in nature.

Local Activation Time Isochronal Maps

Isochronal maps display color-coded activation times for each collected location. The local activation time is the difference in milliseconds between detected activation on the roving waveform and the reference waveform. Colors range from white (early), to red, to yellow, to blue, to purple (late) (Fig. 8-10). It also can be displayed as an animated propagation map.

Voltage Map

A peak-to-peak voltage map displays color-coded voltage values for each collected location. The peak-to-peak voltage is the difference in millivolts between the peak-positive and the peak-negative components of the complex on the mapping catheter. Colors range from gray (low voltage) to purple (high voltage) (Fig. 8-11).

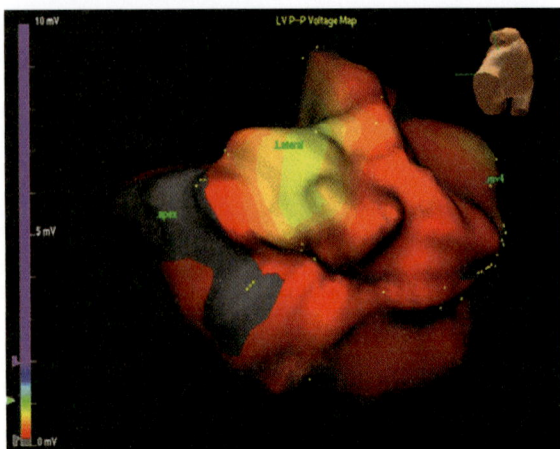

FIGURE 8-11. NavX system. Voltage map of the left ventricle is displayed. The *gray area* is low voltage. The threshold of the low voltage can be adjusted.

Complex Fractionated Electrogram Map

The Fractionation Mapping Tool creates a complex fractionated electrogram (CFE) map that displays a color-coded index of fractionation levels, either as the mean time between fractionated complexes or as the standard deviation on the mean. CFE mean maps provide a fractionation index based on the cycle length between multiple, discrete, local activations in an electrogram. Collected points with a lower value are displayed toward the white end of the color spectrum. CFE standard deviation maps provide a fractionation index based on the cycle length between multiple, discrete, local activations in an electrogram. The CFE standard deviation calculates the standard deviation between tick marks. Collected points with a lower value are displayed toward the white end of the color spectrum.

Fusion with the Preacquired Image

This system also allows the registration of a previously acquired 3D image (such as CT angiogram of the heart chambers and vessels) with the NavX chamber geometry model, which was created using any conventional mapping catheter. Especially detailed models can be created by using a multi-electrode catheter. The reconstructed geometry can be fused with the 3D image by placing fiduciary points on each surface (Fig. 8-12), or images can be displayed side by side.

Ensite Array Mapping System

The Ensite Array system (EnSite 3000, Endocardial Solutions) consists of a multielectrode array catheter (MEA), an amplifier system, and a Silicon Graphics workstation to run specially designed system software (Fig. 8-13). The MEA (a woven braid of 64 electrodes, 0.003-inch diameter wires) is mounted on a 7.6-ml balloon on a 9-French catheter. Each wire has a 0.0025-inch break in insulation, producing a noncontact unipolar electrode. The raw far-field electrographic data from the MEA is acquired and fed into a multichannel recorder and amplifier system, sampled at 1.2 kHz, and filtered with a bandwidth of 0.1 to 300 Hz. The amplifier also has 16 channel inputs for contact catheters and 12 for the surface ECG. A ring electrode located on the proximal shaft of the MEA catheter is used as the reference for unipolar electrogram recordings.

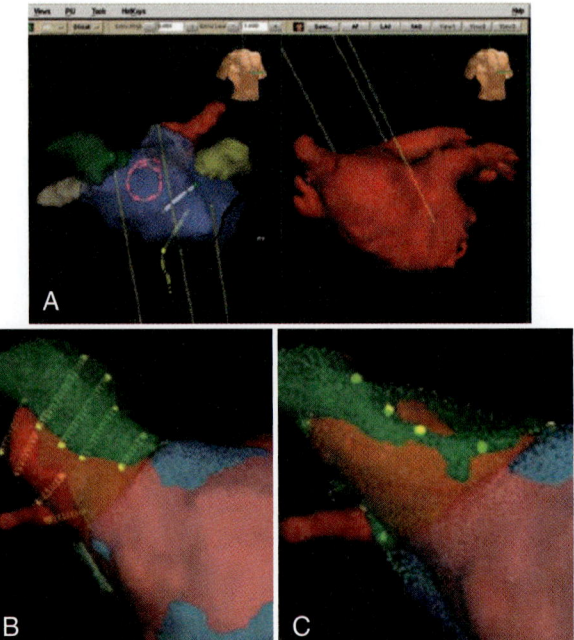

FIGURE 8-12. EnSite fusion registration is the process of aligning the EnSite NavX coordinate system and geometry points to the digital image fusion (DIF) model obtained by computed tomography or magnetic resonance imaging. It uses paired locations between the EnSite navigation field and DIF model to perform registration. Paired fiduciary points are used between the two surfaces as reference points of fused surfaces. **A,** First step is to place fiduciary points to initially register the two surfaces. The correlating locations between the EnSite NavX geometry and the DIF model should be easily identifiable on both images, such as the carina between pulmonary veins and the ridge between the left pulmonary veins and the left atrial appendage. **B** and **C,** Placing the fiduciary point pair will link to the nearest geometry point.

Electrograms recorded from the MEA are analyzed by a boundary-element method to obtain the inverse solution to the Laplace equation and to derive 3360 virtual endocardial electrograms superimposed on the reconstructed cardiac chamber geometry. This geometry is created by contacting the endocardium with a conventional mapping catheter to collect a series of special coordinates. A mathematical constraint (spatial regularization) is placed on the final solution to reduce electrogram noise. These virtual electrograms are displayed on a workstation as color isopotential maps (Clarity Software, Endocardial Solutions).[13,14] A locator signal is used to track the real-time position of any ablation catheter within the virtual geometry.

Accuracy in locating the focal potential using the isopotential map presentation is reduced, however, if the endocardial surface exceeds 50 mm from the surface of the balloon (2.33 ± 0.44 mm verus 7.5 ± 1.13 mm; $P < .01$)[15] by in vitro tank testing. In addition, in vitro electrogram comparison between the computed electrogram and the contact electrogram showed the morphologic correlation of 0.966 (median, 0.984), and most beats (91%) had a correlation higher than 0.90. Timing difference of the electrogram was 0.64 ± 2.48 milliseconds (negative value indicates that computed activation onsets were earlier than those measured from the contact electrograms). Further study showed that the accuracy of electrogram reproduction, including electrogram voltage estimation, decreased at a distance greater than 40 mm. The mean cross-correlation coefficient was 0.82 ± 0.16 for sites

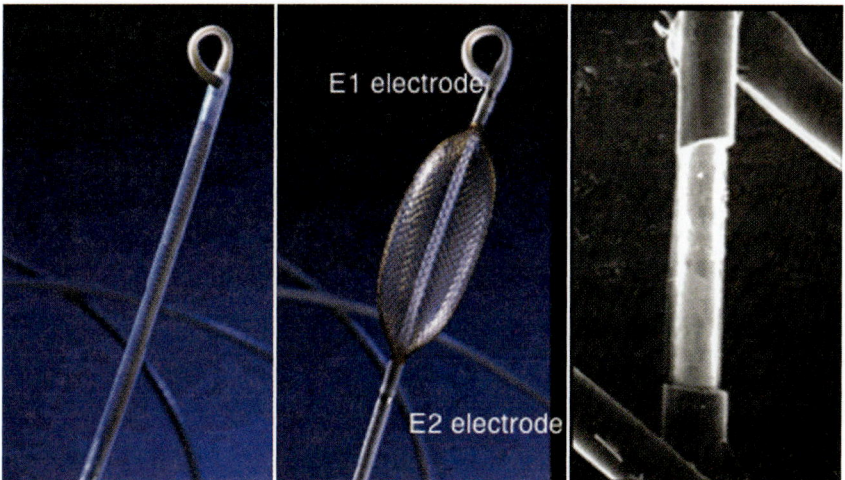

FIGURE 8-13. The Ensite multielectrode array (MEA) is manufactured to have 64 electrodes, which are deployed by expanding the mesh and held in place by an inflated balloon.

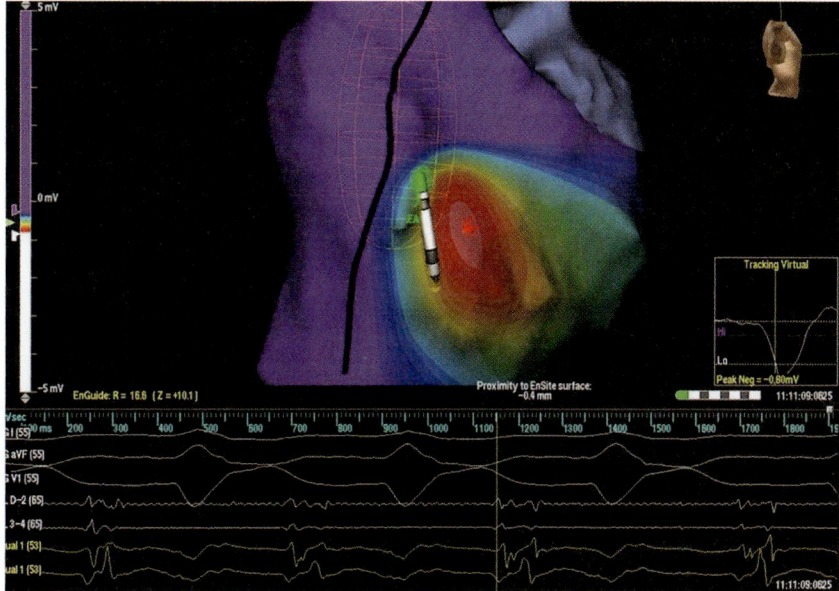

FIGURE 8-14. The activation map obtained with MEA in the right atrium. Atrial tachycardia, which originated (earliest site is shown with *white*) along the crista terminalis (shown with *black line*), is identified. The unipolar recording from the earliest site is shown in the *lower right inset*.

within 40 mm of the balloon center and 0.72 ± 0.16 (*P* < .05) at sites more than 40 mm from the balloon center. The better electrogram reconstruction accuracy at sites close to the balloon was present regardless of the rhythm for which this relationship was evaluated. Therefore, position of the balloon is crucial for precise mapping.

The system displays the activation by quickly processing the signals within the time frame of a single cardiac cycle. In addition, the dynamic substrate mapping tool allows quick, accurate identification of areas of low voltage. The system is ideally suited for activation mapping of unstable and nonsustained arrhythmia because single beat activation can be assessed (Fig. 8-14). In 90% of cases of VT, an exit site may be identified, and in some patients, a portion of the diastolic pathway can be delineated.[16] In a series of VT ablations using the system,[16] the exit site was identified in most VTs by comparison with the time of local activation at adjacent sites and the time of earliest onset of the QRS

complex of the surface ECG. The entire VT circuit was identified in 21% of patients. In addition, activity in some of the diastolic interval could be identified in more than 60% of the VTs. Limitations of the system include the loss of electrogram resolution with distance from the MEA, sensitivity of mapping results on filter settings, and differentiation of ventricular repolarization from late ventricular depolarization and atrial depolarization.

References

1. Gepstein L, Hayam G, Ben-Haim SA. A novel method for nonfluoroscopic catheter-based electroanatomical mapping of the heart. In vitro and in vivo accuracy results. *Circulation.* 1997;95:1611–1622.
2. Tung S, Soejima K, Maisel WH, et al. Recognition of far-field electrograms during entrainment mapping of ventricular tachycardia. *J Am Coll Cardiol.* 2003;42:110–115.
3. Marchlinski FE, Callans DJ, Gottlieb CD, Zado E. Linear ablation lesions for control of unmappable ventricular tachycardia in patients with ischemic and nonischemic cardiomyopathy. *Circulation.* 2000;101:1288–1296.

4. Arenal A, del Castillo S, Gonzalez-Torrecilla E, et al. Tachycardia-related channel in the scar tissue in patients with sustained monomorphic ventricular tachycardias: influence of the voltage scar definition. *Circulation.* 2004;110: 2568–2574.

5. Brunckhorst CB, Delacretaz E, Soejima K, et al. Identification of the ventricular tachycardia isthmus after infarction by pace mapping. *Circulation.* 2004;110:652–659.

6. Soejima K, Suzuki M, Maisel WH, et al. Catheter ablation in patients with multiple and unstable ventricular tachycardias after myocardial infarction: short ablation lines guided by reentry circuit isthmuses and sinus rhythm mapping. *Circulation.* 2001;104:664–669.

7. Brunckhorst CB, Stevenson WG, Soejima K, et al. Relationship of slow conduction detected by pace-mapping to ventricular tachycardia re-entry circuit sites after infarction. *J Am Coll Cardiol.* 2003;41:802–809.

8. Arenal A, Glez-Torrecilla E, Ortiz M, et al. Ablation of electrograms with an isolated, delayed component as treatment of unmappable monomorphic ventricular tachycardias in patients with structural heart disease. *J Am Coll Cardiol.* 2003;41:81–92.

9. Dong J, Dickfeld T, Dalal D, et al. Initial experience in the use of integrated electroanatomic mapping with three-dimensional MR/CT images to guide catheter ablation of atrial fibrillation. *J Cardiovasc Electrophysiol.* 2006;17:459–466.

10. Rossillo A, Indiani S, Bonso A, et al. Novel ICE-guided registration strategy for integration of electroanatomical mapping with three-dimensional CT/MR images to guide catheter ablation of atrial fibrillation. *J Cardiovasc Electrophysiol.* 2009;20:374–378.

11. Okumura Y, Henz B, Johnson S, et al. Three-dimensional ultrasound for image-guided mapping and intervention: methods, quantitative validation, and clinical feasibility of a novel multi-modality image mapping system. *Circulation.* 2008;1:110–119.

12. Patel A, d'Avila A, Neuzil P, et al. Atrial tachycardia after ablation of persistent atrial fibrillation: identification of the critical isthmus with a combination of multielectrode activation mapping and targeted entrainment mapping. *Circulation.* 2008;1:14–22.

13. Kadish A, Hauck J, Pederson B, et al. Mapping of atrial activation with a non-contact, multielectrode catheter in dogs. *Circulation.* 1999;99:1906–1913.

14. Schilling RJ, Peters NS, Davies DW. Simultaneous endocardial mapping in the human left ventricle using a noncontact catheter: comparison of contact and reconstructed electrograms during sinus rhythm. *Circulation.* 1998;98:887–898.

15. Gornick CC, Adler SW, Pederson B, et al. Validation of a new noncontact catheter system for electroanatomic mapping of left ventricular endocardium. *Circulation.* 1999;99:829–835.

16. Schilling RJ, Peters NS, Davies DW. Mapping and ablation of ventricular tachycardia with the aid of a non-contact mapping system. *Heart.* 1999;81: 570–575.

9

Remote Catheter Navigation Systems

Sabine Ernst and Mark A. Wood

Key Points

Remote catheter navigation systems currently comprise magnetic and electromechanical technologies.

Potential advantages of remote navigation include improved catheter stability, enhanced patient safety, automated mapping and catheter navigation, and reduced operator radiation exposure and physical stress.

Early clinical experience with electromechanical mapping has focused on atrial fibrillation and flutter. Magnetic navigation has been applied to all forms of ventricular and supraventricular arrhythmias.

Remote catheter navigation systems have not yet been demonstrated superior to manual catheter navigation in procedural success or total procedure times, although shorter fluoroscopic times are reported.

Catheter ablation of complex arrhythmias can now be performed with good clinical success due largely to the introduction of computerized three-dimensional (3D) mapping systems.[1,2] These systems acquire, organize, and display large volumes of data recorded by intracardiac catheters, but manipulation of the ablation catheter to sites of interest has until recently been performed manually. Conventional ablation catheters are limited in motion, with the ability to deflect in a single plane and generally at a fixed radius. The next technologic "step" in the electrophysiology laboratory after advanced mapping systems has been the introduction of remote navigation systems to improve the precision, stability, and range of motion of ablation catheters. Two robotic catheter navigation systems have been introduced into clinical practice, both enabling remote control of the ablation catheter.[3–8] These systems were introduced with the goals of enhancing the safety and precision of catheter manipulation for

ablation procedures. Computerized navigation may also improve the dexterity for all operators performing catheter manipulation during complex arrhythmia ablations. Reduced operator radiation exposure and physical stress have been demonstrated.

Remote Catheter Navigation Systems

Electromechanical Catheter Navigation
Basic Concepts

The electromagnetic catheter ablation system basically consists of two parts[5,6]: a computerized "master" input device that translates the operator's movement of a handle to an electromechanical patient side "slave" (Fig. 9-1; Table 9-1). This remote catheter manipulator controls the tips of two telescoping guiding sheaths (14-French outer sheath and 11.5-French inner sheath) (Fig. 9-2) that accommodate any conventional ablation catheter otherwise intended for manual manipulation. The outer guiding sheath is controlled by two guidewires that provide deflection at proximal and distal segments of the sheath. The inner sheath is controlled by four guidewires that allow 270 degrees of deflection in any direction (**Video 9-1**). The multiple levels of sheath curvature allow for compound catheter angulation and improved catheter range of motion. The control is provided by the "master-slave" system, which reacts to the hand motion of the user who is situated at a computer console away from the patient (**Video 9-2**). All available 3D mapping systems can be used in conjunction with the electromechanical system. In ex vivo hearts, the robotic system greatly decreased the time needed for precision navigation (to 0.8 mm target) compared with manual navigation.[5]

Clinical Experience Using the Electromechanical System

Most publications report on the use of the system during atrial fibrillation ablation procedures (Table 9-2).[5–12] The use of the system has also been reported for atrial flutter and accessory pathway ablation (Table 9-2, Fig. 9-3). These studies have all reported success rates comparable to manual navigation procedures and frequently reduced

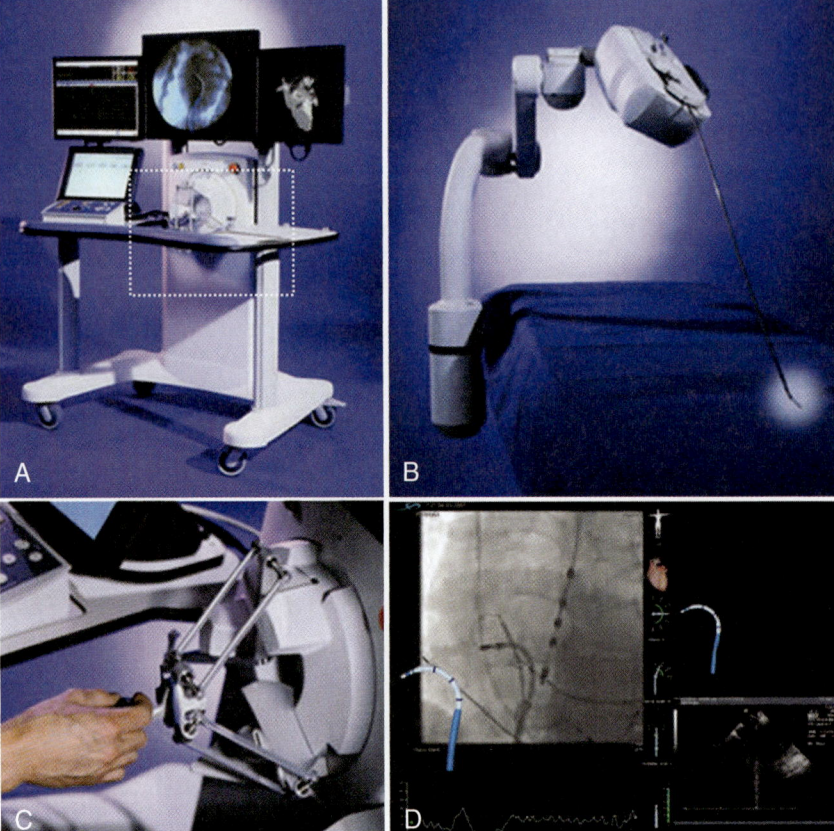

FIGURE 9-1. Electromechanical remote catheter navigation system. **A,** Mobile workstation remote from bedside comprising monitors, electrocardiographic and catheter navigation information, and interface device for manipulation of the catheter. **B,** Bedside unit for steerable sheaths and mechanism to translate remote operator input into catheter motion. **C,** Human interface to direct motion of the steerable sheaths (from *insert* in **A**). **D,** Monitor display for fluoroscopic views and rendering of real-time data for catheter orientation, catheter-tip pressure, and intracardiac echocardiography. *(Courtesy of Hansen Medical, Mountain View, CA.)*

TABLE 9-1

REMOTE CATHETER NAVIGATION SYSTEMS

	Electromechanical Navigation	**Magnetic Navigation**
Concept	Mechanical steering via pullwire-equipped sheaths	Alignment in magnetic field of small magnets embedded in the catheter tip
Potential contraindications	Vascular access (14 French)	Cochlear implants Large metal implants, such as internal cardioverter defibrillator or pacemaker
Available catheters	All ablation catheters and energy types	Standard tip 4 and 8 mm Irrigated tip 3.5 mm platinum (plus Carto sensor) Irrigated gold tip
Compatibility with three-dimensional mapping systems	All	Carto and NavX
Contact force	Significant; contact pressure sensor incorporated	<20 g maximum
Risk for perforation	Yes	Virtually none

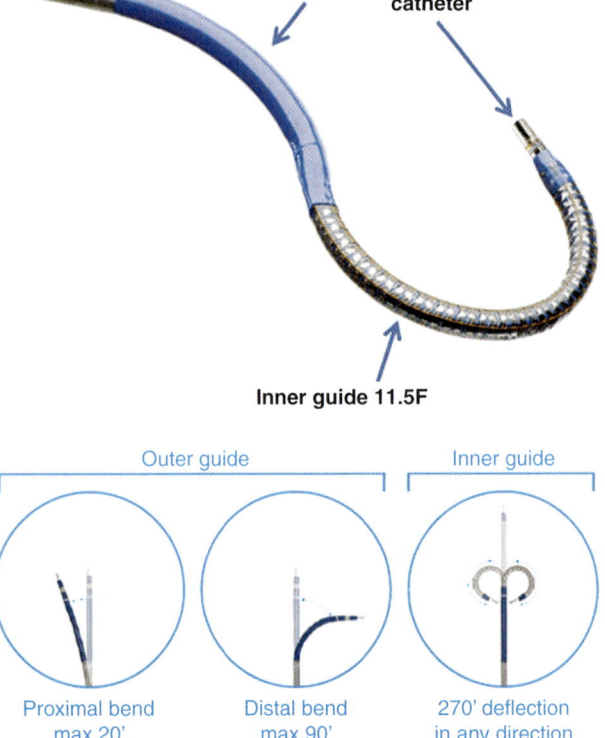

FIGURE 9-2. Deflectable portion of robotic sheath system showing inner and outer sheaths. The range of motion for each sheath is shown. *(Courtesy of Hansen Medical, Mountain View, CA.)*

SELECTED CLINICAL REPORTS ON REMOTE ELECTROMECHANICAL NAVIGATION

Study	No. of Patients	Arrhythmias	Randomized vs. Manual	Success Rate	Procedure Time	Fluoroscopy Time	Complications	Comments
Steven et al, 2008[8]	50	CVTI, AFL	Yes	100% RNS 100% manual	79 ± 31 min RNS 58 ± 18 min* manual	8 ± 5 min RNS 6 ± 4 min* manual	None	Operator radiation exposure and RF time reduced for RNS
Di Biase et al, 2009[9]	390	AF	Yes	85%RNS 81% manual	3 ± 1 hr RNS 3 ± 1 hr manual	49 ± 25 min RNS 58 ± 20 min* manual	2 tamponade, 1 groin hematoma RNS 1 tamponade, 1 groin hematoma Manual	Success measured as absence of AF recurrences at 14 ± 1 mo follow-up
Wazni et al, 2009[7]	71	AF	No	All PV isolated in 90% patients, 76% no AF recurrence at 6 mo	17 ±51 min left atrial instrumentation time	Not given	4 vascular injury, 2 tamponade, 5 severe PV stenosis, 1 gastroparesis	Initial experience, 1 operator for RNS and separate operator for circular mapping catheter
Schmidt et al, 2009[10]	65	AF	No	95% of patients with all PV isolated, 73% without recurrence AF	195 ± 40 min	17 ± 7 min	1 tamponade, 1 air embolism, 1 esophageal ulcer	Median follow-up 239 days (range, 184 to 314), 3D navigation used in all patients
Kanagaratnam et al, 2008[10]	10	1 AP, 2 AFL, 7 AF	No	100% acute success (PV isolation for AF)	106 min AP 70,140 min AFL 180 min mean AF	13 min AP 20,44 min AFL 59 min mean AF	1 pericardial effusion	"Negligible" radiation exposure to robotic operator station

* Statistically significant versus RNS.
AF, atrial fibrillation; AFL, atrial flutter; AP, accessory pathway; CVTI, cavotricuspid isthmus; PV, pulmonary vein; RNS, robotic navigation system.

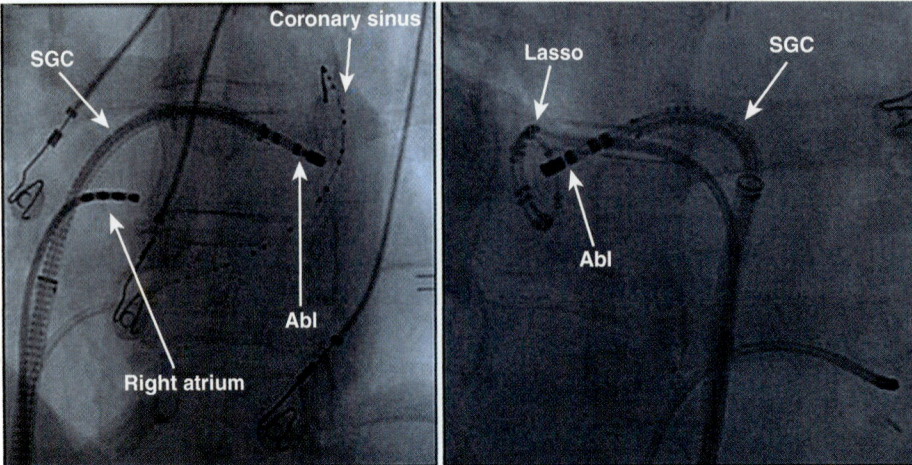

FIGURE 9-3. Fluoroscopic views of robotic sheath system in clinical use. *Left panel,* Left anterior oblique view of robotic sheath system for ablation of a left free wall accessory pathway by the transseptal approach. *Right panel,* Posteroanterior view of robotic sheath system for right superior pulmonary vein isolation through transseptal access. Abl, ablation; SGC, steerable guide sheath. *(From Kanagaratnam P, Koa-Wing M, Wallace DT, et al. Experience of robotic catheter ablation in humans using a novel remotely steerable catheter sheath.* J Interv Card Electrophysiol. *2008;21:19-26.)*

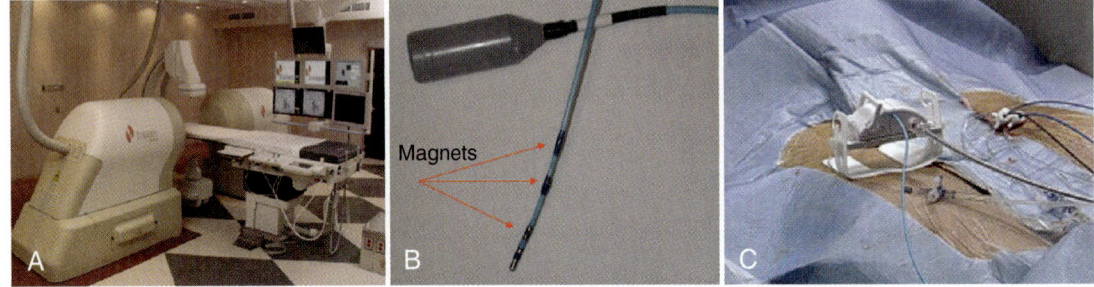

FIGURE 9-4. Magnetic catheter navigation system. **A,** Bedside permanent magnets located on both sides of the examination table. The magnets are shown in the navigation position perpendicular to the table but can be stored in a position rotated parallel to the table. Note the single-plane fluoroscopy unit. **B,** Magnetic mapping and ablation catheter. The catheter body is flaccid and incorporates three magnets in the distal section. **C,** Motorized unit to remotely advance and retract the ablation catheter (right groin). *(Courtesy of Stereotaxis, St. Louis, MO.)*

fluoroscopic times. Neither total procedure time nor the incidence of complications has been reduced by robotic navigation (Table 9-2). In the largest study of ablation using robotic navigation, 390 patients were randomized to manual versus robotic navigation for treatment of atrial fibrillation.[9] Success rates were similar for the two approaches (85% robotic navigation versus 81% manual navigation; $P = .26$), but fluoroscopy time was reduced for the robotic navigation group (49 ± 25 minutes versus 58 ± 20 minutes; $P < .001$). Reduced radiation exposure to the ablation catheter operator has been reported, but manipulations of nonablation catheters (such as circular mapping catheters for atrial fibrillation ablation) still require manual navigation at the bedside. Early experience demonstrated some vascular complications related to the large outer sheath diameter and the enhanced catheter contact with the myocardium.[7] Because of mechanical steering of the catheter, the contact force applied with this system may cause larger than expected radiofrequency lesions, leading to perforations and esophageal trauma (K. H. Kuck, personal communication).[9,13] To correct this problem, a contact force indicator is now available but awaits further assessment of outcomes.

Magnetic Navigation
Basic Concepts
The magnetic navigation system (Niobe, Stereotaxis, St. Louis, MO) consists of two large permanent magnets positioned on either side of the single-plane fluoroscopy table (Fig. 9-4).[3,4] The orientation of the magnets within the housings is under computer control. When in the "navigate" position, the magnets create a relatively uniform spherical magnetic navigation field (0.08 Tesla [T]) about 15 cm in diameter inside the patient's chest. Navigation of the ablation catheter in any direction is possible within the confines of this field. The mapping and ablation catheter is equipped with three small permanent magnets positioned at the tip that align themselves with the externally controlled magnetic field. By changing the orientation of the outer magnets relative to each other, the orientation of the magnetic navigation field vector changes and thereby leads to deflection of the catheter (Fig. 9-5; **Video 9-3**). A motorized computer-controlled catheter advancer system is used to advance and retract the catheter remotely (Fig. 9-4; **Video 9-4**). All catheter movement is under computer control of the operator remote from bedside. The system is controlled by a keyboard or a mouse and allows remote control of the ablation

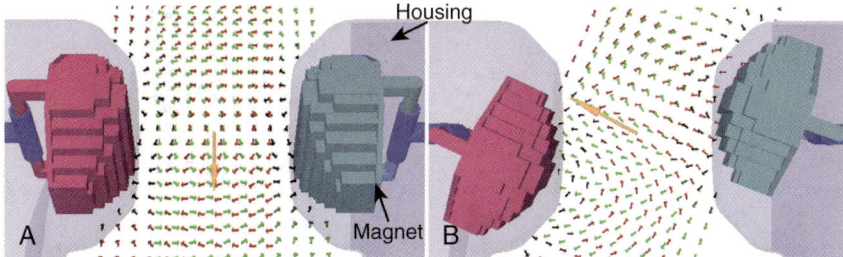

FIGURE 9-5. Schematic animation of the motion of navigational magnets to create a steering vector for the magnetic ablation catheter. The *red* and *green arrows* represent the magnet vectors for each of the bedside magnets. The *large yellow arrow* represents the summation vector created by the two magnets. **A,** The magnet positions create a magnetic field to direct the ablation catheter in a purely cranial direction. **B,** The magnet positions now direct the catheter cranial and toward the patient's right. *(Courtesy of Stereotaxis, St. Louis, MO.)*

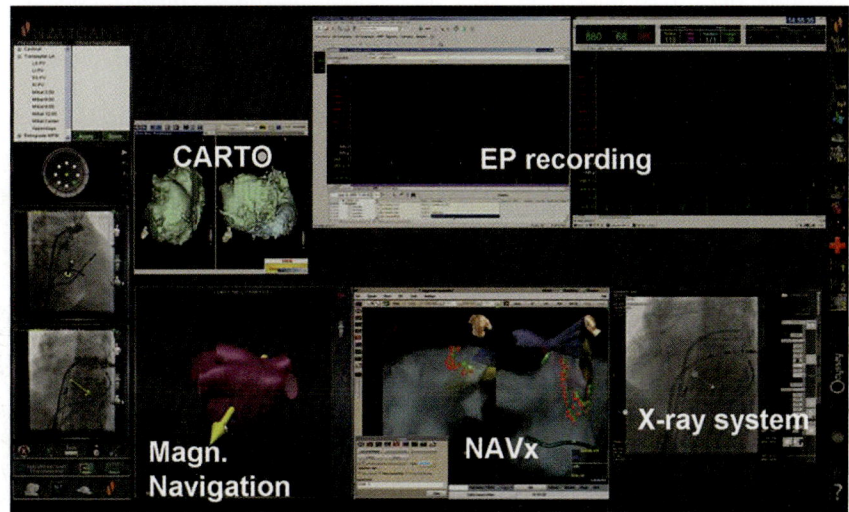

FIGURE 9-6. Combined monitoring screen for the Stereotaxis magnetic navigation system displaying electrophysiologic (EP) recordings, magnetic (MAGN) navigation information, NavX (St. Jude Medical) catheter positions, fluoroscopic views, and Carto (Biosense Webster) imaging.

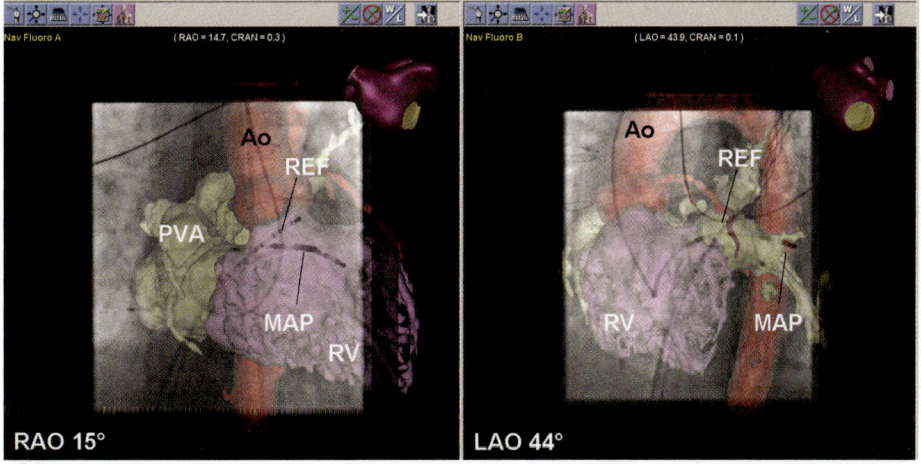

FIGURE 9-7. Example of the Navigant workstation with Carto RMT (Biosense Webster) maps of a patient with an atrial reentrant tachycardia within the pulmonary venous atrium (PVA) after surgical correction (Mustard operation) for transposition of the great arteries. Note the image-integrated map and 3D magnetic resonance images on the fluoroscopic reference images. Lowering the transparency of the 3D images allows depiction of the magnetic catheter (MAP) position within the left inferior pulmonary vein using a retrograde approach. A timing reference (REF) is positioned within the systemic venous atrium. Ao, aorta; RV, right ventricle.

catheter from inside the control room. The operator views by monitors the fluoroscopic screens, real-time catheter orientation data, and electrophysiologic recordings (Fig. 9-6).

Recently, a fully integrated 3D electroanatomic Carto system (Carto RMT, Biosense Webster, Diamond Bar, CA) was introduced that works with its ultralow electromagnetic field (5×10^{-6} to 5×10^{-3} T) and the permanent magnetic field of the navigation system (0.08 T). In addition, integration among the fluoroscopy system, the magnetic navigation system, and the Carto RMT system is enabled such that the information is displayed superimposed on the fluoroscopic reference pictures (Fig. 9-7). The navigation of the mapping and ablation catheter can be performed by designating the desired tip location on registered fluoroscopic reference images, designating points on the Carto electroanatomic map, or controlling the magnetic vector in a virtual cardiac anatomy.

Non-Carto magnetic catheters can be used with the NavX system in the magnetic laboratory (Fig. 9-7). Precise orientation of the catheter by 1-degree deflection increments and by 1- to 3-mm steps in advancement or retraction is possible. All catheter positions (magnetic vector and advanced distance) can be stored and reprogrammed to automatically return the catheter to points of interest. Automated catheter electroanatomic mapping of the cardiac chambers can be performed under computer control. In addition, ablation lines may be designated on the electroanatomic anatomy for the system to automatically follow with the ablation tip. When the external magnet housing is in navigation position (close to the patient), the angulation of the single-plane C arm is limited to about 28 degrees for both right anterior oblique and left anterior oblique projections. The magnets, however, may be canted to allow steeper oblique views in one direction. Magnetic radiofrequency ablation catheters are available with 4 and 8 mm tips and with an open irrigation tip (4-mm tip only).

Clinical Experience with the Magnetic Navigation System

The magnetic navigation system has been used to treat the full range of supraventricular and ventricular arrhythmias that are managed only with difficulty with manual catheter ablation techniques (Table 9-3).[14–32] For atrioventricular (AV) nodal reentry and AV reciprocating tachycardias, magnetic navigation appears to provide comparable success rates and total procedure times but may reduce fluoroscopic time and the number of delivered radiofrequency lesions.[25,31] For slow pathway ablation, the magnetic navigation provides earlier occurrence of junctional rhythm, lower mean electrode temperatures, and less temperature variability than manual navigation, effects attributable to increased catheter stability.[33] Left atrial tachycardias have been approached from retrograde aortic and transseptal access. Complication rates are similar for supraventricular tachycardia ablation with magnetic or manual navigation.[15,25,31] A unique feature of magnetic navigation is the ability to store the magnetic vectors for each catheter position, thus enabling effortless return of the ablation catheter to previous sites of interest.

Pulmonary vein isolation has been performed under magnetic navigation. These early reports, however, used noncooled 4-mm-tip ablation electrodes.[26,27] Catheter navigation around the veins was feasible, but acute success was limited in some cases by inability to create effective lesions. There are currently no large published reports on the use of the irrigated-tip magnetic catheter for pulmonary vein isolation. Theoretically, pulmonary vein isolation should be facilitated by the use of automated catheter movement along prespecified lines designated on 3D virtual anatomic renderings.

Magnetic navigation has been used for ablation of ventricular tachycardias in patients with and without structural heart disease.[24,25,32] In structurally normal hearts, both right ventricular outflow tachycardia (RVOT) and idiopathic left ventricular tachycardia have been ablated. The low perforation risk, catheter stability, and freedom of catheter movement make magnetic navigation an attractive approach to RVOT (Fig. 9-8). Aryana and colleagues reported on the use of magnetic navigation to treat ventricular arrhythmias associated with a variety of heart diseases.[24] Both endocardial mapping and epicardial mapping were performed under magnetic navigation, with high rates of success for selected arrhythmias. Ventricular tachycardia arising from the coronary cusp has also been ablated with magnetic navigation.[22]

Advantages and Disadvantages of Remote Navigation Systems

One of the most obvious advantages of remote-controlled catheter navigation systems is the reduced fluoroscopy exposure for the operator. Documented reduced operator fluoroscopic exposure time has been reported in only one study to date, however.[8] Operators must still position diagnostic and mapping catheters manually so that fluoroscopic exposure cannot be totally eliminated. Both systems have been reported to reduce fluoroscopic time for the patients as well. Although catheter stability and precision are believed to be slightly enhanced by robotic navigation, neither system has been shown superior to manual navigation for procedural success. Each system has its advantages and limitations (Table 9-4). For the electromechanical system, additional benefits are compatibility with all ablation catheters and mapping systems as well as the physical mobility of the system from room to room. Disadvantages are the large external sheath diameter, a risk for vascular or cardiac complications, and the limited access of the system to the coronary sinus, left ventricle, and pericardial space. Early concerns for perforation risk from the system led to the introduction of contact pressure–monitoring algorithms.

For the magnetic navigation system, catheter stability, range of motion, and extremely low perforation risk are major advantages. The disadvantages include a lack of compatibility with some mapping and ablation catheters and systems, the need for continuous "magnet room" precautions, and the limitation to a single-plane fluoroscopy system. The cost of each system is considerable.

TABLE 9-3

SELECTED CLINICAL REPORTS ON REMOTE MAGNETIC NAVIGATION

Study	No. of Patients	Arrhythmias (No. of Patients)	Randomized vs. Manual	Success Rate	Procedure Time	Fluoroscopy Time	Complications	Comments
Kerzner et al, 2006[15]	56	AVNRT	Yes	100% MNS 100% manual	3.4 ± 3 hr MNS 3.4 ± 1 hr manual	17 ± 13 min MNS 16 ± 16 min manual	Transient 2:1 AV block 1 MNS patient	Retrospective controls
Thornton et al, 2006[19]	37	AVNRT	Yes	90% acute success	163 (69–260) min MNS 159 (83–290) min manual	12 (4–37) min MNS 18 (9–51) min manual	None	Retrospective controls
Lactu et al, 2009[20]	84	AVNRT (37) AFL (22) AP (12) VT (7) AT (3)	No	AVNRT: 97% AFL: 54% AP: 67% VT: 85% AT: 100%	169 ± 72 min	14 ± 11 min	1 pericardial effusion	Success with manual navigation in all but one MNS failure
Di Biase et al, 2009[32]	65	RVOT (19) VT with CM (46)	No	RVOT: 86% VT with CM: 36%	4.6 ± 2 hr	57 ± 32 min	2 groin hematomas	Success VT with CM improved with 8-mm-tip catheter
Wood et al, 2008[31]	56 MNS 15 control	MNS: AVNRT (38) AP (12) AVJ EFA (4) Manual: AVNRT (10) AP (5)	Yes	MNS: AVNRT: 95% AP: 75% AVJ RFA: 100% Manual: AVNRT: 90% AP: 80%	151 (111, 221) min MNS 151 (110, 278) min *manual	18 (10, 28) min MNS 27 (19, 48) min *manual	1 pulmonary embolism MNS	Prospective randomized
Kim et al, 2008[25]	127 MNS 594 control	AVNRT AP AF AFL RVOT	Yes	Not given	332 ± 102 MNS 243 ± 95 manual*	51 ± 28 min MNS 51 ± 34 manual	2 tamponade with AF ablation manual	Retrospective controls, fluoroscopy time reduced for AF, AVNRT, and AP with MNS
Chun et al, 2007[16]	59	AP	No	81% overall, 92% with 3-magnet catheter	172 ± 90 min for 3-magnet catheter	4.9 (3.4–8) min for 3-magnet catheter	None	Procedure and fluoroscopy times and success rates all improved with 3-magnet catheter
Aryana et al, 2007[24]	24	VT	No	81%	Not given	21 ± 7 min	1 DVT, 1 pericardial effusion, 1 nerve palsy	Selected VTs targeted for MNS, epicardial mapping performed
Katsiyiannis et al, 2008[29]	40	AF	Yes	75% MNS 80% manual	209 ± 56 min MNS 279 ± 60 min *manual	20 ± 10 min MNS 59 ± 21 min *manual	None	All PVs isolated in both groups, follow-up 1 year

* P < .05 vs. MNS.

AF, atrial fibrillation; AFL, atrial flutter; AP, accesso y pathway; AT, atrial tachycardia; AVJ RFA, atrioventricular junctional radio frequency ablation; AVNRT, atrioventricular nodal reentry tachycardia; DVT, deep venous thrombosis; MNS, magnetic navigation system; RVOT, right ventricular outflow tract tachycardia; VT, ventricular tachycardia.

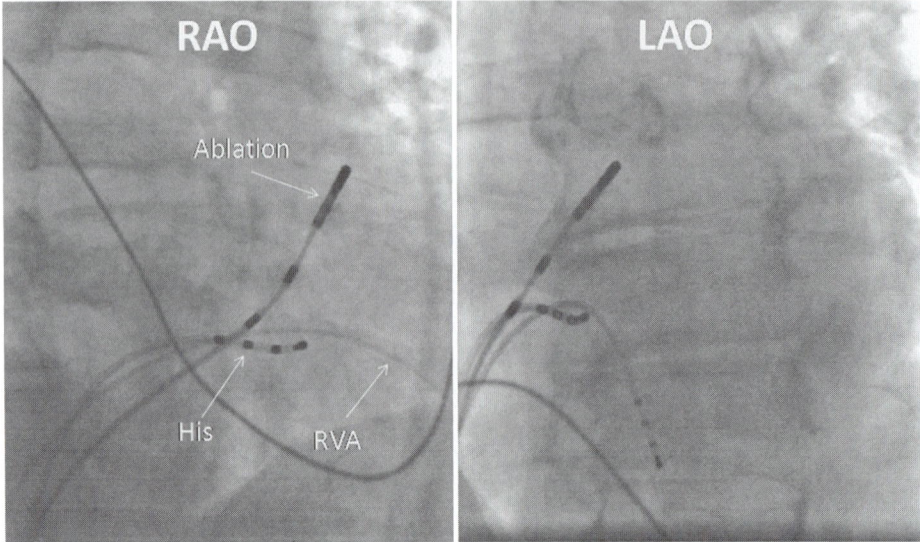

FIGURE 9-8. Magnetic remote navigation of a magnetic-tip ablation catheter for the treatment of right ventricular outflow tract tachycardia. Right anterior oblique (RAO) and left anterior oblique (LAO) views are shown. RVA, right ventricular apex.

TABLE 9-4

ADVANTAGES AND DISADVANTAGES OF NAVIGATION SYSTEMS

	Electromechanical Navigation	**Magnetic Navigation**
Reported applications	Primarily atrial fibrillation and flutter	Supraventricular tachycardia, ventricular tachycardia, atrial tachycardia, atrial fibrillation, atrial flutter
Advantages	Catheter stability Compatable with all ablation catheters Compatable with all mapping systems System is movable, less obtrusive No interference with implanted devices or room precautions Reduced fluoroscopic times	Catheter stability and mobility Minimal perforation risk Automated mapping and ablation Stored magnetic vectors return catheter to previous locations Epicardial mapping possible Reduced fluoroscopic times
Disadvantages	Limited or no access to left ventricle, coronary sinus, or pericardial space Perforation risk Large sheath diameter Cost	Limited to Carto mapping system Single-plane fluoroscopy only Magnetic room precautions always in effect Restricted use in patients with implanted devices Limited catheter contact Pressure generated Cost

References

1. Ben-Haim SA, Osadchy D, Schuster I, et al. Nonfluoroscopic, in vivo navigation and mapping technology. *Nat Med.* 1996;2:1393–1395.
2. Schilling RJ, Peters NS, Davies DW. Simultaneous endocardial mapping in the human left ventricle using a noncontact catheter: comparison of contact and reconstructed electrograms during sinus rhythm. *Circulation.* 1998;98:887–898.
3. Faddis MN, Blume W, Finney J, et al. Novel, magnetically guided catheter for endocardial mapping and radiofrequency catheter ablation. *Circulation.* 2002;106:2980–2985.
4. Ernst S, Ouyang F, Linder C, et al. Initial experience with remote catheter ablation using a novel magnetic navigation system: magnetic remote catheter ablation. *Circulation.* 2004;109:1472–1475.
5. Al-Ahmad A, Grossman JD, Wang PJ. Early experience with a computerized robotically controlled catheter system. *J Interv Card Electrophysiol.* 2005;12:199–202.
6. Saliba W, Reddy VY, Wazni O, et al. Atrial fibrillation ablation using a robotic catheter remote control system: initial human experience and long-term follow-up results. *J Am Coll Cardiol.* 2008;51:2407–2411.
7. Wazni OM, Barrett C, Martin DO, et al. Experience with the Hansen robotic system for atrial fibrillation ablation: lessons learned and techniques modified. Hansen in the real world. *J Cardiovasc Electrophysiol.* 2009; 20:1193–1196.
8. Steven D, Rostock T, Servatius H, et al. Robotic versus conventional ablation for common-type atrial flutter: a prospective randomized trial to evaluate the effectiveness of remote catheter navigation. *Heart Rhythm.* 2008;5:1556–1560.
9. Di Biase L, Wangg Y, Horton R, et al. Ablation of atrial fibrillation utilizing robotic catheter navigation in comparison to manual navigation and ablation: single-center experience. *J Cardiovasc Electrophysiol.* 2009;20:1328–1335.
10. Schmidt B, Tilz RR, Neven K, et al. Remote robotic navigation and electroanatomic mapping for ablation of atrial fibrillation: considerations for navigation and impact on procedural outcome. *Circ Arrhythmia Electrophysiol.* 2009;2:120–128.
11. Kanagaratnam P, Koa-Wing M, Wallace D, et al. Experience of robotic catheter ablation in humans using a novel remotely steerable catheter sheath. *J Interv Card Electrophysiol.* 2008;21:19–26.
12. Schmidt B, Chun KRJ, Tilz RR, et al. Remote navigation systems in electrophysiology. *Europace.* 2008;10:iii57–iii61.
13. Di Biase L, Natale A, Barrett C, et al. Relationship between catheter forces, lesion characteristics, "popping" and char formation: experience with robotic navigation. *J Cardiovasc Electrophysiol.* 2009;20:436–440.
14. Ernst S, Hachiya H, Chun JK, Ouyang F. Remote catheter ablation of parahisian accessory pathways using a novel magnetic navigation system: a report of two cases. *J Cardiovasc Electrophysiol.* 2005;16:659–662.
15. Kerzner R, Sanchez JM, Osborn JL, et al. Radiofrequency ablation of atrioventricular nodal reentrant tachycardia using a novel magnetic guidance system compared with a conventional approach. *Heart Rhythm.* 2006;3:261–267.
16. Chun JK, Ernst S, Matthews S, et al. Remote-controlled catheter ablation of accessory pathways: results from the magnetic laboratory. *Eur Heart J.* 2007;28:190–195.
17. Chun JK, Schmidt B, Kuck KH, Ernst S. Remote-controlled magnetic ablation of a right anterolateral accessory pathway: the superior caval vein approach. *J Interv Card Electrophysiol.* 2006;16:65–68.
18. Arya A, Kottkamp H, Piorkowski C, et al. Initial clinical experience with a remote magnetic catheter navigation system for ablation of cavotricuspid isthmus-dependent right atrial flutter. *Pacing Clin Electrophysiol.* 2008;31:597–603.

19. Thornton AS, Janse P, Theuns DA, et al. Magnetic navigation in AV nodal reentrant tachycardia study: early results of ablation with one- and three-magnet catheters. *Europace*. 2006;8:225–230.
20. Latcu DG, Ricard P, Zarqane N, et al. Robotic magnetic navigation for ablation of human arrhythmias: initial experience. *Arch Cardiovasc Dis*. 2009;102:419–425.
21. Thornton AS, Jordaens LJ. Remote magnetic navigation for mapping and ablating right ventricular outflow tract tachycardia. *Heart Rhythm*. 2006;3:691–696.
22. Burkhardt JD, Saliba WI, Schweikert RA, et al. Remote magnetic navigation to map and ablate left coronary cusp ventricular tachycardia. *J Cardiovasc Electrophysiol*. 2006;17:1142–1144.
23. Thornton AS, Res J, Mekel JM, Jordaens LJ. Use of advanced mapping and remote magnetic navigation to ablate left ventricular fascicular tachycardia. *Pacing Clin Electrophysiol*. 2006;29:685–688.
24. Aryana A, d'Avila A, Heist EK, et al. Remote magnetic navigation to guide endocardial and epicardial catheter mapping of scar-related ventricular tachycardia. *Circulation*. 2007;115:1191–1200.
25. Kim AM, Turakhia M, Lu J, et al. Impact of remote magnetic catheter navigation on ablation fluoroscopy and procedure time. *Pacing Clin Electrophysiol*. 2008;31:1399–1404.
26. Pappone C, Vicedomini G, Manguso F, et al. Robotic magnetic navigation for atrial fibrillation ablation. *J Am Coll Cardiol*. 2006;47:1390–1400.
27. Di Biase L, Fahmy TS, Patel D, et al. Remote magnetic navigation: human experience in pulmonary vein ablation. *J Am Coll Cardiol*. 2007;50:868–874.
28. Ernst S, Berns E. "Two-by-two" pulmonary vein isolation in the presence of a complete situs inversus and dextrocardia: use of magnetic navigation and 3D mapping with image integration. *Europace*. 2009;11:1118–1119.
29. Katisiyiannis WT, Melby DP, Matelski JL, et al. Feasibility and safety of remote-controlled navigation for ablation of atrial fibrillation. *Am J Cardiol*. 2008;102:1674–1676.
30. Thornton AS, Rivero-Ayerza M, Knops P, Jordeans LJ. Magnetic navigation in left-sided AV reentrant tachycardias: preliminary results of a retrograde approach. *J Cardiovasc Electrophysiol*. 2007;18:467–472.
31. Wood MA, Orlov M, Ramaswamy K, et al. Remote magnetic versus manual catheter navigation for ablation of supraventricular tachycardias: a randomized, multicenter trial. *Pacing Clin Electrophysiol*. 2008;31:1313–1321.
32. Di Biase L, Burkhardt JD, Lakkireddy D, et al. Mapping and ablation of ventricular arrhythmias with magnetic navigation: comparison between 4- and 8-mm catheter tips. *J Interv Card Electrophysiol*. 2009;26:133–137.

Videos

Video 9-1. Motion of inner robotic sheath for electromechanical catheter navigation system. (Courtesy of Hansen Medical, Mountain View, CA.)

Video 9-2. Human interface for electromechanical catheter navigation system. Motion of the controller is conveyed to the robotic sheath to deflect the ablation catheter. (Courtesy of Hansen Medical, Mountain View, CA.)

Video 9-3. Schematic animation of the motion of navigational magnets to create a steering vector for the magnetic ablation catheter. The *red* and *green arrows* represent the magnet vectors for each of the bedside magnets. The *large yellow arrow* represents the summation vector created by the two magnets.

Video 9-4. Bedside device to advance and withdraw the ablation catheter remotely during magnetic catheter manipulation. The flaccid ablation catheter is held in a horizontal plane by the navigational magnetic field.

10

Role of Intracardiac Echocardiography in Clinical Electrophysiology

Raphael Rosso, Joseph B. Morton, and Jonathan M. Kalman

Key Points

Catheter technology includes mechanical types (single rotating transducer, 360-degree circumferential imaging, 9 to 12 MHz, near-field clarity, poor tissue penetration) and phased- array types (64-element sector scan, 5 to 10 MHz, steerable, full Doppler capability, good depth penetration).

CartoSound three-dimensional reconstruction of the images obtained by intracardiac echocardiography (ICE) and integration with electroanatomic mapping system helps to identify atrial endocardial structures and to characterize the role of anatomy in arrhythmia mechanism (e.g., crista terminalis, pulmonary veins).

For guidance of radiofrequency (RF) ablation, ICE is used to identify the anatomic location of the catheter tip and to ensure tissue contact (distal tip electrode or linear ablation catheter).

For monitoring RF lesions, ICE is used for real-time assessment of lesion formation and size (mural swelling and increased tissue echodensity).

For AF ablation, ICE assists with transseptal puncture, defines pulmonary vein (PV) anatomy, allows accurate positioning of the lasso catheter at the PV ostium, monitors lesion formation, monitors for complications (e.g., tamponade, thrombus, atrioesophageal fistula), and identifies and possibly predict PV stenosis.

Other uses of ICE include atrial flutter ablation (imaging cavotricuspid isthmus anatomy), ventricular tachycardia (imaging scar border, identifying coronary cusps and left ventricular outflow tract), guidance of transseptal puncture in difficult cases, assessment of left atrial and appendage mechanical function and thrombus, and guidance of atrial septal defect device closure.

The development of intracardiac echocardiography (ICE) has led to an increasing appreciation of the important relationship between arrhythmia mechanism and anatomy. Uses of ICE in the electrophysiology laboratory have included the identification of atrial endocardial structures and the manipulation of mapping and ablation catheters in relation to these structures,[1,2] the creation and quantification of focal[3–9] and continuous[10–12] radiofrequency ablation (RFA) lesions, guidance in the performance of atrial transseptal puncture,[13,14] and identification and prevention of procedural complications.

Although intracardiac echo was critical to our understanding of the importance of cardiac anatomy in arrhythmia mechanism, until recently its clinical utility was limited mostly to guidance of difficult transseptal procedures. However, in recent years, ICE has developed a central role in some centers during catheter ablation procedures for atrial fibrillation (AF). In particular, the development of CartoSound (Biosense Webster, Diamond Bar, CA), which allows three-dimensional (3D) reconstruction of the images obtained by ICE and integration with an electroanatomic mapping system, represents the most recent step in the utility of ultrasound in clinical electrophysiology.

Intracardiac Echocardiography Catheter Design

Technical advances in the construction of compact ultrasound transducers have allowed the development of ICE. Two forms of ICE catheters have been designed that may be described as mechanical ICE and phased-array ICE.

Mechanical ICE catheters have a single ultrasound crystal mounted at the distal end of a 6- to 10-French (F) catheter. Most of these catheters have been non-steerable. The transducer is connected to a motor in the handle of the device through a braided drive shaft. Engagement of the mechanism results in the rapid rotation of the transducer, providing 360-degree circumferential imaging in a plane perpendicular to the long axis of the catheter. Mechanical ICE uses imaging frequencies of

9 to 12 MHz, which provide near-field clarity but poor tissue penetration and far-field resolution (Fig. 10-1). As a result, these systems have not allowed clear imaging of the left atrium and pulmonary veins (PVs) with the catheter located in the right atrium.[2] Imaging with this catheter has been used in experimental and clinical studies to identify endocardial landmarks, guide mapping and ablation catheters in proximity to these landmarks, guide transseptal puncture, and monitor for procedural complications.[1,4,5,13,15–19]

Phased-array ICE is a newer imaging system incorporating a miniaturized 64-element, phased-array, electronically controlled transducer mounted at the distal end of a 90-cm long, steerable, 8F or 10F catheter. Variable imaging frequencies can be used that range from 5 to 10 MHz, and the system permits the full range of two-dimensional (2D), M-mode, and Doppler imaging (including pulsed-wave, color, continuous-wave, and tissue Doppler). The catheter tip can be deflected 160 degrees in two planes (anteroposterior and right-to-left) and then locked in position. Bidirectional steering and locking are performed through three separate controls located in the catheter handle. This catheter produces a wedge-shaped (sector) image, which is displayed on a conventional echocardiographic workstation similar to that used in transthoracic echocardiography or transesophageal echocardiography (TEE).[20]

Phased-array ICE has been shown to provide image quality similar to that obtained with TEE, both for imaging of the interatrial septum during device closure of an atrial septal defect (ASD)[21] and for imaging of the left atrial appendage with Doppler assessment of mechanical function in patients with atrial arrhythmias.[22]

Three-dimensional reconstruction of the images obtained by ICE has further improved the definition of the endocardial structures examined, providing additional benefits in the guidance of ablation procedures. To date, 3D ICE imaging can be obtained by the analysis and reconstruction of 2D images provided by both phased-array and mechanical ICE catheters. The integration between 3D ICE and an electroanatomic mapping system has resulted in the development of the CartoSound. In the CartoSound system, a phased-array ICE catheter uses an embedded position sensor to display location and beam orientation on the Carto XP mapping system (Biosense Webster, Diamond Bar, CA). The merging of 3D ICE images and electrical signals allows the creation of 3D electroanatomic maps. Further improvement in image accuracy can be achieved by integrating the 3D ICE images with previously obtained computed tomography (CT) or magnetic resonance imaging (MRI) studies of the cardiac chamber of interest (Fig. 10-2).

Okumura and colleagues recently evaluated the utility of the CartoSound system for generating anatomically accurate chamber geometry and for accurately guiding ablation to designated anatomical sites.[23] Evaluation was performed in an animal model and subsequently in a clinical series. The animal model consisted of 12 dogs in which clip markers were percutaneously implanted in selected areas of each cardiac chamber. Using actual real-time 2D ICE images of the clip sites for reference, the accuracy of the 3D ICE reconstruction was significantly better compared with the Carto merge CT images. Target ablations delivered at each clip site guided by CartoSound images were within 1.1 ± 1.1 mm of the actual clip position. Circumferential pulmonary

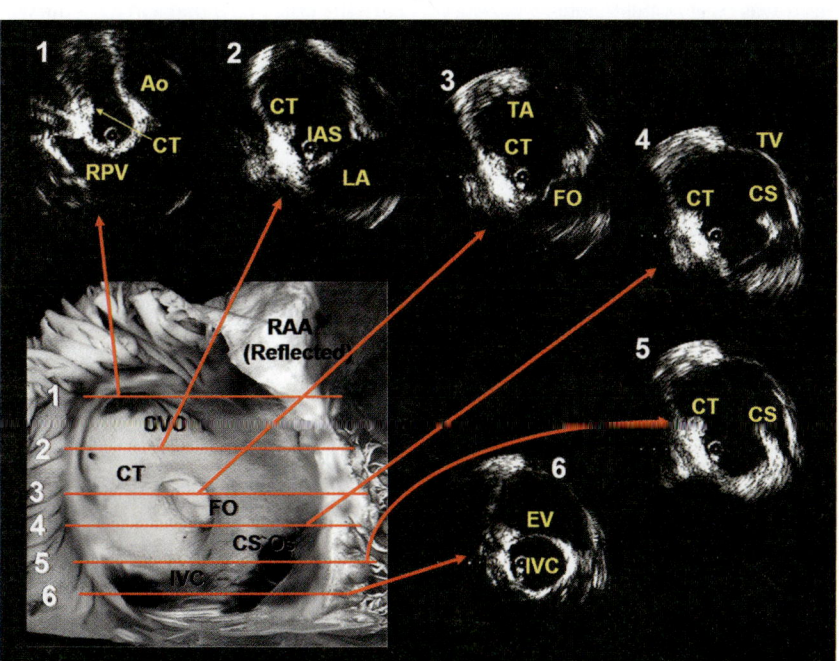

FIGURE 10-1. Serial horizontal slices taken through the right atrium using a conventional 9-MHz mechanical transducer and an intracardiac echocardiography catheter. The *inset* shows an anatomic cut-away view of the right atrium. The catheter has been withdrawn sequentially from the junction of the superior vena cava (SVC) and right atrium to the inferior vena cava (IVC). The anatomy of the crista terminalis (CT) is highlighted through a series of images. Superiorly, the CT is closely related to the right superior pulmonary vein (RPV). The interatrial septum (IAS) then comes into view with the fossa ovalis (FO). The mouth of the coronary sinus (CS) appears superior to the level of the eustachian valve (EV). The eustachian ridge (continuation of caudal CT) passes septally toward the mouth of the CS (CS Os; posterior rim). Ao, aorta; LA, left atrium; TA, tricuspid annulus; TV, tricuspid valve. *(Inset adapted from Anderson RH, Becker AE. The Heart: Structure in Health and Disease. London: Gower Medical, 1992. With permission.)*

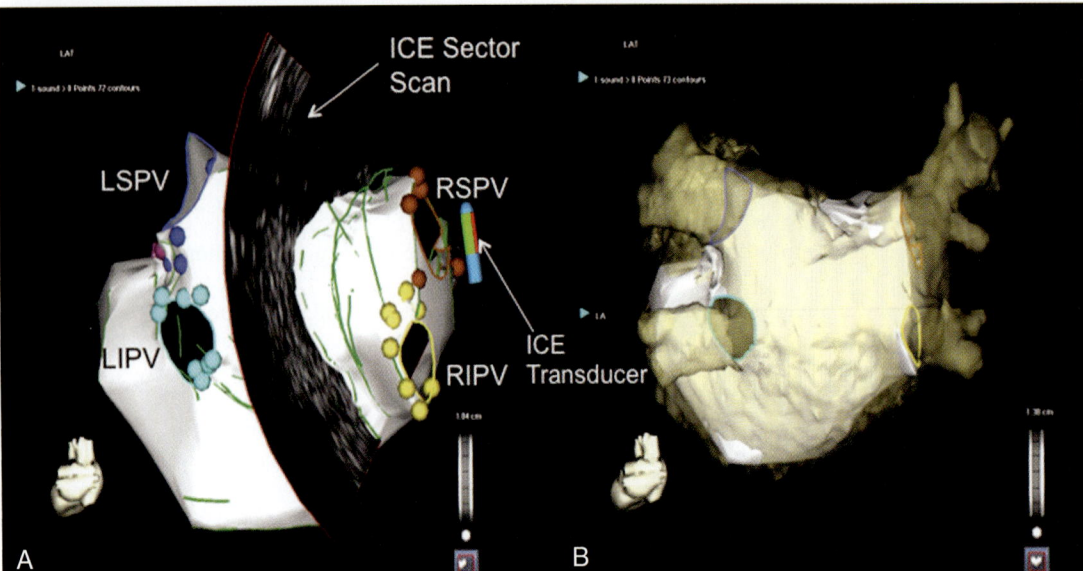

FIGURE 10-2. A, Three-dimensional reconstruction of the left atrium and pulmonary vein ostia with CartoSound. The intracardiac echocardiographic (ICE) transducer has an embedded position sensor to display location and beam orientation on the Carto XP and is located within the right atrium. The ultrasound "fan" projects through the left atrium, allowing the three-dimensional reconstruction of the left atrium and pulmonary veins (PV). **B,** Integration of the CartoSound three-dimensional reconstruction with a previously obtained computed tomography shell of the left atrium and pulmonary veins shows excellent registration.

vein isolation and mitral isthmus ablation performed in dogs resulted in 97% ± 4% circumferentially around the pulmonary veins by gross pathology with 0.6 ± 0.7 gaps of an average size of 2.3 ± 0.7 mm and complete isthmus lines. The lesions appeared to be precisely positioned at the venoatrial junction, with no lesions observed within the pulmonary veins. Importantly, no complications, such as cardiac tamponade or esophageal damage, were observed at gross examination. The CartoSound was then evaluated in 15 patients undergoing circumferential pulmonary vein isolation with additional ablation lines for both persistent and paroxysmal AF. The left atrial volumes and pulmonary vein dimensions created by CartoSound mapping were slightly smaller than those obtained with the electroanatomic mapping, whereas the pulmonary vein orifice areas determined by CartoSound were significantly larger. Again, the accuracy of CartoSound for localization of specific sites such as the venoatrial junction appeared to be superior to that of electroanatomic mapping. Circumferential pulmonary vein isolation with additional lines as needed guided by CartoSound was successfully conducted in all patients without major complications such as cardiac tamponade or esophageal injury. In summary, navigation guided by CartoSound appeared to be 1.5- to 2.5-fold more accurate than with electroanatomic mapping merged with CT images.[23]

Identification of Atrial Endocardial Structures

One of the initial uses of ICE was to identify endocardial structures and the accurate positioning of diagnostic and ablation electrophysiology catheters in relation to this defined anatomy.[24,25] This technology facilitated, for the first time, an understanding of the relationship between anatomy and electrophysiology. Kalman and colleagues[24] and Olgin and associates[1] used conventional ICE to define

the tricuspid annulus, crista terminalis, and eustachian ridge as important anatomic barriers to conduction during typical human atrial flutter (AFL). Subsequently, in a study also using ICE guidance of catheter positioning, Kalman and associates[16] used ICE to assist in the accurate positioning of a multipolar catheter along the crista terminalis, to define this structure as a major focus for atrial tachycardia within the right atrium (cristal tachycardias). ICE was used to identify the crista terminalis in patients with inappropriate sinus tachycardia and to guide modification of sinus pacemaker function.[15] Although the anatomic location of the crista terminalis in the right atrium is well known, Marchlinski and coworkers[26] demonstrated that fluoroscopically guided identification of this structure was frequently inaccurate and was greatly facilitated by the use of ICE.

Guidance of Radiofrequency Ablation Catheter

The creation of lesions during RFA procedures requires stable contact between the ablation catheter electrode and the target tissue. ICE may facilitate this process, leading to more efficient ablation.[4,6,10] RFA catheters can be easily visualized by ICE and have a typical appearance with a bright tip and fan-shaped acoustic shadow.[27] Kalman and colleagues[6] compared traditional criteria for determining tissue contact (stable electrogram signals and fluoroscopic appearance) with conventional ICE-guided ablation in dogs. Without ICE guidance, lateral sliding of the ablation catheter (>5 mm) was frequent (18%), as was poor perpendicular electrode tissue contact (27%), leading to smaller lesion formation and a lower efficiency of heating index (ratio of steady-state temperature to power). For linear ablation arrays, ICE improves the accuracy of positioning and the extent of tissue contact in animal models compared with fluoroscopy alone.[10–12]

Identification of structures on the left side of the heart may be enhanced if the catheter is introduced into the arterial circulation[18,28]; however, this approach may be associated with increased complications. Mangrum and associates[18] introduced a 9F, 9-MHz mechanical ICE catheter into the left atrium and PV mouth through a transseptal sheath. ICE was then used to guide circumferential RFA, ensure good ablation catheter tissue contact, and monitor for PV stenosis. After ablation, the PV wall was observed to be thickened with increased echogenicity. The mean reduction in luminal diameter after ablation was 12%.

Monitoring and Quantification of Radiofrequency Ablation Lesions

In the clinical electrophysiology laboratory, ICE is the only technique available for providing real-time assessment of lesion formation and size. In an excised canine heart model of ablation, Kalman and coworkers used high-frequency ICE imaging (15 MHz) to measure RFA lesion size and demonstrated a high correlation between ultrasonic and pathologic lesion depth.[3] Although other investigators have used ICE to observe lesion formation in vivo, it is less clear that a correlation exists between the endocardial changes (swelling and increased echogenicity) observed in the beating heart and lesion size.[15,27]

In a series of human and porcine studies, Marchlinski and coworkers[29-31] used mechanical ICE to describe the nature of the lesion formed as a result of the application of radiofrequency (RF) energy. They observed the formation of mural swelling and increased tissue echodensity after the application of RF in the right atrium. Furthermore, after transmural linear-lesion formation in the posterior right atrium of pigs, the demonstration by ICE of mural swelling correlated with the finding of mural edema on histopathology.[30] In a study of cavotricuspid isthmus ablation by Morton and colleagues[32] using

phased-array ICE and an imaging frequency of up to 10 MHz, discrete lesion formation, manifesting predominantly as regions of tissue swelling, was observed after RF applications. Interestingly, without additional RF applications, ICE demonstrated a progression over ensuing minutes to more diffuse swelling and lesion coalescence. The significance of this finding is uncertain but again may represent development of tissue edema after the RF application.

This swelling at the region of RF application has in some anatomic locations had important clinical implications. In humans, ICE allowed the identification of narrowing of the superior vena cava–right atrium junction during RFA of the crista terminalis for inappropriate sinus tachycardia.[31] Indeed, superior vena cava syndrome has been described as a potential complication of circumferential ablation at this junction. This observation predated by several years a similar observation of PV narrowing as a result of circumferential ostial ablation (see later).

Role in Atrial Fibrillation Ablation Procedures

Catheter ablation procedures for the treatment of AF have assumed an increasingly important therapeutic role. After initial experience with catheter ablation targeting arrhythmogenic foci within the PV,[33,34] techniques have evolved that electrically isolate the PV by ablation of left atrial–PV connections. Both circumferential ablation[35] and a segmental approach (targeting sites with early activation[36-38]) have been employed.

A key requirement for successful and safe ablation within the left atrium is anatomic characterization of the PVs and accurate localization of the ostia. At the venoatrial junction, the PVs demonstrate considerable anatomic heterogeneity in their ostial diameter, number, location, and pattern of branching (Fig. 10-3).[39] PV imaging can be

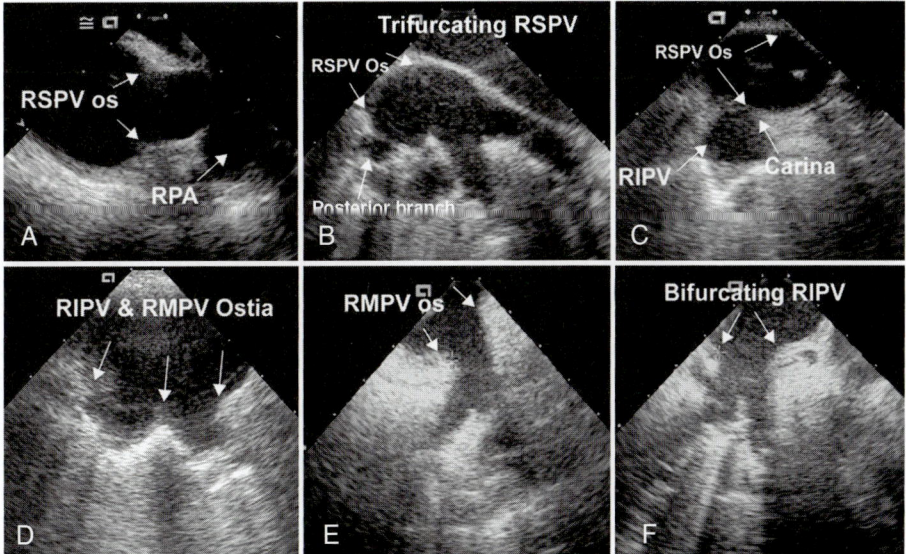

FIGURE 10-3. Intracardiac echocardiographic images demonstrating anatomic variations of the right-sided pulmonary veins (PV): right superior (RSPV), right middle (RMPV), and right inferior (RIPV). **A,** The usual relationship of the RSPV to the right pulmonary artery (RPA). **B,** Posterior RSPV branch. **C,** Carina between RSPV and RIPV. **D** and **E,** RMPV examples. **F,** RIPV early bifurcation. *Small arrows* indicate the pulmonary vein ostia.

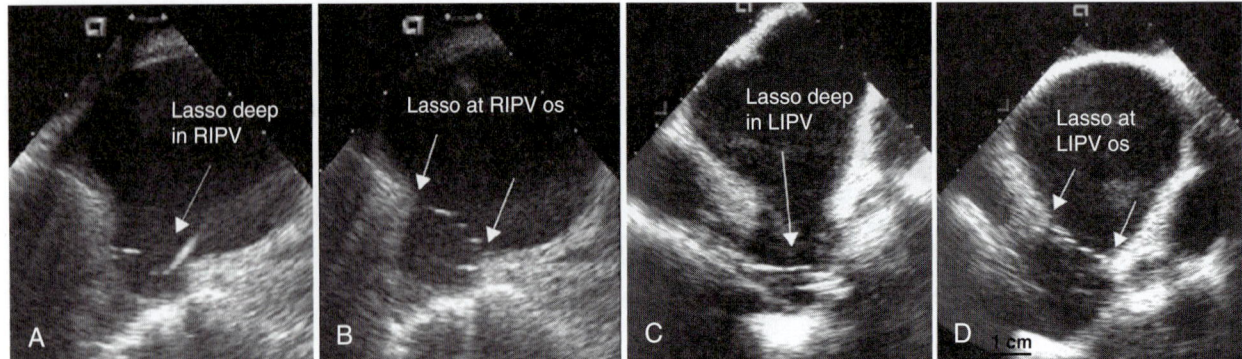

FIGURE 10-4. Positioning of lasso catheter. **A** and **C,** Lasso catheter deep within right and left inferior pulmonary vein (RIPV and LIPV, respectively). **B** and **D,** Correction of lasso position to a true ostial location using intracardiac echocardiography. *Small arrows* indicate lasso catheter.

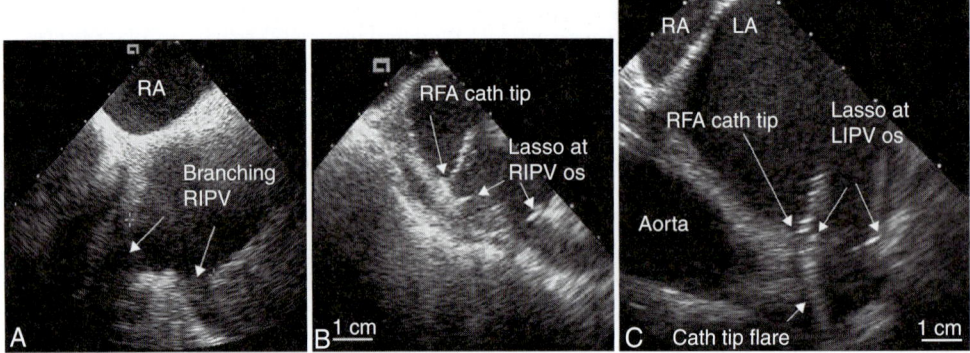

FIGURE 10-5. A and **B,** Complex right inferior pulmonary vein (RIPV) anatomy with two separate branches *(arrows)* opening into a single pulmonary vein (PV) ostium. In **B,** a lasso is positioned at the true ostium of the PV, allowing radiofrequency ablation (RFA) to be delivered to the atrial tissue adjacent to the venoatrial junction. **C,** Lasso catheter and RFA catheter positioned at the true ostium of a left inferior PV (LIPV os). LA, left atrium; RA, right atrium.

performed with the use of contrast venography. However, this may require separate contrast injections and does not allow real-time monitoring of catheter positioning or provide physiologic data. Alternatively, electroanatomic and noncontact mapping systems are used to define anatomy, potentially with a CT or MRI template for the 3D chamber reconstruction.

Phased-array ICE has been shown in experimental and clinical studies[20,40] to provide accurate 2D and Doppler imaging of the left atrium and PVs while positioned in the right atrium. Furthermore, ICE has the potential to accurately guide and monitor the positioning of diagnostic and ablation catheters within the left atrium. A negative aspect of existing ICE imaging using a mechanically rotating 9-MHz transducer is that the field of view is limited. As a result, these systems have not allowed clear imaging of the left atrium and PVs,[2] except when introduced directly into the left atrium and advanced to the PV ostium.[18]

Wood and associates[41] compared measurements of PV diameter by phased-array ICE with those obtained by CT, contrast venography, and TEE. Ostial PV diameters were significantly correlated between each imaging modality; however, several important observations were made. PV values measured by CT and ICE were similar, whereas venography tended to overestimate and TEE underestimate the ostial diameter. Furthermore, CT and ICE identified more PV ostia than either venography or TEE.

In general, phased-array ICE is the system of choice for assisting AF catheter ablation.

The main roles of ICE in left atrium ablation procedures are the following:
1. Assisting with transseptal puncture
2. Defining PV anatomy
3. Allowing accurate positioning of the lasso catheter at the venous ostium
4. Titrating energy delivery
5. Monitoring for complications
6. Identifying and possibly predicting PV stenosis

Accurate Positioning of the Lasso Catheter at the Venous Ostium

ICE has demonstrated that inward migration and misalignment of the lasso catheter are common during AF ablation procedures.[42] ICE allows continuous referencing of the lasso and ablation catheter positions to the PV ostium, permitting frequent readjustment of both before RFA (Figs. 10-4 to 10-6).

Clinical and experimental studies have indicated that triggers for AF frequently arise from a very proximal location in the PV and indeed at the PV–left atrium junction.[37,43,44] Accurate identification of the PV ostium with fluoroscopy alone may be challenging, especially with inexperienced operators. Migration of the lasso catheter into the PV during the course of PV isolation is common and is not readily detectable by fluoroscopy (Fig. 10-6). In a subset of 30 patients specifically monitored for lasso movement, we found that displacement of the lasso by more

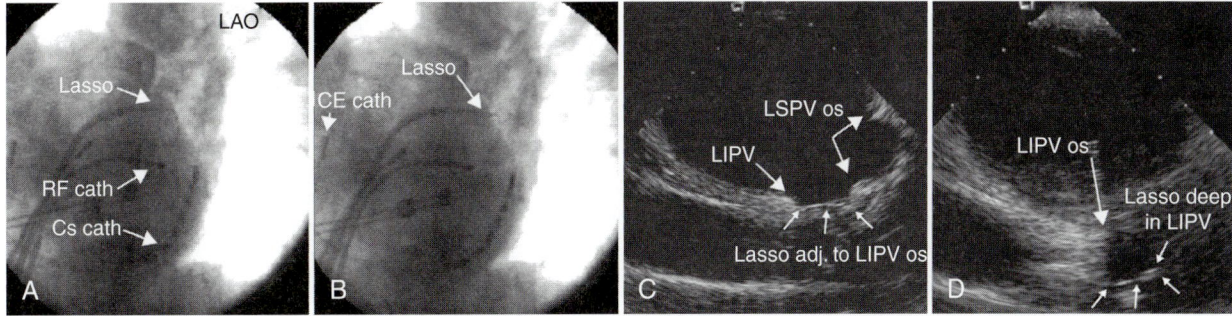

FIGURE 10-6. Left anterior oblique radiographs (**A** and **B**) and corresponding intracardiac echocardiographic (ICE) images (**C** and **D**) of lasso catheter positioning in the left inferior pulmonary vein (LIPV). **A** and **C** demonstrate appropriate positioning at the venous ostium. During the course of the ablation, the lasso migrated more than 1.5 cm into the vein (**D**), with little apparent change in radiographic position (**B**). Cs, coronary sinus; LSPV, left superior pulmonary vein; RF, radiofrequency.

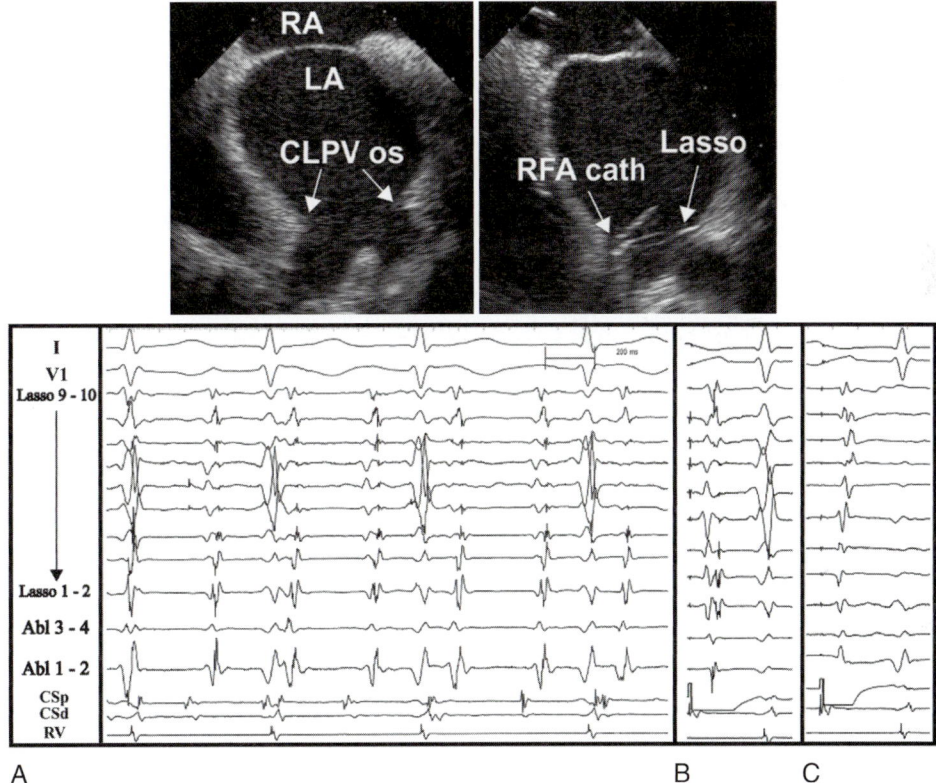

FIGURE 10-7. Intracardiac echocardiographic images of a common left pulmonary vein (CLPV) with superior and inferior divisions. Adjacent image shows lasso and radiofrequency ablation catheter (RFA cath) positioned at the venous ostium. With the lasso in this position, pulmonary vein potentials were recorded from each bipole during spontaneous atrial tachycardia arising from the CLPV (**A**), with the earliest PV potential recorded in lasso 1-2. After several radiofrequency (RF) applications, tachycardia was terminated, but sharp PV potentials were still present on the lasso during coronary sinus pacing (**B**), Further RF applications targeting the remaining PV potentials were given, and venous isolation was achieved (**C**). LA, left atrium; RA, right atrium.

than 1 cm inside the ostium occurred at least once during the course of isolation in 32% of PVs (Morton and Wilber, unpublished data). ICE permitted rapid identification of this problem and guided subsequent repositioning to a more ostial location (Fig. 10-7).

Marrouche found that fluoroscopic guidance for lasso positioning was often misleading, with the circular mapping located a mean of 5 ± 3 mm distal to the true ostium.[45] Similarly, a study comparing the accuracy of preprocedural CT of the left atrium and PVs with phased-array ICE have shown that points taken with electroanatomic mapping alone could be 5 to 10 mm away from points

recorded with ICE.[46] A strategy of pulmonary vein isolation guided by phased-array imaging has been reported by Verma in 400 patients.[47] The success rate with one procedure was 80%, comparable to that of other strategies for AF ablation. Importantly, ICE allowed a very low complication rate.[47]

Singh and colleagues have recently reported their experience with the use of CartoSound as a mapping system in ablation of AF.[48] Sequential images were obtained and merged with preacquired CT or MRI studies. In 15 patients, the 2D ICE images were recorded with the phased-array probe positioned in the right atrium, whereas in other 15 patients, the probe was directly positioned in the left atrium through the transseptal puncture. Imaging directly from the left atrium was feasible, with comparable time required to obtain ICE imaging and integration to a right atrial approach. Moreover, left atrium imaging allowed for a more complete and precise mapping of the left atrium and PVs compared with right atrial mapping.[48] CartoSound mapping was shown to be feasible and safe to guide RFA of AF, with accuracy comparable if not superior to that of electroanatomic mapping based on preacquired CT and MRI studies.[23]

Titrating Energy Delivery

ICE has been used not only to titrate energy delivery during RFA but also to identify potential complications. In an early study in dogs, Kalman and colleagues[6] used ICE to observe coagulum formation (shaggy echodensity) on the ablation catheter tip. This occurrence was usually preceded (by 5 to 10 seconds) by local microbubble formation during the ablation.[6] Marrouche and coworkers[45] have extended these observations and described their clinical utility. These investigators have based the titration of power during RF delivery on the real-time observations obtained from ICE during ablation. They defined type 1 and type 2 microbubbles during RF applications. Type 1 is defined as scattered microbubbles. They are presumed to be caused by early tissue overheating and, when observed, lead the operator to reduce the power delivered by 5-W decrements until the microbubbles disappear. Type 2 microbubbles are defined as dense showers of bubbles. These usually herald an imminent impedance rise, and therefore the RF application is immediately interrupted by the operator. Using this approach, this group achieved a greater success rate than when using ICE without bubble monitoring to direct energy delivery, and with fewer complications. In particular, the incidence of thromboembolic events was significantly reduced. Although these are intriguing and provocative observations, to date they have not been confirmed in a prospective, randomized study. In addition, if externally irrigated catheters are used for AF ablation, type 1 microbubbles cannot be distinguished from the catheter irrigation.

Bunch and coworkers[49] have demonstrated in an animal model of PV ablation using an 8-mm tip catheter that microbubbles are an inconsistent marker of tissue overheating. Using phased-array ICE and implanted atrial thermocouples, this group showed that type 1 and type 2 microbubbles were not seen during some ablations (13% and 40%, respectively) despite tissue temperatures greater than 80°C. Furthermore, in 40% of ablations, type 1 microbubbles did not precede the development of type 2 microbubbles. Overall, however, microbubble formation was correlated with tissue overheating.

Phased-array ICE has also been deployed into the left atrium and coronary sinus to achieve novel views during linear lesion formation between the left inferior pulmonary vein and mitral annulus. In a case report,[50] tissue edema during RF application, together with the appearance of a hypodense region within the atrial musculature, was identified as a prelude to imminent impedance rise and "pop."

Postablation Imaging: Can Pulmonary Vein Stenosis Be Predicted?

PV stenosis remains a significant limiting factor to procedures targeting these structures.[51–57]

Several reports have shown a small but statistically significant decrease in PV dimensions and increase in the PV flow velocity after ablation, as measured by ICE for each of the PVs.[18,58–61] Importantly, Saad and colleagues also demonstrated a lack of relationship between immediate postablation PV measurements and the development of PV stenosis.[59] In a study of 95 patients undergoing PV isolation, the mean preablation and postablation flow velocities were observed to increase, the correlation between flow velocity was observed to increase, and the correlation between flow velocity and PV stenosis was poor. All patients underwent CT of the PVs 3 months after ablation. Of 380 PVs ablated, the CT scans revealed 2 (1%) with severe (>70%) stenosis, 13 (3%) with moderate (51% to 70%) stenosis, and 62 (16%) with mild (>50%) stenosis. The authors concluded that "acute changes in PV flow immediately after ostial PV isolation do not appear to be a strong predictor of chronic PV stenosis."

This observation supports the suggestion that the mechanism of PV stenosis is progressive after ablation[62] and may involve thrombus formation, intimal proliferation, or both.[57] Nonetheless, it would appear reasonable to closely follow any patient with a marked increase (>1.0 m/second) in PV flow velocity after ablation or a significant acute reduction in luminal diameter for the development of late PV stenosis.

Avoidance of Atrioesophageal Fistula

Esophageal injury and atrioesophageal fistula are major concerns during ablation for AF.[63–70] The real incidence of atrioesophageal fistula is unknown but appears to range between 0.05% and 0.2%.[64,71] Esophageal injury of lesser degree can be frequently observed after catheter ablation for AF. In a study published by Schmidt, among 28 patients who underwent RFA for AF, the incidence of any esophageal mucosal damage was 47%, with 18% of the patients showing necrosis and ulcerative lesions.[72] Despite its rarity, atrioesophageal fistula is associated with a very high mortality rate due to air embolism, sepsis, endocarditis, and gastrointestinal exsanguination.[64–67,73–83]

Understanding the relationship between the esophagus and the posterior wall of the left atrium is of paramount importance to avoid this complication.

The thickness of the myocardium at the left atrium–PV junction can be as little as 2 mm, much thinner than the rest of the atrial myocardium, enhancing the possibility of heat transfer to the esophageal wall.[39,83] Suggested strategies to reduce the risk for esophageal injury during RFA of AF are based on titrating the RF energy when ablating in the posterior wall of the left atrium and avoiding RF energy delivering on myocardial sites directly in contact with the esophagus.[64,70,75,84–86] Hence, knowing the location of the esophagus in relationship to the posterior wall of the left atrium and PV ostia before RF application may reduce the risk for esophageal injury. The esophagus can be visualized by different imaging techniques such as CT,[87,88] MRI,[87] intraprocedural barium swallow,[87,89,90] nasogastric tube,[89,90] temperature probe,[91–93] and tagging of the esophagus during electroanatomic mapping with the Carto or NavX (Ensite, St. Jude Medical, St. Paul, MN) system.[87,93–95] ICE offers the advantage of allowing real-time visualization of the esophagus during ablation, thus overcoming the question of the possible shift in position of the esophagus before and during the ablation procedure.[79,82,95–98]

ICE not only allows precise localization of the esophagus in relationship to the posterior wall of the left atrium and PVs but also demonstrates the longitudinal extension of the area of contiguous contact and the thicknesses of the esophageal wall, left atrium posterior wall, and connective and adipose tissue layer separating the esophagus and left atrium[86,93,99–102] (Fig. 10-8). The accuracy of ICE in determining the esophageal course and relationship with the left atrium has been found to be comparable to that of MRI.[97] ICE clearly visualizes morphologic changes related to RF energy to the atrial myocardium and the eventual involvement of the esophagus.[86] Ren and associates have shown that the use of ICE to monitor lesion formation and lesion extension toward the esophageal wall, together with titration of the RF energy level, allowed complete prevention of esophageal injury.[86] Cummings and coworkers used ICE for the monitoring of microbubble formation when using an 8-mm tip ablation catheter during AF ablation.[93] They demonstrated that lesions near the course of the esophagus that generated microbubbles significantly increased esophageal temperature compared with lesions that did not. In that study, power did not correlate with esophageal temperature. However, Marrouche and colleagues found that ICE monitoring of microbubbles during ablation with an 8-mm-tip catheter was not effective in preventing esophageal ulceration.[72,103] This study demonstrated a higher incidence of esophageal erythema and ulceration using ICE to monitor microbubbles during RF with an 8-mm-tip catheter compared with an open irrigated tip catheter. These authors suggested that microbubble formation may have too long latency to allow well-timed cessation of ablation and prevention of esophageal damage. Helms and associates reported the feasibility and accuracy of a strategy to prevent esophageal injury based on the use of a rotational ICE catheter, producing a 360° image around the catheter, directly placed into the left atrium through transseptal puncture in 41 patients referred for ablation of AF.[101] Positioning of the ICE catheter close to the site of ablation provided a precise measurement of the distance and relationship between the tip of the ablation catheter and the esophagus during the procedure.[101]

In conclusion, it appears that ICE has significant value in real-time imaging of the anatomic course of the esophagus and therefore may have value in preventing atrioesophageal fistula during AF ablation. However, the superiority of ICE compared with other strategies to avoid esophageal injury has not been established.

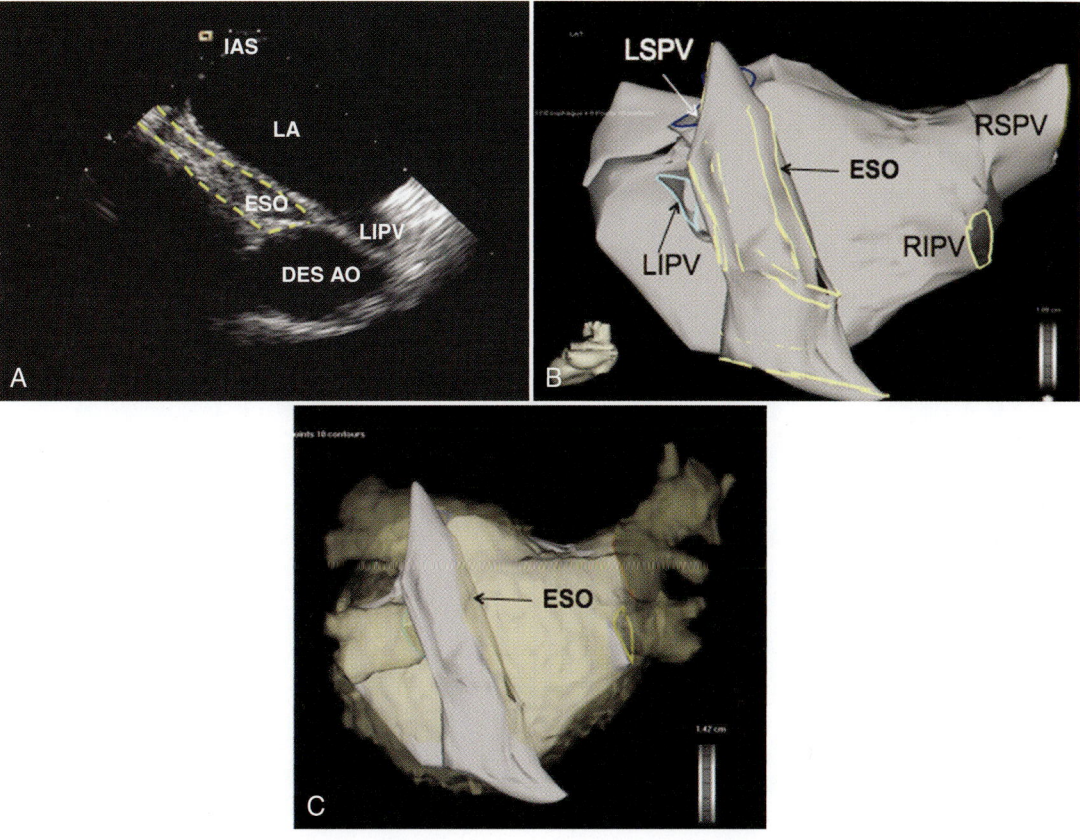

FIGURE 10-8. A, Two-dimensional intracardiac echocardiographic (ICE) view of the left atrium (LA). Short-axis view of the esophagus (ESO, *yellow outline*) in proximity to the ostium of the left inferior pulmonary vein. **B,** Three-dimensional reconstruction of the left atrium, pulmonary veins, and esophagus by CartoSound from a posterior perspective. **C,** Integration of the CartoSound three-dimensional reconstruction with a previously obtained computed tomography shell of the left atrium and pulmonary veins. DES AO, descending aorta; IAS, inter-atrial septum; LIPV, left inferior pulmonary vein; LSPV, left superior pulmonary vein; RIPV, right inferior pulmonary vein; RSPV, right superior pulmonary vein.

Phased-Array Intracardiac Echocardiography and Ablation of Atrial Flutter

RFA for the creation of bidirectional conduction block across the cavotricuspid isthmus has become first-line therapy in the management of typical cavotricuspid isthmus–dependent atrial flutter[104–109] and has a high success rate. However, the complex and variable anatomy of the cavotricuspid region may be an impediment to achieving isthmus block.[110] Large-tip and irrigated-tip catheters facilitate isthmus ablation, but there is still a potential role for a real-time imaging modality that has the capability of accurately defining cavotricuspid anatomy and guiding RFA in difficult cases. The use of ICE for this purpose remains largely experimental. Mechanical ICE has facilitated detailed endocardial mapping of the boundaries to an isthmus-dependent atrial flutter[1,24] but is limited in its discrimination of other cavotricuspid isthmus features.[111] Right atrium angiography may also give a general guide to cavotricuspid anatomy[112] but does not provide detailed endocardial definition or information regarding the thickness of the isthmus.

Morton and associates[32] used phased-array ICE with a high imaging frequency (7.5 to 10 MHz) in 15 patients who were undergoing ablation of typical atrial flutter. With this modality, they were able to perform detailed analysis of the cavotricuspid isthmus in all patients (Fig. 10-9). The boundaries of the cavotricuspid isthmus (tricuspid annulus, eustachian ridge, coronary sinus, and trabeculated free wall of the right atrium) were well visualized, as were the endocardial contour and shape; the presence of pouching, recesses, and trabeculations; and the isthmus thickness along its length before and after ablation. The thickness of the cavotricuspid isthmus measured as follows: anterior cavotricuspid isthmus (at the tricuspid annulus), 4.1 ± 0.8 mm; mid-cavotricuspid isthmus, 3.3 ± 0.5 mm, and posterior cavotricuspid isthmus (at the eustachian ridge), 2.7 ± 0.9 mm $(P < .001)$.

ICE was used to identify the ablation catheter and guide lesion delivery away from deep recesses and prominent trabeculations. After each RF application, a discrete lesion was usually visible. Over time (minutes), these lesions lost their definition and were replaced by a diffuse swelling of the cavotricuspid isthmus. Pouching and recesses were commonly seen and usually deeper in the septal rather than lateral isthmus. In this study, ICE confirmed a long-held clinical impression that there may be no single ideal anatomically determined location in the cavotricuspid isthmus at which to perform ablation.

Intracardiac Echocardiography–Guided Ablation in the Left Ventricle

Experimental studies by Callans and colleagues[113,114] showed the efficacy of conventional ICE for defining scar in a porcine model of healed anterior infarction when the catheter is introduced directly into the left ventricle.

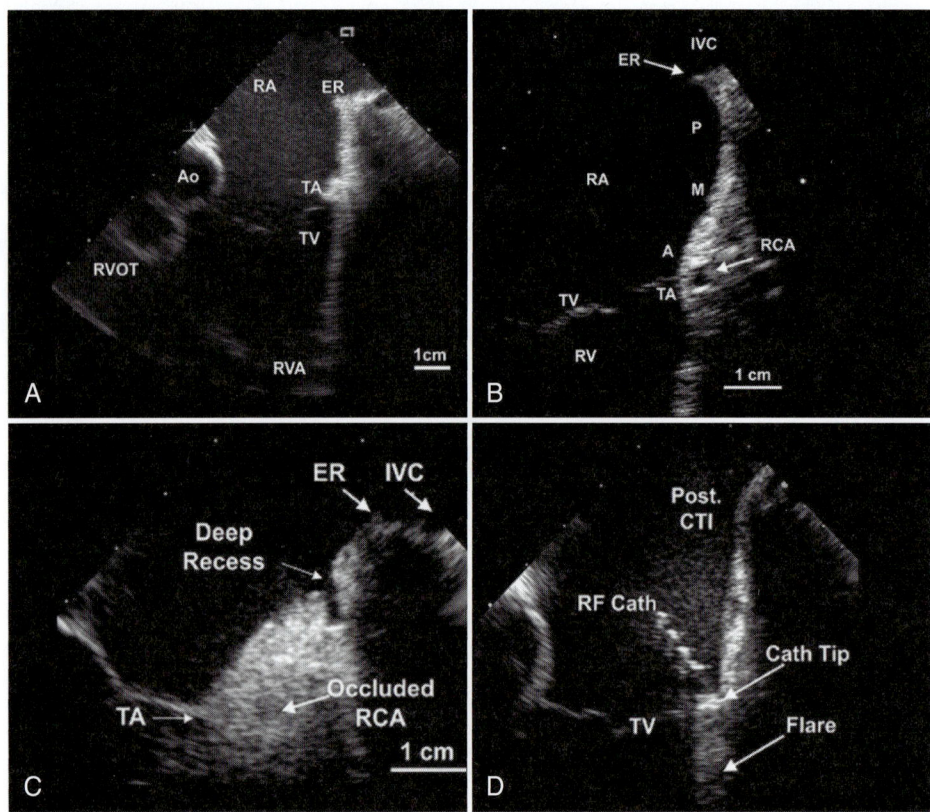

FIGURE 10-9. A, Baseline view of the right atrium (RA), ventricle (RVA), and outflow tract (RVOT), tricuspid valve (TV), and annulus (TA). The eustachian ridge (ER) and aortic root (Ao) can also be seen. **B,** View with higher imaging frequency (8.5 MHz) of the central cavotricuspid isthmus (CTI), identifying the RA; right ventricle (RV); TV; TA; right coronary artery (RCA); ER; inferior vena cava (IVC); and anterior (A), middle (M), and posterior (P) isthmus sectors. **C,** Deep recess within the CTI. Note the chronically occluded RCA. **D,** Radiofrequency ablation of the anterior isthmus. Note the prominent flare of the radiofrequency ablation catheter tip. Cath, catheter; Post, posterior.

As in standard nonintracardiac echocardiography, chronically infarcted scarred myocardium was identified as thinned muscle with increased echodensity. ICE-defined infarction correlated with that defined by electroanatomic mapping and pathologic analysis.

Clinical experience with ICE and ablation of VT is less than with AF ablation. Phased-array ICE can visualize the infarcted area of myocardium when positioned in the RV by the femoral vein approach, and all regions of the left ventricle can be imaged. Under ICE guidance, the ablation catheter can be precisely positioned in contact with specific structures such as the mitral annulus, a "false tendon," the papillary muscles, or the coronary cusps.[115,116] ICE allows monitoring for the development of either microbubble formation (tissue overheating) or pericardial effusion. ICE-detected lesion size tends to overestimate the true pathologic necrotic area, because of the adjacent regions of edema.[117]

Phased-array ICE has also been used to monitor the delivery of RF energy within the left coronary cusp in patients with idiopathic VT arising from this region (Fig. 10-10). Although coronary angiography is the gold standard for identifying the relationship of ablation sites to the left coronary artery, ICE provides real-time visualization of the distance between the RF catheter tip and both the coronary ostium and proximal left main coronary artery, and it monitors for microbubble formation.

Jongbloed and associates evaluated the feasibility of ICE in RF ablation of VT of different etiologies in 11 patients.[116] The underlying causes of VT were idiopathic

right ventricle outflow tract (RVOT) VT in 3, ischemic heart disease in 5, arrhythmogenic right ventricular dysplasia (ARVD) in 2, and hypertrophic cardiomyopathy in 1 patient. ICE successfully identified areas of akinesia or dyskinesia in patients with previous myocardial infarction and areas of focal aneurysm in patients with ARVD. VT could be induced from these areas, which were then targeted during ablation. ICE confirmed adequate catheter-tissue contact during ablation, which was successfully performed in all patients. None of the patients developed complications. Lamberti and colleagues investigated the contribution of ICE to ablation of left ventricle outflow tract (LVOT) VT.[118] In LVOT VT, the site of origin of the tachycardia may be closely related to structures such as the aortic valve leaflets or coronary artery ostia, and RF application in this vicinity is associated with significant risk.[119] These structures, which cannot be identified by fluoroscopy, are clearly imaged with ICE. RF ablation guided by ICE was conducted successfully and without complications in five patients with LVOT VT originating from the aortomitral continuity area. ICE proved effective in delineating the anatomy of the aortic root region and the relationship of ablation sites to the coronary arteries' ostia. Furthermore, ICE was useful in establishing catheter stability and catheter-tissue contact during the procedure.[118]

The papillary muscles may be the origin of VT in patients with or without a previous history of myocardial infarction.[120-122] The mitral valve apparatus and the papillary muscle have a complex anatomic structure, which makes catheter movement and stability difficult. ICE

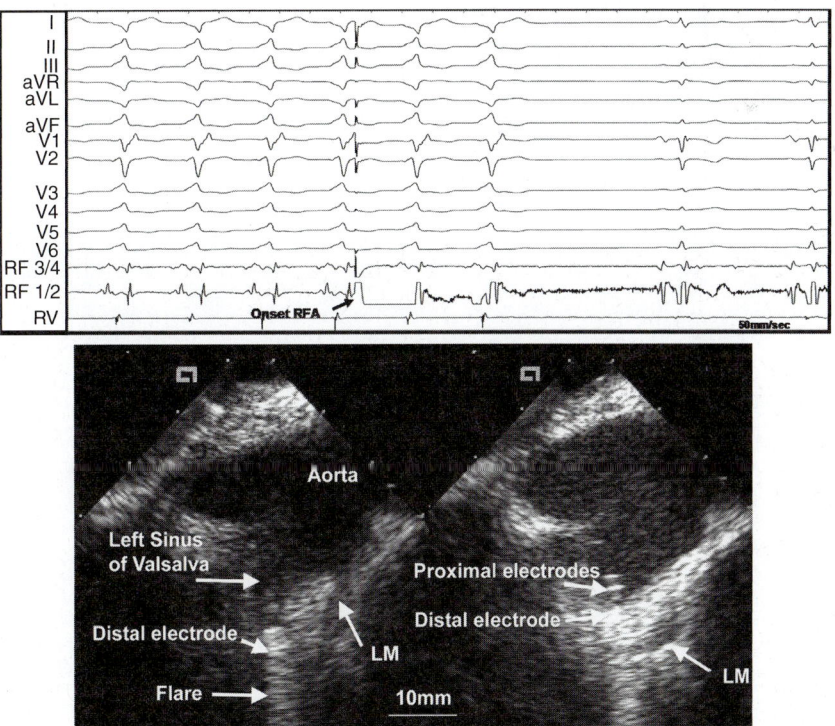

FIGURE 10-10. The *top panel* shows an inferior-axis ventricular tachycardia mapped to the left coronary cusp, with rapid termination during application of radiofrequency ablation (RFA) using a 4-mm-tip ablation catheter. Radiofrequency (RF) energy application was monitored in real time by an intracardiac echocardiographic catheter positioned in the right side of the heart *(bottom two panels)*, which was able to clearly discern the aortic root and valve, distal and proximal ablation catheter electrodes, catheter tip flare, and both the proximal *(bottom left)* and distal *(bottom right)* left main coronary artery (LM). Note the close relationship of both proximal and distal LM to the distal ablation catheter tip (10 to 13 mm). No arterial injury occurred during RFA.

clearly visualizes the papillary muscles (Fig. 10-11) aiding in the endocardial mapping and ablation in relation to these structures. Bogun and colleagues[122] and Good and associates[123] demonstrated the utility of ICE for localizing the ablation catheter in relation to the papillary muscles in patients with ischemic heart disease and in those with no structural heart disease, respectively.

Percutaneous intrapericardial echocardiography (PICE) is a novel application of ICE imaging in VT ablation. Horowitz and coworkers reported their experience in the use of PICE in the ablation of VT requiring an epicardial mapping.[124] A phased-array ICE probe was introduced in the pericardial space through a pericardial sheath. Using two peculiar views, oblique sinus and transverse sinus, detailed imaging of the cardiac chambers could be obtained in addition to observing the location and movement of the epicardial and endocardial catheters. Compared with ICE, PICE allowed a similar if not superior resolution because of better near-field visualization. Compared with TEE,

PICE demonstrated a better resolution of structures frequently not clearly defined with TEE as the lateral wall of the left ventricle, the left pulmonary artery, the right coronary artery, and the posterior left atrial wall. PICE improved on imaging with luminal ICE by demonstrating regions at the limits of luminal ICE resolution. In addition, PICE avoided the relative instability of the endoluminal ICE images and the possible interference with the other endocardial catheters. PICE precisely defined the extent of myocardial scar, and the images obtained were well correlated with the electroanatomic voltage map.[124]

CartoSound has been evaluated in 17 patients with nonidiopathic VT referred for ablation by Khaykin and colleagues.[125] ICE allowed a clear definition of cardiac structures, including the papillary muscles and trabeculations. The scar borders identified by ICE corresponded exactly with the voltage mapping, and ICE aided in achieving optimal tissue-catheter contact in particularly difficult areas such as myocardial crypts, aneurysms, and trabeculations. The precise delineation of the scar borders with ICE may result in a faster analysis of the arrhythmic substrate both in ischemic and dilated cardiomyopathy compared with point-by-point electroanatomic mapping and may facilitate improved definition of potentially critical structures of the VT circuit[125] (Figs. 10-12 and 10-13).

Transseptal Puncture

ICE has been used to accurately guide transseptal puncture both in animal and human studies.[5,13,14,126,127] Daoud and associates[13] characterized the variations in the size, thickness, and anatomy of the fossa ovalis. If the fossa is thick and small or very localized, ICE can be effectively used to guide accurate positioning of the transseptal needle. If the septum in the region of the fossa ovalis is highly mobile, ICE can monitor the distance between the point of maximal tenting and the adjacent lateral left atrium wall,

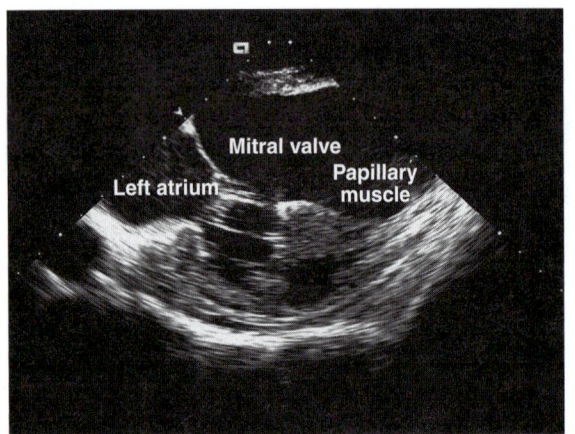

FIGURE 10-11. Two-dimensional long-axis view of the left ventricle and anterolateral papillary muscle.

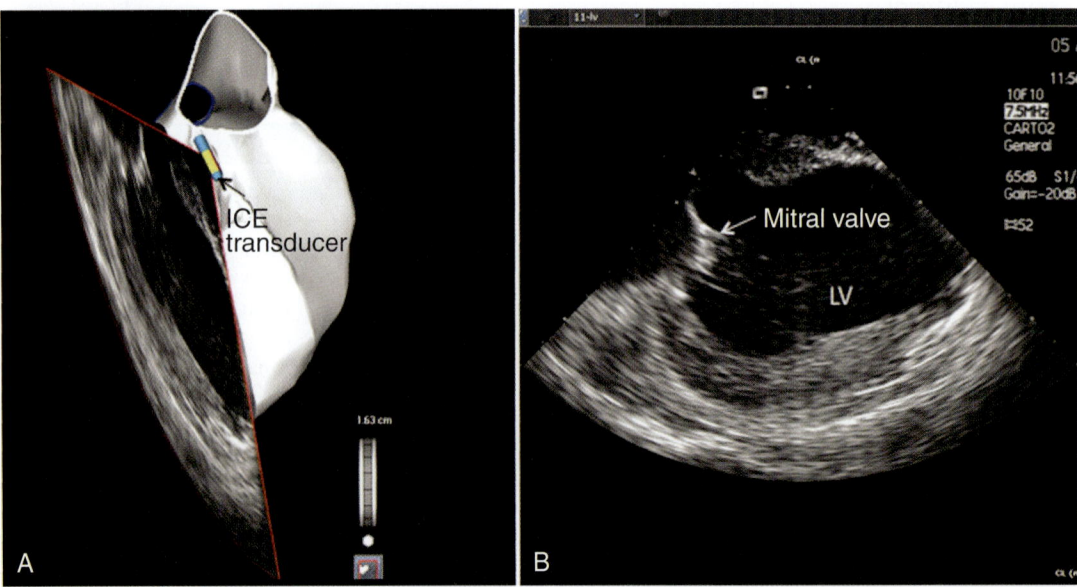

FIGURE 10-12. A, The intracardiac echocardiographic (ICE) transducer is located in the right ventricle. The ultrasound "fan" projects through the left ventricle. **B,** Two-dimensional long-axis view of the left ventricle (LV).

which in the extreme may be impinged by the tented fossa. Without ICE, the transseptal puncture assembly may slide superiorly during the process of advancing the needle. ICE can monitor for excessive sliding with the potential for puncture of the high septum and atrial roof.

Echocardiographic Evaluation of Atrial Mechanical Function

At present, TEE remains the clinical gold standard for assessment of left atrial mechanical function and screening

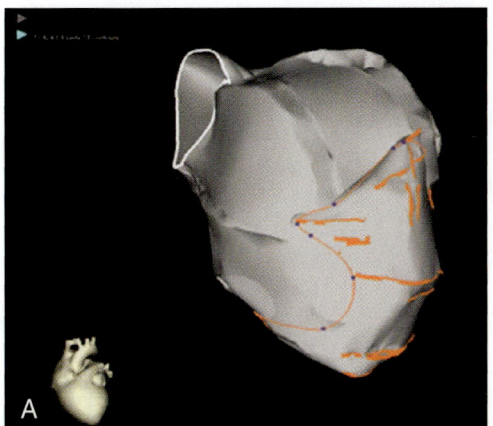

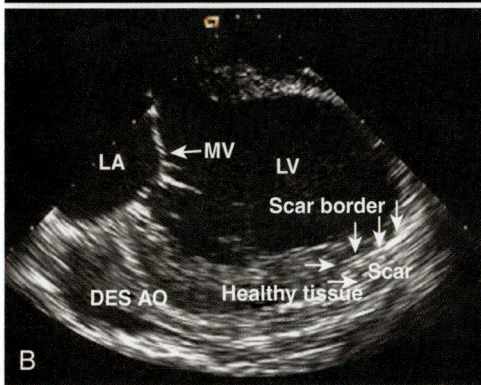

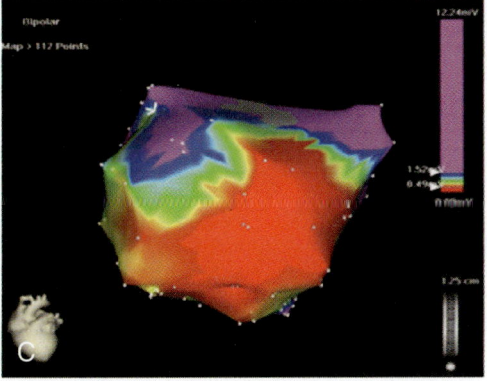

FIGURE 10-13. A, Three-dimensional reconstruction of the left ventricle with delineation of an anteroapical area of scar by CartoSound. **B,** Two-dimensional long-axis view of the left ventricle (LV) showing anteroapical thinning of the myocardium due to a previous myocardial infarction. **C,** Carto electroanatomic voltage map of the left ventricle showing an area of anteroapical scar (area of electrogram amplitude <0.5 mV). CartoSound precisely defined the extent of myocardial scar, and the images obtained were well correlated with the electroanatomic voltage map. DES AO, descending aorta; LA, left atrium; MV, mitral valve.

for the presence of left atrial appendage thrombus. Phased-array ICE has been evaluated against TEE for measuring atrial mechanical function. In a small prospective study, Morton and colleagues[22] compared ICE with multiplane TEE for this purpose in a patient undergoing RFA for atrial flutter, in which atrial mechanical stunning occurs after ablation (Fig. 10-14).

A high correlation and clinically excellent limits of agreement were found to exist between the two imaging modalities for measurement of left atrial appendage emptying velocity, right and left PV flow, mitral E and A wave inflow velocities, severity of left atrial spontaneous echo contrast, and left atrial appendage fractional area change. No patients were identified with left atrial appendage thrombus, and this was a limitation of the study. However, previous animal studies have identified left atrial thrombus with ICE,[40] and small, highly mobile strands of thrombus attached to long vascular sheaths deployed in the left atrium are occasionally seen using ICE.

Therefore, ICE may be an alternative to TEE for the measurement of left atrium mechanical function and surveillance for left atrial thrombus formation in selected patients undergoing atrial catheter ablation procedures.

Suggested Imaging Protocol for Phased-Array Intracardiac Echocardiography

Under fluoroscopic guidance, the catheter is advanced into the body of the right atrium. For inexperienced operators, it is helpful to obtain a view of the tricuspid valve, right ventricle, and right ventricular infundibulum and use this as a reference point for the examination. An imaging frequency of either 5.0 or 7.5 MHz is used. To achieve this view, the catheter is positioned vertically in the mid-right atrium and then simply rotated without either left-right or anterior-posterior steering. Next, clockwise rotation of the catheter brings septal structures into view, and the fossa ovalis is easily visualized. Further clockwise rotation will bring important left atrial structures into view. The mitral annulus and left atrial appendage are imaged with clockwise rotation on a level at or just inferior to the fossa ovalis. To image the mitral valve in a long-axis, two-chamber view (left atrium, mitral valve, and left ventricle), a mild degree of apically directed ICE catheter-tip deflection may be required. At the level of the left atrial appendage, the catheter shaft is rotated and the tip deflected, using the steering mechanism, until the mouth and body of the appendage are clearly visualized. Pulsed-wave Doppler of the left atrial appendage can be performed and an assessment made for spontaneous echo contrast or thrombus.[22]

The PVs are visualized with further clockwise rotation on a level at or immediately superior to the fossa. The left-sided PVs are visualized first, and a common left PV ostium may be seen in up to 25% of patients. A common left PV may be defined by the ICE appearance of a single left-sided PV ostium with a common segment (neck) of at least 5 mm between the left atrium–PV junction and first-order branching. The mean common left PV ostial diameter is about 26 ± 4 mm (range, 20 to 40 mm) with a common venous segment (neck) of variable length (12 ± 4 mm; range, 6 to 23mm).[128]

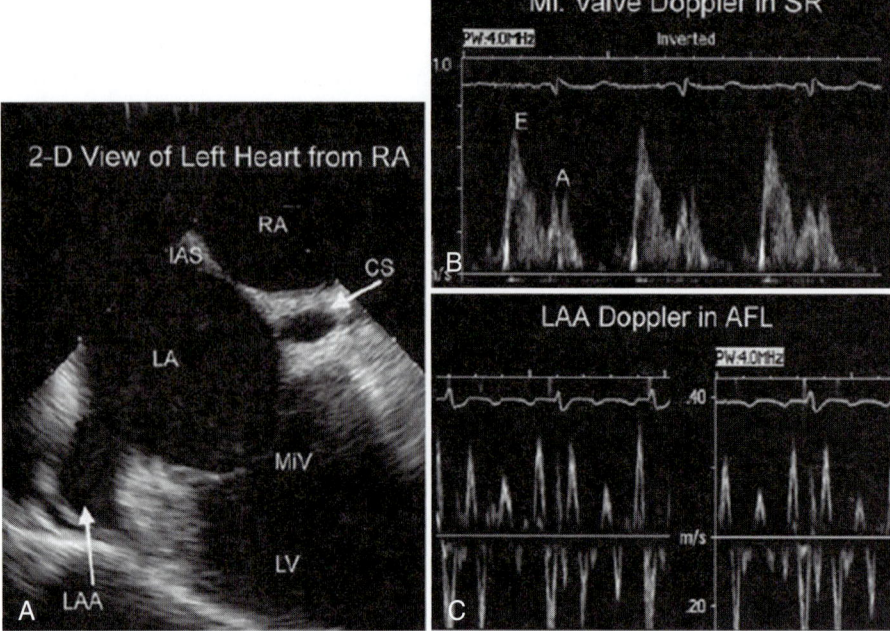

FIGURE 10-14. A, Two-dimensional view of the left side of the heart with the intracardiac echocardiography catheter positioned in the right atrium (RA). The imaging frequency was 7.5 MHz. Visible are the interatrial septum (IAS), left atrium (LA), proximal coronary sinus in cross section (CS), mitral valve (MiV), left ventricle (LV), and left atrial appendage (LAA). The catheter transducer (which is mounted parallel to the long axis of the catheter shaft) has been directed posterolaterally toward the mitral valve. Note the presence of spontaneous echo contrast within the LA and LAA. **B,** Pulsed wave (PW). Doppler trace of the mitral valve (Mi. valve) inflow pattern during sinus rhythm (SR), illustrating the E and A wave components to flow. The mean E wave is 0.7 m/sec, and the mean A wave is 0.4 m/sec. **C,** PW. Doppler trace of the LAA emptying velocity recorded during atrial flutter (AFL). *(From Morton JB, Sanders P, Sparks PB, et al. Usefulness of phased-array intracardiac echocardiography for the assessment of left atrial mechanical "stunning" in atrial flutter and comparison with multiplane transesophageal echocardiography. Am J Cardiol. 2002;90:741–746, with permission of Blackwell Scientific Publishing. With permission.)*

If the ostia are separate, it is usually not possible to clearly discern the left atrium–PV junction of both PVs in the same view, and small amounts of adjustment in steering and rotation are required to distinguish each vein. Occasionally, a third left PV may be identified.

After imaging of the left-sided PVs is complete, further clockwise rotation of the catheter at the same level brings the right inferior PV into view. If the ICE catheter is advanced superiorly and rotated to direct the transducer more posteriorly, the right superior PV (RSPV) can be seen; the right pulmonary artery passes superiorly to it. Variations in right PV anatomy detected by ICE are common. A right middle PV occurs in 5% to 15% of patients, although a posterior branch of the RSPV may be mistaken for a right middle PV if it does actually enter the RSPV just proximal to the PV–left atrium junction. A common right PV may be observed, or, alternatively, there may be closely related right superior and inferior PVs with a discrete carina or ridge between them.

The left and right inferior PVs are easily visualized in their longitudinal axis. Some degree of catheter manipulation is required to visualize the left and right superior PVs in their long axis.

For each PV, the vein diameter at the left atrium–PV junction and maximal PV inflow velocity by pulsed-wave Doppler are acquired before and after ablation (see later discussion). For the PV inflow velocity measurement using pulsed-wave Doppler, the sample volume is placed about 5 mm inside the PV ostium.

To visualize the left ventricle, the ICE catheter is advanced with apically directed tip deflection into the right ventricle and rotated clockwise against the interventricular septum. Excellent images of the left ventricle and mitral valve are obtained, and this view also permits easy and rapid identification of any pericardial effusion. If the catheter is further advanced and rotated, the apex of the right ventricle can be inspected and false tendons identified.

Withdrawing the catheter back to the base of the right ventricle outflow tract and rotating the shaft allow the tract to be seen in its long axis, with a cross-sectional view of the pulmonic valve.

Alternatively, the right and left outflow tracts and aortic root with coronary artery ostia can be imaged by advancing the catheter in the right atrium to the level of the outflow tracts. The aortic valve can also be imaged in its cross section from this region.

References

1. Olgin JE, Kalman JM, Fitzpatrick AP, Lesh MD. Role of right atrial endocardial structures as barriers to conduction during human type I atrial flutter: activation and entrainment mapping guided by intracardiac echocardiography. *Circulation.* 1995;92:1839–1848.
2. Kalman JM, Olgin JE, Karch MR, Lesh MD. Use of intracardiac echocardiography in interventional electrophysiology. *Pacing Clin Electrophysiol.* 1997;20:2248–2262.
3. Kalman JM, Jue J, Sudhir K, et al. In vitro quantification of radiofrequency ablation lesion size using intracardiac echocardiography in dogs. *Am J Cardiol.* 1996;77:217–219.
4. Chu E, Kalman JM, Kwasman MA, et al. Intracardiac echocardiography during radiofrequency catheter ablation of cardiac arrhythmias in humans. *J Am Coll Cardiol.* 1994;24:1351–1357.
5. Ren JF, Schwartzman D, Callans D, et al. Imaging technique and clinical utility for electrophysiologic procedures of lower frequency (9 MHz) intracardiac echocardiography. *Am J Cardiol.* 1998;82:1557–1560, A1558.

6. Kalman JM, Fitzpatrick AP, Olgin JE, et al. Biophysical characteristics of radiofrequency lesion formation in vivo: dynamics of catheter tip-tissue contact evaluated by intracardiac echocardiography. *Am Heart J.* 1997;133:8–18.

7. Chugh SS, Chan RC, Johnson SB, Packer DL. Catheter tip orientation affects radiofrequency ablation lesion size in the canine left ventricle. *Pacing Clin Electrophysiol.* 1999;22:413–420.

8. Kalman JM, Lee RJ, Fisher WG, et al. Radiofrequency catheter modification of sinus pacemaker function guided by intracardiac echocardiography. *Circulation.* 1995;92:3070–3081.

9. Asirvatham SJS, Wahl MR, Packer DL. Superiority of ultrasound over fluoroscopic assessment of electrode tissue contact for optimal lesion formation [abstract]. *Circulation.* 1999;100:1–374.

10. Epstein LM, Mitchell MA, Smith TW, Haines DE. Comparative study of fluoroscopy and intracardiac echocardiographic guidance for the creation of linear atrial lesions. *Circulation.* 1998;98:1796–1801.

11. Olgin JE, Kalman JM, Chin M, et al. Electrophysiological effects of long, linear atrial lesions placed under intracardiac ultrasound guidance. *Circulation.* 1997;96:2715–2721.

12. Roithinger FX, Steiner PR, Goseki Y, et al. Low-power radiofrequency application and intracardiac echocardiography for creation of continuous left atrial linear lesions. *J Cardiovasc Electrophysiol.* 1999;10:680–691.

13. Daoud EG, Kalbfleisch SJ, Hummel JD. Intracardiac echocardiography to guide transseptal left heart catheterization for radiofrequency catheter ablation. *J Cardiovasc Electrophysiol.* 1999;10:358–363.

14. Epstein LM, Smith T, TenHoff H. Nonfluoroscopic transseptal catheterization: safety and efficacy of intracardiac echocardiographic guidance. *J Cardiovasc Electrophysiol.* 1998;9:625–630.

15. Lee RJ, Kalman JM, Fitzpatrick AP, et al. Radiofrequency catheter modification of the sinus node for "inappropriate" sinus tachycardia. *Circulation.* 1995;92:2919–2928.

16. Kalman JM, Olgin JE, Karch MR, et al. "Cristal tachycardias": origin of right atrial tachycardias from the crista terminalis identified by intracardiac echocardiography. *J Am Coll Cardiol.* 1998;31:451–459.

17. Fisher WG, Pelini MA, Bacon ME. Adjunctive intracardiac echocardiography to guide slow pathway ablation in human atrioventricular nodal reentrant tachycardia: anatomic insights. *Circulation.* 1997;96:3021–3029.

18. Mangrum JM, Mounsey JP, Kok LC, et al. Intracardiac echocardiography-guided, anatomically based radiofrequency ablation of focal atrial fibrillation originating from pulmonary veins. *J Am Coll Cardiol.* 2002;39:1964–1972.

19. Ren JF, Schwartzman D, Lighty GW Jr, et al. Multiplane transesophageal and intracardiac echocardiography in large swine: imaging technique, normal values, and research applications. *Echocardiography.* 1997;14:135–148.

20. Bruce CJ, Packer DL, Seward JB. Intracardiac Doppler hemodynamics and flow: new vector, phased-array ultrasound-tipped catheter. *Am J Cardiol.* 1999;83:1509–1512, A1509.

21. Hijazi Z, Wang Z, Cao Q, Koenig P, et al. Transcatheter closure of atrial septal defects and patent foramen ovale under intracardiac echocardiographic guidance: feasibility and comparison with transesophageal echocardiography. *Catheter Cardiovasc Interv.* 2001;52:194–199.

22. Morton JB, Sanders P, Sparks PB, et al. Usefulness of phased-array intracardiac echocardiography for the assessment of left atrial mechanical "stunning" in atrial flutter and comparison with multiplane transesophageal echocardiography. *Am J Cardiol.* 2002;90:741–746.

23. Okumura Y, Henz BD, Johnson SB, et al. Three-dimensional ultrasound for image-guided mapping and intervention: methods, quantitative validation, and clinical feasibility of a novel multimodality image mapping system. *Circ Arrhythm Electrophysiol.* 2008;1:110–119.

24. Kalman JM, Olgin JE, Saxon LA, et al. Activation and entrainment mapping defines the tricuspid annulus as the anterior barrier in typical atrial flutter. *Circulation.* 1996;94:398–406.

25. Friedman PA, Luria D, Fenton AM, et al. Global right atrial mapping of human atrial flutter: the presence of posteromedial (sinus venosa region) functional block and double potentials. A study in biplane fluoroscopy and intracardiac echocardiography. *Circulation.* 2000;101:1568–1577.

26. Marchlinski FE, Ren JF, Schwartzman D, et al. Accuracy of fluoroscopic localization of the crista terminalis documented by intracardiac echocardiography. *J Interv Card Electrophysiol.* 2000;4:415–421.

27. Chu E, Fitzpatrick AP, Chin MC, et al. Radiofrequency catheter ablation guided by intracardiac echocardiography. *Circulation.* 1994;89:1301–1305.

28. Schwartz SL, Gillam LD, Weintraub AR, et al. Intracardiac echocardiography in humans using a small-sized (6F), low frequency (12.5 MHz) ultrasound catheter: methods, imaging planes and clinical experience. *J Am Coll Cardiol.* 1993;21:189–198.

29. Ren JF, Marchlinski FE, Callans DJ, Zado ES. Echocardiographic lesion characteristics associated with successful ablation of inappropriate sinus tachycardia. *J Cardiovasc Electrophysiol.* 2001;12:814–818.

30. Schwartzman D, Ren JF, Devine WA, Callans DJ. Cardiac swelling associated with linear radiofrequency ablation in the atrium. *J Interv Card Electrophysiol.* 2001;5:159–166.

31. Callans DJ, Ren JF, Schwartzman D, et al. Narrowing of the superior vena cava-right atrium junction during radiofrequency catheter ablation for inappropriate sinus tachycardia: analysis with intracardiac echocardiography. *J Am Coll Cardiol.* 1999;33:1667–1670.

32. Morton JB, Sanders P, Davidson NC, et al. Phased-array intracardiac echocardiography for defining cavotricuspid isthmus anatomy during radiofrequency ablation of typical atrial flutter. *J Cardiovasc Electrophysiol.* 2003;14:591–597.

33. Haissaguerre M, Jais P, Shah DC, et al. Spontaneous initiation of atrial fibrillation by ectopic beats originating in the pulmonary veins. *N Engl J Med.* 1998;339:659–666.

34. Chen SA, Hsieh MH, Tai CT, et al. Initiation of atrial fibrillation by ectopic beats originating from the pulmonary veins: electrophysiological characteristics, pharmacological responses, and effects of radiofrequency ablation. *Circulation.* 1999;100:1879–1886.

35. Natale A, Pisano E, Shewchik J, et al. First human experience with pulmonary vein isolation using a through-the-balloon circumferential ultrasound ablation system for recurrent atrial fibrillation. *Circulation.* 2000;102:1879–1882.

36. Haissaguerre M, Jais P, Shah DC, et al. Electrophysiological end point for catheter ablation of atrial fibrillation initiated from multiple pulmonary venous foci. *Circulation.* 2000;101:1409–1417.

37. Marrouche NF, Dresing T, Cole C, et al. Circular mapping and ablation of the pulmonary vein for treatment of atrial fibrillation: impact of different catheter technologies. *J Am Coll Cardiol.* 2002;40:464–474.

38. Oral H, Knight BP, Tada H, et al. Pulmonary vein isolation for paroxysmal and persistent atrial fibrillation. *Circulation.* 2002;105:1077–1081.

39. Ho SY, Sanchez-Quintana D, Cabrera JA, Anderson RH. Anatomy of the left atrium: implications for radiofrequency ablation of atrial fibrillation. *J Cardiovasc Electrophysiol.* 1999;10:1525–1533.

40. Morton JB, Sanders P, Byrne MJ, et al. Phased-array intracardiac echocardiography to guide radiofrequency ablation in the left atrium and at the pulmonary vein ostium. *J Cardiovasc Electrophysiol.* 2001;12:343–348.

41. Wood MA, Wittkamp M, Henry D, et al. A comparison of pulmonary vein ostial anatomy by computerized tomography, echocardiography, and venography in patients with atrial fibrillation having radiofrequency catheter ablation. *Am J Cardiol.* 2004;93:49–53.

42. Packer DL, Darbar D, Bhulm CM, et al. Utility of phased array intracardiac ultrasound for guiding the positioning of the lasso mapping catheter in pulmonary veins undergoing AF ablation [abstract]. *Circulation.* 2001;104:620.

43. Arora R, Verheule S, Scott L, et al. Arrhythmogenic substrate of the pulmonary veins assessed by high-resolution optical mapping. *Circulation.* 2003;107:1816–1821.

44. Mandapati R, Skanes A, Chen J, et al. Stable microreentrant sources as a mechanism of atrial fibrillation in the isolated sheep heart. *Circulation.* 2000;101:194–199.

45. Marrouche NF, Martin DO, Wazni O, et al. Phased-array intracardiac echocardiography monitoring during pulmonary vein isolation in patients with atrial fibrillation: impact on outcome and complications. *Circulation.* 2003;107:2710–2716.

46. Daccarett M, Segerson NM, Gunther J, et al. Blinded correlation study of three-dimensional electro-anatomical image integration and phased array intracardiac echocardiography for left atrial mapping. *Europace.* 2007;9:923–926.

47. Verma A, Marrouche NF, Natale A. Pulmonary vein antrum isolation: intracardiac echocardiography-guided technique. *J Cardiovasc Electrophysiol.* 2004;15:1335–1340.

48. Singh SM, Heist EK, Donaldson DM, et al. Image integration using intracardiac ultrasound to guide catheter ablation of atrial fibrillation. *Heart Rhythm.* 2008;5:1548–1555.

49. Bunch TJ, Bruce GK, Johnson SB, et al. Analysis of catheter-tip (8-mm) and actual tissue temperatures achieved during radiofrequency ablation at the orifice of the pulmonary vein. *Circulation.* 2004;110:2988–2995.

50. Weerasooriya R, Jais P, Sanders P, et al. Images in cardiovascular medicine: early appearance of an edematous tissue reaction during left atrial linear ablation using intracardiac echo imaging. *Circulation.* 2003;108:e80.

51. Scanavacca MI, Kajita LJ, Vieira M, Sosa EA. Pulmonary vein stenosis complicating catheter ablation of focal atrial fibrillation. *J Cardiovasc Electrophysiol.* 2000;11:677–681.

52. Moak JP, Moore HJ, Lee SW, et al. Case report. Pulmonary vein stenosis following RF ablation of paroxysmal atrial fibrillation: successful treatment with balloon dilation.. *J Interv Card Electrophysiol.* 2000;4:621–631.

53. Yang M, Akbari H, Reddy GP, Higgins CB. Identification of pulmonary vein stenosis after radiofrequency ablation for atrial fibrillation using MRI. *J Comput Assist Tomogr.* 2001;25:34–35.

54. Yu WC, Hsu TL, Tai CT, et al. Acquired pulmonary vein stenosis after radiofrequency catheter ablation of paroxysmal atrial fibrillation. *J Cardiovasc Electrophysiol.* 2001;12:887–892.

55. Gerstenfeld EP, Guerra P, Sparks PB, et al. Clinical outcome after radiofrequency catheter ablation of focal atrial fibrillation triggers. *J Cardiovasc Electrophysiol.* 2001;12:900–908.

56. Robbins IM, Colvin EV, Doyle TP, et al. Pulmonary vein stenosis after catheter ablation of atrial fibrillation. *Circulation.* 1998;98:1769–1775.

57. Taylor GW, Kay GN, Zheng X, et al. Pathological effects of extensive radiofrequency energy applications in the pulmonary veins in dogs. *Circulation.* 2000;101:1736–1742.

58. Minich LL, Tani LY, Breinholt JP, et al. Complete follow-up echocardiograms are needed to detect stenosis of normally connecting pulmonary veins. *Echocardiography.* 2001;18:589–592.

59. Saad EB, Cole CR, Marrouche NF, et al. Use of intracardiac echocardiography for prediction of chronic pulmonary vein stenosis after ablation of atrial fibrillation. *J Cardiovasc Electrophysiol.* 2002;13:986–989.

60. Martin RE, Ellenbogen KA, Lau YR, et al. Phased-array intracardiac echocardiography during pulmonary vein isolation and linear ablation for atrial fibrillation. *J Cardiovasc Electrophysiol.* 2002;13:873–879.

61. Swarup V, Azegami K, Arruda MS, et al. Four vessel pulmonary vein isolation guided by intracardiac echocardiography without contrast venography in patients with drug refractory paroxysmal atrial fibrillation. *J Am Coll Cardiol.* 2002;13:873–879.

62. Dill T, Neumann T, Ekinci O, et al. Pulmonary vein diameter reduction after radiofrequency catheter ablation for paroxysmal atrial fibrillation evaluated by contrast-enhanced three-dimensional magnetic resonance imaging. *Circulation.* 2003;107:845–850.

63. Malamis AP, Kirshenbaum KJ, Nadimpalli S. CT radiographic findings: atrio-esophageal fistula after transcatheter percutaneous ablation of atrial fibrillation. *J Thorac Imaging.* 2007;22:188–191.

64. Pappone C, Oral H, Santinelli V, et al. Atrio-esophageal fistula as a complication of percutaneous transcatheter ablation of atrial fibrillation. *Circulation.* 2004;109:2724–2726.

65. Scanavacca MI, D'Avila A, Parga J, Sosa E. Left atrial-esophageal fistula following radiofrequency catheter ablation of atrial fibrillation. *J Cardiovasc Electrophysiol.* 2004;15:960–962.

66. Cummings JE, Schweikert RA, Saliba WI, et al. Brief communication: atrial-esophageal fistulas after radiofrequency ablation. *Ann Intern Med.* 2006;144:572–574.

67. Schley P, Gulker H, Horlitz M. Atrio-oesophageal fistula following circumferential pulmonary vein ablation: verification of diagnosis with multislice computed tomography. *Europace.* 2006;8:189–190.

68. Bunch TJ, Nelson J, Foley T, et al. Temporary esophageal stenting allows healing of esophageal perforations following atrial fibrillation ablation procedures. *J Cardiovasc Electrophysiol.* 2006;17:435–439.

69. D'Avila A, Ptaszek LM, Yu PB, et al. Images in cardiovascular medicine. Left atrial-esophageal fistula after pulmonary vein isolation: a cautionary tale. *Circulation.* 2007;115:e432–e433.

70. Sonmez B, Demirsoy E, Yagan N, et al. A fatal complication due to radiofrequency ablation for atrial fibrillation: atrio-esophageal fistula. *Ann Thorac Surg.* 2003;76:281–283.

71. Dagres N, Hindricks G, Kottkamp H, et al. Complications of atrial fibrillation ablation in a high-volume center in 1,000 procedures: still cause for concern? *J Cardiovasc Electrophysiol.* 2009;20:1014–1019.

72. Schmidt M, Nolker G, Marschang H, et al. Incidence of oesophageal wall injury post-pulmonary vein antrum isolation for treatment of patients with atrial fibrillation. *Europace.* 2008;10:205–209.

73. Mohr FW, Fabricius AM, Falk V, et al. Curative treatment of atrial fibrillation with intraoperative radiofrequency ablation: short-term and midterm results. *J Thorac Cardiovasc Surg.* 2002;123:919–927.

74. Cappato R, Calkins H, Chen SA, et al. Prevalence and causes of fatal outcome in catheter ablation of atrial fibrillation. *J Am Coll Cardiol.* 2009;53:1798–1803.

75. Doll N, Borger MA, Fabricius A, et al. Esophageal perforation during left atrial radiofrequency ablation: is the risk too high? *J Thorac Cardiovasc Surg.* 2003;125:836–842.

76. Gillinov AM, Pettersson G, Rice TW. Esophageal injury during radiofrequency ablation for atrial fibrillation. *J Thorac Cardiovasc Surg.* 2001;122:1239–1240.

77. Sanchez-Quintana D, Cabrera JA, Climent V, et al. Anatomic relations between the esophagus and left atrium and relevance for ablation of atrial fibrillation. *Circulation.* 2005;112:1400–1405.

78. Gillinov AM, McCarthy PM, Pettersson G, et al. Esophageal perforation during left atrial radiofrequency ablation: is the risk too high? *J Thorac Cardiovasc Surg.* 2003;126:1661–1662, author reply, 1662.

79. Lemola K, Sneider M, Desjardins B, et al. Computed tomographic analysis of the anatomy of the left atrium and the esophagus: implications for left atrial catheter ablation. *Circulation.* 2004;110:3655–3660.

80. Hornero F, Berjano EJ. Esophageal temperature during radiofrequency-catheter ablation of left atrium: a three-dimensional computer modeling study. *J Cardiovasc Electrophysiol.* 2006;17:405–410.

81. Ripley KL, Gage AA, Olsen DB, et al. Time course of esophageal lesions after catheter ablation with cryothermal and radiofrequency ablation: implication for atrio-esophageal fistula formation after catheter ablation of atrial fibrillation. *J Cardiovasc Electrophysiol.* 2007;18:642–646.

82. Tsao HM, Wu MH, Higa S, et al. Anatomic relationship of the esophagus and left atrium: implication for catheter ablation of atrial fibrillation. *Chest.* 2005;128:2581–2587.

83. Berjano EJ, Hornero F. What affects esophageal injury during radiofrequency ablation of the left atrium? An engineering study based on finite-element analysis. *Physiol Meas.* 2005;26:837–848.

84. Bahnson TD. Strategies to minimize the risk of esophageal injury during catheter ablation for atrial fibrillation. *Pacing Clin Electrophysiol.* 2009;32:248–260.

85. Benussi S, Nascimbene S, Calvi S, Alfieri O. A tailored anatomical approach to prevent complications during left atrial ablation. *Ann Thorac Surg.* 2003;75:1979–1981.

86. Ren JF, Lin D, Marchlinski FE, et al. Esophageal imaging and strategies for avoiding injury during left atrial ablation for atrial fibrillation. *Heart Rhythm.* 2006;3:1156–1161.

87. Pollak SJ, Monir G, Chernoby MS, Elenberger CD. Novel imaging techniques of the esophagus enhancing safety of left atrial ablation. *J Cardiovasc Electrophysiol.* 2005;16:244–248.

88. Wang SL, Ooi CG, Siu CW, et al. Endocardial visualization of esophageal-left atrial anatomic relationship by three-dimensional multidetector computed tomography "navigator imaging". *Pacing Clin Electrophysiol.* 2006;29:502–508.

89. Martinek M, Bencsik G, Aichinger J, et al. Esophageal damage during radiofrequency ablation of atrial fibrillation: impact of energy settings, lesion sets, and esophageal visualization. *J Cardiovasc Electrophysiol.* 2009;20:726–733.

90. Yamane T, Matsuo S, Date T, Mochizuki S. Visualization of the esophagus throughout left atrial catheter ablation for atrial fibrillation. *J Cardiovasc Electrophysiol.* 2006;17:105.

91. Perzanowski C, Teplitsky L, Hranitzky PM, Bahnson TD. Real-time monitoring of luminal esophageal temperature during left atrial radiofrequency catheter ablation for atrial fibrillation: observations about esophageal heating during ablation at the pulmonary vein ostia and posterior left atrium. *J Cardiovasc Electrophysiol.* 2006;17:166–170.

92. Redfearn DP, Trim GM, Skanes AC, et al. Esophageal temperature monitoring during radiofrequency ablation of atrial fibrillation. *J Cardiovasc Electrophysiol.* 2005;16:589–593.

93. Cummings JE, Schweikert RA, Saliba WI, et al. Assessment of temperature, proximity, and course of the esophagus during radiofrequency ablation within the left atrium. *Circulation.* 2005;112:459–464.

94. Sherzer AI, Feigenblum DY, Kulkarni S, et al. Continuous nonfluoroscopic localization of the esophagus during radiofrequency catheter ablation of atrial fibrillation. *J Cardiovasc Electrophysiol.* 2007;18:157–160.

95. Kottkamp H, Piorkowski C, Tanner H, et al. Topographic variability of the esophageal left atrial relation influencing ablation lines in patients with atrial fibrillation. *J Cardiovasc Electrophysiol.* 2005;16:146–150.

96. Good E, Oral H, Lemola K, et al. Movement of the esophagus during left atrial catheter ablation for atrial fibrillation. *J Am Coll Cardiol.* 2005;46:2107–2110.

97. Kenigsberg DN, Lee BP, Grizzard JD, et al. Accuracy of intracardiac echocardiography for assessing the esophageal course along the posterior left atrium: a comparison to magnetic resonance imaging. *J Cardiovasc Electrophysiol.* 2007;18:169–173.

98. Cury RC, Abbara S, Schmidt S, et al. Relationship of the esophagus and aorta to the left atrium and pulmonary veins: implications for catheter ablation of atrial fibrillation. *Heart Rhythm.* 2005;2:1317–1323.

99. Calkins H. Prevention of esophageal injury during catheter ablation of atrial fibrillation: is intracardiac echocardiography the answer? *Heart Rhythm.* 2006;3:1162–1163.

100. Higashi Y, Shimojima H, Wakatsuki D, et al. Pulmonary vein isolation under direct visual identification of the left atrium-pulmonary vein junction using intra-cardiac echography. *J Interv Card Electrophysiol.* 2006;15:15–20.

101. Helms A, West JJ, Patel A, et al. Real-time rotational ICE imaging of the relationship of the ablation catheter tip and the esophagus during atrial fibrillation ablation. *J Cardiovasc Electrophysiol.* 2009;20:130–137.

102. Oh S, Kilicaslan F, Zhang Y, et al. Avoiding microbubbles formation during radiofrequency left atrial ablation versus continuous microbubbles formation and standard radiofrequency ablation protocols: comparison of energy profiles and chronic lesion characteristics. *J Cardiovasc Electrophysiol.* 2006;17:72–77.

103. Marrouche NF, Guenther J, Segerson NM, et al. Randomized comparison between open irrigation technology and intracardiac-echo-guided energy delivery for pulmonary vein antrum isolation: procedural parameters, outcomes, and the effect on esophageal injury. *J Cardiovasc Electrophysiol.* 2007;18:583–588.

104. Schwartzman D, Callans DJ, Gottlieb CD, et al. Conduction block in the inferior vena caval-tricuspid valve isthmus: association with outcome of radiofrequency ablation of type I atrial flutter. *J Am Coll Cardiol.* 1996;28:1519–1531.

105. Cosio FG, Arribas F, Lopez-Gil M, Gonzalez HD. Radiofrequency ablation of atrial flutter. *J Cardiovasc Electrophysiol.* 1996;7:60–70.

106. Lesh MD, Kalman JM, Olgin JE. New approaches to treatment of atrial flutter and tachycardia. *J Cardiovasc Electrophysiol.* 1996;7:368–381.

107. Shah DC, Haissaguerre M, Jais P, et al. Simplified electrophysiologically directed catheter ablation of recurrent common atrial flutter. *Circulation.* 1997;96:2505–2508.

108. Poty H, Saoudi N, Nair M, et al. Radiofrequency catheter ablation of atrial flutter. Further insights into the various types of isthmus block: application to ablation during sinus rhythm. *Circulation.* 1996;94:3204–3213.

109. Nakagawa H, Lazzara R, Khastgir T, et al. Role of the tricuspid annulus and the eustachian valve/ridge on atrial flutter: relevance to catheter ablation of the septal isthmus and a new technique for rapid identification of ablation success. *Circulation.* 1996;94:407–424.

110. Cabrera JA, Sanchez-Quintana D, Ho SY, et al. The architecture of the atrial musculature between the orifice of the inferior caval vein and the tricuspid valve: the anatomy of the isthmus. *J Cardiovasc Electrophysiol.* 1998;9:1186–1195.

111. Darbar D, Olgin JE, Miller JM, Friedman PA. Localization of the origin of arrhythmias for ablation: from electrocardiography to advanced endocardial mapping systems. *J Cardiovasc Electrophysiol.* 2001;12:1309–1325.

112. Heidbuchel H, Willems R, van Rensburg H, et al. Right atrial angiographic evaluation of the posterior isthmus: relevance for ablation of typical atrial flutter. *Circulation.* 2000;101:2178–2184.

113. Callans DJ, Ren JF, Narula N, et al. Effects of linear, irrigated-tip radiofrequency ablation in porcine healed anterior infarction. *J Cardiovasc Electrophysiol.* 2001;12:1037–1042.

114. Callans DJ, Ren JF, Michele J, et al. Electroanatomic left ventricular mapping in the porcine model of healed anterior myocardial infarction: correlation with intracardiac echocardiography and pathological analysis. *Circulation.* 1999;100:1744–1750.

115. Ren JF, Marchlinski FE. Utility of intracardiac echocardiography in left heart ablation for tachyarrhythmias. *Echocardiography*. 2007;24:533–540.

116. Jongbloed MR, Bax JJ, van der Burg AE, et al. Radiofrequency catheter ablation of ventricular tachycardia guided by intracardiac echocardiography. *Eur J Echocardiogr*. 2004;5:34–40.

117. Doi A, Takagi M, Toda I, et al. Real time quantification of low temperature radiofrequency ablation lesion size using phased array intracardiac echocardiography in the canine model: comparison of two dimensional images with pathological lesion characteristics. *Heart*. 2003;89:923–927.

118. Lamberti F, Calo L, Pandozi C, et al. Radiofrequency catheter ablation of idiopathic left ventricular outflow tract tachycardia: utility of intracardiac echocardiography. *J Cardiovasc Electrophysiol*. 2001;12:529–535.

119. Friedman PL, Stevenson WG, Bittl JA, et al. Left main coronary artery occlusion during radiofrequency catheter ablation of idiopathic outflow tract ventricular tachycardia [abstract]. *Pacing Clin Electrophysiol*. 1997;20:1185.

120. Kim YH, Xie F, Yashima M, et al. Role of papillary muscle in the generation and maintenance of reentry during ventricular tachycardia and fibrillation in isolated swine right ventricle. *Circulation*. 1999;100:1450–1459.

121. Wilde AA, Duren DR, Hauer RN, et al. Mitral valve prolapse and ventricular arrhythmias: observations in a patient with a 20-year history. *J Cardiovasc Electrophysiol*. 1997;8:307–316.

122. Bogun F, Desjardins B, Crawford T, et al. Post-infarction ventricular arrhythmias originating in papillary muscles. *J Am Coll Cardiol*. 2008;51:1794–1802.

123. Good E, Desjardins B, Jongnarangsin K, et al. Ventricular arrhythmias originating from a papillary muscle in patients without prior infarction: a comparison with fascicular arrhythmias. *Heart Rhythm*. 2008;5:1530–1537.

124. Horowitz BN, Vaseghi M, Mahajan A, et al. Percutaneous intrapericardial echocardiography during catheter ablation: a feasibility study. *Heart Rhythm*. 2006;3:1275–1282.

125. Khaykin Y, Skanes A, Whaley B, et al. Real-time integration of 2D intracardiac echocardiography and 3D electroanatomical mapping to guide ventricular tachycardia ablation. *Heart Rhythm*. 2008;5:1396–1402.

126. Cafri C, de la Guardia B, Barasch E, et al. Transseptal puncture guided by intracardiac echocardiography during percutaneous transvenous mitral commissurotomy in patients with distorted anatomy of the fossa ovalis. *Catheter Cardiovasc Interv*. 2000;50:463–467.

127. Mitchel JF, Gillam LD, Sanzobrino BW, et al. Intracardiac ultrasound imaging during transseptal catheterization. *Chest*. 1995;108:104–108.

128. Morton JB, Swarup V, Stobie P, et al. The common left pulmonary vein: intracardiac ultrasound characteristics and impact upon pulmonary vein isolation. *J Am Coll Cardiol*. 2003;41:124A.

Catheter Ablation of Atrial Tachycardias and Flutter

PART III

11
Ablation of Focal Atrial Tachycardias

Nitish Badhwar, Byron K. Lee, and Jeffrey E. Olgin

Key Points

The mechanism of focal atrial tachycardia (AT) can be automatic, triggered, or reentry.

The P-wave morphology on a 12-lead electrocardiogram gives a general idea of the site of origin of the focal AT. Mapping techniques include determining the earliest atrial activation during tachycardia and pace mapping of the P-wave morphology.

Ablation targets comprise abnormal atrial tissue from which the tachycardia originates, as identified by the site of earliest atrial activation and abnormal local atrial electrograms.

Three-dimensional mapping systems are often useful, and intracardiac echocardiography can be helpful, especially for crista terminalis tachycardias. Difficulty arises when the tachycardia is not inducible or is not sustained.

Troubleshooting difficult cases includes the unusual location of the tachycardia focus arising from the coronary sinus, superior or inferior vena cava, ligament of Marshall, appendages, or aortic cusps. Mapping of the left atrium and pulmonary veins is often needed when a left-sided tachycardia is suspected.

Focal atrial tachycardia (AT) is defined as atrial activation starting rhythmically at a small area (focus), from where it spreads out centrifugally and without endocardial activation over significant portions of the cycle length.[1] By definition, AT does not use the atrioventricular (AV) junction or an accessory pathway as an essential portion of its circuit and can continue indefinitely and independently of them.[2] More specifically, *focal atrial tachycardias* are defined as ATs that originate from a single site in either atrium, in contrast to *macroreentrant atrial tachycardias (or flutters)*, which are discussed in Chapters 12 through 14.

Anatomy

Focal atrial tachycardias usually arise from well-defined anatomic regions in the right and the left atrium. They usually occur along the crista terminalis in the right atrium and near the pulmonary veins (PVs) in the left atrium.[3–11] Less frequently, they can arise from the aortic cusps, coronary sinus musculature,[12] coronary sinus ostium,[13] parahisian region,[14] appendages,[15,16] or rarely along the tricuspid[17] or mitral annulus.[18]

Pathophysiology

Chen and colleagues[19] showed that focal AT can occur in any age group, with a greater incidence in the adult middle-aged population and no gender preference. It more commonly arises from the right atrium, and a second focus of AT may be found in up to 17% of the patients.[2]

Focal ATs may have an automatic, triggered, or microreentrant mechanism. Although it can be difficult to precisely define the basic mechanism of a particular AT, understanding the basic principles of focal ATs may help with certain therapeutic decisions.[4,20] The arrhythmogenic mechanisms should not be used with stringency, and flexibility should be used in the judgment of apparent inconsistencies in a particular tachycardia mechanism.

Abnormal automaticity, most likely caused by a positive ionic influx during phase 4 depolarization, is thought to be the most common underlying mechanism for focal ATs. Clinically, automatic tachycardias are characterized by sudden onset with a "warm-up" period and facilitation by adrenergic surge or exogenous catecholamines. Vagal stimulation, β-blockers, and calcium channel blockers may suppress these types of ATs, and adenosine may provoke an ambiguous response.[21] In the electrophysiology laboratory, these tachycardias are not inducible by programmed stimulation and may be suppressed by overdrive pacing.

Triggered activity is the mechanism by which the cardiac cell depolarizes due to afterpotentials. Delayed afterpotentials occur after the repolarization of the cell action potential and are able to depolarize the cell membrane to the depolarization threshold. This triggers activation of the inward ionic currents, causing an action potential. The role of afterdepolarizations in ATs appears to be limited and is inferential from single-cell recordings, but evidence suggests that this mechanism may play a role in AT during digitalis toxicity.[22] Triggered tachycardias usually are inducible by programmed stimulation—commonly, constant-rate pacing. They may have a warm-up period and are facilitated by catecholamines. Overdrive pacing may also accelerate them. Vagal maneuvers, β-blockers, calcium channel blockers, and adenosine may terminate this type of AT.[21,23]

Reentry is another mechanism of focal ATs. In reentry, a self-perpetuating circuit travels around an area of scar or slow conduction that maintains the arrhythmia. If the reentry circuit is discrete (arbitrarily defined as <3 cm in diameter), the AT is still classified as focal. However, if the reentry circuit is larger (>3 cm), it is classified as a macro-reentrant AT. Focal reentrant tachycardias can be ablated with a single ablation lesion, whereas macro-reentrant ATs typically require a series of linear ablation lesions. Macro-reentrant ATs are discussed in detail in Chapters 13 and 14. Focal reentrant atrial tachycardia is characterized by initiation and termination with programmed atrial stimulation. Because of the small circuit size, criteria for entrainment of these tachycardias can be difficult to demonstrate. This form of focal AT has been shown to be insensitive to adenosine.[24] Markowitz and associates have proposed an algorithm to differentiate the mechanism of focal AT based on the response to adenosine.[24]

Although there are no large-scale trials in the medical treatment of focal ATs, it appears, based on the reported data, that β-blockers[25] and calcium channel blockers are at least partially effective, particularly if the underlying mechanism of the tachycardia is abnormal automaticity or triggered activity.[21,26] Because of their safety profile, these drugs are usually first-line medical therapy.

Inappropriate sinus tachycardia is one type of focal AT that deserves special consideration. It is a syndrome characterized by an increased sinus rate, either at rest or with minimal exertion. The P-wave morphology is generally identical to that of normal sinus rhythm. The resting heart rate often is in excess of 100 beats/minute, with an exaggerated response to minimal exertion or postural changes. It is a rare clinical syndrome and usually affects young women. The clinical presentation includes palpitations, easy fatigability, dizziness, lightheadedness, shortness of breath, and sometimes presyncope or syncope.

The mechanism of inappropriate sinus tachycardia is poorly understood. Possible mechanisms have been postulated, among them a depressed cardiovagal reflex with an elevated intrinsic heart rate and β-adrenergic sensitivity,[27] abnormal autonomic control of the sinus node,[28] and a primary abnormality of the sinus node.[29] Although inappropriate sinus tachycardia is often difficult to differentiate from a focal AT, the mechanism appears to be different.[30–32]

Clinically, patients with AT may present with varying degrees of symptoms, from being only mildly symptomatic to having overt congestive heart failure due to tachycardia-induced cardiomyopathy.[33,34] The latter scenario warrants emphasis because patients with incessant ATs and tachycardia-induced cardiomyopathy can be misdiagnosed as having a compensatory sinus tachycardia in the setting of an idiopathic dilated cardiomyopathy. Focal AT-induced cardiomyopathy is more common in male patients, in patients with slower incessant tachycardias and, in those with ATs arising from the atrial appendages. Curative catheter ablation of the tachycardia focus can normalize left ventricular function and reverse the cardiomyopathy.[34]

Diagnosis and Differential Diagnosis

Analysis of the 12-lead scalar electrocardiogram P-wave morphology during AT can be helpful in determining the origin of the tachycardia (Fig. 11-1). Leads aVL and V₁

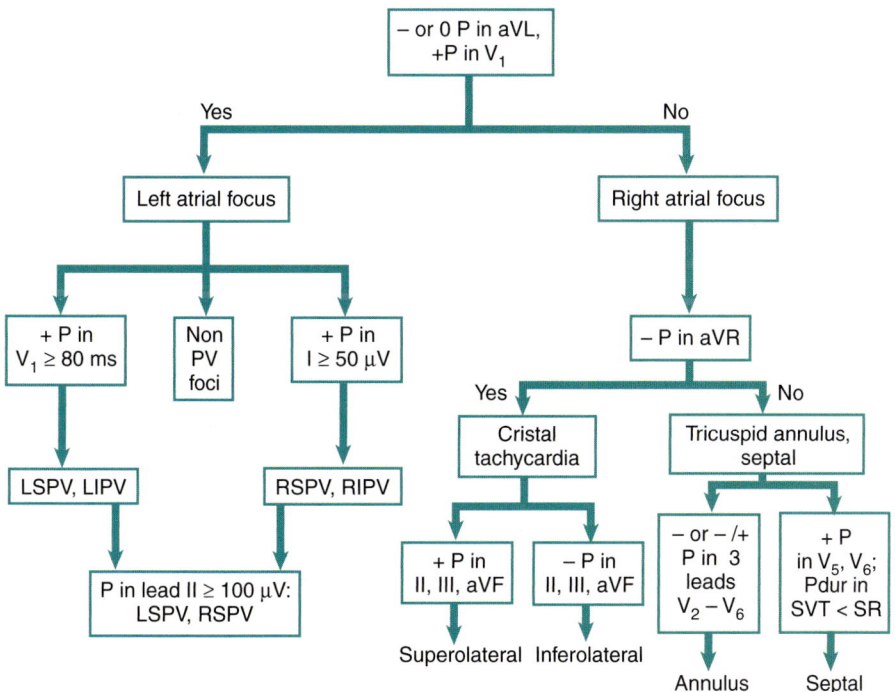

FIGURE 11-1. Algorithm for localization of atrial tachycardia origin based on surface electrocardiogram. +, upright P-wave morphology; −, inverted P-wave morphology; I, inferior; L, left; R, right; Pdur, P wave duration; PV, pulmonary vein; S, superior; SR, sinus rhythm; SVT, supraventricular tachycardia. *(From Ellenbogen KA, Wood MA. Atrial tachycardia. In Zipes DP, Jalife J [eds]: Cardiac Electrophysiology: From Cell to Bedside, 4th ed. Philadelphia: Saunders; 2004:500–511. With permission.)*

are the most useful to distinguish between left and right origin.[9] A positive or biphasic P wave in aVL predicts a right atrial origin of the tachycardia with a sensitivity of 88% and a specificity of 79%. In lead V_1, a negative or biphasic with negative terminal P wave demonstrated a specificity of 100% for a right atrial focus, and a positive or biphasic with positive terminal P wave demonstrated a sensitivity of 100% for a left atrial focus.[35] Tang and colleagues[9] made the important observation that right superior PV foci showed a change in configuration in lead V_1 from biphasic in sinus rhythm to upright in AT, a change not seen in right atrial foci. In addition, leads II, III, and aVF may help differentiate a superior focus (positive P wave) from an inferior one (negative P wave). Furthermore, a negative P wave in lead aVR suggests a right lateral location, specifically the crista terminalis, with 100% sensitivity and 93% specificity, whereas a negative P wave in leads V_5 and V_6 suggests an inferomedial location.[36] AT arising from the apex of the triangle of Koch (parahisian AT) usually demonstrates isoelectric P waves in V_1 and shorter P-wave duration in the inferior leads during AT compared with sinus rhythm.[36] Focal AT arising from the coronary sinus ostium is associated with deep negative P waves in inferior leads, positive P waves in aVL, and –/+ or iso/+ in V_1.[13] Focal AT arising from the right atrial appendage has P-wave morphology similar to sinus rhythm and can be misdiagnosed as inappropriate sinus tachycardia.

In the left atrium, focal AT commonly arises from the PVs and is associated with a characteristic P-wave morphology that is positive in precordial leads and negative in aVR and aVL (right superior PVs can give positive P wave in aVL, as discussed earlier).[37] Left-sided PVs are associated with notched and wider P waves with a lead III/II ratio of greater than 0.8, whereas right-sided PVs are positive in lead I. Focal AT arising from the left-sided coronary sinus musculature gives positive P waves in V_1 with transition to negative P waves in V_3 to V_4, negative P waves in inferior leads, positive P waves in aVR, and biphasic P waves (+/–, +/iso) in aVL.[12] AT arising from the mitral annulus tend to cluster at the superior aspect close to the aortomitral continuity with biphasic (–/+) P waves in V_1, negative or isoelectric in I and aVL, and low-amplitude positive or isoelectric in the inferior leads.[18] AT arising from the left atrial appendage is associated with broad positive P waves in precordial leads, deep negative P waves in lead I and aVL, and positive P waves in inferior leads.[16]

Although these rules generally hold true, there are some limitations to using P-wave vectors for diagnosis. For example, the presence of 1:1 AV conduction can cause distortion of the P waves by the QRS complex or T wave. In such cases, pharmacologic or vagal-induced AV block or induced premature ventricular contractions may be useful to analyze the P wave. Even so, analysis of the origin of the AT based on P-wave morphology alone can be misleading. There is a spatial limitation of morphology that makes P waves indistinguishable if they originate from paced sites 17 mm apart or less.[38] Another frequent problem encountered is the differentiation of left ATs originating in the right pulmonary veins, which anatomically are located behind the right atrium, from those originating from the posterior right atrium. An intracardiac echocardiography (ICE) image can illustrate the close anatomic relationship between these structures (Fig. 11-2). Similarly, AT

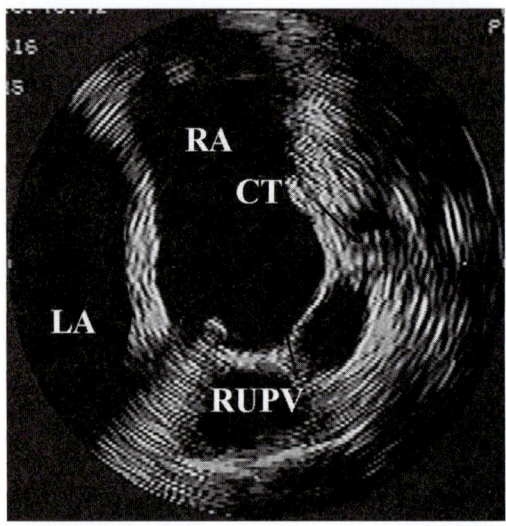

FIGURE 11-2. Intracardiac echocardiogram shows the relationship of the right upper pulmonary vein (RUPV) to the right atrium (RA) and crista terminalis (CT). Atrial tachycardias (ATs) arising from the RUPV may have a very similar activation sequence to those arising from the superior CT. Both areas are common sites for focal ATs. Intracardiac echocardiography may be used to precisely position a mapping catheter in relationship to these structures.

that must be ablated from the noncoronary aortic cusp may be mistaken for a right atrial septal tachycardia because of early activation of this contiguous structure. AT may arise from tissue within or immediately adjacent to the aortic cusps. Large atrial electrograms typically are recorded from the noncoronary cusp due to its position next to the atrial septum. This is the most likely site for ablation of ATs from the aortic cusps. Atrial tachycardia arising from the aortic cusps usually has narrow P waves that are positive in V_1 and tend to be positive or isoelectric in the inferior leads. A short PR interval may be seen.[46]

The R-P relationship is often useful in the differential diagnosis.[39] AT is typically a long R-P supraventricular tachycardia, whereas atrioventricular nodal reentrant tachycardia (AVNRT) and atrioventricular reentrant tachycardia (AVRT) are usually short R-P supraventricular tachycardias. However, in rare circumstances, these expected R-P relationships do not hold. For example, an AT with prolonged AV nodal conduction would be a short R-P tachycardia, whereas atypical AVNRT or AVRT using a slowly conducting accessory pathway would be a long R-P tachycardia. Distinguishing AT from AVNRT or AVRT requires analysis of conventional ICE recordings during tachycardia and the response of the arrhythmia to stimulation maneuvers and pharmacologic manipulation. Spontaneous termination of the tachycardia with an atrial depolarization not followed by a ventricular depolarization makes AT unlikely. Variable AV conduction with more atrial than ventricular signals strongly suggests AT and excludes a reciprocating tachycardia (Fig. 11-3). Conditions such as AV node reentry with block in the lower common pathway are rarely seen.[40] In addition, for ATs originating away from the AV valve annuli or coronary sinus ostium, atrial activation is usually inconsistent with AVRT using an accessory pathway or with AVNRT. However, if there is 1:1 AV conduction and the atrial activation sequence suggests an annular location, differentiation from AVNRT and AVRT can be

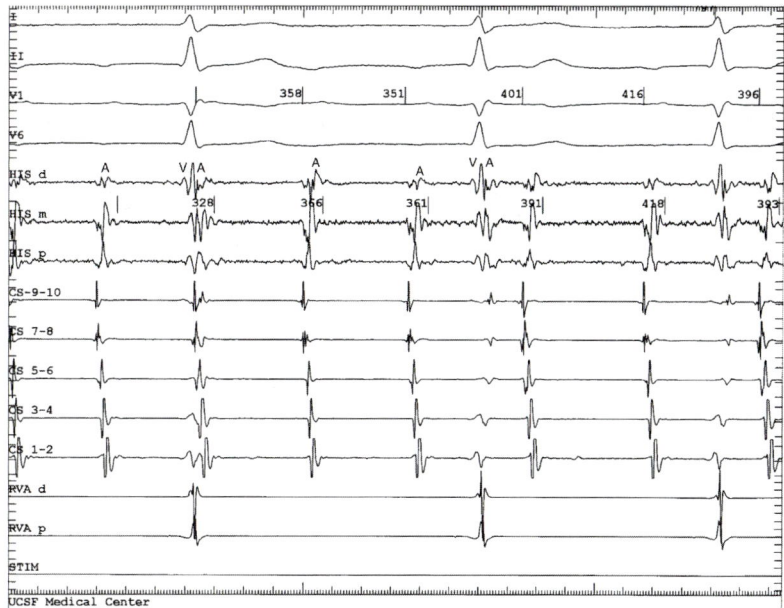

FIGURE 11-3. Variable atrioventricular conduction with more atrial (A) than ventricular (V) signals strongly suggests atrial tachycardia. I, II, V$_1$, V$_6$, surface electrocardiogram leads; CS, coronary sinus; d, distal; m, mid; p, proximal; RVA, right ventricular apex.

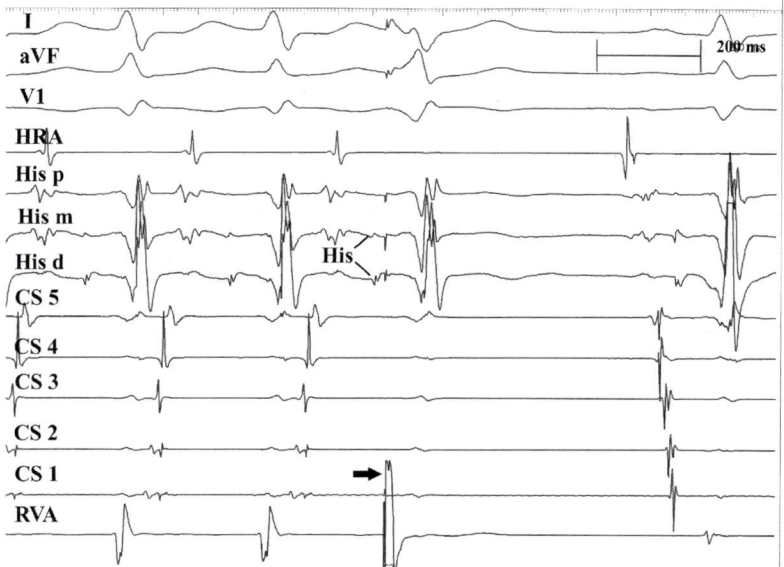

FIGURE 11-4. Reproducible termination of supraventricular tachycardia (SVT) by ventricular stimulation that does not conduct to the atrium excludes an atrial tachycardia. In this figure, SVT occurs with earliest atrial activation in the distal coronary sinus (CS 1). A premature ventricular stimulus (*arrow*) is delivered about 30 msec after activation of the His (labeled), followed by termination of the tachycardia. This finding was reproducible, and the patient underwent successful ablation of a left lateral accessory pathway. CS 5, proximal coronary sinus; d, distal; m, mid; p, proximal; RVA, right ventricular apex.

more difficult, and standard electrophysiologic maneuvers to determine the necessity of the AV node for the arrhythmia are used.

Ventricular pacing maneuvers can be very helpful in differentiating AT from AVNRT and AVRT. If burst pacing in the right ventricle at a rate slightly faster than the tachycardia rate dissociates the ventricle from the tachycardia, AVRT is excluded. If ventricular pacing reproducibly terminates the tachycardia without conduction to the atrium (Fig. 11-4), AT is excluded. If burst pacing in the ventricle entrains the atrium and there is a V-A-A-V response after the last paced beat (Fig. 11-5A), AT is the most likely diagnosis. Care must be taken to exclude the pseudo V-A-A-V response that results from long VA conduction times. In contrast, a V-A-V response (Fig. 11-5B) is more consistent with AVNRT or AVRT.[41]

Atrial pacing maneuvers can also be helpful. One can pace in the atrium at a rate faster than the tachycardia rate. If the VA interval of the return cycle length is within 10 msec of the VA interval during the tachycardia, there is

"VA linking," and AVNRT or AVRT is the most likely diagnosis. If the VA interval is variable, AT is most likely.[42] The difference between the A-H interval during right atrial pacing at the tachycardia cycle length and the A-H interval during tachycardia can be used to differentiate among long R-P tachycardias.[43] If the A-H interval with atrial pacing is less than 20 msec longer than in tachycardia, an AT is most likely. If the difference is between 20 and 40 msec, a reciprocating tachycardia is likely. Differences greater than 40 msec are consistent with AV nodal reentry.

Finally, the response to pharmacologic termination with adenosine also may be helpful. Although adenosine can be useful to dissociate the tachycardia from the AV node and ventricle, some ATs are adenosine sensitive.[44] See Table 11-1 for a list of diagnostic criteria.

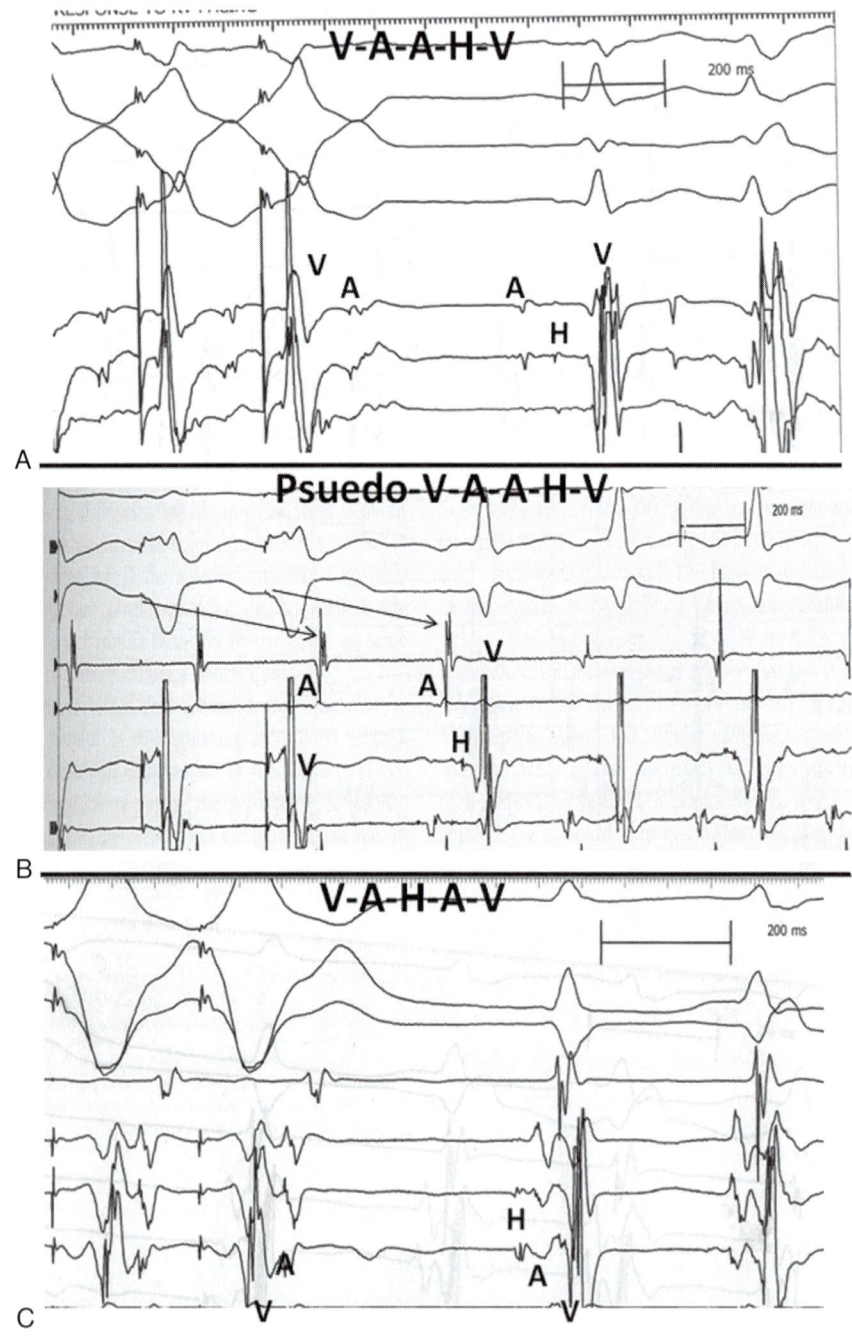

FIGURE 11-5. A, V-A-A-H-V response after the last right ventricular–paced beat suggests atrial tachycardia. To be valid, there must be acceleration of the atrial rate to the ventricular rate during ventricular pacing. Strictly, a V-A-A-H-V response should be seen. B, Pseudo V-A-A-V response after the last right ventricular–paced beat. The second "A" of the V-A-A-V response is entrained by the last paced beat because of long VA conduction times (*arrows*), although a V-A-A-H-V response in the second atrial electrogram does not represent the resumption of tachycardia, and the maneuver is invalid for diagnosing atrial tachycardia. An atypical form of atrioventricular nodal reentry is more likely. C, V-A-H-A-V response due to typical atrioventricular nodal reentry. A relatively long lower common pathway conduction time allows atrial activation before ventricular activation. As such, the first "A" of the V-A-A-V response conducts antegradely in the slow pathway to produce the next "V" after His activation. The second "A" occurs after the His and is not consistent with atrial tachycardia. H, His electrogram.

Mapping

Regardless of the tachycardia mechanism, successful ablation of a focal AT requires precise mapping of the tachycardia focus. Activation mapping, in which the earliest local activation is compared with onset of the tachycardia P wave, is the most common technique for mapping. With this technique, sites with local activation ranging from 15 to 60 msec before P-wave onset are targeted for ablation (Fig. 11-6A). The unipolar atrial electrogram should show QS complex at successful ablation sites (Fig. 11-6B). Often, the electrogram at the earliest site is fractionated (Fig. 11-6). Activation mapping is most effective when there is sustained tachycardia to map. Multielectrode catheters (such as a 20-pole catheter placed along the crista terminalis and a multipolar coronary sinus catheter) can be useful to guide initial mapping.[3] Because most focal ATs originate from the right atrium, a crista terminalis catheter can rapidly identify the best region in which to start mapping (Fig. 11-7). Furthermore, the activation sequence in the multielectrode

TABLE 11-1
DIAGNOSTIC CRITERIA OF FOCAL ATRIAL TACHYCARDIA
Changes in A-A interval precede changes in V-V interval.
Ventricular pacing during tachycardia results in a V-A-A-V response before tachycardia resumes.*
A-H interval during atrial pacing at tachycardia cycle length minus A-H interval during tachycardia is less than 20 msec.
Spontaneous termination of tachycardia with an atrial activation makes atrial tachycardia unlikely.
Ventricle can be dissociated from tachycardia.
Ventricular pacing that reproducibly terminates the tachycardia without conduction to the atrium excludes atrial tachycardia.
Variable VA intervals during sustained tachycardia or with ventricular pacing suggests atrial tachycardia.
Atrial activation occurs over less than 60% of tachycardia cycle length.
Macro-reentrant atrial tachycardia has been excluded.

*Exclude pseudo V-A-A-V response.

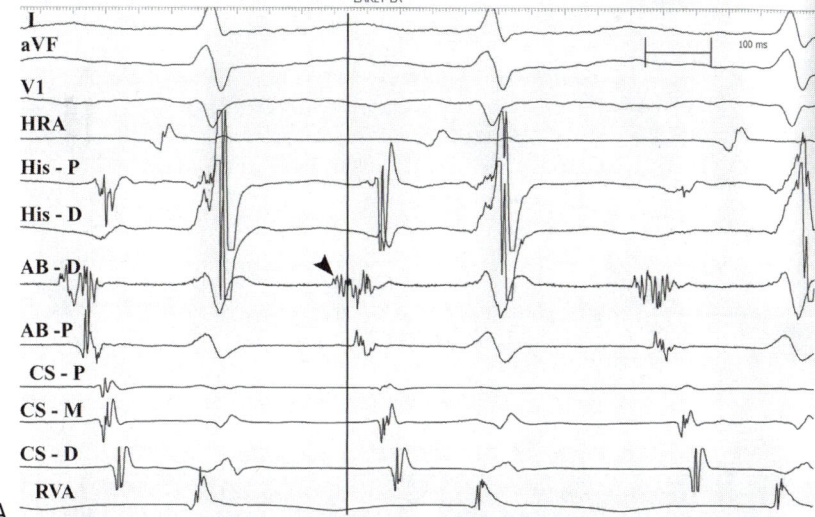

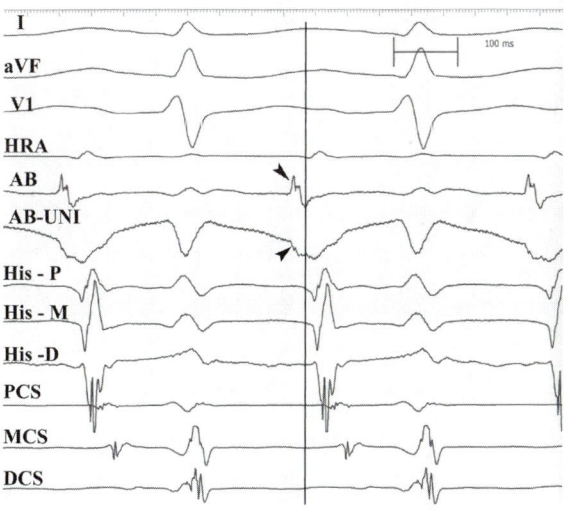

FIGURE 11-6. Electrogram targets for ablation of atrial tachycardias. **A,** The distal ablation electrogram (AB-D) shows electrical activity beginning 30 msec (*arrowhead*) before the surface P-wave onset that is indicated by the *vertical line*. Note the marked fractionation of the electrogram at this site. Ablation at this site terminated an atrial tachycardia in the lateral left atrium. **B,** In this patient with a right atrial tachycardia, the ablation catheter distal bipolar recording (AB) shows local activation 35 msec (*upper arrowhead*) before surface P-wave onset (*vertical line*). The distal ablation unipolar electrogram (AB-UNI) shows a QS morphology with the point of maximal negative dV/dt also 30 msec before P-wave onset (*lower arrowhead*). Ablation at this site terminated the tachycardia and rendered it noninducible. For both figures the time scale (upper left) indicates 100 msec. CS, coronary sinus; D, distal; M, mid; P, proximal; RVA, right ventricular apex.

catheters, in combination with the His atrial signal, can also suggest the location of foci.[37,45] The inability to record early atrial activation should suggest the possibility of AT arising from unusual sites. Coronary sinus musculature tachycardias are rare, and atrial activation may be confusing because of the pattern of electrical attachment between the coronary sinus and atrial musculatures. Also rare are atrial tachycardias that arise from the ligament of Marshall. This epicardial atrial structure is positioned between the left atrial appendage and the left superior pulmonary vein and may be mapped from the distal coronary sinus. Finally, the aortic cusps must also be considered as the source of ATs.[58] The

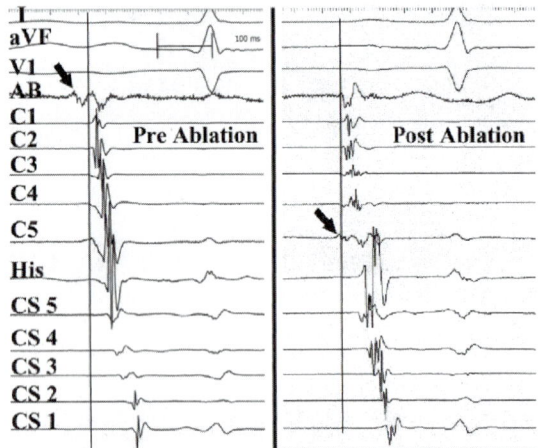

FIGURE 11-7. Ablation of inappropriate sinus tachycardia arising from the crista terminalis using a multipolar crista mapping catheter. *Left panel,* A 10-pole mapping "crista" catheter is positioned along the crista terminalis with the distal bipole (C1) cranial and the proximal bipole (C5) caudal. The activation is cranial to caudal with the ablation electrogram (AB) preceding all other atrial activity (*arrow*) and the surface P-wave onset (*vertical line*). Ablation delivered to this site reduced the atrial rate from 120 to 100 beats/min. *Right panel,* After ablation, the activation of the crista is changed, with the caudal bipole recording the earliest activity. Additional ablation was then performed around this site of early activation to further reduce the atrial rate. The time scale represents 100 msec.

noncoronary cusp is the most common source of ATs, and from this location, large atrial electrograms are recorded in sinus rhythm.[46] The right coronary cusp may also display atrial electrograms, but these usually are accompanied by a ventricular electrogram or a His potential. Large atrial electrograms may sometimes be recorded from the right cusp because of an overlying right atrial appendage. The left cusp is the least intimately related to atrial myocardium because it is adjacent to the aortomitral continuity. The atrial electrograms from the cusps may have a slightly far-field appearance because of the intervening aortic cusp tissue. During ATs, low-voltage fractionated near-field electrograms may precede the larger atrial electrograms. When mapping, the noncoronary cusp is the most posterior of the three (Figs. 11-8 and 11-9).

Tachycardias appearing to arise from the right atrial septum often require mapping of the left atrial septum as well to exclude earlier sites being found in this location. AT arising from the posterior right atrium should initiate mapping of the underlying right superior PV if no satisfactory ablation sites are found.

For instances in which tachycardia is not sustained or is difficult to induce, pace mapping can be useful. It is also useful as an adjunct to activation mapping. Pace mapping is performed by pacing at the lowest capture output; the paced P-wave morphology is then compared with the P wave recorded during tachycardia. This technique has the limitation of requiring a "pure" P wave on the surface 12-lead electrocardiogram, undisturbed by the QRS or T wave. However, use of surrogate markers such as multiple intracardiac recordings has been proposed.[47]

Three-dimensional (3D) mapping systems offer many advantages in the ablation of focal ATs. In general, these systems allow construction of a 3D image of the heart chamber that is suspected to be the source of the tachycardia. If mapping is done during sustained AT, these systems can produce an activation map that identifies the earliest site of atrial activation, which can then be targeted for ablation. The 3D mapping systems can also show the tip of the ablation catheter moving in the generated 3D image. Use

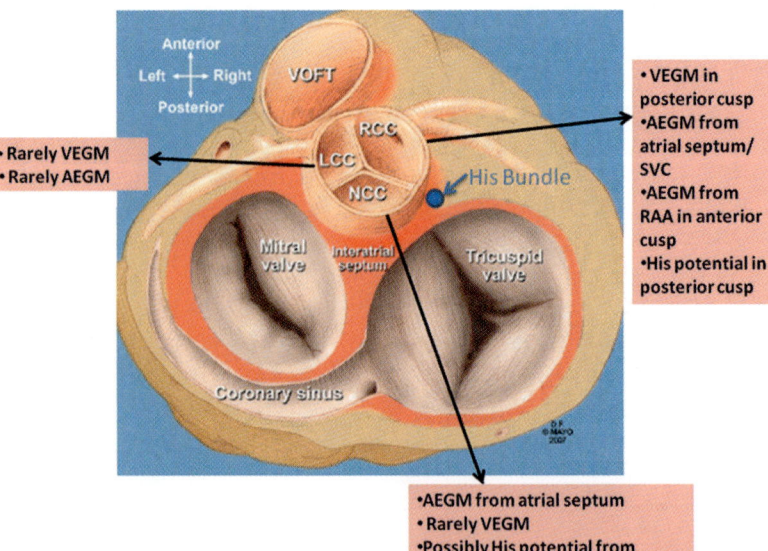

FIGURE 11-8. Anatomy of the aortic valve cusps. Note the posterior location of the noncoronary cusp (NCC) that is the most common site for ablation of atrial tachycardia. The electrogram components typically recorded from each cusp are annotated. AEGM; atrial electrogram; LCC, left coronary cusp; RAA, right anterior artery; RCC, right coronary cusp; VEGM, ventricular electrogram; VOFT, ventricular outflow tract. (*Modified from Sulieman M, Asarvatham S. Ablation above the semilunar valves: when, why and how? Part I. Heart Rhythm. 2008;5:1485–1492. With permission.*)

of this image to guide mapping and ablation minimizes fluoroscopy exposure. Finally, 3D systems allow marking of interesting sites noted during mapping. Marking of the His "cloud" to show areas to avoid during ablation can be helpful, particularly in cases of parahisian AT. If the ablation catheter is unstable during tachycardia, marking of the earliest site during tachycardia facilitates returning to that same site for ablation during sinus rhythm (Table 11-2).

The generated 3D activation map can also be helpful in distinguishing a focal AT from a macro-reentrant tachycardia. In macro-reentrant AT, the activation map spans the entire tachycardia cycle length, and the earliest site meets the latest site. In focal ATs, the activation map typically spans less than 60% of the tachycardia cycle length, and the latest site usually does not meet the earliest site.

Some of the 3D mapping systems have unique features that make them particularly useful. The Carto (Biosense Webster, Diamond Bar, CA) and EnSite NavX (St. Jude Medical, St. Paul, MN) 3D mapping systems can create voltage maps that accurately identify areas of scar with no electrical signal. Voltage maps are more useful for macro-reentrant ATs, in which the circuit often revolves around a scar. The Carto system has been successfully used for ablation of focal ATs with a relatively short mapping time (Fig. 11-10).[48] One of its major limitations is its inability to map transient nonsustained tachycardias. The EnSite array 3D mapping system uses a 64-wire array mounted to a 10-mL balloon-catheter. Once the anatomy has been obtained by tracing of the chamber with a standard catheter, the system superimposes over it the data from 3200 electrograms obtained by mathematical reconstruction simultaneously, to create an isopotential map. The biggest advantage of this system is its ability to map nonsustained tachycardias, and even single beats. The spatial resolution, however, is lost if the system is used in a very large atrium (Fig. 11-11).

Ablation

Although focal ATs may result from automatic, triggered, or micro-reentry mechanisms, their precise mechanism does not affect the mapping technique or the success rate of ablation therapy.

Once mapping identifies the optimal site, 30 to 50 W of radiofrequency energy is delivered for 30 to 60 seconds. Standard ablation catheters with 4-mm tips are usually satisfactory. Large-tip catheters, high-energy generators, or irrigated ablation systems are rarely necessary. Acceleration of the tachycardia before termination suggests that ablation will be successful, as does termination within 10 seconds. A successful ablation is verified by the inability to reinduce the tachycardia after ablation. If isoproterenol was necessary for induction before ablation, it should be used again during attempts at reinduction to confirm success.

Some ATs originate from the coronary sinus or PVs. Lower energy and temperature settings are used in these vascular structures to minimize the risk for perforation and thrombosis. Before ablation in the coronary sinus, angiography of the arterial system can be helpful to rule out proximity to the coronary arteries. The use of irrigated radiofrequency catheters (<45°C at 20 to 30 W) may reduce the risk for impedance rises within the coronary sinus. Aggressive ablation near the coronary arteries can lead to myocardial infarction. Cryoablation may be a safe alternative to radiofrequency ablation for AT arising in the coronary sinus or near the AV conduction system.[49] In the latter situation, cryoablation may greatly reduce the risk for ablation-induced AV block through the reversible nature of cryomapping. Cryoablation may also be a safer alternative to radiofrequency for ablation in the lateral right atrium in proximity to the phrenic nerve. Before ablation in the area of the phrenic nerve, it is recommended to pace at high output (10 mA) from the ablation catheter. If phrenic nerve stimulation is noted on fluoroscopy, the risk for phrenic nerve injury may be substantial. In this situation, use of cryoablation with

TABLE 11-2
TARGET SITES
Atrial electrogram precedes P-wave onset by at least 15 to 60 msec.
Early fractionated electrograms are present.
Pacing from site produces a surface P wave identical to the P wave of tachycardia.
Earliest site identified by three-dimensional mapping.

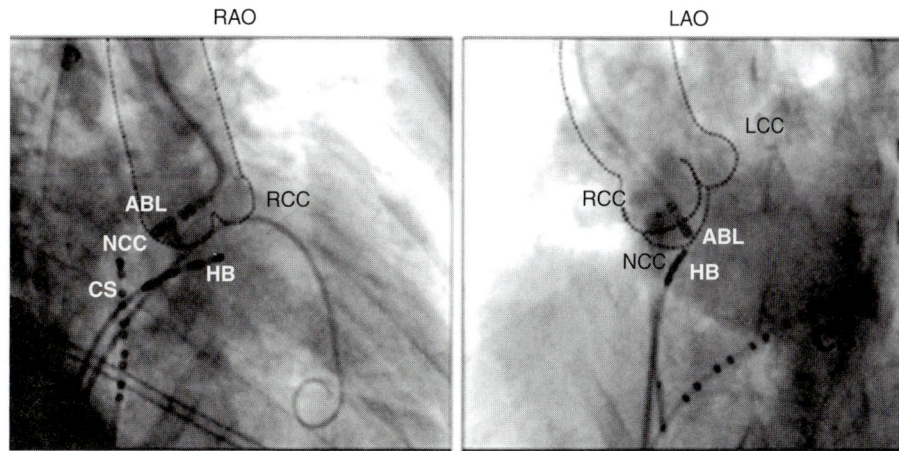

FIGURE 11-9. Left ventriculography to show catheter position for ablation of atrial tachycardia from the noncoronary aortic cusp (NCC). The aortic root is delineated by the *dotted line*. The ablation (ABL) catheter is oriented posteriorly, consistent with the position of the noncoronary cusp. CS, coronary sinus catheter; HB, His bundle catheter; LCC, left coronary cusp; RCC, right coronary cusp. *(Reproduced with permission from Yamada T, Allison JS, McElderry HT et al. Atrial tachycardia initiating atrial fibrillation successfully ablated in the non-coronary cusp of the aorta. J Interv Card Electrophysiol. 2010; 27:123–126. With permission.)*

Right posterior oblique   **Right anterior oblique**

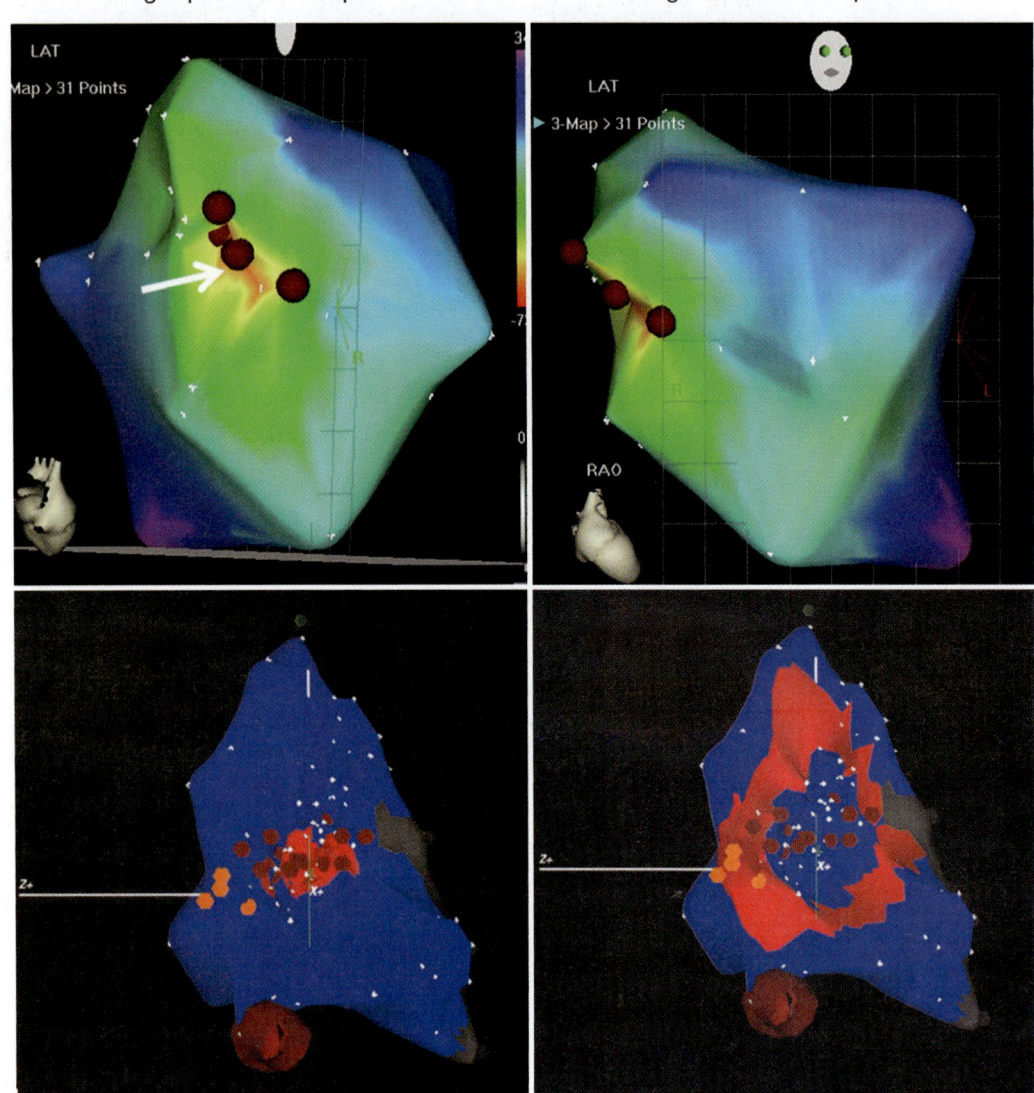

FIGURE 11-10. *Top panels,* Right atrial electroanatomic (Carto) map of a focal atrial tachycardia originating on the posterolateral right atrium in right posterior and right anterior oblique views. The area of earliest activation is shown in *red,* with later activation circumferentially. The site of successful ablation is shown by the *red dot (arrow).* Two additional radiofrequency lesions were given flanking this site. *Bottom panels,* Carto propagation map of atrial tachycardia in another patient. The right lateral view is shown. In the *left panel,* the site of earliest atrial activation is shown. In the *right panel,* the circular concentric wavefront propagates away from the earliest activation.

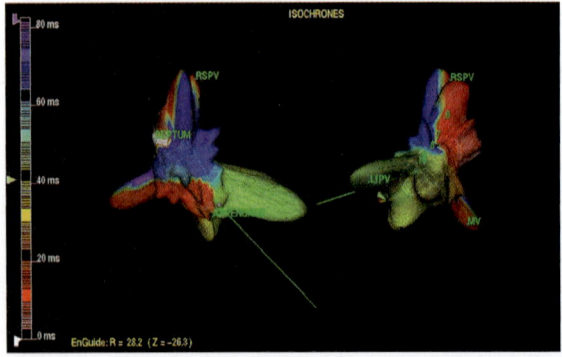

FIGURE 11-11. Endocardial Solutions, Inc. (St. Paul, MN) noncontact activation map of a focal atrial tachycardia originating from the ostium of the right superior pulmonary vein (RSPV). LIPV, left inferior pulmonary vein.

phrenic nerve pacing from a more superior site or displacement of the phrenic nerve away from the atrium using an intrapericardial catheter may be necessary (Fig. 11-12).

ICE (Fig. 11-2) can also help with ablation by localizing anatomic structures, aiding with catheter positioning and catheter-tip contact, and confirming and identifying lesion size and location.[3,50,51] It is particularly useful in helping to guide fine catheter movement between the upper crista terminalis and the right atrial posterior wall opposing the right upper pulmonary vein; in this context, ICE can quickly differentiate a crista terminalis AT from a right upper pulmonary vein AT before a decision for or against transseptal puncture is made. ICE also can help with transseptal puncture in terms of recognizing early complications, such as perforations and clot formation, and with reducing fluoroscopy time.

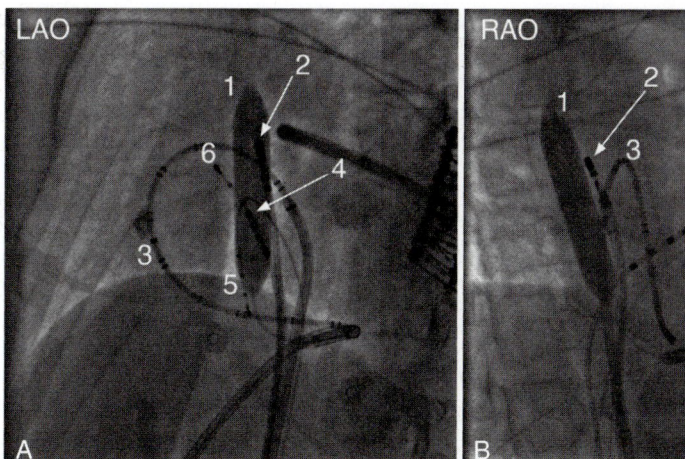

FIGURE 11-12. Displacement of the phrenic nerve from the right atrial wall using an intrapericardial balloon catheter (10 × 40 mm) during ablation of right atrial tachycardia. 1, Balloon catheter; 2, ablation catheter; 3, coronary sinus catheter; 4, His catheter; 5, right ventricular catheter; 6, right atrial catheter. *(From Lee JC, Steven D, Roberts-Thomson KC, et al. Atrial tachycardias adjacent to the phrenic nerve: recognition, potential problems and solutions. Heart Rhythm. 2009;6:1186–1191. With permission)*

Ablation within the aortic cusps may be undertaken with irrigated or nonirrigated catheters. The use of irrigated catheters may minimize the risk for coagulum formation and embolization near the coronary arteries. ICE, aortography, or coronary angiography, or a combination of these, should be used to confirm ablation catheter positions away from coronary artery ostia.

For patients with inappropriate sinus tachycardia, catheter ablation of a portion of the sinus node (sinus node modification) can be offered.[52–54] This technique entails mapping and ablation of a portion of the crista terminalis during isoproterenol infusion. A thorough diagnostic electrophysiologic study must be performed before sinus node modification to rule out another type of tachycardia. Once the diagnosis has been established, a multipolar (20-pole) diagnostic crista terminalis catheter is positioned along the crista terminalis, if possible with ICE guidance to ensure its precise position. The sinus rhythm activation sequence is then analyzed in the crista catheter at baseline and after isoproterenol infusion. A shift of the earliest crista terminalis activation sequence is gradually noted with increased sinus rate. The ablation catheter is then positioned at the more cranial portion of the crista terminalis, and radiofrequency energy is applied in a craniocaudal fashion, again preferably guided by intracardiac ultrasound, along the crista terminalis, shifting the sinus node function and causing a reduction in the sinus rate. This technique has a high acute success rate,[52,53] defined as an increase in the sinus rate cycle length of at least 10%. Others have reported using Carto or EnSite technology to help guide ablation or modification of the sinus node. Although sinus node modification is effective at lowering the sinus rate, the long-term results of symptomatic relief have been at most modest, and this procedure should be considered a measure of last resort.

Catheter ablation for focal ATs has been proved safe and effective,[3,5,8,9,11,19,46,54,55] with reported success rates varying from 77% to 100%. It also has been shown to improve patient quality-of-life scores.[55] Complications are rare and usually reflect the risks of vascular access and intracardiac catheter manipulation. Ablation near the AV node or conduction system may risk heart block. Ablation along the lateral right atrium may damage the phrenic nerve. Therefore, ablation should be indicated for all symptomatic patients who have persistent symptoms despite medical therapy or intolerable side effects from medicines. Patients who are not willing to undergo medical therapy should also be considered.

Troubleshooting the Difficult Case

One of the common problems with ablation of focal ATs is the inability to induce the tachycardia once the patient is in the electrophysiology laboratory. Although the patient may have frequent bouts of tachycardia outside the laboratory, the artificial environment of the laboratory, combined with sedation, may change the milieu enough to make the tachycardia noninducible. Occasionally, the use of high doses of isoproterenol (up to 20 μg/minute) is necessary to induce the tachycardia. Additionally, some ATs are observed during the "washout" phase of isoproterenol. Other adrenergic stimuli, such as norepinephrine or aminophylline, are rarely useful. Minimizing or eliminating sedation may be helpful. For a female patient, scheduling a procedure at a different point in the menstrual cycle may also help.

Sometimes, focal ATs are inducible but not sustained. Occasionally, only one or two beats of the tachycardia can be induced at a time. A nonsustained AT can usually be successfully mapped and ablated with repeated inductions of the nonsustained tachycardia. However, this makes mapping much more time-consuming and painstaking. Pace mapping can be a useful technique in this situation. The EnSite 3D mapping system can also be particularly helpful in this situation because, with even a single beat of tachycardia, it can grossly map and localize the AT origin. If ablation is unsuccessful because the AT was noninducible or nonsustained, it may be necessary to bring the patient back for a repeat procedure at times of frequent tachycardia.

Most difficulties arise from mapping the tachycardia rather than actually ablating a favorable site. If no satisfactory sites are readily apparent in one atrium, mapping of contiguous structures in the other atria should be undertaken. If this is not productive, mapping the coronary sinus, aortic cusps, and atrial appendages should be considered.

Ablation of parahisian ATs, which originate near the AV node or His region, is often difficult and requires careful mapping to avoid ablation-induced complete heart block.

TABLE 11-3

TROUBLESHOOTING THE DIFFICULT CASE

Problem	Causes	Solution
Unable to induce tachycardia	Residual drug effects	Stop antiarrhythmic medicine at least 5 half-lives before the procedure
	Catecholamine dependence	Use isoproterenol, epinephrine
	Sedation	Minimize sedation, hand grip exercise
Tachycardia not sustained long enough for mapping	Characteristic of the tachycardia	Use EnSite three-dimensional mapping
	Catecholamine dependence	High-dose isoproterenol, repeated inductions with multiple roving catheters
Poor catheter stability	Excessive heart motion	Pace during radiofrequency ablation
		Ablate in sinus rhythm
	Poor catheter characteristics	Try alternative catheters or cryoablation
		Use a preformed sheath
Failure despite precise mapping	Poor catheter contact	Adjust catheter
		Try alternative catheters
		Use preformed sheath
	Low temperature or current	High-output or irrigated radiofrequency system
Origin of right-sided focal AT changing with each ablation	Macroreentrant AT	Repeat mapping
	Inappropriate sinus tachycardia	Ablate along crista until tachycardia sinus cycle length increases >10%
AT origin near the AV or His region	Parahisian AT	Map His "cloud" before ablation
		Ablate initially with lower energy and temperature settings
		Use cryoablation
No early atrial sites	Coronary sinus, aortic cusp origin	Map and ablate in coronary sinus, aortic cusps; map "other atrium"

AT, atrial tachycardia; AV, atrioventricular.

Starting ablation with lower energy and temperature settings and stopping immediately if A-H prolongation or heart block occurs may avert permanent damage to the conduction system. Use of a 3D mapping system to create a His cloud can also help delineate areas to avoid ablating. Finally, cryoablation (CryoCath, Montreal, Quebec), which uses cooling to ablate tissue, has been employed successfully to ablate parahisian ATs.[56] Cryoablation allows testing of potential ablation sites by adhering the catheter tip to the target tissue and chilling it to create a reversible electrical effect. If there is no heart block, the catheter tip can be cooled further to create a permanent lesion. Parahisian ATs can also be safely ablated in the noncoronary cusp without the risk for AV block.[57] Damage to the phrenic nerve can be avoided by careful delineation of the location, cryoablation, or displacement of the phrenic nerve.

Troubleshooting difficulties are summarized in Table 11-3.

Conclusion

Advances in the past several years have improved the ability to ablate focal ATs. 3D mapping systems provide a straightforward approach that can identify the origin of focal ATs even if these arrhythmias are unstable or nonsustained. ICE can facilitate mapping and ablation. In addition, 3D mapping of the His cloud and the use of cryoablation have improved the ability to safely ablate parahisian focal ATs. Finally, remote catheter navigation has significantly improved the safety and efficacy of the procedure, including a reduction in fluoroscopy exposure. Although ablation of focal ATs can still be complex and challenging, these advances have allowed safe and successful expansion of the use of curative catheter ablation for these arrhythmias.

References

1. Saoudi N, Cosio F, Waldo A, et al. A classification of atrial flutter and regular atrial tachycardia according to electrophysiological mechanisms and anatomical bases: a Statement from a Joint Expert Group from The Working Group of Arrhythmias of the European Society of Cardiology and the North American Society of Pacing and Electrophysiology. *Eur Heart J*. 2001;22:1162–1182.
2. Hu YF, Higa S, Huang JL, et al. Electrophysiologic characteristics and catheter ablation of focal atrial tachycardia with more than one focus. *Heart Rhythm*. 2009;6:198–203.
3. Kalman JM, Olgin JE, Karch MR, et al. "Cristal tachycardias": origin of right atrial tachycardias from the crista terminalis identified by intracardiac echocardiography. *J Am Coll Cardiol*. 1998;31:451–459.
4. Callans DJ, Schwartzman D, Gottlieb CD, Marchlinski FE. Insights into the electrophysiology of atrial arrhythmias gained by the catheter ablation experience: "learning while burning, part II". *J Cardiovasc Electrophysiol*. 1995;6:229–243.
5. Pappone C, Stabile G, De Simone A, et al. Role of catheter-induced mechanical trauma in localization of target sites of radiofrequency ablation in automatic atrial tachycardia. *J Am Coll Cardiol*. 1996;27:1090–1097.
6. Chen SA, Chiang CE, Yang CJ, et al. Radiofrequency catheter ablation of sustained intra-atrial reentrant tachycardia in adult patients: identification of electrophysiological characteristics and endocardial mapping techniques. *Circulation*. 1993;88:578–587.
7. Walsh EP, Saul JP, Hulse JE, et al. Transcatheter ablation of ectopic atrial tachycardia in young patients using radiofrequency current [see comments]. *Circulation*. 1992;86:1138–1146.
8. Kay GN, Chong F, Epstein AE, et al. Radiofrequency ablation for treatment of primary atrial tachycardias [see comments]. *J Am Coll Cardiol*. 1993;21:901–909.
9. Tang CW, Scheinman MM, Van Hare GF, et al. Use of P wave configuration during atrial tachycardia to predict site of origin. *J Am Coll Cardiol*. 1995;26:1315–1324.
10. Jais P, Shah DC, Haissaguerre M, et al. Atrial fibrillation: role of arrhythmogenic foci. *J Interv Card Electrophysiol*. 2000;4(suppl 1):29–37.
11. Lesh MD, Van Hare GF, Epstein LM, et al. Radiofrequency catheter ablation of atrial arrhythmias: results and mechanisms. *Circulation*. 1994;89:1074–1089.
12. Badhwar N, Kalman JM, Sparks PB, et al. Atrial tachycardia arising from the coronary sinus musculature: electrophysiological characteristics and long-term outcomes of radiofrequency ablation. *J Am Coll Cardiol*. 2005;46:1921–1930.
13. Kistler PM, Fynn SP, Haqqani H, et al. Focal atrial tachycardia from the ostium of the coronary sinus: electrocardiographic and electrophysiological characterization and radiofrequency ablation. *J Am Coll Cardiol*. 2005;45:1488–1493.
14. Iesaka Y, Takahashi A, Goya M, et al. Adenosine-sensitive atrial reentrant tachycardia originating from the atrioventricular nodal transitional area. *J Cardiovasc Electrophysiol*. 1997;8:854–864.
15. Roberts-Thomson KC, Kistler PM, Haqqani HM, et al. Focal atrial tachycardias arising from the right atrial appendage: electrocardiographic and electrophysiologic characteristics and radiofrequency ablation. *J Cardiovasc Electrophysiol*. 2007;18:367–372.

16. Yamada T, Murakami Y, Yoshida Y, et al. Electrophysiologic and electro-cardiographic characteristics and radiofrequency catheter ablation of focal atrial tachycardia originating from the left atrial appendage. *Heart Rhythm.* 2007;4:1284–1291.
17. Morton JB, Sanders P, Das A, et al. Focal atrial tachycardia arising from the tricuspid annulus: electrophysiologic and electrocardiographic characteristics. *J Cardiovasc Electrophysiol.* 2001;12:653–659.
18. Kistler PM, Sanders P, Hussin A, et al. Focal atrial tachycardia arising from the mitral annulus: electrocardiographic and electrophysiologic characterization. *J Am Coll Cardiol.* 2003;41:2212–2219.
19. Chen SA, Tai CT, Chiang CE, et al. Focal atrial tachycardia: reanalysis of the clinical and electrophysiologic characteristics and prediction of successful radiofrequency ablation. *J Cardiovasc Electrophysiol.* 1998;9:355–365.
20. Steinbeck G, Hoffmann E. "True" atrial tachycardia. *Eur Heart J.* 1998;19(suppl E): E10–E12, E48–E49.
21. Engelstein ED, Lippman N, Stein KM, Lerman BB. Mechanism-specific effects of adenosine on atrial tachycardia. *Circulation.* 1994;89:2645–2654.
22. Rosen MR. Cellular electrophysiology of digitalis toxicity. *J Am Coll Cardiol.* 1985;5:22A–34A.
23. Iwai S, Markowitz SM, Stein KM, et al. Response to adenosine differentiates focal from macroreentrant atrial tachycardia: validation using three-dimensional electroanatomic mapping. *Circulation.* 2002;106:2793–2799.
24. Markowitz SM, Nemirovksy D, Stein KM, et al. Adenosine-insensitive focal atrial tachycardia: evidence for de novo micro-re-entry in the human atrium. *J Am Coll Cardiol.* 2007;49:1324–1333.
25. Coumel P, Escoubet B, Attuel P. Beta-blocking therapy in atrial and ventricular tachyarrhythmias: experience with nadolol. *Am Heart J.* 1984;108:1098–1108.
26. Chen SA, Chiang CE, Yang CJ, et al. Sustained atrial tachycardia in adult patients: electrophysiological characteristics, pharmacological response, possible mechanisms, and effects of radiofrequency ablation [see comments]. *Circulation.* 1994;90:1262–1278.
27. Morillo CA, Klein GJ, Thakur RK, et al. Mechanism of "inappropriate" sinus tachycardia: role of sympathovagal balance. *Circulation.* 1994;90:873–877.
28. Bauernfeind RA, Amat YLF, Dhingra RC, et al. Chronic nonparoxysmal sinus tachycardia in otherwise healthy persons. *Ann Intern Med.* 1979;91:702–710.
29. Lowe JE, Hartwich T, Takla M, Schaper J. Ultrastructure of electro-physiologically identified human sinoatrial nodes. *Basic Res Cardiol.* 1988;83:401–409.
30. Lee RJ, Kalman JM, Fitzpatrick AP, et al. Radiofrequency catheter modi-fication of the sinus node for "inappropriate" sinus tachycardia. *Circulation.* 1995;92:2919–2928.
31. Krahn AD, Yee R, Klein GJ, Morillo C. Inappropriate sinus tachycardia: evalu-ation and therapy. *J Cardiovasc Electrophysiol.* 1995;6:1124–1128.
32. Krahn AD, Yee R, Klein GJ, Morillo C. Inappropriate sinus tachycardia: evalu-ation and therapy. *J Cardiovasc Electrophysiol.* 1995;6:1124–1128.
33. Shinbane JS, Wood MA, Jensen DN, et al. Tachycardia-induced cardio-myopathy: a review of animal models and clinical studies. *J Am Coll Cardiol.* 1997;29:709–715.
34. Medi C, Kalman JM, Haqqani H, et al. Tachycardia-mediated cardiomyopathy secondary to focal atrial tachycardia: long-term outcome after catheter ablation. *J Am Coll Cardiol.* 2009;53:1791–1797.
35. Kistler PM, Roberts-Thomson KC, Haqqani HM, et al. P-wave morphology in focal atrial tachycardia: development of an algorithm to predict the anatomic site of origin. *J Am Coll Cardiol.* 2006;48:1010–1017.
36. Tada H, Nogami A, Naito S, et al. Simple electrocardiographic criteria for identi-fying the site of origin of focal right atrial tachycardia. *Pacing Clin Electrophysiol.* 1998;21:2431–2439.
37. Kistler PM, Sanders P, Fynn SP, et al. Electrophysiological and electrocardio-graphic characteristics of focal atrial tachycardia originating from the pulmonary

38. veins: acute and long-term outcomes of radiofrequency ablation. *Circulation.* 2003;108:1968–1975.
38. Man KC, Chan KK, Kovack P, et al. Spatial resolution of atrial pace map-ping as determined by unipolar atrial pacing at adjacent sites. *Circulation.* 1996;94:1357–1363.
39. Kalbfleisch SJ, el-Atassi R, Calkins H, et al. Differentiation of paroxysmal nar-row QRS complex tachycardias using the 12-lead electrocardiogram. *J Am Coll Cardiol.* 1993;21:85–89.
40. Miller JM, Rosenthal ME, Vassallo JA, Josephson ME. Atrioventricular nodal reentrant tachycardia: studies on upper and lower common pathways. *Circulation.* 1987;75:930–940.
41. Knight BP, Ebinger M, Oral H, et al. Diagnostic value of tachycardia features and pacing maneuvers during paroxysmal supraventricular tachycardia. *J Am Coll Cardiol.* 2000;36:574–582.
42. Sarkozy A, Richter S, Chierchia GB, et al. A novel pacing manoeuvre to diag-nose atrial tachycardia. *Europace.* 2008;10:459–466.
43. Man KC, Niebauer M, Daoud E, et al. Comparison of atrial-His intervals during tachycardia and atrial pacing in patients with long RP tachycardia. *J Cardiovasc Electrophysiol.* 1995;6:700–710.
44. Glatter KA, Cheng J, Dorostkar P, et al. Electrophysiologic effects of adenosine in patients with supraventricular tachycardia. *Circulation.* 1999;99:1034–1040.
45. Ashar MS, Pennington J, Callans DJ, Marchlinski FE. Localization of arrhythmogenic triggers of atrial fibrillation. *J Cardiovasc Electrophysiol.* 2000;11:1300–1305.
46. Sulieman M, Asarvatham SJ. Ablation above the semilunar valves: when, why and how? Part II. *Heart Rhythm.* 2008;5:1625–1630.
47. Tracy CM, Swartz JF, Fletcher RD, et al. Radiofrequency catheter ablation of ectopic atrial tachycardia using paced activation sequence mapping [see com-ments]. *J Am Coll Cardiol.* 1993;21:910–917.
48. Hoffmann E, Nimmermann P, Reithmann C, et al. New mapping technology for atrial tachycardias. *J Interv Card Electrophysiol.* 2000;4(suppl 1):117–120.
49. Bastani H, Insulander P, Schwieler J, et al. Safety and efficacy of cryoabla-tion of atrial tachycardia with a high risk of ablation-related injuries. *Europace.* 2009;11:625–629.
50. Lee JC, Steven D, Roberts-Thomson KC, et al. Atrial tachycardias adjacent to the phrenic nerve: recognition, potential problems and solutions. *Heart Rhythm.* 2009;6:1186–1191.
51. Chu E, Kalman JM, Kwasman MA, et al. Intracardiac echocardiography during radiofrequency catheter ablation of cardiac arrhythmias in humans. *J Am Coll Cardiol.* 1994;24:1351–1357.
52. Lesh MD, Kalman JM, Karch MR. Use of intracardiac echocardiography dur-ing electrophysiologic evaluation and therapy of atrial arrhythmias. *J Cardiovasc Electrophysiol.* 1998;9:S40–S47.
53. Lee RJ, Kalman JM, Fitzpatrick AP, et al. Radiofrequency catheter modi-fication of the sinus node for "inappropriate" sinus tachycardia. *Circulation.* 1995;92:2919–2928.
54. Kalman JM, Lee RJ, Fisher WG, et al. Radiofrequency catheter modification of sinus pacemaker function guided by intracardiac echocardiography. *Circulation.* 1995;92:3070–3081.
55. Feld GK. Catheter ablation for the treatment of atrial tachycardia. *Prog Cardiovasc Dis.* 1995;37:205–224.
56. Poty H, Saoudi N, Haissaguerre M, et al. Radiofrequency catheter ablation of atrial tachycardias. *Am Heart J.* 1996;131:481–489.
57. Wong T, Markides V, Peters NS, Davies DW. Clinical usefulness of cryo-mapping for ablation of tachycardias involving perinodal tissue. *J Interv Card Electrophysiol.* 2004;10:153–158.
58. Ouyang F, Ma J, Ho SY, et al. Focal atrial tachycardia originating from the non-coronary aortic sinus: electrophysiological characteristics and catheter ablation. *J Am Coll Cardiol.* 2006;48:122–131.

Ablation of Cavotricuspid Isthmus–Dependent Atrial Flutters

Gregory K. Feld, Uma Srivatsa, and Bobbi Hoppe

Key points

The mechanism of isthmus-dependent atrial flutter is a macro-reentrant circuit around the tricuspid valve (TV) annulus.

The diagnosis is confirmed by demonstration of concealed entrainment from the cavotricuspid isthmus (CTI) or by multielectrode catheter or computerized activation mapping.

The ablation target is the CTI between the TV annulus and the inferior vena cava (IVC).

Special equipment that may be used includes a large-tip catheter with a high-power radiofrequency generator or irrigated ablation catheters and a large-curve catheter with or without preformed sheaths. Electroanatomic or noncontact three-dimensional mapping systems and a multielectrode halo catheter are often useful.

Sources of difficulty may include complex anatomy and topography of the CTI area and failure to achieve isthmus block despite extensive ablation.

Acute success rates range from 90% to 95%, with a 5% to 8% recurrence rate using large-tip or irrigated cathers.

Type 1 (or typical) atrial flutter (AFL) is a common atrial arrhythmia, often occurring in association with atrial fibrillation, that can cause significant symptoms and serious adverse effects, including embolic stroke, myocardial ischemia and infarction, and, rarely, a tachycardia-induced cardiomyopathy resulting from rapid atrioventricular (AV) conduction. The electrophysiologic substrate underlying type 1 AFL has been shown to be a combination of slow conduction velocity in the cavotricuspid isthmus (CTI) and anatomic or functional conduction block along the crista terminalis

and eustachian ridge. This electrophysiologic milieu produces a long enough reentrant path length, relative to the average tissue wavelength around the tricuspid valve (TV) annulus, to allow for sustained reentry. The triggers of AFL may include premature atrial contractions or nonsustained episodes of atrial fibrillation, which originate most commonly in the left atrium and pulmonary veins, respectively, and most likely account for the fact that counterclockwise AFL occurs most frequently clinically. Type 1 AFL is also relatively resistant to pharmacologic suppression.

As a result of the well-defined anatomic substrate and the pharmacologic resistance of type 1 AFL, radiofrequency (RF) catheter ablation has emerged in the past decade as a safe and effective first-line treatment. Although several procedures have been described for ablating type 1 AFL, the most widely accepted and successful technique is an anatomically guided approach targeting the CTI. Recent technologic developments, including three-dimensional (3D) electroanatomic contact and noncontact mapping and the use of large-tip ablation electrode catheters with high-power generators, have produced almost uniform efficacy without increased risk. This chapter reviews the electrophysiology of human type 1 AFL and techniques currently employed for its diagnosis, mapping, and ablation.

Atrial Flutter Terminology

Because of the variety of terms used to describe AFL in humans, including type 1 and type 2 AFL, typical and atypical AFL, counterclockwise (CCW) and clockwise (CW) AFL, and isthmus-dependent and non–isthmus-dependent AFL, the Working Group of Arrhythmias of the European Society of Cardiology and the North American Society of Pacing and Electrophysiology convened and published a consensus document in 2001 in an attempt to develop a generally accepted standardized terminology for AFL.[1] The consensus was that the widely accepted terms "typical" and "type 1" AFL were most commonly used to describe macro-reentrant right atrial tachycardia, using the CTI, in either a CCW or a CW direction as visualized from a left anterior oblique perspective. Therefore, the consensus terminology derived from this working group to describe CTI-dependent, right atrial macro-reentry tachycardia in the CCW direction as "typical" AFL, and a similar tachycardia in the CW direction as "reverse typical" AFL.[1] For the purposes of this book, these two arrhythmias are referred to specifically as *typical* and *reverse typical* AFL when being individually described, but as *type 1* AFL when being referred to jointly. Other isthmus-dependent flutters, including lower loop reentry and partial isthmus-dependent flutter, are also discussed in this chapter.

Anatomy and Pathophysiology

The development of successful RF catheter ablation techniques for human type 1 AFL depended in part on the delineation of its electrophysiologic mechanism. By using advanced electrophysiologic techniques, including intraoperative and transcatheter activation mapping,[2–7] type 1 AFL was determined to be caused by a macro-reentrant circuit rotating in either a CCW (typical) or a CW (reverse typical) direction in the right atrium around the TV annulus, with an area of relatively slow conduction velocity in the low posterior right atrium (Figs. 12-1 and 12-2). The predominant area of slow conduction in the AFL reentry circuit has been shown to be in the CTI, through which conduction times may reach 80 to 100 milliseconds, accounting for one third to one half of the AFL cycle length.[8–10]

The CTI is the target for ablation and warrants special attention. The CTI refers to the quadrilateral portion of the inferior right atrial myocardium between the tricuspid valve and inferior vena cava. In attitudinal orientation, the CTI courses from inferior and lateral to posterior and medial in the low right atrium. Specifically, the CTI is anatomically bounded by the inferior vena cava (IVC) and eustachian ridge posteriorly and by the TV annulus anteriorly (Figs. 12-1 and 12-2). These boundaries form lines of conduction block delineating a protected zone of slow conduction in the reentry circuit.[11–14] The presence of conduction block along the eustachian ridge[11–14] has been confirmed by the demonstration of double potentials along its length during AFL (Fig. 12-3). The superomedial boundary of the CTI is the line between the septal insertion of the eustachian ridge and the most inferior paraseptal insertion of the tricuspid valve (i.e., the base of the triangle of Koch).[15,16] The inferolateral border of the CTI comprises the final ramifications of the pectinate muscles of the crista terminalis, but a precise lateral boundary is not well defined. In attitudinal orientation, the portion of the CTI adjacent to the tricuspid annulus is anterior and sometimes referred to as the *vestibular portion* of the CTI. The portion of the CTI that is adjacent to the IVC is attitudinally posterior and referred to as the *membranous* CTI. The middle portion of the CTI is referred to as the *trabeculated* CTI.[15]

The anatomy of the CTI can be assessed by computed tomography (CT) or magnetic resonance imaging (MRI) before ablation or by angiography, electroanatomic mapping, or echocardiography intraoperatively.[17–19] The CTI is typically 34 ± 5 mm in length when measured angiographically from the IVC to the TV. The CTI is usually subdivided into three sections: septal isthmus, central isthmus, and lateral isthmus (Figs. 12-1 and 12-2).[15,19] In the electrophysiology laboratory, the septal isthmus is defined as that portion between 4 and 5 o'clock when visualized in

the left anterior oblique (LAO) projection fluoroscopically. The central isthmus is that portion located at 6 o'clock, and the lateral isthmus is that starting at 7 o'clock.[15] The central isthmus (6 o'clock) marks the shortest distance between the IVC and tricuspid annulus (19 ± 4 mm, range 13 to 26 mm).[15] In addition, the central isthmus is the thinnest portion, ranging from an average of 3.5 mm near the tricuspid valve to 0.8 mm in the middle portion.[15] The (anterior or vestibular) section of the CTI adjacent to the tricuspid valve is entirely muscular, whereas the posterior portion closest to the inferior vena cava is primarily fibro-fatty tissue.[15] The muscle thickness is least in the central isthmus, greatest at the septal isthmus, and intermediate in the lateral isthmus.[15]

The anatomy of the CTI is highly variable but usually classified into three categories. A flat CTI shows 2 mm or less inferior concavity between the IVC and tricuspid valve and is found in about 28% of patients.[18,19] A concave CTI with inferior concavity more than 2 mm in depth is found in about 20% of patients. In these, the average depth is 3.7 ± 0.8 mm.[19] In up to 83% of patients, the CTI shows a distinct inferior pouch (subeustachian pouch or sinus of Keith) averaging 6.5 ± 2.2 mm in depth but up to 12.4 mm deep (Fig. 12-1 and 12-2).[15–19] The pouch is separated from the tricuspid valve by a smooth vestibular area (Figs. 12-1 and 12-2).[19] The pouch itself may be symmetrical or asymmetrical, with extension toward the atrial septum. In anatomic studies, pouches are confined to the medial or septal CTI but are not seen in the lateral third of the CTI.[20] Other notable anatomic features influencing the ablation of AFL are the presence of a prominent muscular eustachian ridge in about 26% of patients and the extension of pectinate muscles into the CTI in 70% of patients and even into the coronary sinus in 7%.[20] The thickness of the pectinate muscles is greatest laterally and diminishes toward the atrial septum. The presence of pectinate muscles into the CTI may be suggested by recording high voltage electrograms from this area.[20] In autopsy specimens, CTI pectinate muscle extensions and CTI pouches tend to occur together.[20]

The crista terminalis forms another important boundary for type I AFL. The crista leaves the superior right atrial septum to course anterior to the os of the superior vena cava, then descends the posterolateral right atrial free wall. Inferiorly, the crista runs anterior to the inferior vena cava and continues medially in CTI to form the eustachian ridge. Double potentials have also been recorded along the crista terminalis,[11–14] suggesting that it too forms a line of block separating the smooth septal right atrium from the trabeculated right atrial free wall (Fig. 12-3). Such lines of block, which may be either functional or anatomic, are necessary for an adequate path length for reentry to be sustained, even in the presence of an area of slow conduction, and to prevent short-circuiting of the reentrant wavefront.[12–14,21] Thus, during typical AFL, the activation wavefront exits the medial CTI, ascends the atrial septum (possibly bounded posteriorly by the foramen ovale), and then descends the lateral right atrium between the crista terminalis posteriorly and the tricuspid valve anteriorly. Entry of the wavefront into the lateral CTI completes the circuit.[12–14,21]

The medial and lateral CTI, which are contiguous, respectively, with the interatrial septum near the coronary sinus (CS) ostium and with the low lateral right atrium

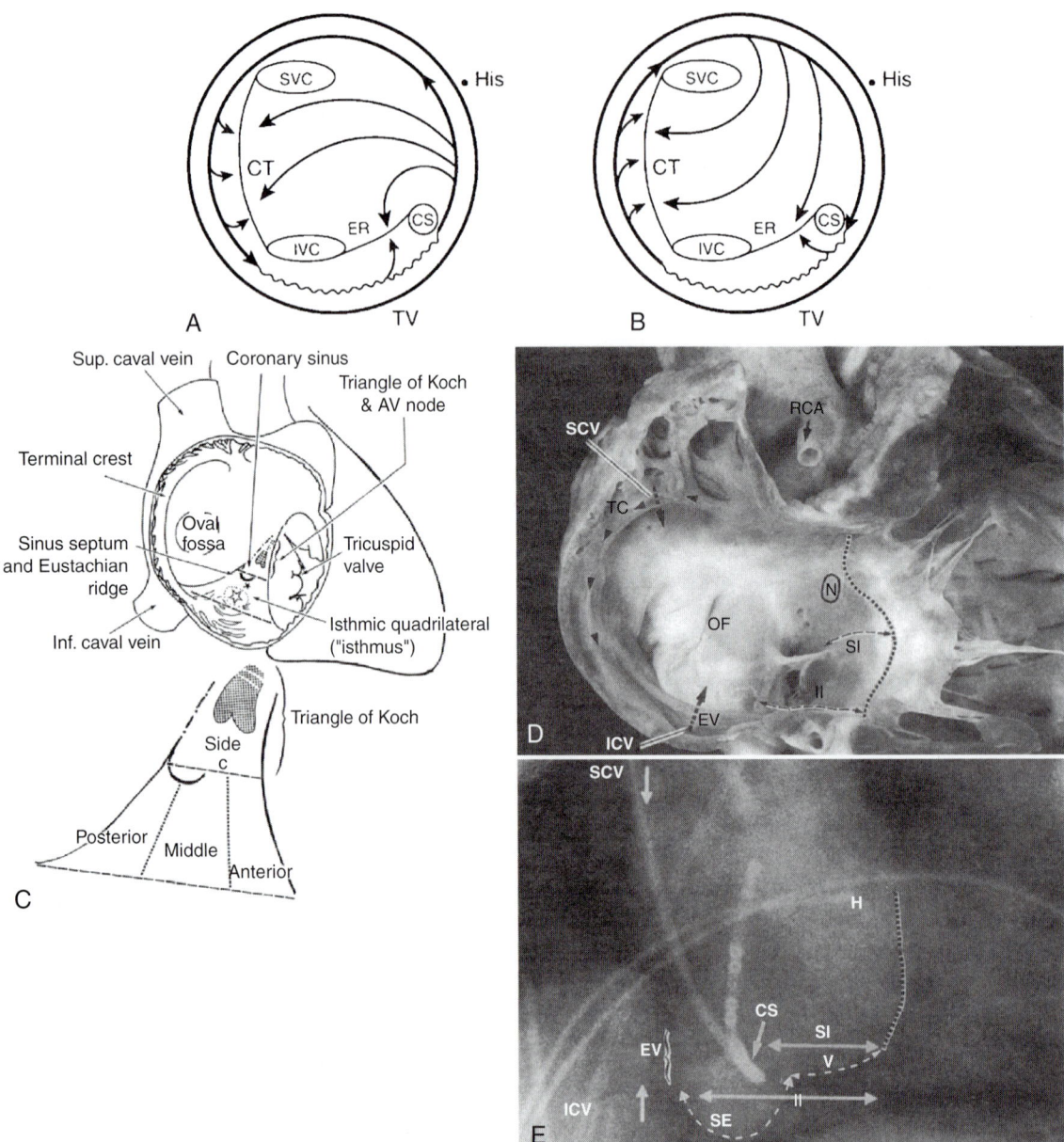

FIGURE 12-1. **A** and **B,** Schematic diagrams showing the activation patterns of human type 1 atrial flutter (AFL), as viewed from below the tricuspid valve (TV) annulus, looking up into the right atrium. In the typical form of AFL (**A**), the reentrant wavefront rotates counterclockwise in the right atrium, but in the reverse typical form (**B**), reentry is clockwise. Note that the eustachian ridge (ER) and crista terminalis (CT) form lines of block and that an area of slow conduction (*wavy line*) is present in the isthmus between the inferior vena cava (IVC) and ER and the TV annulus. CS, coronary sinus ostium; His, His bundle; SVC, superior vena cava. **C** through **E,** Anatomy of the cavotricuspid isthmus area. The schematic diagram of the right atrium (**C**) shows the cavotricuspid isthmus (*expanded insert*), which is posterior and inferior to the triangle of Koch. **D,** Pathologic specimen showing the heart in right anterior oblique (RAO) view. The hinge of the TV is shown by the *dotted line.* Note the complex anatomy along the inferior isthmus line, with a fenestrated thebesian valve present. SI, septal isthmus line; II, inferior isthmus; EV, eustachian valve; OF, foramen ovale; N, AV nodal area; SVC, superior vena cava. **E,** RAO angiogram of the isthmus. A pouchlike subeustachian sinus (SE) is seen adjacent to the vestibule region of the isthmus (V). H, His catheter. *(From Cabrera JA, Sanchez-Quintana D, Ho SY, et al. The architecture of the atrial musculature between the orifice of the inferior caval vein and the tricuspid valve: the anatomy of the isthmus. J Cardiovasc Electrophysiol. 1998;9:1186–1195. With permission.)*

near the IVC (Figs. 12-1 and 12-2), correspond electrophysiologically to the exit and entrance to the zone of slow conduction, depending on whether the direction of reentry is CCW or CW in the right atrium.[2–15] The slower conduction velocity in the CTI, relative to the interatrial septum and right atrial free wall, may be caused by anisotropic fiber orientation in the CTI.[7–10,22,23] This may also predispose to

the development of unidirectional block during rapid atrial pacing, accounting for the observation that typical (CCW) AFL is more likely to be induced when pacing is performed from the CS ostium, and reverse typical (CW) AFL when pacing is from the low lateral right atrium.[24]

Lower loop reentry is an isthmus-dependent flutter in which the caudal-to-cranial limb of the wavefront crosses

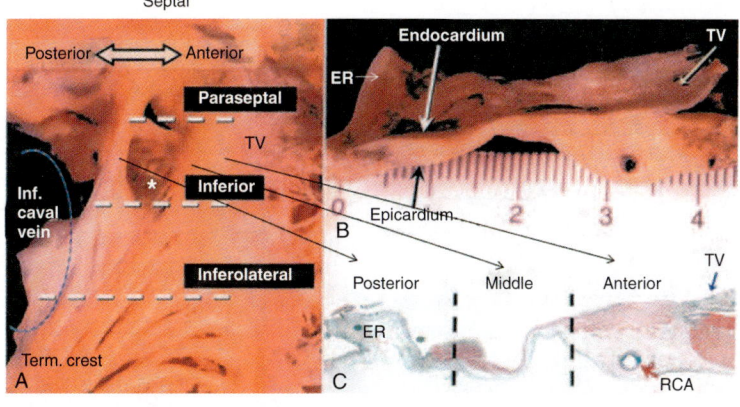

FIGURE 12-2. A, The endocardial surface of the right atrial isthmus is displayed to show the three levels. Note the pouch at the central isthmus and the distal ramifications of the terminal (Term.) crest that feed into the inferolateral isthmus. **B** and **C,** The isthmus viewed in profile. The histologic section shows myocardium in *red* and fibrous tissue in *blue*. The anterior sector corresponds to the vestibule leading to the tricuspid valve (TV) and is related to the right coronary artery (RCA). The posterior sector is closest to the orifice of the inferior caval vein and contains the eustachian valve or ridge (ER) (Masson trichrome stain). *(From Cabrera JA. The inferior right atrial isthmus: further architectural insights for current and coming ablation technologies.* J Cardiovasc Electrophysiol. *2005;16:402–408. With permission.)*

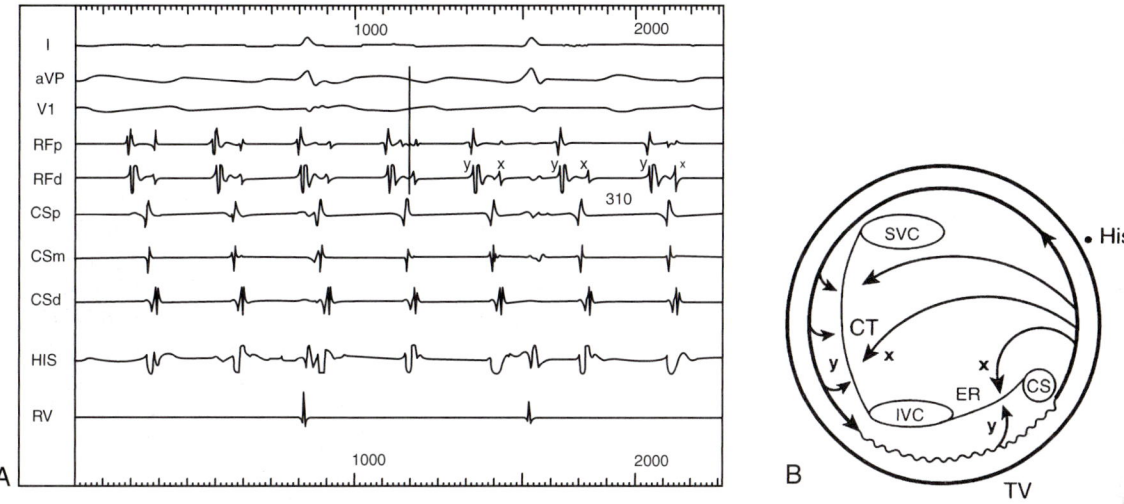

FIGURE 12-3. A, Surface electrocardiographic leads I, aVF, and V₁ and endocardial electrograms in a patient with typical atrial flutter (AFL) demonstrating double potentials (*xy*) recorded along the eustachian ridge (ER) by the ablation catheter (RFd and RFp). Note that the *x* and *y* potentials straddle the onset of the initial downstroke of the F wave in lead aVF *(vertical line)*, indicating that the *x* potential is recorded immediately after the activation wavefront exits the subeustachian isthmus and circulates around the coronary sinus above the ER. The *y* potential is recorded after the activation wavefront has rotated entirely around the atrium and is proceeding through the subeustachian isthmus below the ER. Double potentials may similarly be recorded along the crista terminalis (CT). **B,** A schematic diagram of the right atrium indicates where such double potentials (*xy*) may be recorded along the ER and CT during typical AFL. CSp, CSm, and CSd are electrograms recorded, respectively, from the proximal, middle, and distal electrode pairs on a quadripolar catheter in the coronary sinus (CS) with the proximal pair at the ostium. His, electrogram from the His bundle catheter; IVC, inferior vena cava; RFp and RFd, electrograms from the proximal and distal electrode pairs of the mapping and ablation catheter with the distal pair positioned on the ER; RV, right ventricle electrogram; SVC, superior vena cava; TV, tricuspid valve.

over gaps in the crista terminalis in the inferior to middle right atrium (Fig. 12-4).[25,26] The circuit is essentially around the ostium of the inferior vena cava in the right atrium. The direction of rotation may be CW or CCW. This variant activation sequence may be sustained, or it may interconvert with other forms of AFL.

Partial isthmus flutter is another variant in which the CCW reentrant wavefront "short circuits" through the eustachian ridge barrier to pass between the IVC and the CS ostium (Fig. 12-4).[25] The wavefront then propagates in a CW direction through the medial end of the CTI to collide with the wavefront that is also conducting through the isthmus from its lateral aspect.

Diagnosis

Surface Electrocardiography

The surface 12-lead electrocardiogram (ECG) is helpful in establishing a diagnosis of type 1 AFL, particularly the typical form (Table 12-1). In typical AFL, an inverted sawtooth F-wave pattern is observed in the inferior ECG leads II, III, and aVF, with low-amplitude biphasic F waves in leads I and aVL, an upright F wave in precordial lead V₁, and an inverted F wave in lead V₆ (Fig. 12-5A). In contrast, in reverse typical AFL, the F-wave pattern on the 12-lead ECG is less specific and variable, often with a sine wave pattern in the inferior ECG leads (Fig. 12-5B).

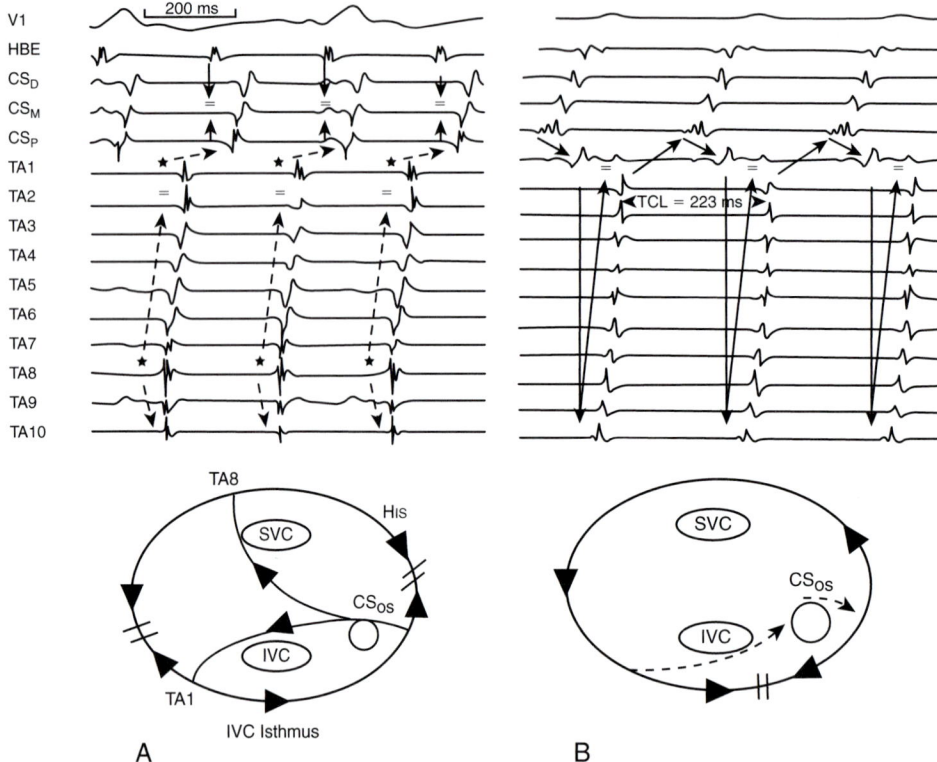

FIGURE 12-4. Electrograms and schematic representation of atrial activation in lower loop reentry and partial isthmus-dependent flutter. **A,** In lower loop reentry, the posterior right atrium is part of the reentry circuit around the inferior vena cava, and wavefronts collide in the lateral right atrium. The electrograms show multiple collisions at recording sites on the lateral right atrial wall TA1 and TA8 *(stars)*. **B,** In partial isthmus-dependent flutter, the wavefront bypasses the anterior cavotricuspid isthmus (CTI) near to the tricuspid valve by passing through the eustachian ridge posterior to the coronary sinus os (CS$_{os}$). The coronary sinus ostium is activated prematurely, and the tachycardia is not entrained from the medial CTI itself. IVC, inferior vena cava; SVC, superior vena cava; TA10, proximal recording electrodes on halo catheter near upper septum; TA1, distal recording electrodes on Halo catheter near lateral aspect of the CTI. *(From Yang Y, Cheng J, Bochoeyer A, et al. Atypical right atrial flutter patterns. Circulation. 2001;103:3092–3098. With permission.)*

TABLE 12-1	
DIAGNOSTIC CRITERIA FOR ISTHMUS-DEPENDENT FLUTTERS	
Type of Flutter	**Criteria**
Surface ECG	
Typical flutter	Saw-tooth inverted F-wave pattern in the inferior ECG leads and upright in V$_1$
Reverse typical flutter	Sine wave or upright F-wave pattern in the inferior ECG leads
Lower loop reentry	Variable; often resembles typical flutter if counterclockwise; clockwise rotation usually yields upright F waves inferiorly and inverted in V$_1$
Partial isthmus-dependent flutter	Poorly described; probably similar to typical flutter
Electrophysiologic Testing	
Isthmus-dependent flutters	Demonstration of entrainment criteria during pacing from the CTI, including the following: First postpacing interval <30 msec longer than tachycardia cycle length Interval of stimulus to F wave equal to interval of electrogram to F wave interval on pacing catheter Identical paced F-wave morphology and atrial activation sequence Macro-reentrant RA activation by standard activation or electroanatomic mapping with entire tachycardia cycle length represented in right atrium
Typical flutter	Concealed entrainment from CTI and counterclockwise macroreentrant RA activation
Reverse typical flutter	Concealed entrainment from CTI and clockwise macro-reentrant RA activation
Lower loop reentry	Concealed entrainment from both CTI *and* low posterior right atrium with clockwise or counterclockwise macro-reentrant RA activation
Partial isthmus-dependent flutter	Concealed entrainment from lateral but *not* medial margin of CTI; early coronary sinus ostium activation during flutter; wavefront collision in CTI; counterclockwise macro-reentrant RA activation

CTI, cavotricuspid isthmus; ECG, electrocardiogram; RA, right atrial.

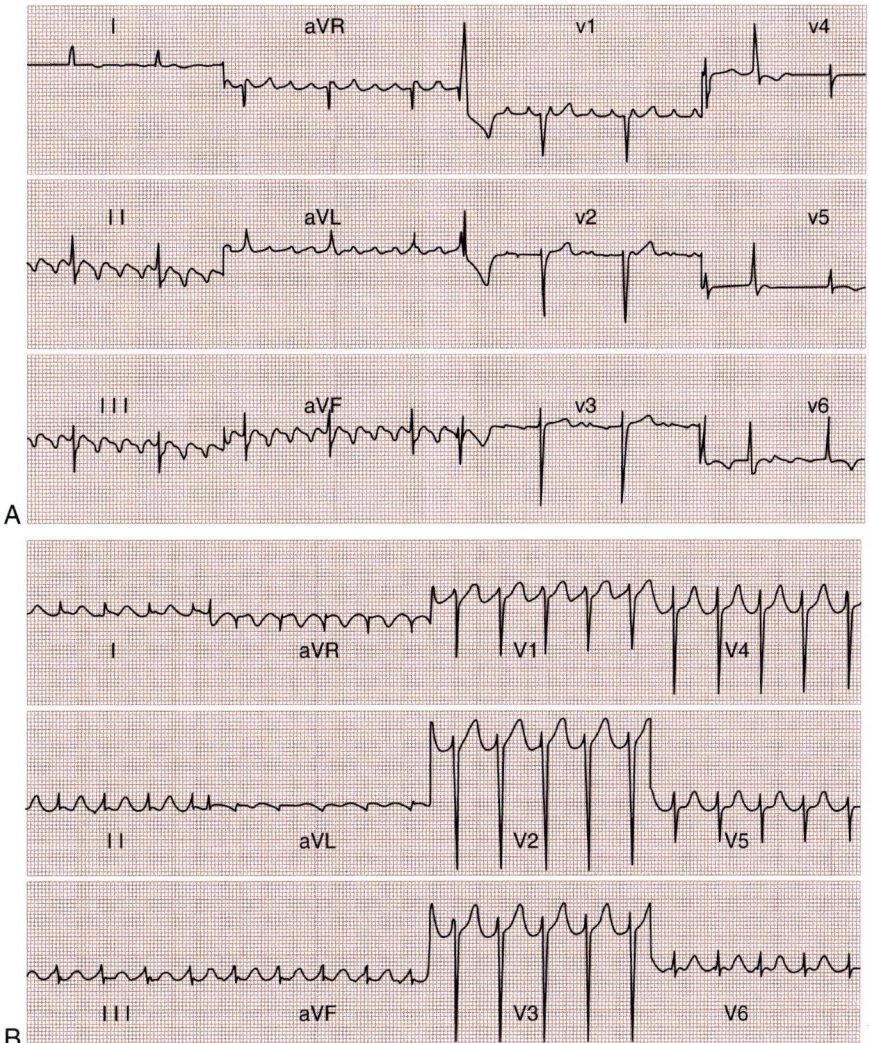

FIGURE 12-5. A, A 12-lead electrocardiogram recorded from a patient with typical atrial flutter (AFL). Note the typical sawtooth pattern of inverted F waves in the inferior leads II, III, and aVF. Typical AFL is also characterized by flat to biphasic F waves in I and aVL, respectively; an upright F wave in V_1; and an inverted F wave in V_6. **B,** A 12-lead electrocardiogram from a patient with the reverse typical AFL. The F wave in the reverse typical form of AFL has a less distinct sine wave pattern in the inferior leads. In this case, the F waves are upright in the inferior leads II, III, and aVF; biphasic in leads I, aVL, and V_1; and upright in V_6.

The determinants of F-wave pattern on ECG are largely dependent on the activation pattern of the left atrium, resulting from reentry in the right atrium. Inverted F waves are inscribed in the inferior ECG leads in typical AFL as a result of activation of the left atrium initially posterior, near the CS, and upright F waves are inscribed in the inferior ECG leads in reverse typical AFL as a result of activation of the left atrium initially anterior, near the Bachmann bundle.[27,28] However, because the typical and reverse-typical forms of type 1 AFL use the same reentry circuit, but in opposite directions, their rates are usually similar. It should be noted that the ECG presentation of typical AFL can be dramatically altered by extensive ablation in the left atrium, as with atrial fibrillation ablation procedures.[29]

The ECG presentation of lower loop reentry is highly variable, depending on the caudal-to-cranial level of wavefront breakthrough across the crista terminalis.[26] CCW lower loop reentry may resemble typical AFL because of similar patterns of activation of the atrial septum and left atrium. A decrease in the late inferior forces may be evident in lower loop reentry as a result of wavefront collision in the lateral right atrium. With multiple or variable wavefront breaks in the lateral atrium, unusual and changing ECG patterns may be observed. Alternation of P-wave polarity from positive to negative in V_1 may occur.[26] CW lower loop reentry typically demonstrates positive flutter waves in the inferior leads and negative flutter waves in V_1.

The ECG description of partial isthmus-dependent flutter is incomplete, but it may be expected to resemble typical AFL, given their similar patterns of atrial activation.[25]

Electrophysiologic Diagnosis

Despite the utility of the 12-lead ECG in making a presumptive diagnosis of typical AFL, an electrophysiologic study with mapping and entrainment must be performed

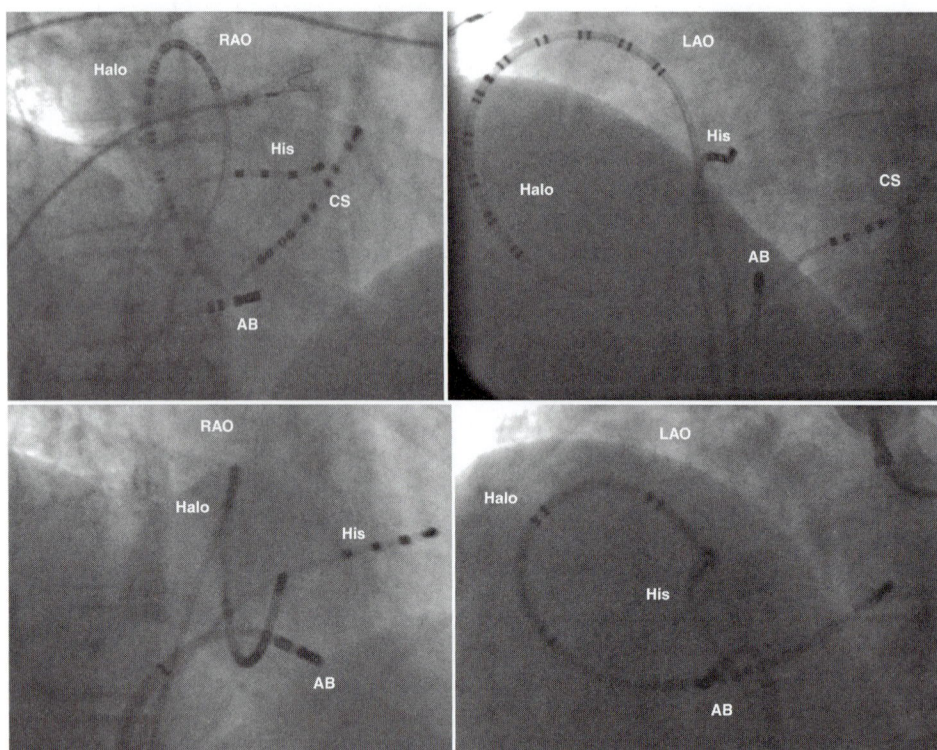

FIGURE 12-6. Right anterior oblique (left panel) and left anterior oblique fluoroscopic (right panel) projections showing the intracardiac positions of the His bundle (His), coronary sinus (CS), halo (Halo), and ablation catheter (AB). Two types of halo catheters are shown. *Top,* This halo design does not reach to the lateral cavotricuspid isthmus (CTI). In this patient, the ablation catheter is very septal and withdrawn near the posterior isthmus near the inferior vena cava. *Bottom,* This halo design spans the CTI with closely spaced electrodes and continues into the coronary sinus. In this patient, the ablation catheter is over the central part of the CTI near the tricuspid valve.

to confirm the underlying mechanism if RF catheter ablation is to be successfully performed (Table 12-1). This is particularly true in the cases of reverse typical AFL or CTI-dependent flutter following extensive left atrial ablation, which are much more difficult to diagnose on 12-lead ECG.

For the electrophysiologic study of AFL, activation mapping may be performed using multielectrode catheters or 3D computerized activation mapping systems. For standard multielectrode catheter mapping, catheters are positioned in the right atrium, His bundle region, and CS. To most precisely elucidate the endocardial activation sequence, a halo 20-electrode (duo-decapolar) mapping catheter is most commonly used in the right atrium, positioned around the TV annulus (Fig. 12-6). These catheters may extend to the lateral CTI or cross the entire CTI into the CS, depending on design. The latter obviates the need for a separate CS catheter. Recordings obtained during AFL from all electrodes are then analyzed to determine the right atrial activation sequence.

For patients who present to the laboratory in sinus rhythm, it is necessary to induce AFL to confirm its mechanism. Induction of AFL is accomplished by atrial programmed stimulation or burst pacing. Preferred pacing sites are the CS ostium and low lateral right atrium; the type of AFL induced (CCW or CW) may depend in part on the pacing site. Burst pacing is the preferred method to induce AFL. Pacing cycle lengths between 180 and 240 milliseconds are typically effective in producing unidirectional CTI block and inducing AFL. Induction of AFL typically

occurs immediately after the onset of unidirectional CTI isthmus block, which can be directly observed during standard electrode catheter mapping, or after a brief period of rapid atrial tachycardia or atrial fibrillation.[24] During electrophysiologic study, a diagnosis of either typical or reverse typical AFL is suggested by observing, respectively, a CCW or CW activation pattern in the right atrium and around the TV annulus. For example, as seen in Figure 12-7A in a patient with typical AFL, the atrial electrogram recorded at the CS ostium is timed with the initial downstroke of the F wave in the inferior surface ECG leads, followed by caudal-to-cranial activation in the interatrial septum-to-His bundle atrial electrogram, then cranial-to-caudal activation in the right atrial free wall from proximal to distal on the halo catheter, and finally signal to the ablation catheter in the CTI, indicating that the underlying mechanism is a CCW macro-reentry circuit with electrical activity in the right atrium encompassing the entire tachycardia cycle length. In a patient with reverse typical AFL, the mirror image of this activation pattern is seen (Fig. 12-7B).

In addition, confirmation that the reentry circuit uses the CTI requires demonstration of the classic criteria for entrainment—specifically, concealed entrainment during pacing from the CTI.[5] Criteria for demonstrating concealed entrainment of AFL include acceleration of the tachycardia to the pacing cycle length without a change in the F-wave pattern on surface ECG or in the endocardial atrial activation pattern and electrogram morphology, as well as immediate resumption of the tachycardia at the original cycle length on termination of

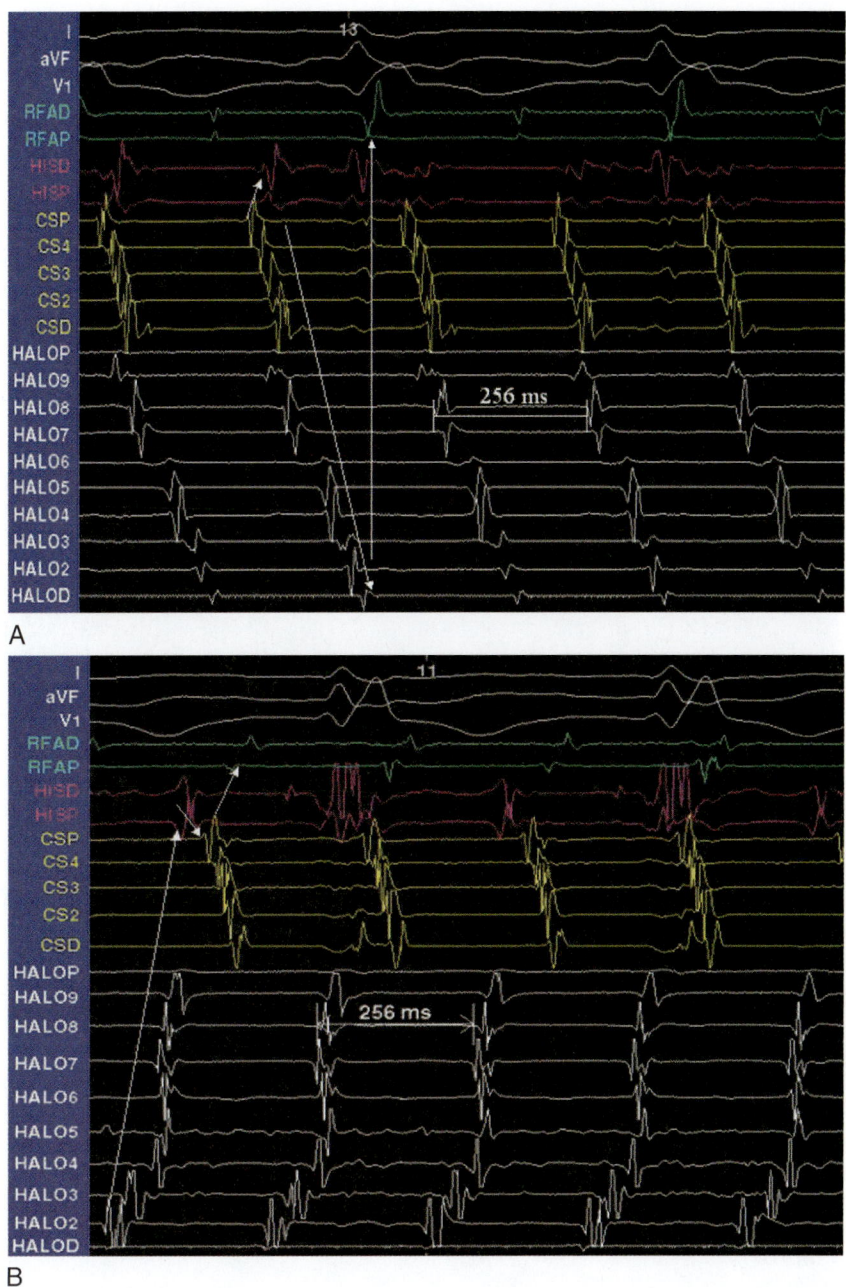

FIGURE 12-7. Endocardial electrograms from the mapping and ablation, halo, coronary sinus (CS), and His bundle catheters and surface electrocardiogram leads I, aVF, and V₁, demonstrating a counterclockwise (CCW) rotation of activation in the right atrium in a patient with typical atrial flutter (AFL) (**A**) and a clockwise (CW) rotation of activation in the right atrium in a patient with reverse typical AFL (**B**). The AFL cycle length was 256 msec for both CCW and CW forms. *Arrows* demonstrate activation sequence. The HALOD through HALOP tracings are 10 bipolar electrograms recorded from the distal (low lateral right atrium) to the proximal (high right atrium) poles of the 20-pole halo catheter positioned around the tricuspid valve annulus with the proximal electrode pair at 1 o'clock and the distal electrode pair at 7 o'clock. CSP electrograms were recorded from the CS catheter proximal electrode pair positioned at the ostium, HISP electrograms from the proximal electrode pair of the His bundle catheter, and RFAD electrograms from the mapping and ablation catheter positioned with the distal electrode pair in the cavotricuspid isthmus.

pacing, including the first postpacing interval (Fig. 12-8). Concealed entrainment is further confirmed, during pacing that is performed within the CTI, if the stimulus-to–F-wave or stimulus-to-reference electrogram interval during pacing and the pacing electrode electrogram-to–F-wave or electrogram-to-reference electrogram interval during AFL are the same (Fig. 12-8). Furthermore, during typical AFL, the stimulus-to–F-wave or stimulus-to-proximal CS electrogram is shorter when the pacing site is medial, near the exit from the CTI (e.g., 30 to 50

milliseconds), and longer when the pacing site is lateral, near the entrance to the CTI (e.g., 80 to 100 milliseconds); the converse is true during reverse typical AFL. In contrast, pacing at sites outside the CTI results in manifest entrainment of AFL, with demonstrable progressive fusion of the F-wave pattern and endocardial atrial electrograms.

The diagnosis of lower loop reentrant AFL is confirmed by the demonstration of concealed entrainment of the tachycardia from not only the CTI but also the inferior-posterior right atrium.[25] Partial isthmus-dependent flutter is confirmed by the demonstration of concealed entrainment from the lateral margin of the CTI but not from the medial portion near the tricuspid valve. In addition, there is early activation of the CS ostium and evidence of collision within the medial CTI. Concealed entrainment should be demonstrable from the area of short circuit between the eustachian ridge and CS ostium.

The differential diagnosis of AFL from other supraventricular arrhythmias is usually apparent given typical ECG manifestations and variable ventricular-atrial relationships. The most likely differential to be made is the exclusion of a focal atrial tachycardia. Rarely, atrial tachycardia in the low posteroseptal right atrium may be confused with AFL if unidirectional CTI block is present. Otherwise, the atrial tachycardia can be recognized by failure to entrain from the CTI and by a radial activation pattern.

Ablation

Ablation of CTI flutters may be performed with the patient on therapeutic doses of warfarin sodium or with bridging anticoagulation using intravenous or subcutaneous heparin. The goal of ablation is to create a line of bidirectional block transecting the CTI from the tricuspid valve to the inferior vena cava.

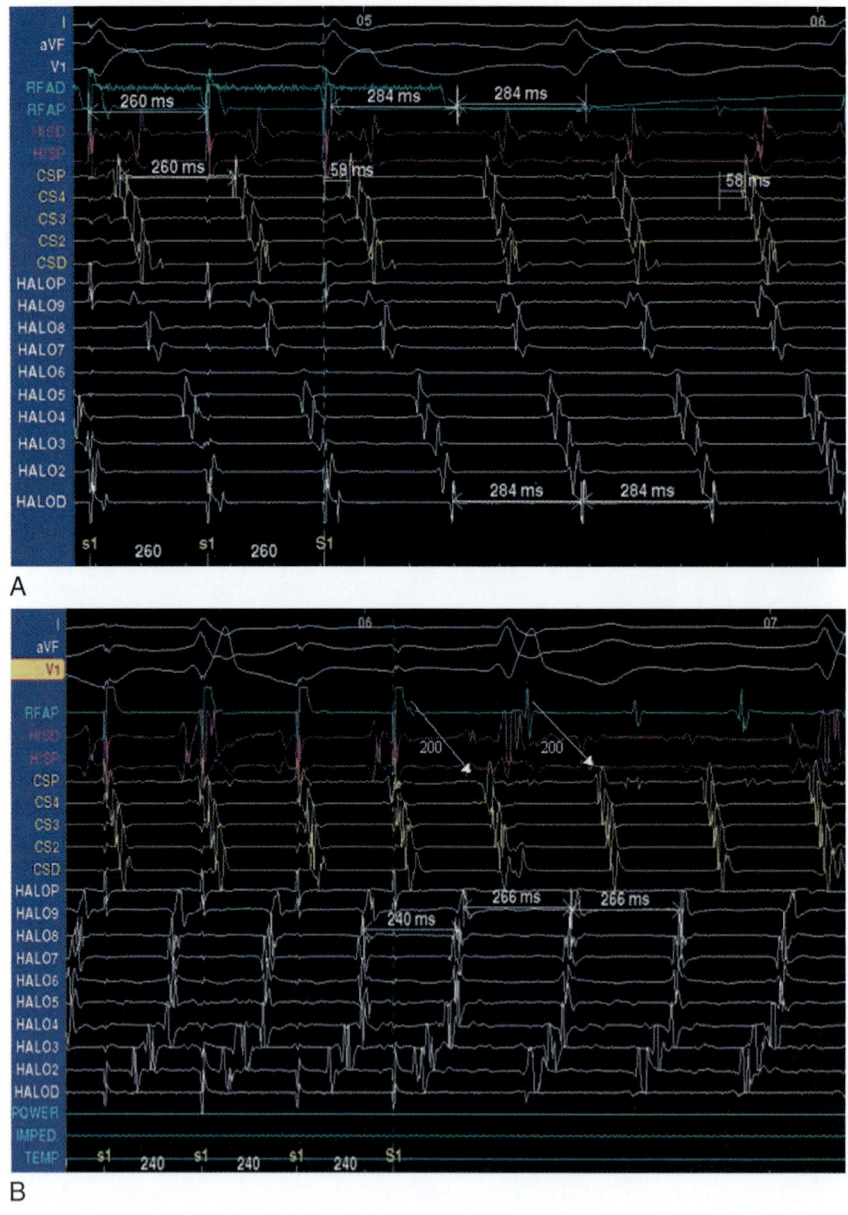

FIGURE 12-8. Surface electrocardiogram (ECG) and endocardial electrogram recordings during pacing entrainment from the cavotricuspid isthmus in patients with typical atrial flutter (AFL) (**A**) and reverse typical AFL (**B**). Note in both examples that the tachycardia is accelerated to the pacing cycle length and that the F-wave morphology on surface ECG and endocardial waveforms and the activation pattern are unchanged during pacing compared with AFL, indicating concealed entrainment. Furthermore, the stimulus-to–F-wave or local electrogram intervals are comparable to the electrogram-to–F-wave or local electrogram intervals recorded on the mapping and ablation catheter (RFAD) during entrainment and AFL in both examples, indicating concealed entrainment. Halo catheter tracings are as described in Figure 12-7. CS, coronary sinus; S1, pacing stimulus artifact.

A variety of mapping and ablation catheters, with different shapes and curve lengths, as well as RF generators, are available from several commercial manufacturers.[2–4,6,30–32] We prefer to use a larger-curve catheter (K2 or mid-distal large curve; EP Technologies, San Jose, CA) to ensure that the ablation electrode will reach the TV annulus, especially in patients with an enlarged right atrium. The use of large-tip (8 to 10 mm) or irrigated ablation electrodes reduces procedure durations and improves success rates compared with standard 4-mm RF electrodes.[33–35] The smaller electrode of irrigated catheter designs provides better near-field electrogram resolution than large-tip electrodes. Long fixed curve or deflectable sheaths (such as an SR0, SL1, or ramp sheath (Daig, Minnetonka, MN) are useful to improve catheter reach, stability, and tissue contact. There is evidence that large-tip ablation catheters are most useful for flat CTI anatomy, whereas irrigated designs may be more advantageous in the presence of CTI pouches.[36] When using formed sheaths, it is important that the curvatures of the sheath and catheter remain coaxial. Paradoxically, rotating the sheath to point into the septum may limit the septal motion of the catheter.

The target for type 1 AFL ablation is the CTI (Table 12-2), which, when standard multipolar electrode catheters are used for mapping and ablation, is localized with a combined fluoroscopically and electrophysiologically guided approach.[2–4,6,30–42] The usual target for the ablation line is the central isthmus because at this point the CTI is at its shortest width (from TV to IVC) and has the thinnest musculature.[15] This site is located at 6 o'clock in the LAO view (Fig. 12-6). The drawback to this site is the frequent occurrence of pouches in the central and medial isthmus. Pouches may be avoided by ablating the lateral isthmus (7 o'clock in LAO projection); however, here thicker right atrial musculature and terminal pectinate muscles are found. The medial isthmus is devoid of pectinate musculature but contains the thickest atrial muscular layer and is nearest to the right coronary artery and AV nodal extensions. Typically, the ablation catheter is positioned fluoroscopically (Fig. 12-6) in the CTI, with the distal ablation electrode on or near the TV annulus in the right anterior oblique (RAO) view, and midway between the septum and low right atrial free wall (6- or 7 o'clock position) in the LAO view. The distal ablation electrode position is then

adjusted toward or away from the TV annulus, based on the ratio of atrial and ventricular electrogram amplitudes (A/V ratio) recorded by the bipolar ablation electrode. An optimal ratio is 1:2 or 1:4 at the TV annulus, as seen in Figure 12-7A on the ablation electrode. After the ablation catheter is positioned on or near the TV annulus, it is very slowly withdrawn during ablation toward the IVC while RF energy is applied continuously; alternatively, it can be withdrawn in a stepwise manner, a few millimeters at a time (usually less than or equal to the length of the distal ablation electrode), with 30- to 60-second pauses at each location, during a continuous or interrupted energy application. For irrigated electrodes, a maximal power of 35 to 50 W and a temperature of 40°C to 45°C should be used.[33–36] In contrast, the large-tip (i.e., 8 to 10 mm) ablation catheters require a higher power, up to 100 W, to achieve target temperatures of 50° to 70°C, because of the greater energy-dispersive effects of the larger ablation electrode, which also requires the use of two grounding pads applied to the patient's skin to avoid skin burns.[36,38–42] Excessive impedance drops should be avoided to prevent tissue overheating and steam pops. CTI can be performed with standard 4-mm-tip RF catheters (50 W, 50° to 65°C); however, these catheters are associated with longer procedure and ablation times, lower acute success rates, and much higher recurrence rates. Electrogram recordings may be employed in addition to fluoroscopy to ensure that the ablation electrode is in contact with viable tissue in the CTI throughout each energy application. Ablation across the entire CTI (Fig. 12-9) may require several sequential 30- to 60-second energy applications during a stepwise catheter pullback, or a prolonged energy application of up to 120 seconds or longer during a continuous catheter pullback. The catheter should be gradually withdrawn until the distal ablation electrode records no atrial electrogram, indicating that it has reached the IVC, or until the ablation electrode is noted to abruptly slip off the eustachian ridge fluoroscopically. RF energy application should be immediately interrupted when the catheter has reached the IVC because ablation in venous structures is known to cause significant pain to patients. Computerized catheter 3D-mapping

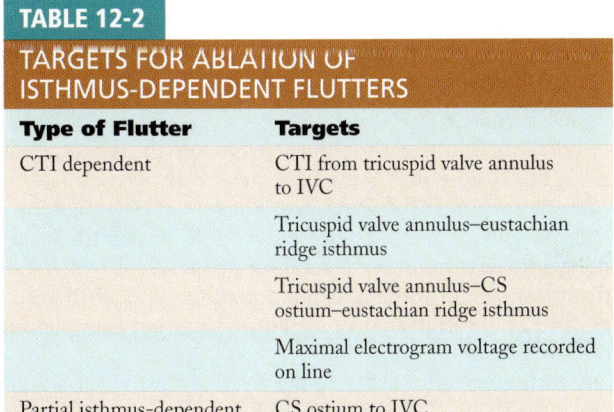

TABLE 12-2	
TARGETS FOR ABLATION OF ISTHMUS-DEPENDENT FLUTTERS	
Type of Flutter	**Targets**
CTI dependent	CTI from tricuspid valve annulus to IVC
	Tricuspid valve annulus–eustachian ridge isthmus
	Tricuspid valve annulus–CS ostium–eustachian ridge isthmus
	Maximal electrogram voltage recorded on line
Partial isthmus-dependent	CS ostium to IVC

CS, coronary sinus; CTI, cavotricuspid isthmus; IVC, inferior vena cava.

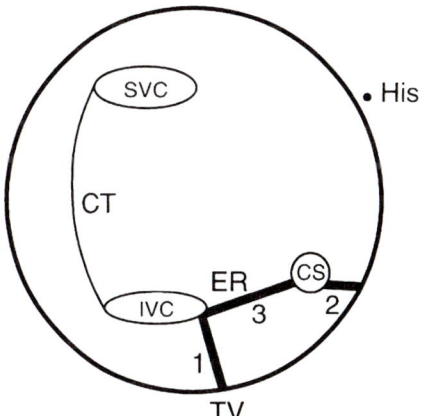

FIGURE 12-9. Schematic diagram of the right atrium in right interior oblique view, showing the typical locations for linear ablation of the cavotricuspid isthmus *(line 1)*, the tricuspid valve (TV)–coronary sinus (CS) isthmus *(line 2)*, and the CS–inferior vena cava (IVC) isthmus *(line 3)*. CT, crista terminalis; ER, eustachian ridge; His, His bundle; SVC, superior vena cava.

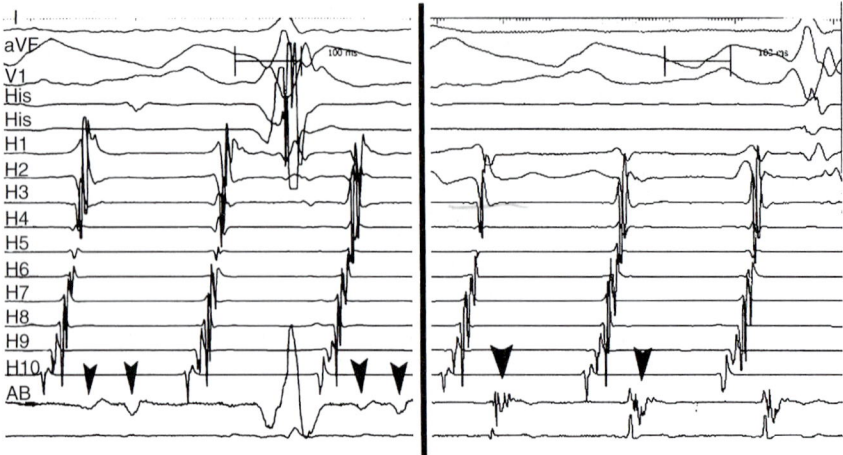

FIGURE 12-10. Mapping for the gap in the ablation line in the cavotricuspid isthmus. In this patient, a previous attempt to terminate typical atrial flutter had failed. *Left panel,* The ablation catheter (AB) records low-amplitude but split electrograms *(arrowheads)* along the prior ablation line. The interval between electrogram components was 70 msec during flutter. *Right panel,* With further interrogation of the ablation line, a site with a single-component but fractionated electrogram *(arrowheads)* was identified. Ablation at this site terminated the flutter in less than 2 sec and created bidirectional block. Surface electrocardiogram leads I, aVF, and V$_1$ are shown. His, His channels; H1 through H10, halo catheter channels from distal to proximal.

systems are useful to document the anatomic placement of ablation lesions.[43] As the ablation catheter approaches the IVC, it is often useful to open the catheter curve slightly and withdraw the sheath and catheter as a unit to allow greater contact between the electrode and eustachian ridge before the catheter falls into the IVC.

Alternatively, ablation of the TV-CS and CS-IVC isthmuses (see Fig. 12-9) may be performed using an approach similar to that used to ablate the CTI.[44] However, for this approach to be successful, it may be necessary to ablate within the CS ostium as well, which may be associated with a higher risk for complications such as AV node block. It has also been reported that type 1 AFL may be cured by ablating between the TV annulus and eustachian ridge only, which is a narrower isthmus than the CTI.[45] During repeat ablation, it may be necessary to rotate the ablation catheter away from the initial line of energy application, either medially or laterally in the CTI, to create new or additional lines of block, or to use a higher power or higher ablation temperature, or both. In addition, if ablation is initially attempted using a standard 4- to 5-mm-tip electrode and fails, repeat ablation with a large-tip electrode catheter or a cooled-tip ablation catheter may be successful.[33–42] Ablation of partial isthmus-dependent flutter requires creation of a block from the CS ostium to the IVC, eliminating conduction across the eustachian ridge. Completion of this line may convert the tachycardia to typical isthmus-dependent flutter, which then requires ablation of the entire CTI.[25]

In many cases, the CTI is composed of discrete muscle bundles embedded within connective tissue. Therefore, a continuous ablation line may be unnecessary to achieve conduction block. To reduce procedure times and unnecessary ablation, the maximal voltage–guided CTI technique has been introduced.[46,47] Bipolar electrograms are recorded from the ablation catheter in the central tricuspid isthmus during AFL or CS pacing at 600-milliseconds cycle length. As the catheter is withdrawn from the tricuspid valve to the inferior vena cava, the site of largest peak-to-peak bipolar voltage is marked. The ablation catheter is returned to the site of maximal voltage, and RF energy is delivered for 60 seconds or until there is more than 50% reduction in the electrogram voltage. The line is then remapped for the largest remaining electrogram voltage and the procedure repeated until isthmus block is confirmed. In randomized trials, the voltage-guided technique has been reported to reduce ablation time, number of lesions, and procedure and fluoroscopic times compared with the conventional anatomic approach.[46,47]

After the termination of flutter, less than half of patients demonstrate bidirectional CTI block, and further ablation is needed.[48] This is most commonly detected during pacing from medial (proximal coronary sinus) or lateral to the ablation line and mapping the line for conduction gaps. The presence of split electrograms with less than 90 milliseconds between electrogram components is highly suggestive of a gap in the line.[48] As the line is systematically mapped, the split electrogram components draw closer together as the gap is approached. The gap itself is identified as a single or fractionated potential along the line bounded by split electrograms (Fig. 12-10).

Cryoablation may also be used for CTI ablation.[49,50,51] Large-tip electrodes (8 mm) should be used and the catheter withdrawn point by point along the CTI as above. Continuous "drag" lesions are not possible owing to electrode adherence to the tissue during ablation. Cryoenergy is delivered for 240 seconds at each location. Cryoablation is painless but may be associated with longer ablation times than RF energy.

Preclinical and early clinical work on the ablation of AFL has begun on the use of a linear microwave ablation catheter system (Medwaves, San Diego, CA) with antenna lengths up to 4 cm.[52] These studies have shown the feasibility of linear microwave ablation of the CTI, which has the advantage of very rapid ablation of the CTI with a single energy application over the entire length of the ablation electrode (Fig. 12-11).

Computerized 3D mapping systems provide several advantages for CTI ablation but are not necessary for the procedure.[43] Electroanatomic mapping before ablation

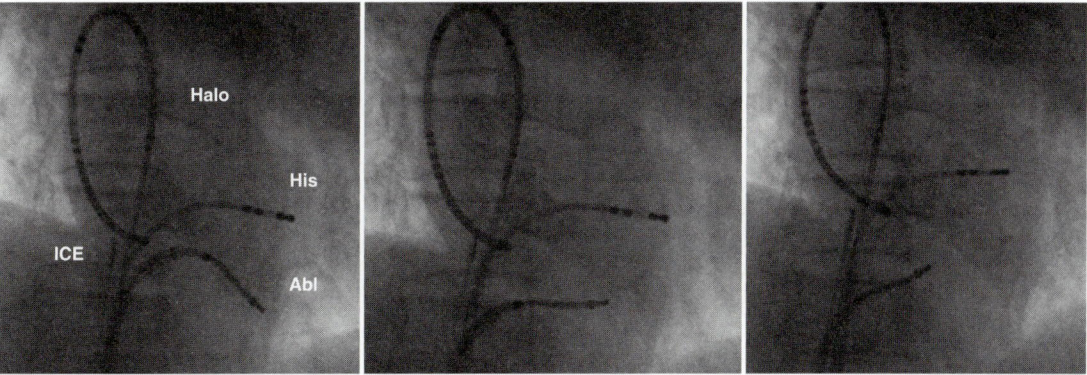

FIGURE 12-11. Fluoroscopic right anterior oblique view of the Medwaves microwave ablation (Abl) antenna positioned across the CTI. *Left panel* shows ablation antenna positioned near the tricuspid valve annulus. *Middle panel* shows ablation antenna at the middle CTI between the tricuspid annulus and eustachian ridge. *Right panel* shows ablation antenna withdrawn near the inferior vena cava. Halo, halo catheter; His, His bundle; ICE, intracardiac echocardiography.

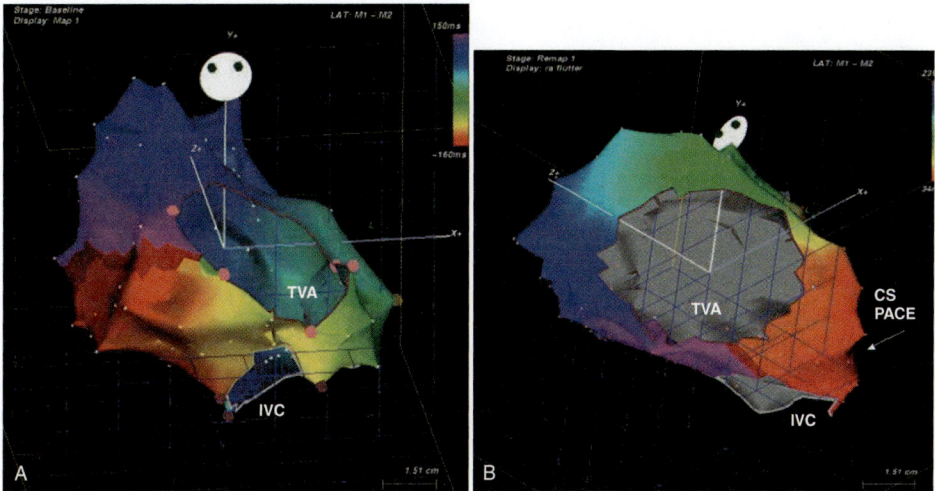

FIGURE 12-12. A three-dimensional electroanatomic (Carto system, Biosense Webster, Diamond Bar, CA) map of the right atrium in a patient with typical atrial flutter (AFL), before (**A**) and after (**B**) cavotricuspid isthmus (CTI) ablation. Note the counterclockwise activation pattern around the tricuspid valve during AFL (**A,** anteroposterior view), which is based on a color scheme indicating activation time from *orange* (early) to *purple* (late). After ablation of the CTI (**B,** left anterior oblique caudal view), during pacing from the coronary sinus (CS) ostium, there is evidence of medial-to-lateral isthmus block, as indicated by juxtaposition of orange and purple color in the CTI. IVC, inferior vena cava; TVA, tricuspid valve annulus.

can demonstrate the reentry circuit, thus confirming the diagnosis (Fig. 12-12). In addition, 3D anatomic reconstruction may identify the presence of a CTI pouch, and high-voltage electrograms may indicate the presence of pectinate muscle extension into the CTI. During ablation, the ability to document the sites of lesion delivery is helpful to complete an anatomically based ablation line and identify areas of anatomic gaps. In this capacity, computerized mapping systems can reduce fluoroscopy times by 50% compared with conventional approaches.[43] After ablation, detailed electroanatomic mapping may be used to confirm the presence of CTI block or slow conduction.

Overcoming Difficult Cavotricuspid Isthmus Anatomy

The anatomy of the CTI may present difficulties for ablation. The most common problems are presence of a large CTI pouch, large pectinate muscles, and a prominent eustachian ridge.[53] The pouch presents a deep recess in the CTI that may

be skirted over by the ablation electrode during pullback (Fig. 12-13). The junction of the IVC and CTI or eustachian ridge, or both, may form a "fulcrum" for the ablation catheter (Fig. 12-13), preventing entry into the pouch. The presence of a pouch may be identified by preprocedure CT or MRI or more commonly by angiography, ICE, or electroanatomic mapping during the procedure. Right atrial angiography is performed by injecting 50 mL of contrast over 3 to 5 seconds through a 5-French pigtail catheter in the upper IVC or IVC–right atrial junction,[18] imaging in the RAO view. The pouch may be avoided by a more lateral ablation line. Ablation within the pouch is accomplished by forming an 180-degree curvature on the ablation catheter in the mid-tricuspid annulus and withdrawing the catheter to enter the pouch perpendicularly (Fig. 12-14). The curvature can be relaxed and tightened to reach the tricuspid valve and IVC ends of the pouch, respectively. Because of the restricted blood flow, ablation within the pouch usually requires cooled ablation (usually irrigated) to achieve target power deliveries. Care should be taken to avoid excessive tissue heating and steam pops. The pouch may extend toward the septum in an asymmetrical fashion.

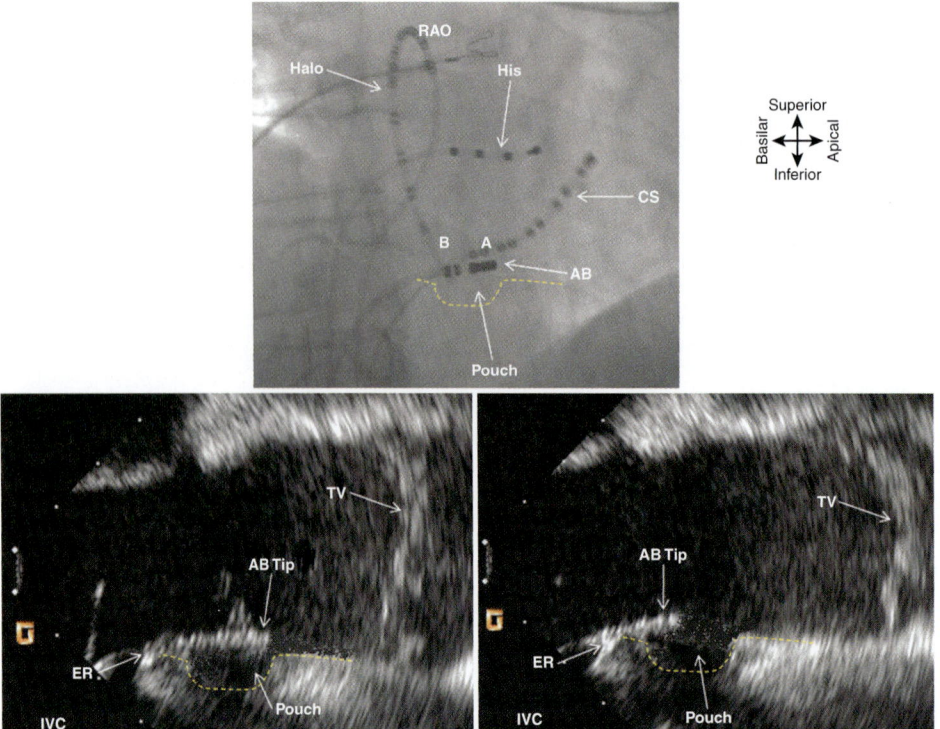

FIGURE 12-13. Cavotricuspid isthmus (CTI) pouch. *Top panel,* Right anterior oblique (RAO) fluoroscopic view of ablation catheters during CTI ablation. The *yellow dashed line* estimates the position of a large pouch visualized in this patient with intracardiac echocardiography (*bottom panels*). As the ablation (AB) catheter is drawn toward the inferior vena cava from point **A** to **B**, the tip of the catheter does not contact the floor of the pouch and is therefore not ablated. *Bottom left panel,* This intracardiac echocardiographic view demonstrates the pouch and ablation catheter skirting over the pouch in position A. The echo view is rotated to correspond to the fluoroscopic orientation. *Bottom right panel,* This echo image corresponds to the ablation catheter at position B. The fulcrum created by the eustachian ridge (ER) prevents the catheter from entering the pouch. CS, coronary sinus catheter; TV, tricuspid valve.

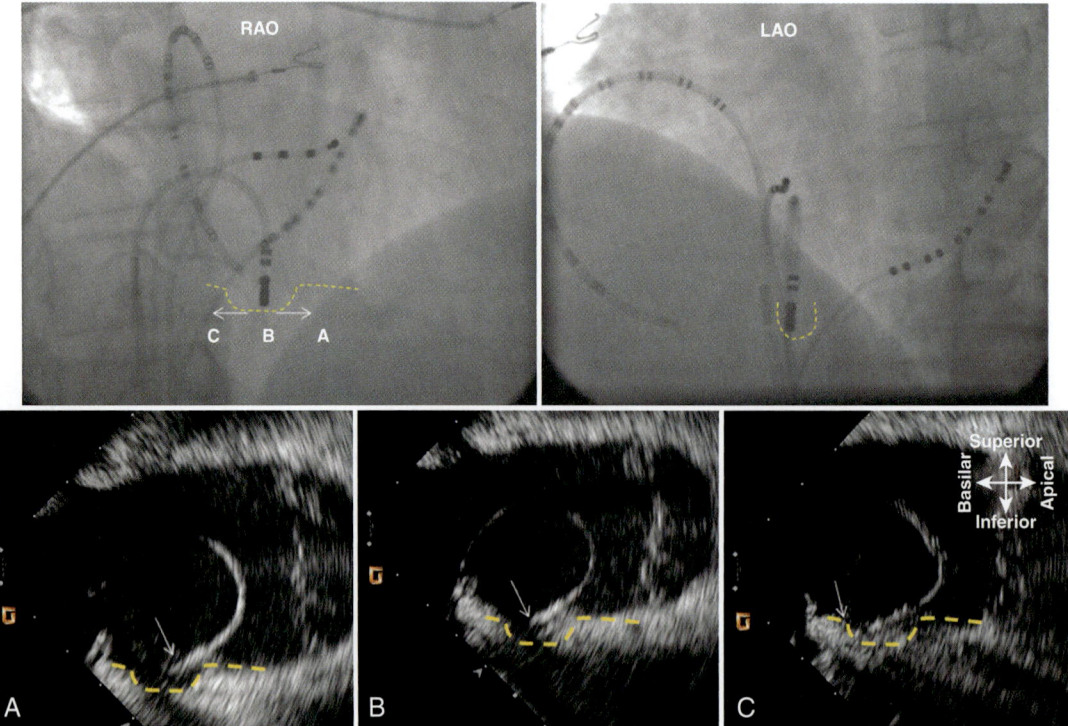

FIGURE 12-14. Ablation within a cavotricuspid isthmus (CTI) pouch. *Top panels* show right anterior oblique (RAO) and left anterior oblique (LAO) fluoroscopic views of the catheter positions. The *dashed yellow line* represents the estimated location of the pouch visualized on intracardiac echocardiography. With a 180-degree angle on the ablation catheter, the ablation electrode contacts the middle floor of the pouch (site B). By opening or closing the curve on the ablation catheter, the tricuspid valve end (site A) and inferior vena cava end (site C) of the pouch can be reached, respectively. *Bottoms panels* visualize the position of the ablation electrode at sites A, B, and C in the pouch. The *arrows* indicate the tip of the ablation catheter. The echo views are rotated to correspond to the RAO fluoroscopic image.

Large pectinate muscles should be suspected on recording high-voltage electrograms within the CTI. These may potentially be avoided by ablation in the medial isthmus. Ablation of the high-voltage areas may require protracted (60 to 120 seconds) RF delivery and possibly fine electrode manipulation to ablate the entire trabeculated region. On the trabecular prominences, the catheter contact may be unstable, whereas in the trabecular valleys, excessive electrode temperatures may result (Fig. 12-15).[53] Preformed or deflectable sheaths may enhance tissue contact, and for irrigated ablation, lesion sizes are maximized with the electrode perpendicular to the tissue. A voltage-guided approach may limit unnecessary ablation.

A prominent eustachian ridge can be detected during surgery by angiography or intracardiac echocardiography (Fig. 12-16). The ridge or adjacent tissue can be conductive and require ablation. In this case, the fulcrum effect of the ridge or the IVC-CTI junction may prevent electrode contact with parts of the ridge, especially the edge facing the tricuspid valve. By forming a tight curvature on the ablation catheter in the middle of the right atrium and withdrawing the catheter, the electrode may be brought into contact with the IVC and tricuspid valve sides of the ridge. Alternatively, the ridge may be compressed with a deflectable sheath and then ablated. The other problem posed by a prominent ridge is that the ridge may limit the motion of the ablation catheter, thereby shielding part of the isthmus.[53] This may be overcome by use of a preformed sheath that directs the catheter anteriorly so that posterior curvature on the catheter body reaches around the obstacle (Fig. 12-17).

Occasionally, multielectrode catheters crossing the CTI map prevent contact between the ablation electrode and cardiac tissue (Fig. 12-18). The mapping catheter can be removed or the ablation catheter positioned beneath the halo.

End Points for Ablation

Ablation may be performed during sustained AFL or during sinus rhythm. If it is performed during AFL, the first end point is its termination during energy application (Fig. 12-19). However, even if AFL terminates, CTI conduction persists in more than half of patients.[48] Therefore, the entire CTI ablation should be completed, after which electrophysiologic testing can be performed. After completion of CTI ablation as determined by fluoroscopic and electrophysiologic criteria described previously, testing can be performed immediately and repeated after at least 20 to 30 minutes to ensure that bidirectional CTI block has been achieved and is persistent (Table 12-3).[2–4,6,30–42,54] Fifty percent of patients demonstrate recurrent CTI conduction during the ablation procedure

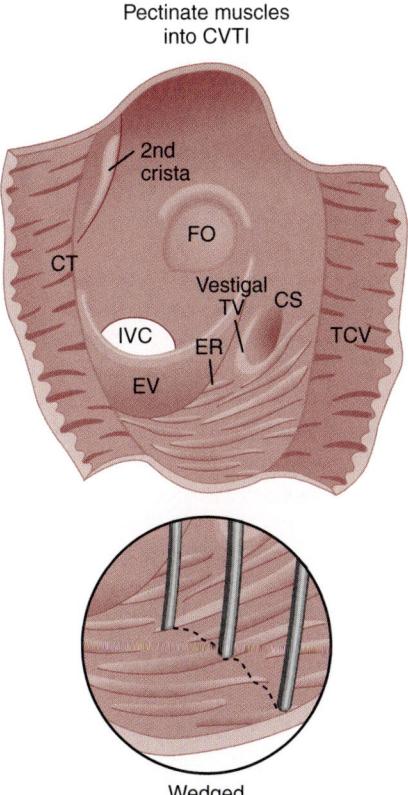

Pectinate muscles into CVTI

Wedged

FIGURE 12-15. Illustration showing difficulties in ablating the lateral isthmus in the presence of prominent pectinate muscles. On the tops of the muscle bundles, the catheter contact may be unstable. In the recesses between bundles, electrode overheating and low power delivery may result because of the absence of convective cooling. CS, coronary sinus; CT, crista terminalis; CVTI, cavotricuspid isthmus; ER, eustachian ridge; EV, eustachian valve; FO, foramen ovale; IVC, inferior vena cava; TCV, tricuspid valve. *(From Asirvatham S. Correlative anatomy and electrophysiology for the interventional electrophysiologist: right atrial flutter.* J Cardiovasc Electrophysiol. *2009;20:113–122. With permission.)*

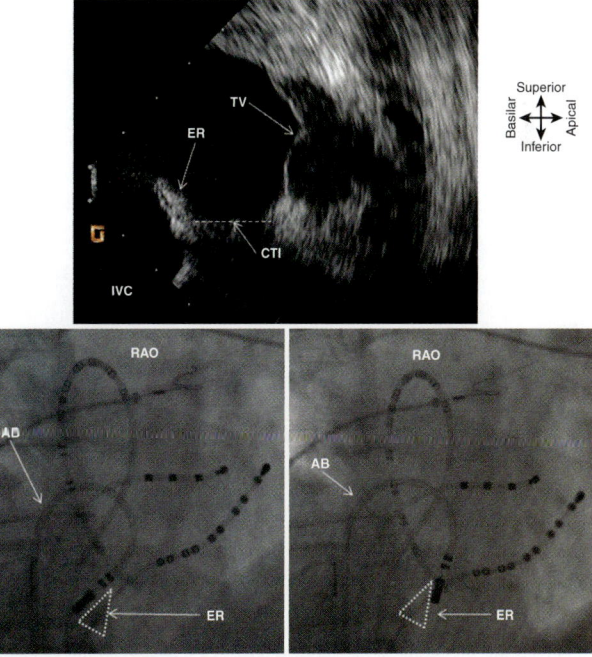

FIGURE 12-16. Ablation of the eustachian ridge. The *top panel* shows a prominent eustachian ridge (ER) on intracardiac echocardiography. The echo views are rotated to correspond to the right anterior oblique (RAO) fluoroscopic image. *Bottom panels* show the estimated location of the ER and acute flexion of the ablation (AB) catheter to ablate both aspects of the ER facing the inferior vena cava (IVC; *lower left*) and tricuspid valve (*lower right*). TV, tricuspid valve.

after CTI bidirectional block is initially documented.[54] Most recurrences occur within 10 minutes of "successful" CTI block, and multiple recurrences after repeat ablation within the same procedure are not uncommon. Isoproterenol infusion may also unmask transient CTI block.[55] If AFL is not terminated during the first attempt at CTI ablation, the activation sequence and isthmus dependence of the AFL should be reconfirmed and ablation repeated.

If AFL is terminated during ablation, pacing should be done at a cycle length of 600 milliseconds or less, depending on the sinus cycle length, to determine whether there is a bidirectional conduction block in the CTI (Figs. 12-20 to 12-23). If ablation is done during sinus rhythm, pacing can also be done during energy application to monitor for the development of conduction block in the CTI (Fig. 12-24). The use of this end point for ablation may be associated

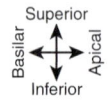

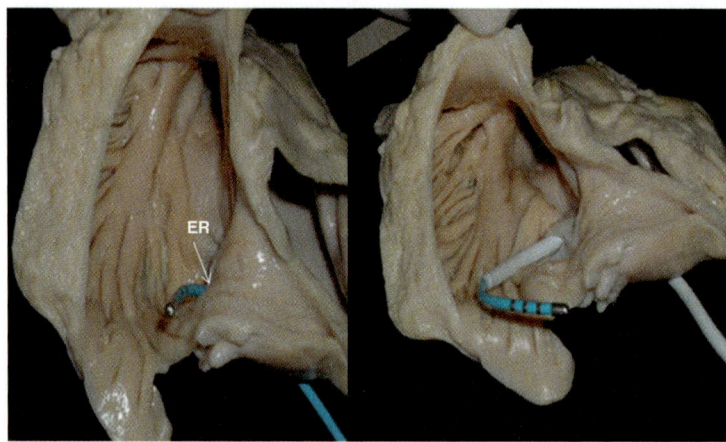

FIGURE 12-17. In this autopsy heart, the catheter excursion toward the septal isthmus is restricted by the eustachian ridge (ER; *left panel*). In the *right panel*, a guiding sheath is used to direct the catheter anteriorly while curving the catheter itself posteriorly to reach around the ridge. *(From Asirvatham S. Correlative anatomy and electrophysiology for the interventional electrophysiologist: right atrial flutter. J Cardiovasc Electrophysiol. 2009; 20:113–122. With permission.)*

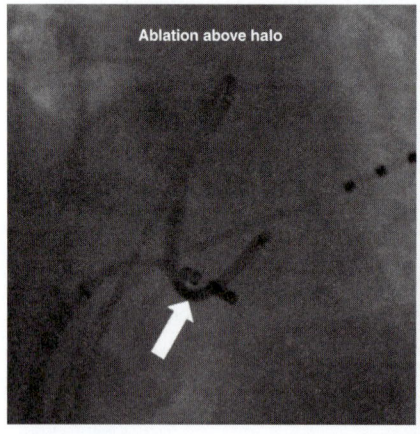
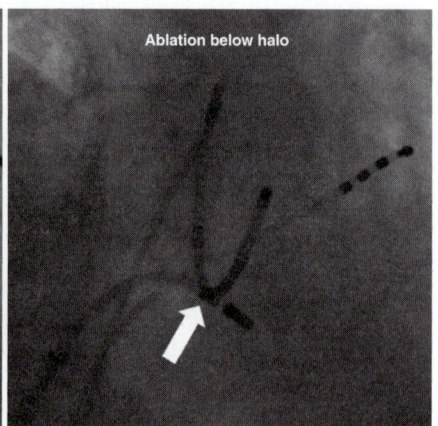

FIGURE 12-18. Shielding of the isthmus by the halo catheter. In this patient, isthmus block could not be achieved after repeated ablation. The ablation catheter repeatedly coursed over the halo catheter that crosses the isthmus (*arrow, left panel*). By delivering lesions beneath the halo catheter (*arrow, right panel*) complete isthmus block was created.

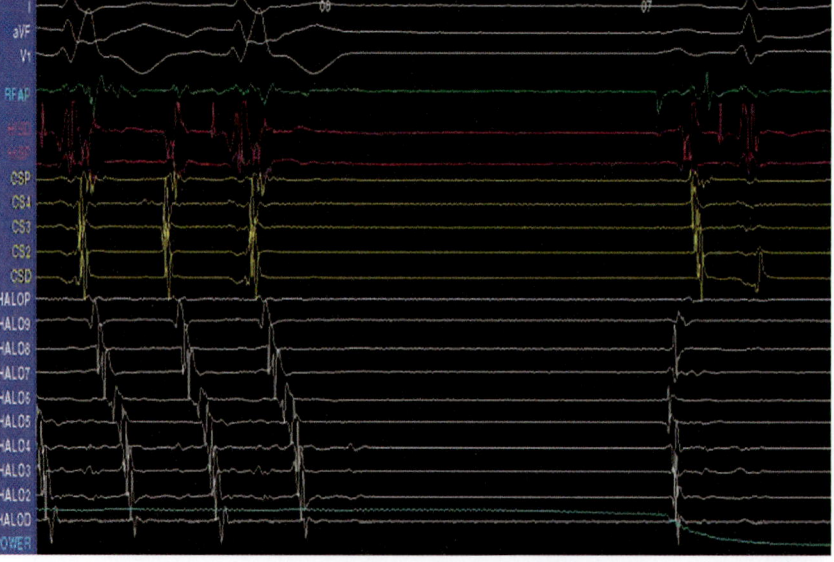

FIGURE 12-19. Termination of typical atrial flutter (AFL) during radiofrequency (RF) energy application using a slow drag technique across the cavotricuspid isthmus (CTI). AFL usually terminates just as the distal ablation electrode on the mapping and ablation catheter (RFAP) approaches the inferior vena cava. Conduction fails at the CTI, as indicated by block developing between the low lateral right atrium and coronary sinus in the typical form, or between the coronary sinus and the low lateral right atrium in the reverse typical form (not shown). The power readout from the RF energy generator is shown in the bottom tracing. CS, coronary sinus.

TABLE 12-3

METHODS FOR CONFIRMING CAVOTRICUSPID ISTHMUS BLOCK

Method	Criteria for CTI Block	Sensitivity/ Specificity (%)	Positive-/Negative- Predictive Values (%)	Comment
Atrial activation sequence	Cranial-to-caudal activation of right atrial inferolateral free wall with PCS pacing Cranial-to-caudal activation of right atrial septum with inferior lateral right atrial pacing			Requires careful mapping adjacent to ablation line on side contralateral to pacing to exclude slow conduction through the line
Widely split electrograms along entire ablation line[48]	Interval between split electrogram components recorded along ablation line ≥90 msec at all sites and ≤15 msec maximal variation among all sites during pacing from PCS	100/80	86/100	Interval between electrogram recordings <90 msec indicates gap in line. Recordings are from ablation catheter
Transisthmus interval[64]	CCW block: ≥50% increase in time interval between pacing stimulus from inferolateral tricuspid annulus to electrogram in PCS CW block: ≥50% increase in time interval between pacing stimulus from PCS to electrogram just lateral to ablation line	100/80	89/100	Minimal transisthmus interval associated with bidirectional CTI block about 140 msec
Differential pacing[66]	Shortening or no change in interval between pacing stimulus and latest component of split electrogram recorded over ablation line when pacing site moved from adjacent to line to 15 mm lateral to line. When pacing close to the edge of ablation line, time to activation of contralateral side of ablation line shortens as pacing site moves away from ablation line	100/75	94/100	First pacing site should be immediately adjacent to ablation line Recording site should be immediately adjacent to ablation line
Electrogram polarity[68,69]	Loss of negative component of unipolar electrogram recorded just lateral to ablation line during PCS pacing, or Reversal of electrogram polarity on two closely spaced bipoles just lateral to ablation line during PCS pacing	89/100	100 (PPV)	Recording must be immediately adjacent to ablation line

CCW, counterclockwise; CW, clockwise; PCS, proximal coronary sinus; PPV, positive-predictive value.

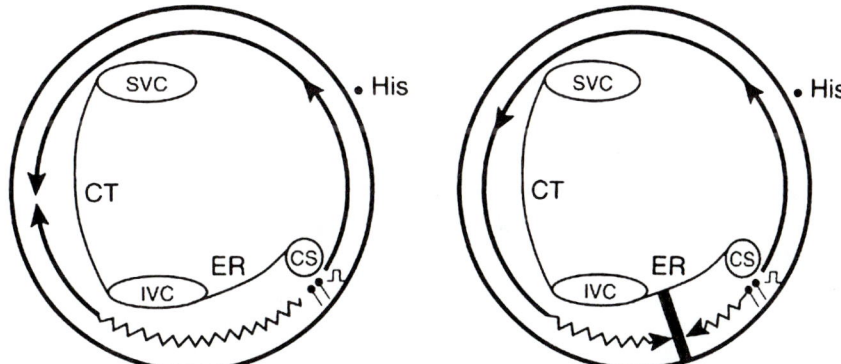

FIGURE 12-20. Schematic diagrams of the expected right atrial activation sequence during pacing in sinus rhythm from the coronary sinus (CS) ostium before *(left panel)* and after *(right panel)* ablation of the cavotricuspid isthmus (CTI). Before ablation, the activation pattern during CS pacing is caudal to cranial in the interatrial septum and low right atrium, with collision of the septal and right atrial wavefronts in the mid-lateral right atrium. After ablation, the activation pattern during CS pacing is still caudal to cranial in the interatrial septum, but the lateral right atrium is now activated in a strictly cranial-to-caudal pattern (i.e., counterclockwise), indicating complete clockwise conduction block in the CTI. CT, crista terminalis; ER, eustachian ridge; His, His bundle; IVC, inferior vena cava; SVC, superior vena cava.

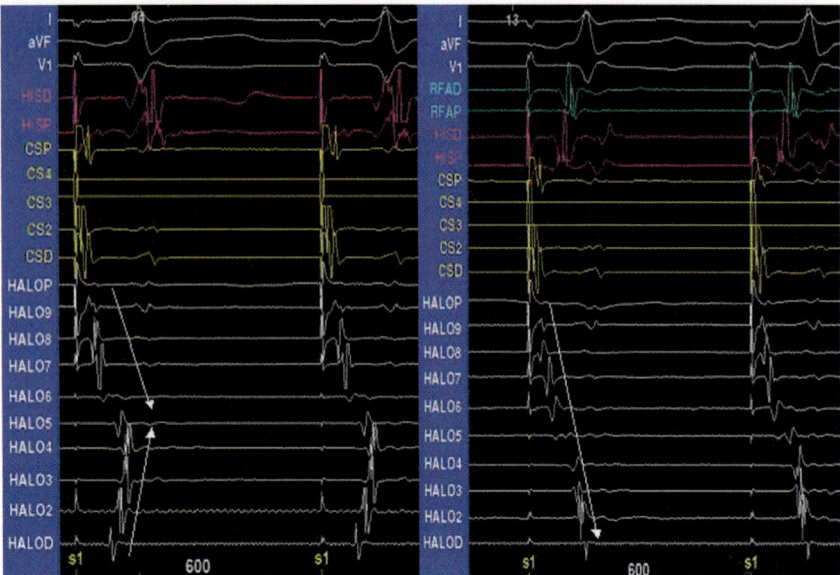

FIGURE 12-21. Surface electrocardiogram (ECG) leads and right atrial endocardial electrograms recorded during pacing in sinus rhythm from the coronary sinus (CS) ostium before *(left panel)* and after *(right panel)* ablation of the cavotricuspid isthmus (CTI). Tracings include surface ECG leads I, aVF, and V₁ and endocardial electrograms from the proximal coronary sinus (CSP), His bundle (HIS), tricuspid valve annulus at 1 o'clock (HALOP) to 7 o'clock (HALOD), and high right atrium (RFA). Before ablation during CS pacing, there is collision of the cranial and caudal right atrial wavefronts in the mid-lateral right atrium (HALO5). After ablation, the lateral right atrium is activated in a strictly cranial-to-caudal pattern (i.e., counterclockwise), indicating complete medial-to-lateral conduction block in the CTI.

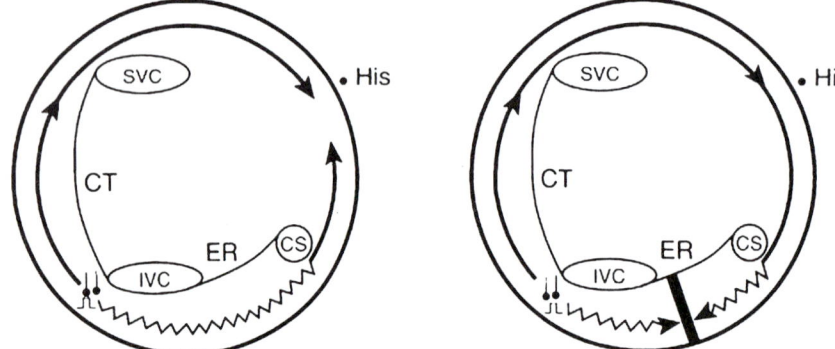

FIGURE 12-22. Schematic diagrams of the expected right atrial activation sequence during pacing in sinus rhythm from the low lateral right atrium before *(left panel)* and after *(right panel)* ablation of the cavotricuspid isthmus (CTI). Before ablation, the activation pattern during coronary sinus (CS) pacing is caudal to cranial in the right atrial free wall, with collision of the cranial and caudal wavefronts (i.e., through the CTI) in the mid-septum; there is simultaneous activation at the His bundle (HISP) and proximal coronary sinus (CSP). After ablation, the activation pattern during low lateral right atrial sinus pacing is still caudal to cranial in the right atrial free wall, but the septum is now activated in a strictly cranial-to-caudal pattern (i.e., clockwise), indicating complete counterclockwise conduction block in the CTI. CT, crista terminalis; ER, eustachian ridge; His, His bundle; SVC, superior vena cava.

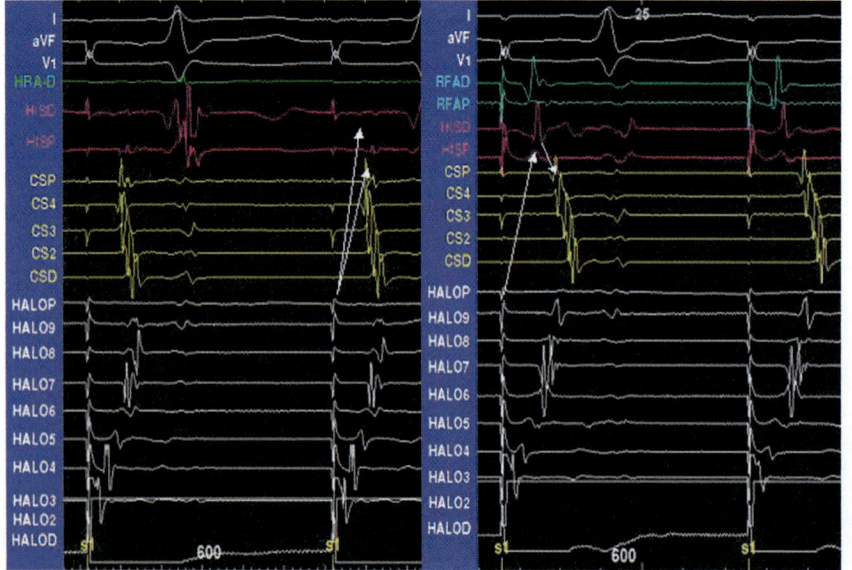

FIGURE 12-23. Surface electrocardiogram (ECG) and right atrial endocardial electrograms during pacing in sinus rhythm from the low lateral right atrium before *(left panel)* and after *(right panel)* ablation of the cavotricuspid isthmus (CTI). Tracings include surface ECG leads I, aVF, and V₁ and endocardial electrograms from the proximal coronary sinus (CSP), His bundle (HIS), tricuspid valve annulus at 1 o'clock (HALOP) to 7 o'clock (HALOD), and high right atrium (HRA or RFA). Before ablation, during low lateral right atrial pacing, there is collision of the cranial and caudal right atrial wavefronts in the mid-septum (HIS and CSP). After ablation, the septum is activated in a strictly cranial-to-caudal pattern (i.e., clockwise), indicating complete lateral-to-medial conduction block in the CTI.

with a significantly lower recurrence rate of type 1 AFL during long-term follow-up.[56–59] Bidirectional CTI block is assessed by mapping the ablation line, atrial activation sequence, or differential pacing maneuvers. The optimal method for clinical use is debated, but most studies have used atrial activation sequence as the standard by which to compare new methodology.

Conduction in the CTI is commonly evaluated by determining the activation sequence in the right atrium while pacing during sinus rhythm at slow rates (i.e., cycle lengths ≥600 milliseconds) from the low lateral right atrium and CS ostium after ablation. It is important to pace at relatively slow rates during assessment for CTI block because conduction block across the CTI may be functional and rate dependent in some patients after ablation. In addition, conduction block across the crista terminalis may be functional in some patients, and at slow pacing rates, conduction across the mid-crista region can result in uncertainty regarding the presence or absence of bidirectional CTI block after ablation.[60–62] Therefore, it may be necessary to pace not only from the proximal CS but also adjacent to the ablation line in the CTI, or in the posterior-inferior right atrial septum, to confirm the presence of CTI isthmus block.[62] Bidirectional conduction block in the CTI is associated with a strictly cranial-to-caudal activation sequence over the lateral right atrium after ablation with pacing from the CS ostium or medial to the ablation line and a cranial to caudal sequence over the right atrial septum with pacing from the lateral edge of the ablation line or the low lateral right atrium[56–58] (Figs. 12-20 to 12-23). This sequence can be documented by multipolar electrode recordings or by electroanatomic mapping. When using a multipolar halo catheter to assess CTI block, it is important that the catheter be properly positioned to record only from within the reentry circuit. Recordings are needed from immediately adjacent to the ablation line to assess for slow conduction through the ablation line. This can be performed from halo electrodes crossing the ablation line or from the ablation catheter. A misleading activation sequence may be recorded if portions of the catheter extend posterior to the crista

terminalis or if the distal electrode is posterior to the eustachian ridge.[53] In addition, during pacing medial to the ablation line, conduction posterior to the IVC can lead to the appearance of both pseudoconduction and pseudoblock through the CTI (Fig. 12-25).[53,63] In the case of pseudoblock, conduction from the medial pacing site (usually proximal coronary sinus) may conduct rapidly posterior to the IVC to activate the lateral CTI from lateral to medial, suggesting medial to lateral isthmus block despite persisting slow conduction through the isthmus. In this case, detailed mapping over or near the ablation line should identify gaps in the line. In the case of pseudoconduction, the posteriorly conducted wavefront activates the distal halo catheter in a CW pattern even if there is CTI block. This is more likely to be seen if the distal halo catheter is displaced laterally and does not record from the immediate edge of the ablation line.[53] Pseudoconduction can be recognized by detailed mapping of sites spanning the ablation line. Theoretically, differential pacing maneuvers (see later) may also unmask these conduction patterns.

The creation of CTI block is accompanied by prolongation of the intervals required for a pacing stimulus on one side of the ablation line to propagate to the opposite side of the line (transisthmus interval).[64] Before ablation, the transisthmus intervals average 99 ± 22 milliseconds and 98 ± 28 milliseconds in the CW and CCW directions, respectively (pacing at 500-milliseconds cycle length). In the presence of bidirectional isthmus block, these times increase to 189 ± 33 milliseconds and 178 ± 31 milliseconds, respectively. Bidirectional CTI block never occurred with less than 50% prolongation in the transisthmus interval. An increase in the transisthmus interval of 50% or greater provided 100% sensitivity, 80% specificity, 89% positive-predictive value, and 100% negative-predictive value in confirming CTI block.

The presence of bidirectional conduction block in the CTI is strongly supported by recording widely spaced double potentials along the entire ablation line during pacing from the low lateral right atrium or CS ostium (Fig. 12-24).[48,65] When pacing from the proximal CS, intervals

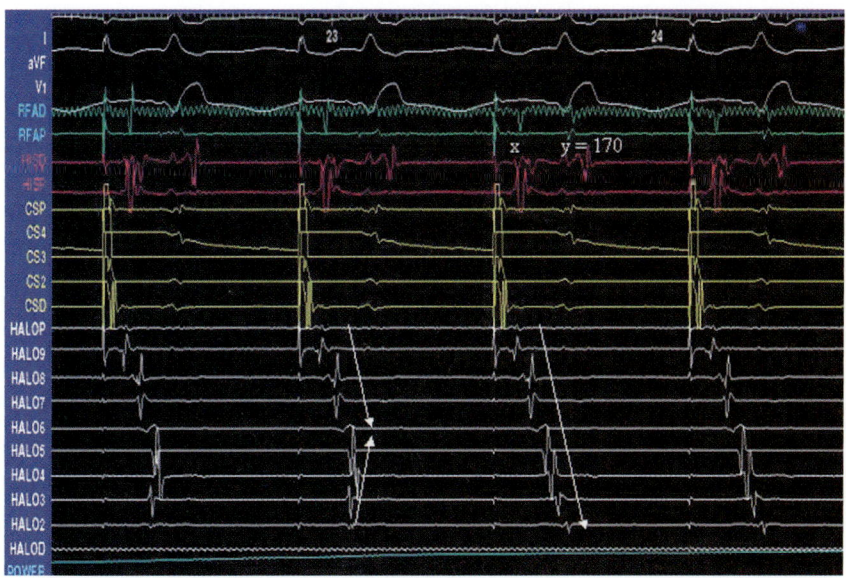

FIGURE 12-24. Surface electrocardiogram leads I, aVF, and V[1], and endocardial electrograms from the coronary sinus (CS), His bundle, halo, mapping and ablation (RF), and right ventricular catheters during radiofrequency catheter ablation of the cavotricuspid isthmus (CTI), while pacing from the CS ostium. Note the change in activation of the lateral right atrium on the Halo catheter from a bidirectional to a unidirectional pattern, indicating the development of clockwise block in the CTI. This was associated with the development of widely spaced (170 msec) double potentials (x and y) on the ablation catheter in the CTI, further confirming medial-to-lateral conduction block. Halo catheter and other tracings are as described in Figure 12-7.

of less than 90 milliseconds between electrogram components anywhere on the ablation line indicates persistent conduction through a gap (Fig. 12-26A).[48] When the interval between electrogram components is more than 90 milliseconds at all points along the ablation line, and maximal variation in the interval is less than 15 milliseconds among all points, it is highly likely that bidirectional CTI is present. When mapping an incomplete ablation line, additional lesions should be given to sites with intervals of less than 90 milliseconds between electrogram components and at sites in which this interval is between 90 and 110 milliseconds if the local electrogram characteristics suggest persistent conduction. These features include the presence of fractionated electrical activity in the interval between electrogram components or if the second electrogram component is positive in polarity. Points along the ablation line with intervals between electrogram components of more than 110 milliseconds do not require further ablation at that site.

Differential pacing maneuvers demonstrate functional linking of local electrograms to a single wavefront passing

through the CTI in the presence of CTI conduction, or dissociation of the local electrograms in the case of conduction block.[66] In this technique, double potentials with an isoelectric interval (>30 milliseconds) are recorded over the ablation line during pacing from just lateral to the line (Fig. 12-27). The times from the stimulus to the initial and terminal components of the split electrograms are measured. The stimulus to first electrogram component represents the time to activation of the ipsilateral side of the ablation line and should be 50 milliseconds or less to demonstrate proximity. The pacing site is then moved about 15 mm further lateral (away from the ablation line) and pacing repeated. In the case of persistent CTI conduction, both components of the split electrogram will be delayed, or linked to the lateral to medial wavefront (Fig. 12-27). In the case of CTI block, however, the time to the first electrogram component is delayed by 20 ± 9 milliseconds, whereas the terminal component is advanced by 13 ± 8 milliseconds, or unchanged in timing (Fig. 12-27). The delay in the terminal component indicates linking of this electrogram, not to the lateral to medial wavefront, but rather to that approaching the ablation line from the medial to lateral direction down the atrial septum. For detection of CTI block, the sensitivity is 100%, specificity 75%, negative-predictive value 94%, and positive-predictive value 100%. It is important that the initial pacing site be as close as possible to the edge of the ablation line and that the more remote pacing site be of limited distance from the first to maintain similar propagation wavefronts. For fractionated electrograms (more than three components) on the ablation line, the first and last component should be measured. This technique may clarify the origin of fractionated potentials as due to a conductive gap or local activation inhomogeneities. Variations on this algorithm have been introduced (Fig. 12-26B).[67]

To expedite the assessment of bidirectional conduction block after CTI ablation and to obviate the need for multipolar electrode catheter recordings, algorithms based on reversal of electrogram polarity near the ablation line and

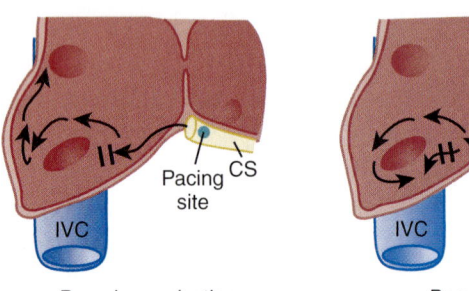

FIGURE 12-25. Patterns of conduction in the low posterior right atrium to create pseudoconduction and pseudoblock after isthmus ablation. See text for details. CS, coronary sinus; IVC, inferior vena cava. *(From Asirvatham S. Correlative anatomy and electrophysiology for the interventional electrophysiologist: right atrial flutter. J Cardiovasc Electrophysiol. 2009;20:113–122. With permission.)*

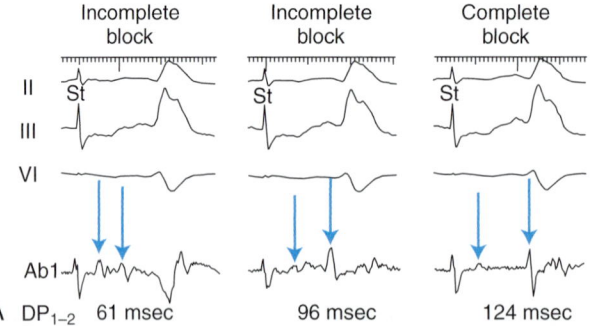

FIGURE 12-26. Methods of determining bidirectional isthmus block after ablation. **A,** Recordings during coronary sinus (CS) pacing before (*left and middle*) and after (*right*) complete isthmus block are shown. Displayed are leads II, III and V1, electrograms recorded by the ablation catheter (Abl). The *arrows* in the electrograms recorded by the Abl point to the components of the double potentials (DPs). The Abl was positioned at exactly the same site in all three panels. *Left,* After several applications of radiofrequency energy along the ablation line, the interval separating the two components of DPs (DP$_{1-2}$) is 61 msec, and there is incomplete block. *Middle,* After an additional application of radiofrequency energy, the DP$_{1-2}$ interval increases to 96 msec, but isthmus block is still incomplete. *Right,* After a final application of radiofrequency energy, the DP$_{1-2}$ interval lengthens to 124 msec, and now there is complete block. Note that when the DP$_{1-2}$ interval was 96 msec, the segment separating the two components of the DP was not isoelectric, providing further evidence that there was a persistent gap in the ablation line. On the transition to complete block, the segment with the DP became isoelectric. St, stimulus artifact.

Methods: Pacing at sites (A, B, C and D) on both sides of ablation line and record bipolar EGM activation times at points A, B, C and D pre- and post ablation.
Measure: Conduction times among sites A, B, C and D
Definition of complete isthmus block: Conduction times A→D > B→D and D→A > C→A after ablation
Reference: Chen. *Circulation* 1999; 100:2507–2513

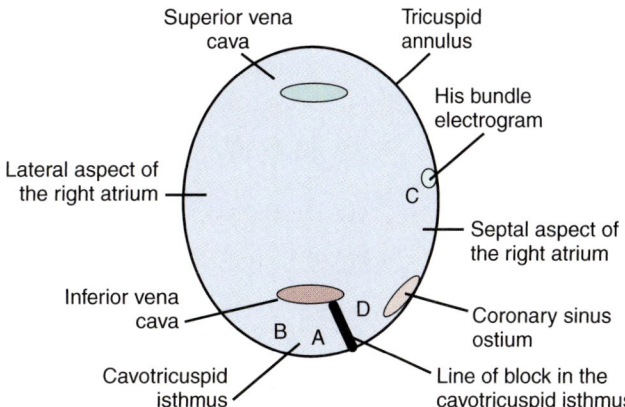

Methods: Pacing PCS and record 2 bipolar EGM (E1 and E2, 2 mm spacing each) 2 mm apart just lateral to ablation line
Measure: Polarity of E1 and E2 during PCS pacing pre- and post ablation
Definition of isthmus block: Transition of EGM polarity from positive to negative at both E1 and E2
Reference: Tada. *JCE* 2001, 12:393–399

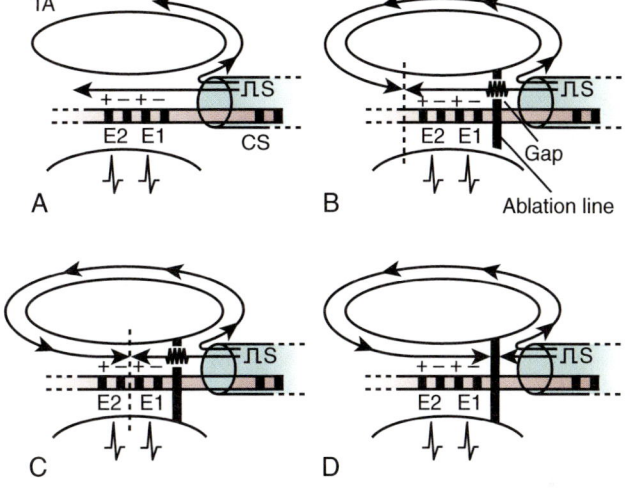

Methods: Unipolar EGM recording during PCS pacing pre- and post ablation
Measure: Unipolar EGM polarity immediately lateral to ablation line
Definition of isthmus complete block: Loss of negative components and development of R or Rs pattern in unipolar EGM
Reference: Villacastin. *Circulation* 2000; 102: 3080–3085

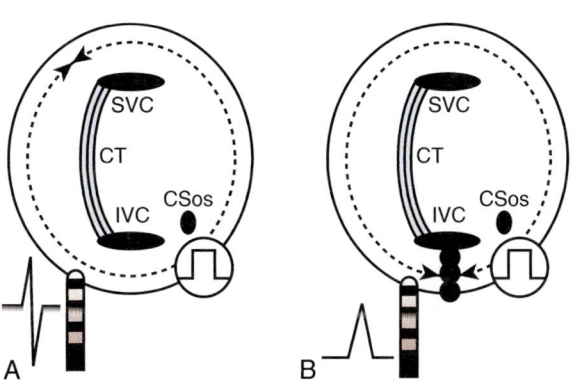

B

FIGURE 12-26, cont'd. B, Additional methods of defining CTI block. *Top,* Use of conduction times needed to cross line of block. In the presence of CTI block, moving the pacing site away from the ablation line shortens the distance to the contralateral side of the line and shortens the conduction time. In the presence of conduction through the line, the distance is prolonged and the conduction times lengthen *Middle,* Bipolar electrograms close to the edge of the ablation line reveal the direction of activation of each bipole. In the presence of CTI block, both bipolar electrogram (EGM) pairs are activated by a wavefront propagating toward the ablation line. In the presence of CTI, one or both bipoles are activated by a wavefront propagating away from the ablation line. *Bottom,* In the presence of CTI block, a unipolar electrogram recorded immediately adjacent to the ablation line records only wavefront activation approaching the electrode and no activation past the edge of the line. In this case, the electrogram is entirely positive. (**A,** From Tada H, Oral H, Sticherling C, et al. Double potentials along the ablation line as a guide to radiofrequency ablation of typical atrial flutter. J Am coll Cardiol, *2001; 38:750–755; B,* top, *from Chen J, de Chilou C, Basiouny T, et al. Cavotricuspid isthmus mapping toassess bidirectional block during common atrial flutter radiofrequency ablation.* Circulation. *1999;100:2507–2513;* **B,** middle, *from Tada H, Oral H, Sticherling C, et al. Electrogram polarity and cavotricuspid isthmus block during ablation of typical atrial flutter.* J Cardiovasc Electroplysiol. *2001m12:393–399,* **B,** bottom, *from Villacastin J, Almendral J, Arenal A, et al. Usefulness of unipolar electrograms to detect isthmus block after radiofrequency ablation of typical atrial flutter.* Circulation, *2000;102:3080–3085. With permission.)*

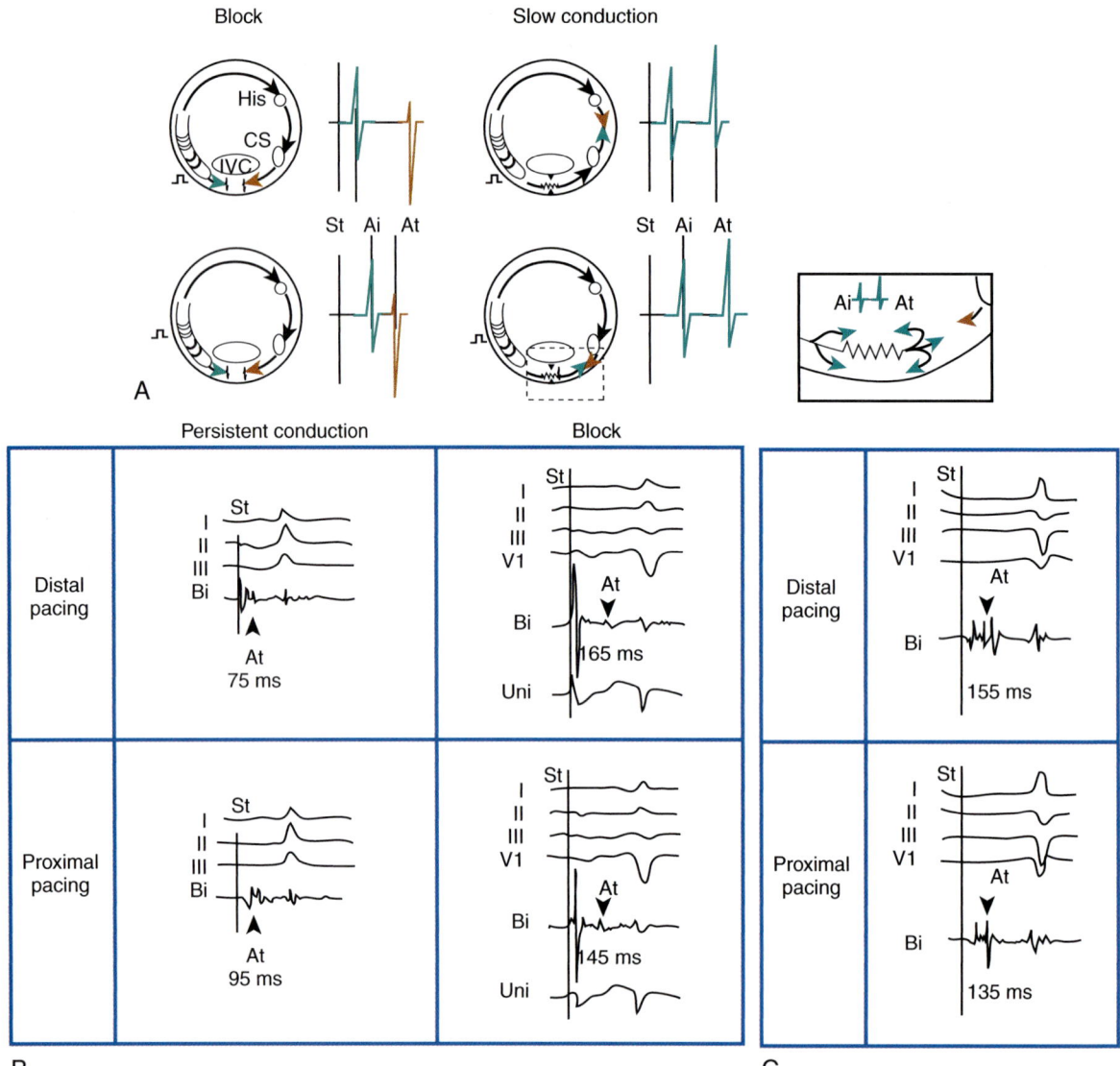

FIGURE 12-27. Differential pacing to assess for isthmus block. **A,** Schematic representation of activation principles on which assessment is based. Right atrium and selected key structures (IVC, His bundle, coronary sinus ostium [Cs]) are shown in a cartoon format. A quadripolar catheter is shown and activation is pictured during distal bipole stimulation (*top row*) and proximal bipole stimulation (*bottom row*). Shown are activation patterns during complete isthmus block (*left*) and during persistent but slow isthmus conduction through a gap in the ablation line (*right*). During complete isthmus block, double potentials separated by an isoelectric interval are recorded on the ablation line as a result of two opposing fronts: a descending front (shown in *blue*) and another that detours around isthmus (in *brown*) give rise to double potentials Ai (initial potential) and At (terminal potential) (*blue* and *brown*, respectively). On changing to a proximal stimulation site, descending wavefront (in *blue*) has to travel a longer distance to reach line of block, whereas detouring wavefront (in *brown*) has a shorter distance to travel; as a result, Ai (*blue* potential) is delayed, and At (*brown* potential) is advanced. During persistent isthmus conduction through a gap in the ablation line, double potentials are recorded as a result of delayed activation of downstream isthmus by the same *blue* front, and therefore both resulting potentials (Ai and At) are shown in *blue* (*inset, far right*). When stimulation is performed from a proximal site, activation pattern does not change, but descending wavefront (in *blue*) has a longer distance to travel to reach isthmus line; as a result, both *blue* potentials (Ai and At) are delayed. St indicates stimulus artifact. **B,** Representative examples of assessment in different patients. *Top left,* double potentials with a stimulus to second potential timing of 75 msec are recorded from isthmus during pacing from distal bipole. The stimulus to first potential timing is 20 msec. As shown in the *bottom left panel,* during pacing from the proximal bipole, both potentials are delayed by 20 msec so that second potential is now activated at 95 msec. This response indicates persistent conduction. Further ablation was performed in cavotricuspid isthmus to complete isthmus block. Surface ECG leads shown are I, II, and III. *Right,* Double potentials with a large first potential and a small second potential are recorded. During distal bipole pacing, as shown in the *top row,* first potential is activated at 15 msec, and second potential is activated at 165 msec after stimulus. During pacing from proximal bipole, below, first potential is delayed by 20 msec and second potential is advanced by 20 msec (145 msec). Note that morphology of both potentials remains unchanged, in bipolar as well as in unipolar electrograms (*lowest trace*). This response indicates complete isthmus block. Surface ECGs include leads I, II, III, and V1. Bi, bipolar electrogram; Uni, unipolar electrogram. Other abbreviations as in **A. C,** Bystander slow conduction and complete block in the presence of a triple potential. A complex triple potential was recorded along the ablation line after documentation of complete isthmus block. Compared with the *top tracing,* which was recorded during stimulation from distal bipole, as shown on *bottom right,* which was recorded during proximal bipole stimulation, the first and second components are delayed identically without a change in their morphology by 25 msec, whereas the third and terminal component, which is also morphologically unchanged, is advanced by 20 msec (155 to 135 msec). This response indicates that complete block exists between second and third components and that first two components are directly linked to each other by a single front of slow or circuitous conduction. Abbreviations as in **A** and **B**. (*From Shah D, Haissaguerre M, Takahashi A, et al. Differential pacing for distinguishing block from persistent conduction through an ablation line.* Circulation. *2000;102:1517–1522. With permission.*)

use of unipolar electrograms have been employed, with varying degrees of accuracy (Fig. 12-26B).[68,69]

Outcomes and Complications

Early reports[1-6] of RF catheter ablation of AFL revealed high initial success rates but with recurrence rates as high as 20% to 45%. However, as experience with RF catheter ablation of AFL has increased, both acute success rates (defined as termination of AFL and bidirectional isthmus block) and chronic success rates (defined as no recurrence of type 1 AFL) have risen to 85% to 95%.[30-42,59] In a large meta-analysis comprising 10,719 patients, the acute success rate for ablation with irrigated or large-tip RF catheters was 94% (95% confidence interval, 90% to 95%) (Table 12-4).[59] Contributing in large degree to these improved results has been the use of cooled irrigation but also the use of bidirectional conduction block in the CTI as a procedural end point.[30-42,59] Randomized comparisons of internally cooled, externally cooled, and large-tip ablation catheters suggest a slightly better acute and chronic success rate with the externally cooled ablation catheters.[33-36,42]

The recurrence rates of AFL after ablation are greatly reduced by the use of irrigated or large-tip ablation catheters (6.7%) compared with standard RF ablation (14%).[59] Most recurrences occur within 6 months of ablation.[59] Individual studies have suggested that the recurrence rates of AFL are higher for cryoablation than for RF ablation.[49] During invasive follow-up 3 months after ablation, 15% of patients undergoing RF CTI ablation had documented recovery of CTI conduction, compared with 34% of patients undergoing cryoablation.[49] In this study, no patient undergoing RF ablation had clinical AFL recurrence, compared with 11% undergoing cryoablation. By meta-analysis, the recurrence rates of AFL were not statistically different for cooled ablation (6.7%) versus cryoablation (11%).[59]

Despite the excellent acute results and long-term outcome after RF catheter ablation for freedom from type 1 AFL, the development of atrial fibrillation or atypical AFL occurs at a high rate in this population of patients (up to 67% over 5 years), especially if there is a history of atrial fibrillation or underlying heart disease.[59,70,71] By meta-analysis, the occurrence rate of atrial fibrillation at 1-2 year follow up was 23% in those without atrial fibrillation before ablation and 53% in those with prior atrial fibrillation.[59] At 5 years' follow-up, the occurrence of atrial fibrillation was similar (60%) regardless of atrial fibrillation history before ablation.[59]

RF catheter ablation of the CTI for type 1 AFL is relatively safe, with complication rates of 2.5% to 3.5%.[59] Most complications are peripheral vascular injury (0.4% of patients), but serious complications can rarely occur, including heart block (0.2% of patients), pericardial effusion and tamponade (0.1% of patients), myocardial infarction from right coronary artery injury, and thromboembolic events, including pulmonary embolism and stroke.[59]

Although conversion of AFL to sinus rhythm is less likely than atrial fibrillation to cause thromboembolic complications (e.g., stroke), there is still a significant risk, and anticoagulation with warfarin before ablation must be considered in patients who have chronic type 1 AFL.[72] This may be particularly important in those patients with depressed left ventricular function, mitral valve disease, or left atrial enlargement with left atrial thrombus or spontaneous contrast on echocardiography. As an alternative, the use of transesophageal echocardiography to rule out left atrial clot or smoke before ablation may be acceptable, but subsequent anticoagulation with warfarin is still recommended because atrial stunning may occur after conversion of AFL, as it does with atrial fibrillation.[72]

Troubleshooting the Difficult Case

With the high acute ablation success rates for AFL reported in most recent series, difficult cases may be encountered only occasionally, but with a large enough caseload, this will eventually happen to most electrophysiologists, and those with a smaller clinical experience may encounter seemingly difficult cases more often. In these cases, several measures can be employed to increase the likelihood of successful ablation (Fig. 12-28; Table 12-5). First and most important, it is critical to ensure that the mechanism of the spontaneous or induced arrhythmia is CTI dependent.

TABLE 12-4

META-ANALYSIS OF ABLATION OUTCOMES BY CATHETER TECHNOLOGY*

Catheter Type	No. of Studies/ No. of Patients	Acute Success (% [95%] CI)	AFL Recurrence (No. of Studies/No. of Patients)	AFL Recurrence (% [95%])†	Atrial Fibrillation Incidence Postablation (% [95%])‡
4-6 mm RF	55/2449	88 (84, 91)	56/2516	14 (11, 17)	21 (13, 33)
8-10 mm or irrigated RF	54/3098	94 (90, 95)	49/3052	7 (5, 8)	25 (19, 31)
Cryoablation	11/489	89 (79, 94)	10/442	11 (8, 16)	31 (14, 54)

*Only studies using cavotricuspid isthmus block as the end point were included.
†Follow-up duration of 14 ± 0.3 months.
‡Data from Perez FJ, Schubert CM, Parvez B, et al. Long-term outcomes after catheter ablation of cavotricuspid isthmus dependent atrial flutter: a meta-analysis. *Circ Arrhythmia Electrophysiol.* 2009;2:393–401. Follow up duration 15 ± 0.4 months and number of studies/patients are 11/231, 24/1936 and 6/325 for 4-6 mm RF, 8-10 mm or irrigated RF and cryoablation, respectively.
AFL, atrial flutter; CI, confidence interval; RF, radiofrequency.

If multielectrode catheter mapping with pacing entrainment is not sufficient to confirm this mechanism, 3D computerized activation may be helpful to rule out other mechanisms of AFL. Occasionally, CTI may terminate into another flutter mechanism that must be recognized.

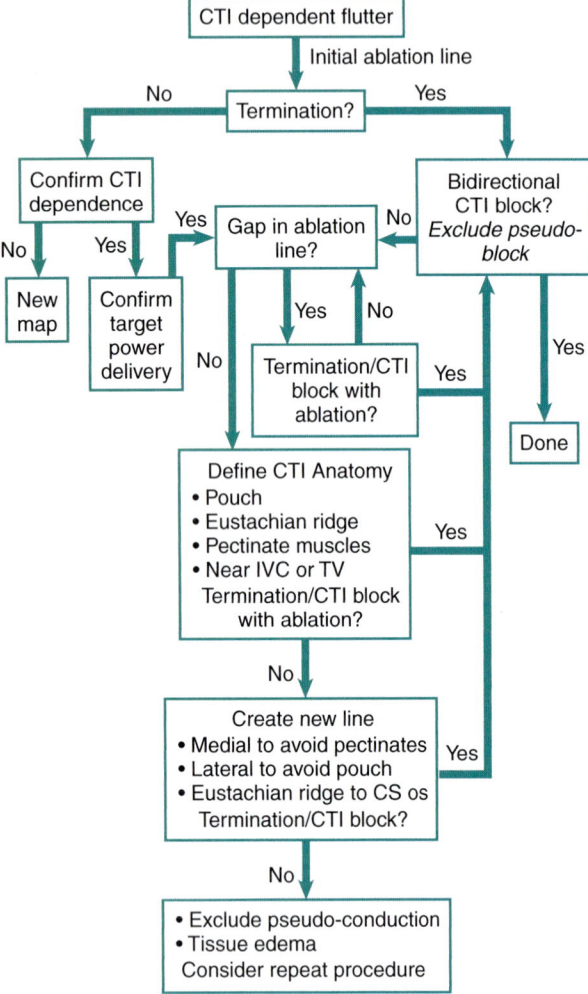

FIGURE 12-28. Schematic diagram for sequence of events during isthmus (CTI) ablation. CS, coronary sinus; IVC, inferior vena cava; TV, tricuspid valve.

Once the CTI dependence of the AFL has been reconfirmed, if initial ablation attempts are unsuccessful, it is essential to ensure that the ablation catheter has reached the extreme borders of the CTI isthmus, including the TV annulus and eustachian ridge or IVC. This again may require the use of large-curve catheters or the use of preformed guiding sheaths, such as the Daig SL1, SRO, or ramp sheaths, to ensure catheter contact across the entire CTI. Careful mapping of the CTI with the appropriate catheter may also help identify a gap in the ablation line by demonstrating an area of narrowly spaced double potentials or continuous fragmented electrical activity, which when ablated may terminate AFL and produce bidirectional CTI conduction block (Fig. 12-10). Persistent CTI conduction after initial failed ablation may also sometimes be identified by 3D computerized activation mapping, if use of standard multielectrode catheters has been unsuccessful. Isthmus pouches are present in most patients in some studies and may not be ablated without specific catheter maneuvers to enter. The presence of a pouch may be visualized by angiography, intracardiac echocardiography, or electroanatomic mapping. The visualization of complex isthmus anatomy early in the case may facilitate a more rapid and successful conclusion.[73]

We recommend that ablation be performed in the 6 o'clock position on the TV annulus initially; if this is unsuccessful and CTI block cannot be achieved even after elimination of gaps in the line, a new ablation line should be created more laterally, at the 7 or 8 o'clock position on the tricuspid annulus. Large right atrial trabeculae may enter the lateral CTI tangentially and require extended ablation to achieve a bidirectional conduction block. If this also is ineffective, an ablation line may be created more medially, at the 5 o'clock position, but care must be taken in this position to monitor AV conduction because the risk for AV block is increased. It is important to give sufficient RF energy at each site. Marked tissue edema may occur after the initial energy delivery, thereby insulating the tissue from further ablation. If new lines fail, voltage-guided ablation of the CTI can be undertaken. Typically, an ablation temperature of 60°C is initially targeted for CTI ablation (non-irrigated catheters), but occasionally, successful ablation requires a temperature as high as 70°C. If standard ablation electrodes of 4 or 5 mm are used initially and ablation fails, the use of either a large-tip (8 to 10 mm) ablation catheter with a high-power generator or an irrigated-tip catheter

TABLE 12-5		
TROUBLESHOOTING DIFFICULT CASES		
Problem	**Cause**	**Solution**
Lack of AFL termination	Non–CTI-dependent AFL as original rhythm or change circuit with ablation	Repeat activation, entrainment mapping

	Incomplete ablation line due to poor tissue contact, low energy delivery, difficult anatomy	Map ablation line for gaps
		  Use steerable or preformed sheath
		  Use large tip or irrigated ablation
		  Angiography, ICE, EA mapping for pouch, large eustachian ridge, pectinate muscles
		  Confirm target energy delivery
		  Deliver new line more lateral or medial
		  Ablate under halo if crosses isthmus

	Partial isthmus reentry	Ablate between IVC and CS os

Continued

TABLE 12-5

TROUBLESHOOTING DIFFICULT CASES—cont'd

Problem	Cause	Solution

Unable to achieve lasting bidirectional CTI	Incomplete ablation line due to poor tissue contact, low energy delivery, difficult anatomy	Map ablation line for gaps
		  Use steerable or preformed sheath
		  Use large tip or irrigated ablation
		  Angiography, ICE, EA mapping for pouch, large eustachian ridge, pectinate muscles
		  Deliver new line more lateral or medial
		  Ablate under halo if crosses isthmus
		  Confirm target energy delivery

	Pseudoconduction posterior to IVC	Detailed mapping with electrodes spanning ablation line, possibly differential pacing maneuvers
	Partial isthmus reentry	Ablate between eustachian ridge and CS os
	Tissue edema after extensive ablation	Create new ablation line, increase power delivery, schedule second procedure after tissue recovery
Low RF energy delivery	Low blood flow due to ablation in pouch, eustachian ridge, or between pectinate muscles	Use irrigated catheter or cryoablation, create new line avoiding unfavorable anatomy
Poor catheter reach, stability, or unable to navigate to target sites	Enlarged right atrium/IVC, large eustachian ridge (limits septal excursion), large pectinate muscles	Use preformed or steerable sheath to stabilize catheter, use longer reach and/or stiffer catheter, angle sheath anteriorly and catheter curvature posteriorly to reach around eustachian ridge, ablation from superior vena cava approach
Failure to attenuate/eliminate local electrograms	Low energy delivery	Increase energy delivery, use irrigated-tip ablation catheter
	Poor tissue contact	Use sheath, increase energy delivery
	Large pectinate muscles in CTI	Increase energy delivery, use sheaths, create new line medially
Painful ablation	Electrical/thermal stimulation Deep sedation of cardiac nerves	Use deep sedation or cryoablation
Changing atrial activation pattern during AFL	Figure-of-eight reentry in right atrium, intermittent crista terminalis breakthrough, intermittent lower loop reentry	Remapping for sustained new activation patterns, use noncontact mapping, reassess after creating CTI block

AFL, atrial flutter; AV, atrioventricular; CS, coronary sinus; CTI, cavotricuspid isthmus; ICE, intracardiac echocardiography; IVC, inferior vena cava; RF, radiofrequency energy

is recommended. We prefer large-tip or cooled-tip catheters as the first-line approach for CTI ablation because they have been shown to have greater efficacy than standard catheters in most studies, or at least to produce CTI block with fewer energy applications and shorter procedure times. The use of temperatures in excess of 70°C with standard or large-tip ablation catheters, or in excess of 50°C with cooled-tip catheters, in an attempt to improve success rates is not recommended because of the increased risk for steam pops, which can cause cardiac rupture.

If CTI block cannot be achieved, the presence of pseudoconduction should be excluded. After extended ablation, tissue edema may make further energy delivery futile, and a second procedure may be necessary.

References

1. Saoudi N, Cosio F, Waldo A, et al. Classification of atrial flutter and regular atrial tachycardia according to electrophysiologic mechanism and anatomic bases: a statement from a joint expert group from the Working Group of Arrhythmias of the European Society of Cardiology and the North American Society of Pacing and Electrophysiology. *J Cardiovasc Electrophysiol.* 2001;12:852–866.
2. Feld GK, Fleck RP, Chen PS, et al. Radiofrequency catheter ablation for the treatment of human type 1 atrial flutter: identification of a critical zone in the re-entrant circuit by endocardial mapping techniques. *Circulation.* 1992;86:1233–1240.
3. Cosio FG, Lopez-Gil M, Goicolea A, et al. Radiofrequency ablation of the inferior vena cava-tricuspid valve isthmus in common atrial flutter. *Am J Cardiol.* 1993;71:705–709.
4. Lesh MD, Van Hare GF, Epstein LM, et al. Radiofrequency catheter ablation of atrial arrhythmias: results and mechanisms. *Circulation.* 1994;89:1074–1089.
5. Cosio FG, Goicolea A, Lopez-Gil M, et al. Atrial endocardial mapping in the rare form of atrial flutter. *Am J Cardiol.* 1990;66:715–720.
6. Tai CT, Chen SA, Chiang CE, et al. Electrophysiologic characteristics and radiofrequency catheter ablation in patients with clockwise atrial flutter. *J Cardiovasc Electrophysiol.* 1997;8:24–34.
7. Olshansky B, Okumura K, Gess PG, et al. Demonstration of an area of slow conduction in human atrial flutter. *J Am Coll Cardiol.* 1990;16:1639–1648.
8. Feld GK, Mollerus M, Birgersdotter-Green U, et al. Conduction velocity in the tricuspid valve-inferior vena cava isthmus is slower in patients with a history of atrial flutter compared to those without atrial flutter. *J Cardiovasc Electrophysiol.* 1997;8:1338–1348.
9. Kinder C, Kall J, Kopp D, et al. Conduction properties of the inferior vena cava-tricuspid annular isthmus in patients with typical atrial flutter. *J Cardiovasc Electrophysiol.* 1997;8:727–737.
10. Da Costa A, Mourot S, Romeyer-Bouchard C, et al. Anatomic and electrophysiological differences between chronic and paroxysmal forms of common atrial flutter and comparison with controls. *Pacing Clin Electrophysiol.* 2004;27:1202–1211.
11. Feld GK, Shahandeh-Rad F. Mechanism of double potentials recorded during sustained atrial flutter in the canine right atrial crush-injury model. *Circulation.* 1992;86:628–641.
12. Olgin JE, Kalman JM, Fitzpatrick AP, et al. Role of right atrial endocardial structures as barriers to conduction during human type 1 atrial flutter: activation and entrainment mapping guided by intracardiac echocardiography. *Circulation.* 1995;92:1839–1848.
13. Olgin JE, Kalman JM, Lesh MD. Conduction barriers in human atrial flutter: correlation of electrophysiology and anatomy. *J Cardiovasc Electrophysiol.* 1996;7:1112–1126.
14. Kalman JM, Olgin JE, Saxon LA, et al. Activation and entrainment mapping defines the tricuspid annulus as the anterior barrier in typical atrial flutter. *Circulation.* 1996;94:398–406.
15. Cabrera JA, Sanchez-Quintana D, Farre G, et al. The inferior right atrial isthmus: further architectural insights for current and coming ablation technologies. *J Cardiovasc Electrophysiol.* 2005;16:402–408.
16. Cabrera JA, Ho SY, Sanchez-Quintana D. How anatomy can guide ablation in isthmic atrial flutter. *Europace.* 2009;11:4–6.
17. Lim K-T, Murray C, Liu H, Weerasooriya R. Pre-ablation magnetic resonance imaging of the cavotricuspid isthmus. *Europace.* 2007;9:149–153.

18. DaCosta A, Romeyer-Bouchard C, Dauphinot V, et al. Cavotricuspid isthmus angiography predicts atrial flutter ablation efficacy in 281 patients randomized between 8 mm- and externally irrigated-tip catheter. *Eur Heart J*. 2006;27:1833–1840.

19. Chang SL, Tai CL, Lin YJ, et al. The electroanatomic characteristics of the cavotricuspid isthmus: implications for the ablation of atrial flutter. *J Cardiovasc Electrophysiol*. 2007;18:18–22.

20. Gami A, Edwards W, Lachman N, et al. Electrophysiological anatomy of typical atrial flutter: the posterior boundary and causes for difficulty with ablation. *J Cardiovasc Electrophysiol*. 2010;21:144–149.

21. Tai CT, Huang JL, Lee PC, et al. High-resolution mapping around the crista terminalis during typical atrial flutter: new insights into mechanisms. *J Cardiovasc Electrophysiol*. 2004;15:406–414.

22. Spach MS, Miller III WT, Dolber PC, et al. The functional role of structural complexities in the propagation of depolarization in the atrium of the dog: cardiac conduction disturbances due to discontinuities of effective axial resistivity. *Circ Res*. 1982;50:175–191.

23. Spach MS, Dolber PS, Heidlage JF. Influence of the passive anisotropic properties on directional differences in propagation following modification of sodium conductance in human atrial muscle: a model of reentry based on anisotropic discontinuous propagation. *Circ Res*. 1988;62:811–832.

24. Olgin JE, Kalman JM, Saxon LA, et al. Mechanisms of initiation of atrial flutter in humans: site of unidirectional block and direction of rotation. *J Am Coll Cardiol*. 1997;29:376–384.

25. Yang Y, Cheng J, Bochoeyer A, et al. Atypical right atrial flutter patterns. *Circulation*. 2001;103:3092–3098.

26. Bochoeyer A, Yang Y, Cheng J, et al. Surface electrocardiographic characteristics of right and left atrial flutter. *Circulation*. 2003;108:60–66.

27. Oshikawa N, Watanabe I, Masaki R, et al. Relationship between polarity of the flutter wave in the surface ECG and endocardial atrial activation sequence in patients with typical counterclockwise and clockwise atrial flutter. *J Interv Card Electrophysiol*. 2002;7:215–223.

28. Okumura K, Plumb VJ, Page PL, et al. Atrial activation sequence during atrial flutter in the canine pericarditis model and its effects on the polarity of the flutter wave in the electrocardiogram. *J Am Coll Cardiol*. 1991;17:509–518.

29. Chugh A, Latchamsetty R, Oral H, et al. Characteristics of cavotricuspid isthmus-dependent atrial flutter after left atrial ablation of atrial fibrillation. *Circulation*. 2006;113:609–615.

30. Fischer B, Haissaguerre M, Garrigues S, et al. Radiofrequency catheter ablation of atrial flutter in 80 patients. *J Am Coll Cardiol*. 1995;25:1365–1372.

31. Kirkorian G, Moncada E, Chevalier P, et al. Radiofrequency ablation of atrial flutter: efficacy of an anatomically guided approach. *Circulation*. 1994;90:2804–2814.

32. Chen SA, Chiang CE, Wu TJ, et al. Radiofrequency catheter ablation of common atrial flutter: comparison of electrophysiologically guided focal ablation technique and linear ablation technique. *J Am Coll Cardiol*. 1996;27:860–868.

33. Jais P, Haissaguerre M, Shah DC, et al. Successful irrigated-tip catheter ablation of atrial flutter resistant to conventional radiofrequency ablation. *Circulation*. 1998;98:835–838.

34. Atiga WL, Worley SJ, Hummel J, et al. Prospective randomized comparison of cooled radiofrequency versus standard radiofrequency energy for ablation of typical atrial flutter. *Pacing Clin Electrophysiol*. 2002;25:1172–1178.

35. Scavee C, Jais P, Hsu LF, et al. Prospective randomized comparison of irrigated-tip and large-tip catheter ablation of cavotricuspid isthmus-dependent atrial flutter. *Eur Heart J*. 2004;25:963–969.

36. Calkins H. Catheter ablation of atrial flutter: do outcomes of catheter ablation with "large-tip" versus "cooled-tip" catheters really differ? *J Cardiovasc Electrophysiol*. 2004;15:1131–1132.

37. Matsuo S, Yamane T, Tokuda M, et al. Prospective randomized comparison of a steerable versus a non steerable sheath for typical atrial flutter ablation. *Europace*. 2010;12:402–409.

38. DaCosta A, Romeyer-Bouchard C, Jamon Y, et al. Radiofreqency catheter selection based on cavotricuspid angiography compared with a control group with an externally irrigated catheter: a randomized pilot study. *J Cardiovasc Electrophysiol*. 2009;20:492–498.

39. Feld GK. Radiofrequency ablation of atrial flutter using large-tip electrode catheters. *J Cardiovasc Electrophysiol*. 2004;15:S18–S23.

40. Feld G, Wharton M, Plumb V, et al, EPT-1000 XP Cardiac Ablation System Investigators. Radiofrequency catheter ablation of type 1 atrial flutter using large-tip 8- or 10-mm electrode catheters and a high-output radiofrequency energy generator: results of a multicenter safety and efficacy study. *J Am Coll Cardiol*. 2004;43:1466–1472.

41. Calkins H, Canby R, Weiss R, et al, 100W Atakr II Investigator Group. Results of catheter ablation of typical atrial flutter. *Am J Cardiol*. 2004;94:437–442.

42. Ventura R, Klemm H, Lutomsky B, et al. Pattern of isthmus conduction recovery using open cooled and solid large-tip catheters for radiofrequency ablation of typical atrial flutter. *J Cardiovasc Electrophysiol*. 2004;15:1126–1130.

43. Hindricks G, Willems S, Kautzner J, et al. Effect of electroanatomically guided versus conventional catheter ablation of typical atrial flutter on the fluoroscopic time and resource use: a prospective randomized multicenter study. *J Cardiovasc Electrophysiol*. 2009;20:734–740.

44. Nakagawa H, Lazzara R, Khastgir T, et al. Role of the tricuspid annulus and the eustachian valve/ridge on atrial flutter: relevance to catheter ablation of the septal isthmus and a new technique for rapid identification of ablation success. *Circulation*. 1996;94:407–424.

45. Nakagawa H, Imai S, Schleinkofer M, et al. Linear ablation from tricuspid annulus to eustachian valve and ridge is adequate for patients with atrial flutter: extending ablation line to the inferior vena cava is not necessary. *J Am Coll Cardiol*. 1997;29:199A.

46. Gula L, Redferarn DP, Veenhuyzen GD, et al. Reduction in atrial flutter ablation time by targeting maximal voltage: Results of a prospective randomized clinical trial. *J Cardiovasc Electrophysiol*. 2009;20:1108–1112.

47. Bauerenfeind T, Kardos A, Foldesi C, et al. Assessment of the maximal voltage-guided technique for cavotricuspid isthmus ablation during ongoing atrial flutter. *J Interv Card Electrophysiol*. 2007;19:195–199.

48. Tada H, Oral H, Sticherling C, et al. Double potentials along the ablation line as a guide to radiofrequency ablation of typical atrial flutter. *J Am Coll Cardiol*. 2001;38:750–755.

49. Kuniss M, Vogtman T, Ventura R, et al. Prospective randomized comparison of durability of bidirectional conduction block in the cavotricuspid isthmus in patients after ablation of common atrial flutter using cryotherapy and radiofrequency energy: the CRYOTIP study. *Heart Rhythm*. 2009;6:1699–1705.

50. Feld GK, Daubert JP, Weiss R, et al, for the Cyoablation Atrial Flutter Efficacy (CAFÉ) Trial Investigators. Acute and long-term efficacy and safety of catheter cryoablation of the cavotricuspid isthmus for treatment of type 1 atrial flutter. *Heart Rhythm J*. 2008;5:1009–1014.

51. Manusama R, Timmermans C, Limon F, et al. Catheter-based cryoablation permanently cures patients with common atrial flutter. *Circulation*. 2004;109:1636–1639.

52. Chan JY, Fung JW, Yu CM, Feld GK. Preliminary results with percutaneous transcatheter microwave: optimizing the detection of bidirectional block across the flutter isthmus for patients with typical isthmus-dependent atrial flutter. *Am J Cardiol*. 2003;91:559–564.

53. Asirvatham SJ. Correlative anatomy and electrophysiology for the interventional electrophysiologist: right atrial flutter. *J Cardiovasc Electrophysiol* 2009;20:113–122.

54. Stovicek P, Fikar M, Wichterle D. Temporal pattern of conduction recurrence during radiofrequency ablation for typical atrial flutter. *J Cardiovasc Electrophysiol* 2006;17:628–641.

55. Nabar A, Rodriguez L, Timmermans C, et al. Isoproterenol infusion to evaluate resumption of conduction after atrial isthmus ablation in Type I atrial flutter. *Circulation* 1999;99:3286–3291.

56. Poty H, Saoudi N, Aziz AA, et al. Radiofrequency catheter ablation of type 1 atrial flutter: Prediction of late success by electrophysiologic criteria. *Circulation* 1995;92:1389–1392.

57. Schwartzman D, Callans D, Gottlieb CD, et al. Conduction block in the inferior caval-tricuspid valve isthmus: association with outcome of radiofrequency ablation of type 1 atrial flutter. *J Am Coll Cardiol* 1996;28:1519–1531.

58. Mangat I, Tschopp DR Jr, Yang Y, et al. Optimizing the detection of bidirectional block across the flutter isthmus for patients with typical isthmus-dependent atrial flutter. *Am J Cardiol* 2003;91:559–564.

59. Perez FJ, Schubert CM, Parvez B, et al. Long-term outcomes after catheter ablation of cavo-tricuspid isthmus dependent atrial flutter: a meta-analysis. *Circ Arrhythmia Electrophysiol*. 2009;2:393–401.

60. Arenal A, Almendral J, Alday JM, et al. Rate-dependent conduction block of the crista terminalis in patients with typical atrial flutter: Influence on evaluation of cavotricuspid isthmus conduction block. *Circulation*. 1999;99:2771–2778.

61. Liu TY, Tai CT, Huang BH, et al. Functional characterization of the crista terminalis in patients with atrial flutter: Implications for radiofrequency ablation. *J Am Coll Cardiol*. 2004;43:1639–1645.

62. Anselme F, Savoure A, Ouali S, et al. Transcristal conduction during isthmus ablation of typical atrial flutter: influence on success criteria. *J Cardiovasc Electrophysiol*. 2004;15:184–189.

63. Scaglione M, Riccardi R, Calo L, et al. Typical atrial flutter ablation: conduction across the posterior region of the inferior vena cava may mimic unidirectional isthmus block. *J Cardiovasc Electrophysiol*. 2000;11:387–395.

64. Oral H, Sticherling C, Tada H, et al. Role of transisthmus intervals in predicting bidirectional block after ablation of typical atrial flutter. *J Cardiovasc Electrophysiol*. 2001;12:169–174.

65. Tai CT, Haque A, Lin YK, et al. Double potential interval and transisthmus conduction time for prediction of cavotricuspid isthmus block after ablation of typical atrial flutter. *J Interv Card Electrophysiol*. 2002;7:77–82.

66. Shah D, Haissaguerre M, Takahashi A, et al. Differential pacing for distinguishing block from persistent conduction through an ablation line. *Circulation*. 2000;102:1517–1522.

67. Chen J, de Chillou C, Basiouny T, et al. Cavotricuspid isthmus mapping to assess bidirectional block during common atrial flutter radiofrequency ablation. *Circulation*. 1999;100:2507–2513.

68. Tada H, Oral H, Sticherling C, et al. Electrogram polarity and cavotricuspid isthmus block during ablation of typical atrial flutter. *J Cardiovasc Electrophysiol*. 2001;12:393–399.

69. Villacastin J, Almendral J, Arenal A, et al. Usefulness of unipolar electrograms to detect isthmus block after radiofrequency ablation of typical atrial flutter. *Circulation.* 2000;102:3080–3085.
70. Gilligan DM, Zakaib JS, Fuller I, et al. Long-term outcome of patients after successful radiofrequency ablation for typical atrial flutter. *Pacing Clin Electrophysiol.* 2003;26:53–58.
71. Tai CT, Chen SA, Chiang CE, et al. Long-term outcome of radiofrequency catheter ablation for typical atrial flutter: risk prediction of recurrent arrhythmias. *J Cardiovasc Electrophysiol.* 1998;9:115–121.
72. Gronefeld GC, Wegener F, Israel CW, et al. Thromboembolic risk of patients referred for radiofrequency catheter ablation of typical atrial flutter without prior appropriate anticoagulation therapy. *Pacing Clin Electrophysiol.* 2003;26:323–327.
73. Da Costa A, Romeyer-Bouchard C, Jamon Y, et al. Radiofrequency catheter selection based on cavotricuspid angiography compared with a control group with an externally cooled-tip catheter: a randomized pilot study. *J Cardiovasc Electrophysiol.* 2009;20:492–498.

13
Ablation of Non–Isthmus-Dependent Flutters and Atrial Macro-Reentry

Steven M. Markowitz and Bruce B. Lerman

Key Points

Atypical atrial flutter requires fixed or functional barriers and regions of slow conduction.

Activation mapping is used to demonstrate early or mid-diastolic potentials, fractionated potentials, and double potentials. Concealed entrainment demonstrates participation in the tachycardia circuit. Electroanatomic mapping is used to visualize the reentrant circuit.

Multipolar electrode (halo) catheter maps right atrial free wall and tricuspid annulus. The electroanatomic mapping system (contact or noncontact) is essential for many cases. An irrigated-tip or large-tip (8-mm) ablation system may be needed.

Sources of difficulty include defining complex reentrant circuits, ablation in the mitral isthmus, and spontaneous conversion of atypical flutter to atrial fibrillation or other arrhythmias.

Atrial macro-reentrant rhythms comprise a heterogeneous group of arrhythmias that arise de novo from both the right and left atria. In many cases, these arrhythmias may also coexist with atrial fibrillation (AF) or play transitional roles in the initiation or termination of AF or in the transformation to typical atrial flutter. In other cases, these rhythms occur late after catheter ablation or surgical treatment of AF.

Historically, there has been confusion over the use of the terms *atrial flutter* and *atrial tachycardia*.[1] It has been proposed that these terms be applied based on rate or the presence of isoelectric intervals on the electrocardiogram. This classification, however, has little clinical relevance because it does not correlate with the mechanism of arrhythmia.[2] In this text, the term *macro-reentrant atrial tachycardia* will be used preferentially to refer to rhythms commonly called

atypical atrial flutters and will comprise a variety of circuits other than right atrial isthmus-dependent flutter.

Macro-reentrant atrial tachycardias may be classified based on their chamber of origin and site within a given atrium (Table 13-1). Subclassification of these arrhythmias is based on type of circuit, such as single or dual loop reentry, and clinical substrate.

Anatomy

The specific configuration of a macro-reentrant circuit is dependent on the anatomy of the atrium as well as its conduction and refractory properties. As a general rule, reentry requires the presence of two limbs, which are anatomically or functionally dissociated, or both. These limbs are dependent on the presence of a central barrier (i.e., atrioventricular annulus, venous ostium, or scar) or a functional line of block. In the right atrium (RA), natural barriers to conduction include the tricuspid valve, inferior vena cava (IVC), superior vena cava (SVC), crista terminalis, eustachian ridge, and fossa ovale. In the left atrium (LA), the mitral annulus and pulmonary venous ostia serve as critical conduction barriers, in addition to electrically silent areas that may be found in myopathic atria or result from prior ablation or surgery.

Pathophysiology

Although atypical macro-reentrant atrial tachycardias can arise in structurally normal hearts, these arrhythmias predominantly occur in patients with organic heart disease or after cardiac surgery or catheter ablation of AF. In patients with organic heart disease, the pathogenesis is thought to involve atrial hypertension, which causes interstitial fibrosis resulting in conduction slowing and block. Left atrial macro-reentry that arises de novo frequently involves regions of patchy scar, which presumably occur as the result of an atrial myopathy. These areas of patchy scar can be identified as electrically silent areas during electroanatomic mapping. Other important features include slowing of atrial conduction velocity, heterogeneity of atrial refractoriness, and a role for initiating or triggering foci.

In response to premature stimuli, arcs of functional block develop and, if of sufficient length, initiate and support reentry. Functional lines of block develop in structures such as the crista terminalis and the eustachian ridge, both of which play a critical role in the formation of typical isthmus-dependent atrial flutter.[3] Gaps in these functional lines of block, as in the crista terminalis, permit atypical circuits to form. Functional lines of block develop in many other locations, including variable sites in the LA. A combination of fixed and functional block has been demonstrated in animal models of lesional tachycardia, in which a line of functional block develops as a extension to a fixed anatomic lesion.[4] In this case, the anatomic lesion might not be large enough to support reentry, but the combined fixed and functional barrier provides the critical path length needed to maintain reentry. Formation and breakdown of these arcs of block are responsible for interconversion of flutter circuits with each other and the transition to AF.

In recent years, macro-reentrant atrial tachycardias have become increasingly frequent after catheter and surgical ablation. Discontinuities in ablation lines result in unidirectional or rate-dependent block as well as conduction slowing.[5] Furthermore, areas of excluded myocardium, such as occurs with wide encircling pulmonary vein isolation, give rise to large central barriers that permit circus movement reentry. Many macro-reentrant atrial tachycardias are complex circuits that involve dual loops ("figure-of-eight" reentry) or, less commonly, triple loops. In multiple loop tachycardias, conduction times are equal around the individual loops, but sometimes a dominant circuit exists as a "driver," which entrains other loops.

Diagnosis

Macro-Reentrant versus Focal Atrial Tachycardia

A fundamental consideration in evaluating an atrial tachycardia is to establish whether the arrhythmia is macro-reentrant or focal in origin. Surface electrocardiographic criteria are not sufficiently sensitive or specific to establish the mechanism of an atrial tachycardia. For example, an isoelectric baseline does not reliably distinguish a focal from a macro-reentrant atrial arrhythmia.[2] When the tachycardia cycle length varies by 15% or more, a focal mechanism is suggested, but a regular cycle length can occur with both focal and macro-reentrant atrial tachycardias.[6] For localization of atypical reentrant circuits, the flutter wave morphology similarly has limited utility. Although "typical" flutter waves (referring to the so-called sawtooth flutter wave pattern with deep negative deflections in the inferior leads and positive deflections in V_1) are usually associated with counterclockwise isthmus-dependent right atrial flutter, other atypical right atrial or even left atrial flutters may demonstrate similar flutter wave morphology. Typical isthmus-dependent right atrial flutter that occurs after left atrial ablation for AF may also present with atypical electrocardiographic morphologies.[7] In the LA, in particular, there is a large overlap in the flutter morphologies among different circuits.

Evidence for a macro-reentrant mechanism can be obtained through manifest entrainment, entrainment with concealed fusion ("concealed entrainment"), or electroanatomic mapping (Table 13-2; see also "Mapping," later). Manifest entrainment is recognized as fixed but progressive fusion with progressively rapid overdrive pacing.[8] Because the surface P-wave morphology may not be visible or may

---

TABLE 13-1

TYPES OF NON–ISTHMUS-DEPENDENT ATRIAL FLUTTERS

Circuit	Boundaries	Clinical Scenarios
Right Atrium		
Upper loop reentry	SVC and crista terminalis	De novo or with CVTI dependent flutter
Right atrial free wall reentry	Right atrial scar with or without crista terminalis	Prior right atriotomy, atrial myopathy
Dual loop reentry (combined lower loop, upper loop, free wall, and/or tricuspid valve)	Combinations of right atrial scar, SVC, crista terminalis with or without CVTI	De novo or with CVTI-dependent flutter, prior right atriotomy, atrial myopathy
Left Atrium		
Perimitral annular reentry	Mitral annulus, left atrial isthmus	After left atrial ablation for atrial fibrillation, de novo
Peripulmonary vein reentry ("roof dependent") or multiple gaps in encircling lesion	Linear ablation lines around left and/or right pulmonary veins, possibly electrically active pulmonary vein tissue	After left atrial ablation for atrial fibrillation with encircling lesions
Periseptal tachycardia	Right pulmonary veins and mitral annulus or fossa ovalis with right pulmonary veins or mitral annulus	After atriotomy, left atrial ablation for atrial fibrillation, de novo
Lesional tachycardias	Surgical scars	After left atriotomy, maze surgery
Miscellaneous		
Coronary sinus–mediated reentry	Coronary sinus with left or right atrial myocardium	De novo

CVTI, cavotricuspid isthmus; SVC, superior vena cava.

be obscured by ventricular depolarization or repolarization, intracardiac electrograms provide a surrogate marker for orthodromic and antidromic capture and the degree of fusion. During entrainment, the last beat of overdrive pacing is entrained at the paced cycle length but is not fused. Manifest entrainment with progressive fusion implies at least two dimensions to the tachycardia circuit and therefore a reentrant mechanism.

If the return cycle length after entrainment is within 30 milliseconds longer than the tachycardia cycle length, the pacing site is considered a critical component of the tachycardia circuit. Entrainment from two opposite quadrants (such as septal and lateral LA, or anterior and posterior

LA), each with return cycle lengths within 30 milliseconds of the tachycardia cycle length, indicates the presence of a macro-reentrant circuit.[6] Thus, "perfect" entrainment from the septal and lateral LA often indicates perimitral reentry; entrainment from the anterior and posterior LA indicates a roof-dependent left atrial flutter.

Manifest entrainment may also give indirect information about the distance of a recording site from the elements of a reentrant circuit.[9] When the pacing site is different from the recording site, a return cycle length equal to the tachycardia cycle length indicates that the recording site is orthodromically captured (and may be within the circuit or outside). A return cycle length longer than the tachycardia cycle length indicates that the site is outside the circuit, with more distant sites having longer return cycle lengths. A short return cycle length is consistent with antidromic capture of the recording site. These general rules may break down if there are separate entrance and exit sites to the reentrant circuit.

Adenosine is useful in distinguishing macro-reentrant from focal atrial tachycardias in that it exerts mechanistic-specific effects on atrial arrhythmias.[10,11] With rare exceptions, adenosine does not terminate most macro-reentrant atrial arrhythmias but either terminates or transiently suppresses focal atrial tachycardias (Fig. 13-1). In a cohort of 84 atrial tachycardias, we found that the sensitivity and specificity of adenosine for identifying a macro-reentrant mechanism were 96% and 95%, respectively. Adenosine-insensitive atrial tachycardias with apparently focal activation patterns show characteristics of localized reentrant circuits, including low amplitude, long-duration fractionated electrograms, and can be entrained.[12] This simple tool provides a reliable means to establish a tachycardia mechanism before mapping (Fig. 13-2).

TABLE 13-2
DIAGNOSTIC CRITERIA
Macro-Reentrant Tachycardia
Entrainment with fusion (with last beat entrained but not fused)
Electroanatomic mapping of >90% of tachycardia cycle length with adjacent early and late areas of activation
Insensitivity to adenosine (in dose sufficient to cause atrioventricular block)
Left Atrial Tachycardias
Passive conduction in the right atrium, with early septal activation and fusion of wavefronts in the right atrial lateral wall
Absence of right atrium activation during long segments of the cycle length (mapping <50% of tachycardia cycle length)
Large variations in the right atrial cycle length with a relatively fixed cycle length in the left atrium
Entrainment pacing at multiple sites in the right atrium yielding postpacing intervals >30 msec

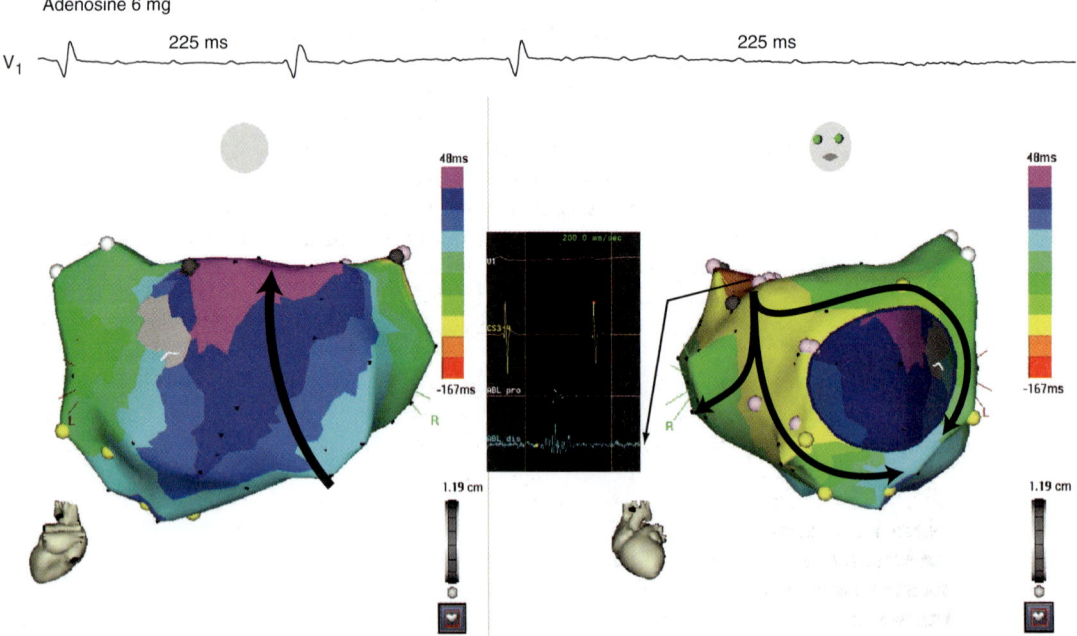

FIGURE 13-1. Left atrial roof-dependent macro-reentry. Adenosine results in transient high-grade atrioventricular block but no change in the atrial tachycardia cycle length or morphology, an effect typical for macro-reentrant atrial tachycardias. Electroanatomic map of this roof-dependent tachycardia shows an ascending wavefront in the posterior wall seen in posteroanterior projection (*left*). The wavefront encircles the right pulmonary veins and fuses around the mitral annulus, as shown in the left anterior oblique projection (*right*). A fractionated, low-amplitude electrogram is present in the roof of the left atrium, the site of successful termination of the tachycardia with radiofrequency ablation. Isochronal maps are displayed with steps of 20 msec.

Localization of Reentry to the Right or Left Atrium

Left atrial tachycardias typically manifest positive deflections in lead V_1. The limb leads are highly variable and depend on the particular circuit and conduction characteristics. They may show inferior or superior axes or low-amplitude oscillating deflections. Some cases of left atrial tachycardia can give rise to morphologies that are similar to typical flutter.

Right atrial tachycardias typically exhibit proximal-to-distal activation in the coronary sinus (CS), unless activation proceeds over the Bachmann bundle, in which case the distal CS may be activated earlier. Left atrial tachycardias show a variety of activation sequences depending on the particular reentrant circuit (Fig. 13-3). Some LA tachycardias, such as clockwise perimitral annular reentry and tachycardias originating near the left pulmonary

veins, exhibit distal-to-proximal CS activation. However, a proximal-to-distal sequence does not necessarily locate the arrhythmia to the RA and may be seen with counterclockwise perimitral reentry or tachycardias involving the septum or right pulmonary veins. Other unusual activation sequences in the CS can be explained by complex wavefront interactions at the mitral annulus. Wavefronts that descend the posterior wall first activate the mid-posterior annulus, whereas wavefronts that descend the anterior LA wall usually demonstrate fusion in the posterior mitral annulus; both patterns occur in LA roof-dependent flutter. It should be recognized that activation of the coronary sinus may be dissociated from the left atrial endocardium because of a muscular sleeve that envelopes the CS and is attached to the LA through discrete connections. Macro-reentry involving the CS musculature as a critical part of the circuit has also been reported.[13,14]

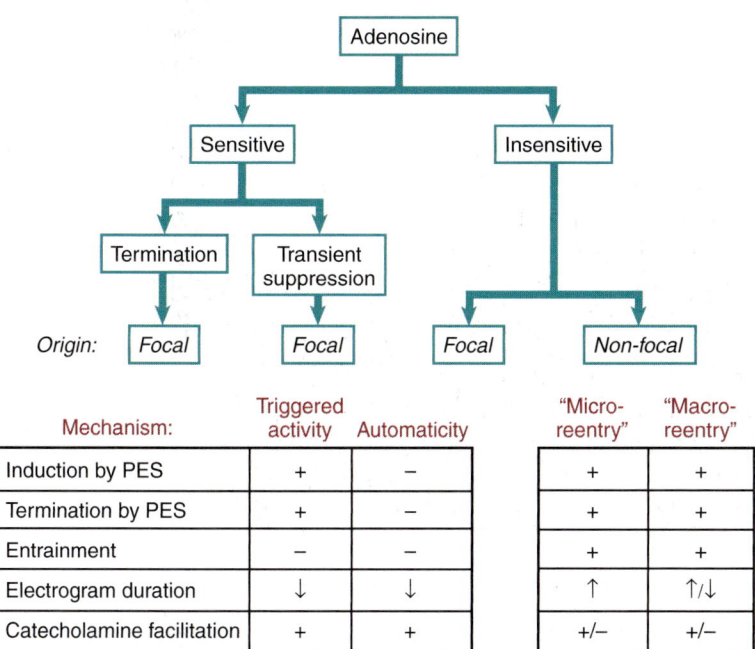

Mechanism:	Triggered activity	Automaticity		"Micro-reentry"	"Macro-reentry"
Induction by PES	+	−		+	+
Termination by PES	+	−		+	+
Entrainment	−	−		+	+
Electrogram duration	↓	↓		↑	↑/↓
Catecholamine facilitation	+	+		+/−	+/−

FIGURE 13-2. Differentiating mechanisms of atrial tachycardia using adenosine and electrophysiologic characteristics. Adenosine-sensitive atrial tachycardia is typically focal in origin and due to triggered activity or, far less commonly, automaticity. Adenosine-insensitive atrial tachycardia is either macro-reentrant or micro-reentrant, depending on circuit size and the resolution of the mapping system. Entrainment with the postpacing interval nearly equal to the atrial tachycardia cycle length is typical for macro- or micro-reentrant tachycardias. Prolonged electrogram durations may be recorded at early sites in micro-reentrant tachycardias but are not typical at the origin of triggered and automatic rhythms. Electrogram durations at sites around a macro-reentrant circuit might vary depending on local conduction characteristics. PES, programmed electrical stimulation. *(Adapted from Markowitz SM, Nemirovksy D, Stein KM, et al. Adenosine-insensitive focal atrial tachycardia: evidence for de novo micro-re-entry in the human atrium. J Am Coll Cardiol. 2007;49:1324-1333. With permission.)*

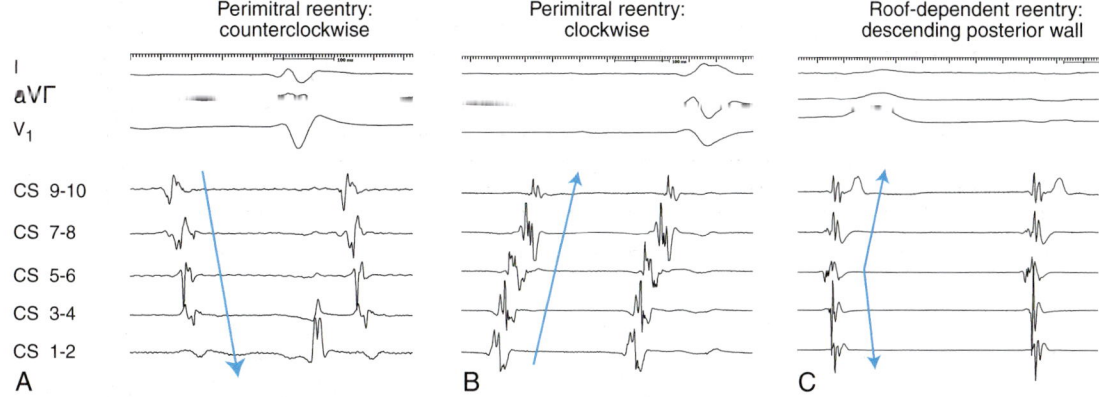

FIGURE 13-3. Activation sequences of the coronary sinus (CS) in various forms of left atrial tachycardia. **A,** Counterclockwise perimitral reentry gives rise to proximal-to-distal CS activation. **B,** Clockwise perimitral reentry produces distal-to-proximal CS activation. **C,** Roof-dependent atrial tachycardia with a descending wavefront in the posterior wall causes early activation in the middle CS, after which the impulse propagates both proximally and distally along the mitral annulus.

It is possible to establish a diagnosis of left atrial tachy-cardia during mapping in the RA and thus to identify the need for transseptal catheterization and LA mapping.[15,16] Criteria for identifying an LA origin through intracardiac mapping include the following:

1. Passive conduction into the RA, which may be demon-strated as fused wavefronts in the lateral wall of the RA
2. Earliest RA activation in the septum, typically in the region of Bachmann bundle or the coronary sinus ostium
3. Absence of RA activation during long segments of the cycle length. In the case of a macro-reentrant rhythm, if less than 50% of the tachycardia cycle length cannot be mapped in the RA, it is highly likely that the origin arises in the LA.
4. Large variations in the RA cycle length with a relatively fixed cycle length in the LA, implying LA and RA dis-sociation or conduction block
5. Entrainment pacing at multiple sites in the RA (includ-ing the cavotricuspid isthmus and the RA free wall) yield-ing postpacing intervals of more than 30 milliseconds

Although fusion of wavefronts in the lateral wall of the RA is common during LA tachycardias, it is possible to record a single wavefront mimicking counterclockwise or clockwise atrial flutter. This situation depends on (1) the location of the multipolar catheter in the lateral wall, (2) the location of conduction breakthrough from the LA (i.e., preferential conduction over Bachmann bundle or the CS), and (3) the presence of conduction block in the cavotricuspid isthmus. Typically, activation time in the RA is substantially less than the tachycardia cycle length. Exceptions occur when the tachycardia cycle length is short or if conduction is substantially slowed in the RA, falsely implying the presence of a right atrial tachycardia.

Mapping

Activation Mapping

Conventional activation mapping with multielectrode cath-eters may be the chief means to define some mechanisms of atypical right atrial flutter, especially if the arrhythmia is transitory. For example, counterclockwise lower loop reen-try reveals lateral-to-septal activation in the cavotricuspid isthmus and areas of "breakthrough" in the lateral RA with fusion of waveforms along the lateral wall (Fig. 13-4).[17]

Double potentials, which usually signify lines of block, may be identified through conventional activation map-ping. If reentry proceeds around a line of block, double potentials are widely split in the middle of the line, and they

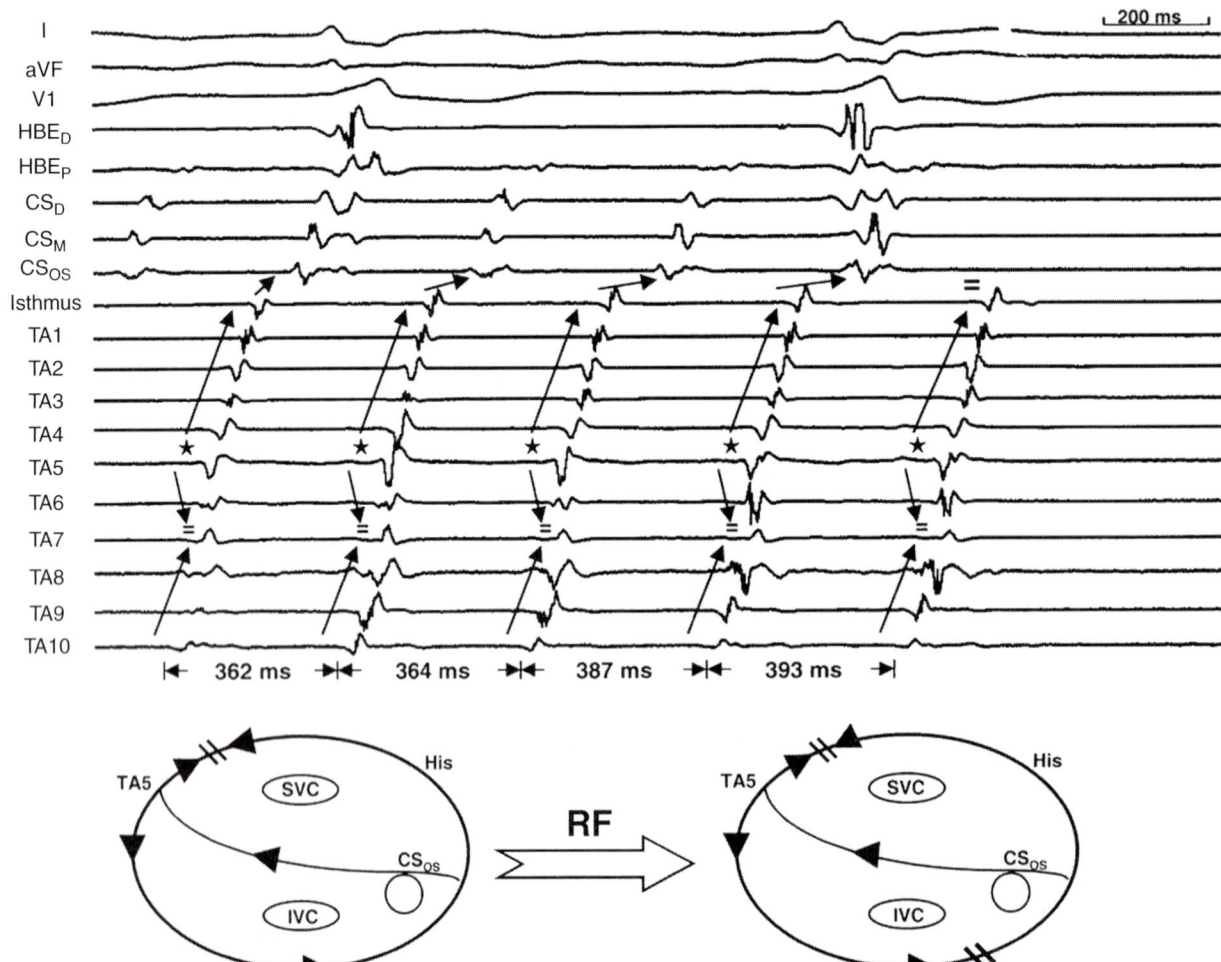

FIGURE 13-4. Lower loop reentry in a patient who also showed counterclockwise right atrial flutter. Early breakthrough is depicted by stars at TA5. Collision of wavefronts occurs over the high/lateral right atrium. During radiofrequency energy (RF) application of the cavotricuspid isthmus, gradual prolongation of the tachycardia cycle length was recorded before block in the isthmus. CS, coronary sinus; HBE, His bundle electrogram; IVC, infe-rior vena cava; SVC, superior vena cava; TA, tricuspid annulus. *(From Yang Y, Cheng J, Bochoeyer A, et al. Atypical right atrial flutter patterns. Circulation. 2001;103:3092–3098. With permission.)*

progressively narrow toward the end of the line where the wavefront pivots.[18] An example of this may be found in right atrial free wall macro-reentry (Fig. 13-5). Mid-diastolic and fragmented potentials are consistent with sites within critical zones of slow conduction, but verification of participation in the tachycardia circuit is required through other means.

Activation mapping in the LA relative to a fixed reference can identify or exclude mitral reentry or roof-dependent flutter.[6] Opposite activation sequences in the superior and inferior mitral annulus (e.g., lateral-to-septal activation along the superior annulus and septal-to-lateral activation along the inferior annulus) identify perimitral reentry. In contrast, similar directions of activation (e.g., lateral-to-septal) in both the anterior and inferior annulus exclude perimitral reentry. Opposite activation along the anterior and posterior walls is seen with roof-dependent reentry.

Entrainment Mapping

Concealed entrainment is an essential tool for identifying sites that participate in a reentrant arrhythmia.[19] Criteria for identifying sites within a circuit are (1) concealed entrainment (with P-wave and intracardiac activation sequences resembling those in tachycardia), (2) a postpacing interval within 30 milliseconds

of the tachycardia cycle recorded at the pacing site, and (3) a stimulus to P-wave interval during pacing equal to the electrogram to P-wave interval during tachycardia. Because the P wave may not be visible in many cases of atypical atrial flutter, identifying the initial inscription of the P wave may be arbitrary, and an intracardiac reference is often used as a surrogate.

Limitations or "pitfalls" in using concealed entrainment must be recognized:

1. Rate-related conduction slowing may occur, and therefore the postpacing interval might not equal the tachycardia cycle length. This can be minimized by pacing 10 to 30 milliseconds less than the tachycardia cycle length.
2. Failure to capture might occur in some critical regions of a reentrant circuit.
3. Acceleration or termination of atrial tachycardia with pacing occurs commonly. Finally, spontaneous variations in the tachycardia cycle length can make the interpretation of entrainment maneuvers difficult.

Electroanatomic Mapping

Electroanatomic mapping provides direct visualization of a reentrant circuit, which is defined as the shortest distance of continuous activation comprising the tachycardia cycle length.

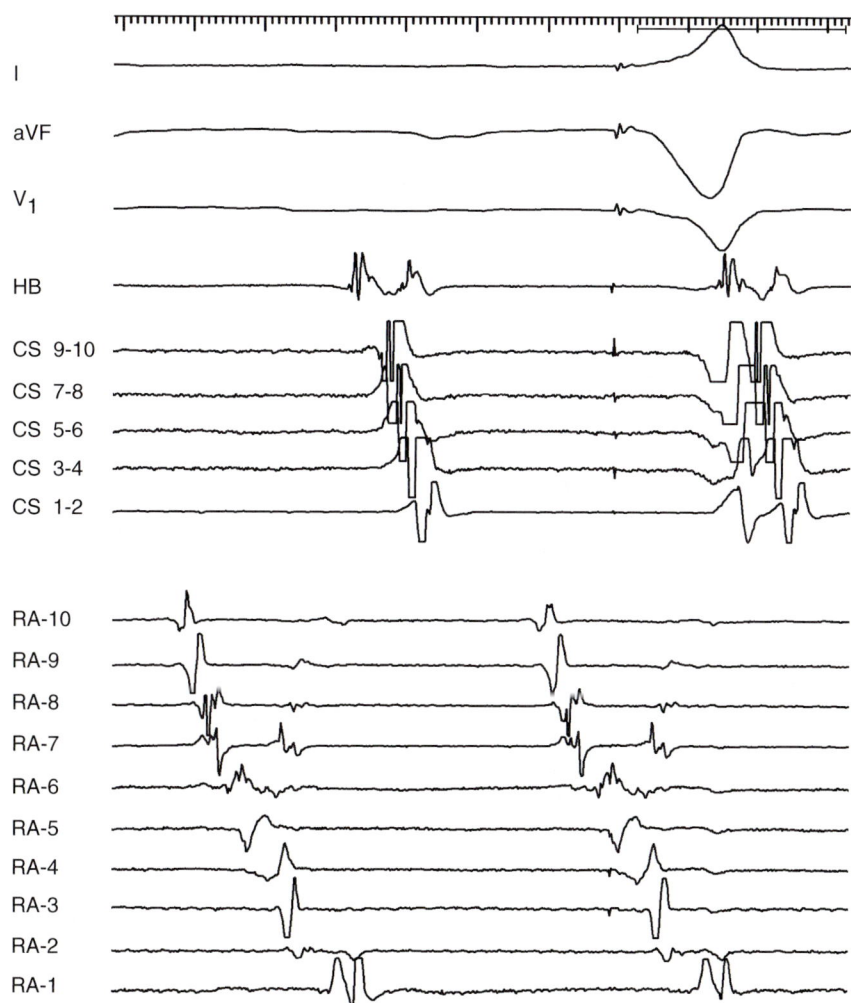

FIGURE 13-5. Right atrial free wall reentry. Double potentials in the lateral wall reflect descending and ascending wavefronts, with narrowing of the intervals between double potentials down the lateral wall and a fragmented electrogram reflecting a "pivot point" in pole RA-6 (RA-1, low lateral RA; RA-10, high lateral RA). HB, His bundle.

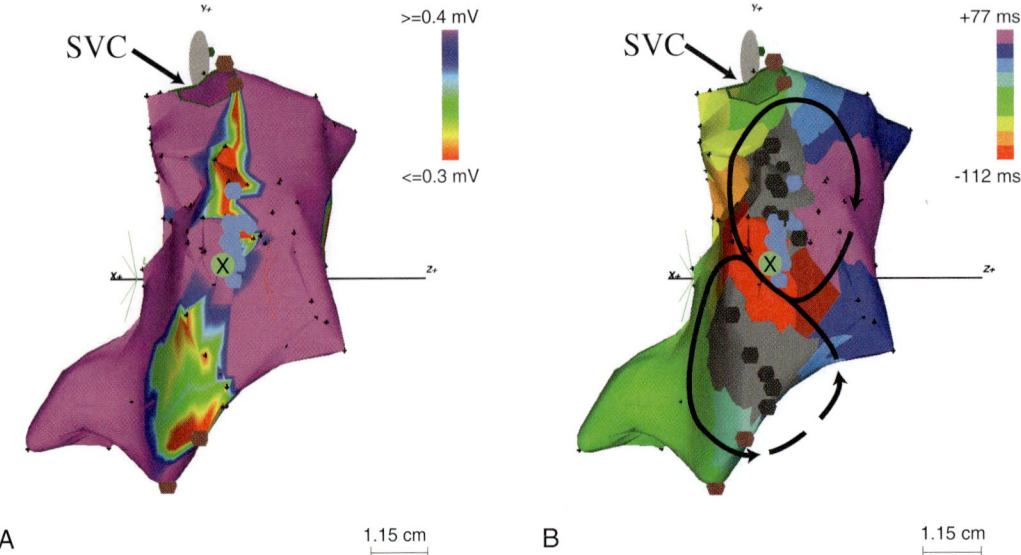

FIGURE 13-6. Dual loop right atrium tachycardia in a patient who had mitral valve surgery, with a separate left atriotomy and reoperation with the superior transseptal approach. **A,** Bipolar electroanatomic voltage map of the right atrium in a right posterolateral projection. A zone of low voltage is present in the lateral wall of the right atrium, extending to the superior vena cava (SVC) and the inferior vena cava. *Blue tags* indicate double potentials. The *green tag* is a site of concealed entrainment where ablation terminated atrial tachycardia. At this site, the stimulus to P-wave interval during pacing was identical to the electrogram to P-wave during tachycardia (125 msec). **B,** Isochronal activation map. Dual loop reentry is present, with a common isthmus between two lesions in the lateral wall. *(From Markowitz SM, Brodman RF, Stein KM, et al. Lesional tachycardias related to mitral valve surgery. J Am Coll Cardiol. 2002;39:1973–1983. With permission.)*

A hallmark of macro-reentrant arrhythmias is the presence of areas of early activation adjacent to late regions, with intermediate values connecting these two regions (Fig. 13-6). In practice, it is necessary to account for at least 90% of the tachycardia cycle length to visualize a reentrant circuit. Many macro-reentrant atrial tachycardias do not require exhaustive electroanatomic mapping to achieve successful ablation because inferences about tachycardia mechanism and location can be drawn from a deductive approach of activation and entrainment mapping. Typically if less than 50% of the tachycardia cycle length is accounted for by mapping of one atrium, the circuit is probably contained in the contralateral atrium.

Contact electroanatomic mapping (Carto, Biosense Webster, Diamond Bar, CA, and NavX, St. Jude Medical, St. Paul, MN) involves the sequential recording of contact bipolar or unipolar electrograms and display on a 3D navigation system. Conceptually, this technique is an extension of conventional activation mapping by graphically displaying activation times. In mapping a reentrant atrial tachycardia, the user defines a window close to the tachycardia cycle length, and activation times are assigned as "early" or "late" relative to a reference. Designating activation times in a macro-reentrant circuit as early or late is arbitrary. In theory, a change in the window or reference would not change the circuit but only results in a phase shift of the map. Displaying activation information as an isochronal map may clearly demonstrate the direction of wavefront propagation, which is perpendicular to the isochronal steps (Figs. 13-1 and Fig. 13-6). About 40 to 50 points are generally required for a useful activation map for each atrial chamber. Atrial scar is defined as voltages of less than 0.05 mV (the noise floor for the Carto system) and the inability to capture at 20 mA of output. The reference electrogram, typically a coronary sinus bipole, should be chosen such that there are no far-field components to confuse mapping.

Entrainment mapping may be combined with electroanatomic mapping to define critical components of a reentrant circuit. This combined technique is especially useful in situations in which the electroanatomic map is ambiguous, and it is difficult to distinguish critical components from bystander regions.

Misinterpretation of electroanatomic maps may occur unless care is taken to avoid the following pitfalls:

1. *Incomplete mapping and low resolution.* It is important to sample different regions in the atrium of interest. Interpolation of activation times in the map may lead to misinterpretation of the rhythm and failure to identify critical components of the circuit.

2. *Fractionated electrograms.* If highly fractionated and wide potentials are present, it might be difficult to assign an activation time. In this case, the critical isthmus might not be identified, and the reentrant arrhythmia might be confused with a focal rhythm.

3. *Central obstacles or conduction block.* Failure to identify areas of scar or central obstacles to conduction may confuse an electroanatomic map because interpolation of activation times through areas of conduction block may give the appearance of wavefront propagation and obscure the reentrant circuit. If this occurs, it is impossible to identify a critical isthmus to target for ablation. A line of conduction block can be inferred if there are adjacent regions with wavefront propagation in opposite directions, separated either by a line of double potentials or dense isochrones.[20]

4. *Conduction delay in either atrium.* Slow conduction or local block may prolong activation in either the right or left atrium, and conduction time in the passively activated chamber may approach the tachycardia cycle length. For example, if conduction block is present in the cavotricuspid isthmus, an LA tachycardia can give rise to a craniocaudal activation pattern of the lateral RA.

Even if conduction is present in the cavotricuspid isthmus, RA activation in the lateral wall may be craniocaudal if conduction occurs over the Bachmann bundle; if the isthmus and septum are not mapped in sufficient detail, the activation pattern may mimic typical counterclockwise flutter. In these situations, entrainment is an important adjunctive tool that would define the RA as a bystander and clarify the electroanatomic map.

By displaying an atrial voltage map, areas of scar can be identified to permit the localization of channels that form potential reentrant circuits. Areas with no detectable voltage (defined as the noise limit of recording systems, usually 0.05 mV) represent a dense scar and thus a region of fixed conduction block.

Noncontact electroanatomic mapping (EnSite, St. Jude Medical) uses a multielectrode array that records intracavitary potentials and software to construct virtual unipolar electrograms on a three-dimensional representation of a chamber. This technique is useful in delineating transitory arrhythmias and has been used to visualize upper loop and RA free wall reentry.[21] Care must be taken to analyze atrial beats without ventricular depolarization or repolarization, which can obscure the atrial unipolar electrograms. The presence of lines of block can be inferred based on activation sequence rather than direct imaging of scar.

Ablation

The guiding principle in ablating macro-reentrant atrial tachycardias is to target a critical isthmus that participates in the tachycardia circuit (Table 13-3). For successful ablation, it is often not necessary to delineate the complete reentrant circuit because interruption of the circuit at any one site will terminate the tachycardia and prevent its initiation. The critical isthmus may be a narrow channel or a relatively broad region, and boundaries may include scar or anatomic structures. Fixed anatomic boundaries are most amenable to this strategy of ablation. In the case of dual-loop tachycardias, it is important to identify the common isthmus or corridor. Ablation can be performed by targeting the common isthmus or each loop separately. The technique of ablation involves the creation of a linear lesion between two boundaries to transect the isthmus. On occasion, a single lesion suffices to interrupt a narrow isthmus.

Standard radiofrequency with 4-mm-tip catheters may be sufficient, but creation of long linear transmural lesions may require the use of larger-tip (8 mm) catheters or irrigated radiofrequency. It is common to see electrogram reduction at sites of effective ablation. Ideally, bidirectional conduction block should be verified after ablation by pacing from either side of the ablation line and recording from the other side. The detour of wavefronts around completed ablation lines can be displayed graphically with a reconstructed electroanatomic map during pacing or sinus rhythm. Widely spaced double potentials along the ablation line, while pacing from one side, provide supporting evidence for conduction block after ablation. Alternatively, electrogram abatement of more than 80% or to less than 0.1 mV has been used as an end point for lesion delivery.

Noninducibility is another end point. However, atypical flutters are frequently associated with other inducible atrial arrhythmias, and judgment is required to decide whether to target other inducible arrhythmias. Strategies that involve

TABLE 13-3

TARGET SITES FOR ABLATION

General Principles

Critical isthmus identified by electroanatomic mapping bounded by two conduction barriers

Entrainment demonstrates orthodromic capture of most of atrium ("concealed entrainment" is present) and postpacing interval minus tachycardia cycle length ≤30 msec

Ablation Strategies for Specific Arrhythmias

Upper Loop Reentry

Gap in crista terminalis

Right Atrial Free Wall Reentry

Linear lesion from conduction barrier to inferior vena cava

Linear lesion from conduction barrier to crista terminalis

Perimitral Reentry

Linear lesion from left inferior pulmonary vein to mitral annulus

Linear lesion from right inferior pulmonary vein to mitral annulus

Linear lesion from anterior mitral valve annulus to roof line

Linear lesion from anterior mitral valve annulus to right pulmonary veins

Peripulmonary Vein Reentry

Linear lesion between left and right superior pulmonary veins (roof line)—preferred strategy

Linear lesion from left pulmonary vein to mitral annulus

Linear lesion from right pulmonary vein to mitral annulus

Left Septal Reentry

Linear lesion from septum primum to mitral annulus or right pulmonary veins to mitral annulus

Lesional Tachycardia

Linear lesion from scar boundary to anatomic barrier

Gap within incomplete incisional lines

ablation of all inducible atrial arrhythmias and channels for potential reentrant circuits have been successful in preventing recurrences, particularly in patients with prior surgery for congenital heart disease.[22] This strategy can be used for multiple interconverting atrial tachycardias that are challenging to define with contact mapping.

In several clinical series, short-term follow-up reveals that most patients are free of symptomatic arrhythmias, including AF. For example, in two series of left atrial flutter, ablation rendered patients free of symptomatic recurrences in 73% and 71% (average follow-up 16 and 14 months, respectively).[15,16] Another series of patients with macro-reentrant atrial tachycardia in the absence of surgical or catheter intervention reported that atrial arrhythmia–free clinical outcome was achieved without antiarrhythmic drugs in 82% of patients with right atrial and 55% with left atrial tachycardias (average follow-up, 37 months).[23] Successful outcome may require up to three staged procedures. For macro-reentrant atrial tachycardias that occur after catheter ablation of AF, success rates of 77% to 95% have been reported.[6,24] In patients with macro-reentrant atrial tachycardia unrelated to AF ablation, the long-term recurrence rates of atrial arrhythmias after ablation is unknown. This issue is of particular importance because atypical flutters are associated with other atrial arrhythmias and AF.

Specific Forms of Atypical Flutter

Upper Loop Reentry

This macro-reentrant circuit involves reentry around the superior vena cava and conduction along the crista terminalis but not the cavotricuspid isthmus.[17,25-29] This arrhythmia occurs in patients who also have isthmus-dependent flutter, but it also occurs in isolation. Upper loop reentry may be observed in the electrophysiology laboratory as a result of pacing maneuvers in patients undergoing ablation of typical isthmus-dependent atrial flutter, or it may occur during spontaneous transitions of isthmus-dependent flutter.

Most examples of upper loop reentry reported in the literature are clockwise. Electrograms show clockwise activation of the high lateral RA (with early "breakthrough" in the lateral RA). Collision of wavefronts may occur in the cavotricuspid isthmus or the low lateral RA. Concealed entrainment may be demonstrated in the septum between the fossa ovale and the SVC.

Most experience with upper loop reentry has used noncontact electroanatomic mapping to define the circuit. Using this technology, the reentrant circuit has been identified as circus movement around a central obstacle, consisting of the crista terminalis, an area of functional block, and the superior vena cava.[21,30]

Although the published literature on upper loop reentry is limited and follow-up is relatively short (between 3 and 17 months), small clinical series reveal that ablation can be accomplished with a low recurrence rate of AF or other atrial flutters (23% in one clinical series).[21] When guided by noncontact electroanatomic mapping, an effective strategy is to create a linear lesion through a gap in the crista terminalis.

Right Atrial Free Wall Flutter

Macro-reentry may occur in the free wall of the RA in patients with an atriotomy but also has been reported in patients without prior cardiac surgery.[18,20,21,31] The pathophysiology of this arrhythmia is reentry around a line of block in the lateral RA, defined by an electrically silent area or a line of double potentials. The conduction barrier in the lateral wall may be discrete from the crista terminalis, but under some circumstances, particularly in patients without an atriotomy, the crista terminalis appears to form a line of rate-related functional block.

Mapping with conventional multipolar catheters reveals a line of double potentials in the lateral wall with single fractionated potentials at the inferior end of the line, reflecting the lower pivot point (Fig. 13-5). Entrainment from both sides of the central line of block results in postpacing intervals within 30 milliseconds of the tachycardia cycle length, but pacing from the cavotricuspid isthmus or the posterior RA results in longer return cycle lengths. The location of the upper pivot point may be in the upper free wall of the RA or involve the SVC.[18,21] Catheter ablation may be performed by creating linear lesions between the lateral RA (the area of double potentials) to the IVC. Alternatively, ablation may be performed in the corridor between the line of block in the lateral wall and the crista terminalis.

Dual Loop Right Atrial Reentry

In dual loop reentry, which may occur in the RA, atypical circuits (described previously) coexist or combine with rotation around the tricuspid annulus.[23,26] For example, entrainment and contact electroanatomic mapping has been used to identify various combinations of reentry around the IVC (lower loop reentry), the tricuspid annulus, and a conduction barrier in the lateral RA (Fig. 13-6). Noncontact mapping has permitted the identification of upper loop reentry combined with lower loop reentry or free wall reentry.[21] Ablation of one component usually transforms the tachycardia to another arrhythmia. For example, free wall reentry coexists with peritricuspid reentry, ablation in the cavotricuspid isthmus transforms the arrhythmia to free wall reentry alone, and complete ablation requires additional treatment in the lateral RA.

Left Atrial Macro-Reentry

A variety of reentrant circuits have been described in the left atria of patients with structural heart disease and after surgery for acquired heart disease.[15,16,20,23] Anatomic obstacles to conduction include the mitral valve orifice, the pulmonary vein ostia, and electrically silent patches. In patients with prior left atrial surgery, low voltage areas may be found in the vicinity of atrial incisions or may be remote from these sites, reflecting an underlying atrial myopathy in this population. Functional block, which can occur adjacent to areas of fixed block, may also play a role in facilitating reentry. Examples of left atrial reentrant circuits include circus movement around the mitral valve, around the pulmonary veins (Fig. 13-7), around electrically silent areas, or involving a variety of these barriers. Dual loop circuits are common, and multiple loops are sometimes encountered. For example, simultaneous reentry can occur around the mitral annulus and a single pair of ipsilateral pulmonary veins.

Because the configurations of LA flutter are highly variable, there is no single anatomic approach to ablation that is universally successful. Typical sites of ablation include the following: (1) from the left pulmonary veins to the mitral annulus, the lateral "mitral isthmus"; (2) along the roof between the pulmonary veins; (3) from the right pulmonary veins to the mitral annulus; (4) from a pulmonary vein to an electrically silent area in the posterior wall; and (5) between two electrically silent areas in the posterior wall or roof of the LA.t

Completion of the ablation line in the mitral isthmus may be difficult to achieve and often requires ablation within the coronary sinus with an irrigated-tip catheter.[32] Ablation within the coronary sinus is performed at power settings of 20 to 30 W with irrigation rates of 17 to 60 mL/minute. When an 8-mm-tip ablation catheter is used, initial power and temperature settings are 35 W and 50°C, and power and temperature can be gradually increased to a maximum of 70 W and 55°C. Verification of a line of block along the mitral isthmus can be demonstrated by pacing on either side of the ablation line using a catheter in the coronary sinus and one in the LA (Fig. 13-8). In addition, the presence of widely separated double potentials (150 to 300 milliseconds apart) along the line supports the existence of conduction block. To distinguish slow conduction from

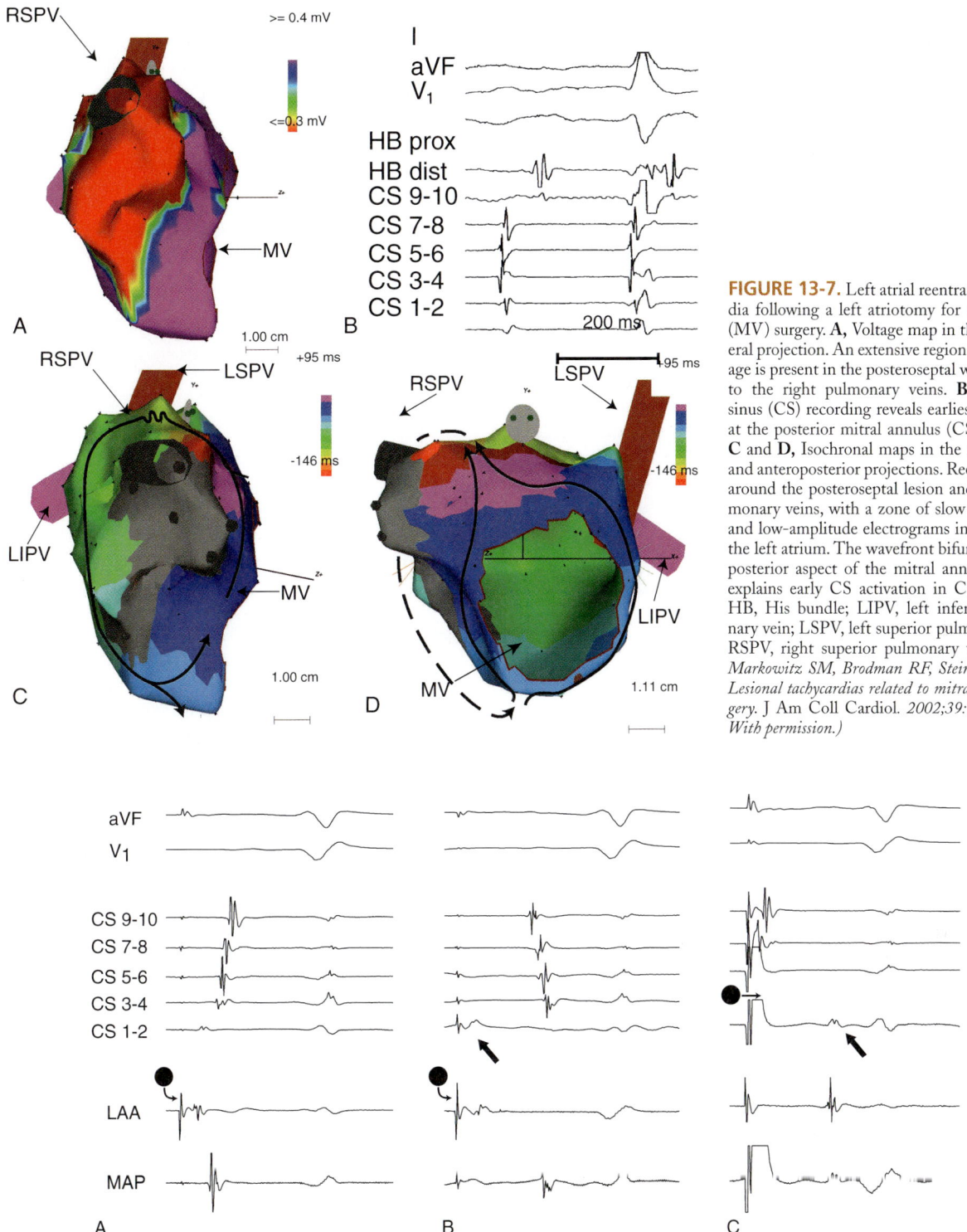

FIGURE 13-7. Left atrial reentrant tachycardia following a left atriotomy for mitral valve (MV) surgery. **A,** Voltage map in the right lateral projection. An extensive region of low voltage is present in the posteroseptal wall adjacent to the right pulmonary veins. **B,** Coronary sinus (CS) recording reveals earliest activation at the posterior mitral annulus (CS pole 5-6). **C** and **D,** Isochronal maps in the right lateral and anteroposterior projections. Reentry occurs around the posteroseptal lesion and right pulmonary veins, with a zone of slow conduction and low-amplitude electrograms in the roof of the left atrium. The wavefront bifurcates at the posterior aspect of the mitral annulus, which explains early CS activation in CS pole 5-6. HB, His bundle; LIPV, left inferior pulmonary vein; LSPV, left superior pulmonary vein; RSPV, right superior pulmonary vein. *(From Markowitz SM, Brodman RF, Stein KM, et al. Lesional tachycardias related to mitral valve surgery. J Am Coll Cardiol. 2002;39:1973–1983. With permission.)*

FIGURE 13-8. Conduction block in the mitral isthmus. **A,** Pacing is performed from the left atrial appendage (LAA) before the ablation line was made between CS 1-2 and CS 3-4. Pacing from the appendage activates the coronary sinus (CS) from distal to proximal. **B,** After the line is completed, conduction block is demonstrated by proximal to distal CS activation from CS 9-10 to CS 3-4. CS 1-2 is on the opposite anterior side of the line (*arrow*). **C,** To assess conduction in the opposite direction, pacing is performed from the distal CS, in this case poles 3-4. After the line is completed, there is late activation of the adjacent distal pole (CS 1-2, *arrow*) and the appendage. MAP, mapping catheter.

complete block, the technique of *differential pacing* may be used, which involves comparing conduction times during pacing from distal and proximal poles of a coronary sinus catheter: If complete conduction block is present, clockwise conduction time around the mitral annulus is

longer with distal pacing compared with proximal pacing (Fig. 13-9). A risk for ablation in the mitral isthmus, as with ablation in other locations in the LA, is cardiac tamponade, which can be avoided by limiting power to 42 W or less during endocardial ablation.[32]

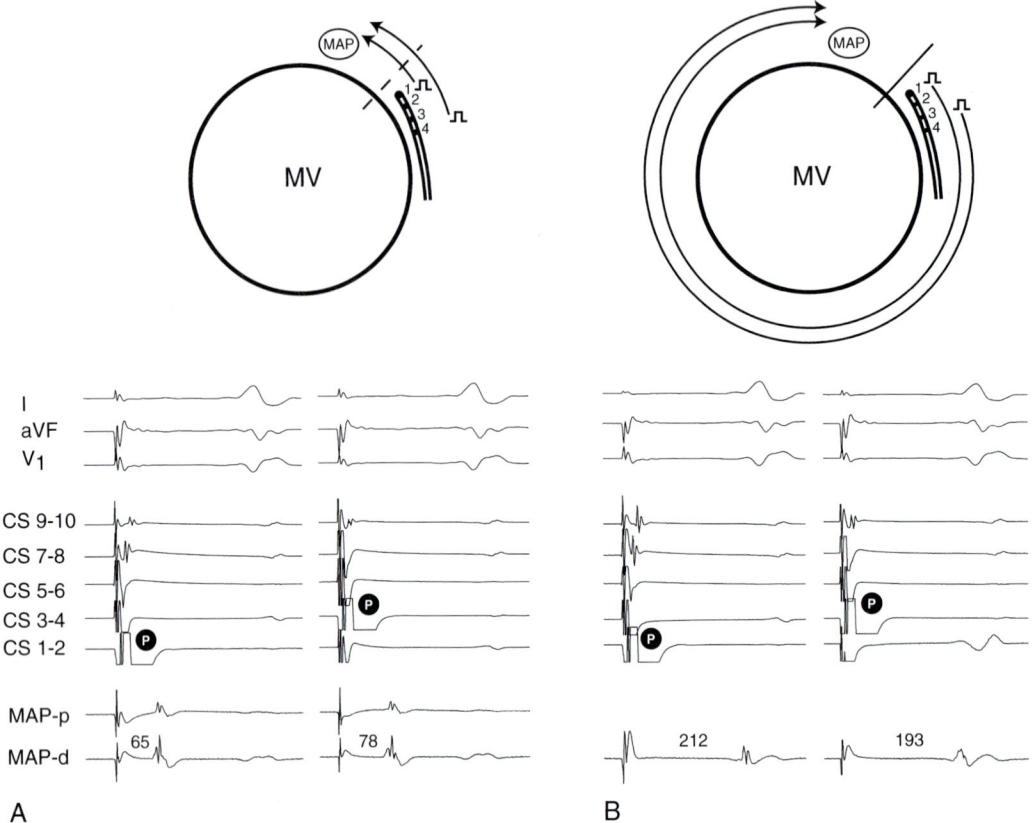

FIGURE 13-9. Differential pacing to demonstrate block in the mitral isthmus. **A,** Pacing (P) from the distal coronary sinus (CS poles 1-2) shows a shorter conduction time to a mapping catheter (MAP) in the anterolateral mitral annulus, compared with pacing from more proximal poles CS 3-4. **B,** After line of block is achieved, pacing from the distal poles CS 1-2 results in a longer conduction time to the anterolateral mitral annulus compared with pacing from CS 3-4. MV, mitral valve.

Roof-dependent macro-reentry is treated with linear ablation along the LA roof between the left and right superior pulmonary veins. Completeness of the line can be demonstrated by recording widely spaced double potentials along the ablation line during pacing from one side of the line.[33] The LA appendage may be selected as a stable pacing site in the anterior segment of the LA. In addition, activation of the posterior wall during appendage pacing should proceed from an inferior to superior direction as the impulse diverts around the pulmonary veins to engage the posterior wall (Fig. 13-10).

If block in the lateral mitral isthmus cannot be achieved, perimitral reentry can be interrupted by creating a linear ablation lesion in the anterior LA between the mitral annulus and a linear lesion in the LA roof or the right pulmonary veins.[34] Conduction block can be verified by the demonstration of double potentials along the line during pacing from the lateral or septal sides, or by the concepts of differential pacing.

Atrial Macro-Reentry after Mitral Valve Surgery

Atypical atrial flutter occurs in both the right and left atria after mitral valve surgery.[15,16,20] The substrate for these arrhythmias involves atriotomy incisions as well as intrinsically diseased myocardium, which give rise to anatomic and functional regions of block as well as slowed conduction. Reentry in the RA may be attributed to several factors, including surgical approaches to the mitral

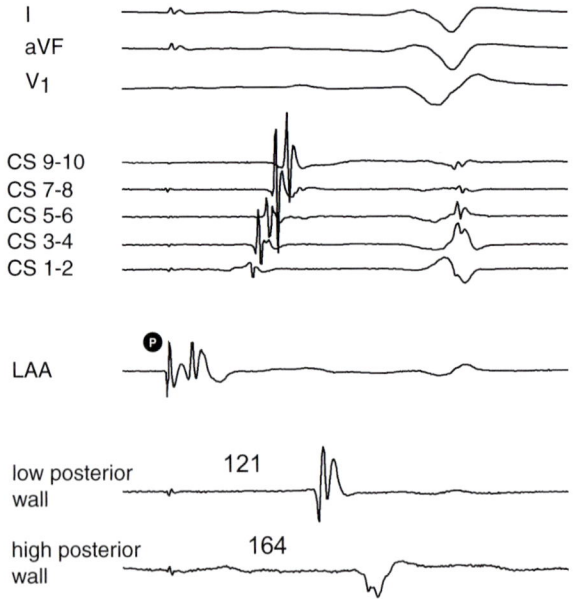

FIGURE 13-10. Assessing line of block in the left atrial roof. During pacing from the anterior left atrium, in this case from the left atrial appendage (LAA), activation to the high posterior wall is delayed and follows activation to the low posterior wall.

valve that involve RA incisions (such as the transseptal or superior septal approaches), cannula insertion in the RA, and underlying myocardial disease. Tachycardias in the RA include single and dual loop circuits that involve

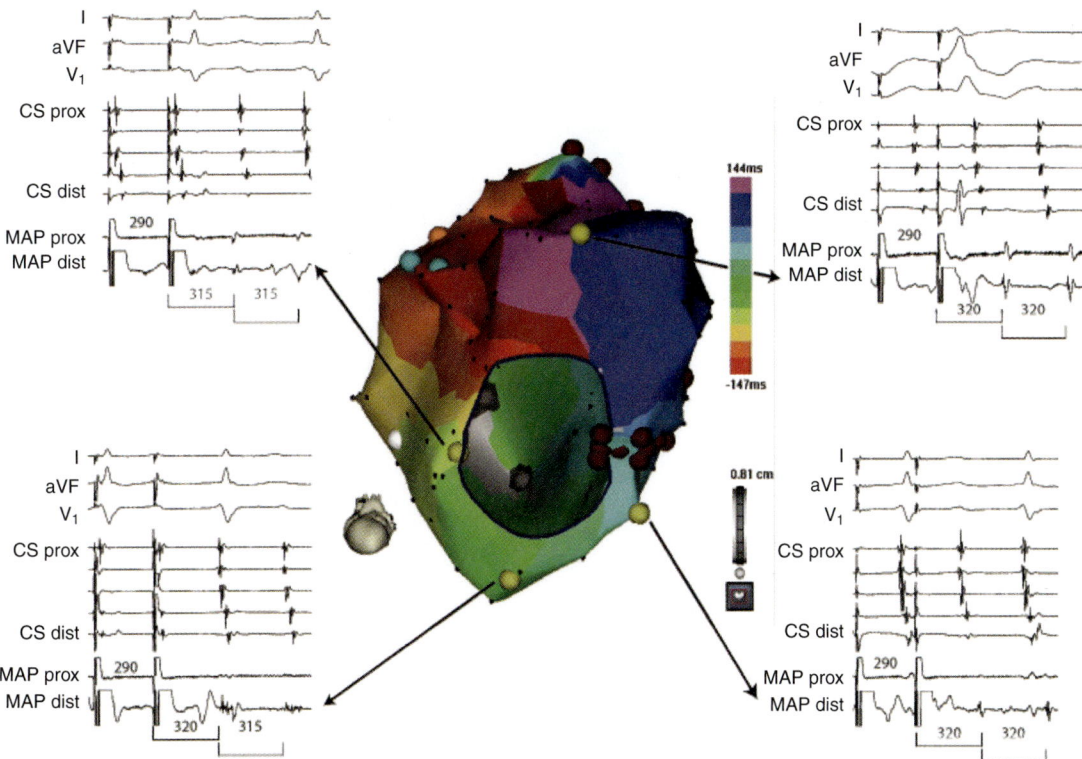

FIGURE 13-11. Perimitral annular reentry that occurred late after catheter ablation of paroxysmal atrial fibrillation. The electroanatomic map shows counterclockwise activation around the mitral annulus. *Red tags* show sites of ablation in the mitral isthmus. *Beige tags* are pacing sites at which entrainment revealed participation in the tachycardia circuit. Entrainment criteria were fulfilled to the anterior and superior mitral annulus, as well as lateral and septal annulus. CS, coronary sinus; MAP, mapping catheter.

the RA free wall (Fig. 13-6). In the LA, areas of low voltage are often identified anterior to the right pulmonary veins, which correspond to left atrial incisions (Fig. 13-7). Reentry around the right pulmonary veins (involving this zone of low voltage) may be present as a single circuit or in a dual loop configuration (one loop around the right pulmonary veins and a second around the left pulmonary veins, a posterior scar, or the mitral annulus). Other variations in this population include single loop reentry around the mitral annulus and around a posterior scar.

Atrial Macro-Reentry after Catheter Ablation for Atrial Fibrillation

With the growing application of wide encircling pulmonary vein isolation and linear left atrial ablation for treatment of AF, it has become apparent that left atrial flutter may present as a late complication in 10% to 30% of patients.[24,35-37] These forms of atypical flutter present as persistent or paroxysmal arrhythmias about 1 to 6 months after AF ablation, often in patients still treated with antiarrhythmic drugs following the procedure. Both focal and macro-reentrant tachycardias occur late after ablation. In addition, macro-reentrant atrial tachycardias often occur during ablation of persistent AF as an intermediate step before conversion to sinus rhythm. The most common forms of macro-reentry occurring after AF ablation are perimitral reentry and roof-dependent reentry (Fig. 13-11). A unique form of reentrant tachycardia can occur after pulmonary vein isolation, in which two gaps in an isolation

line give rise to a circuit involving atrial myocardium and electrically active tissue within a pulmonary vein.[38] This arrhythmia can be treated with reisolation of the involved pulmonary vein.

A deductive stepwise approach using activation and entrainment mapping can be employed to determine the mechanism of the atrial tachycardia and its location.[6] This strategy is based on the recognition that left atrial macroreentry after AF ablation is due to either perimitral reentry or roof-dependent reentry, and basic activation and entrainment mapping can identify or exclude these circuits. It is not necessary to define the specific roof-dependent circuit (e.g., reentry around the right pulmonary veins or left pulmonary veins, or dual loop tachycardia involving both sets of veins) because each variant can be successfully interrupted in the roof.

First, cycle length variation is assessed, and variations of 15% or greater should prompt a search for a focal tachycardia. Before transseptal catheterization, right atrial isthmus-dependent flutter is excluded. Pulmonary vein isolation is confirmed, and reisolation is performed if necessary. Activation mapping around the mitral annulus, supplemented by entrainment mapping from opposite segments (e.g., septal and lateral) is performed to assess for perimitral reentry. Similarly, activation and entrainment mapping of the posterior and anterior LA walls is performed to assess for a roof-dependent flutter. If both perimitral and roof-dependent reentries are excluded, activation and entrainment mapping can be performed to localize a focal source of tachycardia. Gaps in prior

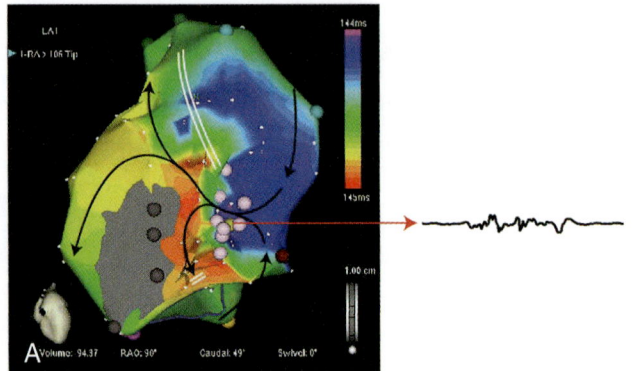

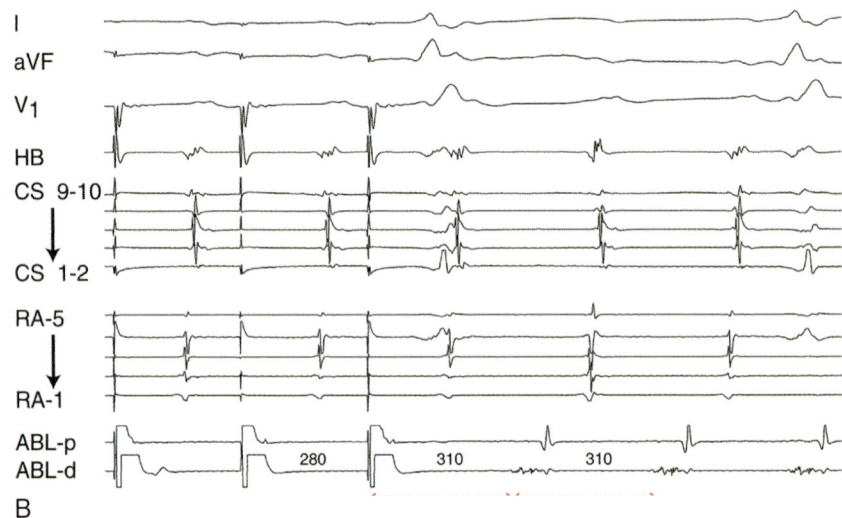

FIGURE 13-12. Reentrant atrial tachycardia after maze surgery. This patient had surgical cryoablation in the cavotricuspid isthmus, an intercaval line, and a line between the right atrial appendage and lateral right atrium (RA), in addition to left atrial lesions. **A,** Right atrial electroanatomic activation map in right lateral caudal view, which demonstrates a line of block in the lateral wall with double potentials (*pink tags*). A gap in this line served as critical isthmus for the reentrant tachycardia. **B,** The electrogram at this ablation site (*green tag in* **A**) was low amplitude and fractionated (ABL-d). Concealed entrainment from this ablation site indicated participation in the tachycardia circuit (postpacing interval of 310 msec, identical to the tachycardia cycle length). Note block in the cavotricuspid isthmus due to prior surgical ablation, thus preventing dual loop tachycardia. ABL, ablation electrodes; CS, coronary sinus; d, distal. HB, His bundle; p, proximal.

ablation lines often demonstrate low-amplitude fragmented electrograms.

During ablation of these lesional atrial tachycardias, attention should be paid to the possibility of dual loop tachycardias, and ablation of one limb might transform the tachycardia rather than convert to sinus rhythm. Clues to the existence of a second circuit include subtle alterations in intracardiac activation sequence, P-wave morphology, or cycle length. Extensive ablation in one line that eliminates voltage but fails to terminate a tachycardia should raise the possibility of a second limb.

With these techniques, such iatrogenic atrial tachycardias can be treated effectively with catheter ablation, targeting the mitral isthmus or other critical components of the circuits, with initial success rates exceeding 85%.

Macro-Reentrant Atrial Tachycardia after Maze Surgery

Atypical flutter may occur later after maze surgery for AF because of gaps in the operative lesions, similar to the situation described for arrhythmias after catheter ablation.[39–41] If lesions are limited to LA, typical right atrial flutter occurs in up to 10% of patients late after surgery. Even if lesions are placed in the cavotricuspid isthmus, reentrant circuits can occur in the RA, possibly related to cannula locations or gaps in the RA ablation lines. An example of a dual loop tachycardia in the RA after maze surgery is shown in Figure 13-12. In the LA, gaps in the posterior wall lesions have been described, resulting in reentrant circuits around the right pulmonary veins.[39] It is not clear whether these gap-related flutters occur more commonly with a particular surgical modality (i.e., conventional incisions, radiofrequency, cryoablation, or microwave energy). Catheter ablation of gap-related atrial flutter after maze surgery is feasible, using the same mapping techniques for other complex atrial reentrant circuits.

Left Septal Flutter

Reentry around the septum primum has been recognized as a mechanism of left atrial flutter in the absence of previous cardiac surgery, in most cases occurring in patients with AF treated with antiarrhythmic drugs.[28,42] The reentrant circuit is bounded by the right pulmonary veins posteriorly (which demonstrate a line of double potentials) and the mitral annulus anteriorly. The electrocardiogram shows positive or negative flutter waves in V_1 and low-amplitude flutter waves in the other leads.

The ablation strategy involves creating a linear lesion between the septum primum and the right pulmonary veins, or between the septum primum and the mitral annulus. The anterior approach appears to have a higher success rate. In one series, 76% of patients were in sinus rhythm after a follow-up of 13 months.

TABLE 13-4

TROUBLESHOOTING PROBLEMS

Problem	Cause	Solution
Unstable rhythm interconverting with atrial fibrillation or other forms of atypical flutter	Instability of lines of block	Limit atrial pacing and entrainment mapping Consider noncontact electroanatomic mapping Consider long linear lesions and/or ablation of atrial fibrillation Low-dose IC or III drug to stabilize reentry
Uninterpretable electroanatomic map	Incomplete map Failure to identify lines of block and areas of scar	Map 80-100 points during tachycardia Review voltage map to identify areas of scar (<0.05-0.1 mV) Review previous surgery and ablation attempts
Failure to achieve conduction block in mitral isthmus	Persistent epicardial conduction	Use irrigated radiofrequency catheter Ablate within coronary sinus
Failure to terminate tachycardia despite complete ablation line	Dual loop reentry Inaccurate mapping of critical isthmus	Re-evaluate cycle length, surface electrocardiogram, and activation sequence Re-evaluate map
Unstable catheter during linear ablation	Large left atrium, limited catheter mobility	Use adjustable or telescoping sheath system, change catheters, linear ablation array, robotic navigation

Troubleshooting the Difficult Case

Cases involving non–isthmus-dependent atrial flutters are typically complex, and the sources of difficulty are many. Perhaps, the most critical difficult aspect of these cases is the accurate mapping and understanding of the reentrant circuit. For most cases, electroanatomic mapping capabilities are invaluable. Even with this capability, problems may arise from interpretation of low-voltage electrograms, frequent termination of the tachycardia of interest, or spontaneous oscillation between different tachycardia circuits. Incomplete maps from an inadequate number of sampled sites can be confusing as well. Meticulous attention to the generation of maps is necessary to minimize confusion. Reassessment of the maps using different system control settings or threshold levels for voltage mapping may clarify channels not previously evident. Once identified, the targets for ablation may be broad channels requiring creation of linear lesions. Ablation to complete lines to the mitral annulus may require extensive endocardial ablation or ablation within the coronary sinus itself. The use of steerable or telescoping sheaths may improve the stability and reach of the ablation catheter to difficult-to-access sites. The inability to complete the preferred ablation line may necessitate targeting an alternative site in the circuit. Failure to terminate a tachycardia despite extensive ablation may represent the "other" circuit in dual loop reentry. Careful attention to changes in cycle length, surface electrocardiogram, and atrial activation sequence may reveal this occurrence. A list of common problems and potential solutions is given in Table 13-4.

References

1. Saoudi N, Cosio F, Waldo A, et al. Classification of atrial flutter and regular atrial tachycardia according to electrophysiologic mechanism and anatomic bases: a statement from a joint expert group from the Working Group of Arrhythmias of the European Society of Cardiology and the North American Society of Pacing and Electrophysiology. *J Cardiovasc Electrophysiol.* 2001;12:852–866.
2. Shah D. ECG manifestations of left atrial flutter. *Curr Opin Cardiol.* 2009;24:35–41.
3. Olgin JE, Kalman JM, Lesh MD. Conduction barriers in human atrial flutter: correlation of electrophysiology and anatomy. *J Cardiovasc Electrophysiol.* 1996;7:1112–1126.
4. Tomita Y, Matsuo K, Sahadevan J, et al. Role of functional block extension in lesion-related atrial flutter. *Circulation.* 2001;103:1025–1030.
5. Perez FJ, Wood MA, Schubert CM. Effects of gap geometry on conduction through discontinuous radiofrequency lesions. *Circulation.* 2006;113:1723–1729.
6. Jais P, Matsuo S, Knecht S, et al. A deductive mapping strategy for atrial tachycardia following atrial fibrillation ablation: importance of localized reentry. *J Cardiovasc Electrophysiol.* 2009;20:480–491.
7. Chugh A, Latchamsetty R, Oral H, et al. Characteristics of cavotricuspid isthmus-dependent atrial flutter after left atrial ablation of atrial fibrillation. *Circulation.* 2006;113:609–615.
8. Waldo AL. Atrial flutter: entrainment characteristics. *J Cardiovasc Electrophysiol.* 1997;8:337–352.
9. Cosio FG, Martin-Penato A, Pastor A, et al. Atypical flutter: a review. *Pacing Clin Electrophysiol.* 2003;26:2157–2169.
10. Markowitz SM, Stein KM, Mittal S, et al. Differential effects of adenosine on focal and macroreentrant atrial tachycardia. *J Cardiovasc Electrophysiol.* 1999;10:489–502.
11. Iwai S, Markowitz SM, Stein KM, et al. Response to adenosine differentiates focal from macroreentrant atrial tachycardia: validation using three-dimensional electroanatomic mapping. *Circulation.* 2002;106:2793–2799.
12. Markowitz SM, Nemirovksy D, Stein KM, et al. Adenosine-insensitive focal atrial tachycardia: evidence for de novo micro-re-entry in the human atrium. *J Am Coll Cardiol.* 2007;49:1324–1333.
13. Olgin JE, Jayachandran JV, Engesstein E, et al. Atrial macroreentry involving the myocardium of the coronary sinus: a unique mechanism for atypical flutter. *J Cardiovasc Electrophysiol.* 1998;9:1094–1099.
14. Chugh A, Oral H, Good E, et al. Catheter ablation of atypical atrial flutter and atrial tachycardia within the coronary sinus after left atrial ablation for atrial fibrillation. *J Am Coll Cardiol.* 2005;46:83–91.
15. Jais P, Shah DC, Haïssaguerre M, et al. Mapping and ablation of left atrial flutters. *Circulation.* 2000;101:2928–2934.
16. Ouyang F, Ernst S, Vogtmann T, et al. Characterization of reentrant circuits in left atrial macroreentrant tachycardia: critical isthmus block can prevent atrial tachycardia recurrence. *Circulation.* 2002;105:1934–1942.
17. Yang Y, Cheng J, Bochoeyer A, et al. Atypical right atrial flutter patterns. *Circulation.* 2001;103:3092–3098.
18. Kall JG, Rubenstein DS, Kopp DE, et al. Atypical atrial flutter originating in the right atrial free wall. *Circulation.* 2000;101:270–279.
19. Stevenson WG, Sager PT, Friedman PL. Entrainment techniques for mapping atrial and ventricular tachycardias. *J Cardiovasc Electrophysiol.* 1995;6:201–216.
20. Markowitz SM, Brodman RF, Stein KM, et al. Lesional tachycardias related to mitral valve surgery. *J Am Coll Cardiol.* 2002;39:1973–1983.
21. Tai CT, Liu TY, Lee PC, et al. Non-contact mapping to guide radiofrequency ablation of atypical right atrial flutter. *J Am Coll Cardiol.* 2004;44:1080–1086.
22. Nakagawa H, Shah N, Matsudaira K, et al. Characterization of reentrant circuit in macroreentrant right atrial tachycardia after surgical repair of congenital heart disease: isolated channels between scars allow "focal" ablation. *Circulation.* 2001;103:699–709.
23. Fiala M, Chovancik J, Neuwirth R, et al. Atrial macroreentry tachycardia in patients without obvious structural heart disease or previous cardiac surgical or catheter intervention: characterization of arrhythmogenic substrates, reentry circuits, and results of catheter ablation. *J Cardiovasc Electrophysiol.* 2007;18:824–832.
24. Chae S, Oral H, Good E, et al. Atrial tachycardia after circumferential pulmonary vein ablation of atrial fibrillation: mechanistic insights, results of catheter ablation, and risk factors for recurrence. *J Am Coll Cardiol.* 2007;50:1781–1787.
25. Cheng J, Cabeen WR, Scheinman MM. Right atrial flutter due to lower loop reentry: mechanism and anatomic substrates. *Circulation.* 1999;99:1700–1705.

26. Zhang S, Younis G, Hariharan R, et al. Lower loop reentry as a mechanism of clockwise right atrial flutter. *Circulation.* 2004;109:1630–1635.

27. Cheng J, Scheinman MM. Acceleration of typical atrial flutter due to double-wave reentry induced by programmed electrical stimulation. *Circulation.* 1998;97:1589–1596.

28. Bochoeyer A, Yang Y, Cheng J, et al. Surface electrocardiographic characteristics of right and left atrial flutter. *Circulation.* 2003;108:60–66.

29. Tai CT, Huang JL, Lin YK, et al. Noncontact three-dimensional mapping and ablation of upper loop re-entry originating in the right atrium. *J Am Coll Cardiol.* 2002;40:746–753.

30. Huang JL, Tai CT, Lin YJ, et al. Substrate mapping to detect abnormal atrial endocardium with slow conduction in patients with atypical right atrial flutter. *J Am Coll Cardiol.* 2006;48:492–498.

31. Iesaka Y, Takahashi A, Goya M, et al. Nonlinear ablation targeting an isthmus of critically slow conduction detected by high-density electroanatomical mapping for atypical atrial flutter. *Pacing Clin Electrophysiol.* 2000;23:1911–1915.

32. Jais P, Hocini M, Hsu LF, et al. Technique and results of linear ablation at the mitral isthmus. *Circulation.* 2004;110:2996–3002.

33. Hocini M, Jais P, Sanders P, et al. Techniques, evaluation, and consequences of linear block at the left atrial roof in paroxysmal atrial fibrillation: a prospective randomized study. *Circulation.* 2005;112:3688–3696.

34. Sanders P, Jais P, Hocini M, et al. Electrophysiologic and clinical consequences of linear catheter ablation to transect the anterior left atrium in patients with atrial fibrillation. *Heart Rhythm.* 2004;1:176–184.

35. Pappone C, Manguso F, Vicedomini G, et al. Prevention of iatrogenic atrial tachycardia after ablation of atrial fibrillation: a prospective randomized study comparing circumferential pulmonary vein ablation with a modified approach. *Circulation.* 2004;110:3036–3042.

36. Gerstenfeld EP, Marchlinski FE. Mapping and ablation of left atrial tachycardias occurring after atrial fibrillation ablation. *Heart Rhythm.* 2007;4:S65–S72.

37. Chugh A, Oral H, Lemola K, et al. Prevalence, mechanisms, and clinical significance of macroreentrant atrial tachycardia during and following left atrial ablation for atrial fibrillation. *Heart Rhythm.* 2005;2:464–471.

38. Satomi K, Bansch D, Tilz R, et al. Left atrial and pulmonary vein macroreentrant tachycardia associated with double conduction gaps: a novel type of man-made tachycardia after circumferential pulmonary vein isolation. *Heart Rhythm.* 2008;5:43–51.

39. Thomas SP, Nunn GR, Nicholson IA, et al. Mechanism, localization and cure of atrial arrhythmias occurring after a new intraoperative endocardial radiofrequency ablation procedure for atrial fibrillation. *J Am Coll Cardiol.* 2000;35:442–450.

40. Duru F, Hindricks G, Kottkamp H. Atypical left atrial flutter after intraoperative radiofrequency ablation of chronic atrial fibrillation: successful ablation using three-dimensional electroanatomic mapping. *J Cardiovasc Electrophysiol.* 2001;12:602–605.

41. McElderry HT, McGiffin DC, Plumb VJ, et al. Proarrhythmic aspects of atrial fibrillation surgery: mechanisms of postoperative macroreentrant tachycardias. *Circulation.* 2008;117:155–162.

42. Marrouche NF, Natale A, Wazni OM, et al. Left septal atrial flutter: electrophysiology, anatomy, and results of ablation. *Circulation.* 2004;109:2440–2447.

14

Ablation of Postoperative Atrial Tachycardia in Patients with Congenital Heart Disease

Edward P. Walsh

Key Points

Activation and entrainment mapping are used to identify macro-reentrant circuits.

Ablation is targeted at critical points or channels in reentrant circuits.

Electroanatomic mapping systems are often helpful. Cooled ablation systems and long preformed sheaths may be needed. Intracardiac or transesophageal echocardiography may be helpful, and angiographic catheters may be needed to delineate anatomy.

Sources of difficulty include complex cardiac anatomy, complex or multiple reentrant circuits, and thick or scarred tissue that is resistant to ablation.

It is hard to imagine a more fertile environment for tachyarrhythmias than the postoperative atria of patients with congenital heart disease (CHD). The pathology begins with chambers that are dilated and thickened because of variable volume or pressure loads of long duration, which then suffer the additional insults of an atriotomy incision, caval cannulation scars, and septal patches with running suture lines. This substrate may be further compromised by sinus node dysfunction and suboptimal hemodynamics, all of which ultimately contribute to a high probability of tachycardia events. It should come as no surprise that recurrent atrial arrhythmias are a major source of morbidity and mortality among the rapidly growing population of adolescent and young adult survivors of CHD.[1-3] Some follow-up studies have placed the risk for long-term sudden death as high as 6% to 10% in association with these tachycardias, due to either acute hemodynamic collapse or thromboembolic complications.[4]

Atrial tachycardias can occur after almost any form of CHD surgery, including uncomplicated closure of a simple atrial septal defect. However, the incidence is clearly highest for patients who have undergone extensive atrial manipulation as part of the Mustard or Senning operation for transposition of the great arteries, or the Fontan operation for single ventricle. The most common tachycardia mechanism is macro-reentry within the right atrial muscle. Unlike typical atrial flutter in an anatomically normal heart, which traverses a very predictable counterclockwise course through the cavotricuspid isthmus (CTI) at a cycle length of about 200 milliseconds, the reentrant circuits in CHD patients tend toward much longer cycle lengths and can follow novel routes related to a wide variety of natural and surgical conduction barriers. It has become customary to distinguish this type of atrial circuit from typical flutter by the label *intra-atrial reentrant tachycardia (IART)*, or *incisional tachycardia*. Less commonly, CHD patients demonstrate *focal atrial tachycardia (FAT)* with gross electrophysiologic behavior consistent with micro-reentry or triggered activity. Atrial fibrillation can also occur in a subset of CHD patients, especially those with left-sided heart defects such as congenital aortic stenosis or mitral valve disease.[5]

The treatment options available for CHD patients with recurrent atrial tachycardias include catheter ablation,[6] pharmacologic therapy,[4,7] atrial antitachycardia pacemakers,[8,9] and arrhythmia surgery.[10,11] Although therapeutic decisions still are largely made on a case-by-case basis, catheter ablation has become a preferred intervention at many centers. It is the purpose of this chapter to review the current techniques and outcome data for radiofrequency (RF) ablation of IART and FAT in the CHD population. Ablation has not yet been extended to atrial fibrillation in any systematic way for these patients but is likely to be considered in the near future.

Anatomic Considerations

With only rare exceptions, atrial tachycardias arise from right atrial tissue in the CHD group. This is easily visualized in patients with relatively straightforward anatomy, such as those who have undergone atrial or ventricular septal

217

defect closures or tetralogy of Fallot repair (Fig. 14-1), in whom caval return to the right atrium (RA) is normal and an obvious CTI can be identified. Most IART circuits found in such patients do not differ fundamentally from typical atrial flutter, and they can usually be ablated by the standard maneuver of blocking conduction through the CTI.[12] Although IART may occasionally involve a circuit around an atriotomy scar along the lateral RA wall, it is more common for these scars to function as modulators of isthmus flutter by simply channeling conduction along the lateral edge of the tricuspid ring. Therefore, IART circuits in CHD patients with simple anatomy can be understood reasonably well by applying the same mapping and ablation principles used for typical flutter.

The situation becomes less intuitive when complex atrial anatomy is considered. Even though embryologic right atrial tissue is still the source of most tachycardias, the exact orientation of the RA can be grossly distorted by abnormalities of atrial situs, atresia of an atrioventricular (AV) valve and ventricle, and surgical septation or baffling, which segregates portions of the RA into the pulmonary venous atrium. A classic example is the patient who has undergone the Mustard or Senning operation, in which vena caval flow is baffled toward the mitral valve by a large atrial patch (Fig. 14-2). As a result of this arrangement, the critical right atrial segment containing the CTI is now on the systemic side of the circulation. The isthmus remains the most likely region for an IART circuit to develop,[12–14] but to reach this site for mapping and ablation, the catheter must be delivered to the left side of the heart by a retrograde arterial approach or a transbaffle puncture.[15]

By far the most difficult atrial anatomy and least predictable IART circuitry occurs in patients with a single ventricle. Surgery for these cases typically involves one of the many modifications of the Fontan operation, in which the RA is connected directly to the pulmonary arteries (Fig. 14-3). Because there is usually no AV valve associated

with the RA, there is no actual CTI. Instead, reentrant circuits tend to propagate through regions of fibrotic right atrial muscle around lateral wall atriotomy scars, atrial septal patches, or the region of anastomosis with the pulmonary artery. Natural conduction barriers, such as the crista terminalis and the superior and inferior caval orifices, also influence these circuits.[12] Often, multiple IART circuits are present in the same patient, making mapping and ablation a challenging exercise in the Fontan population.

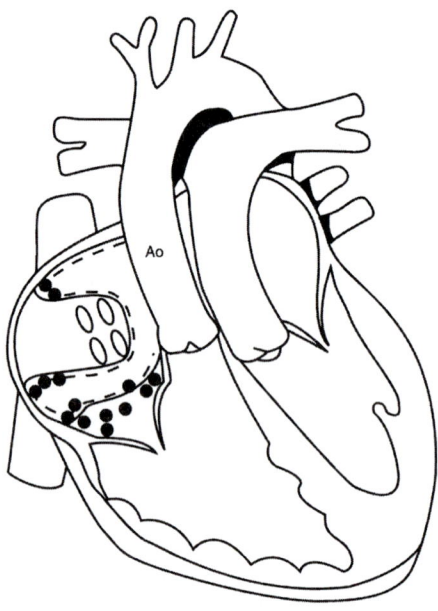

FIGURE 14-2. Diagrammatic view of the Mustard or Senning operation for transposition of the great arteries. The *black dots* represent sites of successful ablation for intra-atrial reentrant tachycardia. The cavotricuspid isthmus is typically the most productive ablation site in this group, although it is located within the left side of the heart and must be approached with a retrograde or transbaffle technique. Ao, aorta.

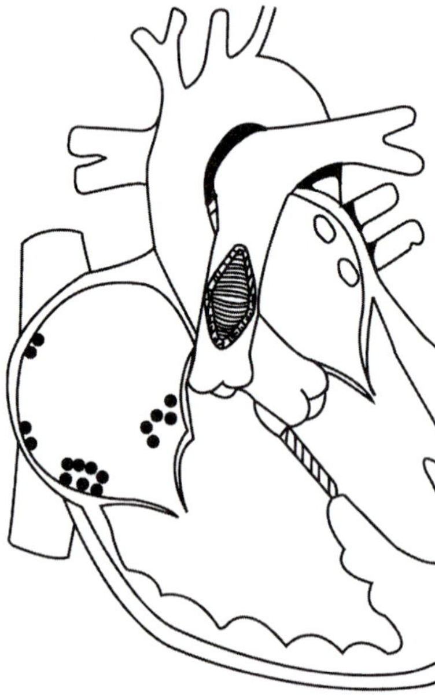

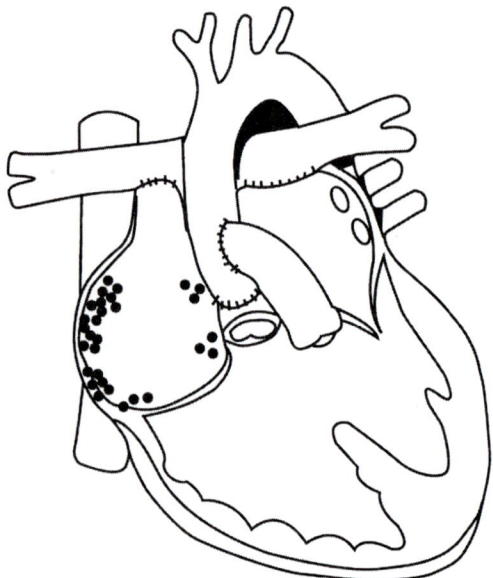

FIGURE 14-3. Diagrammatic view of a single-ventricle heart repaired with an older modification of the Fontan operation, in which the right atrium (RA) is connected directly to the pulmonary arteries. The RA in such cases tends to be very thickened and dilated. The *black dots* represent sites of successful ablation for intra-atrial reentrant tachycardia, which are widely scattered throughout the chamber.

FIGURE 14-1. Diagrammatic view of "simple" congenital heart disease, in this case repaired tetralogy of Fallot. The *black dots* represent sites of successful ablation for intra-atrial reentrant tachycardia. The cavotricuspid isthmus is typically the most productive ablation site in this group of patients.

Atrial anatomy for CHD patients can be further complicated by abnormal wall thickness, chamber dilation, and diffuse fibrosis. The RA in some cases can become hypertrophied almost to the thickness of ventricular muscle, and it may exhibit layered myocytes sandwiched between thick sheets of scar (Fig. 14-4). This adds yet another dimension to the already disordered process of atrial conduction, and it almost certainly increases the potential for reentry. The dramatic wall thickness also confounds the effectiveness of RF ablation because it can be difficult to achieve full transmural tissue destruction with conventional RF techniques.

Pathophysiology

As mentioned, macro-reentry is by far the most common mechanism for atrial tachycardia in the CHD population. These circuits have an excitable gap and tend to rotate around a central obstacle that has either a fixed or a rate-related conduction block.[16] The conduction velocity through atrial muscle can vary from point to point within the circuit, typically including at least one region of slow conduction. However, slow conduction zones are not absolutely required for IART to develop. Animal models of incisional reentry have demonstrated that circuits can be sustained with a uniform velocity[17] if the total conduction

time is prolonged by diffusely abnormal tissue or a physically long path for the circuit.

In general, the atrial rate in IART tends to be much slower than that in typical atrial flutter, with cycle lengths on the order of 270 to 450 milliseconds. Furthermore, the morphology of the P wave on the surface electrocardiogram rarely takes on the classic sawtooth appearance of atrial flutter. Instead, more discrete P waves tend to be seen, with long isoelectric periods between them (Fig. 14-5). The initial deflection of the P wave usually corresponds to the moment of breakout for atrial activation from a zone of slow conduction, whereas atrial activation during the isoelectric period usually corresponds to conduction within the slow zone. These timing features can be of strategic importance during IART mapping because they help localize regions that might be the most productive sites for ablation.

Figure-of-eight reentry circuits using a common narrow corridor with inner and outer loops have been well demonstrated in patients with IART, especially among the Fontan population of patients with massively dilated right atrial chambers and unconventional circuits. Likewise, it is common for a given IART circuit to be capable of supporting both clockwise and counterclockwise patterns of conduction. During ablation, abrupt slowing of IART without interruption can indicate a shift to a slower outer loop of conduction; similarly, an abrupt change in atrial activation pattern and P-wave morphology could represent reversal in direction of propagation through the same tissue rather than a completely novel IART circuit.

The presence of an excitable gap allows IART circuits to be entrained with pacing maneuvers.[18–20] This assists with accurate circuit localization using the principles of postpacing interval analysis and concealed entrainment (Fig. 14-6). Although these techniques have become somewhat less critical in the era of three-dimensional (3D) mapping, they nevertheless represented the mainstay of IART mapping for many years and are still used on a regular basis to help decipher complex circuits.

The focal variety of atrial tachycardia is far less common than IART in the CHD population, representing fewer than 10% of cases in our institutional experience. This paucity of clinical material makes it difficult to characterize

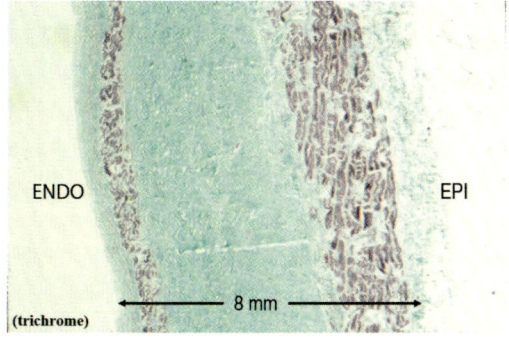

FIGURE 14-4. Microscopic section of the lateral right atrial wall from a patient who had undergone the Fontan operation. A trichrome stain accentuates the diffuse scarring in the atrium. Wall thickness approaches 8 mm. ENDO, endocardial surface; EPI, epicardial surface.

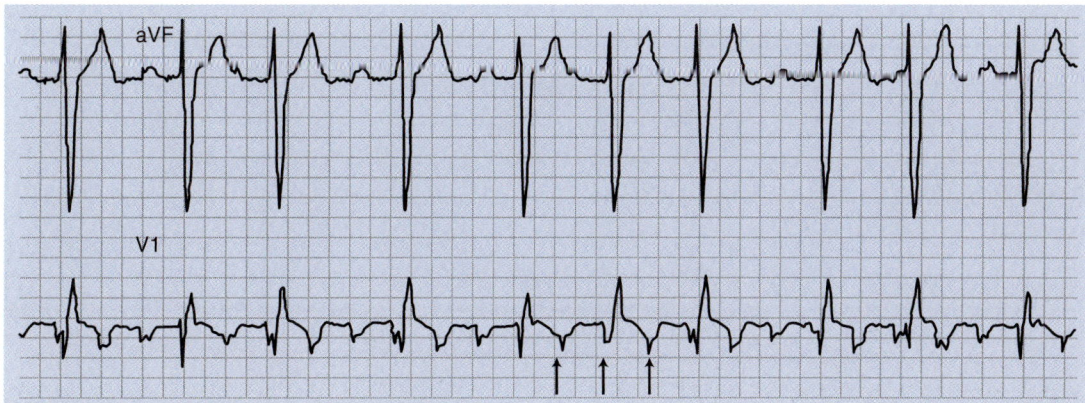

FIGURE 14-5. Rhythm strip (simultaneous electrocardiographic leads aVF and V$_1$) showing intra-atrial reentrant tachycardia at cycle length of 355 msec. The P waves in this case are discrete, with a high-frequency onset and clear isoelectric times.

the mechanism of FAT exactly, and no doubt different mechanisms could be operative in individual patients.[21] However, there are some fairly consistent clinical features that might best be explained by micro-reentry or triggered activity. First, these tachycardias can usually be initiated by programmed atrial stimulation and can be terminated with overdrive pacing and direct-current cardioversion. Second, mapping strongly suggests a point source for tachycardia origin, with atrial activation on 3D maps emanating in all directions from the site. Finally, effective ablation can usually be accomplished by targeting the epicenter of atrial activation with a single RF application. Nothing conclusive can be said beyond these observations, except that FAT frequently maps to atrial tissue that is immediately adjacent to suture lines and sometimes can be terminated with adenosine administration. Although FAT is uncommon in CHD patients, failure to consider its possibility could result in a long and frustrating search for missing segments of a traditional macro-reentry circuit when none really exists.

Why some CHD patients develop atrial tachycardias, whereas others with the same lesion do not, is a difficult question. Certainly the position of surgical scars is important,[17] but there is more to this issue than unfortunate placement of an atriotomy incision or septal patch because otherwise the problem would be ubiquitous and immediate. In fact, these arrhythmias occur only in a subset of CHD patients, and they usually do not surface until a decade or longer after the operation. Clinical series seeking risk factors for IART have identified sinus node dysfunction and older age at time of surgery as two important predictive variables.[22] Sinus bradycardia can result from direct surgical injury to the node or its arterial supply at the time of surgery and may contribute indirectly to the incidence of IART by promoting wider dispersion in atrial muscle refractoriness. The importance of this tachycardia-bradycardia link is underscored by the observation that simple correction of the atrial rate (back to a physiologic range) with a standard pacemaker reduces or even eliminates IART events in many patients.[8] The association of IART with late age at repair may relate to the more advanced degrees of atrial hypertrophy or fibrosis that result from delayed correction of cyanosis and other hemodynamic burdens. Observations such as these have contributed in large measure to revisions in the technical approach and timing for CHD surgery. Nowadays, corrective operations are performed at much younger ages, using techniques that minimize the insult to atrial muscle and the sinus node, including substitution of the arterial switch procedure for the Mustard and Senning operations and new modifications in the Fontan operation that bypass the RA by channeling caval blood flow directly to the pulmonary arteries.[23,24] The incidence of atrial arrhythmias for the current generation of CHD patients has been reduced dramatically by these innovations, but the large population who underwent repair with older techniques will continue to require rhythm interventions.

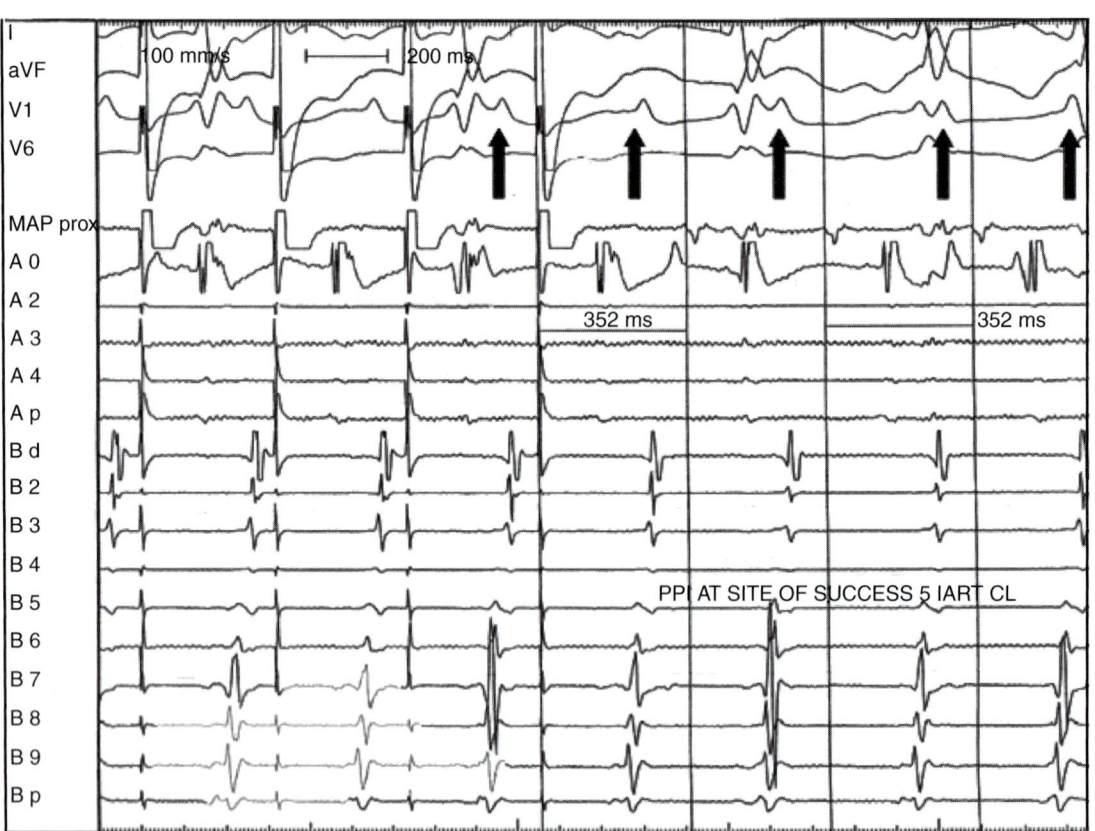

FIGURE 14-6. Recordings from electrophysiologic study of intra-atrial reentrant tachycardia (IART). Shown are surface electrocardiographic leads (I, aVF, V₁, and V₆) along with intracardiac signals from a mapping catheter (MAP) and two multipolar reference catheters (A and B). The tachycardia has a cycle length of 352 msec. Entrainment pacing at cycle length of 320 msec is performed from the mapping catheter at a site that is a critical component of the reentrant circuit. The postpacing interval (PPI) is identical to the tachycardia cycle length (CL), and both the electrogram and P-wave morphologies *(arrows)* are perfectly reproduced by atrial pacing. These two findings prove that the pacing site is involved in the circuit, most likely as part of the zone for slow conduction.

Diagnosis

Making a clinical diagnosis of IART or FAT in CHD patients is not difficult (Table 14-1). The electrocardiographic picture of atrial tachycardia at an unvarying rate is confusing only if there is a 1:1 or 2:1 ratio of atrial and ventricular electrogram amplitudes (A/V ratio) that results in the P waves being obscured by the QRS complex (Fig. 14-7). This is easily clarified whenever necessary by modifying AV conduction with vagal maneuvers or adenosine administration and proving that rapid atrial activity is truly independent of the ventricle. As already implied, P-wave morphology should not be expected to resemble classic flutter waves (Fig. 14-8) and may take on a broad range of appearances. The index of suspicion is usually high enough among physicians caring for CHD patients that these tachycardias are rarely misinterpreted.

The relatively long cycle lengths for atrial tachycardias in the CHD population frequently result in rapid patterns for AV conduction in the absence of medications. This, in conjunction with the fact that many of these patients have suboptimal hemodynamics, accounts for the severe symptoms these arrhythmias tend to produce. Hypotension and

syncope are common, and there are well-documented cases of rapid 1:1 conduction degenerating into ventricular fibrillation.[8] Such concerns cannot be underestimated in the electrophysiology laboratory during a long mapping procedure. Diltiazem should always be readily available to titrate the ventricular response back to a tolerable range should rapid conduction occur in the course of a procedure.

The diagnosis of IART is usually straightforward in the electrophysiology laboratory. These tachycardias can be reliably initiated with pacing maneuvers during electrophysiology study. In our institutional experience, burst pacing appears more productive for inducing IART than conventional extrastimulus testing. Our standard protocol now usually begins with S_2 atrial and ventricular stimulation to assess functional characteristics and rule out alternative tachycardia mechanisms, but then shifts directly to 8-beat atrial bursts at a cycle length that is shortened in 10-millisecond decrements down to a 2:1 pattern of atrial capture. If this fails to induce the tachycardia of interest, an alternative atrial pacing site is chosen. This entire process is then repeated with an isoproterenol infusion if necessary. Nonspecific atrial fibrillation is rarely induced in CHD patients despite such aggressive atrial stimulation, but in the rare case when it does occur, cardioversion is performed and stimulation is reattempted after a loading dose of intravenous procainamide. The diagnosis rests on the demonstration of macro-reentrant atrial arrhythmias by dissociation from the ventricles and AV node and the ability to demonstrate features of entrainment that are consistent with the reentrant nature of the arrhythmia (see Table 14-1). The differential diagnosis is also straightforward, in most cases requiring exclusion of AV nodal reentry and reciprocating tachycardias.

TABLE 14-1
DIAGNOSTIC FEATURES OF INTRA-ATRIAL (MACRO-REENTRY) REENTRY OBSERVED ON ELECTROPHYSIOLOGIC STUDY*
Fixed atrial cycle length (very wide range: 270–450 msec)
Adenosine resistance
Features of macroreentry
• Inducible with programmed stimulation
• Excitable gap
• Entrainment
• Reentrant circuit defined by electroanatomic mapping

*The surface electrocardiogram often is not diagnostic because classic flutter waves are uncommon, and discrete P waves with isoelectric intervals are possible.

Mapping

Anatomic Detail

The underlying anatomy must be extremely well defined before mapping IART or FAT in the CHD population,

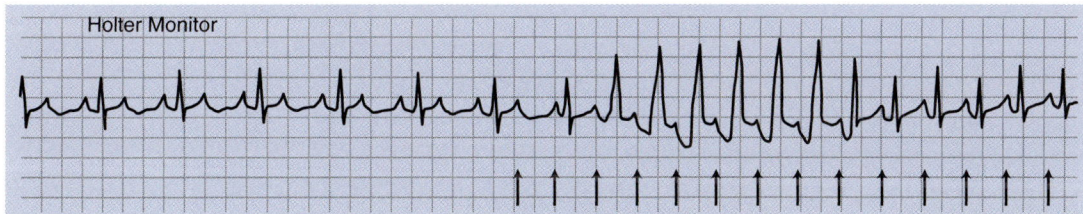

FIGURE 14-7. Holter monitor recording from a patient with intra-atrial reentrant tachycardia at an atrial cycle length of 290 msec. Initially, the ventricle responds in a 2:1 fashion, but then shifts to 1:1 conduction with an initial period of rate-related aberration.

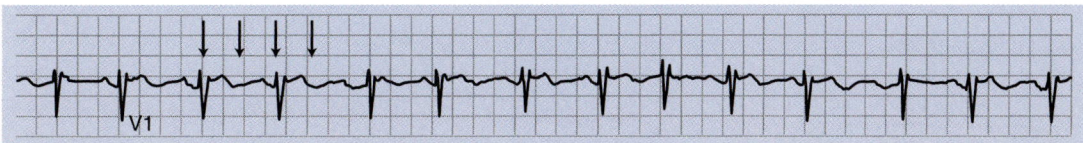

FIGURE 14-8. Rhythm strip (electrocardiographic lead V_1) showing intra-atrial reentrant tachycardia at a cycle length of 360 msec. The P waves do not resemble classic flutter waves. During periods of predominantly 2:1 conduction in this case, the rhythm can be hard to differentiate from mild sinus tachycardia unless the clinical index of suspicion is high.

beginning with careful analysis of all recent echocardiograms, angiograms, or magnetic resonance images. In addition, prior catheterization reports should be reviewed to anticipate potential difficulties with vascular access or redirected vasculature that could thwart catheter positioning at a potential ablation target site. This is particularly true for patients with complicated intra-atrial baffles of the type used for the Mustard, Senning, and Fontan operations. Operative notes should also be reviewed to ascertain the potential location of all patches and suture lines that might serve as a substrate for the tachycardia.

The specific cardiac lesion and surgical details must be understood, not just for anatomic orientation but also as a guide to the position of the specialized conduction tissues. The AV node and His bundle can be displaced far outside the triangle of Koch in some cardiac malformations,[25,26] especially among patients with AV discordance (e.g., "corrected" transposition) and those with AV canal defects. To minimize the chance of inadvertent damage to the AV node or His bundle during ablation of atrial tachycardias, it is essential to have a good working knowledge of conduction system embryology and anatomy in CHD and to spend time carefully locating a high-quality His potential.[27]

Biplane fluoroscopy and angiography are indispensable for mapping and ablation in CHD patients with complex anatomy. As an initial maneuver during these procedures, an angiogram should be performed in the RA to outline gross anatomic landmarks that can serve as a roadmap throughout the mapping process (Figs. 14-9 and 14-10). Such imaging is mandatory whenever conventional electrogram analysis is used as the principal mapping tool,[28] but it is valuable even during sophisticated 3D mapping because it helps ensure that the tip of the mapping catheter has truly sampled the entire endocardial surface of a chamber of interest. Additional imaging with transesophageal echocardiography can be used if specific anatomic questions arise or to help guide difficult Brockenbrough procedures or other forms of transbaffle puncture if necessary. We have not had occasion to use intracardiac ultrasound imaging in our own laboratory during ablation in CHD patients, but we acknowledge its potential utility in experienced hands.

Conventional Electrogram Mapping

The elegant 3D displays that are available with electroanatomic and noncontact mapping technology sometimes appear to overshadow the value of conventional recordings. However, failure to appreciate the importance of standard electrogram analysis and entrainment pacing techniques is likely to result in a high failure rate for ablation in CHD patients. These techniques are all synergistic in localizing circuits and pinpointing potential ablation targets.

Once the anatomy has been clearly delineated and sustained atrial tachycardia has been induced, the electrogram pattern in the RA (or at least those portions of the RA that can be reached) is sampled to generate an activation sequence map.[29,30] Whether this is accomplished with linear catheters, basket catheters, inflatable balloons, or point-by-point mapping is irrelevant. The more critical

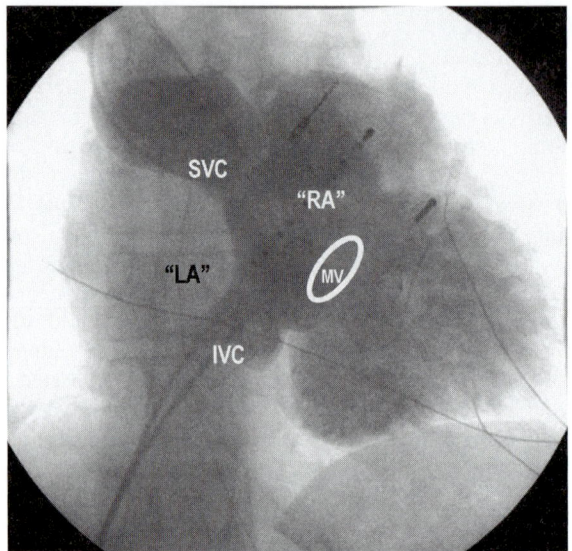

FIGURE 14-9. Angiogram in the modified right atrium ("RA") of a patient who has undergone a Mustard operation, in which blood flow from the inferior vena cava (IVC) and superior vena cava (SVC) is redirected to the mitral valve (MV). "LA," modified left atrium.

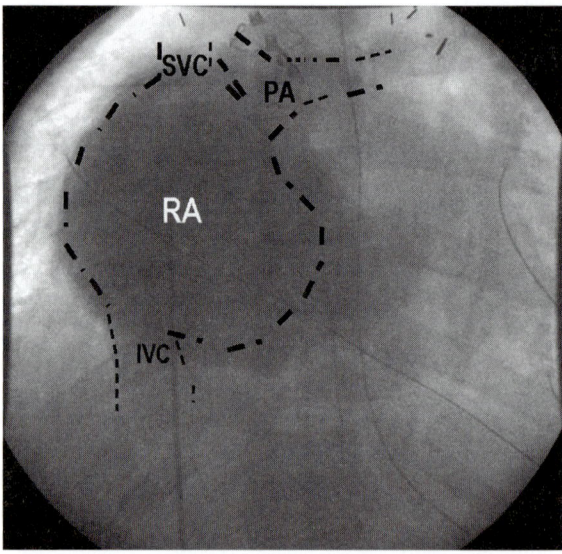

FIGURE 14-10. Angiogram in a patient with tricuspid atresia who underwent a Fontan operation with an old-style connection of the right atrium (RA) directly into the pulmonary artery (PA). The right atrium is severely dilated. IVC, inferior vena cava; SVC, superior vena cava.

issue is compulsive sampling of all possible areas of right atrial endocardium and correct synthesis of this information in the context of the known anatomy.

The electrogram from each sample site is indexed in time against the onset of the surface P wave or, if this is indistinct or uncertain, against some stable atrial reference signal (Fig. 14-11). Electrograms must be collected until sites have been identified to account for the entire duration of the tachycardia cycle length. That is to say, it must be possible to trace out the full path of activation, from the beginning of one P wave to the next, without big gaps in timing.[31] If all electrogram times within the RA cluster

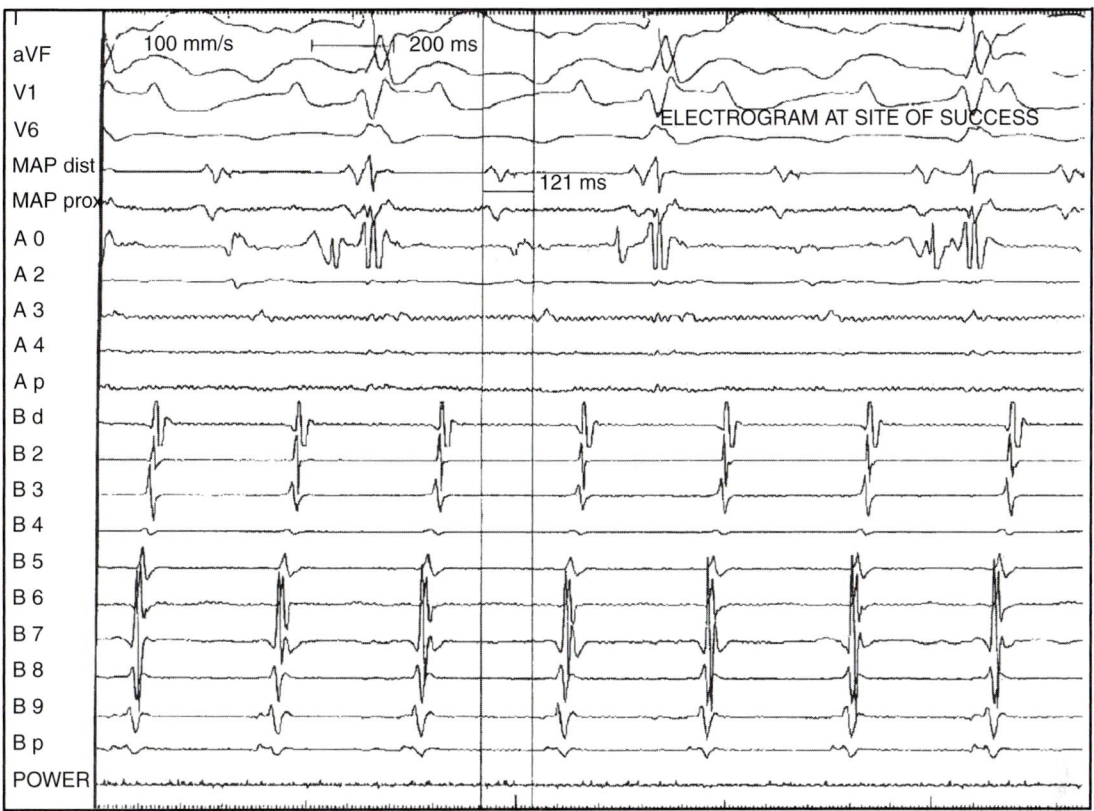

FIGURE 14-11. Recordings from electrophysiologic study of intra-atrial reentrant tachycardia. Shown are surface electrocardiographic leads (I, aVF, V_1, and V_6) along with intracardiac signals from a mapping catheter (MAP) and two multipolar reference catheters (A and B). The atrial cycle length is 365 msec. The mapping catheter is located at a site of successful ablation, where the local electrogram has a fractionated signal that occurs during the isoelectric period between P waves, covering an interval of 60 to 120 msec before P-wave onset. dist, distal; prox, proximal.

toward one end of the tachycardia cycle length, there are only three possible explanations. Most likely, the remaining portion of the circuit is located on the opposite side of the atrial septum or on a surgical baffle, and the other atrial chamber must be entered by transseptal puncture or a retrograde approach to find the missing conduction times. This is a common issue in Mustard or Senning patients, as well as many patients with "lateral tunnel" modifications of the Fontan operation. A second possibility is that a small region of the RA with very slow conduction was inadequately sampled. This option should be considered strongly if the missing portion of the cycle length is confined to the isoelectric or diastolic period between P waves and all other activation times have been clearly accounted for within the RA. A third possibility is that the mechanism of atrial tachycardia is actually FAT, in which activation propagates from a single point rather than involving a large reentry circuit. It usually does not take long to rule in or dismiss this option by brief supplemental mapping in the vicinity of the earliest atrial activation site.

Beyond timing, each electrogram must also be examined for special traits that might indicate an important conduction feature.[32,33] For example, registration of a very-low-amplitude signal from a site where the operator is sure of good endocardial contact strongly suggests a region of scar or a surgical patch. Similarly, a distinctly split electrogram is consistent with recording along the crista terminalis, an old ablation site, an atriotomy incision, or some other suture line (Fig. 14-12). Fractionated electrograms

of long duration (Fig. 14-13) can suggest a zone of slow conduction (although not necessarily one that is critical to the circuit). Finally, a discrete island of entrance block can sometimes be found at which the atrial rate is clearly slower than the underlying tachycardia, and the edges of such an island often correspond to important conduction barriers.

All data regarding atrial anatomy, activation patterns, and conduction features must be combined to generate one or more potential models for IART circuit location. The validity of the model can then be tested by entrainment pacing techniques.[18,34] Although there is always a small risk for interrupting or changing the tachycardia while pacing into an IART circuit, this risk is small as long as the pacing rate is just marginally faster than the tachycardia rate. If circuit localization appears quite firm on the basis of activation sequence and the model makes good anatomic sense, perhaps entrainment pacing might be deferred. However, if there is any ambiguity at all about the circuit, this exercise can be extremely helpful in confirming or refuting the model.

In our electrophysiology laboratory, entrainment is performed with bipolar pacing from the distal electrode pair of the mapping catheter. Some centers perform unipolar pacing from the distal electrode, but we have not found this to be a major advantage for the CHD population. We prefer the reduced pacing artifact that accompanies bipolar pacing over any incremental precision that unipolar pacing might provide. The return atrial signal can usually

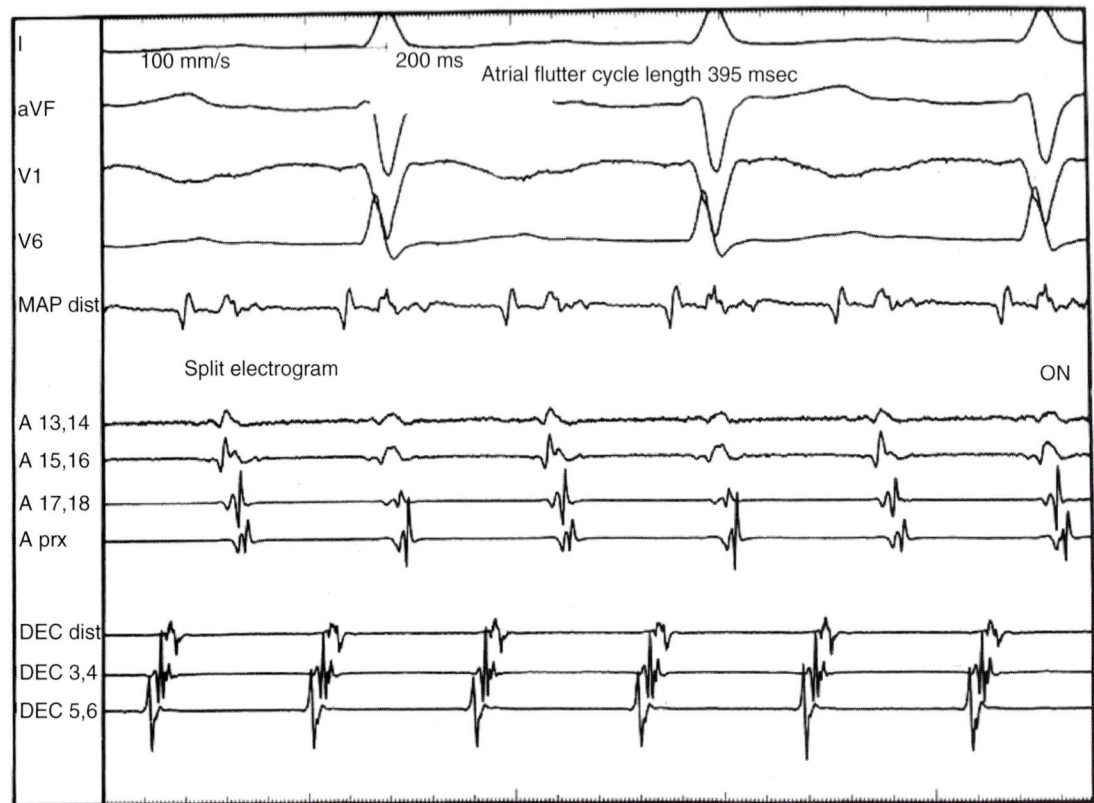

FIGURE 14-12. Recordings from electrophysiologic study of intra-atrial reentrant tachycardia. Shown are surface electrocardiographic leads (I, aVF, V₁, and V₆) along with intracardiac signals from a mapping catheter (MAP) and two multipolar reference catheters (A and DEC). The atrial cycle length is 395 msec. The mapping catheter is located along a presumptive atriotomy scar, showing a split electrogram pattern.

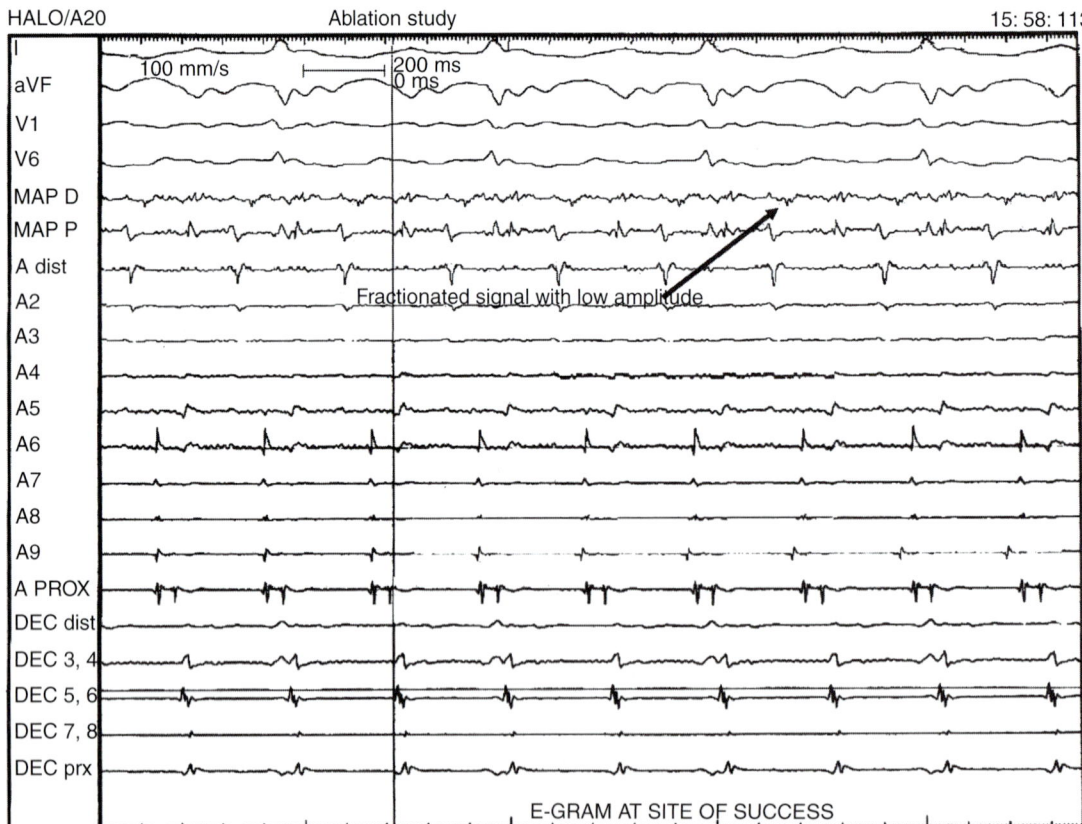

FIGURE 14-13. Recordings from electrophysiologic study of intra-atrial reentrant tachycardia. Shown are surface electrocardiographic leads (I, aVF, V₁, and V₆) along with intracardiac signals from a mapping catheter (MAP) and two multipolar reference catheters (A and DEC). The atrial cycle length is 270 msec. The mapping catheter is located at a site of successful ablation, where the local electrogram has a highly fractionated signal that spans almost the entire duration of atrial diastole. D, distal; dist, distal; prox, proximal.

be measured directly from the pacing electrode pair with modern recording systems (Fig. 14-14), unless the amplitude of the electrogram at the pacing site was exceptionally low to begin with. If the return electrogram from the distal electrode pair is too indistinct for accurate measurement, it is usually sufficient to rely on the proximal electrode pair on the mapping catheter as a proxy, while simply adjusting for the difference in timing between the pacing and recording sites during tachycardia.[35,36] Similar to the experience reported with mapping of reentrant ventricular tachycardia,[18] sites at which the postpacing interval does not exceed the IART cycle length by more than 30 milliseconds tend to indicate tissue within the path of the circuit, and the smaller this difference, the better the localization.

Accurately identifying the full path of an IART circuit does not necessarily imply that one has pinpointed the correct spot to ablate. For RF ablation to succeed, the target area must be as small as possible so that permanent transmural block can be achieved. Therefore, the atrium must be examined for anatomic and electrogram features[37,38] that are most likely to funnel the circuit into a narrow corridor between two conduction barriers (Table 14-2). As it turns out, the narrowest corridor usually translates to the zone of slowest conduction, and this further translates to electrogram timings that occur just before the rapid deflection of the P wave on the surface electrocardiogram. Whenever clear and discrete P-wave activity can be identified during IART, the most optimistic ablation targets usually reg-

ister electrogram times toward the end of the isoelectric period, about 50 to 80 milliseconds before P-wave onset.[6] Electrograms at such a site are quite often fractionated and relatively low in amplitude. Obviously, if the P-wave onset is indistinct on the surface electrocardiogram, slow conduction zones cannot be identified with these simple methods. Instead, one can search for locations within the circuit that

TABLE 14-2
TARGET SITES FOR ABLATION OF INTRA-ATRIAL REENTRY
Sites generally with low-amplitude, fractionated electrograms
If P wave is discrete, local timing precedes P by about 50–80 msec
Sites with entrainment features
• Electrogram-to–P-wave time = stimulus-to–P-wave time
• Postpacing interval - atrial cycle length ≤30 msec
• Perfect concealed entrainment
Physically narrow corridor based on identification of conduction barriers
Common anatomic targets
• Cavotricuspid isthmus (if present)
• Lateral right atrial wall atriotomy area (Fontan patients)

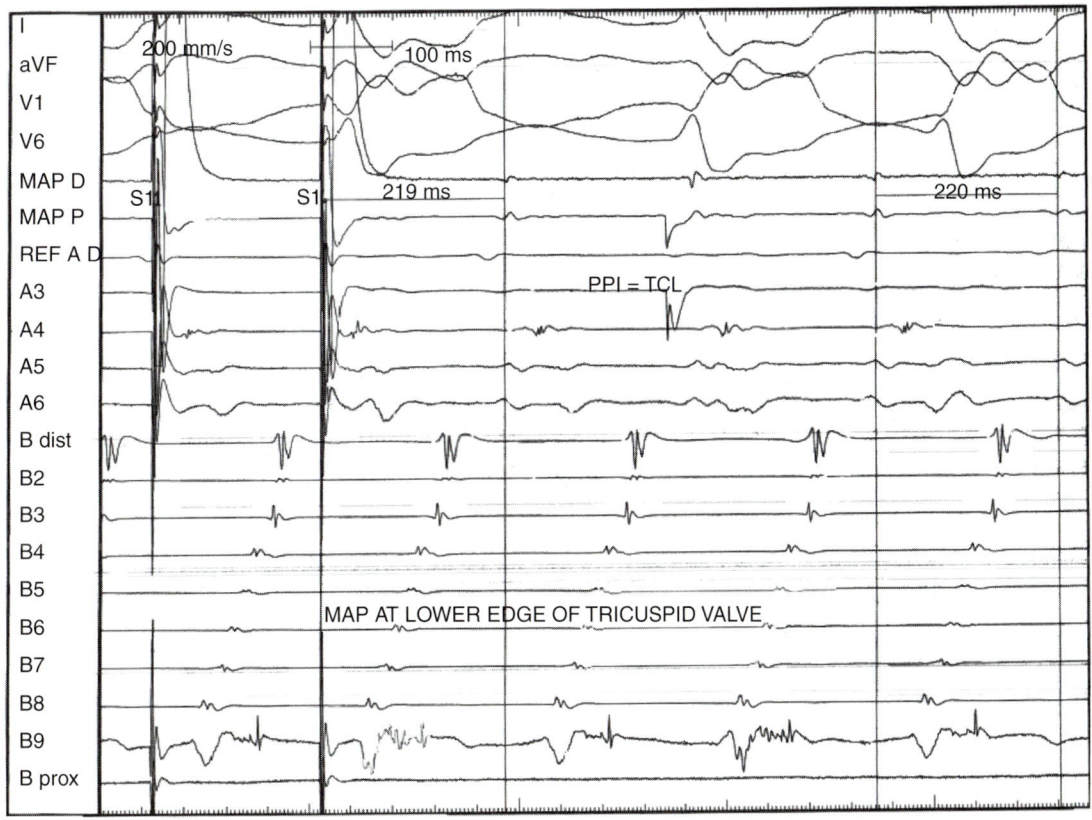

FIGURE 14-14. Recordings from electrophysiologic study of intra-atrial reentrant tachycardia. Shown are surface electrocardiographic leads (I, aVF, V_1, and V_6) along with intracardiac signals from a mapping catheter (MAP) and two multipolar reference catheters (A and B). The tachycardia has a cycle length of 220 msec. Entrainment pacing (S_1) at cycle length of 205 msec is performed from the mapping catheter at a site that is a critical component of the reentrant circuit. The postpacing interval (PPI) measured on the distal MAP electrogram is identical to the tachycardia cycle length (TCL), indicating that the pacing site is involved in the circuit.

generate perfectly concealed entrainment, consisting of a paced P-wave morphology and electrogram patterns that are identical to those observed in spontaneous tachycardia. Such sites should be located in or near a narrow protected conduction corridor. If all else fails, likely corridors of vulnerability can be identified by simply considering the anatomy and picking a region with the narrowest linear dimensions between two well-defined conduction barriers.

Three-Dimensional Mapping

Electroanatomic and noncontact mapping have simplified and improved ablation of atrial tachycardia in CHD patients.[39,40] This is not to say that 3D technologies have revolutionized understanding of the pathophysiology of IART or FAT in any substantial way. Rather, the major benefit has been that electrogram data are presented in a user-friendly format that enhances catheter positioning and keeps track of subtle conduction features that might go unnoticed or become forgotten during the tedious process of mapping with older recording systems. Moreover, these sophisticated mapping tools have greatly improved the ability to confirm complete conduction block across an ablated region in 3D space, a process that formerly was highly prone to error for any site other than the CTI. Once these technologies began to be applied to tachycardia in CHD patients, acute ablation success rates rose, and recurrence rates declined.[41]

Most CHD patients have sustained IART circuits with stable cycle lengths, so that high-quality electroanatomic maps can be achieved reliably with point-by-point sampling of the right atrial endocardial surface and, if necessary, of the left atrium as well (Figs. 14-15 and 14-16).

The ability to tag this 3D display with markers indicating scar regions, split potentials, caval orifices, and valve rings assists greatly in fashioning a rational model for IART propagation.[42] In addition, the ability to project maps of both atrial chambers simultaneously (Fig. 14-17) allows prompt identification of circuits that may have to be ablated from the left side of the heart. Electroanatomic displays also remove most confusion about the differential diagnosis between IART and FAT because radial propagation of the latter usually is readily apparent (Fig. 14-18). With experienced staff, full acquisition of a detailed IART or FAT map in the RA can usually be accomplished in less than 15 minutes.

One important caveat with electroanatomic mapping is that the catheter tip must be in good contact with the endocardial surface for each electrogram collected. In CHD patients with very dilated atria, this can be difficult to ensure. Failure to recognize poor contact could result in collection of phantom data points suggesting a low-amplitude scar region, when in fact the catheter tip was simply floating in the atrial cavity. Using the baseline right atrial angiogram as a guide, the catheter operator must periodically check to ensure that the tip of the mapping electrode has reached the true edge of the atrial silhouette. This sometimes requires the use of a long guiding sheath to extend the reach of the catheter curve.

The major limitation of electroanatomic mapping is that tachycardia must remain stable for the duration of data acquisition. Occasionally, CHD patients, particularly in the Fontan group, have multiple IART circuits, and tachycardias can shift or terminate during the mapping process in response to the mechanical ectopy that

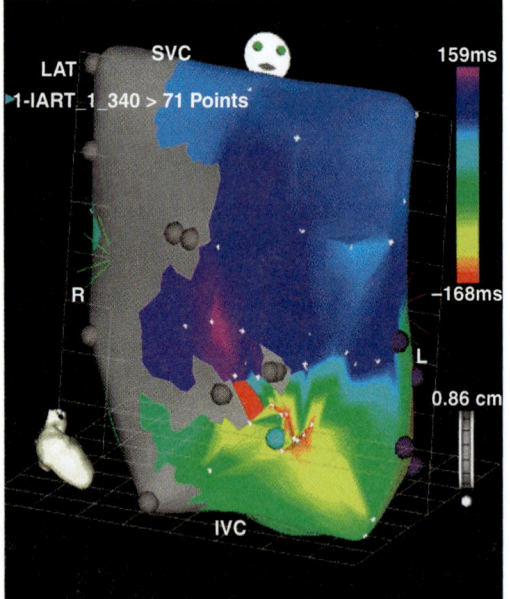

FIGURE 14-15. Electroanatomic map of intra-atrial reentrant tachycardia (cycle length, 330 msec) in a patient with a Fontan operation for tricuspid atresia. This projection shows the lateral wall of the right atrium, with a large area of scar *(gray)* that extends all the way from the superior vena cava (SVC) to the inferior vena cava (IVC), including a small extension that juts forward along the lower half of the right atrial free wall. There was a very narrow conduction channel through this scar extension, and it proved to be a critical part of the tachycardia circuit. Activation proceeds through this channel according to the following color code: blue → purple → red → yellow → green.

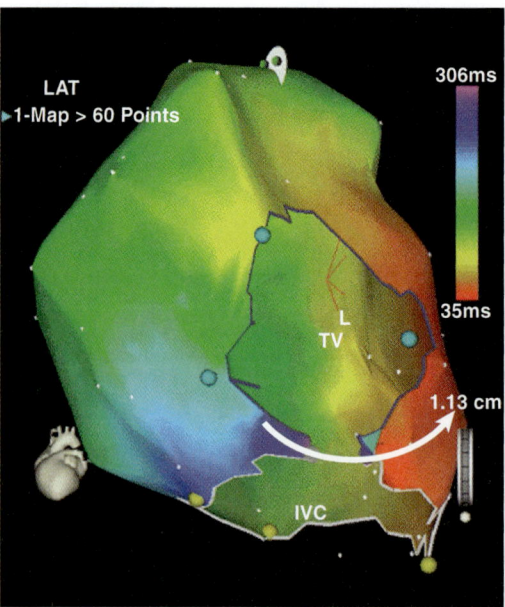

FIGURE 14-16. Electroanatomic map of intra-atrial reentrant tachycardia (cycle length, 340 msec) in the right atrium of a patient with repaired tetralogy of Fallot. This left anterior oblique caudal projection highlights the isthmus between the inferior vena cava (IVC) and the tricuspid valve (TV), which proved to be a critical part of the tachycardia circuit. Activation proceeds through this isthmus *(arrow)* according to the following color code: blue → purple → red.

accompanies catheter manipulation. If this problem repeatedly stymies mapping efforts, it is often useful to revert to a more simple map of sinus rhythm and create a basic anatomic shell of the RA that is focused primarily on the major conduction barriers.[43] This sinus rhythm map can then be examined to identify the most likely narrow conduction corridors, and repeat mapping during any subsequent episodes of tachycardia can concentrate on these regions of interest.

Noncontact mapping[44] may also be used for IART or FAT mapping, and it appears to be particularly well suited to patients with poor hemodynamics, who might not tolerate long episodes of tachycardia, and for those with multiple unstable IART circuits that are too fleeting to map by other techniques (Fig. 14-19). However, this technology has some limitations in CHD patients with very dilated atrial chambers because data quality can suffer to some degree whenever the inflated recording balloon is too far away from the atrial endocardial surface.

Propagation maps of IART generated by either of these 3D techniques must still be viewed critically before deciding exactly where to place ablation lesions. Just because an atrial region displays suspicious conduction features on a 3D map, this does not prove that it is part of a circuit. It may still be helpful to perform entrainment pacing maneuvers to confirm the model before embarking on RF applications.[34]

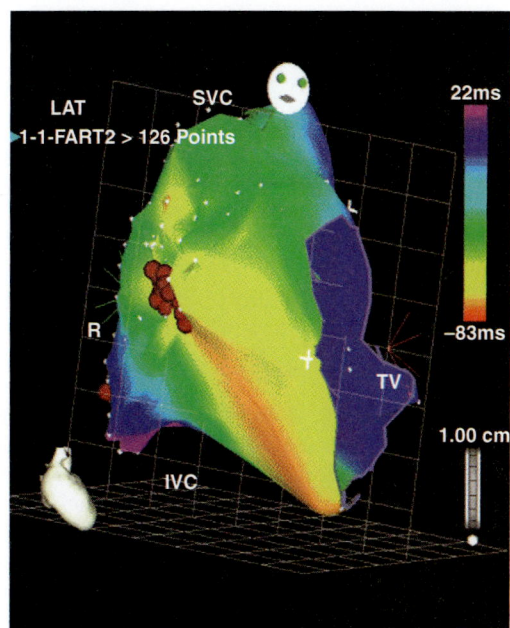

FIGURE 14-18. Electroanatomic map of focal atrial tachycardia in the right atrium of a patient who had undergone closure of atrial and ventricular septal defects. Earliest atrial activation was mapped to the lateral right atrial wall, where electrogram features suggested a nearby atriotomy scar. Activation spread in a radial fashion from this site. The *red dots* mark the site of successful ablation. IVC, inferior vena cava; SVC, superior vena cava; TV, tricuspid valve.

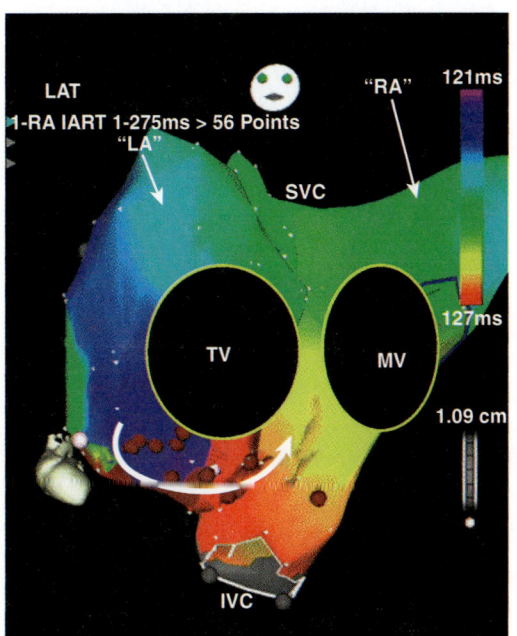

FIGURE 14-17. Electroanatomic map of intra-atrial reentrant tachycardia (cycle length, 255 msec) in a patient who underwent the Mustard operation for transposition of the great arteries. This anteroposterior display combines activation times from both the modified right atrium ("RA") and the modified left atrium ("LA") and highlights the isthmus between the inferior vena cava (IVC) and the tricuspid valve (TV), which proved to be a critical part of the tachycardia circuit. Activation proceeds through this isthmus *(arrow)* according to the following color code: blue → purple → red → yellow. MV, mitral valve; SVC, superior vena cava.

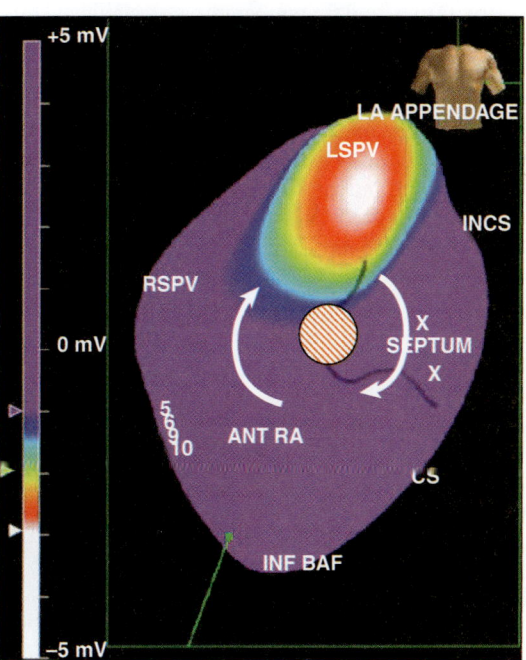

FIGURE 14-19. Noncontact map of intra-atrial reentrant tachycardia in a patient who had undergone a Fontan operation. This projection highlights the atrial septal surface as recorded by the balloon catheter within the left atrium. The activation pattern *(arrows)* indicates a circuit around an atrial septal patch *(nashed area)*. ANT RA, anterior right atrium; CS, coronary sinus; INF BAF, inferior baffle; LA appendage, left atrial appendage; LSPV, left superior pulmonary vein; RSPV, right superior pulmonary vein.

Ablation

Accurate mapping is only half the battle in IART ablation. Even if the tachycardia location is firm, it can still be difficult to create effective ablation lesions in CHD patients using standard RF technology (Table 14-3). The target tissue selected in these cases can be heavily trabeculated and thickened because of hypertrophy or surgical scar, and it almost always has a width greater than that achieved by a single RF application. Multiple overlapping lesions may need to be placed when attempting a line of conduction block, leaving open the possibility of gaps in the line or varying depths of RF penetration that fail to produce full transmural tissue injury. In addition, the biophysics of the RF lesion creation may be compromised in some CHD patients, particularly those who have undergone the Fontan operation and have massively enlarged RAs. These patients can have remarkably low atrial blood flow velocity,[45] as evidenced by the common echocardiographic observation of spontaneous cavitation or "smoke" within the body of the RA. As a consequence, there is low convective cooling of the ablation catheter tip by circulating blood, so that RF power delivery becomes severely limited by high catheter-tip temperatures. This limitation has been dealt with fairly effectively by the widespread adoption of alternative catheter designs for RF delivery in CHD patients, including both large-tip and irrigated-tip catheters.

Ablation efforts can usually begin with a standard 4-mm-tip catheter and a temperature-controlled 50-W RF generator set to a maximum of 70°C. As RF applications are made in a region of interest, careful attention should be given to the biophysical parameters measured from the generator. If maximal tip temperatures are achieved quickly, but peak RF powers register much less than 25W, inadequate tissue injury can usually be predicted. Even if there is an acute tachycardia termination, true conduction block is unlikely to be achieved, and IART will almost always be reinducible (or recur during later follow-up) when these feeble amounts of RF power are applied. It is probably advisable in these cases to switch promptly to either a 6- to 8-mm-tip catheter or an irrigated-tip ablation catheter.

We have had experience with various large-tip designs and several irrigation systems, and so long as improved RF power delivery is accomplished, there does not appear to be any obvious advantage of one technique over the other. However, it is abundantly clear that these alternative catheter techniques can succeed in IART cases after standard ablation with a 4-mm-tip catheter has failed.

The acute response of IART to accurately positioned RF applications varies according to the dimensions and conduction properties of the corridor being targeted. Abrupt termination early into a single RF application may be seen if the corridor is narrow and discrete (Fig. 14-20), but this is actually a fairly rare occurrence in CHD patients. It is far more common to observe a pattern of gradual and progressive cycle length prolongation as cumulative RF applications slowly close off conduction through the critical corridor (Fig. 14-21).

It is important to emphasize that the isolated observation of IART termination is not a sufficient end point for ablation. Granted, interruption of tachycardia is an optimistic sign that the map was correct, but it does not prove that complete conduction block has been achieved. Pacing from both sides of the target zone must be performed, and follow-up propagation maps should be constructed to investigate the possibility of residual gaps through the corridor. If there is any hint of residual conduction, additional RF applications should be delivered at the site (using large-tip or irrigation-tip catheters, if necessary) until unequivocal block has been established.[38,41,46] As mentioned, 3D mapping has greatly improved the accuracy of these follow-up maps for the CHD population (Fig. 14-22).

For the rare CHD patient with FAT, ablation of the focal abnormality with RF current is relatively uncomplicated. The epicenter of early atrial activation can often be ablated with a single application, but, once again, if thermodynamics during RF delivery indicate low wattage because of high tip temperatures, a large-tip or irrigated-tip catheter should be used.

After successful ablation of an IART circuit or FAT focus, repeat atrial stimulation should be performed to rule out additional sources of atrial tachycardia. Among Fontan

TABLE 14-3

TROUBLESHOOTING THE DIFFICULT CASE

Problem	Cause	Solution
Complex anatomy and cardiac access	Congenital malformations, prior surgery with patches, baffles, and so on	Extensive review of prior surgical procedures and all imaging modalities Contrast angiography, intracardiac or transesophageal echocardiography during case
Incomplete reentrant circuit mapped	Small zone of slow conduction missed, portions of atria not mapped, inaccessible Circuit involves "the other" atrium True focal mechanism	High-density mapping and pace-mapping for areas of slow conduction thorough mapping of baffles, pouches, and so on Map contralateral atrium Verify with electroanatomic and/or entrainment mapping
Failure of radiofrequency (RF) ablation at favorable site	Thick tissue from scar, hypertrophy, trabeculae Broad reentry circuit Low-flow area yielding high temperatures/low power	Cooled RF ablation Linear lesions, large-tip ablation catheter Cooled ablation
Multiple reentry circuits and arrhythmias	Extensive scarring and surgical procedures (Fontan)	Noncontact mapping for nonsustained arrhythmias Extensive use of electroanatomic and entrainment mapping

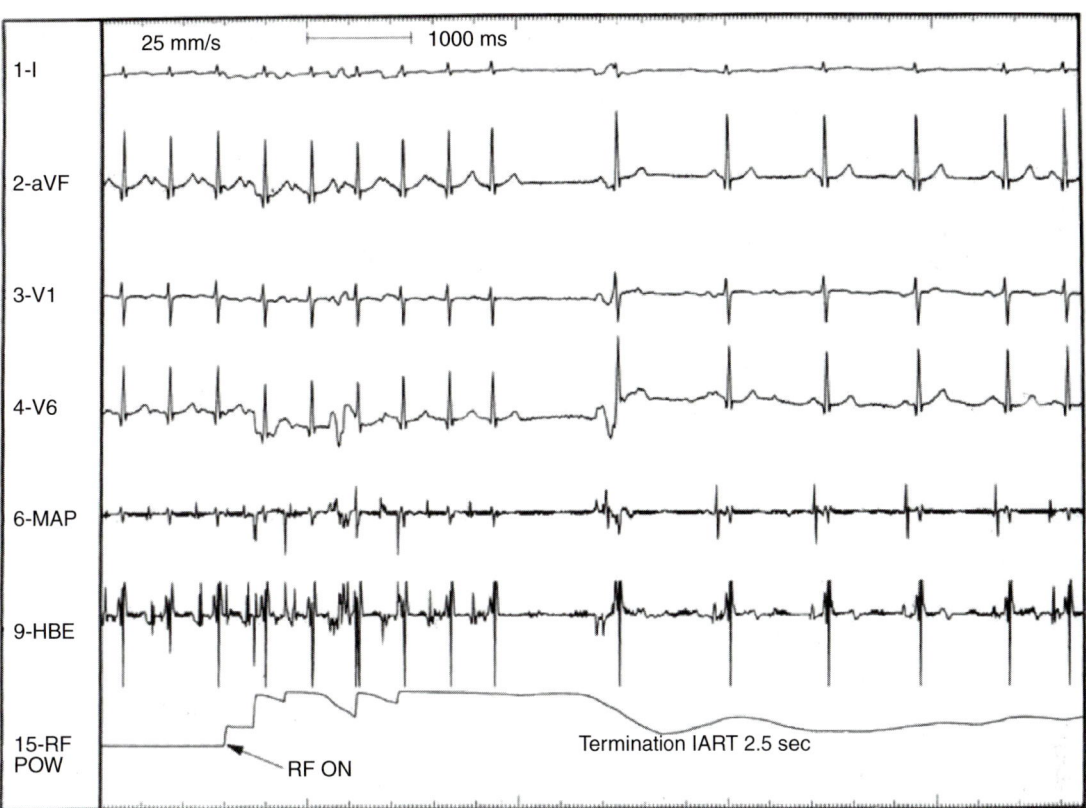

FIGURE 14-20. Recordings from ablation of intra-atrial reentrant tachycardia. Shown are surface electrocardiographic leads (I, aVF, V₁, and V₆) along with intracardiac signals from a mapping catheter (MAP) and a His bundle recording (HBE). In this case, tachycardia terminated promptly on initial radiofrequency application. RF Pow, radiofrequency power.

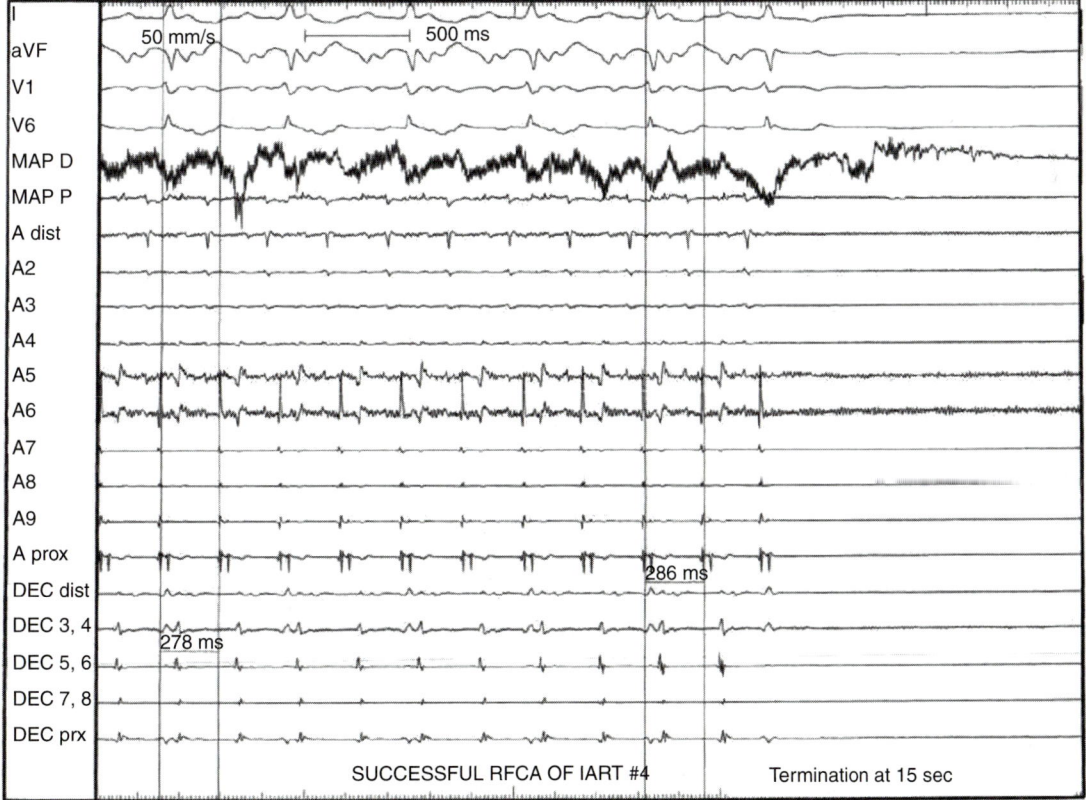

FIGURE 14-21. Recordings from ablation of intra-atrial reentrant tachycardia. Shown are surface electrocardiographic leads (I, aVF, V₁, and V₆) along with intracardiac signals from a mapping catheter (MAP) and two atrial reference catheters (A and DEC). The starting tachycardia cycle length was 260 msec. In this case, tachycardia slowed in a gradual and progressive fashion to 286 msec but did not terminate until 15 seconds into the radiofrequency application. D, distal; dist, distal; prox, proximal.

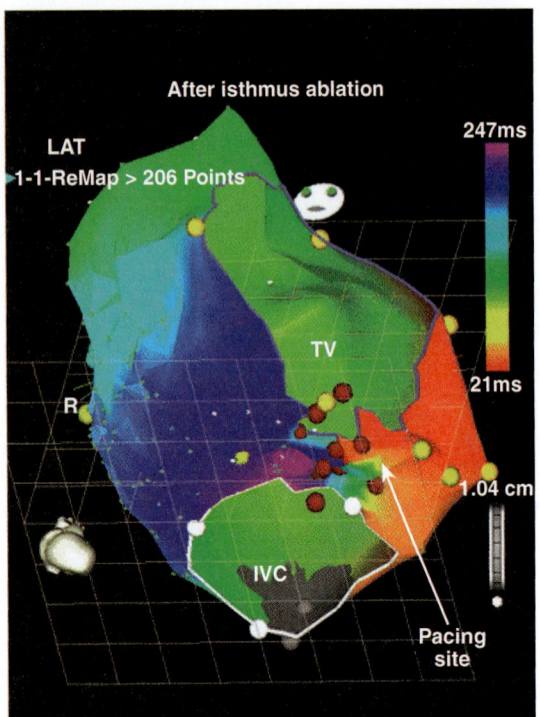

FIGURE 14-22. Electroanatomic map of atrial activation while pacing near the mouth of the coronary sinus in a patient who had just undergone successful interruption of conduction through the cavotricuspid isthmus. The *red dots* mark the sites of radiofrequency applications. The late electrogram times *(blue and purple)* recorded just on the other side of the ablation line suggest that propagation of atrial activation away from the pacing site had to occur in a counterclockwise manner all the way around the tricuspid valve ring, rather than across the isthmus. IVC, inferior vena cava; TV, tricuspid valve.

patients in particular, multiple tachycardias are very common. If the patient has a true CTI that did not participate in the original target arrhythmia, it is probably still wise to close off isthmus conduction as a precaution in the electrophysiology laboratory, even if no tachycardia was identified as involving this site.

Clinical Outcomes

Long-term results for ablation of atrial tachycardias in patients with CHD have been improving steadily as new mapping and ablation technologies have been introduced, but there is still room for improvement. Acute ablation success, defined according to rigorous conduction block criteria, can now be achieved in as many as 90% of cases in the modern era of 3D mapping and aggressive RF lesion creation. This compares with acute success rates of only about 60% that were seen with older mapping technology and standard 4-mm-tip ablation catheters. However, despite generally excellent acute outcomes, recurrence of some form of atrial tachycardia during longer-term follow-up is still disappointingly common. These recurrences can involve return of the original target arrhythmia, but quite often they represent appearance of a totally new atrial substrate. Recurrence is particularly problematic in Fontan patients with multiple IART circuits, as many as 40% of whom achieve acute success but experience at least one

episode of atrial tachycardia within 2 years after the procedure. Recurrence is less common in patients with two ventricles and routine anatomy, in whom ablation can usually be focused on the familiar territory of the CTI. The recurrence risk in this setting is now reasonably low, on the order of 20%.

Contemporary outcome data for atrial tachycardia ablation in CHD patients, although not perfect, may still be viewed as encouraging when compared with the option of pharmacologic therapy,[7] which is associated with a recurrence risk at 2 years as high as 70%. Moreover, even among patients who have a recurrent tachycardia after ablation, global rhythm status is still likely to be improved compared with their preablation condition. This improvement was quantified in a large clinical study from our center using a scoring system that incorporated such items as severity of symptoms, antiarrhythmic drug dependency, the need for cardioversion, and observations on whether tachycardia episodes were sustained or self-terminating.[41] When scored in this fashion, almost all CHD patients (regardless of anatomy) had a substantial improvement in quality of life after ablation for atrial tachycardia.

Conclusion

RF ablation of atrial tachycardia in postoperative CHD patients presents many unique challenges in terms of anatomic complexity, atypical tachycardia substrates, and abnormally thick atrial muscle that can be difficult to ablate. Technologic advances in 3D mapping and the broader availability of ablation catheters designed to make more effective RF lesions have significantly improved outcomes.

Looking forward, it is reasonable to expect a continued reduction in tachycardia recurrence rates with more liberal use of large-tip or irrigated-tip RF ablation catheters, or perhaps the application of novel ablation modalities such as microwave energy or cryoablation.[47] It is anticipated that improved lesion creation, in conjunction with adherence to stringent conduction block criteria for success, may reduce recurrence rates to the range currently seen with ablation of typical atrial flutter in normal hearts.[48] As a spinoff benefit, the clinical experience with catheter ablation of these tachycardias will continue to influence the surgical approach to various forms of CHD. By illustrating the exact spatial relations between scar regions and macro-reentry circuits, certain arrhythmogenic locations for atriotomy incisions and patch placement can now be anticipated and avoided for future generations of CHD patients.[49]

References

1. Flinn CJ, Wolff GS, Dick M, et al. Cardiac rhythm after the Mustard operation for complete transposition of the great arteries. *N Engl J Med.* 1984;3310:1635–1638.
2. Fishberger SB, Wernovsky G, Gentles TL, et al. Factors that influence the development of atrial flutter after the Fontan operation. *J Thorac Cardiovasc Surg.* 1997;113:80–86.
3. Walsh EP. Arrhythmias in patients with congenital heart disease. *Card Electrophysiol Rev.* 2002;4:422–430.
4. Garson A, Bink-Boelkens MTE, Hesslein PS, et al. Atrial flutter in the young: a collaborative study of 380 cases. *J Am Coll Cardiol.* 1985;6:871–878.
5. Kirsh JA, Walsh EP, Triedman JK. Prevalence of and risk factors for atrial fibrillation and intraatrial reentrant tachycardia among patients with congenital heart disease. *Am J Cardiol.* 2002;90:338–340.

6. Triedman JK, Saul JP, Weindling SN, Walsh EP. Radiofrequency ablation of intraatrial reentrant tachycardia following surgical palliation of congenital heart disease. *Circulation*. 1995;91:707–714.

7. Triedman JK. Atrial reentrant tachycardias. In: Walsh EP, Saul JP, Triedman JK, eds. *Cardiac Arrhythmias in Children and Young Adults with Congenital Heart Disease*. Philadelphia: Lippincott Williams & Wilkins; 2001:137–160.

8. Rhodes LA, Walsh EP, Gamble WJ, et al. Benefits and potential risks of atrial antitachycardia pacing after repair of congenital heart disease. *Pacing Clin Electrophysiol*. 1995;18:1005–1016.

9. Stevenson EA, Casavant D, Tuzi J, et al. Efficacy of atrial antitachycardia pacing using the Medtronic AT500 pacemaker in patients with congenital heart disease. *Am J Cardiol*. 2003;92:871–876.

10. Mavroudis C, Backer CL, Deal BJ, et al. Total cavopulmonary conversion and maze procedure for patients with failure of the Fontan operation. *J Thorac Cardiovasc Surg*. 2001;122:863–871.

11. Kreutzer J, Keane JF, Lock JE, et al. Conversion of modified Fontan procedure to lateral atrial tunnel cavopulmonary anastomosis. *J Thorac Cardiovasc Surg*. 1996;111:1169–1176.

12. Collins KK, Love BA, Walsh EP, et al. Location of acutely successful radiofrequency catheter ablation of intraatrial reentrant tachycardia in patients with congenital heart disease. *Am J Cardiol*. 2000;86:969–974.

13. Kanter RJ, Papagiannis J, Carboni MP, et al. Radiofrequency catheter ablation of supraventricular tachycardia substrates after Mustard and Senning operations for d-transposition of the great arteries. *J Am Coll Cardiol*. 2000;35:428–441.

14. Van Hare GF, Lesh MD, Ross BA, et al. Mapping and radiofrequency ablation of intraatrial reentrant tachycardia after the Senning or Mustard procedure for transposition of the great arteries. *Am J Cardiol*. 1996;77:985–991.

15. Perry JC, Boramanand NK, Ing FF. "Transseptal" technique through atrial baffles for 3Dimensional mapping and ablation of atrial tachycardia in patients with d-transposition of the great arteries. *J Interv Card Electrophysiol*. 2003;9:365–369.

16. Waldo AL, MacLean WAH, Karp RB, et al. Entrainment and interruption of atrial flutter with atrial pacing: studies in man following open-heart surgery. *Circulation*. 1977;56:737–745.

17. Bromberg BI, Schuessler RB, Gandhi SK, et al. A canine model of atrial flutter following the intra-atrial lateral tunnel Fontan operation. *J Electrocardiol*. 1998;30:85–93.

18. Khan HH, Stevenson WG. Activation times in and adjacent to reentry circuits during entrainment: implications for mapping ventricular tachycardia. *Am Heart J*. 1994;127:833–842.

19. El-Shalakany A, Hadjis T, Papageorgiou P, et al. Entrainment/mapping criteria for the prediction of termination of ventricular tachycardia by single radiofrequency lesion in patients with coronary artery disease. *Circulation*. 1999;99:2283–2289.

20. Kalman JM, Olgin JE, Saxon LA, et al. Activation and entrainment mapping defines the tricuspid annulus as the anterior barrier in typical atrial flutter. *Circulation*. 1996;94:398–406.

21. Walsh EP. Ablation of ectopic atrial tachycardia in young patients. In: Huang SKS, Wilber DJ, eds. *Radiofrequency Catheter Ablation of Cardiac Arrhythmias*. 2nd ed. Armonk, NY: Futura; 2000:115–138.

22. Fishberger SB, Wernovsky G, Gentles TL, et al. Factors that influence the development of atrial flutter after the Fontan operation. *J Thorac Cardiovasc Surg*. 1997;113:80–86.

23. Rhodes LA, Wernovsky G, Keane JF, et al. Arrhythmias and intracardiac conduction after the arterial switch operation. *J Thorac Cardiovasc Surg*. 1995;109:303–310.

24. Stamm C, Friehs I, Mayer JE, et al. Long-term results of the lateral tunnel Fontan operation. *J Thorac Cardiovasc Surg*. 2001;121:28–41.

25. Levine J, Walsh EP, Saul JP. Catheter ablation of accessory pathways in patients with congenital heart disease including heterotaxy syndrome. *Am J Cardiol*. 1993;72:689–694.

26. Epstein MR, Saul JP, Weindling SN, et al. Atrioventricular reciprocating tachycardia involving twin atrioventricular nodes in patients with complex congenital heart disease. *J Cardiovasc Electrophysiol*. 2001;12:671–679.

27. Mullen MP, VanPraagh R, Walsh EP. Development and anatomy of the cardiac conduction system. In: Walsh EP, Saul JP, Triedman JK, eds. *Cardiac Arrhythmias in Children and Young Adults with Congenital Heart Disease*. Philadelphia: Lippincott Williams & Wilkins; 2001:3–22.

28. Walsh EP. Catheter ablation of ectopic atrial tachycardia. In: Walsh EP, Saul JP, Triedman JK, eds. *Cardiac Arrhythmias in Children and Young Adults with Congenital Heart Disease*. Philadelphia: Lippincott Williams & Wilkins; 2001:355–370.

29. Jenkins JK, Walsh EP, Colan SD, et al. Multipolar endocardial mapping of the right atrium during cardiac catheterization: description of a new technique. *J Am Coll Cardiol*. 1993;22:1105–1110.

30. Triedman JK, Jenkins KJ, Colan SD, et al. Intra-atrial reentrant tachycardia after palliation of congenital heart disease: characterization of multiple macroreentrant circuits using fluoroscopically based three-dimensional endocardial mapping. *J Cardiovasc Electrophysiol*. 1997;8:259–270.

31. Triedman JK, Bergau DM, Saul JP, et al. Efficacy of radiofrequency ablation for control of intraatrial reentrant tachycardia in patients with congenital heart disease. *J Am Coll Cardiol*. 1997;30:1032–1038.

32. De Groot NM, Kuijper AF, Blom NA, et al. Three-dimensional distribution of bipolar atrial electrogram voltages in patients with congenital heart disease. *Pacing Clin Electrophysiol*. 2001;24:1334–1342.

33. Kalman JK, Van Hare GF, Olgin JE, et al. Ablation of "incisional" reentrant atrial tachycardia complication surgery for congenital heart disease. *Circulation*. 1996;93:502–512.

34. Delacretaz E, Ganz LI, Friedman PL, et al. Multiple atrial macroreentry circuits in adults with repaired congenital heart disease: entrainment mapping combined with three-dimensional electroanatomic mapping. *J Am Coll Cardiol*. 2001;37:1665–1676.

35. Triedman JK, Alexander ME, Berul CI, et al. Estimation of atrial response to entrainment pacing using electrograms recorded from remote sites. *J Cardiovasc Electrophysiol*. 2000;11:1215–1222.

36. Hadjis TA, Harada T, Stevenson WG, Friedman PL. Effect of recording site on postpacing interval measurement during catheter mapping and entrainment of postinfarction ventricular tachycardia. *J Cardiovasc Electrophysiol*. 1997;8:398–404.

37. Baker BM, Lindsay BD, Bromberg B, et al. Catheter ablation of intraatrial reentrant tachycardias resulting from previous atrial surgery: locating and transecting the critical isthmus. *J Am Coll Cardiol*. 1996;28:411–417.

38. Poty H, Saoudi N, Nair M, et al. Radio frequency catheter ablation of atrial flutter: further insights into the various types of isthmus block. Application to ablation during sinus rhythm. *Circulation*. 1996;94:3204–3213.

39. Triedman JK, Alexander ME, Berul CI, et al. Electroanatomic mapping of entrained and exit zones in patients with repaired congenital heart disease and intra-atrial reentrant tachycardia. *Circulation*. 2001;103:2060–2065.

40. Nakagawa H, Jackman WM. Use of a three-dimensional, nonfluoroscopic mapping system for catheter ablation of typical atrial flutter. *Pacing Clin Electrophysiol*. 1998;21:1279–1286.

41. Triedman JK, Alexander MA, Love BA, et al. Influence of patient factors and ablative technologies on outcomes of radiofrequency ablation of intra-atrial reentrant tachycardia in patients with congenital heart disease. *J Am Coll Cardiol*. 2002;39:1827–1835.

42. Mandapati R, Walsh EP, Triedman JK. Pericaval and periannular intra-atrial reentrant tachycardias in patients with congenital heart disease. *J Cardiovasc Electrophysiol*. 2003;14:119–125.

43. Love BA, Collins KK, Walsh EP, Triedman JK. Electroanatomic characterization of conduction barriers in sinus/atrial paced rhythm and association with intra-atrial reentrant tachycardia circuits following congenital heart disease surgery. *J Cardiovasc Electrophysiol*. 2001;12:17–25.

44. Schumacher B, Jung W, Lewalter T, et al. Verification of linear lesions using a noncontact multielectrode array catheter versus conventional contact mapping techniques. *J Cardiovasc Electrophysiol*. 1999;10:791–798.

45. Be'eri E, Maier SE, Landzberg MJ, et al. In vivo evaluation of Fontan pathway flow dynamics by multidimensional phase-velocity magnetic resonance imaging. *Circulation*. 1998;98:2873–2882.

46. Willems S, Weiss C, Hoffmann M, Meinertz T. Atrial flutter ablation using a technique for detection of conduction block within the posterior isthmus. *Pacing Clin Electrophysiol*. 1999;22:750–758.

47. Lustgarten DL, Keane D, Ruskin J. Cryothermal ablation: mechanism of tissue injury and current experience in the treatment of tachyarrhythmias. *Prog Cardiovasc Dis*. 1999;41:481–498.

48. Tai CT, Chen SA, Chiang CE, et al. Long-term outcome of radiofrequency catheter ablation for typical atrial flutter: Risk prediction of recurrent arrhythmias. *J Cardiovasc Electrophysiol*. 1998;9:115–121.

49. Collins KK, Rhee EK, Delucca JM, et al. Modification to the Fontan procedure for the prophylaxis of intra-atrial reentrant tachycardia: short-term results of a prospective randomized blinded trial. *J Thorac Cardiovasc Surg*. 2004;127:721–729.

Catheter Ablation
of Atrial Fibrillation

PART IV

15

Pulmonary Vein Isolation for Atrial Fibrillation

Isabelle Nault, Prashanthan Sanders, Ashok Shah, Nick Linton, Amir Jadidi, Sebastien Knecht, Matthew Wright, Andrei Forclaz, Mélèze Hocini, Pierre Jaïs, and Michel Haïssaguerre

Key Points

The pulmonary veins (PVs) play a central role in the genesis of atrial fibrillation through the mechanisms of automaticity, reentry, and possibly triggered activity.

The goal of PV ablation is to produce complete electrical isolation of all PVs. The preferred approach is circumferential antral ablation with PV electrical mapping to confirm entrance block. Exit block is also considered a necessary end point by some centers.

Minimal equipment needed includes apparatus for transseptal access, circular mapping catheters, and an irrigated radiofrequency ablation catheter. Specialized equipment in frequent use includes intracardiac echocardiography (ICE), electroanatomic mapping systems, three-dimensional anatomic renderings of the left atrium, and possibly "single-shot" ablation systems such as the cryoablation balloon.

Acute pulmonary isolation can be achieved in almost all patients. Suppression of atrial fibrillation can be achieved in up to 80% to 85% of patients with paroxysmal atrial fibrillation. Patients with persistent patterns of atrial fibrillation usually require substrate modification in addition to PV isolation.

Complications occur in about 6% of patients, including the risk for PV stenosis, thromboembolism, and rarely, atrioesophageal fistula.

Atrial fibrillation (AF) is the most prevalent cardiac arrhythmia. It affects 1% to 2% of the general population with an important increase in incidence with age.[1] AF has multiple adverse clinical implications. The loss of atrial systole and the irregular, fast heart rate contribute to symptoms such as palpitations and reduced exercise tolerance and also predispose to the development of intracardiac thrombus and systemic thromboembolism. AF can also cause tachycardia-mediated cardiomyopathy or worsening of preexisting heart failure.[2] Moreover, AF is known to increase the mortality risk 1.5- to 2-fold and the risk for stroke 5-fold.[1–4] Whereas anticoagulation treatment reduced the risk for stroke, large randomized trials failed to demonstrate any significant mortality benefit of a pharmacologically based rhythm control strategy even in patients with left ventricular dysfunction when compared with a rate control strategy.[5–8] This has led to a widespread belief that restoration of sinus rhythm (SR) does not improve prognosis. However, in-depth analysis of these trials demonstrated that the restoration of SR was associated with a 47% lower risk for death compared with continuing AF. On the other hand, the use of antiarrhythmic drug (AAD) therapy to restore SR was associated with a 49% increase in mortality rate, nullifying that substantial benefit achieved on establishment of SR from AF.[9] Therefore, pursuing SR by nonpharmacologic means is justified. Besides having a good safety profile, catheter ablation therapy for AF has proved effective in establishing and maintaining SR.

Mechanisms of Atrial Fibrillation: Interplay of Trigger and Substrate

Induction of AF requires an initiating trigger, and perpetuation occurs because triggering activity is sustained or because of the presence of a susceptible atrial substrate. Premature atrial ectopy has been shown to be the most frequent trigger for AF. Observations in patients with dual-chamber pacemakers revealed that 48% of AF episodes were triggered by premature atrial beats, 33% were preceded by bradycardia, and 17% were sudden in onset.[10] Also, continuous cardiac monitoring in postoperative patients demonstrated that supraventricular premature beats induced AF in 72% to 100% of cases.[11]

Arrhythmogenicity of Pulmonary Veins

Endocardial mapping revealed that the origin of ectopic activity initiating AF is located inside the pulmonary veins (PV) in 89% to 94% of cases and that AF is most often triggered by repetitive focal PV discharges[12–14] (Fig. 15-1). Multiple sites inside one PV or multiple PVs can harbor the arrhythmogenic ectopic activity in an individual.[15,16]

Catheter ablation targeting the fascicles, which connect the PVs to the left atrium, leads to electrical isolation of the PVs. Interestingly, after electrical isolation, up to 58% of PVs display slow, dissociated activity, and some sustain ongoing tachycardia dissociated from the left atrium in SR, emphasizing the arrhythmogenic potential of these structures[17,18] (Fig. 15-2). Indeed, besides being triggers for AF, PVs can also be responsible for the perpetuation of AF.

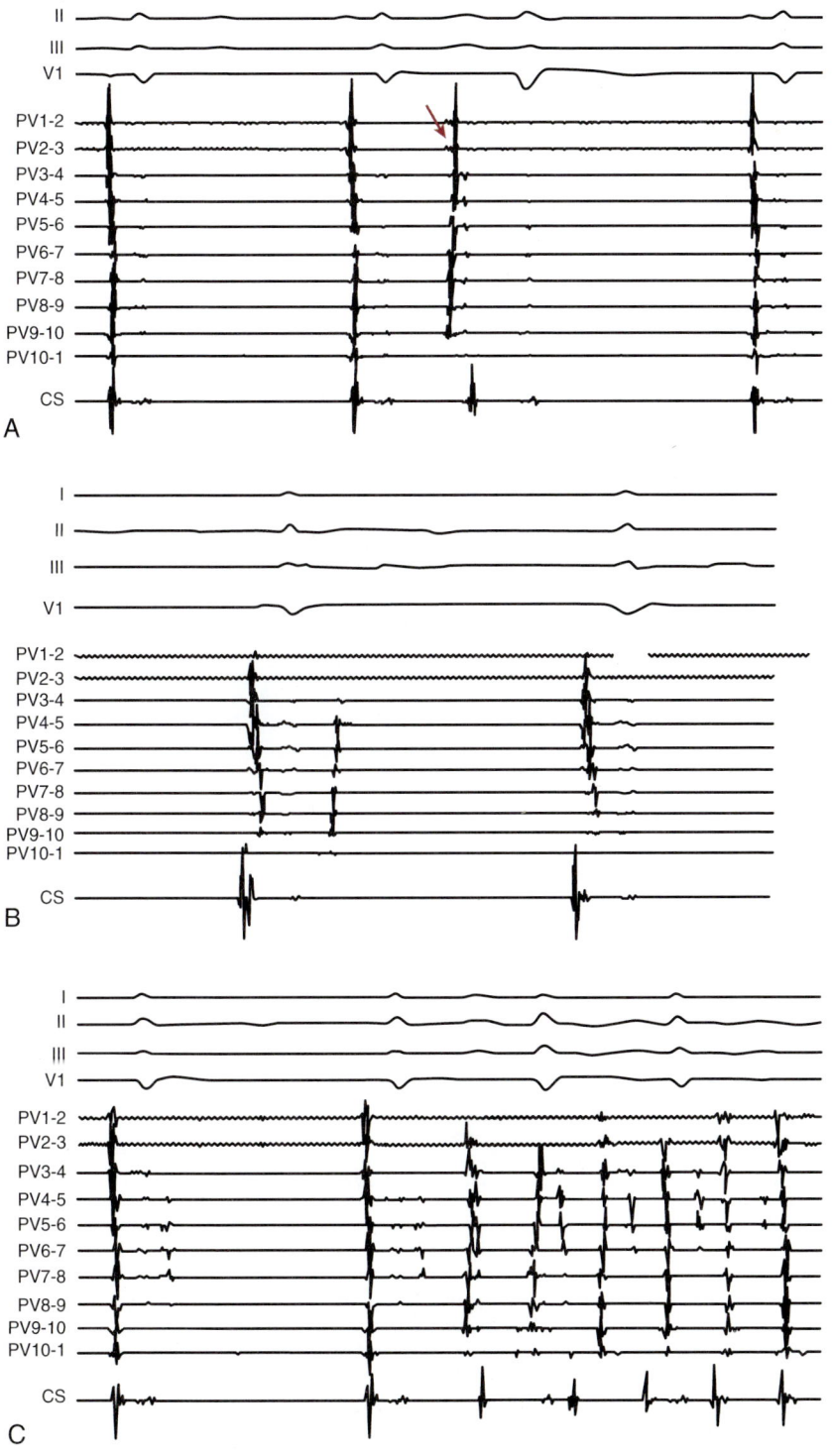

FIGURE 15-1. A, Pulmonary vein (PV) ectopic beat. Surface electrocardiogram (ECG) leads I, II, III and V$_1$, recording from left superior PV and from coronary sinus. The *red arrow* shows an ectopic beat arising from the pulmonary vein and conducted to the left atrium. **B,** Concealed PV ectopy. Surface ECG leads I, II, III and V$_1$, recording from left inferior pulmonary vein (PV) and coronary sinus (CS), showing a concealed atrial premature beat arising from the PV but not conducted to the left atrium. **C,** PV ectopy initiating atrial fibrillation (AF). Surface leads I, II, III, and V$_1$, recording from left superior pulmonary vein (PV) and coronary sinus (CS). A premature beat arising from the left superior pulmonary vein, earliest at PV 9-10, is conducted to the left atrium and initiates AF.

Continued

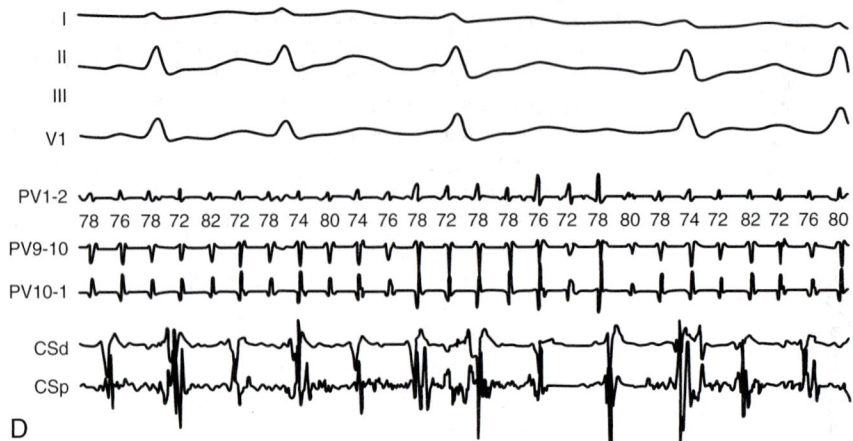

D

FIGURE 15-1, cont'd. D, Extremely fast pulmonary vein activity. In this figure, the left inferior pulmonary vein is firing at a mean cycle length of 76 msec (range, 69-92 msec), whereas the left atrial fibrillating cycle length recorded from the coronary sinus catheter is much slower at 163 msec. Surface ECG leads I, II and III; PV, left inferior pulmonary vein recording; CS, coronary sinus recording distal (d) and proximal (p). *(From Nault I, Wright M, Hocini M, et al. Extreme firing in a pulmonary vein during atrial fibrillation.* J Cardiovasc Electrophysiol. *2009;20:696. With permission.)*

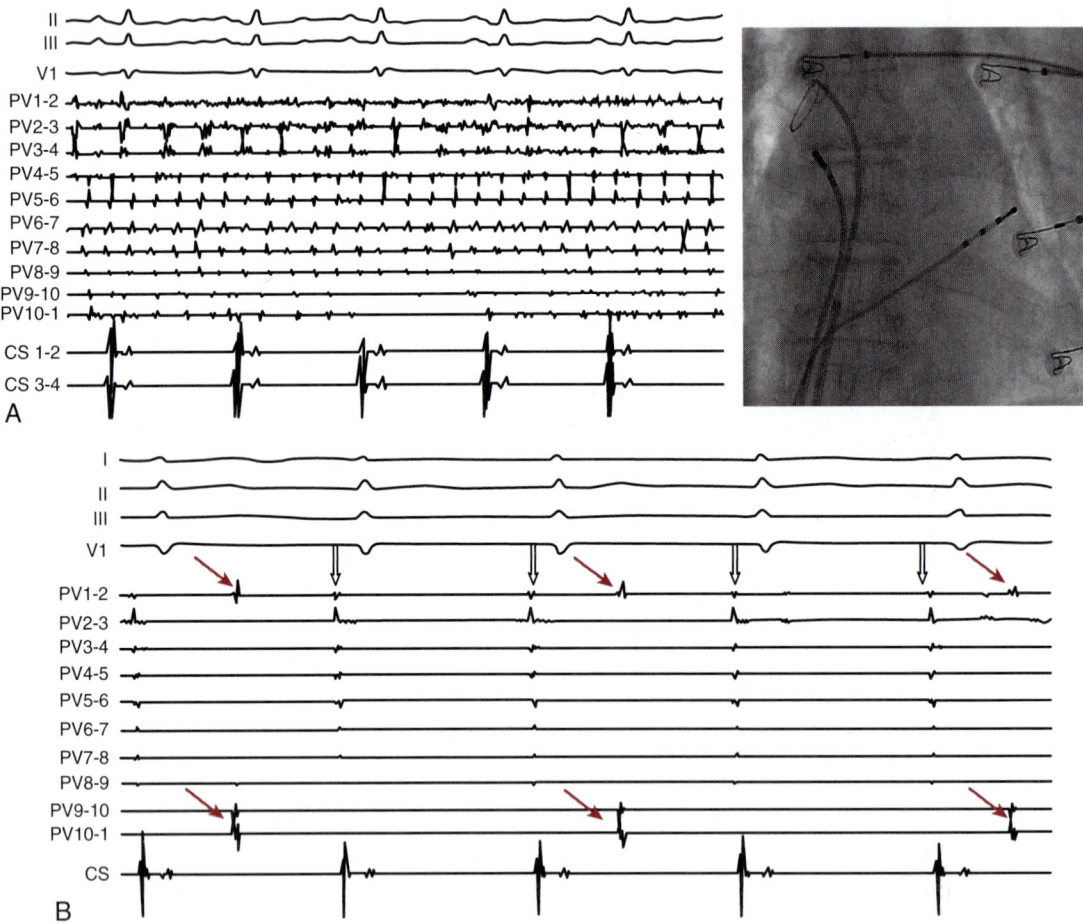

FIGURE 15-2. A, Ongoing fibrillatory activity inside the right superior pulmonary vein (PV) after PV isolation with conversion to sinus rhythm. This demonstrates the arrhythmogenicity of the pulmonary veins and suggests that the right superior pulmonary vein was a significant atrial fibrillation trigger or driver for this patient. The fluoroscopic image shows the position of the circular mapping catheter inside the right upper pulmonary vein, quadripolar inside the coronary sinus and radiofrequency catheter at the lower part of the ostium of the right superior pulmonary vein, where isolation was achieved. **B,** Recording from the right inferior pulmonary vein showing a slow PV rhythm dissociated from left atrial activity *(red arrows).* The *hollow arrows* indicate far field potentials from the adjacent posterior left atrium. Surface electrocardiogram leads I, II, III, V1; PV, right inferior pulmonary vein recording; CS, coronary sinus.

In a small series of patients who had irregular focal discharges initiating and perpetuating AF, foci at the ostium of PVs were found to be the drivers of sustained AF in 66%. Focal radiofrequency (RF) delivery targeting these foci eliminated AF in all these patients.[19] In addition, a spatial gradient in cycle length, with the PVs activating at a higher frequency than the nearest atrial tissue, has been found in some patients, and this reinforces the role of PVs as AF perpetuators[20–23] (see Fig. 15-1D).

The involvement of the PVs in the maintenance of AF was further emphasized by the observation that PV isolation in paroxysmal AF led to a progressive increase in the AF cycle length, culminating in the termination of AF in 75% of patients. PV isolation rendered AF noninducible in 57% of patients and prevented relapse in 74% of patients.[24] These findings led to the *venous wave hypothesis*, postulating a role for PVs in maintenance of AF in most patients with paroxysmal AF.[25] Later, spectral analysis and dominant frequency mapping revealed that the dominant frequency and the highest dominant frequency were spatially distributed in the vicinity of the PVs in most of the patients with paroxysmal AF.[26] Put together, these observations emphatically substantiate the role of PVs in the initiation and maintenance of nonpermanent forms of AF.

Pulmonary Vein Anatomy Relevant to Ablation

Sleeves of myocardium extending from the left atrium (LA) into the PVs constitute the arrhythmogenic substrate for these structures (Figs. 15-3 and 15-4). Myocardial sleeves of variable lengths, extending 2 to 25 mm distally into the vein from the ostium, are more developed in the upper than the lower PVs[27,28] and are thickest at the LA-PV junction, tapering distally in a nonuniform manner. The sleeves tend to be thicker on the inferior aspect of the superior veins and the superior aspect of the inferior veins. Gaps of variable size filled with fibrotic tissue are frequently found at the

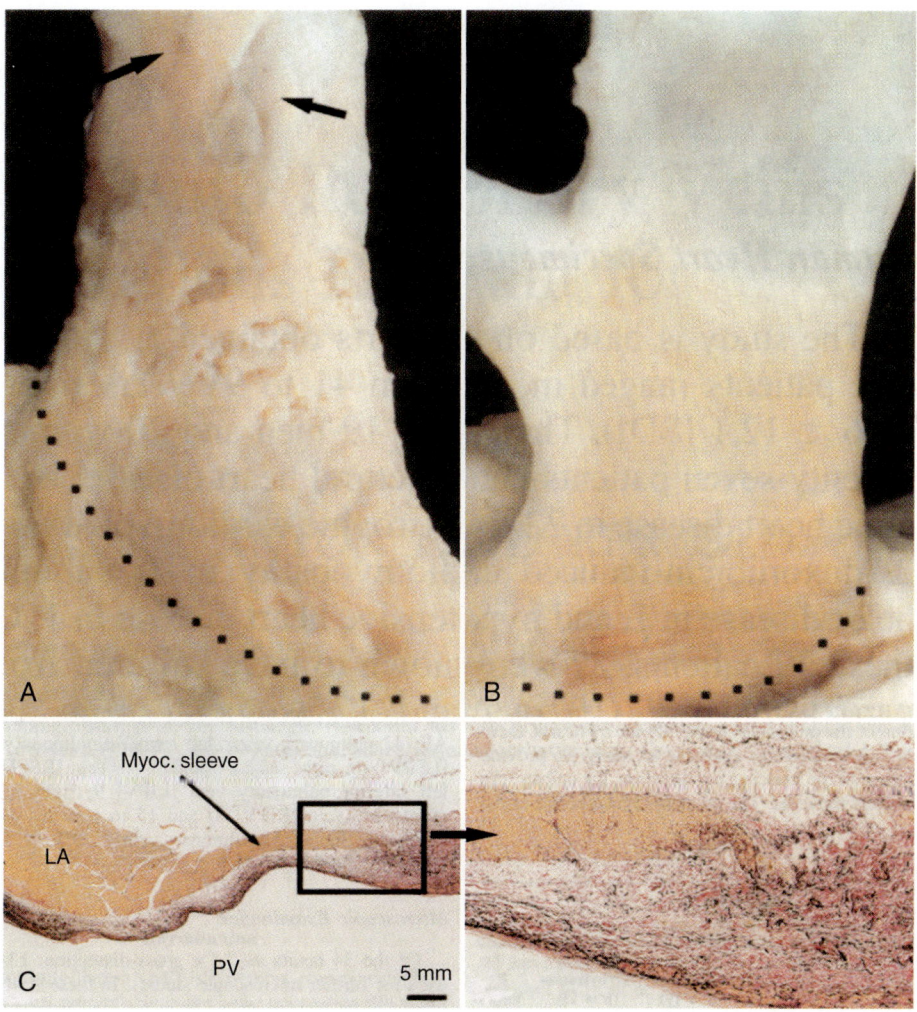

FIGURE 15-3. Gross appearance of myocardial sleeves around the pulmonary veins (PVs). *Dotted lines* indicate the presumed junction between the PV and the left atrium (LA); however, the conical nature of the proximal vein in **A** makes this distinction difficult. In **A,** there is a nonuniform arrangement of the fibers, with terminal finger-like extensions over the vein *(arrows).* In **B,** the myocardial sleeve is smooth and uniform, with a distinct peripheral termination over the vein. **C,** Histologic section of the muscular extension onto the PV. The section highlighted by the *box* is shown at increased magnification on the *right.* The tip of the extension contains atrophic myocardial cells embedded in fibrous tissue. *(From Saito T, Waki K, Becker AE. Left atrial myocardial extensions onto pulmonary veins in humans: anatomic observations relevant for atrial arrhythmias. J Cardiovasc Electrophysiol. 2000;11:888–894. With permission.)*

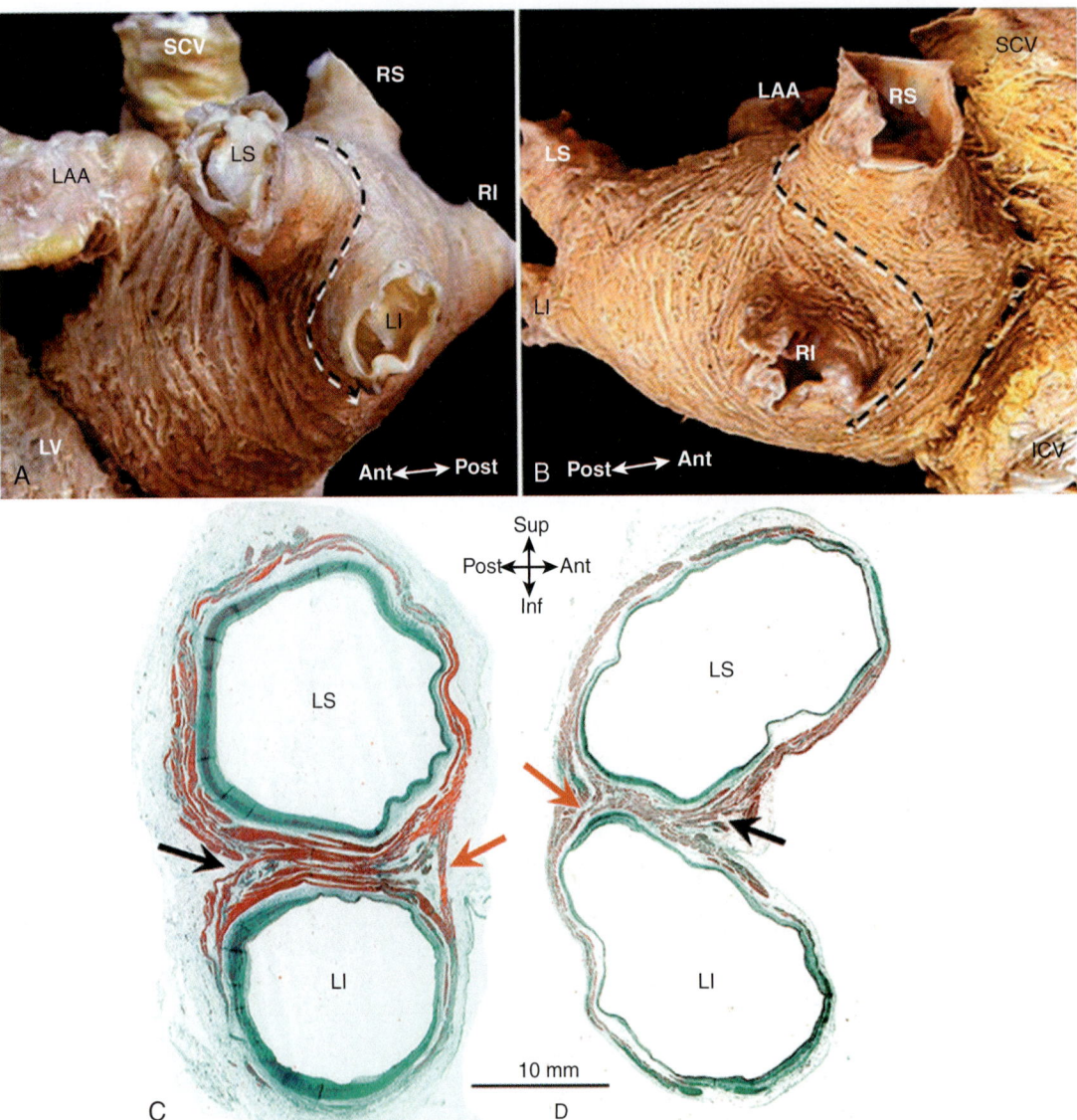

FIGURE 15-4. *Top panels*, Dissections showing the subepicardial myocardial strands viewed from the left (**A**) and right (**B**) lateral aspects. Note that the myocardial strands from the roof (*black–white broken line*) can be traced from the posterior walls of the left or right superior venoatrial junctions to the interpulmonary isthmus and into the anterior margin of the inferior left or right venoatrial junctions. **C** and **D,** Histologic sections of the interpulmonary vein isthmus in transverse plane stained with Masson trichrome technique. They show crossing myocardial strands (*black arrows*) and additional small bridges (*red arrows*) that extended between the epicardial surface of the anterior walls of the left veins in **A** and the posterior walls in **B**. ICV, inferior caval vein; LAA, left atrial appendage; LI, left inferior pulmonary vein; LS, left superior pulmonary vein; RI, right inferior pulmonary vein; RS, right superior pulmonary vein; SCV, superior vena cava. *(From Cabrera JA, Ho SY, Climent V, et al. Morphologic evidence of muscular connections between contiguous pulmonary venous orifices: relevance of the interpulmonary isthmus for catheter ablation in atrial fibrillation.* Heart Rhythm. *2009;6:1192–1198. With permission.)*

LA-PV junction and inside the veins. The alignment of muscle fibers extending into the vein is variable. The fibers are most commonly arranged in a circumferential manner, but some are oriented in either longitudinal or oblique fashion (Fig. 15-4).[29] Therefore, the heterogeneous arrangement of the muscle fibers provides a substrate for reentry and imparts electrical heterogeneity and arrhythmogenicity to PVs. Studies have also suggested that dilation of PVs could translate into greater arrhythmogenicity.[30] Indeed, patients with AF had larger PVs with greater structural heterogeneity (fibrosis, gaps in myocardial tissue, myocyte hypertrophy) than controls.[31–33]

The veins are conical structures without absolute boundaries among the ostium, antrum, and left atrium. Embryologically, the PVs arise from the posterior left atrium.

Therefore, a continuum exists in the anatomy between these structures (Fig. 15-5; see also Fig. 15-3). The boundaries vary somewhat with the imaging modality used. For purposes of PV isolation, however, the ostium may be considered the beginning of the tubular portion of the PV. This is often identified on fluoroscopy or ICE as the point of abrupt departure of the PV from the contour of the left atrial body. Intracardiac echocardiography usually defines the PV ostium at a location more proximal in the vein than does fluoroscopy. The antrum is the outlet of the vein proximal to the ostium and the area of fusion with the left atrial body. In the antrum, both PV potentials and near-field atrial electrograms are recorded. The proximal boundary of the antrum with the left atrium is difficult to define by imaging but may be considered the point at

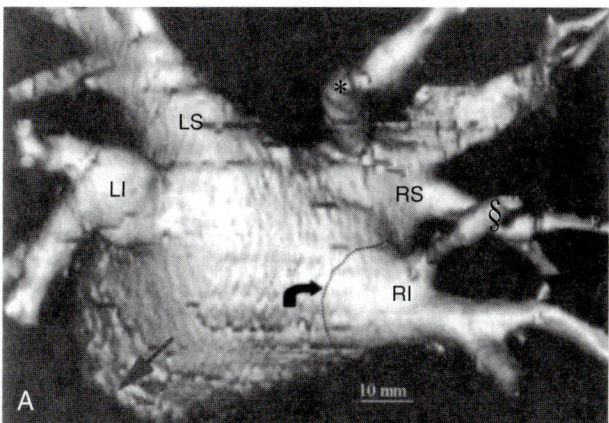

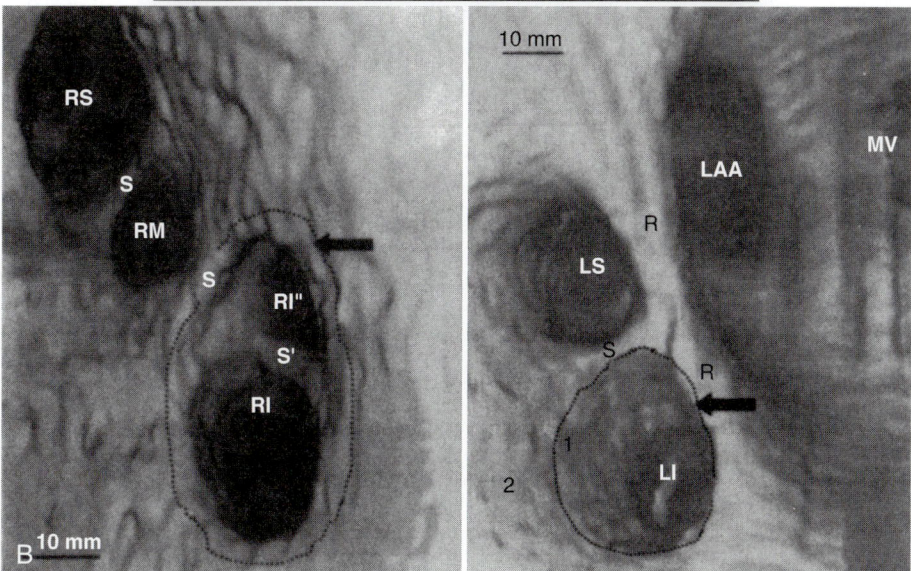

FIGURE 15-5. Computed tomography reconstruction of the atrial and pulmonary vein anatomy. **A,** Three-dimensional reconstruction of the left atrium (LA) and pulmonary veins (PVs) viewed from a posterior perspective. Note the conical nature of the junctions of the veins with the body of the atrium, which makes definition of a true ostium difficult. **B,** Intra-atrial reconstructed views of the posterior LA. Note the "saddles" (S) between adjacent PVs. The complex, funnel-shaped approaches to the veins are apparent. The position of the inferior venous ostia is denoted by the *dotted lines*. In this case, it would be preferable to ablate the right PVs together because they are contiguous. Also demonstrated on the *right panel* is the narrow ridge that separates the left PVs from the left atrial appendage (LAA). Ablation along this ridge in the beating heart frequently is not possible and necessitates infringing on the anterior aspect of the PV to achieve stability for ablation. The *dotted line* and arrows indicate the inferior PVs, but note that particularly on the *right*, the superior and inferior PVs are contiguous and require isolation as a pair. Similarly, the antrum of these PVs is more proximal than indicated by the *dotted lines*. Also note the variation in pulmonary venous anatomy. The *asterisk* indicates the superior early branching of the right superior pulmonary vein. LI, left inferior PV; LS, left superior PV; MV, mitral valve; R, ridge between LAA and PVs; RI and RI", ostia of a complex right inferior PV; RM, right middle PV; RS, right superior PV. *(From Schwartzman D, Lacomis J, Wigginton WG. Characterization of left atrium and distal pulmonary vein morphology using multidimensional computed tomography.* J Am Coll Cardiol. *2003;41:1349–1357. With permission.)*

which PV potentials are lost and only atrial electrograms are recorded. The venous ostia are not circular but are elongated along their cranial-caudal axes.

Electrophysiologic Properties of Pulmonary Veins and Mechanism of Arrhythmogenesis

Experimental evidence supports both reentry and automaticity as the mechanisms of arrhythmogenesis in PVs. In experimental studies in dogs, the complex arrangement of muscle fibers at the PV ostia was also associated with complex conduction patterns, delayed conduction, and

block. These patterns were characteristically seen in areas of abrupt change in the direction of the myocardial fibers or at gaps.[34,35] Significant heterogeneity in the action potential duration was noted inside the PVs compared with the LA.[34-37] Optical mapping in dogs confirmed these findings by demonstrating delay in conduction, heterogeneous depolarization, conduction block, and initiation of reentry in 60% of the preparations. Spontaneous focal activity was also demonstrated in 66% of preparations following isoproterenol infusion and rapid atrial pacing.[36] Other experimental studies have also reported spontaneous or provoked pulmonary venous electrical activity triggered by either early or delayed afterdepolarizations.[38,39] Using a computer model, Cherry and colleagues showed that PV heterogeneity and anisotropy predisposes to reentry and demonstrated that increasing the circumference and the length of the PVs increased the incidence and duration of reentry.[40]

In clinical studies, electrophysiologic properties of PVs have been shown to differ in patients with AF compared with controls without any history of AF. In patients with AF, the PV effective refractory period (ERP) was shorter, and there was a greater difference in PV ERP relative to LA ERP. Decremental PV-LA conduction was more frequent, and a greater decrement was noted than in controls, and AF was preferentially initiated by extrastimuli delivered inside PVs compared with other sites in the LA.[41] In another study, heterogeneity was observed between the ERPs of the distal PV and the PV-LA junction along with anisotropic conduction within these areas. Such diversity in the electrophysiologic properties of PVs favors reentry within the PVs as an arrhythmogenic mechanism. This hypothesis was confirmed clinically using a multielectrode basket catheter to record reentry at the LA-PV junction and within the PV during AF.[42] Indirect evidence of reentry was also provided in a patient in whom a PV tachycardia was inducible by pacing, was amenable to entrainment, and could be terminated by overdrive pacing. On mapping the circumference of the vein during tachycardia, nearly complete cycle length of the tachycardia could be recorded inside the PV.[43] Based on this and similar clinical reports, the role of reentrant circuits limited to the PV or its junction with the LA, or both, has been emphasized. Despite these findings, in humans, the first ectopic discharge in a salvo or initiating AF has never been shown to be reentrant and therefore can be triggered activity or automaticity. Clinical evidence supports PV automaticity as a mechanism of AF arrhythmogenesis. In one report, high-density mapping within the left superior PV revealed the simultaneous presence of two different interacting tachycardias, which were interrupted by adenosine infusion, suggestive of abnormal automaticity as the underlying mechanism.[44] In a study conducted in 35 patients using a 64-pole basket catheter to map spontaneous PV ectopic beats, several discrete foci of abnormal activity were observed, and there was no evidence of reentry.[45] Therefore, in PVs, both the automatic and the reentrant mechanisms may be implicated in the perpetuation of the fibrillatory process in an interactive manner.

Catheter Ablation of Atrial Fibrillation

Current guidelines recommend catheter ablation as a second-line therapy for symptomatic AF, after failure of or intolerance to AADs.[46] Current expert consensus acknowledges the importance of PV targets in the strategy of AF ablation and recommends that when PVs are targeted, *complete electrical isolation should be achieved*.[47] Electrical isolation requires at least entrance block into the vein, with demonstrated exit block also being an important criterion for some centers. PV isolation alone is most likely to benefit patients with a normal heart and short episodes of paroxysmal AF.[17] Patients with longer durations of AF or persistent AF are more likely to require left atrial substrate modification in addition to PV isolation.[48] Atrial ectopy arising from the PV can be suspected from the surface electrocardiogram. Ectopic P waves from any of the PVs share the following general characteristics: positive morphology across all precordial leads (100%), negative or isoelectric in aVL (86%), and negative in aVR (96%). Additional features that localize ectopy to specific PVs are given in Table 15-1.

Initially, PV ablation targeted observed triggers of AF inside the PVs.[12,13,49] However, it was soon observed that RF injury inside the veins carried the risk for PV stenosis[13,50,51] and that the clinical outcome was better when more PVs were isolated.[52,53] Based on such observations, the ablation strategy changed toward achieving systematic isolation of all four PVs by creating more proximal lesions in order to avoid lesions inside the PVs.

Isolation of Pulmonary Veins

Isolation of the PV may be performed segmentally at the level of the venous ostium or circumferentially at the venous antrum or in the atrial tissue surrounding the PV. Currently, most leading centers perform circumferential antral ablation. As discussed previously, the exact anatomic boundaries of the PV antrum are not absolutely defined but may be considered to be the area proximal to the venous ostium where PV potentials can still be recorded. It is this antral area, usually 5 to 10 mm around the perimeter of the PV os, that

TABLE 15-1

P-WAVE MORPHOLOGIES FROM PULMONARY VEINS

P-Wave Morphology	Pulmonary Vein (PV) Origin	Sensitivity (%)	Specificity (%)
+ Leads V$_1$-V$_6$ - or ± Lead aVL - Lead aVR	All PVs All PVs All PVs		
Notching in ≥2 leads (usually inferior leads)	Left-sided PV	100	93
Width 0.12 ± 0.02 mV vs. 0.07 ± 0.02 mV	Wider P wave left-sided veins vs. right-sided veins		
+ Lead I	Right-sided veins	92	87
Markedly + Inferior leads, amplitude >0.1 mV lead II	Superior veins	95	66

+, Positive; −, negative; ±, isoelectric.
From Kistler PM, Sanders P, Fynn SP, et al. Electrophysiologic and electrocardiographic characteristics of focal atrial tachycardia originating from the pulmonary veins: acute and long-term outcomes of radiofrequency ablation. *Circulation.* 2003;108:1968–1975.

is the target for antral PV isolation. Circumferential mapping allows determination of the distribution of PV activity and the pattern of its activation by recording PV potentials arising from the extensions of atrial myocardium into the PVs.[54] On bipolar recordings, PV potentials are characterized as sharp and of high frequency and short duration (<50 milliseconds). In SR, these potentials follow the left atrial potentials; however, with ectopy or pacing from the PV, the order of the potentials is reversed, with the PV potential preceding the atrial electrogram (Fig. 15-6). With PV ectopic activity, the sharp PV potential precedes the surface P-wave onset by 40 to 160 milliseconds (Table 15-2). In comparison, left atrial far-field signals appear blunted, with a slow rise and low frequency within the PV, but they may appear sharper and higher in amplitude proximally in the antrum. Far-field left atrial potentials are advanced in timing with pacing near the source of the potentials (Fig. 15-7).

Access to the left atrium is gained by transseptal puncture. Meticulous attention to anticoagulation throughout the procedure is required from the time of transseptal access. The target activated clotting time is typically 300 to 350 seconds. The procedure can safely be performed on therapeutic anticoagulation with warfarin, but full heparinization is also given intraoperatively. One or two mapping catheters can be placed in addition to the ablation catheter through transseptal access (Fig. 15-8). When performing the transseptal access, crossing the foramen ovale too high or low

or too anterior or posterior can impair catheter manipulation about the PV. Circular mapping catheters are available with a variety of fixed or adjustable diameters and 10 or 20 electrodes. The mapping catheter diameter should be chosen based on venous anatomy defined by angiography, ICE, or preprocedural computed tomography (CT) or magnetic resonance imaging (MRI). For 10-pole catheters, the bipoles are arranged as electrodes 1-2, 2-3, 3-4, and so forth. The wider electrode spacing from 10-pole catheters may produce

TABLE 15-2
ELECTROPHYSIOLOGIC FEATURES OF PULMONARY VEIN POTENTIALS
Rapid, high-frequency initial deflection*
Short duration (<50 msec)*
Follows coronary pacing stimulus by >50 to 70 msec (generally)
Follows far-field atrial electrogram during atrial or coronary sinus pacing*
Precedes far-field atrial electrogram during pulmonary vein pacing or ectopy from vein*
Potentials advanced with pacing within pulmonary vein but not advanced by atrial pacing

*From Tada H, Oral H, Greenstein R, et al. Differentiation of atrial and pulmonary vein potentials recorded circumferentially within pulmonary veins. *J Cardiovasc Electrophysiol.* 2002;13:118–123.

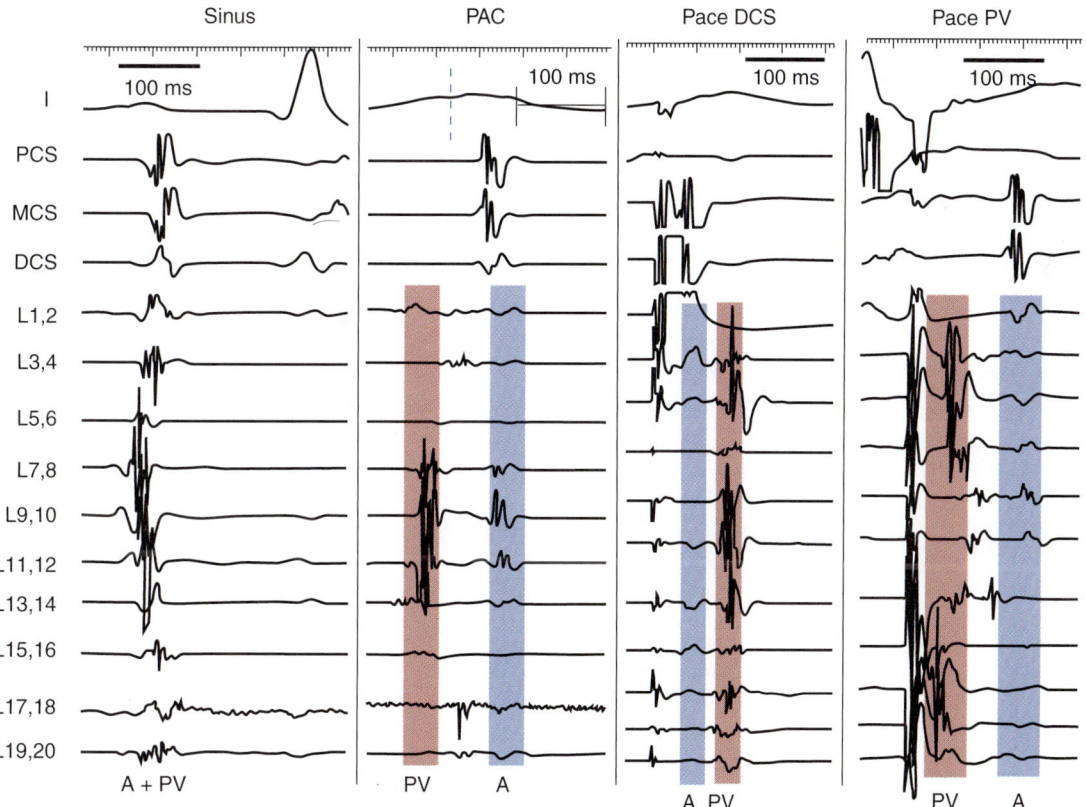

FIGURE 15-6. Pulmonary vein (PV) potentials recorded from the left superior PV in a patient undergoing ablation. The circular mapping lasso (L1,2 through L19,20) catheter is at the os of the PV. In sinus rhythm, the atrial (A) and PV potentials cannot be readily distinguished. With a premature atrial contraction (PAC) originating from the vein, the PV (*shaded red*) and atrial (*shaded blue*) are distinct, with the PV potentials occurring first. The *vertical dashed line* indicates the start of the P wave on the surface electrocardiogram. With pacing from the distal coronary sinus (DCS), the atrial and PV electrogram components are again separated, but the atrial components occur first. With pacing from the ablation catheter deep in the PV, the PV components are advanced, and the atrial components follow.

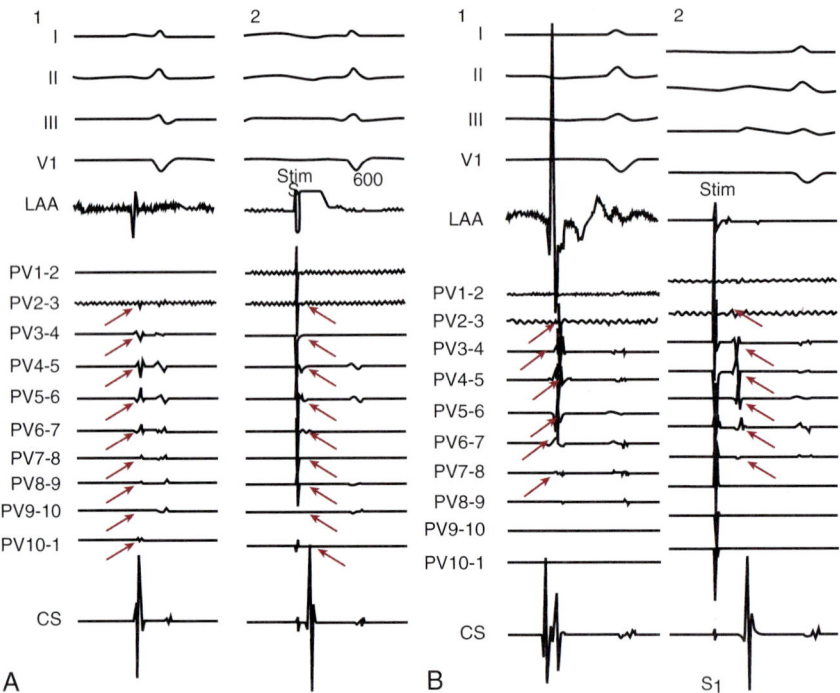

FIGURE 15-7. A, Surface electrocardiogram leads I, II, III and V₁, recording from left inferior pulmonary vein (PV), left atrial appendage (LAA), and coronary sinus (CS). *Panel 1,* Recording on the circular mapping catheter inside left inferior pulmonary vein depicts potentials (*arrows*) concurrent with the left atrial appendage (LAA) recording. *Panel 2,* Pacing (Stim) from the LAA advances the potentials in the PV, with the LAA potentials confirming that the potentials observed in **A** are far-field recordings from LAA and not PV potentials. **B,** The potentials (*arrows*) with the PV in *panel 1* are recorded simultaneously with the LAA in sinus rhythm. *Panel 2,* In this example, pacing from the LAA causes the potentials in the PV to be delayed, proving that they are true PV potentials and not far-field recordings from the appendage.

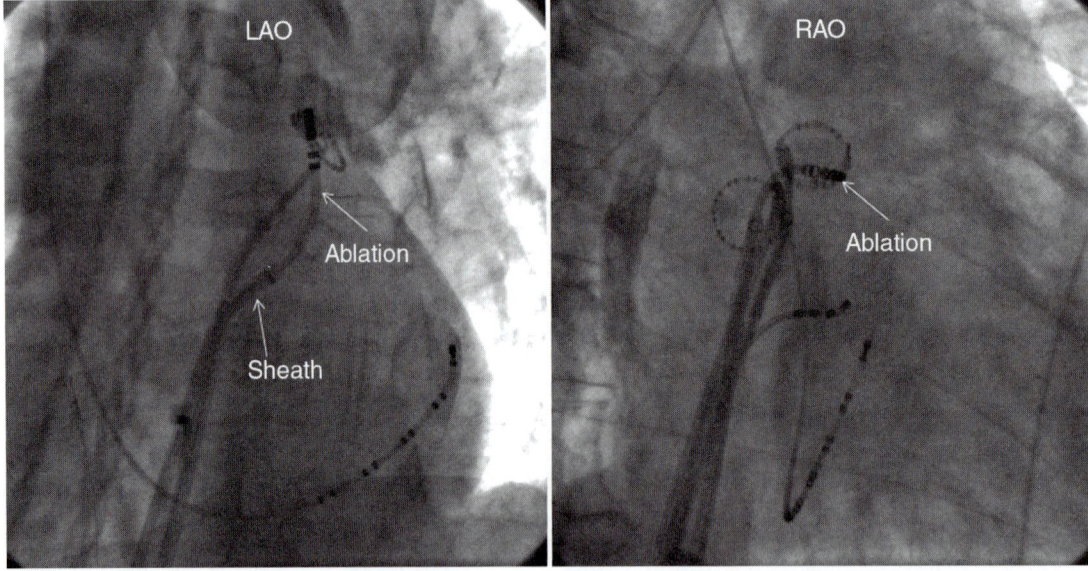

FIGURE 15-8. Transseptal access for single mapping catheter and ablation catheter (*left panel*) and two mapping catheters and ablation catheter (*right panel*). In the *right panel*, the mapping catheters are in the left superior and left inferior veins. In both panels, note the compound curves produced by the catheter and sheaths to reach the superior (*left panel*) and anterior (*right panel*) aspects of the veins. Such curvatures can provide firm, stable contact with the atrial wall. LAO, left anterior oblique; RAO, right anterior oblique.

more far-field signals. For 20-pole catheters, electrodes are organized as 1-2, 2-3, 3-4, and so forth. The smaller bipole spacing of these catheters produces better near-field signal discrimination. The circular mapping catheter should be positioned at the PV antrum or ostium or no more than 5 mm deep into the vein ostium as stability permits (Fig. 15-9). Ablation is directed at the PV antrum regardless of the mapping catheter position. The catheter should be perpendicular to the long axis of the vein to ensure circumferential venous

recordings. It is easier to perform PV mapping in SR or atrial pacing. During AF, the PV potentials are fragmented and diminished, making recognition more difficult. Ablation may be initiated in AF in patients with incessant arrhythmias, but end points should be finally confirmed during SR and atrial pacing.

The veins can be isolated one by one, or ipsilateral veins can be isolated en bloc, two by two, by creating proximal posterior and anterior lines joined distally (Fig. 15-10).[17,54,55]

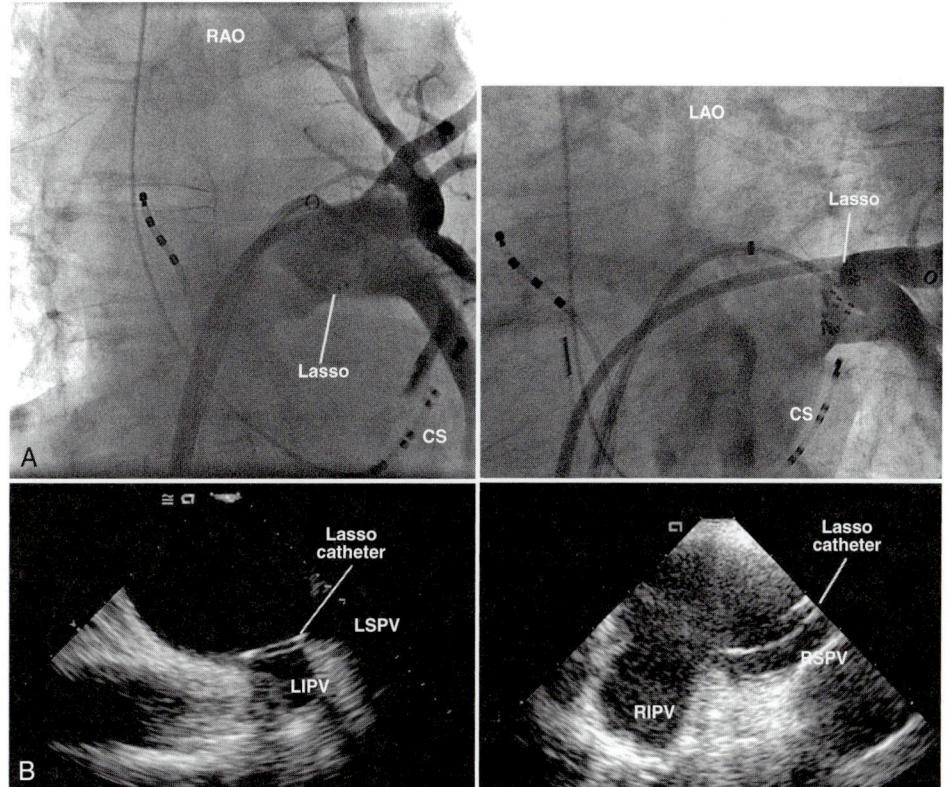

FIGURE 15-9. Methods of maintaining circular mapping catheter at pulmonary vein (PV) ostia. **A,** Venography. Injection of the left inferior pulmonary vein shows the circular mapping catheter at the os of the vein in the right anterior oblique (RAO) and left anterior oblique (LAO) views. **B,** Intracardiac echocardiography. The circular mapping catheter is seen at the os of the left inferior pulmonary vein (LIPV) in the *left panel* and at the os of the right superior pulmonary vein (RSPV) in the *right panel*. CS, coronary sinus.

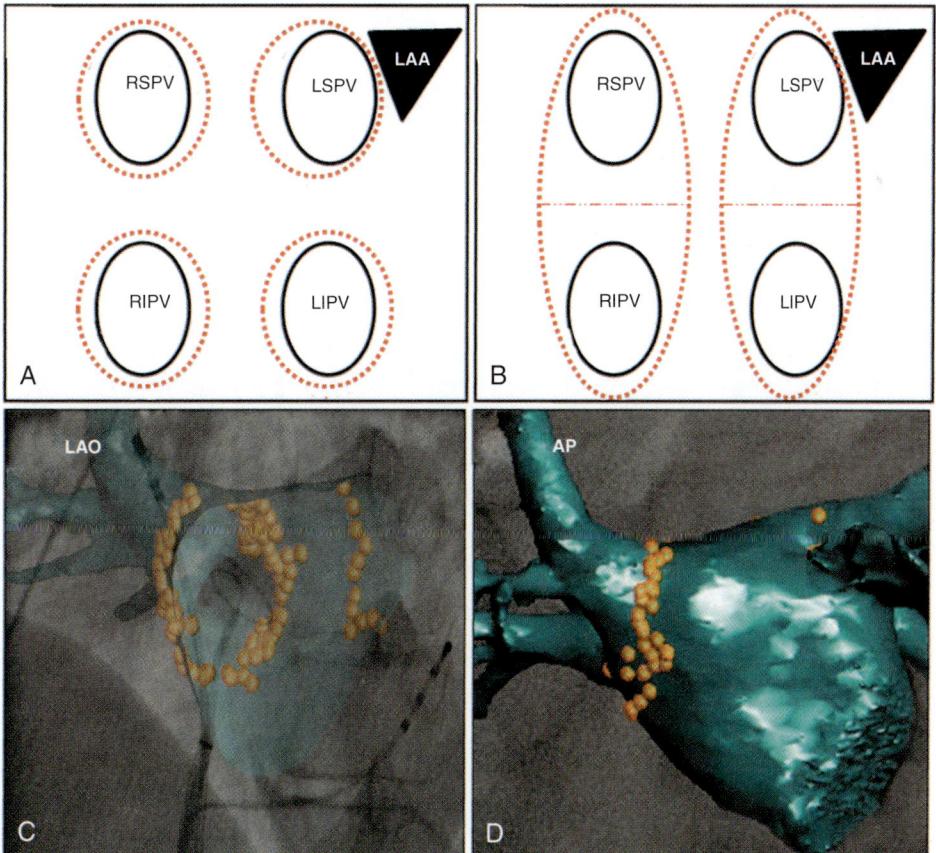

FIGURE 15-10. Schematic illustration of the lesion sets for segmental (**A**) and 2 × 2 (**B**) PV isolation. The *dashed line* in **B** represents optional ablation of the carina between the superior and inferior PVs. Note that for the 2 × 2 lesion set, the ablation line encroaches on the anterior aspect of the left veins due to the ridge between the PV and the left atrial appendage (LAA). **C** and **D,** Left atrial computed tomography overlay on fluoroscopy with PV isolation 2 × 2. In **C**, the cutting plane allows visualization of the endocardium and the lesions (*dots*) on the posterior wall. AP, anteroposterior; LAO, left anterior oblique; LIPV, left inferior pulmonary artery; LSPV, left superior pulmonary artery; RIPV, right inferior pulmonary artery; RSPV, right superior pulmonary artery.

However, when using the latter technique, ablation at the carina between the upper and the lower veins is often necessary to achieve complete isolation. Moreover, when ablation is performed along the anterior portion of the left PVs, infringement of the PV is often necessary to achieve catheter stability because the ridge between the vein and the left atrial appendage is relatively narrow and prohibits catheter stability in the beating heart. Interestingly, fascicles are commonly shared by the upper and the lower veins, and using circumferential mapping catheters in both upper and lower ipsilateral veins, it has been observed that electrical isolation of both veins may occur simultaneously (Fig. 15-4).[17]

By isolating a greater area around the veins, certain arrhythmogenic foci and triggers, which are often located at the venous ostia, can be isolated. With ostial segmental PV isolation, ablation is generally required around only 40% to 80% of the PV circumference. However, proximal ablation often requires more extensive lesion sets because a greater circumference is involved, and the muscular tissue that may be sparse inside the veins becomes more continuous proximally. Proximal lesions also carry the risk for creating corridors capable of supporting reentry on the posterior wall of the atrium.[56] Despite these limitations, it is widely accepted that ablation should be performed as proximal as possible to isolate the PVs and their ostia together.

Navigation

Fluoroscopy, angiography, ICE, and three-dimensional (3D) mapping systems are available and can be used alone or in combination to facilitate catheter navigation and guide ablation.[57–62] In most patients, four PVs can be found; however, anatomic variants such as a middle PV and a common ostium for ipsilateral PVs are frequent (see Fig. 15-5).[27]

Fluoroscopy

The course of the upper veins is superior-posterolateral, and a catheter introduced deep inside an upper vein is seen outside the heart silhouette in posteroanterior view. The lower veins have a more posterior course, more parallel to the x-ray beam in the posteroanterior view. The left anterior oblique (LAO) projection is best for assessing proximal-distal catheter position inside the left-sided veins, and the right anterior oblique (RAO) projection is best for inside the right-sided veins, because these projections are more orthogonal to the axis of the veins (Fig. 15-11). In all fluoroscopic views, the PV ostia are superimposed over the left atrial silhouette (Fig. 15-12). The left veins are accessed by advancing the mapping or ablation catheter laterally in the

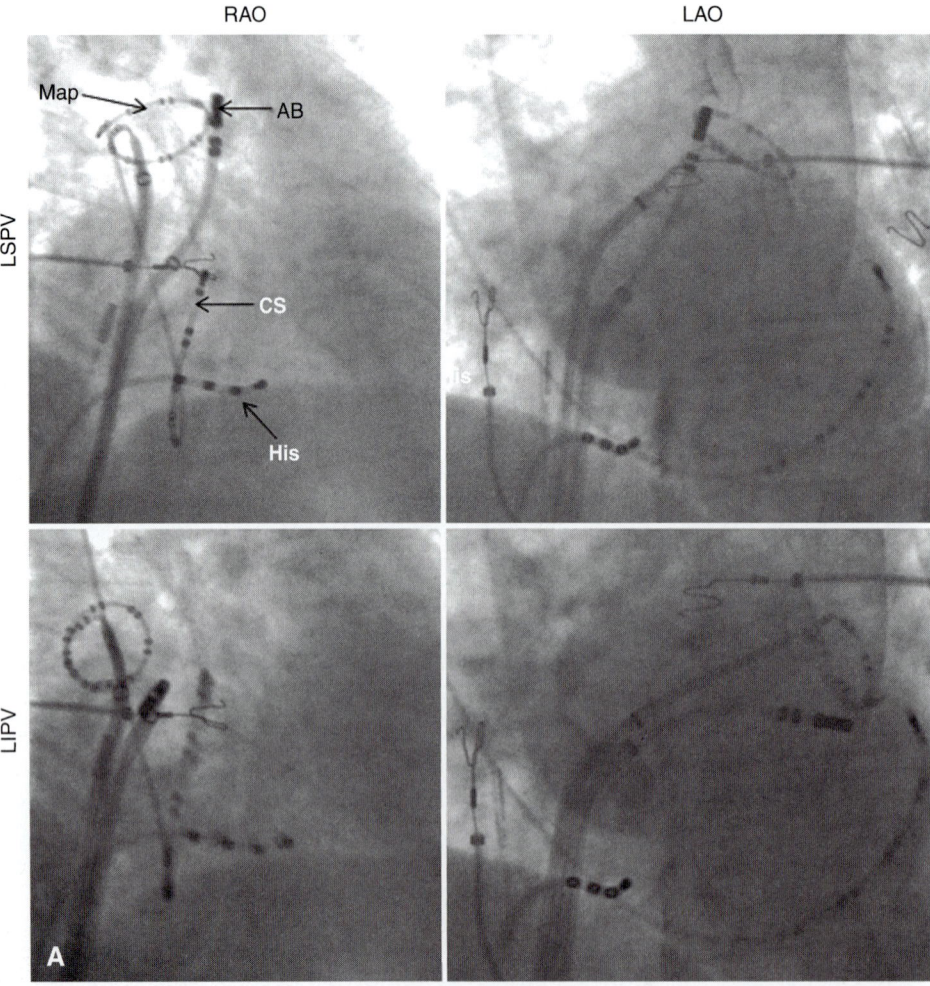

FIGURE 15-11. A and **B,** Circular mapping (Map) and ablation (AB) catheter positions for left superior (LS), left inferior (LI), right superior (RS), and right inferior (RI) pulmonary veins (PVs). Note that the mapping and ablation catheters remain posterior to the coronary sinus (CS) catheter to avoid the left atrial appendage. The positions of the veins shown here are typical of many patients, but marked variation in the vein locations can occur.

LAO projection while remaining posterior to the coronary sinus catheter. After engaging the superior vein, the inferior vein is often accessed by withdrawing the catheter with caudally oriented deflection. From the left inferior vein, the circular mapping catheter often moves easily to the superior vein by withdrawing slightly and opening the curve with clockwise torque. From the body of the left atrium, the right superior PV is engaged with clockwise torque on the catheter and probing the cranial aspect of the atrium posterior to the septum. The right inferior PV is most difficult to cannulate. From the right superior PV, the catheter is withdrawn and deflected caudally while applying slight counterclockwise torque. It is often necessary to engage the right inferior PV by placing a large, caudally directed curve on the catheter in the body of the atrium (Fig. 15-13). The catheter is then rotated clockwise with the tip inferior to the right superior os until oriented perpendicular to the LAO image plane. Here, opening the curve on the catheter will allow engagement of the right inferior vein.

For PV isolation, determination of the ostium is important but difficult to establish because the junction between the vein and the LA is funnel shaped and does not have a clear radiographic demarcation. Using fluoroscopy, the PV ostium can be located by advancing the ablation catheter into the PV, applying downward deflection of the tip, and withdrawing it in the atrium to see the fall-off at the ostial edge (Fig. 15-14; **Video 15-1**) Selective angiography (20 mL contrast during adenosine-induced asystole) can be performed to further delineate the atriovenous junction (Fig. 15-10). The use of a circumferential mapping catheter provides not only electrophysiologic guidance but

also an anatomic reference for PV ablation (Figs. 15-10 and 15-11). Fluoroscopy should be used sparingly to avoid excessive radiation exposure for the patient, the operator, and the laboratory staff. The use of a radiation protection cabin can significantly reduce global radiation dose to the operator, especially to regions left uncovered by a conventional lead apron, like the head.[63] Rotational angiography or CT overlay allows reconstruction of an image of the left atrial volume that can be superimposed on the fluoroscopic image (**Video 15-2**; Fig. 15-12).[64] The volume is either reconstructed from a CT scan previously performed or obtained by performing a left atrial contrast angiography using cinefluoroscopic equipment of the electrophysiology laboratory. The latter allows for timely and precise image acquisition and automatic registration of the reconstructed left atrial image over the fluoroscopic image. The PV ostia can then be localized using cut planes through the atrial volume at different projections.[65,66]

Intracardiac Echocardiography
ICE can be used to locate the venous ostia, position circular mapping catheters, and guide ablation (see Fig. 15-10).[55] It can also visualize the interatrial septum to guide transseptal puncture and monitor for the development of pericardial effusion or the formation of microbubbles. Because irrigated ablation prevents identification of microbubbles, the latter is applicable only when nonirrigated catheters are used. In addition, the position of the esophagus can be determined in real time, and 3D anatomic reconstruction can be performed for navigation alone or registered to CT or MRI reconstructions.

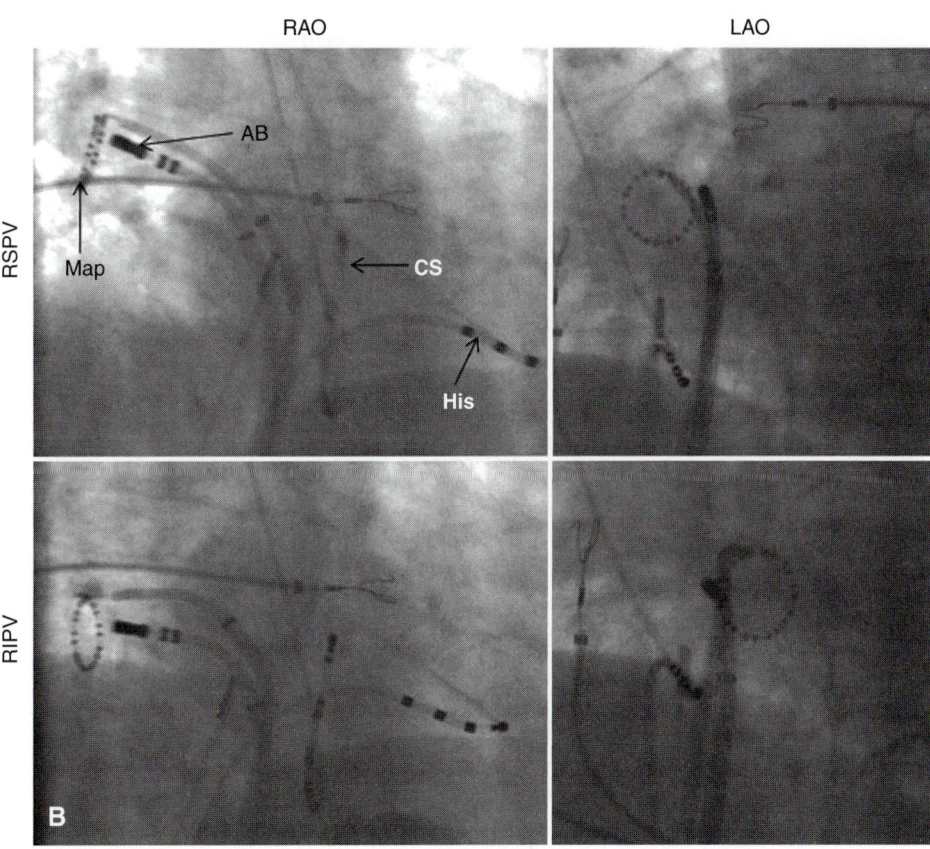

FIGURE 15-11, cont'd.

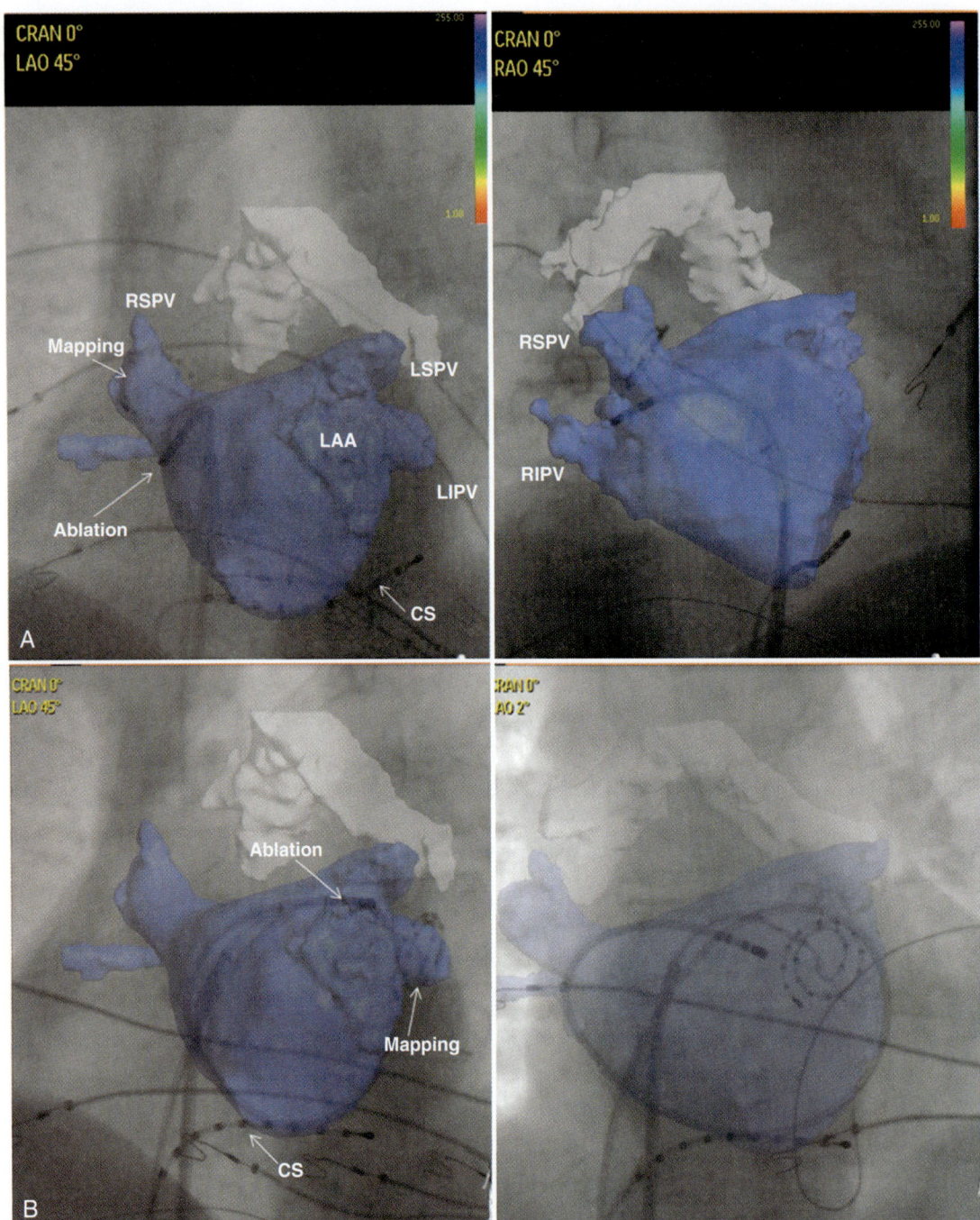

FIGURE 15-12. A, Left atrial anatomy (EP Navigator, Philips Medical Systems, Best, The Netherlands): left anterior oblique (LAO) 45-degree (*left panel*) and right anterior oblique (RAO) 45-degree (*right panel*) projections. **B,** Left atrial angiography or rotational angiography (EP Navigator): LAO 45-degree (*left panel*) and RAO 45-degree (*right panel*) projections. A three-dimensional reconstruction of the left atrium from a computed tomography scan performed at the time of the procedure using the fluoroscopy equipment is overlaid on the fluoroscopic image of the heart. Cut planes allow endocardial visualization, and tagging ablation points is possible. Contrast can be injected from the inferior vena cava, the right atrium, the left atrium, or the pulmonary artery. In this case, contrast was injected from the bottom of the right atrium, and scanning was performed 9 seconds after injection to allow passage through the pulmonary circulation. (See also Video 15-2.) CS, coronary sinus; LAA, left atrial appendage; LIPV, left inferior pulmonary vein; LSPV, left superior pulmonary vein.

Engaging RIPV from LA body

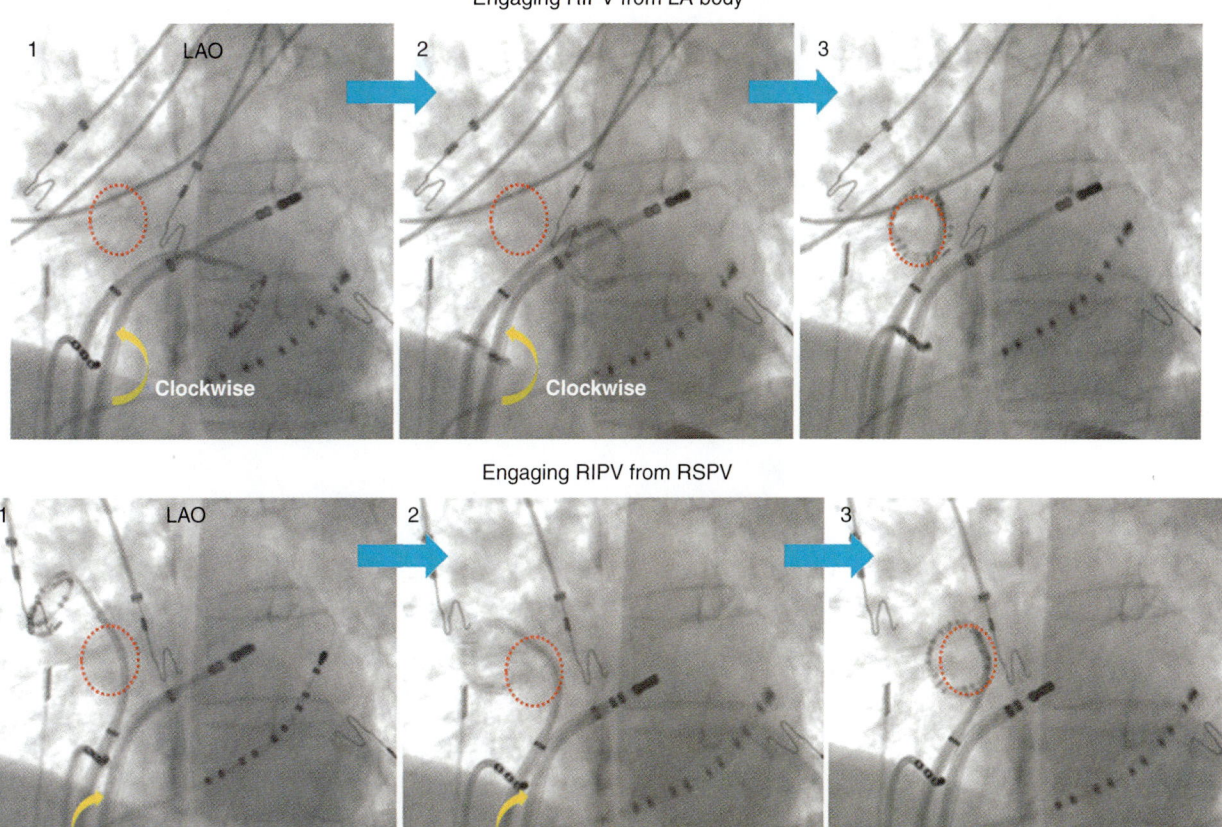

Engaging RIPV from RSPV

FIGURE 15-13. Engaging the right inferior pulmonary vein (RIPV; ostium marked with *red circle*) with the circular mapping catheter. *Top panels 1 to 3,* With the mapping catheter curved in the body of the left atrium (LA), the catheter and sheath are rotated clockwise (posteriorly) until the loop is seen on face. Advancing the catheter slightly will typically engage the os. By then opening the catheter curvature slightly and withdrawing the catheter and sheath, the mapping loop of the catheter will be oriented perpendicular to the axis of the vein. The os may be more inferiorly displaced than shown in this example. *Bottom panels 1 to 3,* From the right superior pulmonary vein (RSPV), the catheter is withdrawn with counterclockwise torque to drive the loop posteriorly into the RIPV os. Both maneuvers work well for the ablation catheter too. LAO, left anterior oblique.

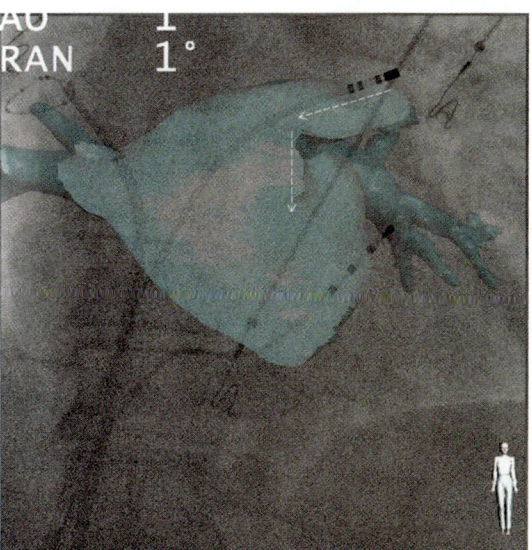

FIGURE 15-14. Determination of the location of the ostium of the left superior pulmonary vein (PV). By inserting the catheter inside the PV, applying downward deflection, and withdrawing the catheter to the atrium, the point at which the catheter falls inferiorly is the venous ostium. (*See also Video 15-1.*)

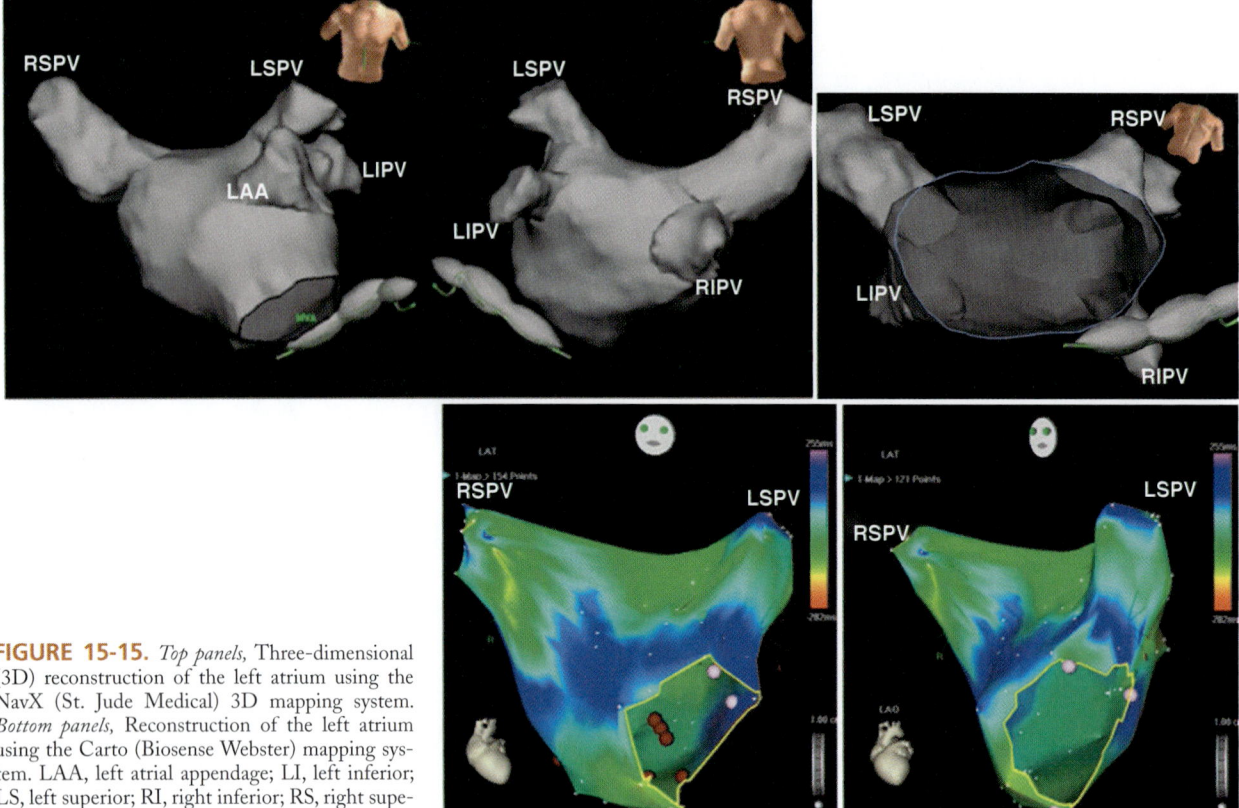

FIGURE 15-15. *Top panels,* Three-dimensional (3D) reconstruction of the left atrium using the NavX (St. Jude Medical) 3D mapping system. *Bottom panels,* Reconstruction of the left atrium using the Carto (Biosense Webster) mapping system. LAA, left atrial appendage; LI, left inferior; LS, left superior; RI, right inferior; RS, right superior; PV, pulmonary vein.

Three-Dimensional Electroanatomic Mapping Systems

Among 3D electroanatomic mapping tools, Carto (Biosense Webster, Diamond Bar, CA) and NavX (St. Jude Medical, St. Paul, MN) systems are commonly used for AF ablation procedures. They allow reconstruction of the left atrial anatomy and help navigation by displaying catheter positions relative to the virtual left atrium anatomy (Fig. 15-15). This electroanatomic reconstruction can be merged with CT or MRI anatomy by the mapping system (Fig. 15-16). These applications reduce patients' exposure to radiation because catheter movement and tracking are possible without the use of fluoroscopy (Fig. 15-17).[57] Images from cardiac CT or MRI can be merged with the electroanatomic map for more precise delineation of the anatomy of interest.[67] It is also possible to mark the sites of ablation. However, studies have shown that even if ablation tags form a coalescent line around the PV ostia, it is observed that the veins are not electrically isolated in 45% of patients.[56] To consistently achieve the electrophysiologic end point of eliminating all the electrical connections, conventional electrical mapping must be used in addition.

Remote Magnetic and Robotic Navigation Systems

Recently, we have seen the development of tools with advanced technologies using magnetic fields (Stereotaxis, St. Louis, MO) and a robotic sheath (Hansen Medical, Mountain View, CA) for remote catheter navigation and ablation.[68-72] The advantages of these systems are good catheter stability, improved catheter steerability, and reduction in operator radiation exposure.[73,74] Most important, the potential advantages of procedure automation using these technologies are of major interest.

Ablation

At our institution, ablation is usually performed circumferentially, using an open irrigated-tip 3.5-mm catheter. The goals are to create a continuous anatomic line of lesions 5 to 10 mm from the PV ostia and to eliminate all PV potentials from within the vein. The complete electrical isolation of the PV may require additional ablation targeting residual PV potentials identified by the mapping catheter on the PV side of the antral ablation line (Fig. 15-18). The use of fixed or adjustable curved sheaths can improve catheter stability. With the ablation catheter directed toward the left veins, clockwise torque on the catheter and sheath will move the tip posteriorly, and counterclockwise torque will move the tip anteriorly (Fig. 15-19). It is important to avoid the left atrial appendage during left-sided PV ablation. To avoid the appendage, the catheter should remain posterior to the coronary sinus catheter. A catheter in the left atrial appendage will record high-amplitude atrial electrograms and fail to pass outside the cardiac border. For the right veins, the movements are opposite: clockwise torque moves the catheter tip anteriorly, whereas counterclockwise torque moves it posteriorly (Fig. 15-19). The catheter tip is moved superiorly or inferiorly by advancing or withdrawing the catheter, respectively, or by opening and closing the

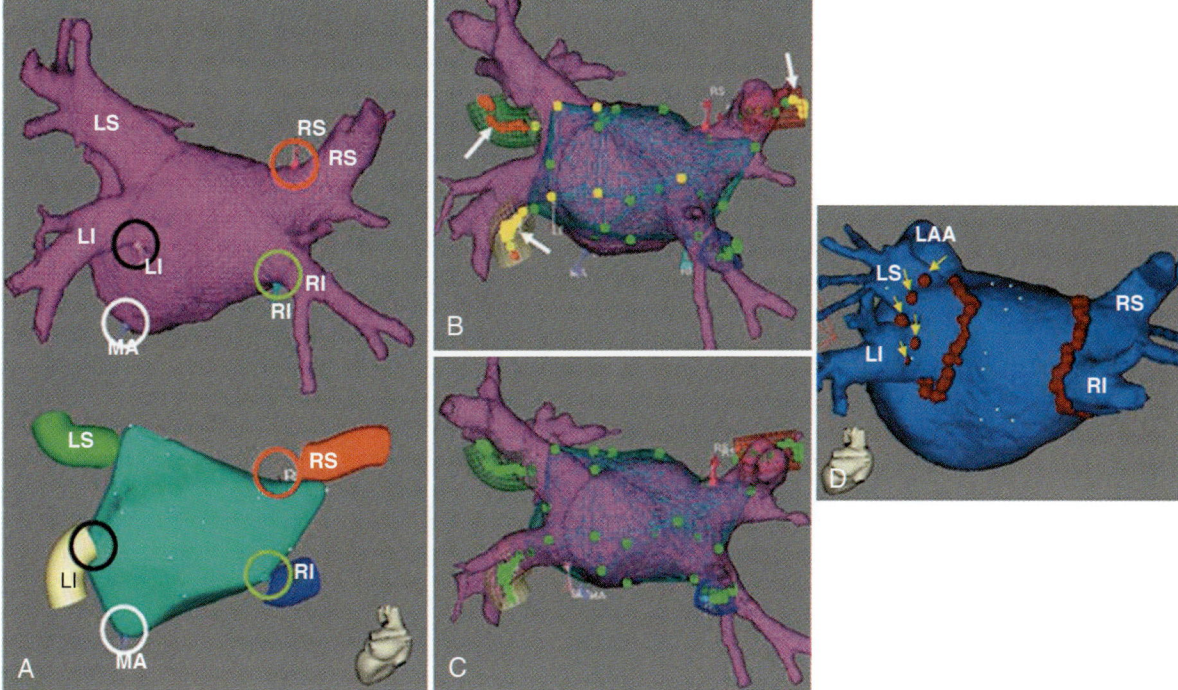

FIGURE 15-16. Left atrium (LA) registration. **A,** Landmark pairs (highlighted with *colored circles*) at the 6-o'clock mitral annulus (MA) position and the junctions of the LA and right superior pulmonary vein (RS), right inferior pulmonary vein (RI), and left inferior pulmonary vein (LI) were annotated on the three-dimensional (3D) computed tomography (CT) LA surface reconstruction (*upper image,* shown as *wire frame*) and the LA electroanatomic map (*lower image,* shown as *solid shell*) with *colored tubes* representing pulmonary veins (PVs). **B,** After landmark registration, the 3D LA surface reconstruction was superimposed on the electroanatomic map (shown as *mesh*). Note the misalignment of the left superior pulmonary artery (LS), LI, and RS between the two image data sets, indicated by the *yellow* or *red* PV points (*arrows*) sampled in those PVs. **C,** After surface registration was executed, the PV alignment between the two image data sets was significantly improved, indicated by the *green* PV points. The *green, yellow,* and *red* on the electroanatomic map points indicate their distance of <5 mm, 5 to 10 mm, and >10 mm, respectively, from the registered CT reconstruction surface. **D,** Tailored radiofrequency (RF) applications to individual left atrium (LA) and pulmonary vein (PV) anatomy. Registered 3D LA surface reconstructions, posteroanterior view, show that the continuous circumferential RF applications (*dark brown tags*) were placed outside the PV-LA junction encircling the left-sided and right-sided PVs in a patient with normal pattern of four PVs. Note, the segmental ablations (*yellow arrows*) guided by electrophysiologic mapping and fluoroscopy were located about 10 mm inside the PVs. LAA, left atrial appendage. (*From Dong J, Dickfeld T, Dalal D, et al. Initial experience in the use of integrated electroanatomic mapping with three-dimensional MR/CT images to guide catheter ablation of atrial fibrillation.* J Cardiovasc Electrophysiol. *2006;17:459–466. With permission.*)

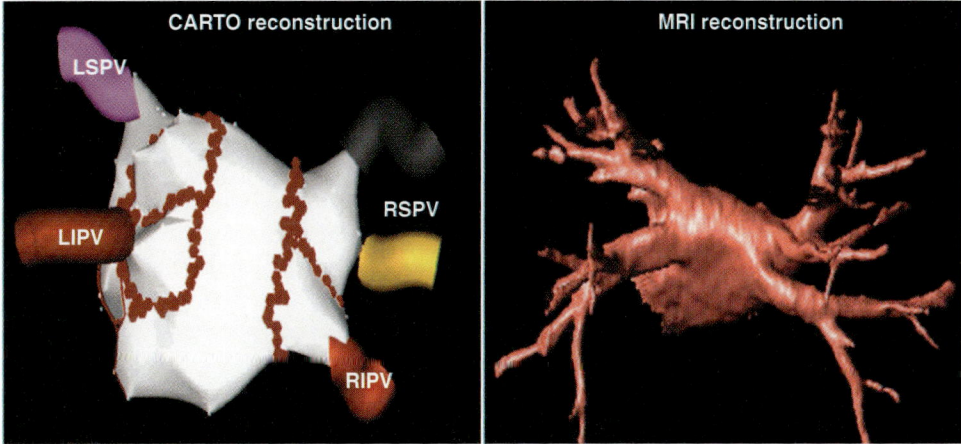

FIGURE 15-17. Comparison between reconstruction of the pulmonary vein–left atrial junction using an electroanatomical guidance system (Carto, Biosense Medical) and contrast magnetic resonance imaging (MRI). Note the high correlation between the two imaging techniques with respect to identification of the antrum and ostium.

catheter curvature, respectively. Compound sigmoid curves created with the catheter and sheath can improve contact in difficult to reach positions (Fig. 15-8). Despite apparent "isolation" of a PV by either continuous lesion delivery or by antral electrogram abatement, remaining connections to the left atrium are often noted deeper in the vein in almost half of the patients (Fig. 15-20).[64] Circumferential

mapping enables targeting the connecting fascicles identified as the earliest site of PV activation during atrial pacing and as sites showing electrogram reversal (Fig. 15-21). Electrogram features suggestive of successful fascicle ablation sites include timing of the electrogram on the ablation catheter equal to or earlier than earliest PV potential on mapping catheter, large PV electrogram amplitude, and

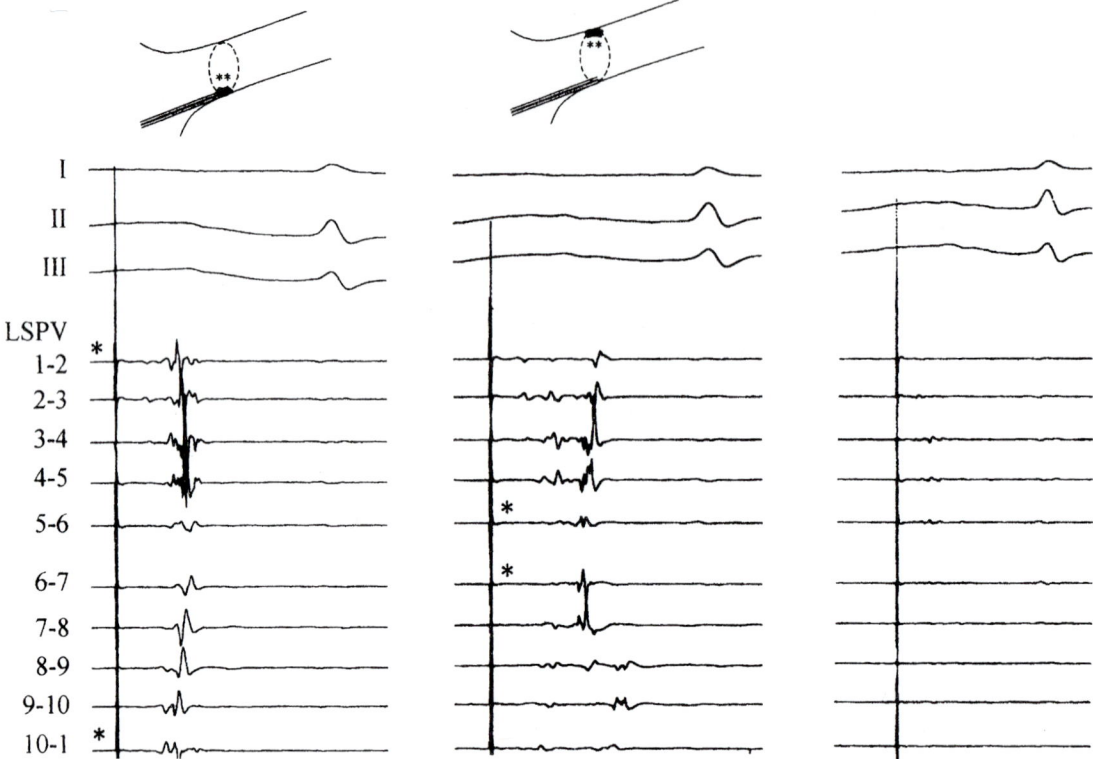

FIGURE 15-18. Change in activation of left superior pulmonary vein (LSPV) potentials with ablation. Bipoles recorded electrograms from the circular mapping catheter at the venous ostium. In the *left panel*, the earliest pulmonary vein (PV) potentials are recorded at the inferior aspect of the vein, from bipoles 10-1 and 1-2 *(asterisks)*. In the *middle panel*, after ablation to the inferior aspect of the vein, the PV activation is delayed by 90 msec, and the sequence is changed so that the earliest activation is now at the superior portion of the vein covered by bipoles 5-6 and 6-7 *(asterisks)*. Ablation to these sites eliminated all PV electrical activity *(right panel)*. *(From Haïssaguerre M, Shah DC, Jais P, et al. Electrophysiologic breakthroughs from the left atrium to the pulmonary veins.* Circulation. *2000;102:2463–2465. With permission.)*

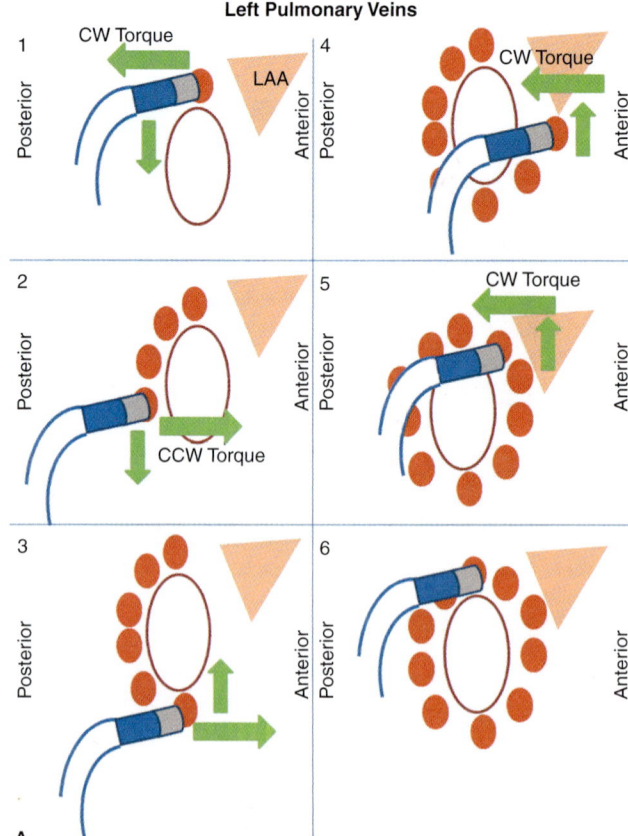

FIGURE 15-19. Catheter movements for circumferential antral pulmonary vein (PV) isolation. **A,** Left veins. The PV ostium is represented by the elongated circular structure. A transseptal sheath is shown in *white,* and the ablation catheter is *blue and gray. Panel 1,* Starting at the superior aspect of the left superior PV, clockwise (CW) torque on the catheter moves the tip posteriorly. Flexing or withdrawing the catheter moves it inferiorly to ablate the posterior wall *(red dots). Panel 2,* Midway down the posterior wall, counterclockwise (CCW) torque becomes necessary to move the catheter tip anteriorly under the vein *(panel 3). Panel 4,* Ascending the anterior wall, clockwise torque is needed to complete the circumferential lesion set. The catheter movements can be performed around each vein separately or around both veins together.

identical morphology of ablation electrogram with the target electrogram on the mapping catheter. Other important sites to target are ectopic foci around PVs and possibly ostial and antral sites displaying fragmented signals (Table 15-3, p. 250).

Energy Source and Catheter Design

Radiofrequency Energy

RF electrical current is the most frequently used modality for ablation. Catheter-tip irrigation can be used to cool the catheter tip and superficial tissues, causing the greatest temperature rises to occur deeper in the tissue. This reduces the risk for char or coagulum formation compared with nonirrigated-tip catheters.[75] In our institution, ablation is performed using an open irrigation catheter in power-controlled mode, using 25 to 30 W around the PVs and the posterior left atrium and up to 30 to 35 W on the septum and the anterior atrium. The irrigation flow is manually adjusted from 10 to 60 mL/minute to keep the temperature below 45°C at the desired power. RF is applied for 30 to 60 seconds at each point or for 60 to 120 seconds at the sites where a significant effect is observed (such as a change in PV activation pattern or PV isolation). Whereas most centers now use irrigated-tip ablation catheters, 8-mm

solid-tip catheters can also be used for AF ablation. For the 8-mm catheter, energy up to 50 to 70 W has been used with target temperatures of 50° to 55°C. Power should be reduced on the posterior atrial wall. With a nonirrigated catheter, the detection of microbubbles on ICE signals excessive tissue heating and can be used to titrate energy delivery.

Before ablation, many centers define the position of the esophagus by contrast swallow, ICE, CT, MR, or placement of a radiopaque nasogastric tube (Fig. 15-22; **Video 15-3**). Esophageal temperature monitoring has been applied as well but does not provide complete protection from esophageal injury. Because the esophagus can move during the ablation procedure, most centers limit power delivery to 25 W and move the catheter frequently (every 20 seconds) for ablation on the entire posterior left atrial wall. Chest pain is a nonspecific marker for esophageal heating.

Specialized RF ablation catheters designed for single-shot circumferential PV ablation are now available (Fig. 15-23). The high-density mesh ablator (HDMA; Bard Electrophysiology, Lowell, MA) is designed with 36 bipoles for high-density circumferential mapping and ablation. The catheter is advanced to the ostium of the vein and deployed. RF energy is then delivered circumferentially or to circumscribed segments of the PV ostia. In clinical trials, the HDMA achieved isolation in 88% (63% to 100%) of PVs.[76-82] The pulmonary vein ablation catheter (PVAC; Ablation Frontiers, Medtronic, Minneapolis, MN) is a nonirrigated decapolar circular mapping and ablation catheter that is advanced over a wire to the PV ostia (Fig. 15-23). It uses bipolar and unipolar RF that can be delivered circumferentially or segmentally. Clinical studies with the PVAC catheter report 88% to 100% acute PV electrical isolation and absence of arrhythmia relapse in 83% of patients at 6 months.[83-85]

Cryogenic Energy

PV isolation using cryoablation was made practical by the development of balloon catheters (Arctic Front, Medtronic CryoCath) designed to create single-shot ostial PV ablation (Fig. 15-23). Contact between the balloon and the tissue is crucial to achieve complete isolation. Complete occlusion of the PV by the balloon is confirmed before ablation by PV angiography distal to the balloon or by color Doppler using ICE (Fig. 15-24).[86] PV electrical isolation needs to be confirmed with a circular mapping catheter because the balloon has no mapping capability. Typically, one to three 4-minute cryoablation applications are required for each vein. Transient phrenic nerve palsy during cryoballoon ablation of the right-sided veins is observed in 7% of patients. Continuous phrenic pacing during cryoablation is recommended to allow for interruption of freezing if phrenic capture is lost. Clinical studies report 93% (84% to 98%) acute PV isolation using cryoballoon ablation and AF freedom in 71% (42% to 86%) of patients at 3 to 33 months.[86-93] The incidence of PV stenosis and esophageal fistula appear very low, although esophageal inflammation can be seen.[89-93]

Focal cryoablation with a 6- or 8-mm catheter can be used for PV connections not eliminated with the balloon. Focal cryoablation can also be used for ablation on the posterior wall near the esophagus and for more distal ablation in the PV when isolation cannot be achieved more proximally with RF.

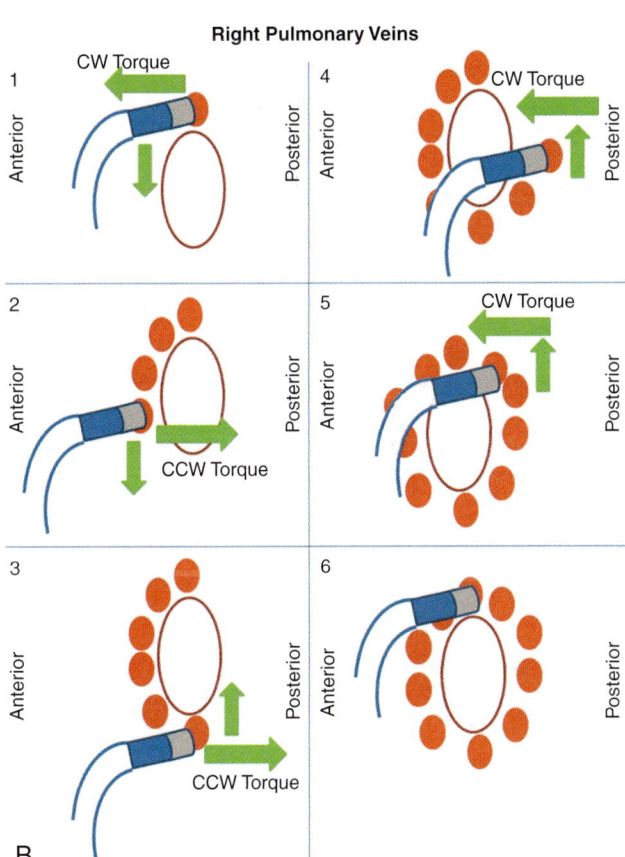

Right Pulmonary Veins

FIGURE 15-19, cont'd. B, For the right veins, the catheter movements are opposite those for the left—clockwise torque moves the catheter tip anteriorly, and counterclockwise torque moves the tip posteriorly. LAA, left atrial appendage.

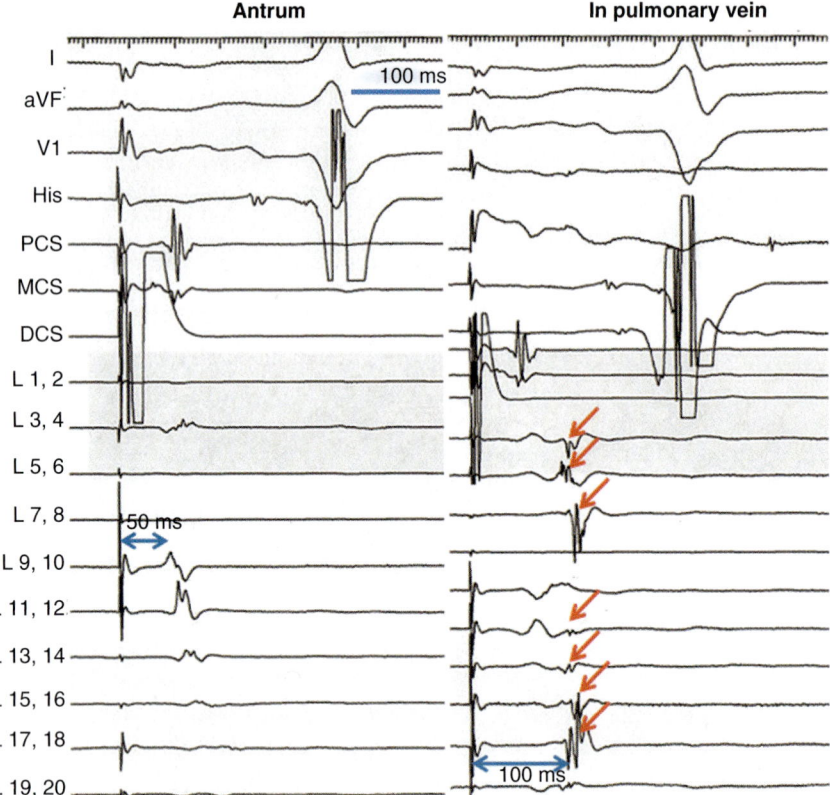

FIGURE 15-20. *Left panel,* After antral ablation of the left inferior pulmonary vein (PV) in this patient, a circular mapping catheter (L1, 2 through L19, 20) records only far-field atrial potentials 50 msec after the pacing stimulus. Without further investigation, the vein would be assumed to be isolated. *Right panel,* Moving the mapping catheter 1 cm inside the vein from the antrum reveals almost circumferential PV potentials (*arrows*), which were shown to conduct out of the vein with pacing. The residual PV potentials deep in the vein after antral ablation probably result from the epicardial course of the myocardial tissue over the vein.

Ultrasound

High-intensity focused ultrasound (HIFU) energy uses ultrasound to create thermal injury. It is delivered by a balloon-type catheter. The mechanism by which the lesion is created is a combination of coagulation necrosis and acoustic cavitation in which vibration, hyperthermia, and pressure changes lead to cellular death. Initial experience with HIFU revealed many problems. Several applications were necessary to obtain PV isolation, making for an unduly time-consuming process. Moreover, damage to collateral structures raised concerns about its safety.[94] Recently, the results of a clinical trial using third generation of HIFU balloons have been published. In this latest version of the catheter, the ultrasound has been defocused so that the energy zone is broader and directed more proximally, closer to the balloon-tissue interface, and the energy density is lower. It has a central lumen allowing the insertion of a hexapolar spiral mapping catheter to record PV potentials and monitor for PV isolation during ablation. In this clinical trial of 22 patients, acute isolation was obtain in 81% of PVs, which could be improved to 90% by using a steerable sheath. After one procedure, 71% of patients remained free from arrhythmia. However, a rise in esophageal temperature was observed in 25% of HIFU applications despite no esophageal injury being reported.[94] Further studies are warranted to evaluate the safety and efficacy of this modality in AF ablation.

Laser

Light amplification by stimulated emission of radiation (laser) is also being studied as an alternative to RF energy. It has been developed for use in balloon catheters for PV isolation. Experimental evidence showed that laser energy created transmural coagulation necrosis.[95-97] A recent clinical trial using a balloon catheter delivering laser energy through an optical fiber and allowing direct endoscopic visualization of the treated area reported 91% success in terms of acute PV isolation and 60% freedom from arrhythmia at 1 year after a single procedure.[98] The plane of ablation with all balloon catheters was found to be more distal than initially expected. Indeed, the extent of the isolated area started from the PV ostia and left the antral region unablated.[99,100] (Table 15-4).

End Points for Ablation

There is general consensus in that complete electrical PV isolation is the optimal end point when ablation is performed at the PV-LA junction (Table 15-5).[101] Entrance block is shown by elimination of all PV potentials within the vein. Exit block is shown by failure to conduct spontaneous PV potential to the left atrium or by the inability to conduct from the vein during high-output pacing (10 mA) from each bipole on a circular mapping catheter in the proximal PV (Fig. 15-25). The demonstration of exit block using high-output pacing

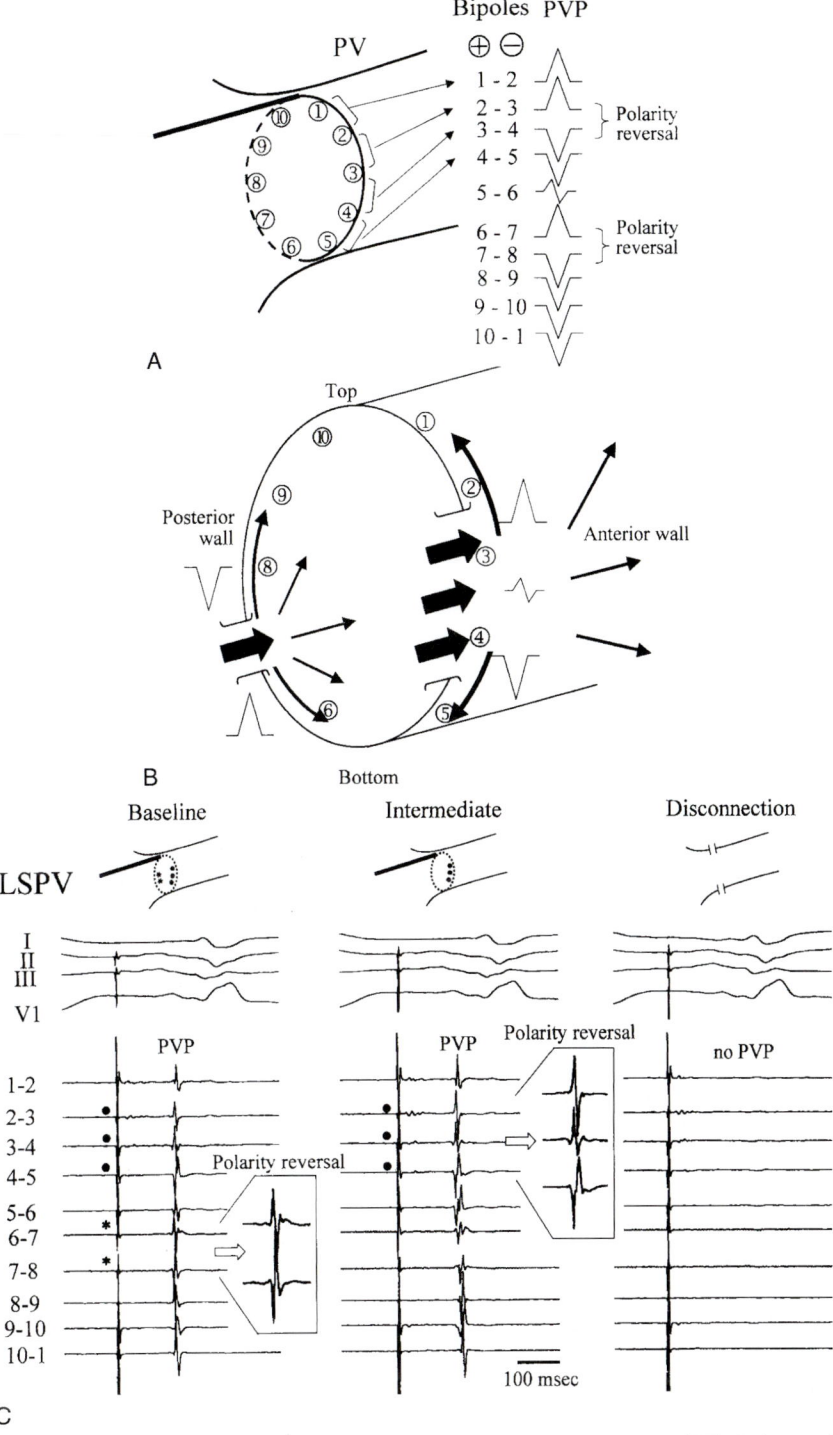

FIGURE 15-21. Electrogram polarity reversal indicating breakthrough from left atrium to pulmonary vein (PV). **A,** A 10-pole circular mapping catheter is represented in the ostium of a PV *(top)*. Polarity reversal is defined as a sudden change in the main deflection of the pulmonary vein potential (PVP). The reversal occurs as the wavefront of activation propagates radially in the PV from its connection with the left atrium *(bottom)*, thus reaching contiguous bipolar recording electrodes in opposing directions. **B** and **C,** Demonstration of use of electrogram reversal to isolate a left superior pulmonary vein (LSPV) with a wide synchronous breakthrough front. At baseline *(left panel)*, electrogram reversal is identified over lasso bipoles 2-3 to 4-5 *(filled circles)* and between 6-7 and 7-8 *(asterisks)*, consistent with two connection sites to the PV. In the *middle panel*, radiofrequency ablation to bipoles 6-7 and 7-8 has delayed activation of these PVPs, leaving the reversal site between bipoles 2-3 to 4-5. Ablation at this site eliminated all PV potentials *(right panel)*. *(From Yamane T, Shah DC, Jais P, et al. Electrogram polarity reversal as an additional indicator of breakthroughs from the left atrium to the pulmonary veins. J Am Coll Cardiol. 2002;39:1337–1344. With permission.)*

TABLE 15-3

TARGETS FOR ABLATION DURING PULMONARY VEIN ISOLATION

Ectopic activity triggering AF
Earliest PV potential activation in PV
All ostial and antral PV potentials
Sites of PV polarity reversal
Antral fragmented potentials
Possibly sites of dominant frequency or rapid activity during AF

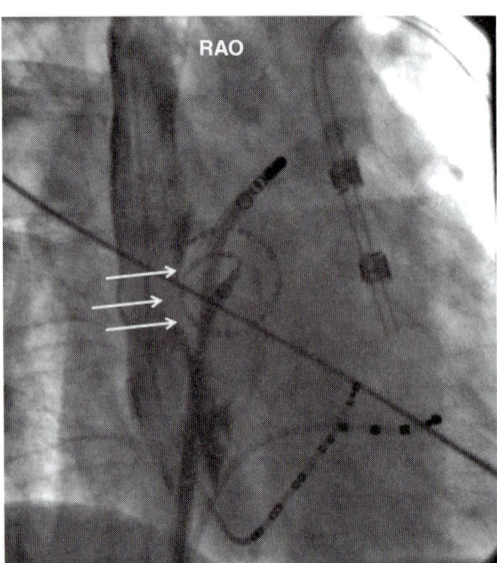

FIGURE 15-22. Esophageal barium contrast swallow with a circular mapping catheter positioned at the os of the left inferior pulmonary vein. The posterior aspect of the catheter indents the esophagus (*arrows*). RAO, right anterior oblique. *(See also Video 15-3.)*

is also considered an important end point by some centers. After initial success, up to one third of patients will have acute reconnection during the index procedure. Therefore, PV isolation should be reconfirmed 20 to 30 minutes after the last energy delivery. The administration of isoproterenol, adenosine, or both to unmask PV reconnection can be useful.[102–104] Residual atrial ectopy may be provoked by isoproterenol (up to 20 μg/minute), adenosine (6 to 24 mg), burst atrial pacing or after termination of AF (spontaneous or cardioversion). If anatomic circumferential ablation is performed, abatement of local bipolar voltage by 90% or 0.05 mV or less within the encircled areas has been suggested as a surrogate end point.[59] As mentioned, the presence of PV potentials within the vein is common despite complete abatement of antral electrograms. The completion of an anatomic encircling lesion set without assessment of the electrical effects does not reliably produce PV isolation and is not recommended. If additional, linear lesions are performed, bidirectional conduction block should be achieved and verified. If the ablation is performed during AF, we believe that AF termination using a stepwise ablation strategy (PV isolation, substrate modification, linear lesion, until conversion directly to SR or to atrial tachycardia and then further mapping and ablation until SR) should be achieved or at least attempted.[105] The role of inducibility testing as a procedural end point is still debated.[101]

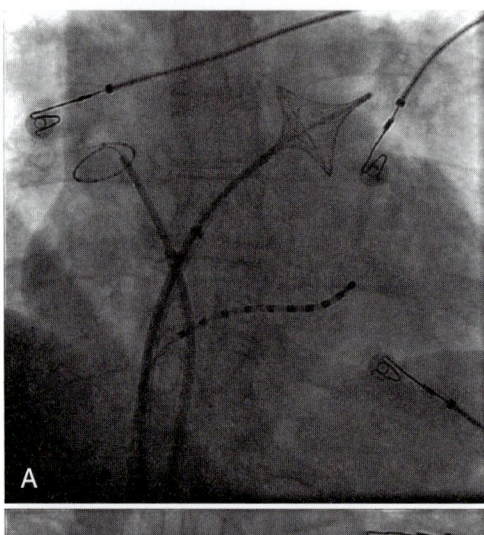

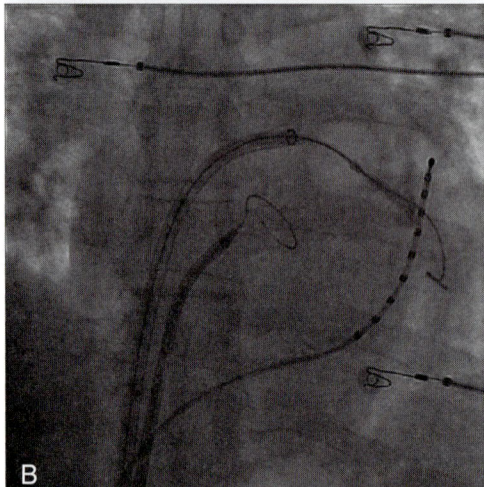

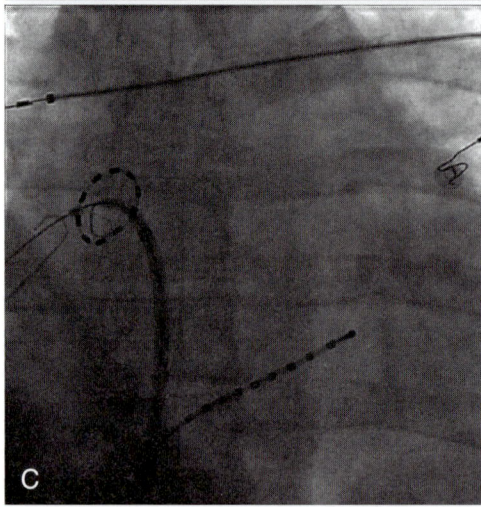

FIGURE 15-23. A, HDMA catheter (Bard Electrophysiology, Lowell, MA) in left superior pulmonary vein (PV), circular mapping catheter in right superior PV. **B,** Arctic Front cryoballoon (Medtronic, Minneapolis, MN) in left inferior PV, circular mapping catheter at fossa. **C,** Pulmonary vein ablation catheter (Ablation Frontiers, Medtronic) in the right superior PV.

Results of Ablation

Acute isolation of the PVs should be achievable in 90% to 100% of cases. PV isolation is reported to achieve durable SR without the need for AADs in 59% to 93% of patients with paroxysmal AF.[1–8,61,99,106–115] Some have advocated the

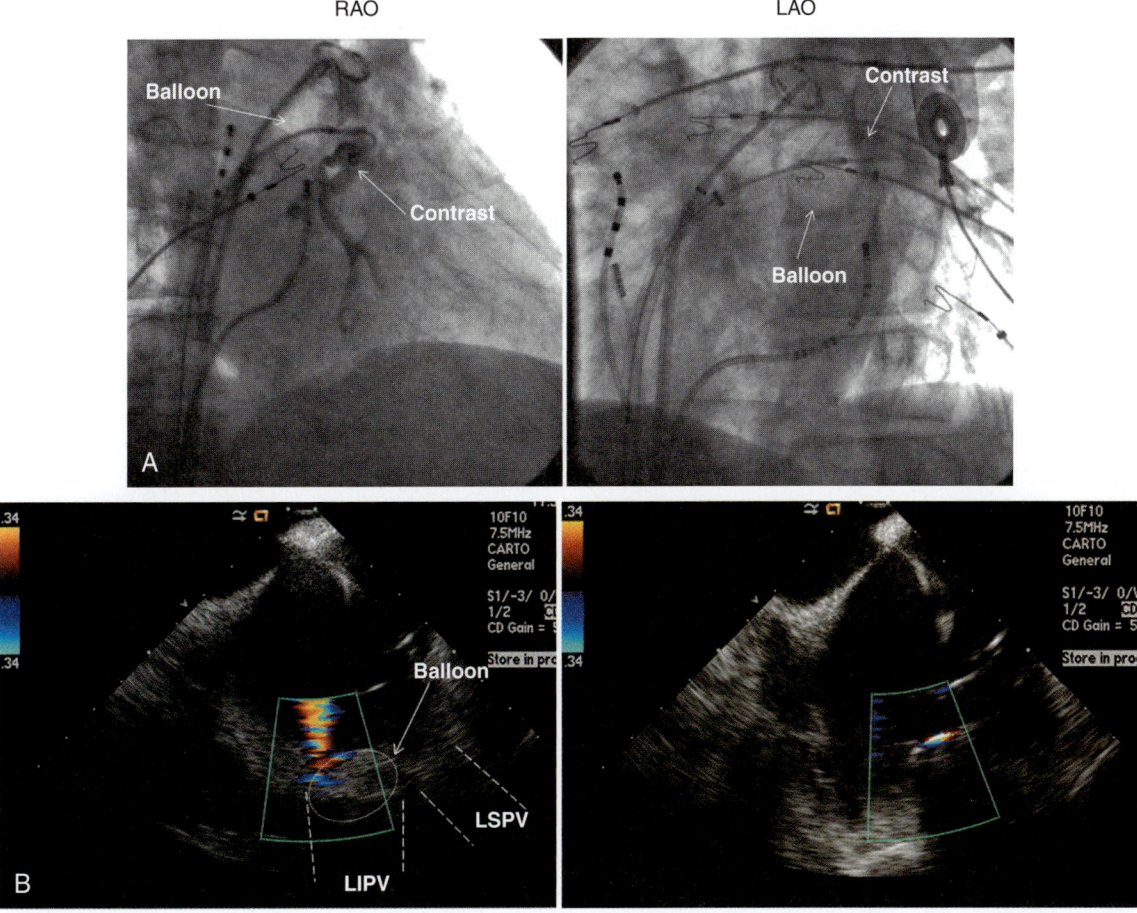

FIGURE 15-24. Contact of cryoballoon with ostium of pulmonary vein (PV) for ablation. **A,** Fluoroscopic views after contrast injection through lumen of a 28-mm balloon catheter after seating in the left inferior PV. Note that the contrast is retained in the vein after injection, indicating a complete seal of the PV ostium. The circular mapping catheter is in the left superior PV. **B,** Assessment of balloon contact with the ostium of the left inferior pulmonary vein (LIPV) using intracardiac echocardiography. In this patient, a 23-mm balloon is deployed. *Top panel,* Color Doppler demonstrates a high-velocity jet around the inferior aspect of the balloon, indicating a "leak" from incomplete occlusion of the PV. *Bottom panel,* After adjusting the catheter curvature, there is complete seal of the PV by the balloon. LSPV, left superior pulmonary vein. LAO, left anterior oblique; RAO, right anterior oblique.

addition of linear lesions (roof or mitral lines) in patients with ongoing or inducible AF despite PV isolation and have reported long-term success in 82% to 91% of patients with this approach.[106–112] Other techniques involving PV isolation and substrate modification have reported long-term freedom from arrhythmia without AADs in 41% to 94% of cases. It is still debated whether additional lesions should be delivered after PV isolation in patients with paroxysmal AF. If extra-PV triggers are spontaneously observed, they should be ablated. However, whether AF should be rendered noninducible by pharmacologic means or rapid pacing is unclear. Indeed, when using noninducibility as the procedural end point, 43% of paroxysmal AF cases required additional ablation in one study.[107] In these patients, linear lesions were created. However, half of the cases required a subsequent procedure for recurrent AF (50%) and new-onset left atrial tachycardia (50%). After the final procedure, 91% of patients remained free from atrial arrhythmia without the need for AADs during a follow-up period of 1.5 years.[107] Therefore, the benefits of additional ablation need to be balanced with the proarrhythmic risk from additional left atrial lesions (Table 15-6).

In patients with persistent AF, PV isolation alone achieved successful restoration of SR in 20% to 61% of patients in most of the serial studies,[91,109,113–118] although

TABLE 15-4
TOOLS USED DURING PULMONARY VEIN ISOLATION FOR ATRIAL FIBRILLATION
Mapping
Point-by-point mapping using a roving catheter
Circular mapping catheter
Basket catheter mapping
Navigation
Fluoroscopy
Three-dimensional reconstruction from tomography overlaid on fluoroscopy
Electroanatomic mapping
Intracardiac echocardiography
Remote navigation systems (robotic or magnetic)
Ablation
Cooled ablation by internal or external irrigation (preferred)
Ablation with 8-mm-tip
Cryoballoon ablation
Duty-cycled radiofrequency ablation using a circular mapping and ablation catheter
Radiofrequency ablation using a high-density mesh ablator catheter

some reported success rates as high as 95%.[119,120] For most persistent AF cases, ablation of PV targets alone appears insufficient,[53] and strategies combining PV isolation and substrate modification are often adopted, achieving SR without AADs in 42% to 95% patients, with most cen-ters reporting success rates of more than 70%.[105,109,111,121–129] In persistent AF, more than one ablation procedure is often needed to abolish AF; therefore, patients should be informed that about half of them will require more than one procedure (Table 15-7).

TABLE 15-5

END POINTS FOR PULMONARY VEIN ISOLATION

End Point	Definition	Comment
Pulmonary vein (PV) entrance block	Elimination of all PV potentials on detailed mapping within proximal PV during sinus rhythm and atrial/coronary sinus pacing	Most widely accepted end point and minimal criteria for electrical isolation; confirm 30 min after last ablation and possibly with isoproterenol and/or adenosine challenge
PV exit block	Failure to conduct from PV to affect atrial capture with high output (10 mA) pacing from all bipoles on circular mapping catheter in proximal PV Failure to conduct spontaneous PV activity to the left atrium (PV dissociation)	Importance stressed by many centers; conduction from PV may persist despite meeting criteria for entrance block; confirm 30 min after last ablation and possibly with isoproterenol and/or adenosine challenge
Voltage abatement	Reduction of antral bipolar electrogram voltage by ≥90% or to <0.05 mV within areas encircled by ablation	Electrogram abatement does not equate with PV isolation; demonstration of entrance/exit block required
Atrial fibrillation inducibility	Failure to initiate atrial fibrillation with atrial burst pacing with or without isoproterenol	Methods empirical and not standardized; validity questioned
Atrial fibrillation termination	Restoration of sinus rhythm or conversion to organized atrial tachycardia/flutter by ablation	Accumulating data showing better long-term outcome when ablation successfully converts atrial fibrillation
Elimination of spontaneous and evoked atrial ectopy	Absence of atrial ectopy in response to: Isoproterenol, ≤20 µg/min Adenosine, 6-24 mg Atrial burst pacing up to 200 beats/min (postpause ectopy) Termination of induced atrial fibrillation by cardioversion or spontaneously	Adjunctive end point in addition to PV isolation

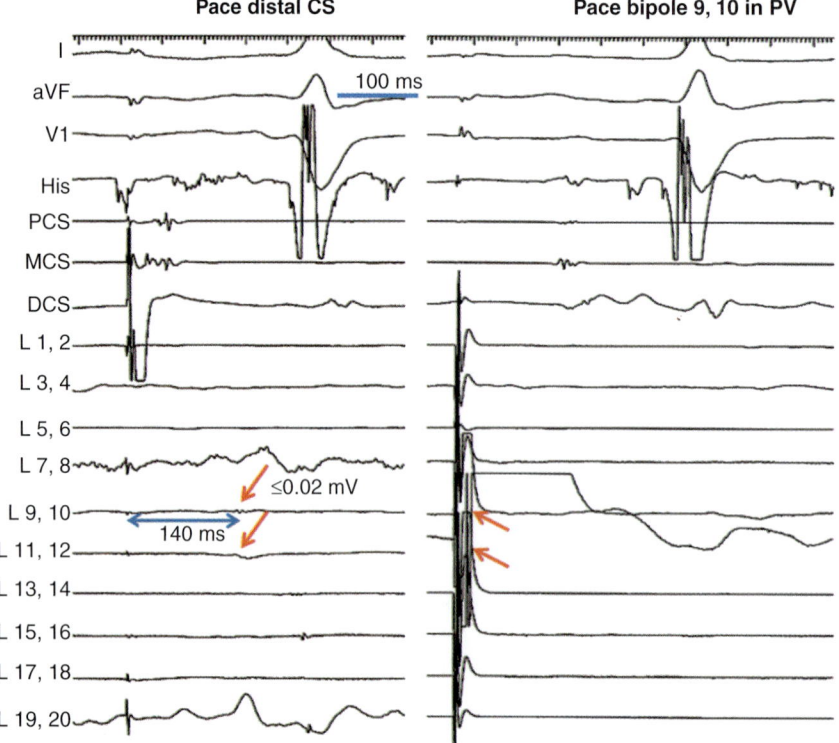

FIGURE 15-25. Intact conduction from within a pulmonary vein (PV) despite miniscule PV potentials. *Left panel,* After combined antral and ostial ablation, extremely small potentials (≤0.02 mV) are recorded with a circular mapping catheter (L1,2 through L19,20) in the PV (*arrows*). The electrogram on bipoles L11,12 are barely discernible. *Right panel,* Pacing from bipoles L9,10 (shown) and L11,12 (not shown) advanced the small PV potentials and resulted in conduction out of the vein. Further ablation proximal to these sites produced complete exit block. CS, coronary sinus.

TABLE 15-6

CATHETER ABLATION FOR PAROXYSMAL ATRIAL FIBRILLATION

Study	No. of Subjects	Strategy	Follow-Up (mo)	No. of Procedures	Antiarrhythmic Drug	Atrial Fibrillation Freedom (%)
Della Bella et al, 2009[124]	207	Conventional ablation vs. image integration (CartoMerge, Biosense Webster)	14 ± 12	1.3*	58%	88
Van Belle et al, 2008[93]	141	PVI cryoablation	15 ± 8	1.2	No	59
Jais et al, 2008[110]	53	PVI ± lines ± defragmentation	12	1.8	No	89
Kettering et al, 2008[154]	43	PVI	6	1	12%	82
Fiala et al, 2008[111]	59	PVI ± substrate	31 ± 14	27% repeat ablation	No	90
Yoshida et al, 2008[117]	32	Antral PVI	10 ± 2	1	No	69
Wang et al, 2008[155]	106	CPVI vs. CPVI + SVC isolation	12	1.2	5%	93 vs. 94
Fiala et al, 2008[156]	110	PVI vs. CPVA	48 ± 8	1.3	No	80
Corrado et al, 2008[157]	96 PAF, 78 PsAF	PVI antrum + SVC	20 ± 14	1.1	No	82
Chen et al, 2008[125]	18	PVI + posterior wall isolation	20 ± 4	1 repeat ablation	43%	94
Dixit et al, 2008[158]	77 PAF, 28 PsAF	4 PVI, arrhythmogenic PVI only	12	1	No	59
Arentz et al, 2007[114]	67	PVI vs. large PVI	15 ± 4	1.2	No	54 vs. 72
Chang et al, 2007[112]	88	PVI ± lines/inducibility testing	12 ± 6	1	Yes	45 vs. 82 (noninducible)
Verma et al, 2007[123]	120	PVI ± anterior line	12	1	No	85 vs. 87
Sheikh et al, 2006[108]	100	PVI vs. PVI + lines	9	1	Yes	82 vs. 90
Cheema et al, 2006[159]	92 PAF, 108 PsAF	CPVA vs. PVI + lines	26 ± 11	1	No	28, 41 after redo*
Stabile et al, 2006[160]	42 PAF, 26 PsAF	CPVA + mitral line + CTI	13	1	No	56
Jais et al, 2006[107]	74	PVI ± lines/inducibility testing	18 ± 4	1.3	No	91
Wazni et al, 2005[161]	97 PAF 1 PsAF	PVI (33)	12	1	No	85
Pappone et al, 2006[162]	99 PAF	CPVA + CTI + mitral line (99)	12	1	No	85
Hocini et al, 2005[106]	90	PVI vs. PVP + roof line	15 ± 4	3 repeat ablation	No	69 vs. 87
Fassini G et al., 2005[109]	126	PVI vs. PVI + Mitral line	12	1	~50%	62 vs. 76

CPVA, circumferential pulmonary veins ablation; CPVI, circumferential pulmonary veins isolation; CTI, cavotricuspid isthmus; PAF, paroxysmal atrial fibrillation; PsAF, persistent atrial fibrillation; PVI, pulmonary vein isolation; SVC, superior vena cava.

TABLE 15-7

CATHETER ABLATION FOR PERSISTENT ATRIAL FIBRILLATION

Study	No. of Subjects	Strategy	Follow-Up (mo)	No. of Procedures	Antiarrhythmic Drug	Atrial Fibrillation Freedom (%)
O'Neill et al, 2009[105]	153	PVI + CFAE + lines ± RA ablation	34	52% repeat ablation	13	89
Della Bella et al, 2009[124]	83	Conventional ablation vs. image integration (CartoMerge, Biosense Webster)	14 ± 12	1.3*	61	69
Forleo et al, 2009[163]	19 PsAF, 16 PAF Diabetic patients	PVI + CTI ± roof and mitral lines	12	1	No	80
Neumann et al, 2008[91]	53	PVI with cryoablation	12	1	No	42
Estner et al, 2008[126]	35	PVI + CFAE	19 ± 12	1.26	No	74
Elayi et al, 2008[115]	47	CVPA	16	1	No	11
	48	PVAI	16	1	No	40
	49	PVAI + CFAE	16	1	No	61
Fiala M, 2008[111]	135	PVI + substrate	30	1.4	No	70
Yoshida et al, 2008[117]	45	PVAI	10 ± 2	1	No	49
Chen et al, 2008[125]	24	PVI + isolation of posterior wall	20 ± 4	1.2	43	75
Arentz et al, 2007[114]	43	PVI vs. large PVI	15 ± 4	1.2*	No	40 vs. 61
Verma et al, 2007[123]	80	PVAI ± anterior line	12	1	No	78 vs. 82
Seow et al, 2007[129]	53	PVI + line (roof, MI)	21.6 ± 8.8	1.5	No	62.5
Sanders et al, 2007[127]	27	PVI + posterior LA isolation	21 ± 5	1.33	63	59
Willems et al, 2006[116]	62	PVI, PVI + roof + MI	16	1	No	20, 69
Oral et al, 2006[164]	77	CPVA	12	1.26	No	74
Lim et al, 2006[118]	51	PVI	17 ± 9	1.7 ± 0.9	17	45
Calo et al, 2006[165]	80	CPVI + mitral and CTI lines ± RA ablation	14 ± 5	1	50	61 L ablation vs. 85 L + R ablation
Oral et al, 2005[128]	80	LACA vs. LA lines	9 ± 4	1.4	No	72 vs. 75
Haïssaguerre et al, 2005[122]	60	PVI + CFAE + lines	11 ± 6	1.45	12	95
Ouyang et al, 2005[120]	40	2 × 2 PVI	8 ± 2	1.35	No	95
Fassini G et al, 2005[109]	61	PVI vs. PVI + Mitral line	12	1	~50%	36 vs. 74
Cappato R et al, 2005[140]	1619	Multiple	12		No	66, 90
			24		Yes	43, 70

CFAE, complex fractionnated atrial electrogram; CPVA, circumferential pulmonary veins ablation; CPVI, circumferential pulmonary veins isolation; CTI, cavotricuspid isthmus; LA, left atrium; LACA, left atrial circumferential ablation; MI, mitral isthmus; PAF, paroxysmal atrial fibrillation; PsAF, persistent atrial fibrillation; PVAI, pulmonary veins antral isolation; PVI, pulmonary vein isolation; R, right; RA, right atrium; SVC, superior vena cava.

The benefits of AF ablation are not judged solely by the absence of arrhythmia at follow-up. Many patients with a reduction of AF burden report symptomatic improvement, demonstrate better exercise tolerance, and have higher quality-of-life scores. The subgroup of patients with heart failure represents a population in whom AF ablation is particularly beneficial, with substantial improvement in quality of life and functional class associated with significant increase in left ventricular function.[130–132]

Arrhythmia Relapses after Ablation for Atrial Fibrillation

Arrhythmia recurrences after PV isolation are mostly due to PV reconnection. When a repeat procedure is performed because of AF recurrence, 95% to 100% of patients have resumption of conduction at the PV-LA junction (Fig. 15-26).[133–137] In contrast, among the patients who remain free from arrhythmia, 81% have no PV reconnection.[137] Predictors of acute reconnection include old age, large atrial size, high blood pressure, sleep apnea, and persistent AF.[138] Reisolation of PVs can lead to AF control in most cases (reported as 86% in one study).[135] Wide area ablation can be associated with atrial flutter around the PVs or mitral annulus. In addition, right atrial cavotricuspid isthmus–dependent flutter can occur and present with atypical electrocardiogram patterns due to extensive left atrial ablation.

Complications

Mortality after catheter ablation of AF occurs in 1 per thousand procedures according to an international survey analyzing cases from 162 centers worldwide over more than 10 years, from 1995 to 2006.[139] In 2005, a similar survey reported an overall complication rate of 6% for AF ablation procedures, including a 1 in 2000 risk for procedural death, 1.2% risk for tamponade, 1% risk for stroke or transient ischemic attack, and less than 2% risk for PV stenosis, including 0.6% risk for symptomatic PV stenosis (Fig. 15-27).[140] Others have reported higher rates (up to 28%) of PV stenosis; however, severe reduction (>70% reduction in lumen) occurred in only 1% to 3% of patients.[141–144] Proximal ablation reduces the risk for PV stenosis. In the presence of severe symptomatic PV stenosis, PV stenting has been attempted with an acute angiographic success rate of 95%, and long-term patency of the PV was associated with the resolution of symptoms.[142,145] Concerning the occurrence of stroke or transient ischemic attack, it is important to maintain an adequate level of anticoagulation throughout the procedure (activated clotting time, >300 seconds) and continue anticoagulation after ablation to minimize the risk. Expert consensus suggests that warfarin be continued indefinitely in patients with a CHADS2 score of 2 or higher. It is feasible to perform the ablation without interruption of preoperative warfarin sodium therapy.

Atrioesophageal fistula is one of the most feared complications of catheter ablation and is often fatal. It is rare and has an incidence of about 0.01%,[9,146] although the exact incidence is difficult to establish. Different strategies are advocated to prevent this fatal complication, but a very low event rate makes it difficult to evaluate their efficacy. Esophageal imaging, temperature monitoring, and opacification of the esophagus with barium paste before the procedure have been used as means of avoiding injury.[147–151] It has been recently reported that the use of conscious sedation is associated with significantly less endoscopic esophageal lesions compared with general anesthesia during ablation.[152] Vascular access–related complications occur in about 0.5% of cases. Hemidiaphragmatic paralysis consequent to phrenic nerve injury occurred in 0.1% of patients in a large survey when ablation was performed with conventional RF catheters. However, the incidence of transient phrenic nerve injury is much higher when using balloon catheters, especially cryoballoon (7%). The right phrenic nerve is most vulnerable because of its proximity to the right superior PV. As previously mentioned, phrenic pacing during cryoablation of the right veins allows for rapidly interruption of ablation if capture is lost and for recovery of phrenic function in most cases.[86,88–93] Other complications, such as mitral valve damage secondary to catheter entrapment, sepsis, pneumothorax, and aortic dissection, have been reported but are rare (<0.1%).[140]

Troubleshooting the Difficult Case

Difficulties in isolating the PVs occur in certain patients, and some few frequent challenges confronting the electrophysiologist are presented next (Table 15-8).

Distinguishing between PV potential and far-field signal or left atrial electrogram can sometimes be difficult. Knowing from which part of the atria far-field signal can be recorded in a given structure helps to recognize and confirm the true nature of the recordings. Recordings from the right superior PV can detect far-field signal originating from the superior vena cava, posterior LA (in the posterior part of the vein), right inferior or right middle PV, or right atrium (in the anterior portion of the vein). Likewise, recordings from the right inferior PV can detect far-field activity from the posterior left or right atria. A signal recorded on the anterior portion of the right veins timed with the beginning of the surface P wave is strongly suggestive of right atrial far-field recording. Left-sided veins, especially the left superior, classically display far-field signals from the adjacent left atrial appendage, ipsilateral PV, left atrium, or ligament of Marshall. The observation that the recorded potential inside the vein is concomitant with the activation of an adjacent structure (e.g., superior vena cava or left atrial appendage) is suggestive of far-field signal recording. Pacing maneuvers can help confirm the nature of the recorded signal: pacing the structure from which the signal is believed to have originated will advance and synchronize far-field signals with pacing and delay local PV potentials.[153] In left-sided veins, distal coronary sinus pacing separates far field activity from PV potentials as the left atrial appendage is activated earlier and PV potentials occur later.

Some veins or fascicles can be recalcitrant to ablation. Unstable catheter contact with the atrial wall is a common cause of failure to eliminate PV potentials. Every effort

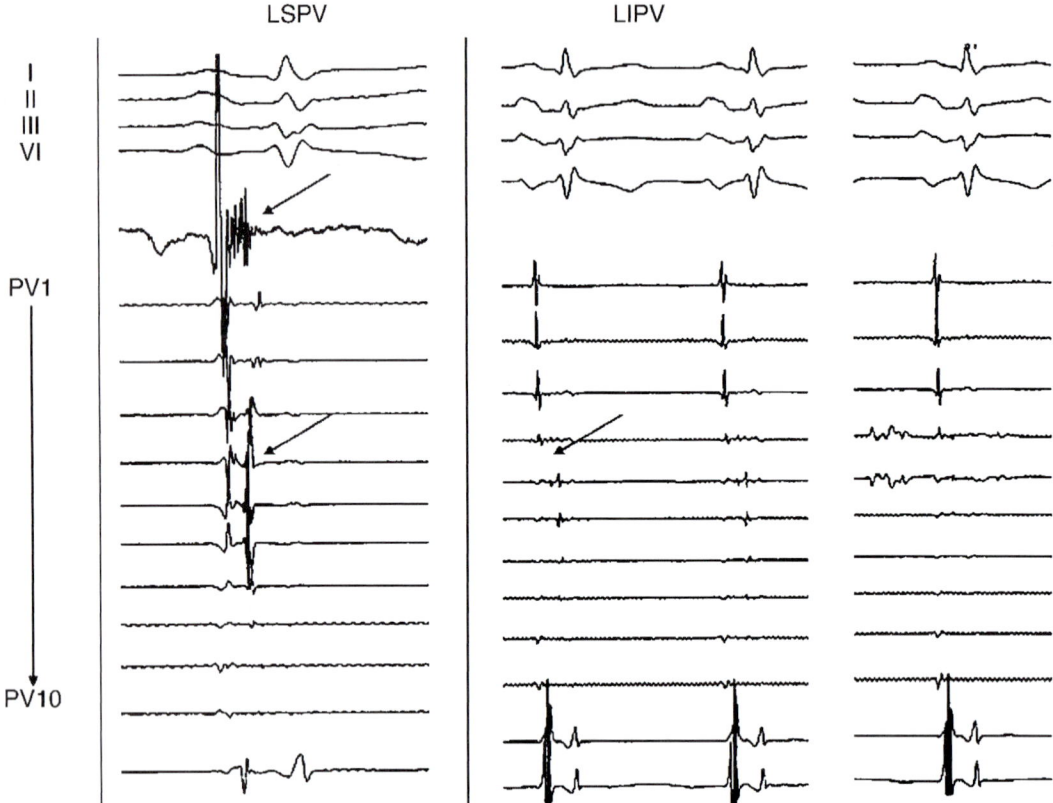

LSPV   LIPV

I
II
III
VI

PV1

PV10

FIGURE 15-26. Mapping of pulmonary veins (PV) in a patient with recurrence of atrial fibrillation (AF) 2 months after PV isolation. In this patient, both the left superior pulmonary vein (LSPV) and the left inferior pulmonary vein (LIPV) demonstrate recovery. The tracing of the LSPV demonstrates the typical appearance of PV conduction slowing, separating the far-field atrial component from the PV potential without the need for pacing the left atrial appendage. Note the continuous slowed activity detected on the ablation catheter at the site of the conduction gap *(arrows)*. A similar finding is observed in the LIPV. The *panel on the far right* demonstrates ablation at the site of gap (noise on electrograms) and the loss of PV potentials with isolation of the LIPV. Since isolation of both PVs, this patient has not had further AF.

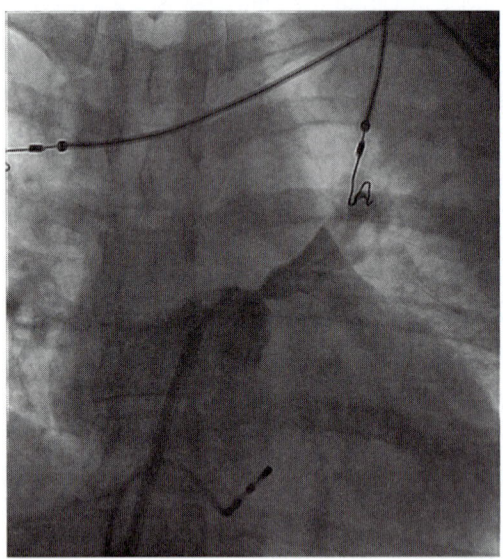

FIGURE 15-27. Angiography of the left superior pulmonary vein showing severe narrowing in a patient with previous pulmonary vein isolation for atrial fibrillation.

should be made to ensure stable contact by changing the catheter orientation or using a different sheath. It is also important to confirm that the nature of the signal recorded is PV potential. Then, if increasing power delivery does not result in isolation, it is often worthwhile to map the adjacent PV because, as previously mentioned, the upper and lower PVs often share common fascicles, and ablation in one vein can lead to isolation of both ipsilateral veins. If the catheter is unstable or unable to reach certain areas, the use of a steerable sheath, visualization of the catheter using ICE or a 3D mapping system, or the use of robotic or magnetic remote navigation systems may help achieve the end point. Ablation at more distal sites within the PV with focal cryoablation may achieve PV isolation when RF fails.[91]

Patients with persistent AF despite PV isolation may benefit from additional left atrial ablation to restore SR (see Chapters 17 and 18). Finally, in cases in which acute PV reconnection is observed during the index procedure, reisolation is necessary to prevent recurrences. Reassessment of PV isolation after 30 minutes of waiting allows for detection of reconnection in more patients. Adenosine infusion can also detect dormant PV-LA conduction. Repeat ablation at areas of reconnection is associated with a better long-term outcome.[103]

Conclusion

The PVs play a central role in the genesis of AF. PV isolation can be achieved in all patients and leads to atrial arrhythmia suppression in 80% to 85% of patients with

TABLE 15-8

TROUBLESHOOTING THE DIFFICULT CASE

Problem	Causes	Solutions
Difficult to identify pulmonary vein (PV) potentials	Fusion with atrial electrogram	Differential pacing from coronary sinus, atrium, or appendage
	Prominent far-field electrogram	Differential pacing
	Intractable atrial fibrillation	Perform ablation in atrial fibrillation and cardiovert, use ibutilide, etc., to maintain sinus rhythm, confirm end points in sinus/atrial pacing
PV potentials persist after ablation	Broad/thick PV connection	Prolonged RF delivery, improve catheter contact/orientation, segmental ablation at os, distal ablation with cryocatheter
	Connection inserts into contiguous PV	Map/ablate contiguous PV
	Far-field electrogram	Differential pacing to identify true PV potentials
Unstable catheter positions	Unfavorable PV anatomy	Visualize catheters with intracardiac echocardiography or mapping system, use steerable sheath
Recurrent atrial fibrillation after PV isolation	Non-PV triggers	Map and ablate all triggers
	Arrhythmogenic atrial substrate	Substrate modification with linear lesions or target dominant frequency sources

paroxysmal AF and about 50% of patients with persistent AF. It is an essential first step in all the catheter ablation strategies for AF. The need for further ablation beyond the PVs is frequent in patients suffering from persistent AF. In patients with paroxysmal AF, electrical isolation of the PVs is a required end point, but the need for further substrate modification, with further end points such as inducibility testing, is not yet clear. Active research in the field will bring answers to resolve the debates, and technologic innovations will help to achieve more efficient, widely accessible, and safer procedures in the future.

References

1. Kannel WB, Abbott RD, Savage DD, et al. Epidemiologic features of chronic atrial fibrillation: the Framingham study. *N Engl J Med.* 1982;306:1018–1022.
2. Grogan M, Smith HC, Gersh BJ, et al. Left ventricular dysfunction due to atrial fibrillation in patients initially believed to have idiopathic dilated cardiomyopathy. *Am J Cardiol.* 1992;69:1570–1573.
3. Wolf PA, Abbott RD, Kannel WB. Atrial fibrillation as an independent risk factor for stroke: the Framingham Study. *Stroke.* 1991;22:983–988.
4. Benjamin EJ, Wolf PA, D'Agostino RB, et al. Impact of atrial fibrillation on the risk of death: the Framingham Heart Study. *Circulation.* 1998;98:946–952.
5. Wyse DG, Waldo AL, DiMarco JP, et al. A comparison of rate control and rhythm control in patients with atrial fibrillation. *N Engl J Med.* 2002;347:1825–1833.
6. Roy D, Talajic M, Nattel S, et al. Rhythm control versus rate control for atrial fibrillation and heart failure. *N Engl J Med.* 2008;358:2667–2677.
7. Van Gelder IC, Hagens VE, Bosker HA, et al. A comparison of rate control and rhythm control in patients with recurrent persistent atrial fibrillation. *N Engl J Med.* 2002;347:1834–1840.
8. Hohnloser SH, Kuck KH, Lilienthal J. Rhythm or rate control in atrial fibrillation. Pharmacological Intervention in Atrial Fibrillation (PIAF): a randomised trial. *Lancet.* 2000;356:1789–1794.
9. Corley SD, Epstein AE, DiMarco JP, et al. Relationships between sinus rhythm, treatment, and survival in the Atrial Fibrillation Follow-Up Investigation of Rhythm Management (AFFIRM) Study. *Circulation.* 2004;109:1509–1513.
10. Hoffmann E, Sulke N, Edvardsson N, et al. New insights into the initiation of atrial fibrillation: a detailed intraindividual and interindividual analysis of the spontaneous onset of atrial fibrillation using new diagnostic pacemaker features. *Circulation.* 2006;113:1933–1941.
11. Jideus L, Kesek M, Joachimsson PO, et al. The role of premature atrial contractions as the main triggers of postoperative atrial fibrillation. *J Electrocardiol.* 2006;39:48–54.
12. Haïssaguerre M, Jais P, Shah DC, et al. Spontaneous initiation of atrial fibrillation by ectopic beats originating in the pulmonary veins. *N Engl J Med.* 1998;339:659–666.
13. Chen SA, Hsieh MH, Tai CT, et al. Initiation of atrial fibrillation by ectopic beats originating from the pulmonary veins: electrophysiological characteristics, pharmacological responses, and effects of radiofrequency ablation. *Circulation.* 1999;100:1879–1886.
14. Valles E, Fan R, Roux JF, et al. Localization of atrial fibrillation triggers in patients undergoing pulmonary vein isolation: importance of the carina region. *J Am Coll Cardiol.* 2008;52:1413–1420.
15. Hocini M, Haïssaguerre M, Shah D, et al. Multiple sources initiating atrial fibrillation from a single pulmonary vein identified by a circumferential catheter. *Pacing Clin Electrophysiol.* 2000;23:1828–1831.
16. Haïssaguerre M, Jais P, Shah DC, et al. Electrophysiological end point for catheter ablation of atrial fibrillation initiated from multiple pulmonary venous foci. *Circulation.* 2000;101:1409–1417.
17. Ouyang F, Bansch D, Ernst S, et al. Complete isolation of left atrium surrounding the pulmonary veins: new insights from the double-Lasso technique in paroxysmal atrial fibrillation. *Circulation.* 2004;110:2090–2096.
18. Weerasooriya R, Jais P, Scavee C, et al. Dissociated pulmonary vein arrhythmia: incidence and characteristics. *J Cardiovasc Electrophysiol.* 2003;14:1173–1179.
19. Jais P, Haïssaguerre M, Shah DC, et al. A focal source of atrial fibrillation treated by discrete radiofrequency ablation. *Circulation.* 1997;95:572–576.
20. Kumagai K, Yasuda T, Tojo H, et al. Role of rapid focal activation in the maintenance of atrial fibrillation originating from the pulmonary veins. *Pacing Clin Electrophysiol.* 2000;23:1823–1827.
21. O'Donnell D, Furniss SS, Bourke JP. Paroxysmal cycle length shortening in the pulmonary veins during atrial fibrillation correlates with arrhythmogenic triggering foci in sinus rhythm. *J Cardiovasc Electrophysiol.* 2002;13:124–128.
22. Oral H, Ozaydin M, Tada H, et al. Mechanistic significance of intermittent pulmonary vein tachycardia in patients with atrial fibrillation. *J Cardiovasc Electrophysiol.* 2002;13:645–650.
23. Nault I, Wright M, Hocini M, et al. Extreme firing in a pulmonary vein during atrial fibrillation. *J Cardiovasc Electrophysiol.* 2008;9:1236–1241.
24. Haïssaguerre M, Sanders P, Hocini M, et al. Changes in atrial fibrillation cycle length and inducibility during catheter ablation and their relation to outcome. *Circulation.* 2004;109:3007–3013.
25. Haïssaguerre M, Sanders P, Hocini M, et al. Pulmonary veins in the substrate for atrial fibrillation: the "venous wave" hypothesis. *J Am Coll Cardiol.* 2004;43:2290–2292.
26. Sanders P, Berenfeld O, Hocini M, et al. Spectral analysis identifies sites of high-frequency activity maintaining atrial fibrillation in humans. *Circulation.* 2005;112:789–797.
27. Ho SY, Sanchez-Quintana D, Cabrera JA, et al. Anatomy of the left atrium: implications for radiofrequency ablation of atrial fibrillation. *J Cardiovasc Electrophysiol.* 1999;10:1525–1533.
28. Nathan H, Eliakim M. The junction between the left atrium and the pulmonary veins: an anatomic study of human hearts. *Circulation.* 1966;34:412–422.
29. Ho SY, Cabrera JA, Tran VH, et al. Architecture of the pulmonary veins: relevance to radiofrequency ablation. *Heart.* 2001;86:265–270.
30. Yamane T, Shah DC, Jais P, et al. Dilatation as a marker of pulmonary veins initiating atrial fibrillation. *J Interv Card Electrophysiol.* 2002;6:245–249.
31. Hassink RJ, Aretz HT, Ruskin J, et al. Morphology of atrial myocardium in human pulmonary veins: a postmortem analysis in patients with and without atrial fibrillation. *J Am Coll Cardiol.* 2003;42:1108–1114.
32. Lin WS, Prakash VS, Tai CT, et al. Pulmonary vein morphology in patients with paroxysmal atrial fibrillation initiated by ectopic beats originating from the pulmonary veins: implications for catheter ablation. *Circulation.* 2000;101:1274–1281.
33. Tsao HM, Yu WC, Cheng HC, et al. Pulmonary vein dilation in patients with atrial fibrillation: detection by magnetic resonance imaging. *J Cardiovasc Electrophysiol.* 2001;12:809–813.
34. Hocini M, Ho SY, Kawara T, et al. Electrical conduction in canine pulmonary veins: electrophysiological and anatomic correlation. *Circulation.* 2002;105:2442–2448.
35. Hamabe A, Okuyama Y, Miyauchi Y, et al. Correlation between anatomy and electrical activation in canine pulmonary veins. *Circulation.* 2003;107:1550–1555.

36. Arora R, Verheule S, Scott L, et al. Arrhythmogenic substrate of the pulmonary veins assessed by high-resolution optical mapping. *Circulation.* 2003;107:1816–1821.

37. Po SS, Li Y, Tang D, et al. Rapid and stable re-entry within the pulmonary vein as a mechanism initiating paroxysmal atrial fibrillation. *J Am Coll Cardiol.* 2005;45:1871–1877.

38. Chen YJ, Chen SA, Chang MS, et al. Arrhythmogenic activity of cardiac muscle in pulmonary veins of the dog: implication for the genesis of atrial fibrillation. *Cardiovasc Res.* 2000;48:265–273.

39. Chen YJ, Chen SA, Chen YC, et al. Effects of rapid atrial pacing on the arrhythmogenic activity of single cardiomyocytes from pulmonary veins: implication in initiation of atrial fibrillation. *Circulation.* 2001;104:2849–2854.

40. Cherry EM, Ehrlich JR, Nattel S, et al. Pulmonary vein reentry—properties and size matter: insights from a computational analysis. *Heart Rhythm.* 2007;4:1553–1562.

41. Jais P, Hocini M, Macle L, et al. Distinctive electrophysiological properties of pulmonary veins in patients with atrial fibrillation. *Circulation.* 2002;106:2479–2485.

42. Kumagai K, Ogawa M, Noguchi H, et al. Electrophysiologic properties of pulmonary veins assessed using a multielectrode basket catheter. *J Am Coll Cardiol.* 2004;43:2281–2289.

43. Drewitz I, Steven D, Lutomsky B, et al. Persistent, isolated pulmonary vein re-entry: inducibility, entrainment, and overdrive termination of a sustained tachycardia within an isolated pulmonary vein. *Europace.* 2008;10:261–264.

44. Rostock T, O'Neill MD, Takahashi Y, et al. Interactions between two simultaneous tachycardias within an electrically isolated pulmonary vein. *J Cardiovasc Electrophysiol.* 2007;18:441–445.

45. Arentz T, Haegeli L, Sanders P, et al. High-density mapping of spontaneous pulmonary vein activity initiating atrial fibrillation in humans. *J Cardiovasc Electrophysiol.* 2007;18:31–38.

46. Fuster V, Ryden LE, Cannom DS, et al. ACC/AHA/ESC 2006 Guidelines for the Management of Patients with Atrial Fibrillation: a report of the American College of Cardiology/American Heart Association Task Force on Practice Guidelines and the European Society of Cardiology Committee for Practice Guidelines (Writing Committee to Revise the 2001 Guidelines for the Management of Patients With Atrial Fibrillation). Developed in collaboration with the European Heart Rhythm Association and the Heart Rhythm Society. *Circulation.* 2006;114:e257–e354.

47. Calkins H, Brugada J, Packer DL, et al. HRS/EHRA/ECAS expert consensus statement on catheter and surgical ablation of atrial fibrillation: recommendations for personnel, policy, procedures and follow-up. A report of the Heart Rhythm Society (HRS) Task Force on Catheter and Surgical Ablation of Atrial Fibrillation developed in partnership with the European Heart Rhythm Association (EHRA) and the European Cardiac Arrhythmia Society (ECAS); in collaboration with the American College of Cardiology (ACC), American Heart Association (AHA), and the Society of Thoracic Surgeons (STS). Endorsed and approved by the governing bodies of the American College of Cardiology, the American Heart Association, the European Cardiac Arrhythmia Society, the European Heart Rhythm Association, the Society of Thoracic Surgeons, and the Heart Rhythm Society. *Europace.* 2007;9:335–379.

48. Matsuo S, Lellouche N, Wright M, et al. Clinical predictors of termination and clinical outcome of catheter ablation for persistent atrial fibrillation. *J Am Coll Cardiol.* 2009;54:788–795.

49. Haïssaguerre M, Jais P, Shah DC, et al. Catheter ablation of chronic atrial fibrillation targeting the reinitiating triggers. *J Cardiovasc Electrophysiol.* 2000;11:2–10.

50. Robbins IM, Colvin EV, Doyle TP, et al. Pulmonary vein stenosis after catheter ablation of atrial fibrillation. *Circulation.* 1998;98:1769–1775.

51. Yu WC, Hsu TL, Tai CT, et al. Acquired pulmonary vein stenosis after radiofrequency catheter ablation of paroxysmal atrial fibrillation. *J Cardiovasc Electrophysiol.* 2001;12:887–892.

52. Oral H, Chugh A, Scharf C, et al. Incremental value of isolating the right inferior pulmonary vein during pulmonary vein isolation procedures in patients with paroxysmal atrial fibrillation. *Pacing Clin Electrophysiol.* 2004;27:480–484.

53. Oral H, Knight BP, Tada H, et al. Pulmonary vein isolation for paroxysmal and persistent atrial fibrillation. *Circulation.* 2002;105:1077–1081.

54. Haïssaguerre M, Shah DC, Jais P, et al. Electrophysiological breakthroughs from the left atrium to the pulmonary veins. *Circulation.* 2000;102:2463–2465.

55. Marrouche NF, Martin DO, Wazni O, et al. Phased-array intracardiac echocardiography monitoring during pulmonary vein isolation in patients with atrial fibrillation: impact on outcome and complications. *Circulation.* 2003;107:2710–2716.

56. Hocini M, Sanders P, Jais P, et al. Prevalence of pulmonary vein disconnection after anatomical ablation for atrial fibrillation: consequences of wide atrial encircling of the pulmonary veins. *Eur Heart J.* 2005;26:696–704.

57. Estner HL, Deisenhofer I, Luik A, et al. Electrical isolation of pulmonary veins in patients with atrial fibrillation: reduction of fluoroscopy exposure and procedure duration by the use of a non-fluoroscopic navigation system (NavX). *Europace.* 2006;8:583–587.

58. Pappone C, Oreto G, Lamberti F, et al. Catheter ablation of paroxysmal atrial fibrillation using a 3D mapping system. *Circulation.* 1999;100:1203–1208.

59. Pappone C, Rosanio S, Oreto G, et al. Circumferential radiofrequency ablation of pulmonary vein ostia: a new anatomic approach for curing atrial fibrillation. *Circulation.* 2000;102:2619–2628.

60. Kistler PM, Earley MJ, Harris S, et al. Validation of three-dimensional cardiac image integration: use of integrated CT image into electroanatomic mapping system to perform catheter ablation of atrial fibrillation. *J Cardiovasc Electrophysiol.* 2006;17:341–348.

61. Kettering K, Greil GF, Fenchel M, et al. Catheter ablation of atrial fibrillation using the NavX-/EnSite-system and a CT-/MRI-guided approach. *Clin Res Cardiol.* 2009;98:285–296.

62. Richmond L, Rajappan K, Voth E, et al. Validation of computed tomography image integration into the EnSite NavX mapping system to perform catheter ablation of atrial fibrillation. *J Cardiovasc Electrophysiol.* 2008;19:821–827.

63. Dragusin O, Weerasooriya R, Jais P, et al. Evaluation of a radiation protection cabin for invasive electrophysiological procedures. *Eur Heart J.* 2007;28:183–189.

64. Knecht S, Skali H, O'Neill MD, et al. Computed tomography-fluoroscopy overlay evaluation during catheter ablation of left atrial arrhythmia. *Europace.* 2008;10:931–938.

65. Kriatselis C, Tang M, Nedios S, et al. Intraprocedural reconstruction of the left atrium and pulmonary veins as a single navigation tool for ablation of atrial fibrillation: a feasibility, efficacy, and safety study. *Heart Rhythm.* 2009;6:733–741.

66. Li JH, Haim M, Movassaghi B, et al. Segmentation and registration of three-dimensional rotational angiogram on live fluoroscopy to guide atrial fibrillation ablation: a new online imaging tool. *Heart Rhythm.* 2009;6:231–237.

67. Bertaglia E, Bella PD, Tondo C, et al. Image integration increases efficacy of paroxysmal atrial fibrillation catheter ablation: results from the CartoMerge Italian Registry. *Europace.* 2009;11:1004–1010.

68. Katsiyiannis WT, Melby DP, Matelski JL, et al. Feasibility and safety of remote-controlled magnetic navigation for ablation of atrial fibrillation. *Am J Cardiol.* 2008;102:1674–1676.

69. Di Biase L, Fahmy TS, Patel D, et al. Remote magnetic navigation: human experience in pulmonary vein ablation. *J Am Coll Cardiol.* 2007;50:868–874.

70. Pappone C, Vicedomini G, Manguso F, et al. Robotic magnetic navigation for atrial fibrillation ablation. *J Am Coll Cardiol.* 2006;47:1390–1400.

71. Kautzner J, Peichl P, Cihak R, et al. Early experience with robotic navigation for catheter ablation of paroxysmal atrial fibrillation. *Pacing Clin Electrophysiol.* 2009;32(suppl 1):S163–S166.

72. Saliba W, Reddy VY, Wazni O, et al. Atrial fibrillation ablation using a robotic catheter remote control system: initial human experience and long-term follow-up results. *J Am Coll Cardiol.* 2008;51:2407–2411.

73. Davis DR, Tang AS, Gollob MH, et al. Remote magnetic navigation-assisted catheter ablation enhances catheter stability and ablation success with lower catheter temperatures. *Pacing Clin Electrophysiol.* 2008;31:893–898.

74. Kim AM, Turakhia M, Lu J, et al. Impact of remote magnetic catheter navigation on ablation fluoroscopy and procedure time. *Pacing Clin Electrophysiol.* 2008;31:1399–1404.

75. Macle L, Jais P, Weerasooriya R, et al. Irrigated-tip catheter ablation of pulmonary veins for treatment of atrial fibrillation. *J Cardiovasc Electrophysiol.* 2002;13:1067–1073.

76. Arruda MS, He DS, Friedman P, et al. A novel mesh electrode catheter for mapping and radiofrequency delivery at the left atrium-pulmonary vein junction: a single-catheter approach to pulmonary vein antrum isolation. *J Cardiovasc Electrophysiol.* 2007;18:206–211.

77. Mansour M, Forleo GB, Pappalardo A, et al. Initial experience with the mesh catheter for pulmonary vein isolation in patients with paroxysmal atrial fibrillation. *Heart Rhythm.* 2008;5:1510–1516.

78. Meissner A, Plehn G, Van Bracht M, et al. First experiences for pulmonary vein isolation with the high-density mesh ablator (HDMA): a novel mesh electrode catheter for both mapping and radiofrequency delivery in a single unit. *J Cardiovasc Electrophysiol.* 2009;20:359–366.

79. Pratola C, Notarstefano P, Artale P, et al. Paroxysmal atrial fibrillation ablation with the multipolar mapping and ablation catheter (Mesh-Bard). *Pacing Clin Electrophysiol.* 2008;31:753–756.

80. Pratola C, Notarstefano P, Artale P, et al. Radiofrequency ablation of paroxysmal atrial fibrillation by mesh catheter. *J Interv Card Electrophysiol.* 2009;25:135–140.

81. Steinwender C, Honig S, Leisch F, et al. Acute results of pulmonary vein isolation in patients with paroxysmal atrial fibrillation using a single mesh catheter. *J Cardiovasc Electrophysiol.* 2009;20:147–152.

82. De Filippo P, He DS, Brambilla R, et al. Clinical experience with a single catheter for mapping and ablation of pulmonary vein ostium. *J Cardiovasc Electrophysiol.* 2009;20:367–373.

83. Wijffels MC, Van Oosternhout M, Boersma LV, et al. Characterization of in vitro and in vivo lesions made by a novel multichannel ablation generator and a circumlinear decapolar ablation catheter. *J Cardiovasc Electrophysiol.* 2009;20:1142–1148.

84. Fredersdorf S, Weber S, Jilek C, et al. Safe and rapid isolation of pulmonary veins using a novel circular ablation catheter and duty-cycled RF generator. *J Cardiovasc Electrophysiol.* 2009;20:1097–1101.

85. Boersma LV, Wijffels MC, Oral H, et al. Pulmonary vein isolation by duty-cycled bipolar and unipolar radiofrequency energy with a multielectrode ablation catheter. *Heart Rhythm.* 2008;5:1635–1642.

86. Siklody CH, Minners J, Allgeier M, et al. Cryoballoon pulmonary vein isolation guided by transesophageal echocardiography: novel aspects on an emerging ablation technique. *J Cardiovasc Electrophysiol.* 2009;20:1197–1202.

87. Chun KR, Schmidt B, Metzner A, et al. The 'single big cryoballoon' technique for acute pulmonary vein isolation in patients with paroxysmal atrial fibrillation: a prospective observational single centre study. *Eur Heart J.* 2009;30:699–709.

88. Klein G, Oswald H, Gardiwal A, et al. Efficacy of pulmonary vein isolation by cryoballoon ablation in patients with paroxysmal atrial fibrillation. *Heart Rhythm.* 2008;5:802–806.
89. Malmborg H, Lonnerholm S, Blomstrom-Lundqvist C. Acute and clinical effects of cryoballoon pulmonary vein isolation in patients with symptomatic paroxysmal and persistent atrial fibrillation. *Europace.* 2008;10:1277–1280.
90. Moreira W, Manusama R, Timmermans C, et al. Long-term follow-up after cryothermic ostial pulmonary vein isolation in paroxysmal atrial fibrillation. *J Am Coll Cardiol.* 2008;51:850–855.
91. Neumann T, Vogt J, Schumacher B, et al. Circumferential pulmonary vein isolation with the cryoballoon technique results from a prospective 3-center study. *J Am Coll Cardiol.* 2008;52:273–278.
92. Van Belle Y, Janse P, Rivero-Ayerza MJ, et al. Pulmonary vein isolation using an occluding cryoballoon for circumferential ablation: feasibility, complications, and short-term outcome. *Eur Heart J.* 2007;28:2231–2237.
93. Van Belle Y, Janse P, Theuns D, et al. One year follow-up after cryoballoon isolation of the pulmonary veins in patients with paroxysmal atrial fibrillation. *Europace.* 2008;10:1271–1276.
94. Schmidt B, Antz M, Ernst S, et al. Pulmonary vein isolation by high-intensity focused ultrasound: first-in-man study with a steerable balloon catheter. *Heart Rhythm.* 2007;4:575–584.
95. Fried NM, Tsitlik A, Rent KC, et al. Laser ablation of the pulmonary veins by using a fiberoptic balloon catheter: implications for treatment of paroxysmal atrial fibrillation. *Lasers Surg Med.* 2001;28:197–203.
96. Lemery R, Veinot JP, Tang AS, et al. Fiberoptic balloon catheter ablation of pulmonary vein ostia in pigs using photonic energy delivery with Diode laser. *Pacing Clin Electrophysiol.* 2002;25:32–36.
97. Reddy VY, Houghtaling C, Fallon J, et al. Use of a diode laser balloon ablation catheter to generate circumferential pulmonary venous lesions in an open-thoracotomy caprine model. *Pacing Clin Electrophysiol.* 2004;27:52–57.
98. Reddy VY, Neuzil P, Themistoclakis S, et al. Visually-guided balloon catheter ablation of atrial fibrillation: experimental feasibility and first-in-human multicenter clinical outcome. *Circulation.* 2009;120:12–20.
99. Reddy VY, Neuzil P, d'Avila A, et al. Balloon catheter ablation to treat paroxysmal atrial fibrillation: what is the level of pulmonary venous isolation? *Heart Rhythm.* 2008;5:353–360.
100. Phillips KP, Schweikert RA, Saliba WI, et al. Anatomic location of pulmonary vein electrical disconnection with balloon-based catheter ablation. *J Cardiovasc Electrophysiol.* 2008;19:14–18.
101. Natale A, Raviele A, Arentz T, et al. Venice Chart international consensus document on atrial fibrillation ablation. *J Cardiovasc Electrophysiol.* 2007;18:560–580.
102. Hachiya H, Hirao K, Takahashi A, et al. Clinical implications of reconnection between the left atrium and isolated pulmonary veins provoked by adenosine triphosphate after extensive encircling pulmonary vein isolation. *J Cardiovasc Electrophysiol.* 2007;18:392–398.
103. Matsuo S, Yamane T, Date T, et al. Reduction of AF recurrence after pulmonary vein isolation by eliminating ATP-induced transient venous re-conduction. *J Cardiovasc Electrophysiol.* 2007;18:704–708.
104. Jiang CY, Jiang RH, Matsuo S, et al. Early detection of pulmonary vein reconnection after isolation in patients with paroxysmal atrial fibrillation: a comparison of ATP-induction and reassessment at 30 minutes postisolation. *J Cardiovasc Electrophysiol.* 2009;20:1382–1387.
105. O'Neill MD, Wright M, Knecht S, et al. Long-term follow-up of persistent atrial fibrillation ablation using termination as a procedural endpoint. *Eur Heart J.* 2009;30:1105–1112.
106. Hocini M, Jais P, Sanders P, et al. Techniques, evaluation, and consequences of linear block at the left atrial roof in paroxysmal atrial fibrillation: a prospective randomized study. *Circulation.* 2005;112:3688–3696.
107. Jais P, Hocini M, Sanders P, et al. Long-term evaluation of atrial fibrillation ablation guided by noninducibility. *Heart Rhythm.* 2006;3:140–145.
108. Sheikh I, Krum D, Cooley R, et al. Pulmonary vein isolation and linear lesions in atrial fibrillation ablation. *J Interv Card Electrophysiol.* 2006;17:103–109.
109. Fassini G, Riva S, Chiodelli R, et al. Left mitral isthmus ablation associated with PV Isolation: long-term results of a prospective randomized study. *J Cardiovasc Electrophysiol.* 2005;16:1150–1156.
110. Jais P, Cauchemez B, Macle L, et al. Catheter ablation versus antiarrhythmic drugs for atrial fibrillation: the A4 study. *Circulation.* 2008;118:2498–2505.
111. Fiala M, Chovancik J, Nevralova R, et al. Termination of long-lasting persistent versus short-lasting persistent and paroxysmal atrial fibrillation by ablation. *Pacing Clin Electrophysiol.* 2008;31:985–997.
112. Chang SL, Tai CT, Lin YJ, et al. The efficacy of inducibility and circumferential ablation with pulmonary vein isolation in patients with paroxysmal atrial fibrillation. *J Cardiovasc Electrophysiol.* 2007;18:607–611.
113. Arentz T, von Rosenthal J, Blum T, et al. Feasibility and safety of pulmonary vein isolation using a new mapping and navigation system in patients with refractory atrial fibrillation. *Circulation.* 2003;108:2484–2490.
114. Arentz T, Weber R, Burkle G, et al. Small or large isolation areas around the pulmonary veins for the treatment of atrial fibrillation? Results from a prospective randomized study. *Circulation.* 2007;115:3057–3063.
115. Elayi CS, Verma A, Di Biase L, et al. Ablation for longstanding permanent atrial fibrillation: results from a randomized study comparing three different strategies. *Heart Rhythm.* 2008;5:1658–1664.
116. Willems S, Klemm H, Rostock T, et al. Substrate modification combined with pulmonary vein isolation improves outcome of catheter ablation in patients

117. Yoshida K, Ulfarsson M, Tada H, et al. Complex electrograms within the coronary sinus: time- and frequency-domain characteristics, effects of antral pulmonary vein isolation, and relationship to clinical outcome in patients with paroxysmal and persistent atrial fibrillation. *J Cardiovasc Electrophysiol.* 2008;19:1017–1023.
118. Lim TW, Jassal IS, Ross DL, et al. Medium-term efficacy of segmental ostial pulmonary vein isolation for the treatment of permanent and persistent atrial fibrillation. *Pacing Clin Electrophysiol.* 2006;29:374–379.
119. Chen MS, Marrouche NF, Khaykin Y, et al. Pulmonary vein isolation for the treatment of atrial fibrillation in patients with impaired systolic function. *J Am Coll Cardiol.* 2004;43:1004–1009.
120. Ouyang F, Ernst S, Chun J, et al. Electrophysiological findings during ablation of persistent atrial fibrillation with electroanatomic mapping and double lasso catheter technique. *Circulation.* 2005;112:3038–3048.
121. Haïssaguerre M, Sanders P, Hocini M, et al. Catheter ablation of long-lasting persistent atrial fibrillation: critical structures for termination. *J Cardiovasc Electrophysiol.* 2005;16:1125–1137.
122. Haïssaguerre M, Hocini M, Sanders P, et al. Catheter ablation of long-lasting persistent atrial fibrillation: clinical outcome and mechanisms of subsequent arrhythmias. *J Cardiovasc Electrophysiol.* 2005;16:1138–1147.
123. Verma A, Patel D, Famy T, et al. Efficacy of adjuvant anterior left atrial ablation during intracardiac echocardiography-guided pulmonary vein antrum isolation for atrial fibrillation. *J Cardiovasc Electrophysiol.* 2007;18:151–156.
124. Della Bella P, Fassini G, Cireddu M, et al. Image integration-guided catheter ablation of atrial fibrillation: a prospective randomized study. *J Cardiovasc Electrophysiol.* 2009;20:258–265.
125. Chen J, Off MK, Solheim E, et al. Treatment of atrial fibrillation by silencing electrical activity in the posterior inter-pulmonary-vein atrium. *Europace.* 2008;10:265–272.
126. Estner HL, Hessling G, Ndrepepa G, et al. Acute effects and long-term outcome of pulmonary vein isolation in combination with electrogram-guided substrate ablation for persistent atrial fibrillation. *Am J Cardiol.* 2008;101:332–337.
127. Sanders P, Hocini M, Jais P, et al. Complete isolation of the pulmonary veins and posterior left atrium in chronic atrial fibrillation: long-term clinical outcome. *Eur Heart J.* 2007;28:1862–1871.
128. Oral H, Chugh A, Good E, et al. Randomized comparison of encircling and nonencircling left atrial ablation for chronic atrial fibrillation. *Heart Rhythm.* 2005;2:1165–1172.
129. Seow SC, Lim TW, Koay CH, et al. Efficacy and late recurrences with wide electrical pulmonary vein isolation for persistent and permanent atrial fibrillation. *Europace.* 2007;9:1129–1133.
130. Gentlesk PJ, Sauer WH, Gerstenfeld EP, et al. Reversal of left ventricular dysfunction following ablation of atrial fibrillation. *J Cardiovasc Electrophysiol.* 2007;18:9–14.
131. Hsu LF, Jais P, Sanders P, et al. Catheter ablation for atrial fibrillation in congestive heart failure. *N Engl J Med.* 2004;351:2373–2383.
132. Khan MN, Jais P, Cummings J, et al. Pulmonary-vein isolation for atrial fibrillation in patients with heart failure. *N Engl J Med.* 2008;359:1778–1785.
133. Rajappan K, Kistler PM, Earley MJ, et al. Acute and chronic pulmonary vein reconnection after atrial fibrillation ablation: a prospective characterization of anatomical sites. *Pacing Clin Electrophysiol.* 2008;31:1598–1605.
134. Lo LW, Tai CT, Lin YJ, et al. Characteristics and outcome in patients receiving multiple (more than two) catheter ablation procedures for paroxysmal atrial fibrillation. *J Cardiovasc Electrophysiol.* 2008;19:150–156.
135. Callans DJ, Gerstenfeld EP, Dixit S, et al. Efficacy of repeat pulmonary vein isolation procedures in patients with recurrent atrial fibrillation. *J Cardiovasc Electrophysiol.* 2004;15:1050–1055.
136. Shah AN, Mittal S, Sichrovsky TC, et al. Long-term outcome following successful pulmonary vein isolation: pattern and prediction of very late recurrence. *J Cardiovasc Electrophysiol.* 2008;19:661–667.
137. Verma A, Kilicaslan F, Pisano E, et al. Response of atrial fibrillation to pulmonary vein antrum isolation is directly related to resumption and delay of pulmonary vein conduction. *Circulation.* 2005;112:627–635.
138. Sauer WH, McKernan ML, Lin D, et al. Clinical predictors and outcomes associated with acute return of pulmonary vein conduction during pulmonary vein isolation for treatment of atrial fibrillation. *Heart Rhythm.* 2006;3:1024–1028.
139. Cappato R, Calkins H, Chen SA, et al. Prevalence and causes of fatal outcome in catheter ablation of atrial fibrillation. *J Am Coll Cardiol.* 2009;53:1798–1803.
140. Cappato R, Calkins H, Chen SA, et al. Worldwide survey on the methods, efficacy, and safety of catheter ablation for human atrial fibrillation. *Circulation.* 2005;111:1100–1105.
141. Dixit S, Marchlinski FE. How to recognize, manage, and prevent complications during atrial fibrillation ablation. *Heart Rhythm.* 2007;4:108–115.
142. Prieto LR, Schoenhagen P, Arruda MJ, et al. Comparison of stent versus balloon angioplasty for pulmonary vein stenosis complicating pulmonary vein isolation. *J Cardiovasc Electrophysiol.* 2008;19:673–678.
143. Arentz T, Jander N, von Rosenthal J, et al. Incidence of pulmonary vein stenosis 2 years after radiofrequency catheter ablation of refractory atrial fibrillation. *Eur Heart J.* 2003;24:963–969.

144. Dill T, Neumann T, Ekinci O, et al. Pulmonary vein diameter reduction after radiofrequency catheter ablation for paroxysmal atrial fibrillation evaluated by contrast-enhanced three-dimensional magnetic resonance imaging. *Circulation.* 2003;107:845–850.

145. Qureshi AM, Prieto LR, Latson LA, et al. Transcatheter angioplasty for acquired pulmonary vein stenosis after radiofrequency ablation. *Circulation.* 2003;108:1336–1342.

146. Doll N, Borger MA, Fabricius A, et al. Esophageal perforation during left atrial radiofrequency ablation: is the risk too high? *J Thorac Cardiovasc Surg.* 2003;125:836–842.

147. Ren JF, Lin D, Marchlinski FE, et al. Esophageal imaging and strategies for avoiding injury during left atrial ablation for atrial fibrillation. *Heart Rhythm.* 2006;3:1156–1161.

148. Kuwahara T, Takahashi A, Kobori A, et al. Safe and effective ablation of atrial fibrillation: importance of esophageal temperature monitoring to avoid periesophageal nerve injury as a complication of pulmonary vein isolation. *J Cardiovasc Electrophysiol.* 2009;20:1–6.

149. Kobza R, Schoenenberger AW, Erne P. Esophagus imaging for catheter ablation of atrial fibrillation: comparison of two methods with showing of esophageal movement. *J Interv Card Electrophysiol.* 2009;26:159–164.

150. Good E, Oral H, Lemola K, et al. Movement of the esophagus during left atrial catheter ablation for atrial fibrillation. *J Am Coll Cardiol.* 2005;46:2107–2110.

151. Helms A, West JJ, Patel A, et al. Real-time rotational ICE imaging of the relationship of the ablation catheter tip and the esophagus during atrial fibrillation ablation. *J Cardiovasc Electrophysiol.* 2009;20:130–137.

152. Biase L, Burkhardt DJ, Vacca M, et al. Atrial fibrillation: documented higher risk of luminal esophageal damage with general anesthesia as compared with conscious sedation. *Circ Arrhythmia Electrophysiol.* 2009;2:108–112.

153. Shah D, Haïssaguerre M, Jais P, et al. Left atrial appendage activity masquerading as pulmonary vein potentials. *Circulation.* 2002;105:2821–2825.

154. Kettering K, Weig HJ, Busch M, et al. Segmental pulmonary vein ablation: success rates with and without exclusion of areas adjacent to the esophagus. *Pacing Clin Electrophysiol.* 2008;31:652–659.

155. Wang XH, Liu X, Sun YM, et al. Pulmonary vein isolation combined with superior vena cava isolation for atrial fibrillation ablation: a prospective randomized study. *Europace.* 2008;10:600–605.

156. Fiala M, Chovancik J, Nevralova R, et al. Pulmonary vein isolation using segmental versus electroanatomical circumferential ablation for paroxysmal atrial fibrillation: over 3-year results of a prospective randomized study. *J Interv Card Electrophysiol.* 2008;22:13–21.

157. Corrado A, Patel D, Riedlbauchova L, et al. Efficacy, safety, and outcome of atrial fibrillation ablation in septuagenarians. *J Cardiovasc Electrophysiol.* 2008;19:807–811.

158. Dixit S, Gerstenfeld EP, Ratcliffe SJ, et al. Single procedure efficacy of isolating all versus arrhythmogenic pulmonary veins on long-term control of atrial fibrillation: a prospective randomized study. *Heart Rhythm.* 2008;5:174–181.

159. Cheema A, Vasamreddy CR, Dalal D, et al. Long-term single procedure efficacy of catheter ablation of atrial fibrillation. *J Interv Card Electrophysiol.* 2006;15:145–155.

160. Stabile G, Bertaglia E, Senatore G, et al. Catheter ablation treatment in patients with drug-refractory atrial fibrillation: a prospective, multi-centre, randomized, controlled study (Catheter Ablation For The Cure Of Atrial Fibrillation Study). *Eur Heart J.* 2006;27:216–221.

161. Wazni OM, Marrouche NF, Martin DO, et al. Radiofrequency ablation vs antiarrhythmic drugs as first-line treatment of symptomatic atrial fibrillation: a randomzed trial. *JAMA.* 2005;293:2634–2640.

162. Pappone C, Augello G, Sala S, et al. A randomized trial of circumferential pulmonary vein ablation versus antiarrhythmic drug therapy in paroxysmal atrial fibrillation: the APAF Study. *J Am Coll Cardiol.* 2006;48:2340–2347.

163. Forleo GB, Mantica M, De Luca L, et al. Catheter ablation of atrial fibrillation in patients with diabetes mellitus type 2: results from a randomized study comparing pulmonary vein isolation versus antiarrhythmic drug therapy. *J Cardiovasc Electrophysiol.* 2009;20:22–28.

164. Oral H, Pappone C, Chugh A, et al. Circumferential pulmonary-vein ablation for chronic atrial fibrillation. *N Engl J Med.* 2006;354:934–941.

165. Calo L, Lamberti F, Loricchio ML, et al. Left atrial ablation versus biatrial ablation for persistent and permanent atrial fibrillation: a prospective and randomized study. *J Am Coll Cardiol.* 2006;47:2504–2512.

Videos

Video 15-1. An ablation catheter is withdrawn from a position deep in the left superior vein. The point at which the catheter falls inferiorly defines the ostium of the vein.

Video 15-2. Left atrial angiography or angiorotation (EP Navigator, Philips). A three-dimensional reconstruction of the left atrium from a tomography performed at the time of the procedure using the fluoroscopy. The sweep of the fluoroscopic image is shown.

Video 15-3. A circular mapping catheter in the os of the left inferior pulmonary vein is seen to deeply indent the esophagus during this barium swallow.

16

Catheter Ablation of Paroxysmal Atrial Fibrillation Originating from the Non–Pulmonary Venous Foci

Satoshi Higa, Yenn-Jiang Lin, Li-Wei Lo, Shih-Lin Chang, Ching-Tai Tai, and Shih-Ann Chen

Key Points

The mechanism of paroxysmal atrial fibrillation (AF) originating from the non–pulmonary vein areas are automaticity, triggered activity, and microreentry.

Diagnosis is made on the basis of spontaneous onset of ectopic beats initiating AF during baseline or after provocative maneuvers.

Ablation targets are the earliest activation sites for focal ablation and the myocardial sleeve surrounding the ostium of vena cava for isolation.

Special equipment includes the circular catheter, basket catheter, noncontact balloon catheter, and three-dimensional mapping.

The success rates are greater than 95% for vena cava, 95% for the crista terminalis, 50% for the left atrial posterior wall, 50% for the ligament of Marshall.

The pulmonary veins (PVs) are a major source of ectopies initiating atrial fibrillation (AF), and isolation of PVs from the left atrium (LA) can cure paroxysmal AF.[1–3] On the other hand, several laboratories have demonstrated that ectopies originating from non-PV areas can also be AF initiators.[1–34] Previous work has reported that non-PV ectopies caused AF recurrence in more than 24% patients after isolation of four PVs.[7] Several institutions have reported a lower recurrence rate and a higher cure rate of AF in patients for whom non-PV ablation was added after multiple AF ablation procedures.[16,33] Those findings support the important role of non-PV ectopies in AF initiation and recurrence, as was previously proposed by our laboratory.[2,4–6,26] The aim of this chapter is to review the current state of knowledge about the electrophysiologic features, mapping and ablation strategy, safety, and efficacy associated with catheter ablation of AF initiated by ectopic foci originating from non-PV areas.

Characteristics of Atrial Fibrillation Originating from Non–Pulmonary Vein Areas

Incidence of Non–Pulmonary Vein Atrial Fibrillation Initiators

Our group has proposed several important concepts regarding the role of non-PV ectopy in initiating AF.[2,4–6,26] Other investigators also have demonstrated ectopies initiating AF that originated from non-PV areas, with an incidence as great as 47%.[3,7–9,35–38] Recent data have shown that 14% to 28% of patients have non-PV AF initiators. In addition, most non-PV ectopic beats initiating AF have a characteristic anatomic distribution, with the preferential distribution in the left atrial posterior free wall and the superior vena cava (SVC), followed by crista terminalis, coronary sinus (CS) ostium, ligament of Marshall, and interatrial septum (Table 16-1).[6–12] Our previous study demonstrated that the incidence of non-PV ectopic beats initiating AF is increased in women and patients with left atrial enlargement.[39]

Pathophysiology of Non–Pulmonary Vein Atrial Fibrillation Initiators

Embryonic sinus venosus tissue has been found in the musculature of the SVC, CS, and crista terminalis of the mammalian heart.[40–42] Several investigators have demonstrated that

TABLE 16-1

INCIDENCE OF ATRIAL FIBRILLATION ORIGINATING FROM NON-PULMONARY VEIN AREAS

| Study | No. of Patients | | Age (yr) (Mean ± SD) and Gender | No. of Ectopic Foci | | Mapping Tool | Location of Ectopy (No. of Foci) | | | | | | | |
	Total	Non-PV Ectopy		Total	Non-PV		RA	SVC	CS	IAS	LA	LOM	SVT	Other
Lin et al, 2003[6]	240	68 (28%)	61 ± 13, 43M/25F	358	73 (20%)	C, basket, ICE	CT (10)	27	1	1	PW (28)	6	—	—
Shah et al, 2003[7]	160†	36 (24%)	53 ± 11, 130M/30F	NA	85	C	5	3‡	4	—	PW (30), PV os (39), others (5)	—	—	—
Beldner et al, 2004[8]	401	68 (17%)	NA	NA	83	C, ICE, Carto	CT (11), TA (4), ER (13)	4	3	FO (4)	PW (15), MA (7)	—	20*	2
Suzuki et al, 2004[9]	127§	18 (14%)	53 ± 11, 106M/21F	NA	20	C	CT (4)	5	1	7	2	1	—	—
Kurotobi et al, 2006[10]	97	63 (65%)	59 ± 11, 71M/26F	269	99 (37%)**	C	CT (3)	28 (6)	10 (2)	—	42 (17)	11	—	—
Yamada et al, 2007[11]	147	31 (21%)	NA	NA	38	Basket	CT (5)	12	2	5	9	—	—	5†
Valles et al, 2008[12]	45	NA	56 ± 9, 35M/10F	57	6	C	CT (2)	2	1	—	1	—	—	—
Total	1217	284 (24.2%)	—	—	404	—	62 (15.3%)	81 (20.0%)	22 (5.3%)	17 (4.2%)	178 (44.1%)	18 (4.5%)	20 (5.0%)	7 (1.7%)

*Atrioventricular nodal reentrant tachycardia (19) and atrioventricular reentrant tachycardia (1) triggered atrial fibrillation.
†After isolation of one to four PVs, non-PV triggers were identified, but at least 16 foci were of unknown origin.
‡Includes persistent left superior caval vein.
§After isolation of four PVs, non-PV triggers were identified in the first and second sessions.
**In this study, 53% of arrhythmogenic foci were the direct initiators of atrial fibrillation shown in parentheses, and 47% of foci showed reproductive premature beats or repetitive firing.
††In this study, five foci were speculated to be located epicardially.

Basket, basket catheter; C, conventional mapping; Carto, electroanatomic mapping; CS, coronary sinus; CT, crista terminalis; ER, eustachian ridge; F, female; FO, fossa ovalis; IAS, interatrial septum; ICE, intracardiac echocardiography; LA, left atrium; LOM, ligament of Marshall; M, male; MA, mitral annulus; NA, data not available; PV, pulmonary vein; PV os, ostia of ablated pulmonary vein including the zone between ipsilateral veins; PW, left atrial posterior wall; RA, right atrium; SVC, superior vena cava; SVT, supraventricular tachycardia; TA, tricuspid annulus.

the SVC is one of the major foci for causing AF.[5,7,13–16,21] We also found that heterogeneity in the myocardial sleeve is present in the SVC and that cardiomyocytes isolated from the SVC show spontaneous depolarization.[41,42] The myocardial fibers of the SVC sleeve are connected to the right atrium (RA), and atrial excitation can conduct to the SVC.[43–45] Previous reports showed that sustained tachyarrhythmias are induced by abnormal automaticity or triggered activity in human atrial fibers.[46–48] The diseased human atria may show hypopolarized behavior compared with normal atria.[47,48] This may account for abnormal electrical activity arising from the posterior free wall of the left atrium (LA). The crista terminalis, which is an area with abnormal automaticity, anisotropy, and slow conduction, may serve as an arrhythmogenic substrate for developing microreentry.[49,50] We have demonstrated catecholamine-sensitive ectopy from the crista terminalis that showed very fast depolarization with fibrillatory conduction in the atrium.[6] The ligament of Marshall is an embryologic remnant of the left SVC, and the myocardial fibers of this structure may connect with the LA and CS musculatures. Recently, several investigators have reported the presence of catecholamine-sensitive tissue within the ligament of Marshall that has abnormal automaticity and therefore could be a potential source of AF.[6,29,51,52] Myocardial fibers within the CS also have been reported to have the capability of spontaneous depolarization associated with catecholamine.[53,54]

Diagnosis of Non–Pulmonary Vein Atrial Fibrillation Initiators

Provocative Maneuvers

In our laboratory, we first try to record the spontaneous onset of ectopic beats initiating AF during baseline monitoring or after isoproterenol infusion (up to 8 mg/minute). If ectopy does not occur, a short duration of atrial pacing with intermittent pause (8 to 12 beats at a cycle length of 200 to 300 milliseconds) is applied to induce the ectopy with AF initiation. If AF still does not appear, burst atrial pacing is used to induce AF. If pacing-induced AF is sustained for longer than 5 minutes, external cardioversion is performed to terminate the AF, and spontaneous reinitiation of AF is monitored. If a consistent location of ectopy and onset pattern of spontaneous AF are confirmed, the earliest activation site during ectopy is defined as the AF initiator.[2,4–6,26]

Mapping Techniques

An ectopic focus can be localized by detailed endocardial mapping using several multipole catheters, during frequent atrial ectopies initiating burst AF. We have demonstrated that the use of endocardial activation sequences in the high RA, His bundle, and CS ostium can predict the location of AF ectopic foci (Fig. 16-1).[2,4–6,26]

Predicting the Location of Atrial Fibrillation Initiators

With the difference in time interval between high RA and His bundle atrial activation during sinus rhythm

and the time interval between high RA and His bundle atrial activation with an ectopic beat of less than 0 milliseconds, the accuracy for discriminating ectopy in the SVC or upper portion of the crista terminalis from PV ectopy is 100% (Fig. 16-1).[55] Because of the close spatial opposition, potentials from the right superior pulmonary vein (RSPV) can be recorded from a contiguous area of the RA, and ectopies from both areas show similar P-wave morphologies. Therefore, if the ectopy originates from the upper portion of the crista terminalis or from the RA-SVC junction, ectopy from the RSPV should be excluded.[49,56,57] If far-field potentials from the right PV are recorded at the high posteromedial RA wall, the true origin of ectopy can be clarified by simultaneous mapping of the SVC and the RSPV using two multipolar catheters.[5] Another concern to be raised is ectopy from the left side of the interatrial septum. Atrial ectopy may originate from either side of the interatrial septum.[58] If the earliest atrial activation site is suspected to be from the interatrial septum, LA mapping should be considered before ablation of the right-sided septum in cases with a shorter activation time (≤15 milliseconds) preceding the P-wave onset or with a monophasic positive P wave in lead V_1 during ectopy, or in those in which the earliest site is near the area of the putative Bachmann bundle.[58,59] If the earliest endocardial activation site is around the posterolateral mitral annulus or the left PV ostium, a ligament of Marshall potential may be identified by differential pacing or by detailed epicardial mapping through the distal CS, or both (Table 16-2).[26,60]

Atrial Fibrillation Initiators from the Right Atrium. Analysis of P-wave polarity of the AF ectopy has been a useful method to predict the approximate location of the AF ectopy.[61] Ectopy originating from the SVC or upper portion of the crista terminalis exhibits upright P waves in the inferior leads; ectopy from the CS ostium produces a negative P-wave polarity in the inferior leads; and ectopy from the middle portion of crista terminalis causes biphasic P waves. If RA AF ectopy is being considered, we place a duo-decapolar catheter (1-mm electrode length and 2-mm interelectrode spacing) from the crista terminalis to the SVC with the most distally recorded electrogram amplitude larger than 0.05 mV.[2,4–6,26] The intracardiac recordings from the proximal portion of the SVC usually show a blunted atrial potential followed by a discrete SVC potential (Fig. 16-2). The activation sequence of these double potentials is reversed during SVC ectopy. Intracardiac recordings from the distal portion of the SVC usually show double potentials: the first one represents the SVC potential, and the second one, the RSPV far-field potential. During SVC ectopy, the activation sequence of these double potentials remains unchanged. Simultaneous recordings from the SVC and RSPV demonstrate double potentials. Intracardiac recordings along the crista terminalis also show double potentials during sinus rhythm, with a high-to-low activation sequence, and the activation sequence of the double potentials reverses during crista terminalis ectopy (Fig. 16-3). To identify the ectopic foci and the mechanism of AF, three-dimensional mapping is also useful (Fig. 16-4).[62]

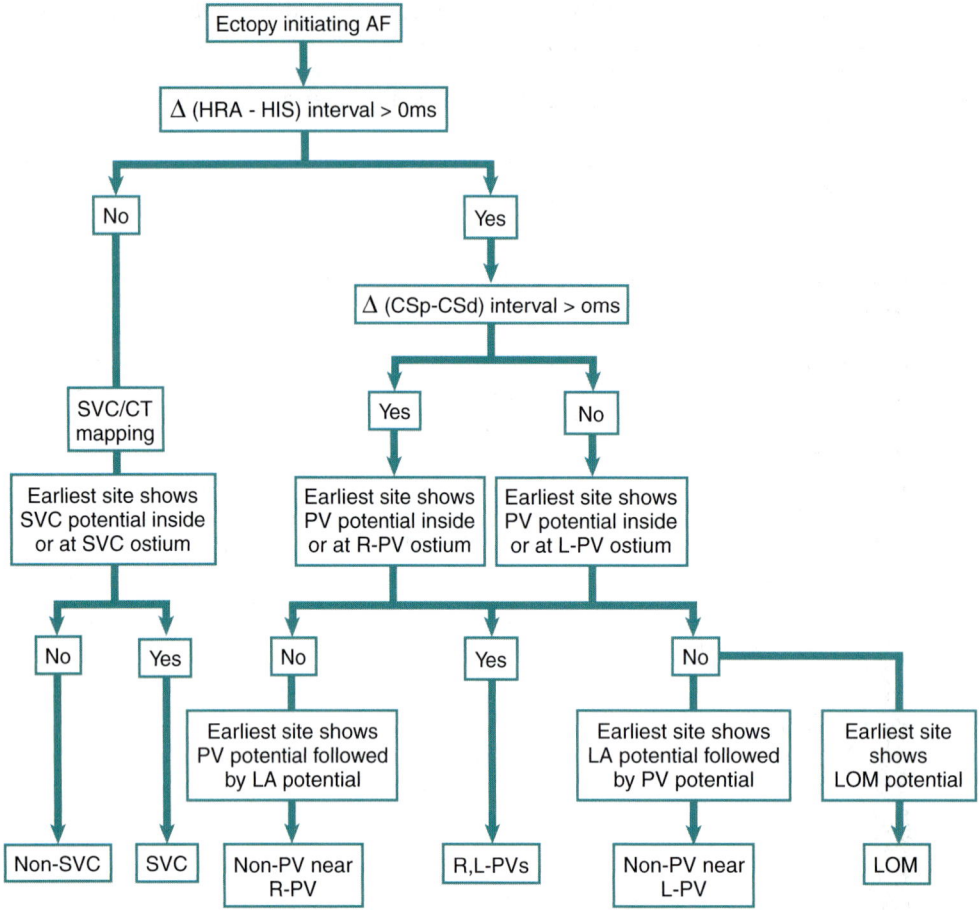

FIGURE 16-1. An algorithm for differential diagnosis of the non–pulmonary vein (non-PV) ectopy initiating atrial fibrillation (AF) and reentrant-type AF. CSd, distal portion of coronary sinus; CSp, proximal portion of coronary sinus; CT, crista terminalis; HBE, His bundle area; HRA, high right atrium; LOM, ligament of Marshall; L-PV, left pulmonary vein; R-PV, right pulmonary vein; SVC, superior vena cava. Δ (HRA-His) represents the time interval from the high right trial electrogram onset to the onset of the His atrial electrogram during sinus beats minus the same interval measured during ectopic atrial activity. CSp-CSd represents the difference in time of activation between the proximal and distal CS atrial electrograms during an ectopic atrial beat. *(Modified from Higa S, Tai CT, Chen SA. Catheter ablation of atrial fibrillation originating from extrapulmonary vein areas: Taipei approach.* Heart Rhythm. *2006;3:1388. With permission.)*

TABLE 16-2

DIAGNOSTIC CRITERIA FOR THE NON–PULMONARY VEIN ECTOPY INITIATING ATRIAL FIBRILLATION

Location	Criteria
AF initiators from RA	Difference in time interval between atrial activation at high RA and His bundle area during sinus rhythm and ectopy < 0 msec
IVC, SVC	Positive (SVC) and negative (IVC) P waves in the inferior leads, positive or biphasic P waves in V_1 (SVC) Earliest ectopic activity in the VC during simultaneous mapping of VC and right PV Reversal of the double-potential sequence during ectopy (VC potentials with a rapid deflection to far-field atrial potential sequence; distal-to-proximal venous activation sequence)
Crista terminalis (CT)	Polarity of P waves in the inferior leads: upper portion of CT, positive; middle portion, biphasic; lower portion, negative
	Earliest ectopic activity along the CT during simultaneous mapping of CT, VC, and right PV
Coronary sinus (CS) ostium	Negative P waves in the inferior leads Earliest ectopic activity in the CS ostium
AF initiators from LA	Difference in time interval between atrial activation at high RA and His bundle area during sinus rhythm and ectopy > 0 msec
Left atrial free wall or left atrial appendage	Atrial potentials with a rapid-deflection PV potential found after the earliest atrial activation
Ligament of Marshall (LOM)	Earliest activation site along the vein of Marshall, posterolateral portion of mitral annulus, or the left PV ostium Reversal of the triple-potential sequence; LOM potential is earlier than LA or left PV potential (LOM-LA-PV potentials sequence)

AF, atrial fibrillation; IVC, inferior vena cava; LA, left atrium; PV, pulmonary vein; RA, right atrium; SVC, superior vena cava; VC, vena cava.

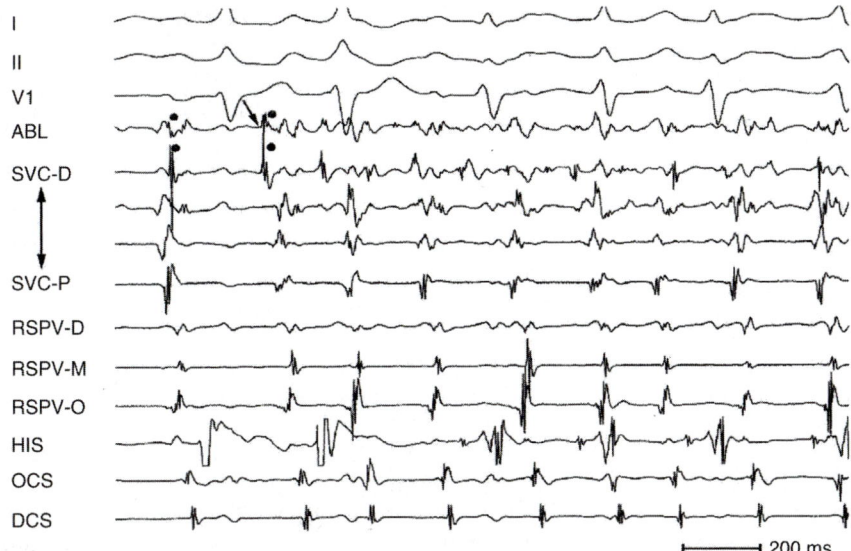

FIGURE 16-2. Spontaneous initiation of atrial fibrillation (AF) originated from the superior vena cava (SVC) after the first sinus beat *(arrow)*. It was marked by the rapid deflection potential preceding the lower-amplitude, slower, far-field atrial activities *(black dots)*. Note that the SVC potential follows the atrial potential during sinus rhythm, in contrast to the onset of AF. *Black dots* represent local SVC potentials. I, II, and V1, surface electrocardiographic leads; ABL, ablation catheter; -D, distal; DCS, distal coronary sinus; HIS, His bundle; -M, middle portion; ms, microseconds; -O, ostial portion; OCS, coronary sinus ostium; -P, proximal; RSPV, right superior pulmonary vein. *(Adapted from Tsai CF, Tai CT, Hsieh MH, et al. Initiation of atrial fibrillation by ectopic beats originating from the superior vena cava: electrophysiological characteristics and results of radiofrequency ablation. Circulation. 2000;102:72. With permission.)*

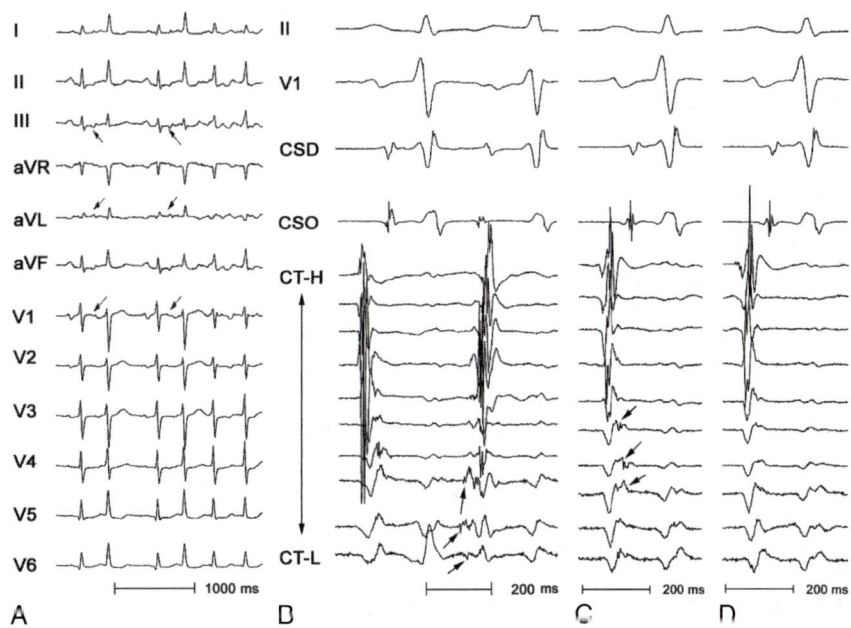

FIGURE 16-3. **A,** The tracings on the *left* show ectopic beats *(arrows)* followed by initiation of atrial fibrillation (AF) in the 12-lead electrocardiogram (ECG). Intracardiac recordings on the *right* show crista terminalis potentials *(arrows)* during ectopic beat originating from the lower portion of the crista terminalis (**B**) and during sinus rhythm before ablation (**C**). **D,** The final tracing on the *right* shows the disappearance of crista terminalis potentials after ablation. CSD, distal coronary sinus; CSO, coronary sinus ostium; CT-H, high crista terminalis; and CT-L, low crista terminalis; ms, microseconds. *(Adapted from Lin WS, Tai CT, Hsieh MH, et al. Catheter ablation of paroxysmal atrial fibrillation initiated by non-pulmonary vein ectopy. Circulation. 2003;107:3180. With permission.)*

Atrial Fibrillation Initiators from the Left Atrium. After RA ectopy is excluded by the surface P-wave polarity and endocardial activation sequence, we start to map the LA free wall ectopy using two multipolar catheters introduced through the interatrial septum. The major sites of the ectopies are distributed in the area between the four PVs or near the PV ostial edge.

The interval between atrial activation of the decapolar catheter in the proximal CS and that in the distal CS during ectopy is useful to predict ectopic foci located near the right PV ostium (> 0 milliseconds) or near the left PV ostium (< 0 milliseconds; Fig. 16-1).[55] During sinus rhythm, the left posterior free wall atrial potential with a rapid deflection is recognized; it may be

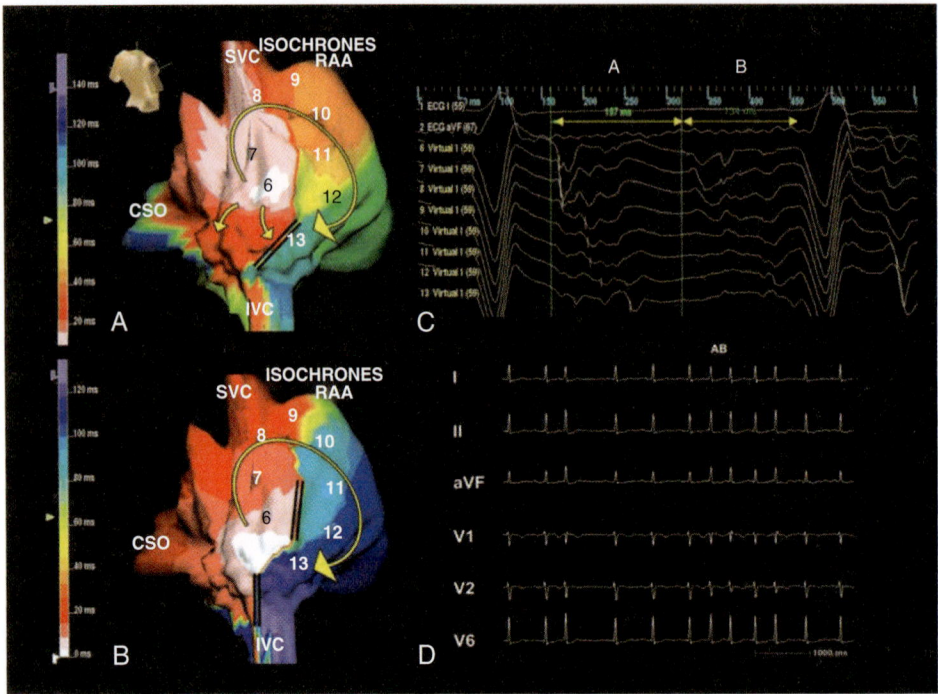

FIGURE 16-4. Noncontact mapping system demonstrating the propagation pattern during initiation of atrial fibrillation (AF). Isochronal maps on the *left* show the first *(top)* and second *(bottom)* beats initiating reentry in the modified right posterior oblique view. At the *upper right* is the unipolar virtual electrogram along the activation followed by the ectopy. At the *lower right* is the surface electrocardiogram recorded during initiation of AF. On the isochronal maps, the color scale ranges from white for the earliest activation to purple for the latest activation site. At first, the wavefront propagated centrifugally from the earliest site of the middle portion of crista terminalis *(top, yellow long arrow)*. Then, unidirectional block occurred in the lower portion of crista terminalis *(yellow short arrows)*, and the activation wavefront spread around the upper portion of crista terminalis to initiate reentry into the second cycle of AF *(bottom, yellow long arrow)*. Note that the unipolar virtual signal from the ectopic foci (virtual 6) demonstrates a "QS" morphology in the first cycle and "rS" morphology in the second cycle. CSO, coronary sinus ostium; IVC, inferior vena cava; RAA, right atrial appendage; SVC, superior vena cava. *(Adapted from Lin YJ, Tai CT, Liu TY, et al. Electrophysiological mechanisms and catheter ablation of complex atrial arrhythmias from crista terminalis: insight from three-dimensional noncontact mapping. Pacing Clin Electrophysiol. 2004;27:1239. With permission.)*

fused with the local PV potential around the edge of PV ostium. An atrial-PV fusion potential can be found in the earliest activation site during the ectopy preceding AF. An alternating pattern of atrial and PV potentials can also be recognized during ectopy (Fig. 16-5A).[6] For ectopy from the ligament of Marshall, the earliest Marshall potential preceding AF is the ablation target site (Fig. 16-5B).[26-28] It has been suggested that this ligament has multiple electrical connections with the LA posterior free wall, near or inside the PV ostium. Therefore, it is necessary to differentiate a Marshall potential from a PV or LA posterior free wall potential. Differential pacing or direct recording of the ligament of Marshall potential using the microelectrode catheter cannulated in the vein of Marshall can distinguish a Marshall potential from a PV potential to avoid misdiagnosis and inappropriate radiofrequency (RF) energy application (Tables 16-3 and 16-4).[26,29] According to the HRS/EHRS/ECAS expert consensus statements, ablation of complex fractionated atrial electrograms (CFAEs) after PV isolation may improve the long-term outcomes of AF ablation.[63] Those CFAE sites may be AF drivers. Recently, we demonstrated a close relationship between the spatial distribution of non-PV AF initiators and CFAEs (Fig. 16-6).[64,65] Lo and colleagues demonstrated that all of the non-PV ectopy initiating AF and atrial tachycardia distributed to the area with continuous CFAEs were detected by automatic algorithm (EnSite NavX, St. Jude Medical, St. Paul, MN). Furthermore, ablation of those continuous CFAEs sites terminated AF and atrial tachycardia and showed good outcomes without recurrence of non-PV ectopy.[65]

Assessing the Geometry around the Atrial-Venous Junctions

Selective PV angiography, venous phase imaging after pulmonary artery angiography, and intracardiac echocardiography help to identify the PV ostium, locate mapping catheters at the PV ostium, and map ectopy from the LA posterior free wall.[2,4-6,26] SVC angiography using a pigtail catheter injection of 40 mL of a contrast medium and intracardiac echocardiography help to determine the SVC orifice and the RA-SVC junction. Balloon-occluded CS angiography using appropriate fluoroscopic views also helps to visualize the vein of Marshall.[8] Integration of three-dimensional computed tomography, magnetic resonance imaging, or intracardiac ultrasound (CartoMerge and CartoSound, Biosense Webster, Diamond Bar, CA) with the LA-PV geometry is the best way to identify the true locations of ectopies and ablation sites.[66,67]

Ablation Techniques

In general, the ablation target site of non-PV ectopy is the site that shows the earliest bipolar deflection or a unipolar QS pattern recorded from the ectopic foci preceding AF.[2,4-6,26] RF energy with temperature control (nonirrigated 50° to 55° C) is delivered for 20 to 40 seconds but should be discontinued immediately if the ablation catheter moves or the patient complains of chest pain, coughs, or shows a Bezold-Jarisch–like reflex.[2,4-6,26] For irrigated RF catheters, energy delivery is restricted to less

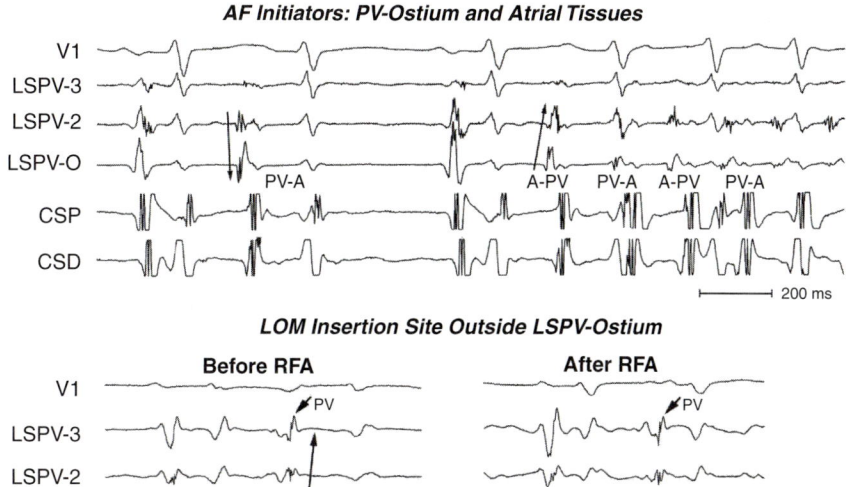

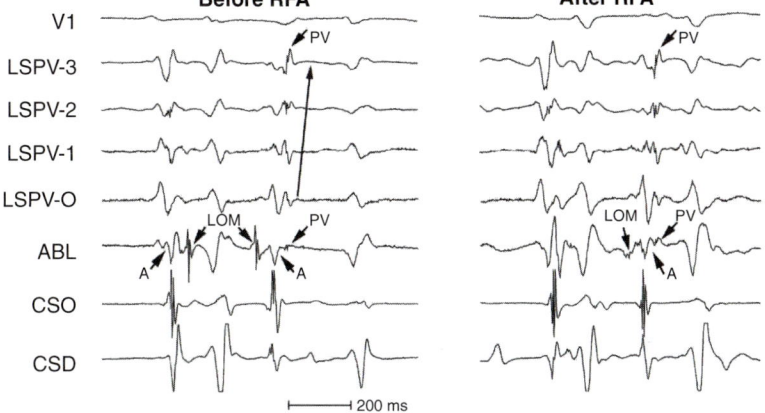

FIGURE 16-5. *Top panel,* Initiation of atrial fibrillation (AF) from the pulmonary vein (PV) and left atrial posterior free wall. The first beat is a sinus beat. The second beat is an ectopic beat originating from the left superior pulmonary vein (LSPV), recorded at the second pair of electrodes in the LSPV (LSPV-2), with conduction to the atrial tissue. The third beat is a sinus beat, and the fourth beat is an ectopic beat originating from A with conduction to the PV. Alternating activation from the PV ostium and the atrial wall was noted. *Bottom left,* Ectopic beat originating from the ligament of Marshall (LOM) before radiofrequency ablation (RFA). The LOM potential can be found in the ablation catheter (ABL), which is outside the ostium of the LSPV (LSPV-O). The typical triple potentials (LOM-A-PV) were noted. *Bottom right,* Diminished LOM potential amplitude after RFA. ABL, ablation catheter; CSO, coronary sinus ostium; CSD, distal coronary sinus; V₁, electrocardiographic surface lead. *(Adapted from Lin WS, Tai CT, Hsieh MH, et al. Catheter ablation of paroxysmal atrial fibrillation initiated by non-pulmonary vein ectopy.* Circulation. *2003;107:3178. With permission.)*

TABLE 16-3

TARGETS FOR ABLATION OF ATRIAL FIBRILLATION ORIGINATING FROM NON–PULMONARY VEIN AREAS

AF Initiators	Target Sites	Mapping Tools
Right Side		
IVC, SVC	Breakthrough sites around RA-VC junction for isolation	Circular, basket, 3D mapping system*
Crista terminalis (CT)	Earliest CT activation site for focal ablation	Unipolar recording with multipolar catheter, basket, 3D mapping system*
Coronary sinus (CS)	Connection sites between CS and atrial musculature for isolation	3D mapping system*
Left Side		
LA atrial free wall, septum, appendage, mitral annulus	Earliest activation site for focal ablation	Unipolar recording with multipolar catheter, basket, 3D mapping system*
Ligament of Marshall (LOM)	Earliest LOM potential for focal ablation	Multipolar recording of triple potentials during ectopy, direct mapping of LOM potentials by microelectrode catheter, Basket, 3D mapping system*
	Connection sites between LA and LOM for isolation	Multipolar recording of triple potentials during ectopy, direct mapping of LOM potentials by microelectrode catheter, basket, 3D mapping system*

*3D mapping either with Carto or EnSite system. AF, atrial fibrillation; basket, basket catheter; IVC, inferior vena cava; LA, left atrium; RA, right atrium; SVC, superior vena cava; VC, vena cava.

TABLE 16-4

TROUBLESHOOTING THE DIFFICULT CASE WITH ATRIAL FIBRILLATION ORIGINATING FROM THE NON–PULMONARY VEIN AREAS

Problem	Causes	Solutions
Unable to induce ectopy initiating AF	Inconsistent ectopic activation or mechanical trauma of ectopy	Repeat the provocative maneuvers Isolation of SVC without provocation of ectopy Ablation of the left atrial wall with Marshall potential
Unable to localize ectopy initiating AF	Misinterpretation of ectopic beat electrogram	Exclude far-field potentials by simultaneous mapping of SVC, CT, and RSPV Exclude far-field potentials by simultaneous mapping of LSPV, LIPV, LA, and LOM, and apply differential pacing method to identify PV or atrial potential
	Immediate degeneration to AF	Use 3D noncontact mapping system Perform atrial substrate ablation (the ectopic activation will become stable atrial tachycardia, without degeneration to AF, and mapping will become easier) Use CFAE mapping or dominant frequency mapping
	Outside the mapping area	Use 3D noncontact mapping system
Refractory to focal ablation	Epicardial foci	Use 8-mm-tip or irrigated-tip catheter, or use the epicardial approach

3D, three-dimensional; AF, atrial fibrillation; CFAE, complex fractionated atrial electrogram; CT, crista terminalis; LA, left atrium; LIPV, left inferior pulmonary vein; LOM, ligament of Marshall; LSPV, left superior pulmonary vein; PV, pulmonary vein; RSPV, right superior pulmonary vein; SVC, superior vena cava.

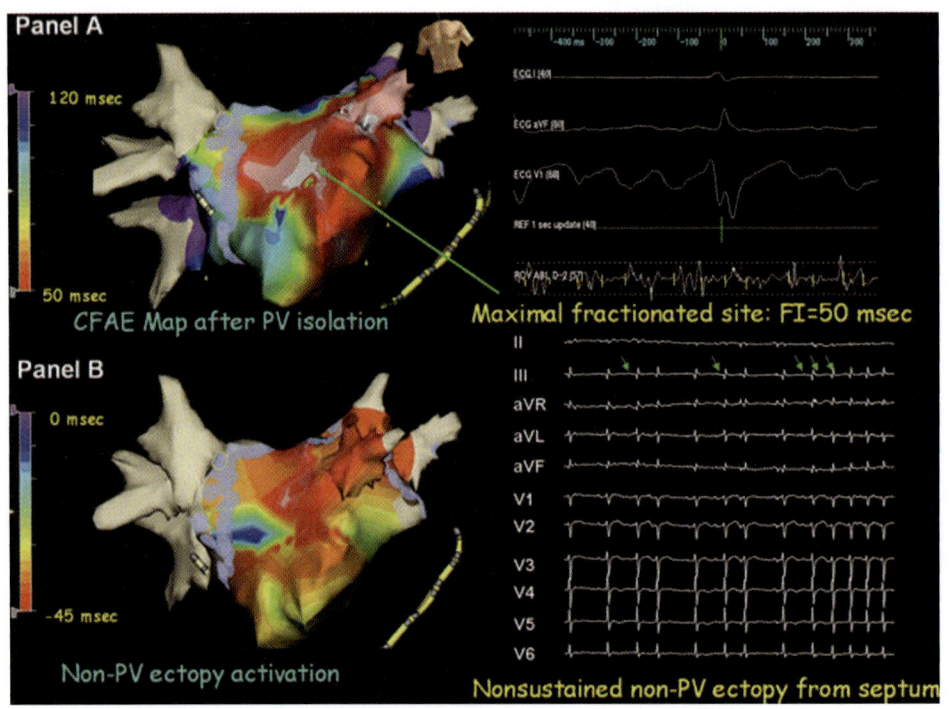

FIGURE 16-6. A, Distribution of the fraction interval (FI) using automated detection algorithm of complex fractionated atrial electrograms (CFAEs) after pulmonary vein (PV) isolation (*left*) and bipolar electrogram tracing at the most fractionated area (*right*). **B,** An isochronal mapping during non-PV ectopy initiating atrial fibrillation (AF) (*left*). Surface electrocardiogram during non-PV ectopy initiating AF (*right*). The area with maximal fractionation (FI: 50 msec) in the high septal wall of the LA was compatible with the origin of the non-PV ectopic beat initiating AF. (*Reproduced from Lin YJ, Tai CT, Chang SL, et al. Efficacy of additional ablation of complex fractionated atrial electrograms for catheter ablation of nonparoxysmal atrial fibrillation.* J Cardiovascular Electrophysiol. 2009;20:611.)

than 25 W on the posterior left atrium. The protocols for facilitating AF initiation before ablation are repeated afterward to assess the effects of ablation.

Superior Vena Cava

For patients with SVC AF, isolation of the SVC from the RA (below the level of the RA-SVC junction) is a preferable approach to avoid recurrence and SVC stenosis. The end point is electrical conduction block between the RA and the SVC. Exit block of the focal repetitive activity inside the SVC may be observed before and after ablation (Fig. 16-7).[5,13] Circular catheter, basket catheter, and three-dimensional mapping, including the Carto system (Biosense Webster) and the EnSite NavX system (St. Jude Medical) can guide the electrical isolation of the SVC.[6,15,16,18,19,21,68,69]

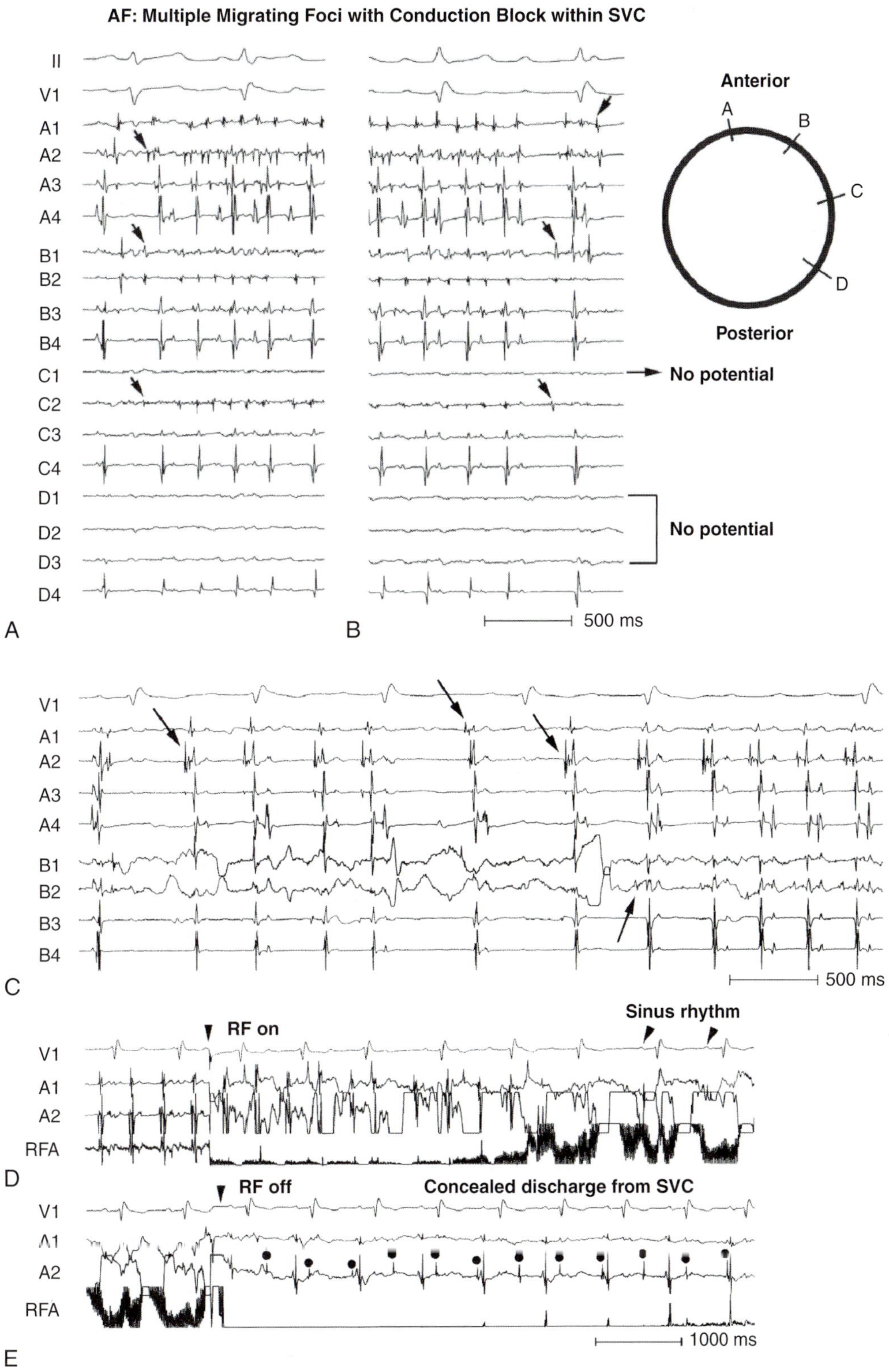

AF: Multiple Migrating Foci with Conduction Block within SVC

FIGURE 16-7. Multiple migrating foci with conduction block during superior vena cava (SVC) atrial fibrillation (AF) recorded by a basket catheter (*upper panel*s). **A,** The first beat is a sinus beat, and the second beat is an ectopic beat from spline B1 and C2, followed by A2 *(arrowheads)*. **B,** Spontaneous early reinitiation of ectopic beats from spline B1, C2, and A1 *(arrowheads)*. As shown in the diagram on the far right, A through D indicate the wall of the SVC from anterior to posterolateral; 1, 2, 3, and 4 are the bipolar recordings from each spline located along the distal to proximal SVC. **C,** Ectopies from the SVC recorded by a basket catheter in a different patient. The earliest activation sites during ectopic beats changed from spline A2, A1, and A2 to B2 *(arrows)*. **D** and **E,** AF termination during segmental isolation of the SVC sleeve by radiofrequency ablation (RFA). After termination, concealed discharge from the SVC is still present *(black dots)*. *(Adapted from Lin WS, Tai CT, Hsieh MH, et al. Catheter ablation of paroxysmal atrial fibrillation initiated by non-pulmonary vein ectopy. Circulation. 2003;107:3179. With permission.)*

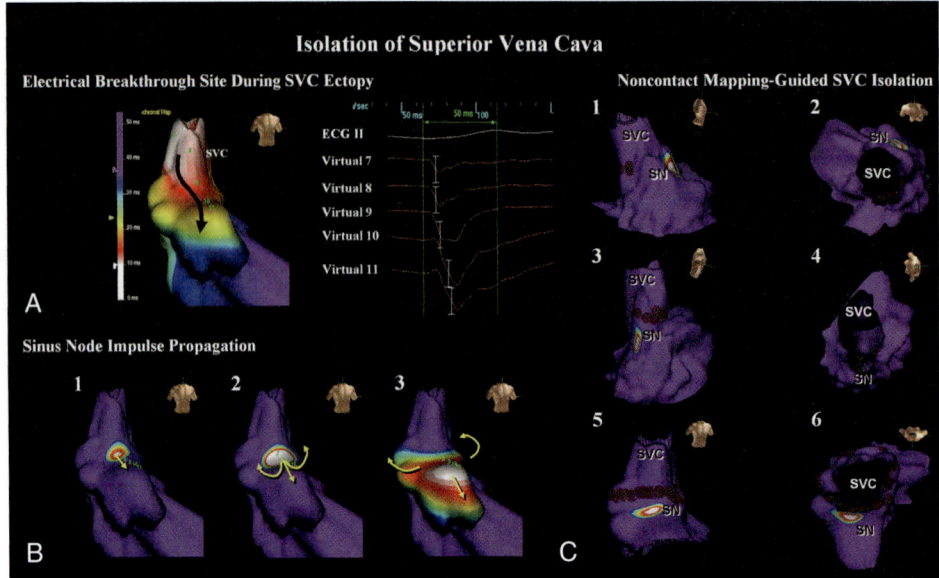

FIGURE 16-8. A, An isochronal map during the superior vena cava (SVC) ectopy. The ectopic beat originates from the SVC and conducts to the right atrium (RA) through an electrical breakthrough site. Virtuals 7 and 8 show a QS pattern at the ectopic focus, and virtuals 9 to 11, an rS pattern. **B,** The sinus node impulse origin is located at the anterior portion of the RA-SVC junction near the electrical breakthrough site (frame 1). The activation wavefront proceeds toward the high anterior RA (frame 2) and spreads out to the rest of the entire RA (frame 3). **C,** Noncontact mapping–guided SVC isolation. Frames 1 to 6 show the endocardial geometry of the RA-SVC complex. The radiofrequency (RF) lesions are indicated as *brown circles*. In frames 1 and 2, the electrical breakthrough site is located at the posterolateral portion of the RA-SVC junction, and the sinus node impulse origin is located on the anterolateral RA wall below the RA-SVC junction. In frames 3 and 4, the electrical breakthrough site is located at the anterolateral portion of the RA-SVC junction, and the sinus node impulse origin is located just below the electrical breakthrough site. In this case, we carefully applied the RF energy to the anterolateral portion of the RA-SVC junction just close to the sinus node impulse origin and successfully isolated the SVC without any sinus node injury. In frames 5 and 6, the electrical breakthrough sites are widely distributed along the full circumferential of the entire RA-SVC junction, and the sinus node impulse origin is located at the anterior portion of the RA-SVC junction. In this case, care must be taken for RF application to the anterior portion of the RA-SVC junction close to the sinus node impulse origin to avoid the sinus node injury. SN, sinus node; SVC superior vena cava. *(From Higa S, Tai CT, Chen SA. Catheter ablation of atrial fibrillation originating from extrapulmonary vein areas: Taipei approach.* Heart Rhythm. *2006;3:1388. With permission.)*

Noncontact mapping can localize the electrical breakthroughs at the RA-SVC junction and guide ablation of SVC AF (Fig. 16-8).[18,19,69] When the noncontact balloon catheter is deployed, only 3mL of saline-contrast medium solution is infused, to reduce balloon size and allow positioning closer to the SVC surface. The atriocaval junction can be confirmed by an SVC venogram, intracardiac echocardiography, and electrical signals. In our previous study, we used these three tools simultaneously to identify the RA-SVC junction.[5,6] Recently, we also divided the SVC into three parts. The first part extends from the junction of the right and left brachiocephalic veins to the upper end of the right pulmonary artery. The second part is the part of SVC that is crossed posteriorly by the right pulmonary artery (i.e., from the upper border of the right pulmonary artery to the lower border of the right pulmonary artery). The third part begins from the lower end of the second part and extends to the site of the RA-SVC junction. The RA-SVC junction is defined as the point below which the cylindrical SVC flares into the RA.[68,69] Before energy delivery to the SVC or lateral right atrium, it is necessary to pace at high output from the distal ablation electrodes to exclude phrenic nerve stimulation. It is also advisable to monitor the right hemidiaphragm fluoroscopically during ablation to avoid phrenic nerve injury.

Crista Terminalis

For ectopy from the crista terminalis, we perform focal ablation of the earliest activation site of the ectopy until there is total elimination of the ectopy initiating AF or greater than 50% reduction in the initial electrogram amplitude of the ectopic focus.[6] The crista terminalis ectopy is usually located around the transverse gap conduction region in the crista terminalis. For patients who have accompanying RA atypical flutter involving the transverse gap conduction region in the crista terminalis, we perform linear ablation around the gap to eliminate the ectopy and to block transverse conduction through this gap (Fig. 16-4).[62] Intracardiac echocardiography is helpful to clarify the anatomic relation between the crista terminalis and the catheter position during ablation.

Coronary Sinus

For patients with CS AF, electrical disconnection of the CS from the atrium by endocardial or epicardial ablation, or both, is a preferable approach to avoid recurrence. A circular catheter or three-dimensional mapping system is useful for the ablation procedure. The disappearance or isolation of the CS potential is the end point.[31] Irrigated RF energy is recommended for ablation within the CS to allow for effective RF delivery and to minimize the risk for impedance. In general, RF is delivered at 10 to 15 W in the distal CS and 10 to 20 W in the proximal CS.

Left Atrial Wall

For ectopy from the LA posterior free wall, we perform focal ablation of the earliest activation site during ectopy (Fig. 16-9).

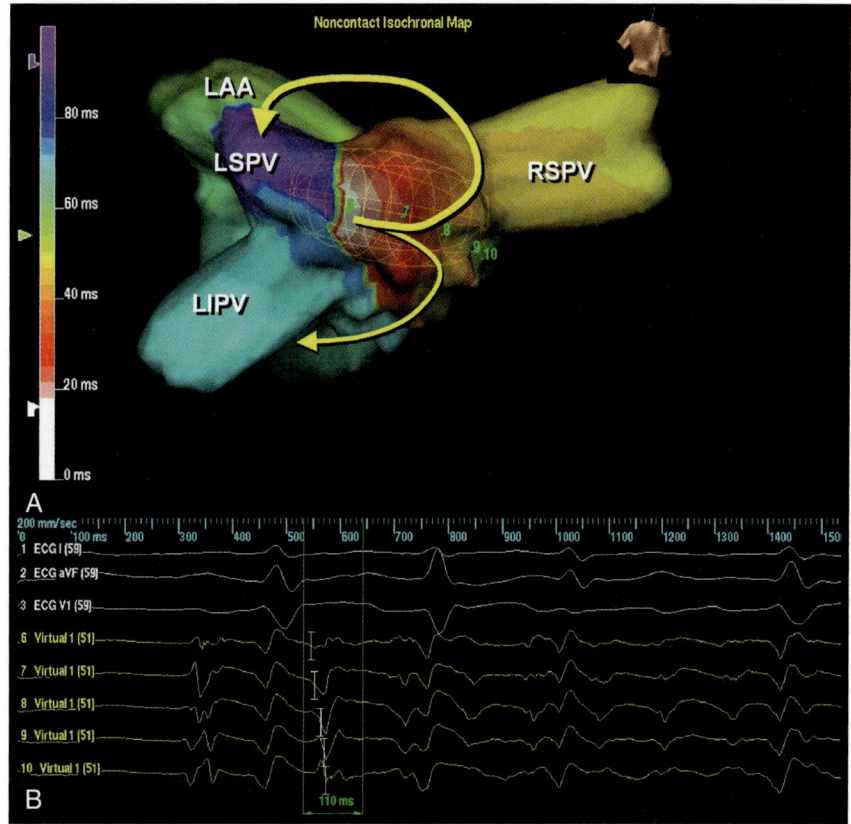

FIGURE 16-9. **A,** An isochronal map during ectopic beat initiating atrial fibrillation (AF). The ectopic beat originates from the left atrial middle posterior wall accompanying unidirectional block on the left side of the posterior wall, and the activation wavefront proceeds toward the right pulmonary veins and spreads out to the rest of the entire left atrium (*yellow arrows*), then initiates AF. **B,** The unipolar virtual signals demonstrate a "QS" morphology at the ectopic focus (virtual 6, from the second beat) and an "rS" morphology (virtual 8, from the second beat) at the breakout site. LAA, left atrial appendage; LIPV, left inferior pulmonary vein; LSPV, left superior pulmonary vein; RIPV, right inferior pulmonary vein; RSPV, right superior pulmonary vein. *(From Higa S, Lin YJ, Tai CT, et al. Noncontact mapping. In Calkin H, Jais P, Steinberg J (eds):* A Practical Approach to Catheter Ablation of Atrial Fibrillation. *Philadelphia, Lippincott Williams & Wilkins; 2008:126. With permission.)*

If ectopy still remains, a box-shaped linear ablation (1.5- × 1.5-cm²) is added around the ectopy.[6] The end point is total elimination of the ectopy initiating AF or a reduction in electrogram amplitude of the ectopic focus to less than 50% of the initial amplitude.[70] RF energy is restricted to less than 25 W on the posterior LA, and the catheter should be moved frequently (about every 20 seconds) to avoid esophageal injury.

Ligament of Marshall

For patients with ligament of Marshall AF, the earliest ligament of Marshall potential preceding onset of AF is targeted for ablation by an endocardial or epicardial approach, or both. Both the ligament of Marshall and the left PVs can be isolated from the LA with guidance by simultaneous mapping of ligament of Marshall and left PV ostia (Fig. 16-5).[27,29]

Efficacy and Safety

Ablation Results and Recurrences

The success rate for catheter ablation of non-PV ectopy depends on the origin of the ectopy.[6] RA non-PV ectopy was eliminated with a higher success rate and a lower recurrence rate than LA non-PV ectopy. Rates of success, recurrences, and complications reported in journals have been 98.6%, 7.0%, and 0%, respectively, for AF originating from the vena cava, and 81.6%, 10.2%, and 2.0% for ligament of Marshall AF (Tables 16-5 to 16-7). In our study, a higher success rate was demonstrated for AF initiated from the RA, including the SVC and crista terminalis.[6] On the other hand, AF initiated from the LA had a higher recurrence rate. Recently, we reported that patients with metabolic syndrome showed higher incidence of recurrent AF and non-PV AF source.[71] Oakes and associates reported that patients who had a greater extent of delayed enhancement on magnetic resonance imaging of the LA wall had a higher recurrence rate after PV isolation, suggesting the existence of a non-PV AF source.[72]

Avoiding Complications

Several issues are discussed here on the efficacy and safety of ablation procedures. RF energy application around the atrial-venous junction and the LA posterior wall can cause sick sinus syndrome, SVC and PV stenosis, phrenic nerve injury, atrioesophageal fistulas, and pyloric spasm.[73–77] Use of a lower power level of RF energy, with a temperature of 50° to 55° C, can avoid these acute and late complications. Pacing to capture

TABLE 16-5

RESULTS OF RADIOFREQUENCY CATHETER ABLATION OF ATRIAL FIBRILLATION ORIGINATING FROM THE VENA CAVA

Study	No. of Patients	Mean Age (yr) by Gender	Mapping Tool	Location of Ectopies	Ablation Method (No. of Patients)	Multiple Foci	Acute Success	Complications	Recurrence	Follow-Up (mo)
Chang et al, 2001[14]	2	57 (F), 50 (M)	C	SVC	Focal	NA	Yes	NA	No	6, 3
Ooie et al, 2002[15]	1	42 (F)	Circular	SVC	Isolation	NA	Yes	No	No	7
Goya et al, 2002[16]	16	59±5	Carto, circular	SVC*	Isolation	NA	16 (100%)	0 (0%)	NA†	13±1
Shah et al, 2003[7]	1	50 (M) 60 (F),	Basket	SVC	Isolation	NA	Yes	NA	No	12
Mansour et al, 2002[17]	2	22 (M)	EnSite, C	IVC–os PL	Focal	No	Yes	No	No	9, 2
Liu et al, 2003[18]	2	57 (F), 73 (M)	EnSite	SVC	Isolation	NA	Yes	No	No	2, 2
Weiss et al, 2003[19]	1	54 (M)	EnSite	SVC	Isolation	NA	Yes	NA	No	4
Lin et al, 2003[6]	27	57±12	Basket, C	SVC	Focal (20) Isolation (7)	12 (44%)	27 (100%)	0 (0%)	3 (11%)	NA
Scavee et al, 2003[20]	1	44 (NA)	Circular	IVC–os PM	Isolation	No	Yes	No	No	14
Jayam et al, 2004[21]	1	39 (M)	Basket	SVC	Isolation	NA	Yes	NA	NA	NA
Hsu et al, 2004[22]	5	46±11, 1F/4M	Carto, circular	PLSVC	Isolation	NA	4 (75%)‡	No	1 (25%)	15±10
Elayi et al, 2006[23]	6	50±6, 2F / 4M	Carto, circular	PLSVC	Isolation	NA**	6 (100%)	No	No	13±7
Pastor et al, 2007[24]	3	50±11, 2F / 1M	C, Circular	SVC	Focal (2) Isolation (1)	Yes††	3 (100%)	NA	No	29±17
Liu et al, 2007[25]	4	50±11, 4M	Carto, circular	PLSVC	Isolation	NA	4 (100%)§	No	1 (25%)	18±7
Total	72	—	—	—	—	—	71 (98.6%)	0 (0%)	5 (7.0%)	—

*This study included patients with or without SVC ectopy.
†Sinus rhythm was maintained in 13 of 16 patients, but the authors did not specify the true recurrence rate of SVC atrial fibrillation.
‡Successful isolation of PLSVC in 4 patients.
**All patients received pulmonary vein antrum isolation.
††One case received pulmonary vein isolation for atrial fibrillation originating from pulmonary vein as a second session.
§All patients received multiple procedures due to acute recurrence of atrial fibrillation.
Basket, basket catheter; C, conventional mapping; Carto, electroanatomic contact mapping system; circular, circular catheter; EnSite, noncontact mapping system; F, female; focal, focal ablation of ectopic focus; isolation, electrical isolation of caval vein; IVC–os PL, posterolateral wall of ostial portion of inferior vena cava; IVC–os PM, posteromedial wall of ostial portion of inferior vena cava; M, male; NA, data not available; PLSVC, persistent superior vena cava; SVC, superior vena cava.

TABLE 16-6

RESULTS OF RADIOFREQUENCY CATHETER ABLATION OF ATRIAL FIBRILLATION ORIGINATING FROM THE LIGAMENT OF MARSHALL

Study	No. of Patients	Mean Age (yr) by Gender	Mapping Tool	Mapping Site	Ablation Sites (No. of Patients)	Ablation Method	Multiple Foci	Acute Success	Complications	Recurrence	Follow-Up (mo)
Katritsis et al, 2001[27]	10*	54.2±9.4 (NA)	C	LA, CS	LA (4), CS (1), LA/CS (5)	Focal	Yes	7 (70.0%)†	1 (10%) ‡	NA	11±5
Polymeropoulos et al, 2002[28]	1	66 (F)	Carto	LA, CS	LA	Focal	Yes	Yes	No	No	3
Lin et al, 2003[6]	6	66±13 (NA)	C	LA, CS	LSPV-os (5), -inside (1)	Focal	5 (83%)	3 (50.0%)	No	3 (50.0%)	NA
Hwang et al, 2004[29]	21	43.2±8.7 (5F/16M)	Microelectrode	VOM	VOM insertion sites	Focal	Yes	18 (85.7%)	No	2 (11.1%)	19±10
Kurotobi et al, 2006[10]	11	NA	C	LA	Distal end of VOM (LA posterior 5, lateral 4, roof 2)	Focal	NA	11 (100%)	NA	NA	NA
Total	49	—	—	—	—	—	—	40 (81.6%)	1 (2.0%)	5 (10.2%)	—

*Ten out of 18 patients received catheter ablation.
†Seven patients showed symptomatic improvement after LOM ablation.
‡One patient showed pericardial effusion requiring pericardiocentesis.
C, conventional mapping–guided radiofrequency ablation; Carto, electroanatomic mapping, CS, coronary sinus; F, female; focal, focal ablation of ectopic focus; LA, left atrium; LSPV-os, left superior pulmonary vein ostium; LSPV-inside, inside the left superior pulmonary vein; M, male; NA, data not available; VOM, vein of Marshall.

TABLE 16-7

RESULTS OF RADIOFREQUENCY CATHETER ABLATION OF ATRIAL FIBRILLATION ORIGINATING FROM THE CORONARY SINUS

Study	No. of Patients	Mean Age (yr) by Gender	Mapping Tool	Location of Ectopies	Ablation Method	Multiple Foci	Acute Success	Complications	Recurrence	Follow-Up (mo)
Lin et al, 2003[6]	1	67 (M)	C	CS-os	Focal	No	Yes	No	No	NA
Rotter et al, 2004[31]	1	59 (M)	C	CS-mid to os	Isolation	Yes	Yes	NA	NA	NA
Sanders et al, 2004[32]	1	53 (M)	C	CS-dis to os	Focal, Isolation	Yes	Yes	No	No	2

C, conventional mapping–guided radiofrequency ablation; CS-dis, distal portion of coronary sinus; CS-mid, middle portion of coronary sinus; CS-os, ostial portion of coronary sinus; focal, focal ablation of ectopic focus; isolation, electrical isolation of coronary sinus; M, male; NA, data not available.

the phrenic nerve before ablation can predict phrenic nerve injury. Acceleration of the sinus rate during ablation around the RA-SVC junction is a sign predicting sinus node injury. Avoiding the application of high RF energy on the LA posterior wall and CS close to the esophagus line is also essential to avoid the fatal complication of LA esophageal fistula.[78] Recently, several protecting system to avoid thermal esophageal injury have been described.[79,80]

Conclusion

In most cases, AF is initiated by ectopic beats originating from the PV; however, it can be initiated from non-PV areas. Considering the high incidence (about 20%) of non-PV AF before and after isolation of four PVs, provocation of non-PV ectopy initiating AF should be considered in both the primary procedure and repeat procedures. Catheter ablation in non-PV areas is safe and effective in eliminating initiators for AF originating from non-PV areas.[35,69]

References

1. Haïssaguerre M, Jais P, Shah DC, et al. Spontaneous initiation of atrial fibrillation by ectopic beats originating in the pulmonary veins. *N Engl J Med.* 1998;339:659–666.
2. Chen SA, Hsieh MH, Tai CT, et al. Initiation of atrial fibrillation by ectopic beats originating from the pulmonary veins: electrophysiological characteristics, pharmacological responses, and effects of radiofrequency ablation. *Circulation.* 1999;100:1879–1886.
3. Oral H, Knight BP, Tada H, et al. Pulmonary vein isolation for paroxysmal and persistent atrial fibrillation. *Circulation.* 2002;105:1077–1081.
4. Chen SA, Tai CT, Yu WC, et al. Right atrial focal atrial fibrillation: electrophysiologic characteristics and radiofrequency catheter ablation. *J Cardiovasc Electrophysiol.* 1999;10:328–335.
5. Tsai CF, Tai CT, Hsieh MH, et al. Initiation of atrial fibrillation by ectopic beats originating from the superior vena cava: electrophysiological characteristics and results of radiofrequency ablation. *Circulation.* 2000;102:67–74.
6. Lin WS, Tai CT, Hsieh MH, et al. Catheter ablation of paroxysmal atrial fibrillation initiated by non-pulmonary vein ectopy. *Circulation.* 2003;107:3176–3183.
7. Shah DC, Haïssaguerre M, Jais P, Hocini M. Nonpulmonary vein foci: do they exist? *Pacing Clin Electrophysiol.* 2003;26:1631–1635.
8. Beldner SJ, Zado ES, Lin D, et al. Anatomic targets for nonpulmonary triggers: identification with intracardiac echo and magnetic mapping. *Heart Rhythm.* 2004;1(suppl):S237.
9. Suzuki K, Nagata Y, Goya M, et al. Impact of non-pulmonary vein focus on early recurrence of atrial fibrillation after pulmonary vein isolation. *Heart Rhythm.* 2004;1(suppl):S203–S204.
10. Kurotobi T, Ito H, Inoue K, et al. Marshall vein as arrhythmogenic source in patients with atrial fibrillation: correlation between its anatomy and electrophysiological findings. *J Cardiovasc Electrophysiol.* 2006;17:1062–1067.
11. Yamada T, Murakami Y, Okada T, et al. Non-pulmonary vein epicardial foci of atrial fibrillation identified in the left atrium after pulmonary vein isolation. *Pacing Clin Electrophysiol.* 2007;30:1323–1330.
12. Valles E, Fan R, Roux JF, et al. Localization of atrial fibrillation triggers in patients undergoing pulmonary vein isolation: importance of the carina region. *J Am Coll Cardiol.* 2008;52:1413–1420.
13. Ino T, Miyamoto S, Ohno T, Tadera T. Exit block of focal repetitive activity in the superior vena cava masquerading as a high right atrial tachycardia. *J Cardiovasc Electrophysiol.* 2000;11:480–483.
14. Chang KC, Lin YC, Chen JY, et al. Electrophysiological characteristics and radiofrequency ablation of focal atrial tachycardia originating from the superior vena cava. *Jpn Circ J.* 2001;65:1034–1040.
15. Ooie T, Tsuchiya T, Ashikaga K, Takahashi N. Electrical connection between the right atrium and the superior vena cava, and the extent of myocardial sleeve in a patient with atrial fibrillation originating from the superior vena cava. *J Cardiovasc Electrophysiol.* 2002;13:482–485.
16. Goya M, Ouyang F, Ernst S, et al. Electroanatomic mapping and catheter ablation of breakthroughs from the right atrium to the superior vena cava in patients with atrial fibrillation. *Circulation.* 2002;106:1317–1320.
17. Mansour M, Ruskin J, Keane D. Initiation of atrial fibrillation by ectopic beats originating from the ostium of the inferior vena cava. *J Cardiovasc Electrophysiol.* 2002;13:1292–1295.
18. Liu TY, Tai CT, Lee PC, et al. Novel concept of atrial tachyarrhythmias originating from the superior vena cava: insight from noncontact mapping. *J Cardiovasc Electrophysiol.* 2003;14:533–539.
19. Weiss C, Willems S, Rostock T, et al. Electrical disconnection of an arrhythmogenic superior vena cava with discrete radiofrequency current lesions guided by noncontact mapping. *Pacing Clin Electrophysiol.* 2003;26:1758–1761.
20. Scavee C, Jais P, Weerasooriya R, Haïssaguerre M. The inferior vena cava: an exceptional source of atrial fibrillation. *J Cardiovasc Electrophysiol.* 2003; 14:659–662.
21. Jayam VK, Vasamreddy C, Berger R, Calkins H. Electrical disconnection of the superior vena cava from the right atrium. *J Cardiovasc Electrophysiol.* 2004;15:614.
22. Hsu LF, Jais P, Keane D, et al. Atrial fibrillation originating from persistent left superior vena cava. *Circulation.* 2004;24:109:828–832.
23. Elayi CS, Fahmy TS, Wazni OM, et al. Left superior vena cava isolation in patients undergoing pulmonary vein antrum isolation: impact on atrial fibrillation recurrence. *Heart Rhythm.* 2006;3:1019–1023.
24. Pastor A, Núñez A, Magalhaes A, et al. The superior vena cava as a site of ectopic foci in atrial fibrillation. *Rev Esp Cardiol.* 2007;60:68–71.
25. Liu H, Lim KT, Murray C, et al. Electrogram-guided isolation of the left superior vena cava for treatment of atrial fibrillation. *Europace.* 2007;9:775–780.
26. Tai CT, Hsieh MH, Tsai CF, et al. Differentiating the ligament of Marshall from the pulmonary vein musculature potentials in patients with paroxysmal atrial fibrillation: electrophysiological characteristics and results of radiofrequency ablation. *Pacing Clin Electrophysiol.* 2000;23:1493–1501.
27. Katritsis D, Ioannidis JP, Anagnostopoulos CE, et al. Identification and catheter ablation of extracardiac and intracardiac components of ligament of Marshall tissue for treatment of paroxysmal atrial fibrillation. *J Cardiovasc Electrophysiol.* 2001;12:750–758.
28. Polymeropoulos KP, Rodriguez LM, Timmermans C, Wellens HJ. Images in cardiovascular medicine: radiofrequency ablation of a focal atrial tachycardia originating from the Marshall ligament as a trigger for atrial fibrillation. *Circulation.* 2002;105:2112–2113.
29. Hwang C, Chen PS. Clinical electrophysiology and catheter ablation of atrial fibrillation from the ligament of Marshall. In: Chen SA, Haïssaguerre M, Zipes DP, eds. *Thoracic Vein Arrhythmias: Mechanisms and Treatment.* Malden, MA: Blackwell Futura; 2004:226–284.
30. Tuan TC, Tai CT, Lin YK, et al. Use of fluoroscopic views for detecting Marshall's vein in patients with cardiac arrhythmias. *J Interv Card Electrophysiol.* 2003;9:327–331.
31. Rotter M, Sanders P, Takahashi Y, et al. Images in cardiovascular medicine: coronary sinus tachycardia driving atrial fibrillation. *Circulation.* 2004;110: e59–e60.
32. Sanders P, Jais P, Hocini M, Haïssaguerre M. Electrical disconnection of the coronary sinus by radiofrequency catheter ablation to isolate a trigger of atrial fibrillation. *J Cardiovasc Electrophysiol.* 2004;15:364–368.
33. Cappato R, Negroni S, Pecora D, et al. Prospective assessment of late conduction recurrence across radiofrequency lesions producing electrical disconnection at the pulmonary vein ostium in patients with atrial fibrillation. *Circulation.* 2003;108:1599–1604.
34. Higa S, Tai CT, Chen SA. Catheter ablation of atrial fibrillation originating from extrapulmonary vein areas: Taipei approach. *Heart Rhythm.* 2006;3:1386–1390.
35. Mangrum JM, Mounsey JP, Kok LC, et al. Intracardiac echocardiography-guided, anatomically based radiofrequency ablation of focal atrial fibrillation originating from pulmonary veins. *J Am Coll Cardiol.* 2002;39:1964–1972.
36. Natale A, Pisano E, Beheiry S, et al. Ablation of right and left atrial premature beats following cardioversion in patients with chronic atrial fibrillation refractory to antiarrhythmic drugs. *Am J Cardiol.* 2000;85:1372–1375.
37. Jais P, Weerasooriya R, Shah DC, et al. Ablation therapy for atrial fibrillation (AF): past, present and future. *Cardiovasc Res.* 2002;54:337–346.
38. Schmitt C, Ndrepepa G, Weber S, et al. Biatrial multisite mapping of atrial premature complexes triggering onset of atrial fibrillation. *Am J Cardiol.* 2002;89:1381–1387.
39. Lee SH, Tai CT, Hsieh MH, et al. Predictors of non-pulmonary vein ectopic beats initiating paroxysmal atrial fibrillation: implication for catheter ablation. *J Am Coll Cardiol.* 2005;46:1054–1059.
40. Keith A, Flack M. The form and nature of the primary divisions of the vertebrate heart. *J Anat.* 1907;41:189.
41. Chen YJ, Chen YC, Yeh HI, et al. Electrophysiology and arrhythmogenic activity of single cardiomyocytes from canine superior vena cava. *Circulation.* 2002;105:2679–2685.
42. Yeh HI, Lai YJ, Lee SH, et al. Heterogeneity of myocardial sleeve morphology and gap junctions in canine superior vena cava. *Circulation.* 2001;104:3152–3157.
43. Spach MS, Barr RC, Jewett PH. Spread of excitation from the atrium into thoracic veins in human beings and dogs. *Am J Cardiol.* 1972;30:844–854.
44. Zipes DP, Knope RF. Electrical properties of the thoracic veins. *Am J Cardiol.* 1972;29:372–376.
45. Hashizume H, Ushiki T, Abe K. A histological study of the cardiac muscle of the human superior and inferior venae cavae. *Arch Histol Cytol.* 1995;58:457–464.
46. Mary-Rabine L, Hordof AJ, Danilo P Jr, et al. Mechanisms for impulse initiation in isolated human atrial fibers. *Circ Res.* 1980;47:267–277.
47. Gelband H, Bush HL, Rosen MR, et al. Electrophysiologic properties of isolated preparations of human atrial myocardium. *Circ Res.* 1972;30:293–300.
48. Ten Eick RE, Singer DH. Electrophysiological properties of diseased human atrium. *Circ Res.* 1979;44:545–557.

49. Kalman JM, Olgin JE, Karch MR, et al. "Cristal tachycardias": origin of right atrial tachycardias from the crista terminalis identified by intracardiac echocardiography. *J Am Coll Cardiol.* 1998;31:451–459.

50. Boineau JP, Canavan TE, Schuessler RB, et al. Demonstration of a widely distributed atrial pacemaker complex in the human heart. *Circulation.* 1988;77:1221–1237.

51. Scherlag BJ, Yeh BK, Robinson MJ. Inferior interatrial pathway in the dog. *Circ Res.* 1972;31:18–35.

52. Doshi RN, Wu TJ, Yashima M, et al. Relation between ligament of Marshall and adrenergic atrial tachyarrhythmia. *Circulation.* 1999;100:876–883.

53. Erlanger J, Blackman JR. A study of relative rhythmicity and conductivity in various regions of the auricles of the mammalian heart. *Am J Physiol.* 1907;19:125–174.

54. Andrew LW, Paul FC. Triggered and automatic activity in the canine coronary sinus. *Circ Res.* 1977;41:435–445.

55. Lee SH, Tai CT, Lin WS, et al. Predicting the arrhythmogenic foci of atrial fibrillation before atrial transseptal procedure: implication for catheter ablation. *J Cardiovasc Electrophysiol.* 2000;11:750–757.

56. Belhassen B, Viskin S. Atrial tachycardia and "kissing catheters". *J Cardiovasc Electrophysiol.* 2000;11:233.

57. Soejima K, Stevenson WG, Delacretaz E, et al. Identification of left atrial origin of ectopic tachycardia during right atrial mapping: analysis of double potentials at the posteromedial right atrium. *J Cardiovasc Electrophysiol.* 2000;11:975–980.

58. Frey B, Kreiner G, Gwechenberger M, Gossinger HD. Ablation of atrial tachycardia originating from the vicinity of the atrioventricular node: significance of mapping both sides of the interatrial septum. *J Am Coll Cardiol.* 2001;38:394–400.

59. Marrouche NF, Sippens-Groenewegen A, Yang Y, et al. Clinical and electrophysiologic characteristics of left septal atrial tachycardia. *J Am Coll Cardiol.* 2002;40:1133–1139.

60. Katritsis D, Giazitzoglou E, Korovesis S, et al. Epicardial foci of atrial arrhythmias apparently originating in the left pulmonary veins. *J Cardiovasc Electrophysiol.* 2002;13:319–323.

61. Kuo JY, Tai CT, Tsao HM, et al. P wave polarities of an arrhythmogenic focus in patients with paroxysmal atrial fibrillation originating from superior vena cava or right superior pulmonary vein. *J Cardiovasc Electrophysiol.* 2003;14:350–357.

62. Lin YJ, Tai CT, Liu TY, et al. Electrophysiological mechanisms and catheter ablation of complex atrial arrhythmias from crista terminalis: insight from three-dimensional noncontact mapping. *Pacing Clin Electrophysiol.* 2004;27:1232–1239.

63. Calkins H, Brugada J, Packer DL, et al. HRS/EHRA/ECAS expert consensus statement on catheter and surgical ablation of atrial fibrillation: recommendations for personnel, policy, procedures and follow-up. A report of the Heart Rhythm Society (HRS) Task Force on catheter and surgical ablation of atrial fibrillation. European Heart Rhythm Association (EHRA); European Cardiac Arrhythmia Society (ECAS); American College of Cardiology (ACC); American Heart Association (AHA); Society of Thoracic Surgeons (STS). *Heart Rhythm.* 2007;4:816–861.

64. Lin YJ, Tai CT, Chang SL, et al. Efficacy of additional ablation of complex fractionated atrial electrograms for catheter ablation of nonparoxysmal atrial fibrillation. *J Cardiovasc Electrophysiol.* 2009;20:607–615.

65. Lo LW, Lin YJ, Tsao HM, et al. Characteristics of complex fractionated electrograms in non-pulmonary vein ectopy initiating atrial fibrillation/atrial tachycardia. *J Cardiovasc Electrophysiol.* 2009;20:1305–1312.

66. Tops LF, Bax JJ, Zeppenfeld K, et al. Fusion of multislice computed tomography imaging with three-dimensional electroanatomic mapping to guide radiofrequency catheter ablation procedures. *Heart Rhythm.* 2005;2:1076–1081.

67. Okumura Y, Henz BD, Johnson SB, et al. Three-dimensional ultrasound for image-guided mapping and intervention: methods, quantitative validation, and clinical feasibility of a novel multimodality image mapping system. *Circ Arrhythmia Electrophysiol.* 2008;1:110–119.

68. Huang BH, Wu MH, Tsao HM, et al. Morphology of the thoracic veins and left atrium in paroxysmal atrial fibrillation initiated by superior caval vein ectopy. *J Cardiovasc Electrophysiol.* 2005;16:411–417.

69. Chen SA, Tai CT. Catheter ablation of atrial fibrillation originating from the non-pulmonary vein foci. *J Cardiovasc Electrophysiol.* 2005;16:229–232.

70. Higa S, Lin YJ, Tai CT, et al. Noncontact mapping. In: Calkin H, Jais P, Steinberg J, eds. *A Practical Approach to Catheter Ablation of Atrial Fibrillation.* Philadelphia: Lippincott Williams & Wilkins; 2008:118–133.

71. Chang SL, Tuan TC, Tai CT, et al. Comparison of outcome in catheter ablation of atrial fibrillation in patients with versus without the metabolic syndrome. *Am J Cardiol.* 2009;103:67–72.

72. Oakes RS, Badger TJ, Kholmovski EG, et al. Detection and quantification of left atrial structural remodeling with delayed-enhancement magnetic resonance imaging in patients with atrial fibrillation. *Circulation.* 2009;119:1758–1767.

73. Lee RJ, Kalman JM, Fitzpatrick AP, et al. Radiofrequency catheter modification of the sinus node for "inappropriate" sinus tachycardia. *Circulation.* 1995;92:2919–2928.

74. Callans DJ, Ren JF, Schwartzman D, et al. Narrowing of the superior vena cava-right atrium junction during radiofrequency catheter ablation for inappropriate sinus tachycardia: analysis with intracardiac echocardiography. *J Am Coll Cardiol.* 1999;33:1667–1670.

75. Man KC, Knight B, Tse HF, et al. Radiofrequency catheter ablation of inappropriate sinus tachycardia guided by activation mapping. *J Am Coll Cardiol.* 2000;35:451–457.

76. Pappone C, Oral H, Santinelli V, et al. Atrio-esophageal fistula as a complication of percutaneous transcatheter ablation of atrial fibrillation. *Circulation.* 2004;109:2724–2726.

77. Shah D, Dumonceau JM, Burri H, et al. Acute pyloric spasm and gastric hypomotility: an extracardiac adverse effect of percutaneous radiofrequency ablation for atrial fibrillation. *J Am Coll Cardiol.* 2005;46:327–330.

78. Tsao HM, Wu MH, Higa S, et al. Anatomic relationship of the esophagus and left atrium: implication for catheter ablation of atrial fibrillation. *Chest.* 2005;128:2581–2587.

79. Tsuchiya T, Ashikaga K, Nakagawa S, et al. Atrial fibrillation ablation with esophageal cooling with a cooled water-irrigated intraesophageal balloon: a pilot study. *J Cardiovasc Electrophysiol.* 2007;18:145–150.

80. Arruda MS, Armaganijan L, di Biase L, et al. Feasibility and safety of using an esophageal protective system to eliminate esophageal thermal injury: implications on atrial-esophageal fistula following AF ablation. *J Cardiovasc Electrophysiol.* 2009;20:1272–1278.

17

Substrate-Based Ablation for Atrial Fibrillation

Thomas Crawford, Mark A. Wood, and Hakan Oral

Key Points

Atrial substrate modification is required for a successful outcome in a minority of patients with paroxysmal atrial fibrillation (AF) but in most of the patients with persistent AF.

Substrate modification is considered when AF persists despite effective elimination of pulmonary vein (PV) arrhythmogenicity by extraostial PV isolation, antral PV isolation, or wide area circumferential ablation.

Substrate modification strategies include linear ablation, ablation guided by complex fractionated atrial electrograms, and ablation of ganglionated plexuses.

Termination of AF to sinus rhythm or to an atrial tachycardia is considered the most favorable procedural end point for substrate modification.

Complete bidirectional conduction block should be confirmed when linear ablation is performed.

Mechanisms of Atrial Fibrillation and Rationale for Substrate Ablation

The pathogenesis of atrial fibrillation (AF) is complex and multifactorial. Pulmonary vein (PV) tachycardias have been demonstrated to play a critical role in both initiation and perpetuation of AF.[1-4]

Although elimination of PV arrhythmogenicity has been highly effective for paroxysmal AF, it has modest efficacy for persistent AF,[5,6] suggesting that mechanisms beyond the PVs also contribute to perpetuation of AF in these patients.

AF promotes diffuse electroanatomic remodeling. AF results in a nonhomogeneous decrease in atrial refractoriness and slowing of intra-atrial conduction.[7] Histologic

examinations of atrial tissue in patients with AF show patchy fibrosis, which may contribute to the nonhomogeneity of conduction. Atrial biopsies from patients undergoing cardiac surgery show increase in cell size, loss of sarcoplasmic reticulum and atrial myofibrils, changes in mitochondrial shape, accumulation of glycogen granules, alteration in connexin expression, and increase in extracellular matrix.[7-10] Structural changes in response to AF may be a consequence of a physiologic adaptation to chronic Ca^{2+} overload and metabolic stress. Reduction of atrial compliance and contractility during AF may enhance atrial dilation, which may add to the persistence of AF.

In the multiple-wavelet hypothesis proposed by Moe, multiple randomly propagating and self-perpetuating "daughter wavelets" act as a mechanism for perpetuation of AF.[11] Critical to the multiple-wavelet hypothesis is a minimal left atrial size that can accommodate the wavelength as determined by the product of the conduction velocity and the effective refractory period. More recently, high-frequency sources (i.e., rotors), as a result of anisotropic reentry, have been demonstrated to perpetuate AF in experimental and simulation models.[12-14] Modulation of the autonomic innervation of the atria through ganglionated plexuses has also been suggested to play a role in AF because an increase in vagal tone is associated with a decrease in the effective refractory period (ERP) and in an increase in spontaneous depolarizations from the PVs and elsewhere in the atria.[15,16] Thus, atrial structures outside the PV may initiate and sustain AF or serve to perpetuate AF once initiated by any means. A number of ablation strategies have been proposed, alone or in combination, to target these substrate-related mechanisms beyond the PV arrhythmogenicity, particularly in patients with persistent AF (Table 17-1).

Antral Pulmonary Vein Isolation

Pathophysiology

The pathophysiologic basis for PV isolation is covered in detail in Chapter 15. The PVs may serve as critical sources of rapid repetitive depolarizations, referred to as *intermittent PV tachycardias*, due to triggered activity,

TABLE 17-1				
STRATEGIES FOR SUBSTRATE ABLATION				
Ablation Strategy	**Targets**	**Mapping**	**Substrate Altered**	**End Point**
PV isolation	PV antrum and encircling tissue	Anatomic with or without 3D mapping	PV arrhythmogenicity CFAE Autonomics Micro-reentry Rotors Debulking	Complete PV and antral electrical isolation
Linear ablation	LA roof Mitral isthmus Posterior wall isolation	Anatomic with or without 3D mapping	Macro-reentry CFAEs with or without autonomics Rotors	Conduction block across lines
Electrogram-guided ablation	CFAEs Frequency gradient Activation gradient	Electrogram features with or without computerized analysis	Slow conduction Rotors, high-frequency sources Autonomics	AF termination Elimination of CFAE
Autonomics	Parasympathetic ganglionated plexuses atrial LOM	High-frequency pacing (plexuses) Angiography (LOM)	Autonomics with or without CFAE	Absence of vagal response

AF, atrial fibrillation; CFAE, complex fractionated atrial electrograms; LA, left atrium; LOM, ligament of Marshall; PV, pulmonary vein.

automaticity, and reentry that both initiate and sustain AF. In addition to a direct role of the PVs, the atrial tissue around the PVs may harbor complex myofibril arrays, ganglionated plexuses, and areas of slow conduction and fractionated electrical activity that also contribute to AF. In addition to eliminating PV arrhythmogenicity, PV isolation may affect ablation of anchor points for rotors, which are more prevalent in the antral regions of the PVs; debulking of the left atrium; ablation of ganglionated plexuses; and ablation of arrhythmogenic foci other than the PVs, such as the ligament of Marshall (LOM) and posterior left atrium.

Mapping and Ablation

Circumferential PV ablation (CPVA) encircles the PVs 1 to 2 cm from the ostium except at the anterior aspect of the left-sided PVs, where ablation is performed along the ostial aspect of the ridge between the left atrial appendage and the PVs (Figs. 17-1 and 17-2).[17-20] By extending the encircling lesions outside the PV into the antral or atrial tissue, critical sites of complex atrial electrograms and autonomic innervations may simultaneously be eliminated. Thus, PV isolation is generally considered a cornerstone of current catheter ablative therapy for AF. The end point of ablation is complete electrical isolation of the PV, confirmed preferably with a circular mapping catheter.

Outcomes

The clinical outcomes after PV isolation are reviewed in Chapter 15. PV isolation is generally considered an appropriate stand-alone procedure for patients with paroxysmal AF. Patients with nonparoxysmal forms of AF typically require additional ablation, specifically for substrate modification, to achieve maximal benefit from ablation procedures.[21,22]

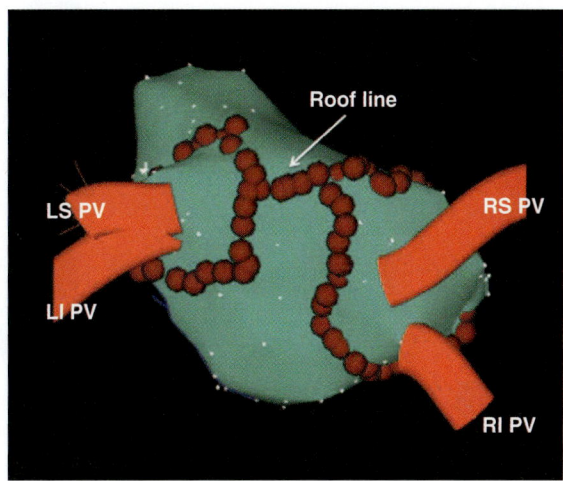

FIGURE 17-1. A three-dimensional electroanatomic depiction of the left atrium and the pulmonary veins (PVs) is shown in a right posterior oblique projection with cranial angulation. Two encircling PV lesions were created. A roof line was added. LI, left inferior; LS, left superior; RI, right inferior; RS, right superior. *(From Oral H, Pappone C, Chugh A, et al. Circumferential pulmonary-vein ablation for chronic atrial fibrillation.* N Engl J Med. *2006;354:934–941. With permission.)*

Problems and Limitations

PV isolation is a complex and technically demanding procedure, although new technology promises to simplify the ablation process.

An important safety consideration during ablation along the posterior left atrial wall is the risk for inadvertent collateral injury to the esophagus. Atrioesophageal fistula is a rare but often fatal complication.[22,23] Ingestion of barium paste[24-28] and esophageal temperature monitoring[26-28] have both been employed to prevent injury to the esophagus during ablation. However, esophageal luminal temperature measurement may underestimate the true esophageal tissue temperature.[29]

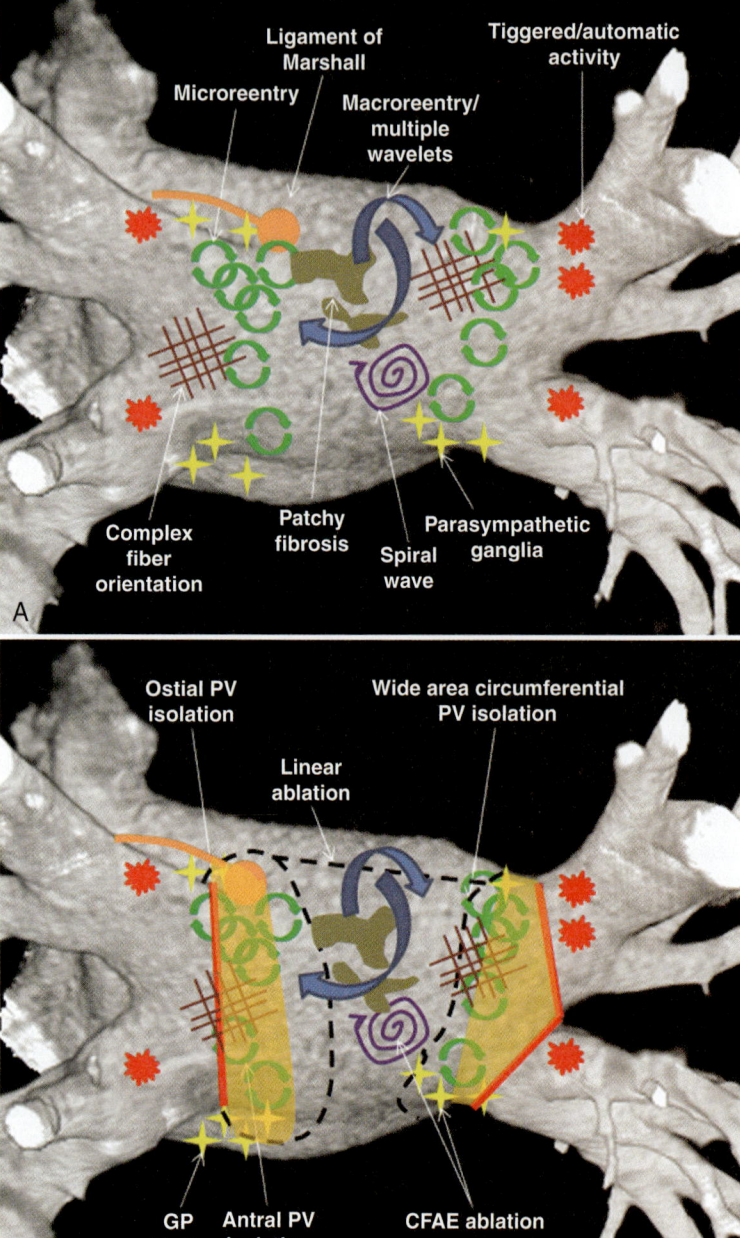

FIGURE 17-2. A, Possible atrial substrates responsible for the initiation and maintenance of atrial fibrillation (posteroanterior atrial view shown). Note the concentrated distribution of important substrates near the pulmonary veins (PVs) and posterior left atrial wall. **B,** Potential effects of PV isolation and linear ablation on left atrial substrate for atrial fibrillation. Ostial PV isolation may eliminate PV arrhythmogenicity but little else. Antral (*orange highlight*) and wide area PV isolation may also eliminate arrhythmia mechanisms near the PV. Linear ablation (roof line shown) may interrupt macro-reentry circuits with variable collateral effects on fractionated electrograms and autonomics. CFAE, complex fractionated atrial electrogram; GP, ganglionated plexus.

Linear Ablation

Pathophysiology

Catheter ablation for AF initially consisted of linear ablation to emulate the Cox surgical maze procedure.[30,31] Linear catheter ablation was first limited to the right atrium and had low efficacy. Later, linear ablation was performed in the left atrium. Linear ablation has been performed both as a stand-alone strategy and as an adjunctive strategy to other ablation techniques targeting the PV antrum and complex electrograms.[32,33] Recent studies have demonstrated that additional linear ablation improves the clinical efficacy of catheter ablation in patients with paroxysmal and persistent AF.[32,34,35] The original intent of linear ablation for AF was to interrupt macro-reentrant circuits.[36,37] Other pos-

sible mechanisms by which linear ablation may improve outcomes of AF ablation are interruption of micro-reentrant circuits, elimination of anchor points for high-frequency sources, and atrial debulking. Complex fractionated atrial electrograms (CFAEs) may also be prevalent along the course of linear lesions such as the septum or the roof. Finally, autonomic ganglia may be eliminated during linear ablation at certain sites, such as the left atrial roof.

Linear lesions may be a necessary step in conversion of AF to sinus rhythm, often through an intermediate step of atrial tachycardia. In a recent study that used a stepwise ablation strategy including isolation of thoracic veins, ablation of CFAEs, and linear ablation until AF terminated, linear ablation was necessary in more than 80% of the patients with persistent AF for termination.[38]

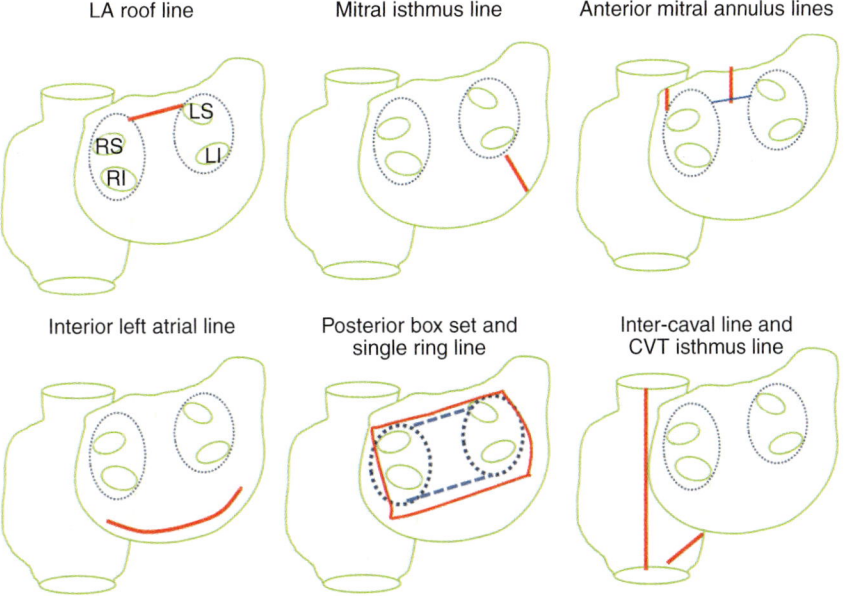

LA roof line   Mitral isthmus line   Anterior mitral annulus lines

Interior left atrial line   Posterior box set and   Inter-caval line and
                             single ring line   CVT isthmus line

FIGURE 17-3. Linear ablation lesions for the left and right atria. The view perspective is anteroposterior. Pulmonary vein (PV) encircling lesions are shown in *blue broken lines* and linear lesions in *solid red lines*. The posterior box set is shown in *blue*, and the single ring lesion set is shown in *red*. CVT, cavotricuspid isthmus; LA, left atrium; LI, left inferior; LS, left superior; RI, right inferior; RS, right superior.

Mapping and Ablation

Linear ablation has been performed along the roof of the left atrium between the contralateral superior PVs, along the lateral mitral isthmus between the ostium of the left inferior PV and the lateral mitral annulus, along the left atrial septum, from the anterior aspect of the right PV antrum to the septal mitral annulus, along the posterior mitral annulus parallel to the coronary sinus, anteriorly between a roof line and anterior mitral annulus, and along the right atrial aspect of the interatrial septum from the superior vena cava (SVC) to the inferior vena cava (IVC) (Fig. 17-3). In addition, a "box set" of lesions to isolate the posterior left atrium has been performed with variable efficacy.[38,39] Currently, the left atrial roof and the mitral isthmus are the most commonly targeted sites. Although completeness of conduction block along a linear lesion has not been uniformly assessed in all prior studies, it is always desirable to confirm complete bidirectional conduction block. Incomplete block with slow conduction promotes reentry and may facilitate proarrhythmia, often in the form of persistent or recurrent atrial flutters. Prior studies have suggested that macro-reentrant circuits may be present during AF. Elimination of high-frequency drivers that lead to fibrillatory conduction often results in termination of AF to a macro-reentrant tachycardia.[36,37] Therefore, linear ablation may interrupt these macro-reentrant circuits that coexist with AF.

Left Atrial Roof Line

The goal of the roof line is to produce a line of block between the left and right superior PVs (Fig. 17-4; also Figs. 17-2 and 17-3). The line should be directed as cranially as possible, avoiding the posterior wall where esophageal injury may result. It is efficient to perform this ablation after encircling PV isolation such that the roof line connects the gap between the PV isolation lines. A long fixed curve (Daig SL0) or steerable sheath can

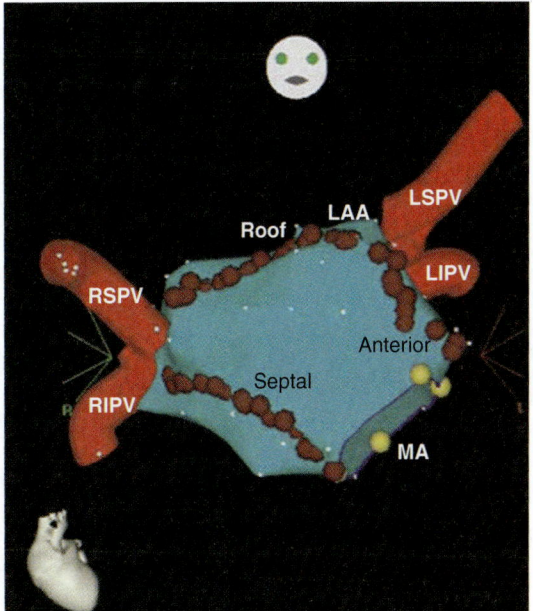

FIGURE 17-4. Three-dimensional anteroposterior electroanatomic map of the left atrium showing nonencircling ablation lesions. Anterior, septal, and roof lines were created in this patient. LAA, left atrial appendage; LIPV, left inferior pulmonary vein; LSPV, left superior pulmonary vein; MA, mitral annulus; RIPV, right inferior pulmonary vein; RSPV, right superior pulmonary vein. *(From Oral H, Chugh A, Good E, et al. Randomized comparison of encircling and nonencircling left atrial ablation for chronic atrial fibrillation.* Heart Rhythm. *2005;2:1165–1172. With permission.)*

greatly improve catheter contact and stability. Two techniques for creation of this line have been described.[40] In the first method, the catheter is positioned at the margin of the left superior PV and dragged to the right superior PV. The catheter tip is maintained in a perpendicular orientation to the atrial wall (Fig. 17-5). The sheath extends almost to the distal electrode to support and steer the catheter. Energy is delivered for 30 to 60 seconds at each site, moving the catheter by about 5-mm increments between locations. Catheter temperature and impedance should be closely monitored because of the perpendicular electrode orientation that may predispose to tissue overheating, steam pops, and perforation.

The second approach positions the catheter at the right superior PV with the catheter retroflexed over the sheath (Fig. 17-6).[40] The electrode is parallel to the tissue with this technique. The sheath and catheter are then advanced, driving the electrode toward the left superior PV. Releasing the catheter deflection will also advance the catheter toward the left vein.

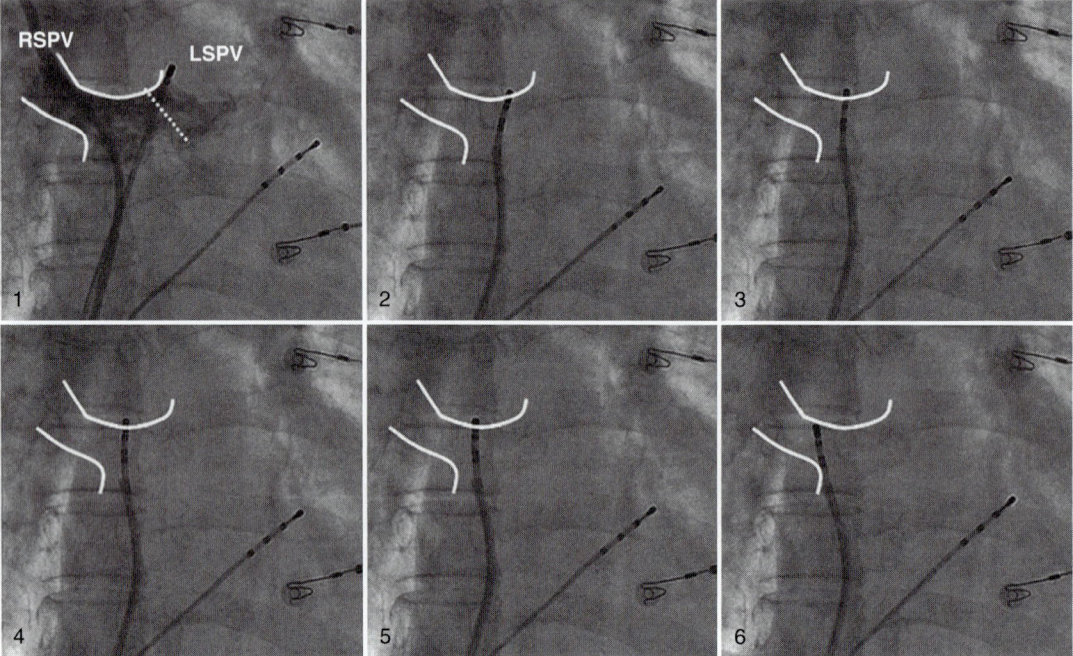

FIGURE 17-5. Anteroposterior views of ablation catheter position during ablation at the left atrial roof. *Panel 1,* The right superior (RS) and left superior (LS) pulmonary veins (PVs) are opacified by contrast injection, showing a concave orientation of the roof. Ablation is started at the ostium of the left superior pulmonary vein *(panel 2)* and progressively moved to the ostium of the right superior pulmonary vein *(panel 6).* Note that the ablation catheter is almost entirely in the long sheath, ensuring good control and tissue contact. Extra care is needed because any sudden push may result in perforation. *(From Jais P, Hocini M, O'Neill MD, et al. How to perform linear lesions. Heart Rhythm. 2007;4:803–809. With permission.)*

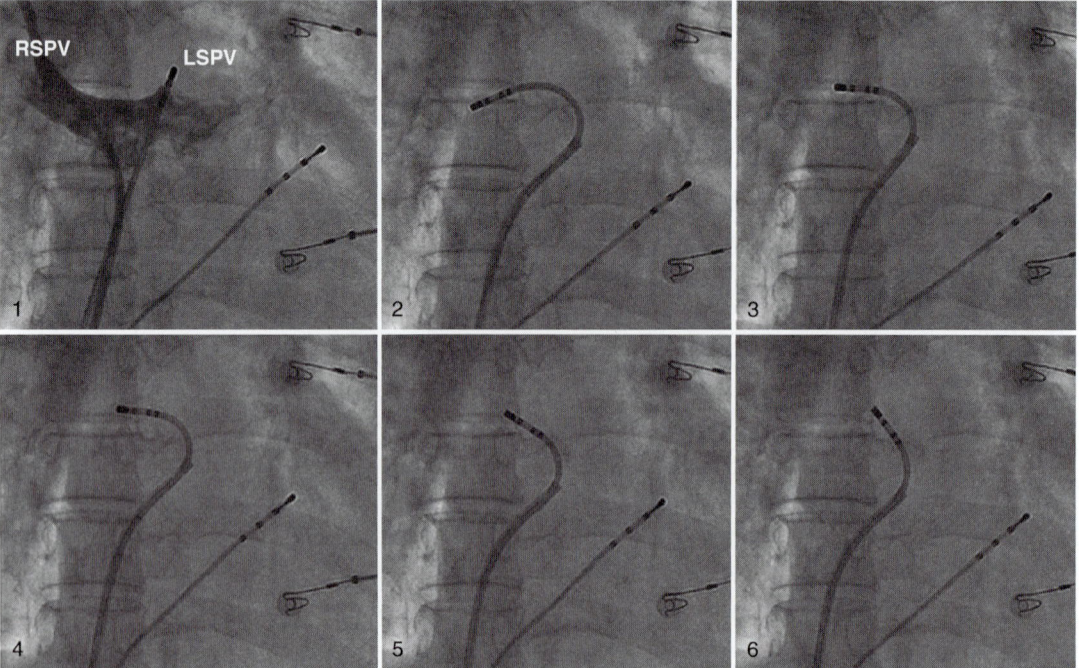

FIGURE 17-6. Alternative approach to creation of the roof line. The ablation catheter placed in the right superior pulmonary vein (RSPV) is deflected, and the sheath and catheter assembly are progressively pushed toward the left superior pulmonary vein (LSPV; *panels 2-5). (From Jais P, Hocini M, O'Neill MD, et al. How to perform linear lesions. Heart Rhythm. 2007;4:803–809. With permission.)*

Assessment of Conduction Block. A complete linear lesion should result in widely separated double potentials along the length of the line (Table 17-2).[40] A delay of more than 100 milliseconds is usually indicative of complete block, but reliance on conduction time alone may be misleading.[40] During left atrial appendage pacing, posterior left atrial activation should proceed in a caudal-to-cranial direction. Differential pacing maneuvers are also useful to detect slow residual conduction through the line. As the pacing site moves away from the edge of the line, the conduction time from the stimulus to the electrogram on the opposite side of the line will shorten with complete block but prolong in the presence of residual slow conduction through the line (Fig. 17-7).[40]

TABLE 17-2

ASSESSING CONDUCTION BLOCK ACROSS LINEAR ABLATION LINES

Finding/Maneuver	Finding Indicative of Complete Block	Comment
Widely split electrograms	>100 msec generally indicates block	Absolute time between electrogram components depends on local conduction velocities Block may be present with shorter times and conduction persistent with longer times
Differential pacing	Pacing site close to edge line produces longer conduction times from stimulus to opposite side of line than pacing at site away from line	Must pace from immediate edge of line
Propagation from pacing adjacent to line	Pacing on either side of line produces two wavefronts, each propagating toward the ablation line from opposite directions	Roof line: pace LAA and confirm that posterior wall is activated from caudal to cranial direction Mitral isthmus line: pacing CS lateral to line produces proximal to distal CS activation and pacing CS medial to the line produces distal-to-proximal CS activation Anterior mitral isthmus line: pacing lateral to line produces atrial septal activation from the posterior and lateral directions Posterior wall isolation: entrance and exit block within "box"

CS, coronary sinus; LAA, left atrial appendage.

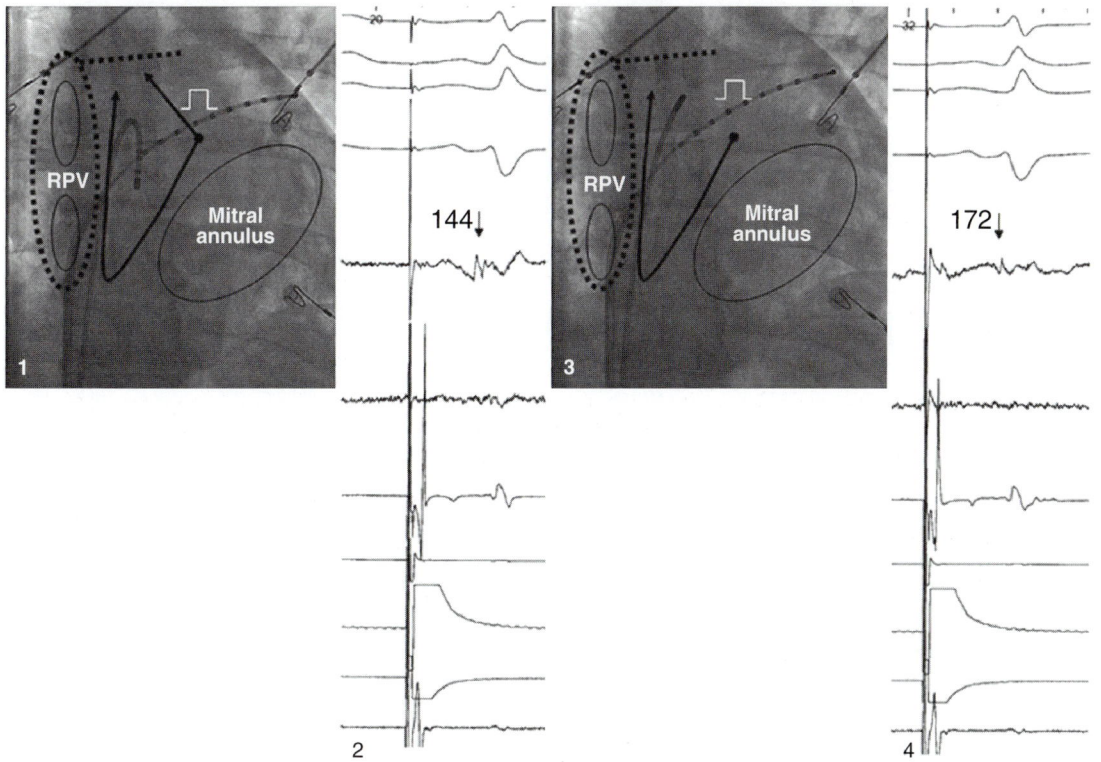

FIGURE 17-7. Roof line and encircling lesion around the right pulmonary veins (RPV, *dashed line, panels 1 and 3*). The encircling lesion around the left pulmonary veins is not shown. The roof line is assessed during pacing from the anterior left atrium from a decapolar catheter across the anterior-superior left atrium. The distal decapolar bipole is located in the left atrial appendage; the proximal bipole is located at the septum. The ablation catheter is used to map the low posterior left atrium (*panel 1*), where a 144-msec delay is recorded (*panel 2*). In the high posterior left atrium, closer to the roof line (*panel 3*), a 172-msec delay (*panel 4*) is recorded, demonstrating an activation front from the caudal to cranial direction. (*From Jais P, Hocini M, O'Neill MD, et al. How to perform linear lesions.* Heart Rhythm. *2007;4:803–809. With permission.*)

Mitral Isthmus Line

The goal of this procedure is to produce a continuous line of block from the lateral mitral isthmus to the left inferior PV.[40,41] It is recommended that a multipolar catheter be placed in the coronary sinus spanning the linear lesion to serve as an anatomic reference and to monitor the effects of ablation.[40,41] Up to 70% of patients require ablation within the distal coronary sinus to achieve conduction block.[41] If ablation within the coronary sinus is not possible or unacceptable to the operator, the creation of this line should be carefully considered. As with any linear ablation, the creation of incomplete linear lesions is often counterproductive by prolonging procedure time, increasing the risk for complications, and possibly creating a proarrhythmic substrate. Using a long sheath, the ablation electrode is positioned at the lateral mitral annulus to record an atrial-to-ventricular (A/V) ratio of 1:1 or 1:2 (Fig. 17-8).[40,41] The electrode can be perpendicular or parallel to the tissue (Fig. 17-8). The site on the annulus can be selected to result in the shortest distance to the left inferior vein and its previously created encircling lesion. Lesions are delivered at each site for 1 to 2 minutes with a power limit of 30 to 35 W.[40,41] Starting at the mitral annulus, the catheter and sheath are rotated with clockwise torque to move the electrode toward the PV in 5-mm steps.[40,41] Care should be taken to detect inadvertent catheter displacement abruptly into the left inferior PV or appendage. Progress during ablation is gauged by splitting of the ablation electrogram and by delay in conduction across the lesion on the coronary sinus catheter during pacing proximal or distal to the line. Conduction times longer than 100 milliseconds from the stimulus to the electrogram on the opposite side of the line are often associated with conduction block across the line.[40] A more lateral line from the base of the appendage to the annulus may produce

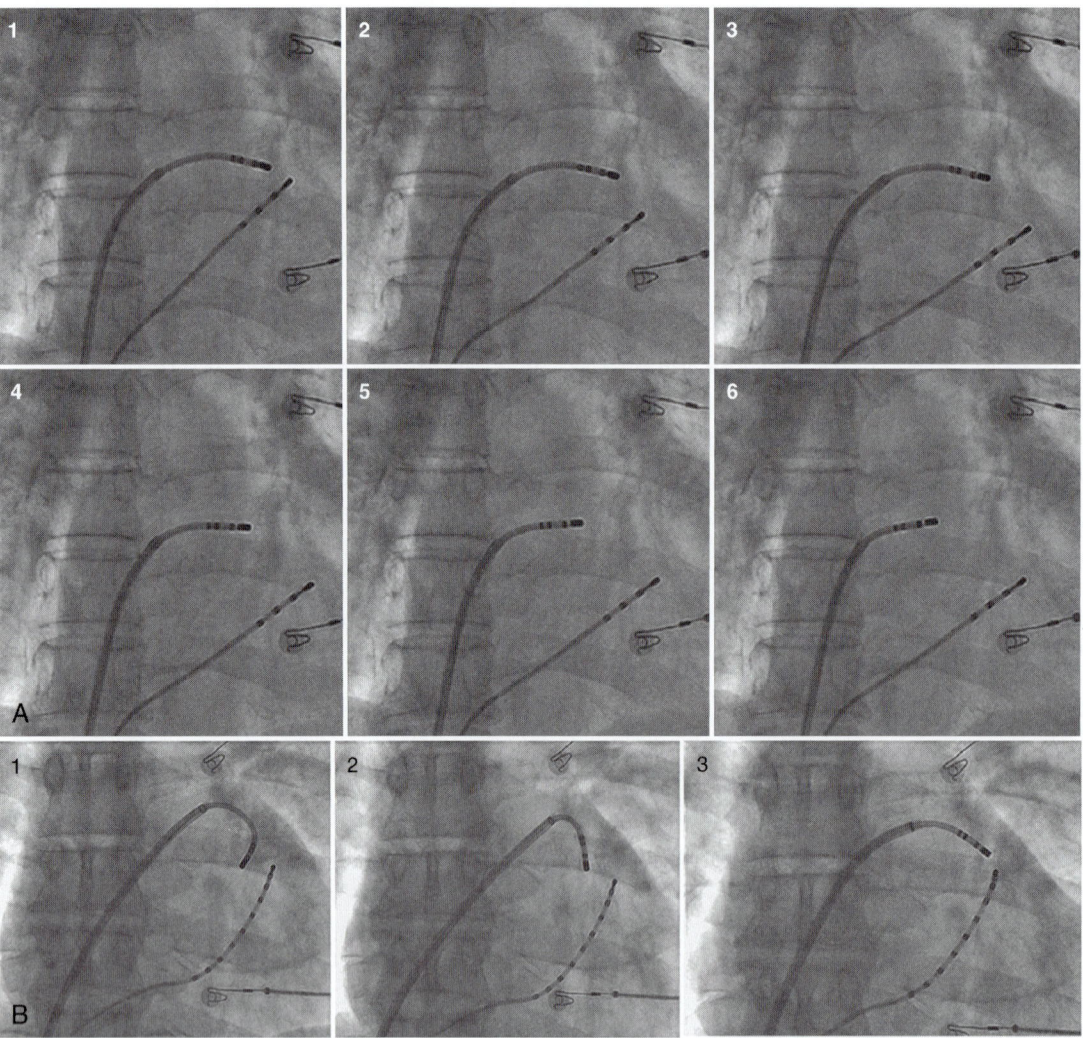

FIGURE 17-8. Mitral isthmus ablation line. Anteroposterior views are shown. **A,** *Panel 1,* Ablation of the mitral isthmus starts at the lateral mitral isthmus. *Panels 1-6,* The sheath and catheter are rotated clockwise to extend the lesion posteriorly to the ostium of the left inferior pulmonary vein. During this movement, the ablation catheter is progressively pulled back in the sheath. **B,** *Panels 1-2,* The sheath and catheter are used to increase tissue contact at the mitral isthmus, with an almost 180-degree curve of the ablation catheter. Despite good contact, the resulting lesion is insufficient in some patients. Moreover, the tip of the catheter may abruptly dislodge into the left atrial appendage and perforate. Therefore, although this approach is useful in some patients, it should not be used in the first instance because it carries a greater risk than the method described in **A.** *Panel 3,* Ablation catheter tip at the ostium of the left atrial appendage. This is the only position where the orientation is truly perpendicular to the tissue. In some patients, this is the only method for achieving complete isthmus block. *(From Jais P, Hocini M, O'Neill MD, et al. How to perform linear lesions. Heart Rhythm. 2007;4:803–809. With permission.)*

block when the initial line fails. Despite up to 30 minutes of delivered endocardial radiofrequency energy, isthmus block results in only 32% of patients. Most patients, therefore, require ablation within the coronary sinus to produce isthmus block.[40,41] Ablation in the coronary sinus should be limited to use of irrigated catheters with maximal power of 20 to 25 W.[40,41] The catheter should deflected toward the endocardium to avoid the left circumflex artery. An average of 5 ± 4 minutes of radiofrequency delivered in the coronary sinus completes isthmus block in 84% of patients.[40,41]

Assessing Conduction Block. Achieving complete conduction block along the mitral isthmus can be challenging. With complete isthmus block, widely separated electrograms, usually by more than 100 milliseconds, should be recorded along the length of the ablation line.[40,41] Pacing the coronary sinus or appendage distal to the ablation line results in proximal-to-distal coronary sinus activation on the septal side of the line (Fig. 17-9). Likewise, coronary sinus pacing proximal to the line results in distal-to-proximal coronary sinus activation lateral to the line. As the pacing site is moved away from the edge of the ablation line, the conduction time from the stimulus to the electrograms recorded on the opposite side of the line decreases in the setting of conduction block but increases in the setting of slow conduction across the line (Fig. 17-10). To accurately assess conduction block, it is important to position the catheters as close as possible to the mitral isthmus line.[40]

Anterior Left Atrial Line

The goal of this procedure is to create a line of block from either the right superior PV or roof line to the anterior mitral annulus (Fig. 17-2).[40] This line serves as an alternative to the mitral isthmus line and also interrupts more localized reentry circuits in this area. It is recommended that the line start at the anterior mitral isthmus (Fig. 17-11). The ablation catheter is withdrawn with counterclockwise torque to maintain contact with the anterior or anteroseptal left atrial wall.[40] When the ablation electrode reaches the level of the transseptal puncture, clockwise torque is begun, and the catheter advanced to reach the right superior PV or

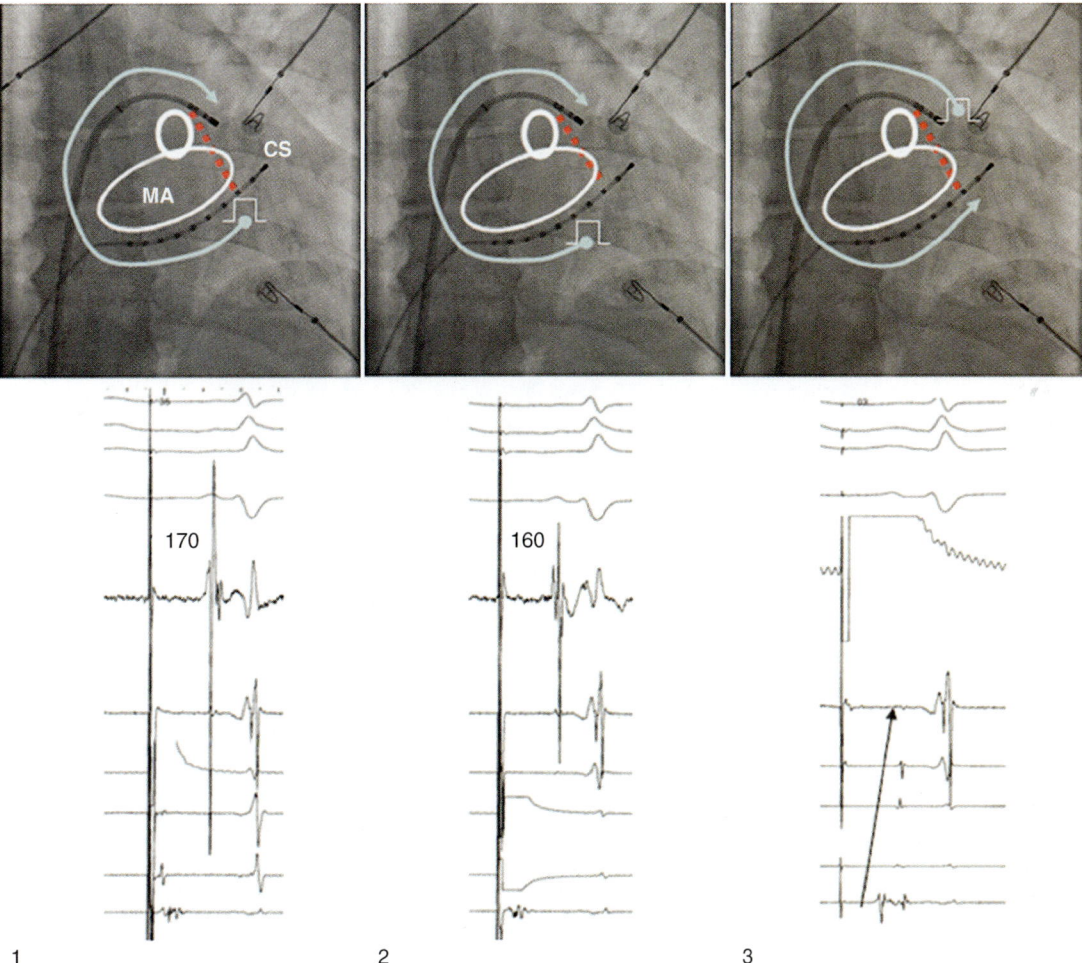

FIGURE 17-9. Mitral isthmus line *(dashed)* connecting the mitral annulus (MA) to the left inferior pulmonary vein *(continuous white lines)*. Panel 1, Pacing from bipole 3-4 of the coronary sinus (CS) catheter, immediately septal to the linear lesion, is associated with a 170-msec delay recorded with the ablation catheter at the lateral edge of the line. *Panel 2,* When pacing is performed more proximally from bipole 5-6, the activation route in the presence of complete block is shortened; accordingly, the delay at the ablation catheter is shorter (160 msec). *Panel 3,* Bidirectional block is demonstrated because pacing lateral to the line of the ablation catheter is associated with proximal-to-distal CS activation. The double potentials observed at the CS ostium are the result of previous CS ablation required to convert this patient with persistent atrial fibrillation. *(From Jais P, Hocini M, O'Neill MD, et al. How to perform linear lesions. Heart Rhythm. 2007;4:803–809. With permission.)*

roof line. The anterior line may lead to a significant delay in atrial conduction and left atrial appendage activation and may adversely affect left atrial transport function.[40–43]

Assessing Conduction Block. With complete conduction block, widely separated electrograms should be recorded along the entire length of the line. In addition, pacing the anterior left atrium just lateral to the line results in left atrial activation proceeding from lateral and posterior directions to activate the left atrial septum. As the pacing site is moved away from the edge of the ablation line, the conduction time from the stimulus to the electrograms recorded on the opposite side of the line decreases in the setting of conduction block but increases in the setting of slow conduction across the line.

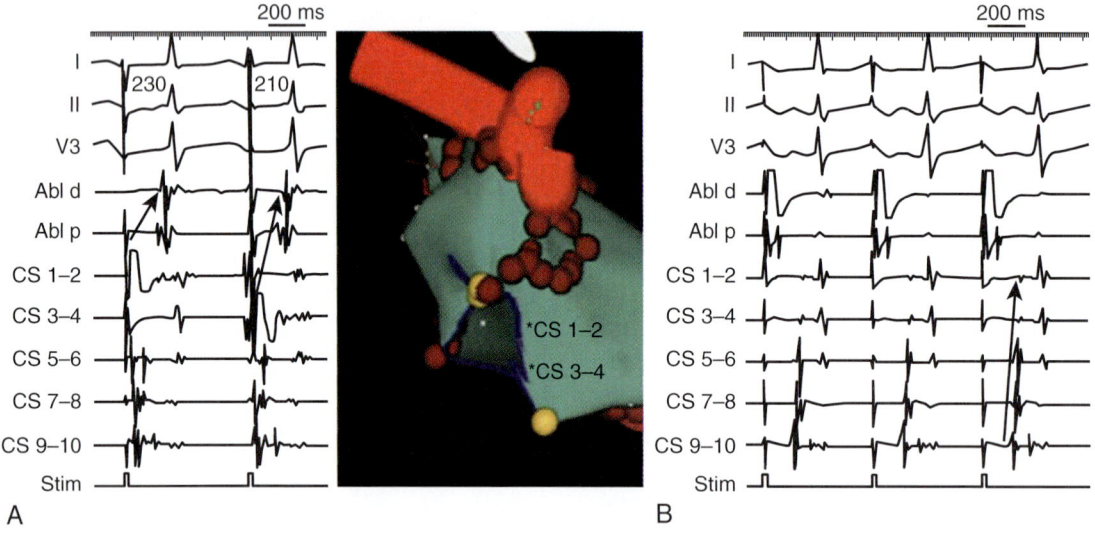

FIGURE 17-10. Mitral isthmus block. **A,** Differential pacing to assess counterclockwise block across an ablation line in the mitral isthmus. The ablation catheter is positioned medial to the ablation line in the left atrium. Pacing was performed in the coronary sinus, and as the pacing site was switched from the distal electrodes (CS 1-2) to a more proximal pair of electrodes (CS 3-4), the interval between the pacing stimulus and the local electrogram recorded from the ablation catheter shortened from 230 to 210 msec. **B,** Clockwise conduction block along the mitral isthmus. Note that atrial activation progresses from the proximal (CS 9-10) to distal (CS 1-2) electrodes during left atrial pacing medial to the ablation line. Abl d and Abl p: distal and proximal bipolar recordings from the ablation catheter, respectively; Stim, stimulus. *(Morady F, Oral H, Chugh A. Diagnosis and ablation of atypical atrial tachycardia and flutter complicating atrial fibrillation ablation. Heart Rhythm. 2009;6:S29–S32. With permission.)*

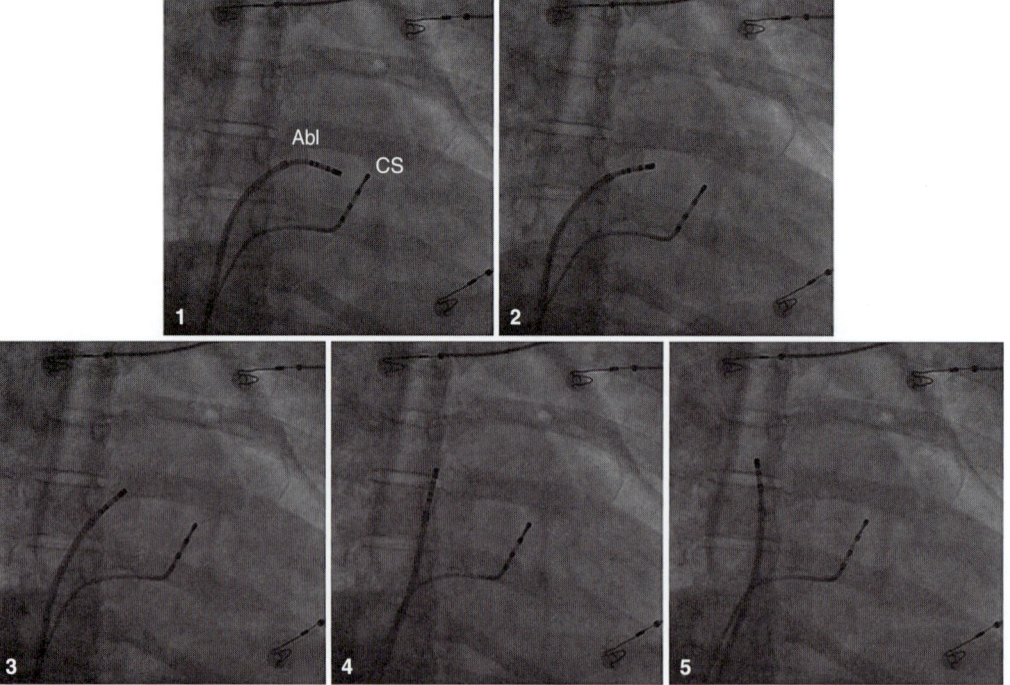

FIGURE 17-11. Position of the ablation catheter during anterior line ablation. An anteroposterior view is shown. The lesion is started at the superior-medial mitral annulus (*panel 1*). The ablation catheter and long sheath are progressively withdrawn with counterclockwise torque to reach the level of the fossa ovale. At this point (*panel 3*), the catheter torque should be clockwise, and the catheter is advanced to connect the line either to the lesion encircling the right pulmonary veins or to the roof line (*panels 4 and 5*). *(From Jais P, Hocini M, O'Neill MD, et al. How to perform linear lesions. Heart Rhythm. 2007;4:803–809. With permission.)*

Inferior Mitral Annulus Line

Ablation along the inferior mitral isthmus parallel to the coronary sinus may be performed to interrupt muscular connections between the atrium and coronary sinus and other foci that may perpetuate AF.[44] This line is generally used within the strategy of ablation of complex atrial electrograms. This line is begun with the catheter forming a loop in the left atrium and directed back toward the atrial septum (Fig. 17-12). The electrode is then withdrawn from the 7- to 4-o'clock position as viewed in the left anterior oblique projection.[44] Opening the catheter curvature as the tip moves laterally will improve tissue contact. Ablation within the coronary sinus is needed to eliminate all complex atrial activity and to produce maximal slowing of the AF rate (Fig. 17-12). The end point for this ablation line is the elimination and organization of complex atrial electrograms within the coronary sinus or significant slowing of the atrial cycle length.[44]

Posterior Left Atrial Isolation

The goal of this lesion set is complete electrical isolation of the left atrial posterior wall.[38,39] Two techniques are described (Fig. 17-3). In the left atrial box set, the PVs are isolated by antral encircling ablations, and a roof line is created as described previously. A linear lesion is then created between the left and right inferior PV to complete the set.[38] Alternatively, the continuous single ring linear lesion extends up the ridge between the left PV and the atrial appendage, across the roof, inferiorly along the interatrial septum between the foramen ovale

and right PVs, then inferior to the right PV and lateral across the atrium to meet the start of the line by ascending lateral to the left inferior PVs.[39] Completion of this line isolates the PV and posterior left atrial wall en bloc (Fig. 17-13).[39]

Assessing Conduction Block. The end point for both approaches is the absence or dissociation of electrograms within the lesion box and exit block during pacing from the posterior wall. The PV should be isolated as well with the single-ring approach.[38,39]

Outcomes

Mitral and left atrial roof lines increase AF cycle length to an extent similar to PV isolation, and AF cycle length prolongation is associated with improved outcome.[45] Linear lesions may be a necessary step in conversion of AF to sinus rhythm, often through an intermediate step of atrial tachycardia. In a recent study that used a stepwise ablation strategy, including isolation of thoracic veins, ablation of CFAEs, and linear ablation until AF was terminated, linear ablation was necessary in more than 80% of the patients for termination of persistent AF.[36,46] For patients with persistent AF, the addition of linear lesions to PV isolation at the initial procedure reduces the incidence of subsequent macro-reentrant arrhythmias.[47] In patients with paroxysmal AF, the addition of *confirmed* mitral isthmus ablation reduces the recurrence rate of AF to 13% at 1 year, compared with 31% for those undergoing PV isolation alone.[41] The addition of mitral isthmus ablation also improves outcomes in patients with persistent AF.[47]

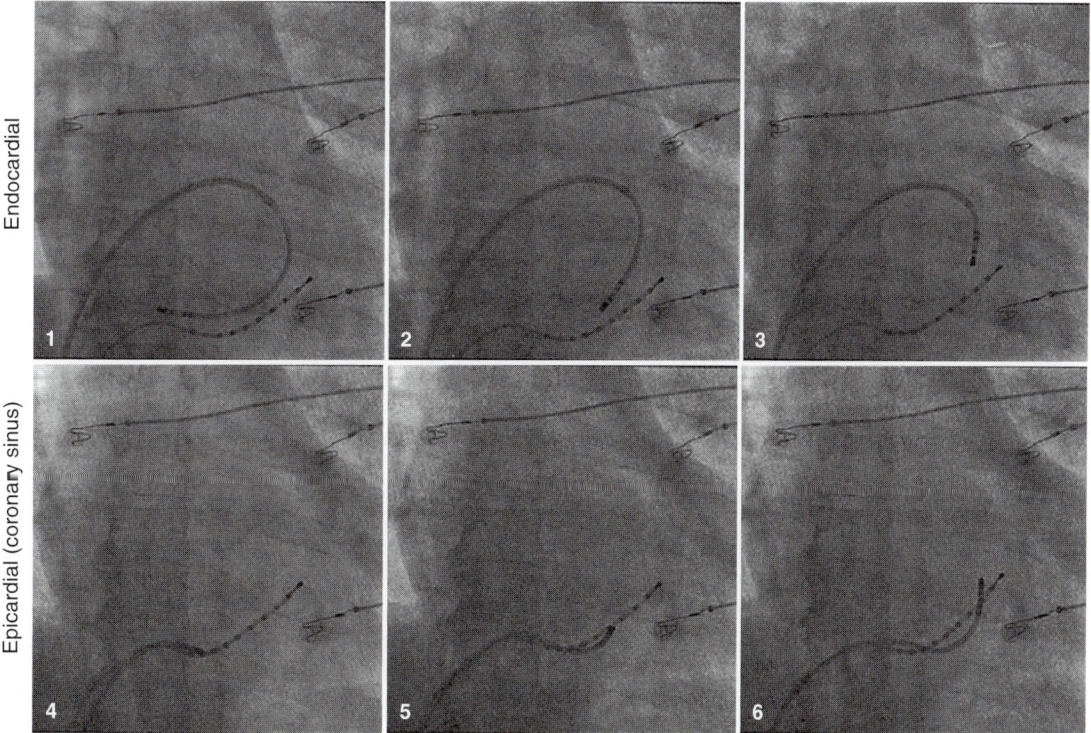

FIGURE 17-12. Anteroposterior fluoroscopic visualization of the catheter positions during ablation of the inferior left atrium (*top panels*) and coronary sinus (*bottom panels*). *Top panels,* After looping the catheter into the atrium facing the coronary sinus ostium (*left*), the catheter is gradually withdrawn parallel to the coronary sinus along the posterior mitral annulus toward the lateral left atrium (*middle* and *right* images) to ablate the left atrial endocardium. *Bottom panels,* Corresponding catheter position at the ostial, middle, and distal segments within the coronary sinus to ablate the epicardial aspects of the left atrial to coronary sinus connections. (*From O'Neill MD, Kim KT, Jais P, et al. Ablation strategies in chronic atrial fibrillation. In Aliot E, Haïssaguerre M, Jackman WM [eds]: Catheter Ablation of Atrial Fibrillation. Malden, MA: Blackwell Futura; 2008:163-189. With permission.*)

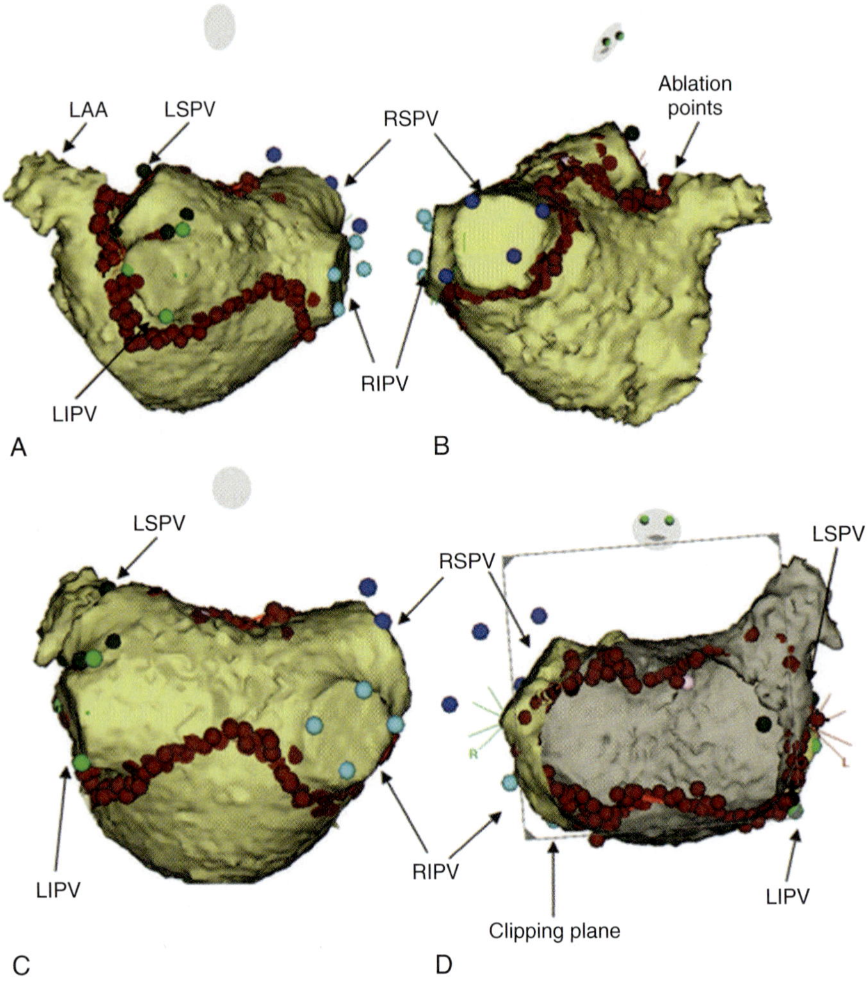

FIGURE 17-13. Isolation of left atrial posterior wall and all four pulmonary veins using a single ring of ablation. The radiofrequency lesions are shown as *red dots* on the volume-rendered computed tomographic image. **A,** Left posterior oblique view. **B,** Right anterior oblique cranial view. **C,** Posterior-anterior view. **D,** Anterior-posterior caudal view with clipping plane to display posterior left atrium shows the ring of ablation encircling the posterior left atrial wall. LAA, left atrial appendage; LIPV, left inferior pulmonary vein (*light green dots*); LSPV, left superior pulmonary vein (*dark green dots*); RIPV right inferior pulmonary vein (*light blue dots*); and RSPV, right superior pulmonary vein (*dark blue dots*). *From Lim TW, Koay CH, McCall R, et al. Atrial arrhythmias after single-ring isolation of the posterior left atrium and pulmonary veins for atrial fibrillation.* Circ Arrhythmia Electrophysiol. *2008;1:120–126. With permission.)*

After the single-ring lesion, macro-reentrant atrial arrhythmias may occur in 34% of patients after the procedure, and recurrent AF may be noted in 35% of patients.[39] Gaps in the ring lesion were found in all patients undergoing repeat ablation for AF after the single-ring approach. Gaps in the ring lesion and mitral annular flutter are responsible for most atrial flutters.[39] The most frequent site of ring gaps is along the left atrial appendage ridge.[39] In a randomized trial, the completion of the box set did not improve outcomes compared with antral PV isolation and roof line alone.[38]

Problems and Limitations

The optimal indications and sites for placement of linear lesions are not known. The greatest difficulty with linear ablation is in achieving and confirming complete block across the lesions. This is particularly difficult for the mitral isthmus line, which may require extensive ablation within the coronary sinus to accomplish. Incomplete linear lesions may be proarrhythmic and may lead to refractory atrial flutters that are often highly symptomatic. The additional catheter manipulation and ablation may also increase the risk for procedural complications.[41]

Electrogram-Guided Atrial Ablation

Pathophysiology

An intraoperative epicardial mapping study in humans suggested that areas of CFAEs may indicate sites of slow conduction, conduction block, wavefront collision, or anchor points for reentrant circuits that can perpetuate AF.[48,49] CFAEs may also indicate sites of high-frequency sources (rotors), fibrillatory conduction, and sites of autonomic innervation.[50–52] CFAEs have been targeted for ablation to eliminate both paroxysmal and persistent AF.[48] CFAEs are quite prevalent and can be found at many sites in both

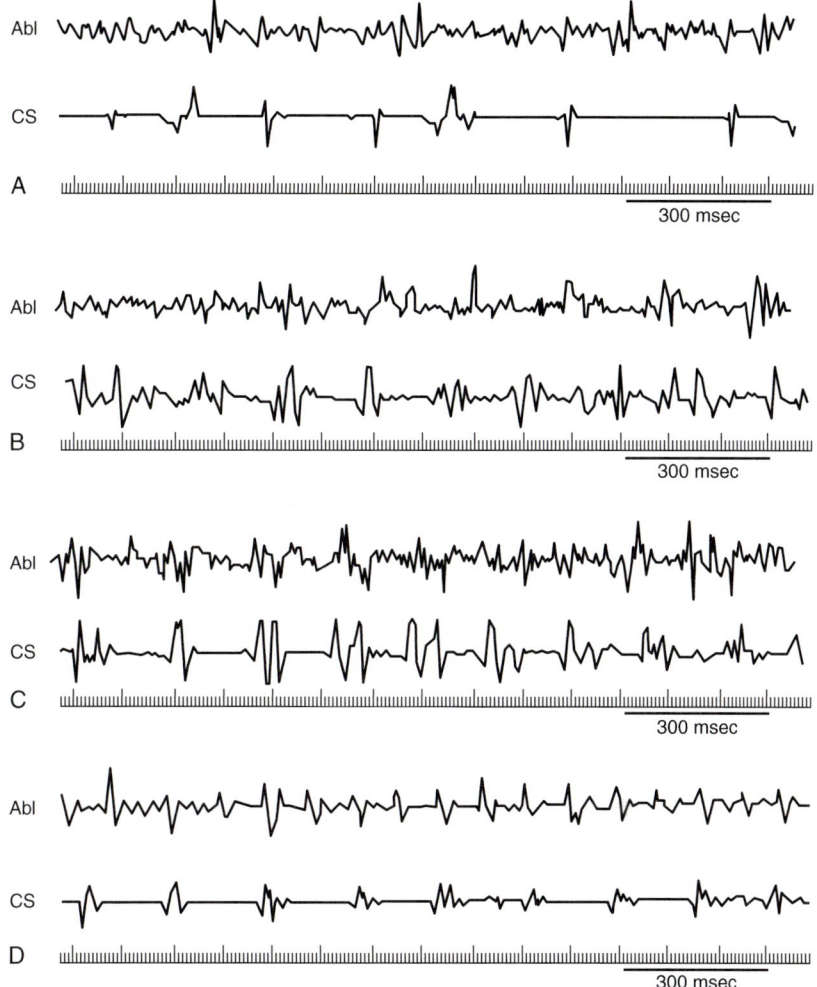

FIGURE 17-14. Examples of complex fractionated atrial electrograms. Abl, distal bipole of the ablation catheter; CS, distal bipole of the coronary sinus catheter. *(From Oral H, Chugh A, Good E, et al. Radiofrequency catheter ablation of chronic atrial fibrillation guided by complex electrograms. Circulation. 2007;115:2606–2612.)*

atria but are most extensively studied in the left atrium. They appear to be spatially stable over time within individual patients. The sites most commonly demonstrating CFAEs are the interatrial septum, left atrial roof, left atrial appendage, near the PVs, and along the crista terminalis in the right atrium.[48,53] Clustering of CFAE sites near the PVs appears to be more pronounced in patients with paroxysmal compared with nonparoxysmal forms of AF.[53–59] CFAEs may be recorded over 38% to 56% of the left atrial endocardium.[53–59]

Mapping and Ablation

CFAEs are identified during AF by visual assessment or by automated computerized algorithms (Fig. 17-14, later).[48,53] In the original description by Nadamanee and associates, CFAEs were defined as (1) atrial electrograms that are fractionated and composed of two or more deflections, and/or have perturbation of the baseline with continuous deflections of a prolonged activation complex over a 10-second recording period; or (2) atrial electrograms with a very short cycle length (≤120 milliseconds) averaged over a 10-second period.[48] In addition, these electrograms are usually considered to be low voltage

(<0.15 mV). Other electrogram characteristics that have been targeted for ablation include sites with a large (>70 milliseconds) temporal gradient between activation of the proximal and distal ablation bipoles, sites with continuous electrical activity without isoelectric intervals, sites with a cycle length less than the mean left atrial cycle length, and sites demonstrating centrifugal activation (Fig. 17-15; Table 17-3).[44,46]

For automated algorithms, samples of 2.5 to 10 seconds are acquired.[55,56] For optimal spectral analysis, windows of 5 seconds duration or longer have been recommended.[57] In addition, automated algorithms incorporate voltage parameters (low voltage < 0.1 to 0.2 mV, high voltage > 1.0 mV) and refractory periods of 50 to 60 milliseconds.[56] Seventy to 120 points are generally acquired to produce the color-coded map to display electrogram frequency or degree of fractionation (Fig. 17-16).[55,56] There appears to be good agreement between visually and automated CFAE classification; however, more sites are characterized as CFAEs with visual than with automated assessment.

Ablation of CFAEs is performed in AF (Fig. 17-17). Local energy delivery is continued until there is elimination of the local electrogram, loss of the fractionated high-

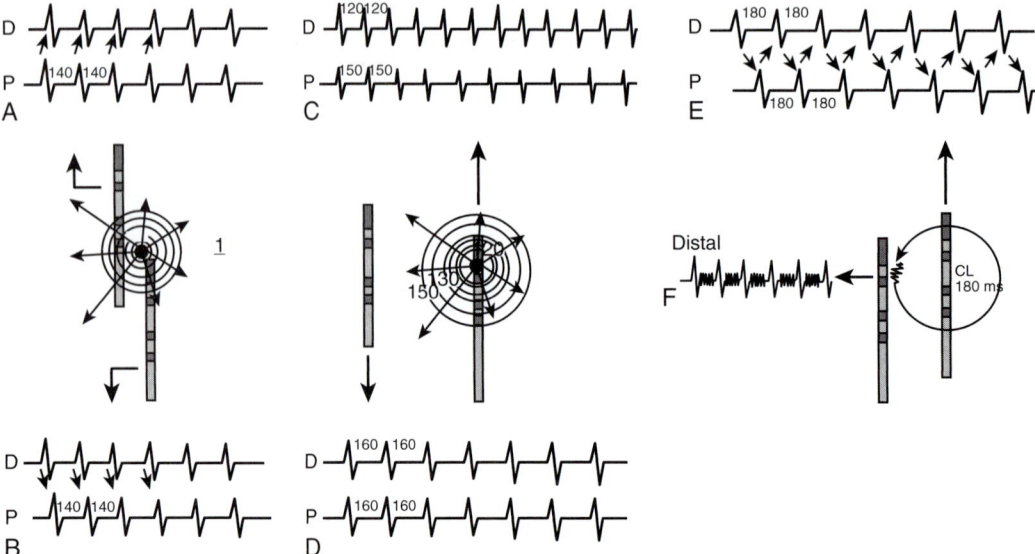

FIGURE 17-15. Depiction of electrograms recorded near or at differing hypothetical focal sources. **A,** Proximal-to-distal activation sequence (*arrows*) consistent with the catheter position relative to a focal source of cycle length (CL) of 140 msec with 1:1 activation of the surrounding tissue. **B,** Distal-to-proximal activation sequence. **C,** Electrograms recorded with the distal (D) catheter bipole positioned over a high-frequency source (shortest cycle length, 120 msec) with a frequency gradient to the surrounding tissue, as indicated by the cycle length of 150 msec recorded on the proximal (P) bipole. **D,** When the catheter is moved away from the source, simultaneous activation at the proximal and distal bipoles is seen, with no discernible difference in cycle length. **E,** Temporal gradient between the proximal and distal bipoles when the catheter is positioned directly over a hypothetical local circuit of cycle length 180 msec. **F,** A fractionated signal is recorded with the distal bipole at a hypothetical zone of slow conduction within the circuit. *(From O'Neill MD, Kim KT, Jais P, et al. Ablation strategies in chronic atrial fibrillation. In Aliot E, Haïssaguerre M, Jackman WM [eds]: Catheter Ablation of Atrial Fibrillation. Malden, MA: Blackwell Futura; 2008:163–189. With permission.)*

TABLE 17-3

COMPLEX ATRIAL ELECTROGRAM TARGETS FOR ABLATION

Electrogram Feature (Reference)	Definition	Possible Pathophysiology
Complex fractionated atrial electrogram (CFAE)[48]	Atrial electrograms that are fractionated and composed of two or more deflections, and/or have perturbation of the baseline with continuous deflections of a prolonged activation complex over a 10-sec recording period, or atrial electrograms with a very short cycle length (≤120 msec) averaged over a 10-sec period	Slow conduction Pivot points Autonomic innervations Rotor Fibrillatory conduction Wavefront collision
Continuous electrical activity[53]	Absence of isoelectric intervals for ≥1 sec recording period	Local reentry Anisotropy Summation overlapping electrograms High-frequency depolarization
Temporal activation gradient[44]	>70-msec interval between activation of proximal and distal ablation electrodes	Local reentry
Frequency gradient[46]	Electrogram cycle length < mean left atrial cycle length	Focal reentry/automaticity or triggered activity
Centrifugal activation[44]	Radial spread of activation from a focus	Focal reentry/automaticity or triggered activity

frequency electrogram components, or increase in the atrial cycle length. In the original description of the technique, an average of 64 ± 36 sites were ablated per patient.[48] The average duration of RF delivery is reported at 36 ± 13 minutes.[58] Antral ablation for PV isolation targets many of the sites that frequently harbor CFAEs. Antral PV isolation may greatly reduce the CFAE distribution over the left atrial endocardium from 56% before PV isolation to 23% after ablation.[59] For patients undergoing PV isolation and CFAE ablation, completion of PV isolation first may reduce the total amount of radiofrequency energy delivered. Once CFAEs are eliminated from the left atrium, the right atrium may then be mapped. Complex atrial electrograms are frequently recorded within the coronary sinus as well. Ablation along the left atrial endocardium abutting the coronary sinus prolongs left atrial cycle length in patients with persistent AF. Ablation within the coronary sinus further prolongs atrial cycle length. The techniques for ablation along and within the coronary sinus were described previously. The end point for electrogram-guided ablation is termination of AF into sinus rhythm or into an organized atrial tachycardia, elimination of all complex atrial electrograms or for patients with paroxysmal AF, and noninducibility of AF (Table 17-4). Termination of AF most commonly occurs during ablation at the interatrial septum near the PV ostia and at the atrial roof near the left atrial appendage (Fig. 17-18).[60]

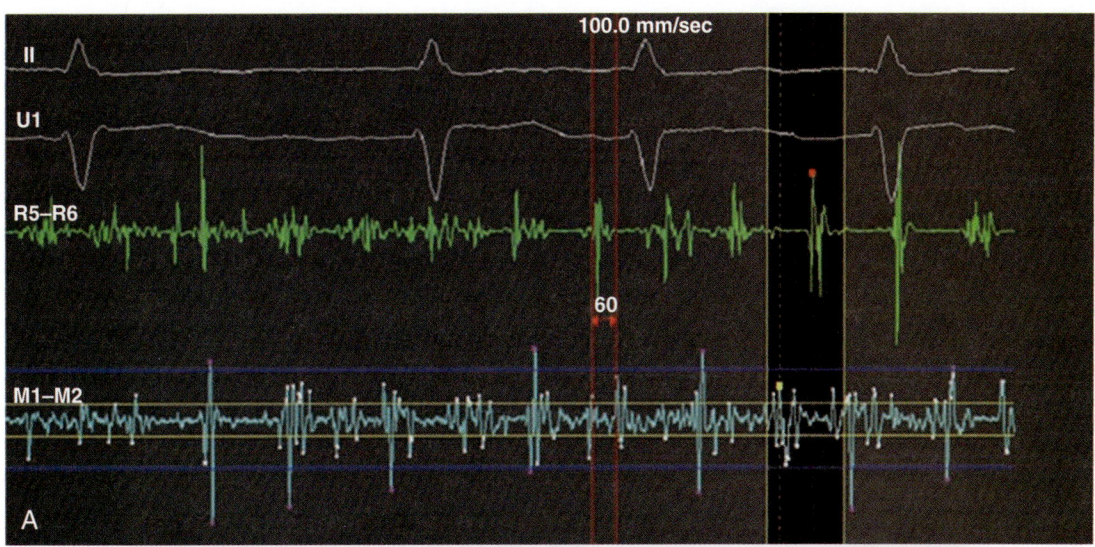

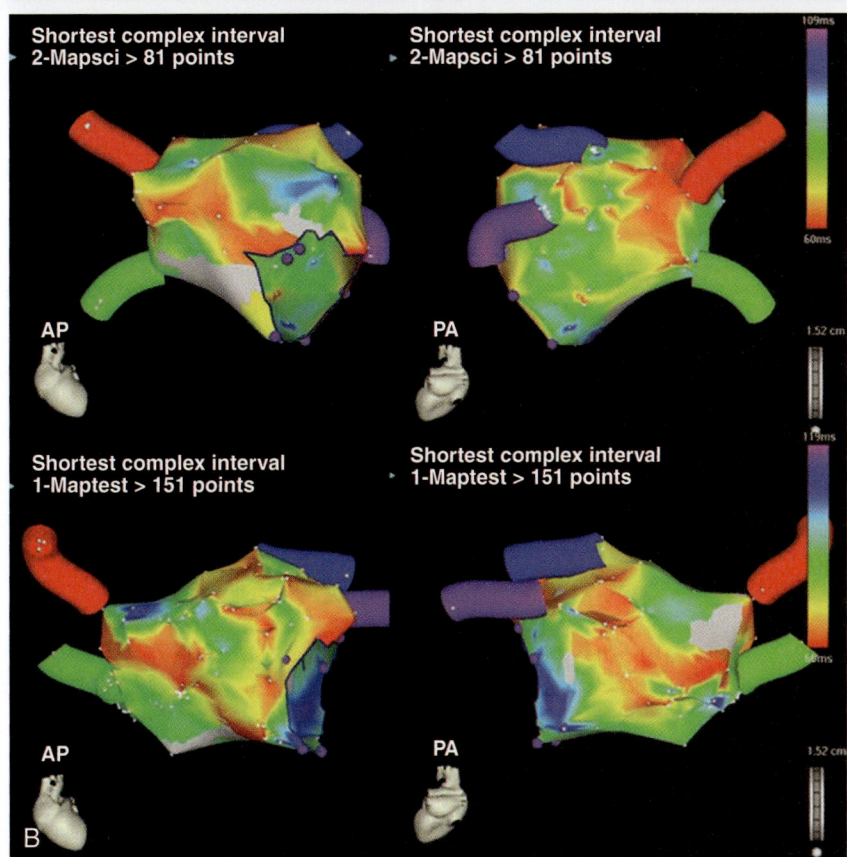

FIGURE 17-16. A, Annotation window for automatic detection of complex fractionated atrial electrograms (CFAEs) by the CFAE software CartoXP (Biosense Webster). Recording channels, from *top* to *bottom*, are surface electrocardiogram lead II, V₁, bipolar electrograms recorded within coronary sinus (R5-R6), and bipolar electrograms of the mapping/ablation catheter (M1-M2) recorded in endocardial locations of the left atrium. The duration of the window in which the local endocardial electrograms recorded by the mapping catheter will be computed is 2.5 sec (predefined by the system). First, the voltage amplitude of the peaks will be computed. The peaks with amplitude over 0.05 mV (*horizontal lines in yellow*) will be tagged with *white points* and the peaks with amplitude over 0.15 mV (*horizontal lines in blue*) will be tagged with *pink points*. Peaks with amplitude lower than 0.05 mV (noise level) will not be analyzed by the software. Peak-to-peak intervals between tagged points will be calculated. For the shortest complex interval (SCI) map, the shortest measured interval (in a preset range of 60-120 msec) will be identified as the local SCI. The local SCI is demonstrated in the annotation viewer with *red lines*. In this example, the SCI was 60 msec. If there is no measured interval found in the preset range of 60-120 msec, the site will be identified as a site without CFAE. **B,** CFAE distribution in the SCI map. *Top panels,* SCI map of a patient with paroxysmal atrial fibrillation (AF) in anterior-posterior (AP) and posterior-anterior (PA) views. The sites with local SCI from 60 to 120 msec are represented as areas colored from *red* to *violet*. Areas without CFAE are in *gray*. The highest density of CFAE was found around the pulmonary vein ostia. *Bottom panels,* SCI maps of a patient with persistent AF in AP and PA views. SCI color-coded as above. CFAE are located in all left atrial regions. *Violet points* indicate the mitral annulus. *(From Wu J, Estner H, Luik A, et al. Automatic 3D mapping of complex fractionated atrial electrograms [CFAE] in patients with paroxysmal and persistent atrial fibrillation. J Cardiovasc Electrophysiol. 2008;19:897–903. With permission.)*

Outcomes

In the original study by Nademanee and associates, ablation of CFAEs without routine isolation of the PVs was reported to result in freedom from AF in 91% of the 121 patients with paroxysmal or chronic AF.[48] AF terminated during ablation in 63% and 95% of the patients without and with infusion of ibutilide, respectively. In a follow-up study of 674 patients, 89% of patients with paroxysmal AF, 85% of patients with persistent AF, and 71% of patients with permanent AF were reported to be in sinus rhythm at 2 years.[52] In a study of 100 patients with chronic AF who underwent CFAE ablation in the left atrium and the coronary sinus, only 33% and 57% of patients were in sinus rhythm without antiarrhythmic medications after single and repeat procedures, respectively.[58] In a randomized study, ablation of CFAEs after antral PV isolation was not found to be associated with a superior efficacy

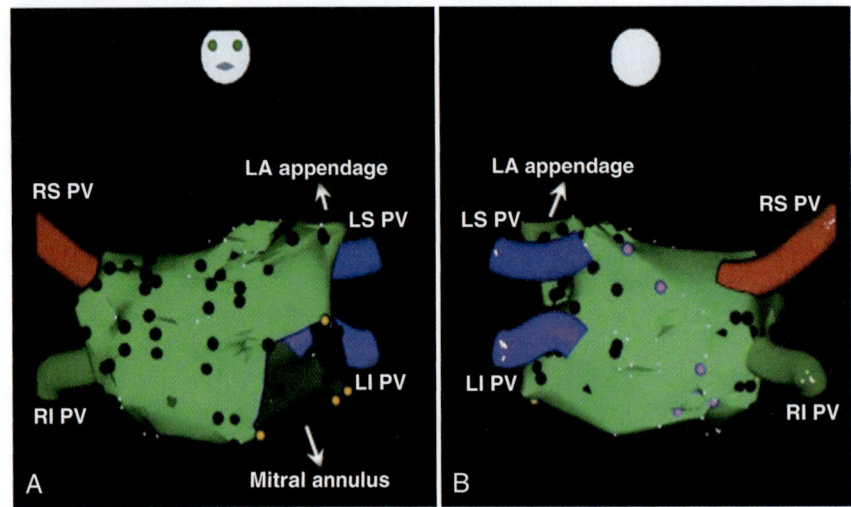

FIGURE 17-17. Example of radiofrequency ablation guided by complex fractionated atrial electrograms. Shown are anteroposterior (**A**) and posteroanterior (**B**) projections of a three-dimensional electroanatomic depiction of the left atrium (LA). *Black tags* indicate ablation sites. The *pink tags* indicate the course of the esophagus along the posterior left atrial wall. LI, left inferior; LS, left superior; PV, pulmonary vein; RI, right inferior; RS, right superior. *(From Oral H, Chugh A, Good E, et al. Radiofrequency catheter ablation of chronic atrial fibrillation guided by complex electrograms. Circulation. 2007;115:2606–2612. With permission.)*

TABLE 17-4	
END POINTS FOR ABLATION COMPLEX ATRIAL ELECTROGRAMS	
For Individual Ablation Sites	**For Electrogram-Guided Strategy**
Electrogram elimination	Termination AF into sinus rhythm
Loss of fractionated components	Termination AF into organized atrial tachycardia or macro-reentry
Prolongation of atrial cycle length	Elimination of all complex electrograms
	Noninducibility of AF (paroxysmal AF patients)

AF, atrial fibrillation.

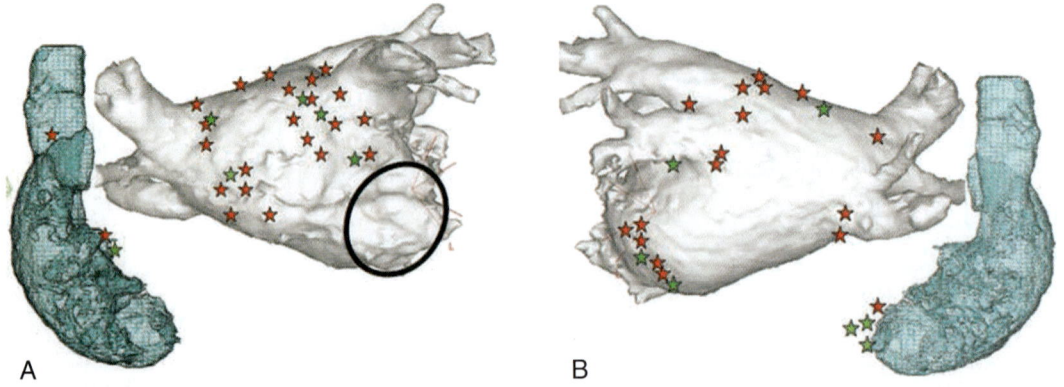

FIGURE 17-18. Sites of atrial fibrillation termination during electrogram-guided ablation in patients with paroxysmal (*red stars*) and persistent (*green stars*) atrial fibrillation. The left atrium is shown in *gray* and the right atrium in *blue.* **A,** Anteroposterior view. **B,** Posteroanterior view. Data from 56 patients are shown. *(From Schmitt C, Estner H, Hecher B, et al. Radiofrequency ablation of complex fractionated atrial electrograms [CFAE]: preferential sites of acute termination and regularization in paroxysmal and persistent atrial fibrillation. J Cardiovasc Electrophysiol. 2007;18:1039–1046. With permission.)*

to antral PV isolation alone in patients with persistent AF.[61] However, ablation of CFAEs was limited to a maximum of 2 hours because the goal of the study was to determine whether AF could be terminated within a practical time frame. AF terminated in only a minority of patients in this study, suggesting that ablation of CFAE for up to 2 hours may not have been sufficient to eliminate most of the residual drivers of AF. Because of the high incidence of recurrences caused by residual PV tachycardias, CFAEs may be best used as a target after routine systematic antral isolation of PVs with or without additional linear lesions.

Problems and Limitations

A difficulty in targeting CFAEs is that most may be due to passive activation and lack specificity to indicate drivers of AF. Thus, primary CFAE-guided ablation may lead to excessive and unnecessary ablation in the left atrium. As mentioned, the target sites for antral PV isolation overlap considerably with CFAE sites in many patients. Currently, most CFAE ablation is performed as an adjunctive step following PV isolation.

Ablation of Intrinsic Cardiac Autonomics

Fluctuations in autonomic tone have been associated with initiation of AF in human subjects and animal models.[63] Vagal stimulation may facilitate spontaneous premature depolarizations in the atria, shorten the atrial and PV ERP, and increase heterogeneity of refractoriness.[64] Changes in autonomic tone may contribute to development of CFAEs.[16,51]

The intrinsic cardiac autonomic system includes autonomic ganglia within epicardial fat pads and the LOM.[65] These ganglionated plexuses (GPs) contain neuronal input from atrial myocardium and the extrinsic autonomic nervous system as well as cholinergic and adrenergic neurons. In addition, there is an extensive network of interconnecting neurons among the ganglia themselves and between the ganglia and atrial and PV myocardium.[65] GPs are located in six major regions of the atria, mostly within the antrum of the PVs, in the crux of the heart, and at the junction of the right atrium and SVC.[66,67] GPs that are targeted for endocardial ablation are often located (1) at the anterior aspect of the right superior PV, (2) posteriorly and inferiorly near the right inferior PV, (3) at the left upper PV GP between the left atrial appendage and left PVs (Marshall tract plexus), and (4) at the left lower PV GP located in the posterior and inferior aspect of the left inferior PV (Figs. 17-19 and 17-20). Because of the proximity of the GPs to the PVs, ablation approaches that do not directly target the GPs have been observed to also modify the autonomic substrate.[60,68] It is postulated that autonomic activation initiates AF by facilitating afterdepolarizations in atrial and PV tissue.[65] In addition, autonomic activation dramatically shortens atrial action potential duration, especially in the PV myocardium. Stimulation of GP may produce remote effects such as PV depolarizations or electrogram fractionation at a distance, suggesting active communication among the ganglia.[65]

Mapping of GPs is performed by high-frequency stimulation. Programmed electrical nerve stimulation has been used to determine the location of the GPs in the heart.[65,69] Mapping can be performed from the cardiac endocardium or epicardially by pericardial access.[70] Typically, stimulation is performed at 20 Hz (1200 ppm), at 5 to 100 V, and with a pulse width of 10 msec.[69,70] This is usually performed under general anesthesia because of poor patient tolerance. Sites showing a vagal response are usually mapped in the antral regions of the PVs. The locations of the targeted plexuses are given in Table 17-5 and in Figures 17-19, 17-20, and 17-21. Patients in sinus rhythm may develop AF during programmed electrical nerve stimulation. High-frequency stimulation of

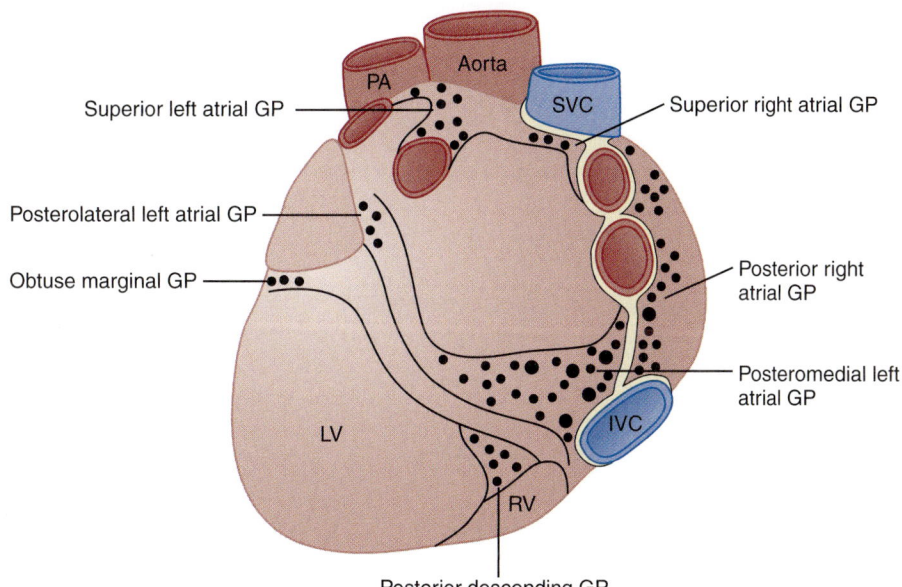

FIGURE 17-19. Drawing of a posterior view of the human heart and major vessels illustrating the locations of posterior atrial and ventricular ganglionated plexuses (GP). Note the mediastinal nerves coursing adjacent to the aortic root and joining the two superior atrial ganglionated plexuses. Positions of the superior vena cava (SVC), inferior vena cava (IVC), right ventricle (RV), pulmonary artery (PA), and left ventricle (LV) are shown. *(Redrawn from Armour JA, Murphy DA, Yuan BX, et al. Gross and microscopic anatomy of the human intrinsic cardiac nervous system. Anat Rec. 1997;247:289–298. With permission.)*

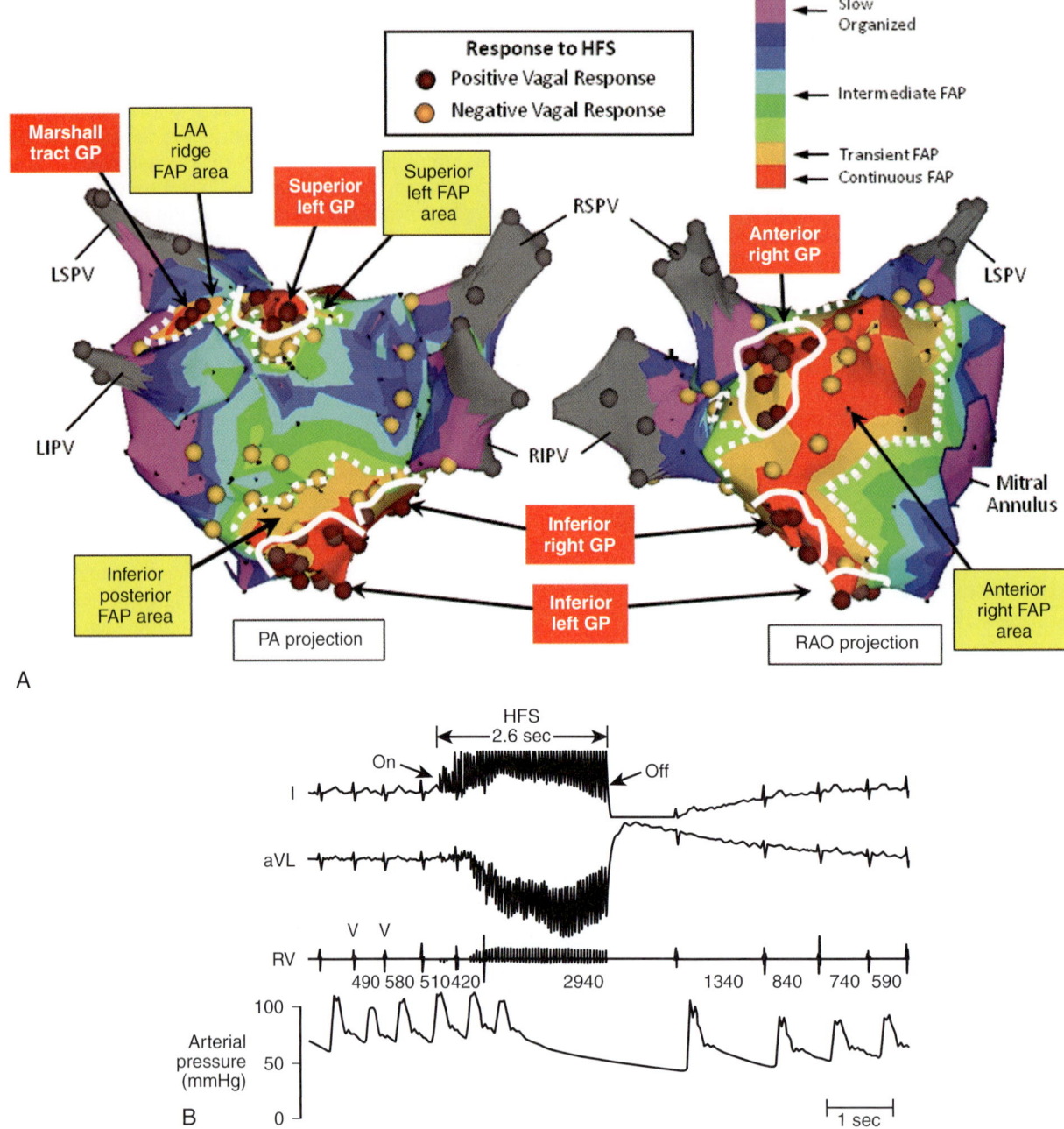

FIGURE 17-20. Correlation between locations of fractionated atrial potentials (FAP) and ganglionated plexuses (GP) in patients undergoing catheter ablation of atrial fibrillation. **A,** Electroanatomic map of FAP in a patient with paroxysmal atrial fibrillation. Electrograms were recorded for 2.5 sec at each site. Sites exhibiting FAP for the entire 2.5 sec were classified as continuous FAP and are colored *red*. Sites with FAP for >0.5 sec but with organized atrial potentials for the remainder of the 2.5 sec were classified as transient FAP and are colored *orange*. Sites exhibiting periods of irregular amplitude, polarity, and cycle length, but not rapid, were classified as "intermediate FAP" and are colored *green–light blue*. Sites exhibiting high-amplitude, discrete atrial potentials with average cycle length of 180 msec or more were classified as "slow organized atrial potentials" and are colored *purple*. An FAP area was defined as a contiguous area of fractionated atrial potentials (continuous or transient FAP). Four FAP areas were identified: left atrial appendage (LAA) ridge FAP area, superior left FAP area, inferior-posterior FAP area, and anterior right FAP area. Sites where endocardial high-frequency stimulation (HFS) produced a vagal response (see **B**) are marked by *brown tags*, corresponding the five major GP areas: (1) Marshall tract GP, (2) superior left GP, (3) inferior left GP, (4) inferior right GP, and (5) anterior right GP. HFS failed to produce a vagal response at the sites marked by *orange tags*. Note that all five GPs are located within the four FAP areas (see **C**). **B,** Tracings shown from top to bottom are electrocardiogram leads I and aVL, electrogram from the right ventricle (RV), and arterial pressure. During atrial fibrillation, endocardial high-frequency stimulation (cycle length, 50 msec; pulse width, 10 msec) in the posterior left atrium, 2.5 cm inferior to the ostium of the left inferior pulmonary vein (LIPV), results in transient complete atrioventricular block (R-R interval, 2940 msec) and hypotension (vagal response), identifying the inferior left GP.

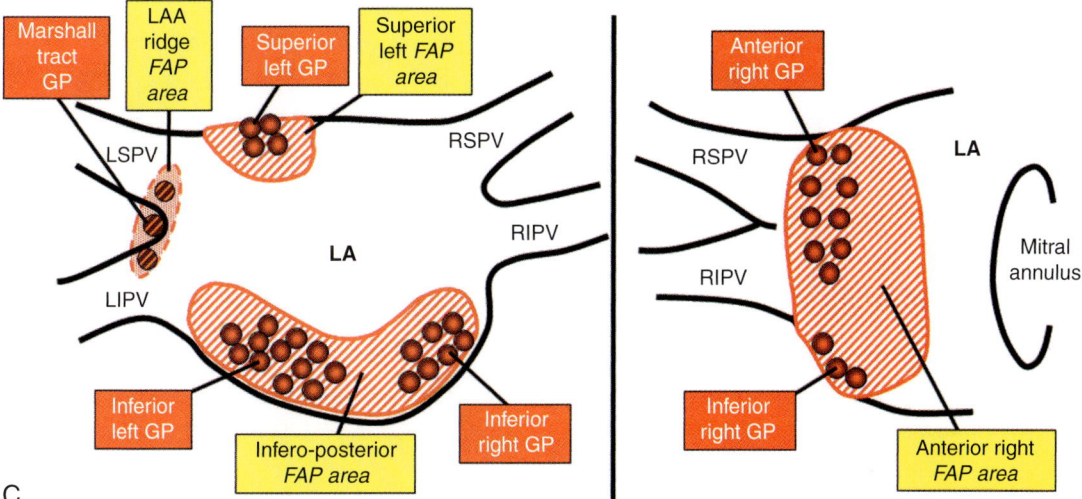

FIGURE 17-20, cont'd. C, Schematic representation of the relationship between the FAP areas and GP locations. *Red tags* indicate sites with a positive HFS response. *Red crossed-hatch* areas indicate FAP areas. LAA ridge FAP area and Marshall tract GP are located anterior to the left pulmonary veins. All five GPs are located within one of the four FAP areas. LSPV, left superior pulmonary vein; PA, posteroanterior; RAO, right anterior oblique; RIPV, right inferior pulmonary vein; RSPV, right superior pulmonary vein. *(Redrawn from Nakagawa H, Scherlag BJ, Patterson E, et al. Pathophysiologic basis of automatic ganglionated plexus ablation in patients with atrial fibrillation.* Heart Rhythm. *2009;6:S26–S34. With permission.)*

TABLE 17-5

TARGET SITES FOR AUTONOMIC ABLATION

Target Site	Location
Right superior GP	Anterior to RSPV
Right inferior GP	Inferior and posterior to RIPV
Left superior GP	Anterior and/or posterior to LSPV
Left Inferior GP	Posterior and inferior to LIPV
Ligament of Marshall	Inferior-anterior aspect of left atrial lateral ridge inferior to LIPV

GP, ganglionated plexus; I, inferior; L, left; PV, pulmonary vein; R, right; S, superior.

GPs results in sympathetic and parasympathetic activation; however, the parasympathetic response occurs immediately, whereas the sympathetic response is delayed.[69,70] During AF, a vagal response is defined as atrioventricular (AV) block with a 50% or greater increase in mean R-R interval within 5 to 10 seconds, associated with hypotension or induced AV block of more than 2 seconds duration (Fig. 17-20B).[65,70] Occasionally, GP stimulation results in firing from the adjacent PVs, and rarely, a predominantly sympathetic hypertensive response may occur.[65] Stimulation mapping may fail to induce vagal responses in up to 30% of patients, even when selected for characteristics of vagally induced AF.[70] In patients with positive endocardial and epicardial responses, 5 ± 2.4 sites are targeted per patient.[70]

Endocardial ablation is delivered at each site demonstrating a positive response to stimulation. Percutaneous catheter epicardial mapping and ablation for GPs have also been performed (Fig. 17-21).[65,69,70] Typically, three to eight radiofrequency applications are needed per site.[65,70] Vagal responses are rarely evoked during radiofrequency energy delivery.[70] The end point for ablation is the elimination of all vagal responses within the left atrium. Occasionally, AV block is not seen during ganglia stimulation. AV block is mediated by vagal output from the crux GP located between the inferior vena cava

and coronary sinus ostium.[65] Loss of interconnecting neurons from other GPs to the crux fat pad may result in failure to elicit vagal responses.[65] A specific order of ablation has been recommended to minimize the loss of vagal response from ablation: first Marshall tract GP, then left superior GP, anterior right GP, inferior left GP, and finally inferior right GP.[65] The sites for autonomic ablation overlap with those incorporated in PV antral ablation, and PV isolation produces changes in Holter-derived indices of autonomic tone similar to endocardial and epicardial parasympathetic catheter denervation.[70]

Ligament of Marshall

The LOM is the remnant of the left SVC and contains autonomic innervations and myocardial muscle bundles.[71] This structure can demonstrate automatic firing during catecholamine infusion and has been implicated as a source of AF initiation and perpetuation. The LOM arises from the coronary sinus musculature and passes laterally and anterior to the left PVs to join with the ridge between the left superior PV and appendage. The structure then continues for variable length medial to the left PVs. The ligament shares muscle fibers with the left atrial and PV epicardium. The ligament contains sympathetic and parasympathetic nerve fibers and a central vein of Marshall that can be visualized with angiography.[71]

The role of the LOM in AF genesis is not clear. It has been suggested that the LOM be targeted for ablation in young (male) patients with the pattern of adrenergic paroxysmal AF.[71] In the laboratory these patients often have AF triggered by high dose isoproterenol (10-20 mcg/min) infusion. In addition, it is suggested that if the earliest endocardial activation is located within a left PV but local activity is less than 45 msec before atrial activity, then mapping of the LOM should be considered.[71] Also, if no early PV sites can be identified for apparent left PV triggers of AF, the LOM should be suspected.[71]

The vein of Marshall can be identified by coronary sinus angiography in about 75% of patients (Fig. 17-22).[72] The

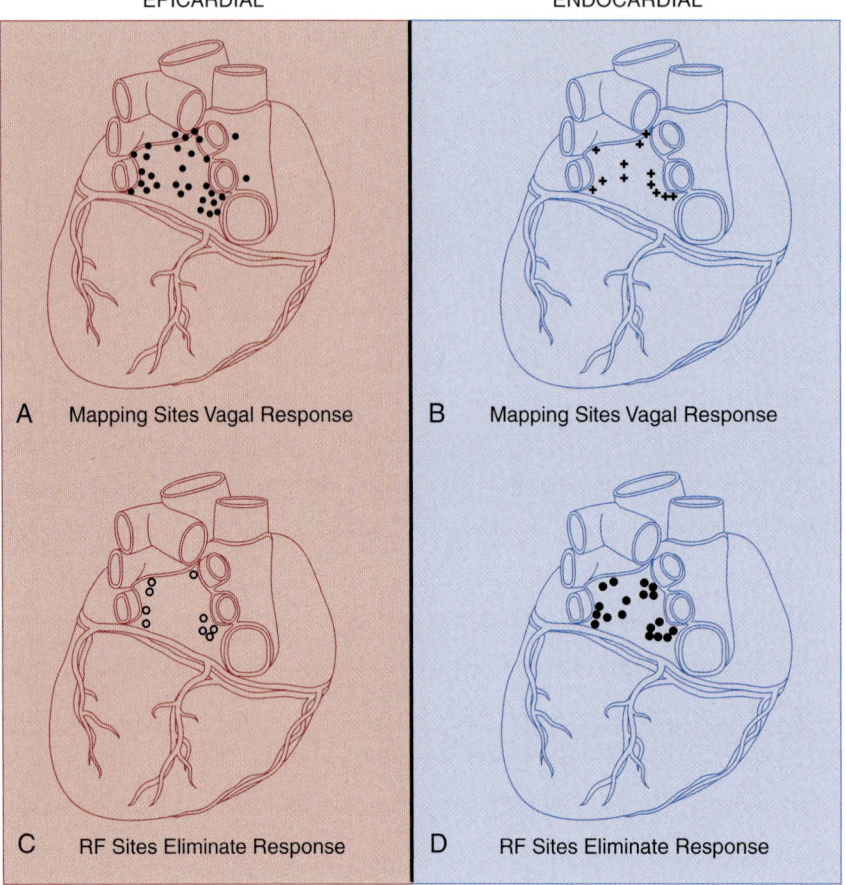

FIGURE 17-21. Atrial epicardial (**A**) and endocardial (**B**) sites where high-frequency stimulation evoked a vagal response in 10 patients. Epicardial (**C**) and endocardial (**D**) sites where radiofrequency (RF) ablation abolished the evoked vagal response. *(Redrawn from Scanavacca M, Pisani D, Lara S, et al. Selective atrial vagal denervation guided by evoked vagal reflex to treat patients with paroxysmal atrial fibrillation.* Circulation. *2006;114:876–885. With permission.)*

vein ostium can be subselected with a 6- or 7-French catheter that then allows passage of a 1.4-French mapping catheter (Cardima, Fremont, CA) Pacing from the left atrial appendage or distal coronary sinus may allow discrimination between LOM and PV potentials. The catheter serves as an anatomic reference to target ablation. The recommended approach is ablation to the mid-ligament from the inferior-anterior aspect of the lateral ridge under the left inferior PV ostium (Fig. 17-23).[71] The end point for ablation is exit block between the muscular portion of the ligament and the left atrium. Typically, there is disappearance of all muscle potentials within the ligament with successful ablation as well.[71] Reportedly, ablation as described produces successful LOM ablation in 90% of patients.[71] Alternatively, the LOM can be ablated by ethanol infusion.[71] The vein of Marshall arises from the posterior aspect of the coronary sinus and is cannulated with a left internal mammary artery guide catheter or a coronary vein subselection catheter (Rapido IC-90, Boston Scientific, Natick, MA). An angioplasty balloon (8 × 2 mm) is advanced over a guidewire for selective angiography of the vein of Marshall. For ablation, two separate injections of 1 mL 100% ethanol are given 2 minutes apart. Ethanol injection creates areas of low atrial electrogram voltage on the lateral wall of the left atrium between the lateral coronary sinus and left PV and anterior to the PV (Fig. 17-24).[73] In addi-

tion, the ethanol injection alone produces partial or complete electrical isolation of the left PV in most patients.

Outcomes

The role of ablation of GPs in patients with AF is not clear. There are limited data on the effect of autonomic ablation on outcomes after catheter ablation.[70,71] The results of the reports on the effect of ablation of fat pads during cardiac surgery on recurrent AF are conflicting.[74–76] GP ablation may reduce PV depolarizations and AF inducibility independent of PV isolation procedures. It appears that PV isolation further reduces AF inducibility after GP ablation in relatively small series.[77] Of 10 patients with vagally induced paroxysmal AF, vagal mapping identified target sites in only 7 patients.[70] Of the 7 undergoing epicardial and endocardial catheter ablation for denervation without PV isolation, 5 had AF recurrences in follow-up. Of interest, the 3 patients without vagal reflexes invoked had PV isolation alone, but none had AF recurrence. As described, PV isolation has significant effects on cardiac autonomic function. In animal models, there is significant return of cardiac parasympathetic function 4 weeks after initial successful ablation, suggesting that reinnervation occurs.[76] There is also evidence of returning autonomic function after parasympathetic modification

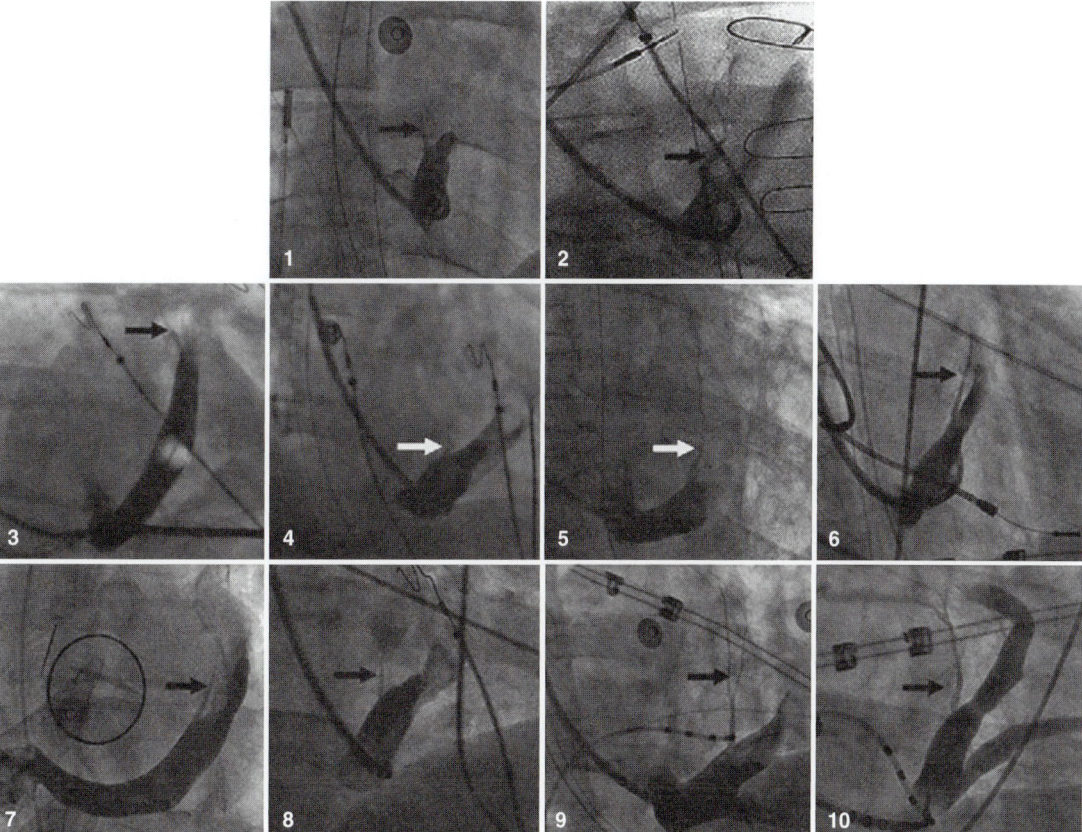

FIGURE 17-22. Vein of Marshall subselective venograms in 10 patients. Right anterior oblique fluoroscopic projections (except for patient #7, left anterior oblique). *(From Hwang C, Chen P-S. Ligament of Marshall: why it is important for atrial fibrillation ablation.* Heart Rhythm. *2009;6:S35-S40. With permission.)*

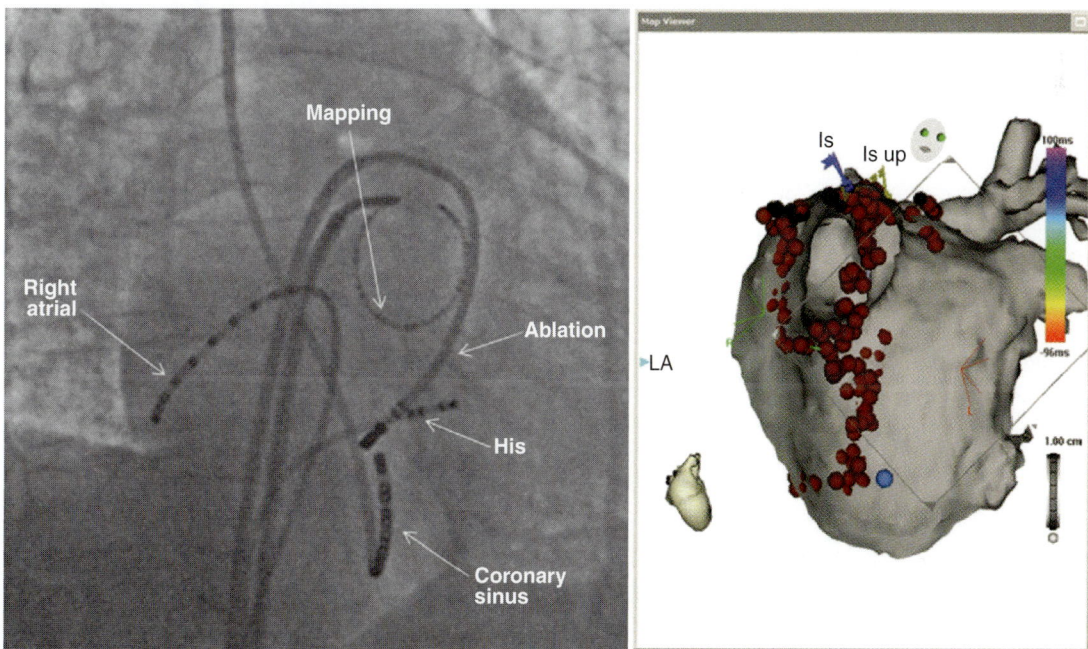

FIGURE 17-23. Ablation of ligament of Marshall (LOM) connections. *Left panel,* Right anterior oblique view of catheters for LOM ablation. The ablation catheter tip is inferior and anterior to the left inferior pulmonary vein. The catheter will be directed along the ridge between the left veins and the left atrial appendage. *Right panel,* Electroanatomic mapping merged with three-dimensional magnetic resonance imaging to document sites of ablation along the ridge between the left veins and the left atrial appendage. LA, left atrium. *(Courtesy of Dr. Chun Hwang.)*

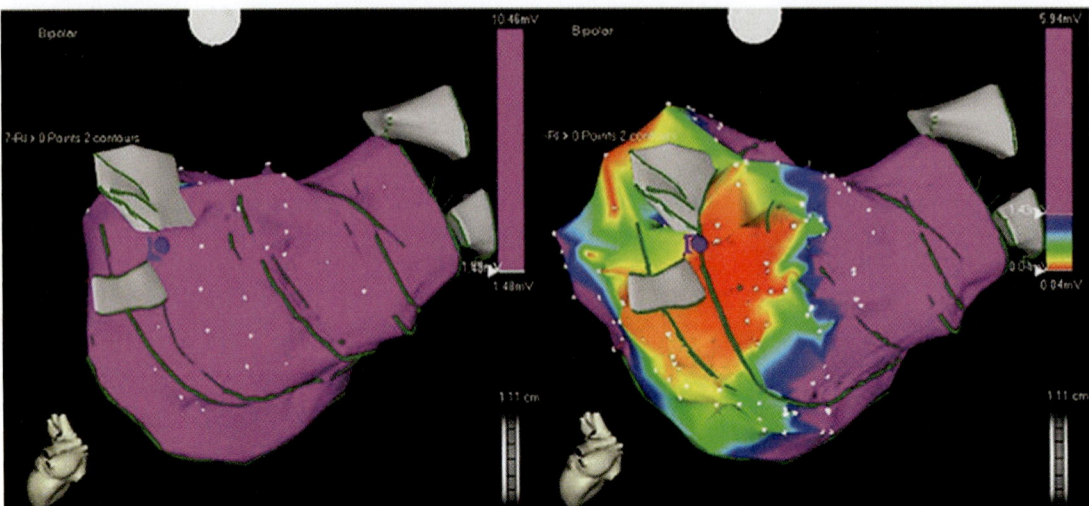

FIGURE 17-24. Three-dimensional bipolar voltage maps before (*left*) and after (*right*) vein of Marshall ethanol infusion. Minor differences in the left atrial geometry are caused by increased density of the postinfusion mapping. The maps were obtained with the Carto (Biosense Webster) system. Posterior view of the left atrium showing a new large area of low bipolar voltage amplitude (*red color*, <0.04 mV) in the areas corresponding to the left pulmonary vein antrum after ethanol infusion. *(From Valderrabano M, Liu X, Sasaridis C, et al. Ethanol infusion in the vein of Marshall: adjunctive effects during ablation of atrial fibrillation. Heart Rhythm. 2009;6:1552–1558. With permission.)*

by catheter ablation.[78] There are few data on the efficacy of LOM ablation for the management of AF.[73]

Problems and Limitations

Significant complications that are specifically related to autonomic ablation for AF have not been reported; however, the clinical experience with these ablation targets is limited. In addition, autonomic targets are usually adjunctive to PV isolation and other ablation strategies, making attribution of complications to one set of targets difficult. Gastric hypomotility occurred in 1 of 10 patients treated with epicardial and endocardial ablation by Scanavacca and colleagues.[70] The completeness of parasympathetic denervation achieved by catheter ablation may be insufficient to prevent arrhythmia recurrences. Complications of LOM ablation appear uncommon and are limited to dissection of the vein of Marshall during cannulation. This event is described as inconsequential.[70,71]

Role of Right Atrial Ablation

Initial attempts of catheter AF ablation targeted the right atrium but demonstrated limited benefit from right atrial linear ablation alone.[79–82] However, it is recognized that right atrial foci such as the SVC, crista terminalis, and coronary sinus ostium may play a role in initiation of AF.[82,83] Ablation in the right atrium is necessary to terminate AF in up to 15% of patients.[84]

Linear ablation in the right atrium is now limited to the cavotricuspid isthmus either as a standard part of the procedure or in response to documented typical atrial flutter. CFAEs can also be found in the right atrium. In a recent randomized study, routine ablation of CFAEs in the right atrium was not associated with an improvement in clinical efficacy of left atrial catheter ablation of AF.[85] Ablation of right atrial CFAEs is usually deferred until ablation is completed in the left atrium without termina-

tion of AF. Once left atrial drivers with the highest frequency are eliminated, residual right atrial drivers may continue to perpetuate AF, particularly in patients with persistent AF.[14] Monitoring right atrial cycle length in comparison with left atrial cycle length may be helpful to determine when to proceed with right atrial ablation during left atrial ablation of AF. Autonomic innervations are found within the fat pads around the SVC and coronary sinus os (crux).

End Points for the Substrate-Based Approach to Atrial Fibrillation Ablation

When antral PV isolation is employed as the primary ablation strategy, elimination of antral potentials and complete PV isolation is the procedural end point. The end point of linear ablation is complete conduction block across the ablation lines. CFAE ablation aims at elimination of all CFAEs and termination of AF. For autonomic ablation, elimination of all induced vagal responses is the goal.

Noninducibility of AF is a conceptually appealing end point for AF ablation. Inducibility of sustained AF after PVI may indicate the presence of an atrial substrate capable of maintaining AF and may identify a subgroup of patients in whom additional substrate modification is required. Termination and noninducibility of AF may indicate effective elimination of the mechanisms needed for the arrhythmia perpetuation. In patients with paroxysmal AF, termination and noninducibility of AF in response to rapid atrial pacing predicts better clinical outcome than when AF persists after ablation.[2,32,45]

Noninducibility of AF by high-dose isoproterenol infusion (up to 20 μg/minute) may be a more clinically useful end point for catheter ablation of AF than noninducibility of AF by rapid atrial pacing. In a recent study, isoproterenol had higher specificity (97% versus 72%) and better diagnostic accuracy (83% versus 64%) than rapid atrial pacing for predicting recurrent AF.[86] Because AF is easily inducible by pacing after cardioversion of persistent AF, reinduction of AF is usually not attempted in patients with persistent AF. In patients with persistent AF, termination of AF during ablation is, however, associated with higher probability of long-term maintenance of sinus rhythm.[33,36,85]

Troubleshooting the Difficult Case

Problems with PV isolation are covered in Chapter 15. For any ablation strategy, difficulty in catheter navigation may be indicative of the inaccuracy of the electroanatomic map due to limited number of registered points or patient movement during the case. Preprocedure image acquisition with computed tomography or cardiac magnetic resonance imaging may aid in identifying variations in the individual atrial and PV anatomy. Phased-array intracardiac echocardiography has been used to provide accurate two-dimensional imaging and three-dimensional reconstruction of the left atrium and the PVs. In addition to defining the PV anatomy, intracardiac echocardiography can confirm catheter position at the venous ostium.

Inability to create continuous transmural lesions is a common challenge during linear substrate modification. Potential causes are poor catheter stability and insufficient power delivery. Switching to a different catheter or a preformed sheath may be helpful. Steerable sheaths may offer better catheter stability; however, caution should be exercised to avoid myocardial perforation. When confronted with an incomplete linear ablation, the first step should be careful remapping of the line for conduction gaps. For the mitral isthmus, gaps most frequently occur at the ostium of the left inferior PV and epicardially near the mitral annulus. Epicardial gaps should be suspected when left atrial ablation results in endocardial conduction delay recorded on the ablation catheter but not on the adjacent bipoles on the coronary sinus catheter.[41] Also, the finding of early or fractionated potentials from the coronary sinus catheter may indicate epicardial gaps. For the roof line, the most frequent sites of gaps are near the superior PV.[44] A more anteriorly positioned line can be considered if all initial attempts fail. For patients undergoing a second procedure after posterior left atrial isolation, gaps are found at any point along the ablation lines but most frequently at the left atrial appendage ridge, at the roof line, and near the PVs.[39]

For electrogram-guided ablation, recognition of CFAE by visual inspection can be tedious and subjective. The use of automated algorithms provides consistency and usually identifies fewer CFAE sites than by physician interpretation. The optimal settings for these algorithms have not yet been established, however. Extensive ablation may be required to eliminate CFAEs. Antral PV isolation greatly reduces the CFAE burden and should be performed first in a stepwise approach to AF ablation. Complete elimination of electrograms may not be necessary, but local organization and loss of fractionated components may be sufficient.

For autonomic ablation, patient discomfort may be an issue during high-frequency stimulation mapping unless the patient is deeply sedated. Prior ablation may interrupt neural interconnections from peripheral sites needed to manifest AV block during stimulation. A specific sequence of ablation has been described previously to minimize this effect. A summary of problems encountered during substrate ablation and possible solutions is given in Table 17-6.

TABLE 17-6

TROUBLESHOOTING THE DIFFICULT CASE

Problem	Causes	Solutions
Linear Ablation		
Difficult catheter manipulation	Atrial enlargement, difficult anatomy	Change sheath angulation or use steerable sheath
Unable to produce block across lines	Gaps from noncontiguous lesions Nontransmural lesions	Careful mapping of ablation line for gaps, especially near PV ostia and left atrial appendage ridge, create new line parallel to first attempt, epicardial ablation (in CS for mitral isthmus line)
	Tissue edema from preceding ablation Esophagus near ablation lines	Create new line parallel to first Redirect line, monitor esophageal temperature, displace esophagus with TEE probe, displace heart with intrapericardial balloon or steerable sheath
Electrogram-Guided Ablation		
CFAE sites difficult to identify	Poor tissue contact Variable electrogram characteristics	Change sheath Average analysis over 5- to 10-sec window, use automated algorithm
	Diffuse, extensive CFAE sites	Linear ablation and antral PV isolation
Ablation of Cardiac Autonomics		
Unable to elicit vagal reflex with mapping	Prior ablation interrupts neural interconnections	Perform autonomic mapping before other ablation
	Ganglia remote from endocardial sites Patient unresponsive to electrical stimulation	Map epicardial sites Perform empirical antral PV isolation

CFAE, complex fractionated atrial electrogram; CS, coronary sinus; PV, pulmonary vein; TEE, transesophageal echocardiogram.

References

1. Haïssaguerre M, Jais P, Shah DC, et al. Spontaneous initiation of atrial fibrillation by ectopic beats originating in the pulmonary veins. *N Engl J Med.* 1998;339:659–666.

2. Oral H, Ozaydin M, Tada H, et al. Mechanistic significance of intermittent pulmonary vein tachycardia in patients with atrial fibrillation. *J Cardiovasc Electrophysiol.* 2002;13:645–650.

3. Douglas YL, Jongbloed MR, Gittenberger-de Groot AC, et al. Histology of vascular myocardial wall of left atrial body after pulmonary venous incorporation. *Am J Cardiol.* 2006;97:662–670.

4. Kalifa J, Tanaka K, Zaitsev AV, et al. Mechanisms of wave fractionation at boundaries of high-frequency excitation in the posterior left atrium of the isolated sheep heart during atrial fibrillation. *Circulation.* 2006;113:626–633.

5. Oral H, Knight BP, Tada H, et al. Pulmonary vein isolation for paroxysmal and persistent atrial fibrillation. *Circulation.* 2002;105:1077–1081.

6. Kanagaratnam L, Tomassoni G, Schweikert R, et al. Empirical pulmonary vein isolation in patients with chronic atrial fibrillation using a three-dimensional nonfluoroscopic mapping system: long-term follow-up. *Pacing Clin Electrophysiol.* 2001;24:1774–1779.

7. Allessie M, Ausma J, Schotten U. Electrical, contractile and structural remodeling during atrial fibrillation. *Cardiovasc Res.* 2002;54:230–246.

8. Aime-Sempe C, Folliguet T, Rucker-Martin C, et al. Myocardial cell death in fibrillating and dilated human right atria. *J Am Coll Cardiol.* 1999;34:1577–1586.

9. Mary-Rabine L, Albert A, Pham TD, et al. The relationship of human atrial cellular electrophysiology to clinical function and ultrastructure. *Circ Res.* 1983;52:188–199.

10. Polontchouk L, Haefliger JA, Ebelt B, et al. Effects of chronic atrial fibrillation on gap junction distribution in human and rat atria. *J Am Coll Cardiol.* 2001;38:883–891.

11. Moe GK, Abildskov JA. Atrial fibrillation as a self-sustaining arrhythmia independent of focal discharge. *Am Heart J.* 1959;58:59–70.

12. Jalife J. Rotors and spiral waves in atrial fibrillation. *J Cardiovasc Electrophysiol.* 2003;14:776–780.

13. Jalife J, Berenfeld O, Mansour M. Mother rotors and fibrillatory conduction: a mechanism of atrial fibrillation. *Cardiovasc Res.* 2002;54:204–216.

14. Sanders P, Berenfeld O, Hocini M, et al. Spectral analysis identifies sites of high-frequency activity maintaining atrial fibrillation in humans. *Circulation.* 2005;112:789–797.

15. Patterson E, Po SS, Scherlag BJ, Lazzara R. Triggered firing in pulmonary veins initiated by in vitro autonomic nerve stimulation. *Heart Rhythm.* 2005;2:624–631.

16. Scherlag BJ, Yamanashi W, Patel U, et al. Autonomically induced conversion of pulmonary vein focal firing into atrial fibrillation. *J Am Coll Cardiol.* 2005;45:1878–1886.

17. Pappone C, Oreto G, Rosanio S, et al. Atrial electroanatomic remodeling after circumferential radiofrequency pulmonary vein ablation: efficacy of an anatomic approach in a large cohort of patients with atrial fibrillation. *Circulation.* 2001;104:2539–2544.

18. Pappone C, Rosanio S, Oreto G, et al. Circumferential radiofrequency ablation of pulmonary vein ostia: a new anatomic approach for curing atrial fibrillation. *Circulation.* 2000;102:2619–2628.

19. Ouyang F, Ernst S, Chun J, et al. Electrophysiological findings during ablation of persistent atrial fibrillation with electroanatomic mapping and double Lasso catheter technique. *Circulation.* 2005;112:3038–3048.

20. Oral H, Pappone C, Chugh A, et al. Circumferential pulmonary-vein ablation for chronic atrial fibrillation. *N Engl J Med.* 2006;354:934–941.

21. Oral H, Scharf C, Chugh A, et al. Catheter ablation for paroxysmal atrial fibrillation: segmental pulmonary vein ostial ablation versus left atrial ablation. *Circulation.* 2003;108:2355–2360.

22. Sonmez B, Demirsoy E, Yagan N, et al. A fatal complication due to radiofrequency ablation for atrial fibrillation: atrio-esophageal fistula. *Ann Thorac Surg.* 2003;76:281–283.

23. Pappone C, Oral H, Santinelli V, et al. Atrio-esophageal fistula as a complication of percutaneous transcatheter ablation of atrial fibrillation. *Circulation.* 2004;109:2724–2726.

24. Pollak SJ, Monir G, Chernoby MS, Elenberger CD. Novel imaging techniques of the esophagus enhancing safety of left atrial ablation. *J Cardiovasc Electrophysiol.* 2005;16:244–248.

25. Good E, Oral H, Lemola K, et al. Movement of the esophagus during left atrial catheter ablation for atrial fibrillation. *J Am Coll Cardiol.* 2005;46:2107–2110.

26. Redfearn DP, Trim GM, Skanes AC, et al. Esophageal temperature monitoring during radiofrequency ablation of atrial fibrillation. *J Cardiovasc Electrophysiol.* 2005;16:589–593.

27. Cummings JE, Schweikert RA, Saliba WI, et al. Assessment of temperature, proximity, and course of the esophagus during radiofrequency ablation within the left atrium. *Circulation.* 2005;112:459–464.

28. Hornero F, Berjano EJ. Esophageal temperature during radiofrequency-catheter ablation of left atrium: a three-dimensional computer modeling study. *J Cardiovasc Electrophysiol.* 2006;17:405–410.

29. Cummings JE, Barrett CD, Litwak KN, et al. Esophageal luminal temperature measurement underestimates esophageal tissue temperature during radiofrequency ablation within the canine left atrium: comparison between 8 mm tip and open irrigation catheters. *J Cardiovasc Electrophysiol.* 2008;19:641–644.

30. Swartz JFPG., Silvers J. A catheter-based curative approach to atrial fibrillation in humans [abstract]. *Circulation.* 1994;90:I–335.

31. Haïssaguerre M, Jais P, Shah DC, et al. Right and left atrial radiofrequency catheter therapy of paroxysmal atrial fibrillation. *J Cardiovasc Electrophysiol.* 1996;7:1132–1144.

32. Oral H, Chugh A, Lemola K, et al. Noninducibility of atrial fibrillation as an end point of left atrial circumferential ablation for paroxysmal atrial fibrillation: a randomized study. *Circulation.* 2004;110:2797–2801.

33. Haïssaguerre M, Hocini M, Sanders P, et al. Catheter ablation of long-lasting persistent atrial fibrillation: clinical outcome and mechanisms of subsequent arrhythmias. *J Cardiovasc Electrophysiol.* 2005;16:1138–1147.

34. Jais P, Hocini M, Hsu LF, et al. Technique and results of linear ablation at the mitral isthmus. *Circulation.* 2004;110:2996–3002.

35. Hocini M, Jais P, Sanders P, et al. Techniques, evaluation, and consequences of linear block at the left atrial roof in paroxysmal atrial fibrillation: a prospective randomized study. *Circulation.* 2005;112:3688–3696.

36. Haïssaguerre M, Sanders P, Hocini M, et al. Catheter ablation of long-lasting persistent atrial fibrillation: critical structures for termination. *J Cardiovasc Electrophysiol.* 2005;16:1125–1137.

37. Waldo AL. The interrelationship between atrial fibrillation and atrial flutter. *Prog Cardiovasc Dis.* 2005;48:41–56.

38. Tamborero D, Mont L, Berruezo A, et al. Left atrial posterior wall isolation does not improve outcome of circumferential pulmonary vein ablation for atrial fibrillation: a prospective randomized study. *Circ Arrhythmia Electrophysiol.* 2009;2:35–40.

39. Lim TW, Koay CH, McCall R, et al. Atrial arrhythmias after single-ring isolation of the posterior left atrium and pulmonary veins for atrial fibrillation. *Circ Arrhythmia Electrophysiol.* 2008;1:120–126.

40. Jais P, Hocini M, O'Neill MD, et al. How to perform linear lesions. *Heart Rhythm.* 2007;4:803–809.

41. Jais P, Hocini M, Hsu L-F, et al. Technique and results of linear ablation at the mitral isthmus. *Circulation.* 2004;110:2996–3002.

42. Verma A, Patel D, Famy T, et al. Efficacy of adjuvant anterior left atrial ablation during intracardiac echocardiography-guided pulmonary vein antrum isolation for atrial fibrillation. *J Cardiovasc Electrophysiol.* 2007;18:151–156.

43. Sanders P, Jais P, Hocini M, et al. Electrophysiologic and clinical consequences of linear catheter ablation to transect the anterior left atrium in patients with atrial fibrillation. *Heart Rhythm.* 2004;1:176–184.

44. O'Neill MD, Kim KT, Jais P, et al. Ablation strategies in chronic atrial fibrillation. In: Aliot E, Haïssaguerre M, Jackman WM, eds. *Catheter Ablation of Atrial Fibrillation.* Malden, MA: Blackwell Futura; 2008:163–189.

45. Haïssaguerre M, Sanders P, Hocini M, et al. Changes in atrial fibrillation cycle length and inducibility during catheter ablation and their relation to outcome. *Circulation.* 2004;109:3007–3013.

46. Knecht S, Hocini M, Wright M, et al. Left atrial linear lesions are required for successful treatment of persistent atrial fibrillation. *Eur Heart J.* 2008;29:2359–2366.

47. Fassini G, Riva S, Chiodelli R, et al. Left mitral isthmus ablation associated with PV isolation: long-term results of a prospective randomized study. *J Cardiovasc Electrophysiol.* 2005;16:1157–1159.

48. Nademanee K, McKenzie J, Kosar E, et al. A new approach for catheter ablation of atrial fibrillation: mapping of the electrophysiologic substrate. *J Am Coll Cardiol.* 2004;43:2044–2053.

49. Konings KT, Smeets JL, Penn OC, et al. Configuration of unipolar atrial electrograms during electrically induced atrial fibrillation in humans. *Circulation.* 1997;95:1231–1241.

50. Sahadevan J, Ryu K, Peltz L, et al. Epicardial mapping of chronic atrial fibrillation in patients: preliminary observations. *Circulation.* 2004;110:3293–3299.

51. Lin J, Scherlag BJ, Zhou J, et al. Autonomic mechanism to explain complex fractionated atrial electrograms (CFAE). *J Cardiovasc Electrophysiol.* 2007;18:1197–1205.

52. Nademanee K, Schwab MC, Kosar EM, et al. Clinical outcomes of catheter substrate ablation for high-risk patients with atrial fibrillation. *J Am Coll Cardiol.* 2008;51:843–849.

53. Tada H, Yoshida K, Chugh A, et al. Prevalence and characteristics of continuous electrical activity in patients with paroxysmal and persistent atrial fibrillation. *J Cardiovasc Electrophysiol.* 2008;19:606–612.

54. Scherr D, Dalal D, Cheema A, et al. Automated detection and characterization of complex fractionated atrial electrograms in human left atrium during atrial fibrillation. *Heart Rhythm.* 2007;4:1013–1020.

55. Wu J, Estner H, Luik A, et al. Automatic 3D mapping of complex fractionated atrial electrograms (CFAE) in patients with paroxysmal and persistent atrial fibrillation. *J Cardiovasc Electrophysiol.* 2008;19:897–903.

56. Park JH, Pak H-N, Kim SK, et al. Electrophysiologic characteristics of complex fractionated atrial electrograms in patients with atrial fibrillation. *J Cardiovasc Electrophysiol.* 2009;20:266–272.

57. Stiles MK, Brooks AG, John B, et al. The effect of electrogram duration on quantification of complex fractionated atrial electrograms and dominant frequency. *J Cardiovasc Electrophysiol.* 2008;19:252–258.

58. Oral H, Chugh A, Good E, et al. Radiofrequency catheter ablation of chronic atrial fibrillation guided by complex electrograms. *Circulation.* 2007;115:2606–2612.

59. Roux J-F, Gojraty S, Bala R, et al. Effect of pulmonary vein isolation on the distribution of complex fractionated electrograms in humans. *Heart Rhythm.* 2009;6:156–160.

60. Schmitt C, Estner H, Hecher B, et al. Radiofrequency ablation of complex fractionated atrial electrograms (CFAE): preferential sites of acute termination and regularization in paroxysmal and persistent atrial fibrillation. *J Cardiovasc Electrophysiol.* 2007;18:1039–1046.

61. Oral H, Chugh A, Yoshida K, et al. A randomized assessment of the incremental role of ablation of complex fractionated atrial electrograms after antral pulmonary vein isolation for long-lasting persistent atrial fibrillation. *J Am Coll Cardiol.* 2009;53:782–789.

62. Jais P, O'Neill MD, Takahashi Y, et al. Stepwise catheter ablation of chronic atrial fibrillation: importance of discrete anatomic sites for termination. *J Cardiovasc Electrophysiol.* 2006;17:s28–s36.

63. Tomita T, Takei M, Saikawa Y, et al. Role of autonomic tone in the initiation and termination of paroxysmal atrial fibrillation in patients without structural heart disease. *J Cardiovasc Electrophysiol.* 2003;14:559–564.

64. Wang J, Liu L, Feng J, Nattel S. Regional and functional factors determining induction and maintenance of atrial fibrillation in dogs. *Am J Physiol.* 1996;271:H148–H158.

65. Nakagawa H, Scherlag BJ, Patterson E, et al. Pathophysiologic basis of automatic ganglionated plexus ablation in patients with atrial fibrillation. *Heart Rhythm.* 2009;6:S26–S34.

66. Pauza DH, Skripka V, Pauziene N, Stropus R. Morphology, distribution, and variability of the epicardiac neural ganglionated subplexuses in the human heart. *Anat Rec.* 2000;259:353–382.

67. Armour JA, Murphy DA, Yuan BX, et al. Gross and microscopic anatomy of the human intrinsic cardiac nervous system. *Anat Rec.* 1997;247:289–298.

68. Lemery R, Birnie D, Tang AS, et al. Feasibility study of endocardial mapping of ganglionated plexuses during catheter ablation of atrial fibrillation. *Heart Rhythm.* 2006;3:387–396.

69. Lemery R. How to perform ablation of the parasympathetic ganglia of the left atrium. *Heart Rhythm.* 2006;3:1237–1239.

70. Scanavacca M, Pisani D, Lara S, et al. Selective atrial vagal denervation guided by evoked vagal reflex to treat patients with paroxysmal atrial fibrillation. *Circulation.* 2006;114:876–885.

71. Hwang C, Chen P-S. Ligament of Marshall: why it is important for atrial fibrillation ablation. *Heart Rhythm.* 2009;6:S35–S40.

72. Kurotobi T, Ito H, Iwakura K, et al. Marshall vein as arrhythmogenic source in patients with atrial fibrillation: correlation between its anatomy and electrophysiologic findings. *J Cardiovasc Electrophysiol.* 2006;17:1062–1067.

73. Valderrabano M, Liu X, Sasaridis C, et al. Ethanol infusion in the vein of Marshall: adjunctive effects during ablation of atrial fibrillation. *Heart Rhythm.* 2009;6:1552–1558.

74. Bagge L, Blomstrom P, Nilsson L, et al. Epicardial off-pump pulmonary vein isolation and vagal denervation improve long-term outcome and quality of life in patients with atrial fibrillation. *J Thorac Cardiovasc Surg.* 2009;137:1265–1271.

75. Rossi P, Bianchi S, Barretta A, et al. Post-operative atrial fibrillation management by selective epicardial vagal fat pad stimulation. *J Interv Card Electrophysiol.* 2009;24:37–45.

76. Sakamoto SI, Schuessler RB, Lee AM, et al. Vagal denervation and reinnervation after ablation of ganglionated plexi. *J Thorac Cardiovasc Surg.* 2010;139:444–452.

77. Nakagawa H, Scherlag BL, Wu R, et al. Addition of selective ablation of autonomic ganglia to pulmonary vein antrum isolation for treatment of paroxysmal and persistent atrial fibrillation [abstract]. *Circulation.* 2004;110:III-543.

78. Oh S, Zhang Y, Bibevski S, et al. Vagal denervation and atrial fibrillation inducibility: epicardial fat pad ablation does not have long term effects. *Heart Rhythm.* 2006;3:701–708.

79. Chugh A, Oral H, Lemola K, et al. Prevalence, mechanisms, and clinical significance of macroreentrant atrial tachycardia during and following left atrial ablation for atrial fibrillation. *Heart Rhythm.* 2005;2:464–471.

80. Jais P, Shah DC, Takahashi A, et al. Long-term follow-up after right atrial radiofrequency catheter treatment of paroxysmal atrial fibrillation. *Pacing Clin Electrophysiol.* 1998;21:2533–2538.

81. Natale A, Leonelli F, Beheiry S, et al. Catheter ablation approach on the right side only for paroxysmal atrial fibrillation therapy: long-term results. *Pacing Clin Electrophysiol.* 2000;23:224–233.

82. Chen SA, Tai CT, Yu WC, et al. Right atrial focal atrial fibrillation: electrophysiologic characteristics and radiofrequency catheter ablation. *J Cardiovasc Electrophysiol.* 1999;10:328–335.

83. Lin YJ, Tai CT, Liu TY, et al. Electrophysiological mechanisms and catheter ablation of complex atrial arrhythmias from crista terminalis. *Pacing Clin Electrophysiol.* 2004;27:1231–1239.

84. O'Neill MD, Jais P, Takahashi Y, et al. The stepwise approach for chronic atrial fibrillation: evidence for a cumulative effect. *J Interv Card Electrophysiol.* 2006;16:153–167.

85. Oral H, Chugh A, Good E, et al. A randomized evaluation of right atrial ablation after left atrial ablation of complex fractionated atrial electrograms for chronic atrial fibrillation. *Circ Arrhythm Electrophysiol.* 2008;1:6–13.

86. Crawford T, Chugh A, Good E, et al. Clinical value of noninducibility by high-dose isoproterenol versus rapid atrial pacing after catheter ablation of paroxysmal atrial fibrillation. *J Cardiovasc Electrophysiol.* 2010;21:13–20.

18

Stepwise Approach for Ablation of Persistent Atrial Fibrillation

Matthew Wright, Shinsuke Miyazaki, and Michel Haïssaguerre

Key Points

The stepwise approach to atrial fibrillation ablation is to sequentially target all foci potentially contributing to the initiation and maintenance of the arrhythmia.

The three major steps in this strategy are (1) pulmonary vein isolation, (2) electrogram-based ablation, and (3) linear ablation.

Special equipment needed includes apparatus for transseptal access and a circular mapping catheter. Computerized mapping systems may be used for image-guided pulmonary vein isolation and computerized determination of atrial cycle lengths.

Termination of atrial fibrillation occurs in 82% to 87% of patients during ablation. About 25% of terminations are directly to sinus rhythm; however, the remainder convert to one or more atrial tachycardias that also require ablation.

Up to 50% of patients require repeat procedures for recurrent atrial arrhythmias.

Atrial fibrillation (AF) is the most frequent sustained human arrhythmia. The incidence and prevalence of AF in the general population are rising,[1] and it is estimated that 15.9 million people will have AF by 2050 in the USA alone[2] if the incidence continues to rise at it has in the past two decades. The overall prevalence of AF in the Framingham Heart Study was 6%, and in people older than 40 years, there was a 16% lifetime chance of developing AF without a history or precedent of heart failure or myocardial infarction. In those older than 75 years, the prevalence is estimated at 10%.[3] AF is associated with an increased risk for all-cause mortality, heart failure, and stroke,[1,4,5] and it is also responsible for about one third of all hospitalizations with cardiac rhythm disturbance.[6] As a consequence, AF constitutes a major socioeconomic and health care problem.

It has been calculated that for the aging United Kingdom population, more than 0.9% of the entire National Health Service budget is already spent on managing AF and its consequences, principally stroke,[7] and in the United States, an estimated $6 to $7 billion is spent on AF management per year.[8]

Although no difference in mortality has been proved to result from using antiarrhythmic medication,[9] a rhythm or a rate control strategy has to be considered in symptomatic patients.[10] If a rhythm control strategy is preferred, the first step still consists of trying at least one antiarrhythmic drug.[6] In patients with symptomatic persistent AF, maintenance of sinus rhythm at 1 year varies between 41% and 62% for sotalol and amiodarone, respectively.[11] In the combined results from EURIDIS and ADONIS, which enrolled a combination of patients with typical atrial flutter, paroxysmal and persistent AF, only 38% had remained in sinus rhythm at 1 year with dronedarone.[12] In comparison, catheter ablation for paroxysmal AF has a 1-year success rate of between 69% and 87%,[13-18] and many groups report success rates of more than 70% for persistent AF,[19-32] including in patients with long-standing persistent AF, off antiarrhythmic drugs.

From these data, it seems clear that catheter ablation is superior to antiarrhythmic drugs in restoring and maintaining sinus rhythm over the long term in patients with both paroxysmal and persistent AF. However, it has to be emphasized that the end points were not all the same in the different studies. In ablation studies, success is defined as the absence of arrhythmia recurrences (AF and atrial tachycardia [AT]), whereas in several pharmacologic studies, the presence of sinus rhythm at the final follow-up has been considered a success regardless of any intervening periods of AF. For example, in AF-related congestive heart failure, 73% of patients in the antiarrhythmic group were in sinus rhythm at last follow-up, but 58% of patients in this same group had experienced at least 1 episode of AF during the study period.[33] Additionally, patients in ablation studies are for the most part attempting second-line therapy, as opposed to those in antiarrhythmic drug trials, a significant proportion of whom were enrolled after a first episode and may represent a lower risk and more easily treated population.

Great efforts are being made to improve the success rates of catheter ablation for AF, which, correctly, are not deemed good enough when compared with ablation of other cardiac arrhythmias. However, the success rates of antiarrhythmic drugs in preventing AF are poor when judged by similar standards. The current HRS/EHRA/ECAS guidelines on catheter ablation of AF support catheter ablation for symptomatic patients in whom at least one antiarrhythmic drug has failed or has not been tolerated.[34]

Electrophysiologic Mechanisms of Atrial Fibrillation Based on Early Ablative Experiences

In the 1990s, early attempts at curing AF with catheter ablation by a percutaneous approach were inspired by the surgical maze technique and its subsequent modifications.[35,36] These early attempts were based on the *multiple-wavelet hypothesis*, proposed by Moe and colleagues,[37] with contributory experimental work by Allessie and associates.[38] The hypothesis was that by compartmentalizing the atria using linear lesions, the critical mass of atrial tissue required for reentrant wavelets would no longer exist, thus curing AF. Schwartz and coworkers were the first to try to replicate biatrial surgical linear approaches, with a high procedural success rate; however, this was at the cost of unacceptable complications.[39] Replication of the surgical procedure by making linear lesions within the right atrium (RA) was unsuccessful.[40]

In the late 1990s, the pivotal role of the pulmonary veins (PVs) in triggering paroxysmal AF was recognized.[41] This led to attempts at treating focal sources that triggered AF rather than compartmentalizing the atria.[42] By mapping the atria, it was observed that paroxysmal AF was triggered by ectopic beats originating from within the PVs, and that by electrically isolating the PVs, AF was eliminated.[43] Other reports also demonstrated the importance of PVs for AF perpetuation through automatic or reentrant mechanisms.[44,45] A *venous wave hypothesis* has therefore been proposed as the main electrophysiologic mechanisms of paroxysmal AF, implicating PVs as the exclusive sources of venous waves and drivers maintaining the atria in fibrillation.[46] For both paroxysmal and persistent AF, isolated sources maintaining AF within the left atrium (LA) and coronary sinus have been observed.[18,47–49]

Ablation for Persistent Atrial Fibrillation

Although pulmonary vein isolation (PVI) without additional ablation has been attempted for patients with persistent AF, the success rates with this approach are disappointing. PV isolation without additional ablation has been reported successful in 20% to 61% of cases, and ablation at sites of complex fractionated atrial electrograms (CFAEs) alone has been reported successful in 9% to 85% of cases,[21,28,29,50–59] although some investigators have reported success rates of up to 95% with PVI alone (Table 18-1).[60,61] For most patients with persistent AF, however, PVI alone is insufficient.[62] Strategies that have combined

two techniques, such as PVI and CFAE ablation, or PVI and linear ablation, or PVI, CFAE ablation, and linear lesions, have achieved success rates between 42% and 95% without antiarrhythmic drugs, with most centers reporting success rates of more than 70% in the short to medium term.[19–32] Importantly, two or more procedures are often necessary to treat persistent AF or secondary AT, and patients considering ablative treatment should be aware that about half require more than one procedure.[19]

Technique of Stepwise Ablation

The stepwise approach to AF ablation has three primary stages (Fig. 18-1). The first step is electrical isolation of the thoracic veins, that is, the PVs with or without the superior vena cava. The second step is to induce local electrogram organization by electrogram-based atrial ablation, including the atrial bodies, coronary sinus, and appendages. The third step is to create linear ablation lines primarily targeting the LA roof, mitral isthmus, and cavotricuspid isthmus. Thus, during persistent AF, stepwise catheter ablation sequentially targets all structures potentially contributing to initiation and maintenance of AF: (1) PVs, (2) LA tissue and RA targets, and (3) LA roof and mitral isthmus (using linear ablation). Each region is ablated following a sequential approach until AF termination, and the impact of ablation is assessed by measurement of AF cycle length in both appendages. Each step is accompanied by an increase in AF cycle length until conversion of AF directly to sinus rhythm or more often to multiple ATs that are then systematically ablated.[19,30,31] A fourth step is ablation of these residual ATs.

This sequential approach has resulted in unprecedented success in maintaining sinus rhythm in the medium term with recovery of atrial mechanical function in patients with long-standing persistent AF.[63] Termination of AF occurs in 82% to 87% of patients,[19,64] with 95% of the patients in sinus rhythm at 1 year and 90% after more than 2 years[19]; however, a second procedure is needed in about 50% of patients, mainly for AT.[19,64]

Atrial Fibrillation Cycle Length: A Real-Time Guide to Ablation

Both the impact of ablation at each region and the amount of work remaining can be followed by monitoring the AF cycle length. The AF cycle length can be reliably monitored during the procedure by averaging 30 consecutive cycles at the LA and RA appendages, which display unambiguous high-voltage and reproducible electrograms (Fig. 18-2).[65] This can be measured with computer software and is relatively stable, with less than 5 milliseconds of variation between repeated measures in most patients. Studies have shown that AF cycle length correlates with the local refractory period, that it shortens in parallel with the duration of AF, and that drugs may affect it.[66] However, AF cycle length prolongation during ablation at remote sites is evidence that the AFCL is not just a representation of the local refractory period.[67] A study using advanced computer simulation demonstrated that the AF cycle length, as measured in the LA appendage, represents the sum of all fibrillatory activities converging to this area.[65] The higher the number

TABLE 18-1

CLINICAL OUTCOME OF PATIENTS UNDERGOING PERSISTENT ATRIAL FIBRILLATION ABLATION DEPENDING ON THE STRATEGY

Study	No. of Patients with Persistent Atrial Fibrillation	Duration of Follow-Up (mo)	Technique	PV Electrical Isolation	LA Linear Lesions	Electrical Block at the Linear Lesions	CFAE Ablation	RA Ablation	Success in Persistent AF Patients (%)	Percentage of Antiarrhythmic Drugs in Persistent AF Patients
Pappone et al, 2000[112]	12	9 ± 3	CPVA	No	No	No	No	No	83	25
Oral et al, 2005[32]	80	9 ± 4	CPVA	No	Yes	No	Yes	No	68	0
Willems et al, 2006[28]	32	14-17	PVI + linear lesions	Yes	Yes	Yes	No	No	69	0
Beukema et al, 2005[113]	53	15 ± 5	CPVA + linear lesions	No	Yes	No	No	No	77	44
Oral et al, 2006[111]	146	12	CPVA + linear lesions	No	Yes	No	No	No	74	0
Bertaglia et al, 2006[114]	74	20 ± 6	CPVA + linear lesions	No	Yes	Yes	No	No	70	64
Calo et al, 2006[27]	80	14 ± 5	CPVA + linear lesions	No	Yes	No	No	Yes	85	52
Nademanee et al, 2004[57]	64	12	CFAE	NA	No	NA	Yes	Yes	88	13
Oral et al, 2007[54]	100	13 ± 7	CFAE	NA	No	NA	Yes	Yes	57	0
Estner et al, 2008[115]	23	13 ± 10	CFAE	No	No	NA	Yes	No	9	0
Estner et al, 2008[59]	54	13 ± 10	PVI + CFAE	Yes	No	NA	Yes	No	41	0
Haïssaguerre et al, 2005[116]	60	11 ± 6	PVI + CFAE + linear lesions	Yes	Yes	Yes	Yes	Yes	95	8
Estner et al, 2008[117]	35	19 ± 12	PVI + CFAE	Yes	No*	NA	Yes	No	74	26
O'Neill et al, 2009[19]	153	30 ± 11	PVI + CFAE + linear lesions	Yes	Yes	Yes	Yes	Yes	89	21
Rostock et al, 2008[96]	88	20 ± 4	PVI + CFAE + linear lesions	Yes	YES	Yes	Yes	Yes	81	5

*Linear lesions were performed if a macro re-entrant atrial tachycardia was mapped.
AF: atrial fibrillation; CFAE, complex fractionated atrial electrogram; CPVA, circumferential pulmonary vein ablation; LA, left atrium; PV, pulmonary vein; PVI, pulmonary vein isolation; RA, right atrium.

of elements participating in the AF process, the shorter the AF cycle length and the more complex the ablation. Of note, the surface AF cycle length is also a marker for resistance to antiarrhythmic drugs and DC cardioversion.[68–70]

After each step of ablation, a gradual prolongation of AF cycle length is observed.[30] More than a 5-millisecond increase in mean AF cycle length is considered significant for any intervention. Conversion to sinus rhythm or AT usually occurs when AF cycle length reaches 180 and 200

milliseconds in patients off drugs (Fig. 18-3).[30] If AF persists during ablation of the LA despite a prolonged LA appendage cycle length, a lesser prolongation of the RA appendage cycle length would suggest that the RA may contain independent elements that participate in the AF process.[65]

Step 1: Thoracic Vein Isolation

PV isolation is described in detail in Chapter 15. PV isolation (antral, ostial, or circumferential) invariably results in a better clinical prognosis in patients with paroxysmal compared with persistent AF.[30,71–74] Despite these poor results when used as a stand-alone strategy, PVI is performed as the initial ablation step in all patients with persistent AF because spared PVs can lead to arrhythmia recurrence due to triggering foci.[75] A circumferential catheter is used to map and guide ablation of PVs, which can be isolated individually or as ipsilateral pairs depending on venous anatomy, catheter stability, and the operator's preference. In all cases, ablation is performed at least 0.5 to 1 cm away from the PV ostia to avoid the risk for PV stenosis when possible. However, it is sometimes necessary to go more distally to achieve PVI; for example, at the anterior part of the left superior PV, catheter stability is sometimes extremely difficult, necessitating ablation at the ostium and even just inside the vein. For all veins, isolation is assessed by either electrical elimination or dissociation of the PV potentials.[76] The superior vena cava may be targeted in this step. After thoracic vein isolation, the cycle length is simultaneously measured in the RA and LA appendages and followed to access the effects of subsequent ablation on the cycle lengths in both chambers.

Step 2: Electrogram-Based Ablation

In the second step of the stepwise approach, targets for electrogram-based ablation are areas with continuous electrical activity, complex fractionated activity, local cycle lengths between 70 and 120 milliseconds, and temporal gradient between adjacent bipoles (Fig. 18-4).[77–88] The techniques for electrogram-based ablation of AF are described in detail in Chapter 17. All parts of the left atrium are mapped; however, the base of the appendage and inferior left atrium–coronary sinus interface are often important sites for cycle length slowing. Other sites requiring particular attention may be the interatrial

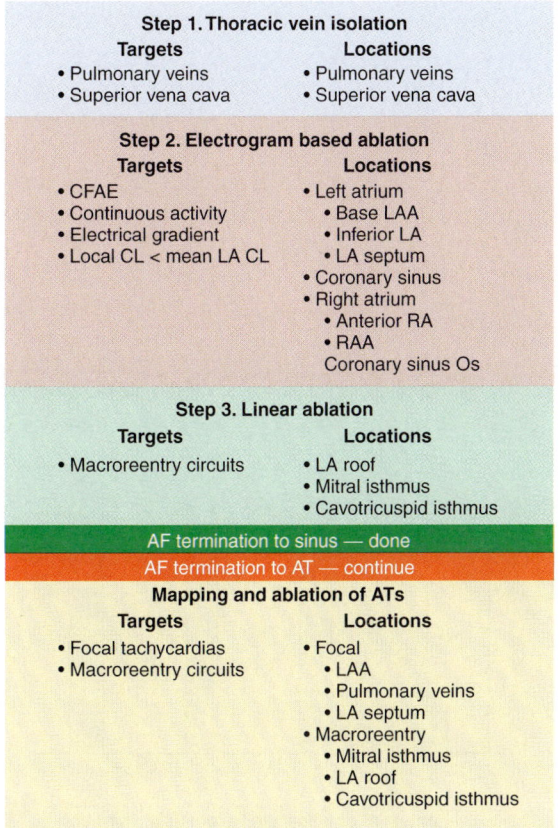

STEPWISE APPROACH TO ATRIAL FIBRILLATION ABLATION

Step 1. Thoracic vein isolation

Targets	Locations
• Pulmonary veins	• Pulmonary veins
• Superior vena cava	• Superior vena cava

Step 2. Electrogram based ablation

Targets	Locations
• CFAE	• Left atrium
• Continuous activity	• Base LAA
• Electrical gradient	• Inferior LA
• Local CL < mean LA CL	• LA septum
	• Coronary sinus
	• Right atrium
	• Anterior RA
	• RAA
	Coronary sinus Os

Step 3. Linear ablation

Targets	Locations
• Macroreentry circuits	• LA roof
	• Mitral isthmus
	• Cavotricuspid isthmus

AF termination to sinus — done

AF termination to AT — continue

Mapping and ablation of ATs

Targets	Locations
• Focal tachycardias	• Focal
• Macroreentry circuits	• LAA
	• Pulmonary veins
	• LA septum
	• Macroreentry
	• Mitral isthmus
	• LA roof
	• Cavotricuspid isthmus

FIGURE 18-1. Stepwise approach to atrial fibrillation ablation. The first three steps terminate atrial fibrillation to sinus rhythm or more commonly an atrial tachycardia. The final stage addresses these postconversion arrhythmias. AT, atrial tachycardia; CFAE, complex fractionated atrial electrograms; CL, cycle length; LA, left atrium; LAA, left atrial appendage; RA, right atrium; RAA, right atrial appendage.

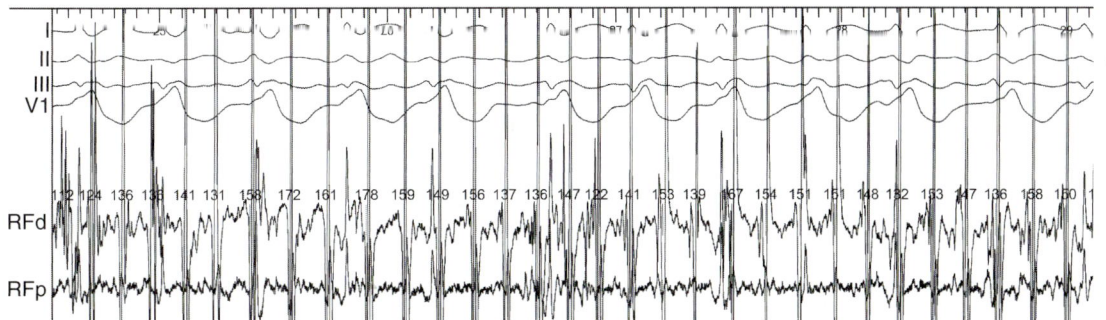

FIGURE 18-2. Atrial fibrillation (AF) cycle length. The AF cycle length can be easily assessed from both the left and right atrial appendages, where an unambiguous signal is recorded. Either using automated software (as shown here, Bard Electrophysiology, Haverhill, MA) or by averaging 10 or more cycles, left and right AF cycle length is worked out (146 msec in this case for the left atrial appendage) and gives an indication of the difficulty of ablation and likelihood of procedural termination. d, distal; RF, radiofrequency; p, proximal.

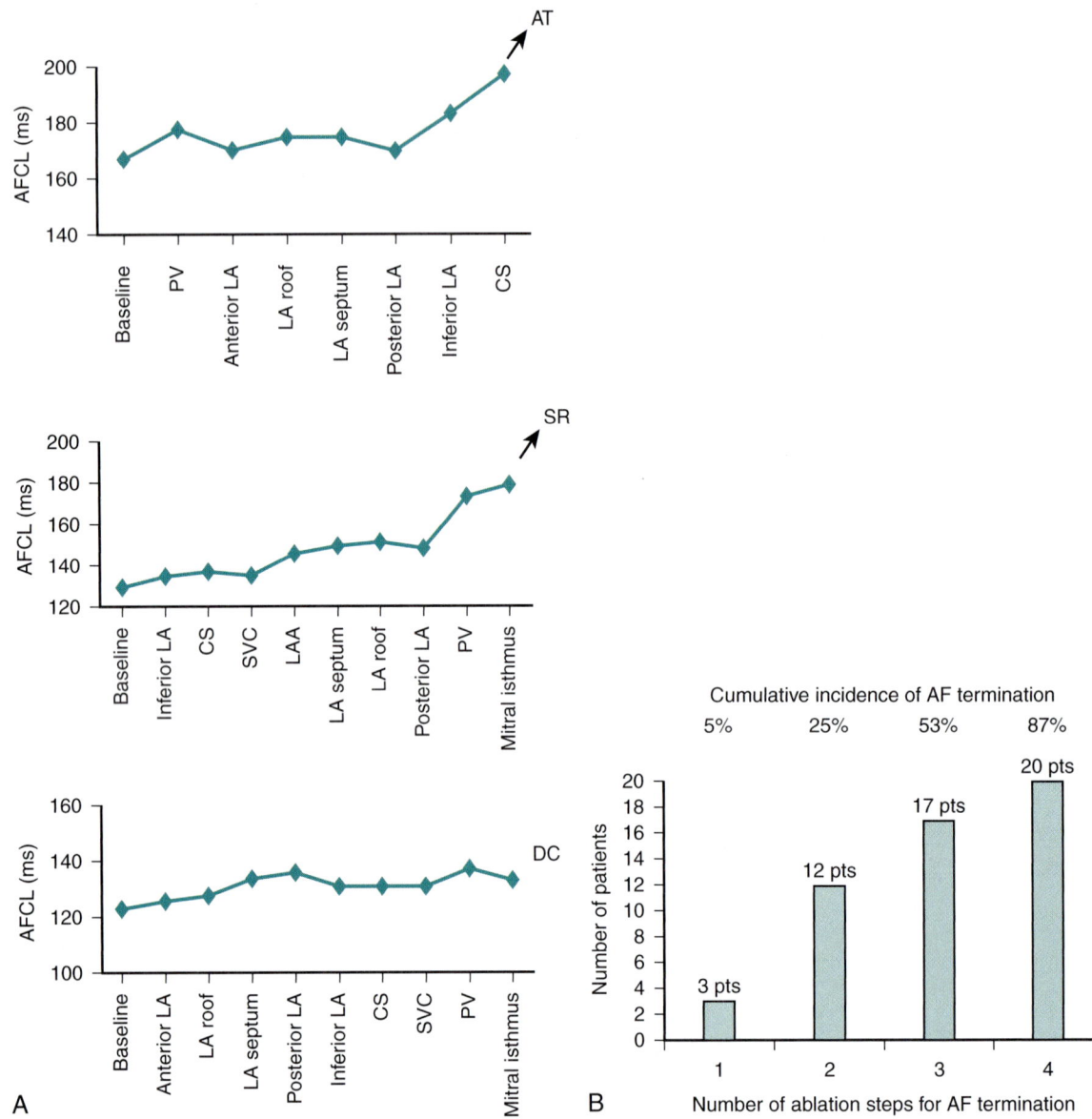

FIGURE 18-3. A, Evolution of the changes in atrial fibrillation cycle length (AFCL) in the left atrial appendage during each ablation step in three patients. The first two patients (*top* and *middle*) converted to atrial tachycardia (AT) or sinus rhythm (SR) after a gradual or sudden increase in AFCL, whereas the third patient (*bottom*) had minimal increase in AFCL and required electrical cardioversion **B,** The figure demonstrates the number and cumulative percentage of patients terminating with each step of ablation. Of note, the first three steps (PV isolation, atrial ablation, and CS/SVC ablation) were performed in a randomized order, whereas the final step was linear ablation in all cases. AF, atrial fibrillation; CS, coronary sinus; LA, left atrium; PV, pulmonary vein; SVC, superior vena cava. (*From Haïssaguerre M, Sanders P, Hocini M, et al. Catheter ablation of long-lasting persistent atrial fibrillation: critical structures for termination. J Cardiovasc Electrophysiol. 2005;16:1125-1137. With permission.*)

septum around the foramen ovale, the posterior atrium, and the anterior left atrium. The perimeter around the foramen ovale for 1 to 2 cm is targeted by turning the ablation catheter posteriorly from the transseptal access site. Ablation of the anterior septum near the His bundle is avoided. The anterior left atrium is ablated along the collar of the appendage and extending superiorly to the roof. A second, more medial line in this area can be performed.

Ablation of the LA endocardium adjacent to the coronary sinus typically slows and organizes electrical activity (Fig. 18-5). Ablation of the inferior LA is accomplished by a linear ablation line along the coronary sinus between 7 and 4 o'clock in the left anterior oblique view

(see Chapter 17). The medial starting position is along the interatrial septum. By looping the catheter in the atrium with the tip directed toward the atrial septum, the line can be created by steadily withdrawing the catheter. Additional ablation within the coronary sinus may also be needed with the goals of eliminating or slowing sharp potentials remaining in the coronary sinus electrical activity and to eliminate residual areas of rapid activation. This is performed with an irrigated catheter within the coronary sinus beginning at the 4-o'clock position and withdrawing to the os. A maximum of 25 W is used within the coronary sinus. Ablation in the RA around the coronary sinus ostium is performed to dissociate the proximal coronary sinus musculature from the atria.

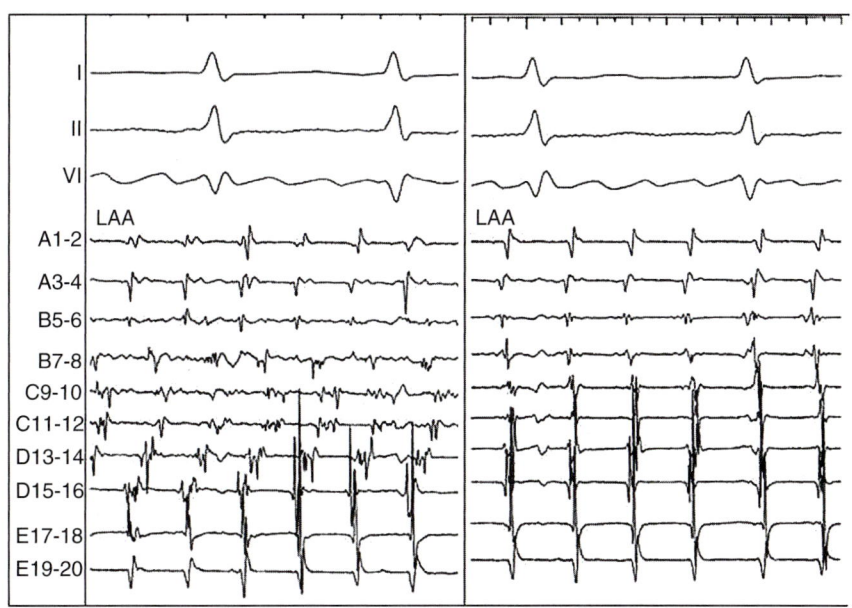

FIGURE 18-4. The figure demonstrates the slowing (from 145 to 170 msec, locally) and organization of local activity (*right*) with ablation at the anterior collar of the left atrial appendage (LAA). Note the activation gradient and activity spanning the entire cycle length observed on spines C and D of a multiple spline catheter (PentaRay, Biosense Webster, Diamond Bar, CA) at the site before ablation (*left*). *(From Haïssaguerre M, Sanders P, Hocini M, et al. Catheter ablation of long-lasting persistent atrial fibrillation: critical structures for termination.* J Cardiovasc Electrophysiol. *2005;16:1125-1137. With permission.)*

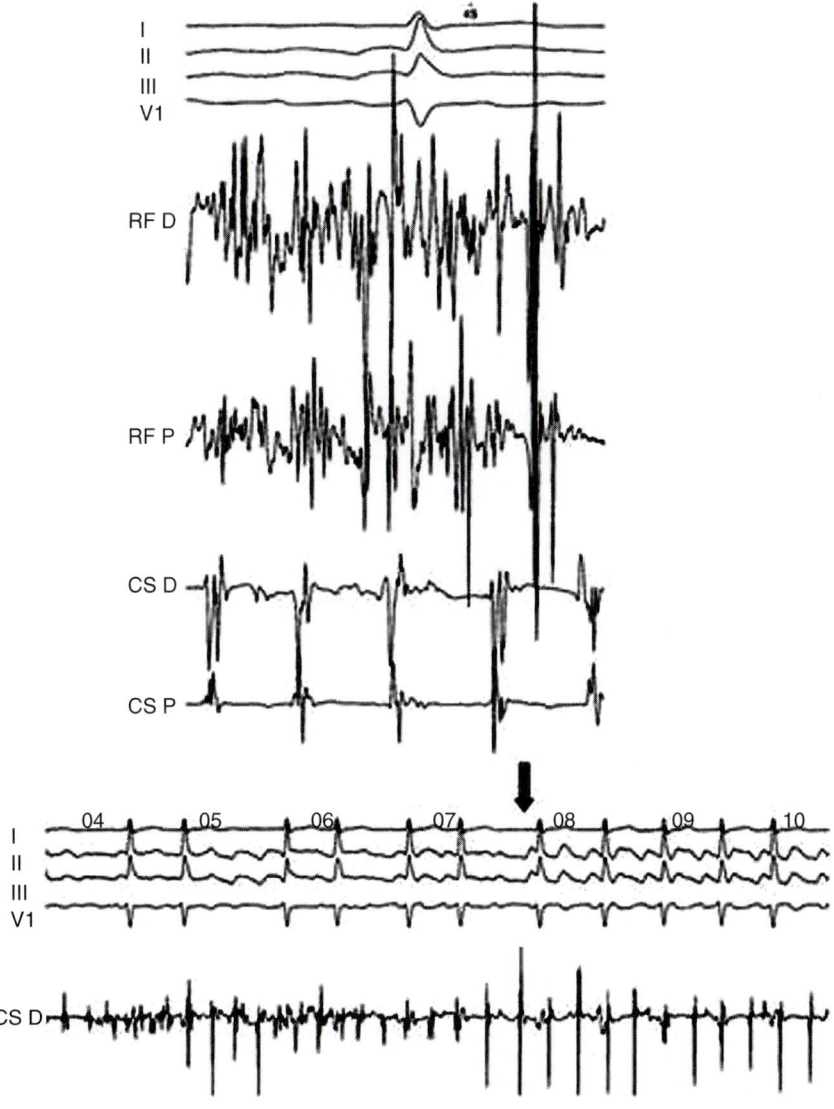

FIGURE 18-5. The ablation catheter (radiofrequency [RF], distal [D], and proximal [P]) placed in the distal coronary sinus (CS) records a typical example of continuous electrical activity. The quadripolar reference catheter is proximal to the ablation catheter in the CS. Ablation at that discrete site terminates the fibrillation, transforming it into an atrial tachycardia (*arrow, lower panel*). *(From Jais P, O'Neill MD, Takahashi Y, et al. Stepwise catheter ablation of chronic atrial fibrillation: importance of discrete anatomic sites for termination.* J Cardiovasc Electrophysiol. *2006;17:S28-S36. With permission.)*

Step 3: Linear Lesions

The third step is the creation of linear lesions to form areas of conduction block (see Chapter 17). The first such linear lesion consists of the roof line, which connects the two superior PVs (Fig. 18-6).[16] The immediate end point is electrogram abolition along the line with verification of conduction block performed after the restoration of sinus rhythm. The mitral isthmus line, which joins the mitral annulus to the PV either anteriorly or laterally,[15,16,89] is reserved for patients whose AF is not terminated with prior ablation steps and those with perimitral macro-reentry after termination of AF. The mitral isthmus line is technically difficult and usually requires ablation within the coronary sinus (see Chapter 17). Incomplete ablation lines may be proarrhythmic. A recent study highlights that although PVI and electrogram-based ablation without linear lesions may be effective in terminating persistent AF in a significant number of patients, macro-reentrant AT requiring LA linear ablation is likely to occur during the overall follow-up period.[64] In this study, 96% of patients ultimately required a roof line and 86% a mitral line after a mean follow-up of 2 years, despite attempts to avoid LA linear lesions. These data suggest that at least the roof line (which is easier and simpler to perform than the mitral isthmus line) could be used in the case of AF persistence after PVI and CFAE ablation. This study also confirmed the high risk for AT recurrence in cases of incomplete conduction block at LA lines.

Right Atrial Ablation

There is accumulating evidence that in a subset of patients, possibly up to 20% of patients with long-lasting persistent AF, the RA plays an active role in the perpetuation of AF.[90] Ablation within the RA may be incorporated into previous steps or, as outlined here for clarity, as a separate process. Prolongation of the left atrial cycle length to more than 170 milliseconds with persistently shorter (<140 millisecond) cycle lengths in the RA suggests that structures within the RA serve to maintain the arrhythmia. Ablation within the RA is directed at electrogram-based targets wherever they occur; however, these are most often localized to the anterior RA or the base of the appendage. The superior vena cava should be explored for evidence of high-frequency activity if not already done. In the current scheme, all patients undergo cavotricuspid isthmus ablation at the end of the procedure. The total procedure time for this strategy (including mapping of ATs) has been reported at 264 ± 77 minutes with 84 ± 30 minutes of fluoroscopic time.[30]

Procedural End Point for Stepwise Ablation

The end point for the stepwise approach to AF ablation is termination of AF. Termination is defined as direct restoration of sinus rhythm or transition to an AT showing a stable cycle length, morphology, and activation sequence of both atria. The ATs are subsequently mapped and ablated. For patients without termination of AF during the

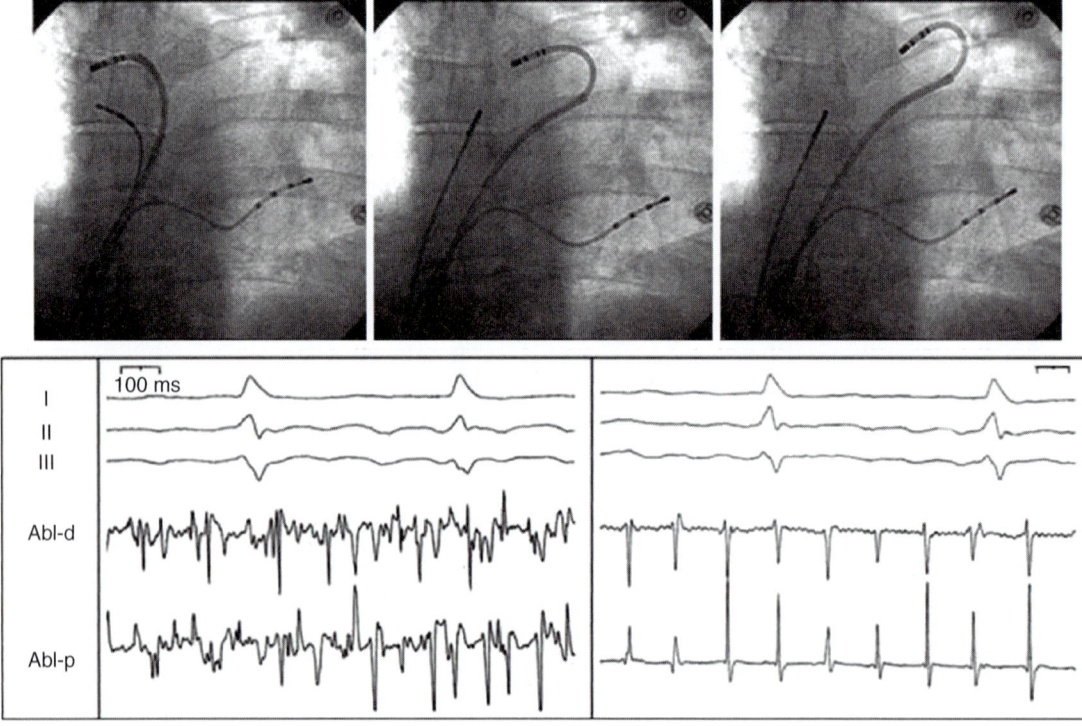

FIGURE 18-6. Linear and atrial ablation at the left atrial (LA) roof. Ablation (Abl) is performed in the most cranial location and extended from the right superior pulmonary vein (PV) to the left superior PV. Although complete roof ablation could be performed as illustrated here with the catheter parallel to the tissue, radiofrequency applications are often necessary with the tip perpendicular to the tissue. The *lower panels* show the local effect of ablation at the LA roof; the rapid disorganized activity (*left*) is converted by ablation locally to organized activity (*right*). d, distal; p, proximal. (*From Haïssaguerre M, Sanders P, Hocini M, et al. Catheter ablation of long-lasting persistent atrial fibrillation: critical structures for termination. J Cardiovasc Electrophysiol. 2005;16:1125-1137. With permission.*)

procedure, cardioversion is performed. After restoration of sinus rhythm, confirmation of PV isolation and the completeness of ablation lines should be demonstrated.

Mapping Atrial Tachycardias

In the stepwise approach, the end point of ablation is restoration of sinus rhythm; however, sinus rhythm is restored directly in less than 30% of patients. In more than 70% of patients, AF terminates by conversion to AT (Fig. 18-7).[30] These ATs are often multiple in number and mechanisms and add significantly to the complexity of ablation. They are considered the last step of persistent and long-standing AF ablation, and results of their mapping and ablation will achieve either subsequent success or failure of the procedure for patients. Mechanisms of AT after an AF ablation vary with the ablation approach.[91-94] Although three-dimensional electroanatomic mapping systems may assist in mapping AT, using these technologies is often impractical because of AT instability or multiple ATs that each require mapping. For this reason, a deductive diagnostic electrophysiologic approach has recently been validated,[95] based on the common mechanisms of ATs that are encountered. Macro-reentrant circuits (either around the ipsilateral veins, and thus roof dependent, or around the mitral or tricuspid valve annulus) are diagnosed by activation mapping and con-

firmed with entrainment at two opposite parts of the circuit. Macro-reentry accounts for about 50% of all ATs after AF ablation; the other 50% are "focal," which again can be mapped using a combination of activation and entrainment mapping.

Focal AT is defined as centrifugal activation from a localized region. These ATs may be true discrete points of tachycardia origin in 26% of patients but more commonly are thought to be localized reentry. In the latter case, the entire tachycardia cycle length may be recorded in an area of several centimeters.[96] A macro-reentrant AT is defined as one in which the entire cycle length can be mapped to a single chamber with entrainment at two or more sites with postpacing intervals that are 20 milliseconds or less in length than the tachycardia cycle length.

A deductive stepwise approach to ablation of these ATs has been described[95] (Fig. 18-8). The first step is the assessment of cycle length variability. When measured from the coronary sinus or LA appendage, ATs with more than 15% variability are very likely to be focal and are mapped accordingly (see later). If ambiguous variation is present, macro-reentry is initially explored.

The second step is to diagnose or exclude macro-reentry. The most common macro-reentrant circuits are perimitral (68%) and roof dependent (around the right or left

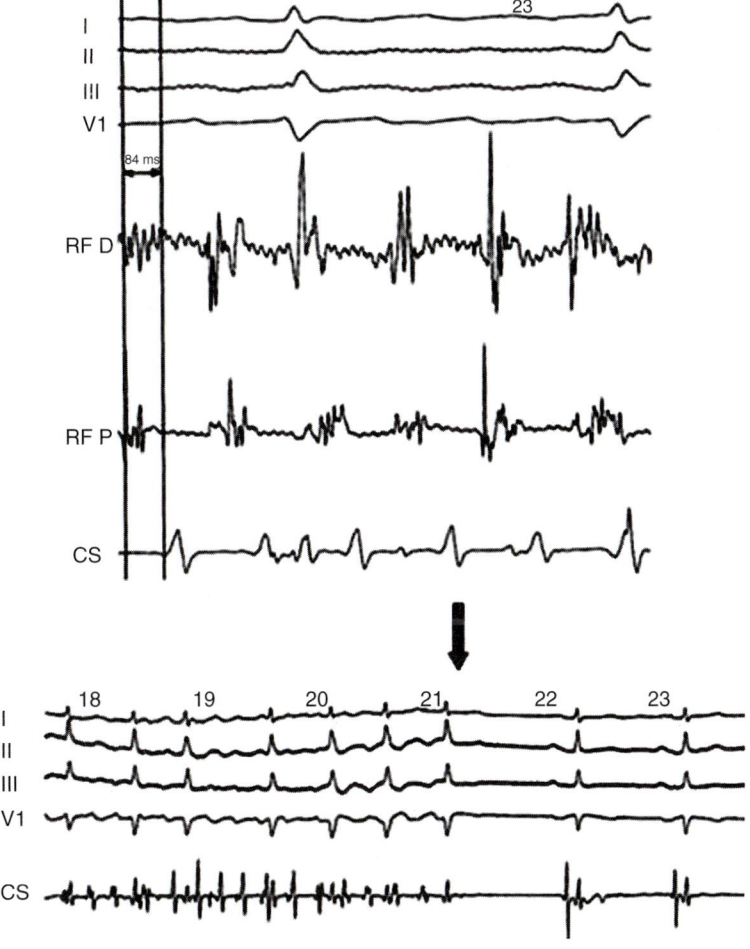

FIGURE 18-7. These fractionated potentials were recorded with the ablation catheter (RF) at the posterior left atrium. Ablation at that site directly terminated atrial fibrillation to sinus rhythm (*lower panel, arrow*). CS, coronary sinus; D, distal; P, proximal. *(From Jais P, O'Neill MD, Takahashi Y, et al. Stepwise catheter ablation of chronic atrial fibrillation: importance of discrete anatomic sites for termination. J Cardiovasc Electrophysiol. 2006;17:S28-S36. With permission.)*

DEDUCTIVE APPROACH TO ATRIAL TACHYCARDIA ABLATION

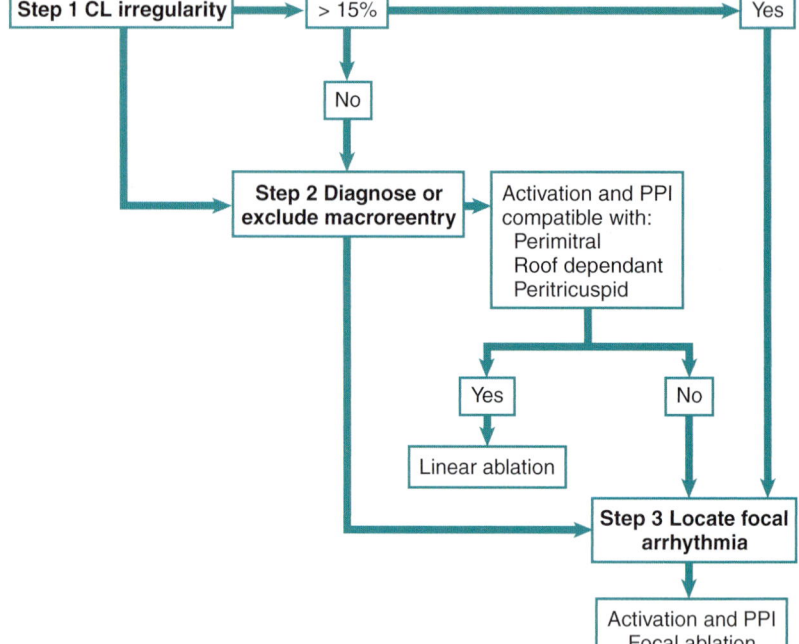

FIGURE 18-8. Deductive approach to mapping and ablation of atrial tachycardias after atrial fibrillation ablation. CL, cycle length; PPI, postpacing interval. *(Reproduced with permission from: Jais P, et al. A deductive mapping strategy for atrial tachycardia following atrial fibrillation ablation: Importance of localized reentry. J Cardiovasc Electrophysiol 2009;20:480–491. With permission.)*

PVs, 28%).[96] Cavotricuspid isthmus–dependent re-entry is noted in 16% of macro-reentrant ATs. Perimitral reentry can be suspected by a circumferential activation pattern simultaneously recorded from the coronary sinus, septal, and lateral atrial sites. Entrainment mapping may further support the presence of perimitral reentry. If perimitral reentry is excluded, roof-dependent reentry is investigated by examining the sequence of atrial activation on the anterior and posterior LA walls. The demonstration of opposite activation patterns (e.g., ascending on the anterior wall and descending on the posterior wall) is consistent with a roof-dependent circuit. Conversely, activation of both walls in a similar direction excludes this mechanism. If LA macro-reentry is excluded, cavotricuspid isthmus–dependent flutter should be explored. Once a specific macro-reentrant circuit is suspected, judicious entrainment mapping is undertaken from limited sites to prevent transformation or termination of the AT. For perimitral reentry, pacing is performed from septal and lateral mitral isthmus sites, and for roof-dependent reentry, pacing is performed on the anterior and posterior walls. Postpacing intervals should be less than 30 milliseconds longer than the tachycardia cycle length within the reentrant circuits. Longer return cycles exclude an LA macro-reentrant circuit and prompt the next step in the process.

The third step is to define the origin of a focal AT after exclusion of a macro-reentrant AT. Mapping is first directed at the LA, then the RA. The direction of coronary sinus activation may direct LA mapping to the septal or lateral atrium. The mapping then seeks to identify the site of earliest centrifugal activation. The most common sites for focal ATs are LA appendage, PVs, and atrial septum (Fig. 18-9). When a favorable site cannot be defined by activation mapping, determining the postpacing interval from various sites may localize the area of interest. Areas with postpacing intervals that are more than 50 milli-

SITES OF ORIGIN OF FOCAL ATRIAL TACHYCARDIA

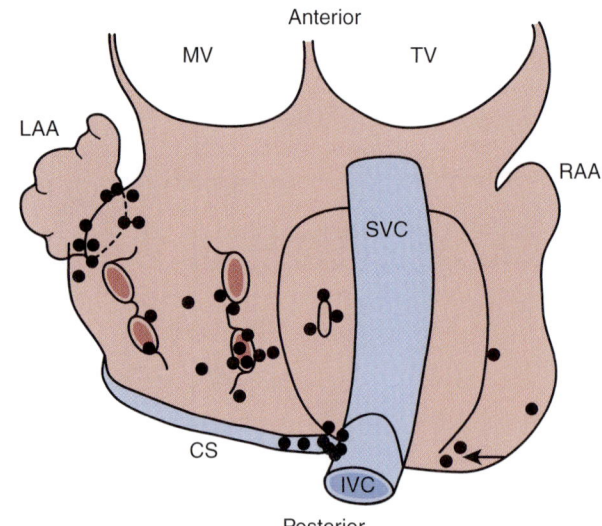

FIGURE 18-9. Location of focal atrial tachycardias ablated during the index procedure. The two points marked with an *arrow* were foci (giving centrifugal activation) located at the cavotricuspid isthmus. CS, coronary sinus; IVC, inferior vena cava; LAA, left atrial appendage; MV, mitral valve; RAA, right atrial appendage; SVC, superior vena cava; TV, tricuspid valve. *(From Haïssaguerre M, Sanders P, Hocini M, et al. Catheter ablation of long-lasting persistent atrial fibrillation: critical structures for termination. J Cardiovasc Electrophysiol. 2005;16:1125-1137. With permission.)*

seconds longer than the tachycardia cycle length should prompt mapping in other areas of the atrium.

Ablation is directed at the source of origin for focal ATs using irrigated ablation at 30 W and 42°C target temperature. Energy is delivered for 30 to 60 seconds at each location. If tachycardia does not terminate or transform, further mapping is performed. Macro-reentry is treated with linear ablation as described in Chapter 17.

Predictors of Success

During the procedure, when AF can be terminated by catheter ablation (without drug or external cardioversion), only 5% of these patients will have recurrent AF[19,96]; however, almost 50% will have AT recurrence, which may be more symptomatic than AF.[19,31] In experienced centers, however, catheter ablation of subsequent ATs is associated with high success rate.[95] Other important predictors of success have been reported by investigators: preexisting LA scarring,[97] voltage abatement,[98] the percentage of LA ablated or vagal denervation,[99] and electrical block at linear lesions.[19,64,100]

More specifically, the main predictors of success before the ablation procedure are AF cycle length more than 140 milliseconds,[65] duration of continuous AF less than 5 years,[19,64,100] no history of hypertension, and smaller LA dimensions.[101]

We have evaluated the clinical predictors of success in 90 consecutive patients with persistent AF followed during 2 years.[70] The duration of AF, LA dimensions, presence of structural heart disease, and surface electrocardiogram (ECG) AF cycle length were assessed before ablation and analyzed with respect to long-term clinical outcome. Long-term maintenance of sinus rhythm was associated with a shorter duration of continuous AF ($P < .0001$), a longer surface ECG AF cycle length ($P < .001$), and a smaller LA ($P < .05$) compared with those with recurrent arrhythmia. In multivariate analysis, the surface ECG AF cycle length and the AF duration predicted clinical success of persistent AF ablation ($P < .01$ and $P < .05$, respectively). Furthermore, using a receiver operating characteristic curve, the optimal cutoff for the AF cycle length as a predictor of AF termination was 142 milliseconds, with specificity and sensitivity of 92.9 % and 69.7 %, respectively. On the other hand, the optimal cutoff point for the duration of continuous AF was 21 months for AF termination (specificity, 92.9 %; sensitivity, 61.8 %). The combined cutoff using a surface ECG AF cycle length of more than 142 milliseconds and duration of continuous AF of less than 21 months had 100% specificity in predicting procedural termination of AF (sensitivity, 39.5 %; positive-predictive value; 100.0%; negative-predictive value; 23.3%).

Complications and Potential Benefits

Complications related to catheter ablation of persistent AF occur in 1% to 2% of the patients and mainly include stroke, which is fortunately rare, and pericardial tamponade.[102] Stroke and transient ischemic attacks are mainly the consequences of thrombi adherent to catheters and sheaths, endocardial disruption from the ablation lesions, and air passing through transseptal sheaths. For this reason, it is important to have ready access to vascular imaging of the brain and protocols for acute thrombolysis for stroke. Anticoagulation is used to prevent thrombi from forming, but this increases the risk for pericardial tamponade. Other possible complications are PV stenosis, which is dramatically reduced with a more proximal ablation strategy compared with the initial reports of isolation within the vein,[103] atrioesophageal fistula (exceedingly rare but almost always fatal),[104] and phrenic nerve paralysis, from which the patient almost always recovers.[105]

On the other hand, catheter ablation of persistent AF has shown promising results in terms of improved morbidity[106,107] and quality of life[108,109](especially in patients with preexisting heart failure),[107,110] but also potential benefits in term of mortality[53,106]

Indications for Persistent Atrial Fibrillation Ablation

The latest guidelines published by the ACC/AHA/ESC societies have recommended not differentiating between patients on the basis of the duration of AF.[34] Briefly, patients are considered for ablation in case of symptomatic recurrent AF after failure of at least one antiarrhythmic drug, electrical cardioversion, or both. Importantly, as mentioned earlier, one has to consider that catheter ablation for patients with AF of very long duration (especially >5 years), very short cycle length on a 12-lead ECG, and extremely dilated LA has very poor chance of clinical success.

Of note, data have indicated that patients with heart failure (New York Heart Association class II or higher) or evidence of left ventricular dysfunction without an alternative explanation have the most to gain from catheter ablation,[107] even if the success rate is lower compared with patients with normal left ventricular function. It has been suggested that asymptomatic patients with AF-related thromboembolism should be treated by catheter ablation,[111] even though no trials have reported a reduction in events after ablation, owing to the large number of patients who would need to be recruited. Therefore the ACC/AHA/ESC recommendations for anticoagulation remain the same after catheter ablation.[34]

Acknowledgments
Matthew Wright receives financial support from the Department of Health via the National Institute for Health Research (NIHR) comprehensive Biomedical Research Centre award to Guy's & St. Thomas' NHS Foundation Trust in partnership with King's College London and King's College Hospital NHS Foundation Trust.

References

1. Stewart S, Hart CL, Hole DJ, et al. Population prevalence, incidence, and predictors of atrial fibrillation in the Renfrew/Paisley study. *Heart*. 2001;86:516–521.
2. Miyasaka Y, Barnes ME, Gersh BJ, et al. Secular trends in incidence of atrial fibrillation in Olmsted County, Minnesota, 1980 to 2000, and implications on the projections for future prevalence. *Circulation*. 2006;114:119–125.
3. Hobbs FD, Fitzmaurice DA, Mant J, et al., The SAFE study. A randomised controlled trial and cost-effectiveness study of systematic screening (targeted and total population screening) versus routine practice for the detection of atrial fibrillation in people aged 65 and over. *Health Technol Assess*. 2005;9:iii-iv, ix-x, 1–74 .
4. Benjamin EJ, Wolf PA, D'Agostino RB, et al. Impact of atrial fibrillation on the risk of death: the Framingham Heart Study. *Circulation*. 1998;98:946–952.
5. Stewart S, Hart CL, Hole DJ, et al. A population-based study of the long-term risks associated with atrial fibrillation: 20-year follow-up of the Renfrew/Paisley study. *Am J Med*. 2002;113:359–364.
6. Fuster V, Ryden LE, Cannom DS, et al. ACC/AHA/ESC 2006 Guidelines for the Management of Patients with Atrial Fibrillation: a report of the American College of Cardiology/American Heart Association Task Force on Practice Guidelines and the European Society of Cardiology Committee for Practice Guidelines (Writing Committee to Revise the 2001 Guidelines for the Management of Patients With Atrial Fibrillation). Developed in collaboration with the European Heart Rhythm Association and the Heart Rhythm Society. *Circulation*. 2006;114:e257–e354.
7. Stewart S, Murphy NF, Walker A, et al. Cost of an emerging epidemic: an economic analysis of atrial fibrillation in the UK. *Heart*. 2004;90:286–292.
8. Kozak LJ, Lees KA, DeFrances CJ. National Hospital Discharge Survey: 2003 annual summary with detailed diagnosis and procedure data. *Vital Health Stat*. 2006;13:1–206.

9. Wyse DG, Waldo AL, DiMarco JP, et al. A comparison of rate control and rhythm control in patients with atrial fibrillation. *N Engl J Med*. 2002;347:1825–1833.

10. Van Gelder IC, Hagens VE, Bosker HA, et al. A comparison of rate control and rhythm control in patients with recurrent persistent atrial fibrillation. *N Engl J Med*. 2002;347:1834–1840.

11. Singh BN, Singh SN, Reda DJ, et al. Amiodarone versus sotalol for atrial fibrillation. *N Engl J Med*. 2005;352:1861–1872.

12. Singh BN, Connolly SJ, Crijns HJ, et al. Dronedarone for maintenance of sinus rhythm in atrial fibrillation or flutter. *N Engl J Med*. 2007;357:987–999.

13. Oral H, Knight BP, Ozaydin M, et al. Clinical significance of early recurrences of atrial fibrillation after pulmonary vein isolation. *J Am Coll Cardiol*. 2002;40:100–104.

14. Oral H, Veerareddy S, Good E, et al. Prevalence of asymptomatic recurrences of atrial fibrillation after successful radiofrequency catheter ablation. *J Cardiovasc Electrophysiol*. 2004;15:920–924.

15. Jais P, Hocini M, Hsu LF, et al. Technique and results of linear ablation at the mitral isthmus. *Circulation*. 2004;110:2996–3002.

16. Hocini M, Jais P, Sanders P, et al. Techniques, evaluation, and consequences of linear block at the left atrial roof in paroxysmal atrial fibrillation: a prospective randomized study. *Circulation*. 2005;112:3688–3696.

17. Gerstenfeld EP, Sauer W, Callans DJ, et al. Predictors of success after selective pulmonary vein isolation of arrhythmogenic pulmonary veins for treatment of atrial fibrillation. *Heart Rhythm*. 2006;3:165–170.

18. Mainigi SK, Sauer WH, Cooper JM, et al. Incidence and predictors of very late recurrence of atrial fibrillation after ablation. *J Cardiovasc Electrophysiol*. 2007;18:69–74.

19. O'Neill MD, Wright M, Knecht S, et al. Long-term follow-up of persistent atrial fibrillation ablation using termination as a procedural endpoint. *Eur Heart J*. 2009;30:1105–1112.

20. Della Bella P, Fassini G, Cireddu M, et al. Image integration-guided catheter ablation of atrial fibrillation: a prospective randomized study. *J Cardiovasc Electrophysiol*. 2009;20:258–265.

21. Estner HL, Hessling G, Ndrepepa G, et al. Electrogram-guided substrate ablation with or without pulmonary vein isolation in patients with persistent atrial fibrillation. *Europace*. 2008;10:1281–1287.

22. Chen J, Off MK, Solheim E, et al. Treatment of atrial fibrillation by silencing electrical activity in the posterior inter-pulmonary-vein atrium. *Europace*. 2008;10:265–272.

23. Fiala M, Chovancik J, Wojnarova D, et al. Results of complex left atrial ablation of long-lasting persistent atrial fibrillation. *J Interv Card Electrophysiol*. 2008;23:189–198.

24. Verma A, Patel D, Famy T, et al. Efficacy of adjuvant anterior left atrial ablation during intracardiac echocardiography-guided pulmonary vein antrum isolation for atrial fibrillation. *J Cardiovasc Electrophysiol*. 2007;18:151–156.

25. Seow SC, Lim TW, Koay CH, et al. Efficacy and late recurrences with wide electrical pulmonary vein isolation for persistent and permanent atrial fibrillation. *Europace*. 2007;9:1129–1133.

26. Sanders P, Hocini M, Jais P, et al. Complete isolation of the pulmonary veins and posterior left atrium in chronic atrial fibrillation. Long-term clinical outcome. *Eur Heart J*. 2007;28:1862–1871.

27. Calo L, Lamberti F, Loricchio ML, et al. Left atrial ablation versus biatrial ablation for persistent and permanent atrial fibrillation: a prospective and randomized study. *J Am Coll Cardiol*. 2006;47:2504–2512.

28. Willems S, Klemm H, Rostock T, et al. Substrate modification combined with pulmonary vein isolation improves outcome of catheter ablation in patients with persistent atrial fibrillation: a prospective randomized comparison. *Eur Heart J*. 2006;27:2871–2878.

29. Fassini G, Riva S, Chiodelli R, et al. Left mitral isthmus ablation associated with PV isolation: long-term results of a prospective randomized study. *J Cardiovasc Electrophysiol*. 2005;16:1150–1156.

30. Haïssaguerre M, Sanders P, Hocini M, et al. Catheter ablation of long-lasting persistent atrial fibrillation: critical structures for termination. *J Cardiovasc Electrophysiol*. 2005;16:1125–1137.

31. Haïssaguerre M, Hocini M, Sanders P, et al. Catheter ablation of long-lasting persistent atrial fibrillation: clinical outcome and mechanisms of subsequent arrhythmias. *J Cardiovasc Electrophysiol*. 2005;16:1138–1147.

32. Oral H, Chugh A, Good E, et al. Randomized comparison of encircling and nonencircling left atrial ablation for chronic atrial fibrillation. *Heart Rhythm*. 2005;2:1165–1172.

33. Roy D, Talajic M, Nattel S, et al. Rhythm control versus rate control for atrial fibrillation and heart failure. *N Engl J Med*. 2008;358:2667–2677.

34. Calkins H, Brugada J, Packer DL, et al. HRS/EHRA/ECAS expert Consensus Statement on catheter and surgical ablation of atrial fibrillation: recommendations for personnel, policy, procedures and follow-up. A report of the Heart Rhythm Society (HRS) Task Force on catheter and surgical ablation of atrial fibrillation. *Heart Rhythm*. 2007;4:816–861.

35. Cox JL, Boineau JP, Schuessler RB, et al. Five-year experience with the maze procedure for atrial fibrillation. *Ann Thorac Surg*. 1993;56:814–823.

36. Haïssaguerre M, Jais P, Shah DC, et al. Right and left atrial radiofrequency catheter therapy of paroxysmal atrial fibrillation. *J Cardiovasc Electrophysiol*. 1996;7:1132–1144.

37. Moe GK, Abildskov JA. Atrial fibrillation as a self-sustaining arrhythmia independent of focal discharge. *Am Heart J*. 1959;58:59–70.

38. Allessie MA, Lammers W.J.E.P., Bonke FIM, et al. Experimental evaluation of Moe's multiple wavelet hypothesis of atrial fibrillation. In: Zipes DP, Jalife J, eds. *Cardiac Electrophysiology and Arrhythmias*. New York: Grune & Stratton; 1985:265–275.

39. Schwartz JF, Pellersels G, Silvers J. A catheter-based curative approach to atrial fibrillation in humans. *Circulation*. 1993;90:I–335.

40. Jais P, Shah DC, Takahashi A, et al. Long-term follow-up after right atrial radiofrequency catheter treatment of paroxysmal atrial fibrillation. *Pacing Clin Electrophysiol*. 1998;21:2533–2538.

41. Haïssaguerre M, Jais P, Shah DC, et al. Spontaneous initiation of atrial fibrillation by ectopic beats originating in the pulmonary veins. *N Engl J Med*. 1998;339:659–666.

42. Haïssaguerre M, Jais P, Shah DC, et al. Catheter ablation of chronic atrial fibrillation targeting the reinitiating triggers. *J Cardiovasc Electrophysiol*. 2000;11:2–10.

43. Haïssaguerre M, Jais P, Shah DC, et al. Electrophysiological end point for catheter ablation of atrial fibrillation initiated from multiple pulmonary venous foci. *Circulation*. 2000;101:1409–1417.

44. Hocini M, Ho SY, Kawara T, et al. Electrical conduction in canine pulmonary veins: electrophysiological and anatomic correlation. *Circulation*. 2002;105:2442–2448.

45. Jais P, Hocini M, Macle L, et al. Distinctive electrophysiological properties of pulmonary veins in patients with atrial fibrillation. *Circulation*. 2002;106:2479–2485.

46. Haïssaguerre M, Sanders P, Hocini M, et al. Pulmonary veins in the substrate for atrial fibrillation: the "venous wave" hypothesis. *J Am Coll Cardiol*. 2004;43:2290–2292.

47. Rostock T, Rotter M, Sanders P, et al. Fibrillating areas isolated within the left atrium after radiofrequency linear catheter ablation. *J Cardiovasc Electrophysiol*. 2006;17:807–812.

48. Haïssaguerre M, Hocini M, Sanders P, et al. Localized sources maintaining atrial fibrillation organized by prior ablation. *Circulation*. 2006;113:616–625.

49. Knecht S, O'Neill MD, Matsuo S, et al. Focal arrhythmia confined within the coronary sinus and maintaining atrial fibrillation. *J Cardiovasc Electrophysiol*. 2007;18:1140–1146.

50. Yoshida K, Ulfarsson M, Tada H, et al. Complex electrograms within the coronary sinus: time- and frequency-domain characteristics, effects of antral pulmonary vein isolation, and relationship to clinical outcome in patients with paroxysmal and persistent atrial fibrillation. *J Cardiovasc Electrophysiol*. 2008;19:1017–1023.

51. Neumann T, Vogt J, Schumacher B, et al. Circumferential pulmonary vein isolation with the cryoballoon technique results from a prospective 3-center study. *J Am Coll Cardiol*. 2008;52:273–278.

52. Elayi CS, Verma A, Di Biase L, et al. Ablation for longstanding permanent atrial fibrillation: results from a randomized study comparing three different strategies. *Heart Rhythm*. 2008;5:1658–1664.

53. Nademanee K, Schwab M, Kosar EM, et al. Clinical outcomes of catheter substrate ablation for high-risk patients with atrial fibrillation. *J Am Coll Cardiol*. 2008;51:843–849.

54. Oral H, Chugh A, Good E, et al. Radiofrequency catheter ablation of chronic atrial fibrillation guided by complex electrograms. *Circulation*. 2007;115:2606–2612.

55. Arentz T, Weber R, Burkle G, et al. Small or large isolation areas around the pulmonary veins for the treatment of atrial fibrillation? Results from a prospective randomized study. *Circulation*. 2007;115:3057–3063.

56. Lim TW, Jassal IS, Ross DL, et al. Medium-term efficacy of segmental ostial pulmonary vein isolation for the treatment of permanent and persistent atrial fibrillation. *Pacing Clin Electrophysiol*. 2006;29:374–379.

57. Nademanee K, McKenzie J, Kosar E, et al. A new approach for catheter ablation of atrial fibrillation: mapping of the electrophysiologic substrate. *J Am Coll Cardiol*. 2004;43:2044–2053.

58. Arentz T, von Rosenthal J, Blum T, et al. Feasibility and safety of pulmonary vein isolation using a new mapping and navigation system in patients with refractory atrial fibrillation. *Circulation*. 2003;108:2484–2490.

59. Estner HL, Hessling G, Ndrepepa G, et al. Acute effects and long-term outcome of pulmonary vein isolation in combination with electrogram-guided substrate ablation for persistent atrial fibrillation. *Am J Cardiol*. 2008;101:332–337.

60. Ouyang F, Ernst S, Chun J, et al. Electrophysiological findings during ablation of persistent atrial fibrillation with electroanatomic mapping and double Lasso catheter technique. *Circulation*. 2005;112:3038–3048.

61. Chen MS, Marrouche NF, Khaykin Y, et al. Pulmonary vein isolation for the treatment of atrial fibrillation in patients with impaired systolic function. *J Am Coll Cardiol*. 2004;43:1004–1009.

62. Oral H, Knight BP, Tada H, et al. Pulmonary vein isolation for paroxysmal and persistent atrial fibrillation. *Circulation*. 2002;105:1077–1081.

63. Takahashi Y, O'Neill MD, Hocini M, et al. Effects of stepwise ablation of chronic atrial fibrillation on atrial electrical and mechanical properties. *J Am Coll Cardiol*. 2007;49:1306–1314.

64. Knecht S, Hocini M, Wright M, et al. Left atrial linear lesions are required for successful treatment of persistent atrial fibrillation. *Eur Heart J*. 2008;29:2359–2366.

65. Haïssaguerre M, Lim KT, Jacquemet V, et al. Atrial fibrillatory cycle length: computer simulation and potential clinical importance. *Europace*. 2007;9(suppl 6):vi64–vi70.

66. Kim KB, Rodefeld MD, Schuessler RB, et al. Relationship between local atrial fibrillation interval and refractory period in the isolated canine atrium. *Circulation*. 1996;94:2961–2967.

67. Haïssaguerre M, Sanders P, Hocini M, et al. Changes in atrial fibrillation cycle length and inducibility during catheter ablation and their relation to outcome. *Circulation.* 2004;109:3007–3013.

68. Biffi M, Boriani G, Bartolotti M, et al. Atrial fibrillation recurrence after internal cardioversion: prognostic importance of electrophysiological parameters. *Heart.* 2002;87:443–448.

69. Fujiki A, Tsuneda T, Sakabe M, et al. Maintenance of sinus rhythm and recovery of atrial mechanical function after cardioversion with bepridil or in combination with aprindine in long-lasting persistent atrial fibrillation. *Circ J.* 2004;68:834–839.

70. Matsuo S, Lellouche N, Wright M, et al. Clinical predictors of termination and clinical outcome of catheter ablation for persistent atrial fibrillation. *J Am Coll Cardiol.* 2009;54:788–795.

71. Pappone C, Radinovic A, Manguso F, et al. Atrial fibrillation progression and management: a 5-year prospective follow-up study. *Heart Rhythm.* 2008;5:1501–1507.

72. Ouyang F, Bansch D, Ernst S, et al. Complete isolation of left atrium surrounding the pulmonary veins: new insights from the double-Lasso technique in paroxysmal atrial fibrillation. *Circulation.* 2004;110:2090–2096.

73. Marrouche NF, Martin DO, Wazni O, et al. Phased-array intracardiac echocardiography monitoring during pulmonary vein isolation in patients with atrial fibrillation: impact on outcome and complications. *Circulation.* 2003;107:2710–2716.

74. Kanagaratnam L, Tomassoni G, Schweikert R, et al. Empirical pulmonary vein isolation in patients with chronic atrial fibrillation using a three-dimensional nonfluoroscopic mapping system: long-term follow-up. *Pacing Clin Electrophysiol.* 2001;24:1774–1779.

75. Gerstenfeld EP, Callans DJ, Dixit S, et al. Mechanisms of organized left atrial tachycardias occurring after pulmonary vein isolation. *Circulation.* 2004;110:1351–1357.

76. Haïssaguerre M, Shah DC, Jais P, et al. Electrophysiological breakthroughs from the left atrium to the pulmonary veins. *Circulation.* 2000;102:2463–2465.

77. Cosio FG, Palacios J, Vidal JM, et al. Electrophysiologic studies in atrial fibrillation. Slow conduction of premature impulses: a possible manifestation of the background for reentry. *Am J Cardiol.* 1983;51:122–130.

78. Jais P, Haïssaguerre M, Shah DC, et al. Regional disparities of endocardial atrial activation in paroxysmal atrial fibrillation. *Pacing Clin Electrophysiol.* 1996;19:1998–2003.

79. Spach MS, Miller WT, Dolber PC, et al. The functional role of structural complexities in the propagation of depolarization in the atrium of the dog: cardiac conduction disturbances due to discontinuities of effective axial resistivity. *Circ Res.* 1982;50:175–191.

80. Konings KT, Smeets JL, Penn OC, et al. Configuration of unipolar atrial electrograms during electrically induced atrial fibrillation in humans. *Circulation.* 1997;95:1231–1241.

81. Rostock T, Rotter M, Sanders P, et al. High-density activation mapping of fractionated electrograms in the atria of patients with paroxysmal atrial fibrillation. *Heart Rhythm.* 2006;3:27–34.

82. Kalifa J, Tanaka K, Zaitsev AV, et al. Mechanisms of wave fractionation at boundaries of high-frequency excitation in the posterior left atrium of the isolated sheep heart during atrial fibrillation. *Circulation.* 2006;113:626–633.

83. Scherlag BJ, Yamanashi W, Patel U, et al. Autonomically induced conversion of pulmonary vein focal firing into atrial fibrillation. *J Am Coll Cardiol.* 2005;45:1878–1886.

84. Sharifov OF, Zaitsev AV, Rosenshtraukh LV, et al. Spatial distribution and frequency dependence of arrhythmogenic vagal effects in canine atria. *J Cardiovasc Electrophysiol.* 2000;11:1029–1042.

85. Lemery R, Birnie D, Tang AS, et al. Feasibility study of endocardial mapping of ganglionated plexuses during catheter ablation of atrial fibrillation. *Heart Rhythm.* 2006;3:387–396.

86. Schauerte P, Scherlag BJ, Pitha J, et al. Catheter ablation of cardiac autonomic nerves for prevention of vagal atrial fibrillation. *Circulation.* 2000;102:2774–2780.

87. Knecht S, Wright M, Matsuo S, et al. Impact of pharmacological autonomic blockade on complex fractionated atrial electrograms. *J Cardiovasc Electrophysiol.* 2010; 21:766–772.

88. Verma A, Novak P, Macle L, et al. A prospective, multicenter evaluation of ablating complex fractionated electrograms (CFEs) during atrial fibrillation (AF) identified by an automated mapping algorithm: acute effects on AF and efficacy as an adjuvant strategy. *Heart Rhythm.* 2008;5:198–205.

89. Sanders P, Jais P, Hocini M, et al. Electrophysiologic and clinical consequences of linear catheter ablation to transect the anterior left atrium in patients with atrial fibrillation. *Heart Rhythm.* 2004;1:176–184.

90. Wright M, Haïssaguerre M, Knecht S, et al. State of the art: catheter ablation of atrial fibrillation. *J Cardiovasc Electrophysiol.* 2008;19:583–592.

91. Ouyang F, Antz M, Ernst S, et al. Recovered pulmonary vein conduction as a dominant factor for recurrent atrial tachyarrhythmias after complete circular isolation of the pulmonary veins: lessons from double Lasso technique. *Circulation.* 2005;111:127–135.

92. Mesas CE, Pappone C, Lang CC, et al. Left atrial tachycardia after circumferential pulmonary vein ablation for atrial fibrillation: electroanatomic characterization and treatment. *J Am Coll Cardiol.* 2004;44:1071–1079.

93. Pappone C, Manguso F, Vicedomini G, et al. Prevention of iatrogenic atrial tachycardia after ablation of atrial fibrillation: a prospective randomized study comparing circumferential pulmonary vein ablation with a modified approach. *Circulation.* 2004;110:3036–3042.

94. Deisenhofer I, Estner H, Zrenner B, et al. Left atrial tachycardia after circumferential pulmonary vein ablation for atrial fibrillation: incidence, electrophysiological characteristics, and results of radiofrequency ablation. *Europace.* 2006;8:573–582.

95. Jais P, Matsuo S, Knecht S, et al. A deductive mapping strategy for atrial tachycardia following atrial fibrillation ablation: importance of localized reentry. *J Cardiovasc Electrophysiol.* 2009;20:480–491.

96. Rostock T, Steven D, Hoffmann B, et al. Chronic atrial fibrillation is a biatrial arrhythmia: data from catheter ablation of chronic atrial fibrillation aiming arrhythmia termination using a sequential ablation approach. *Circ Arrhythmia Electrophysiol.* 2008;1:344–353.

97. Verma A, Wazni OM, Marrouche NF, et al. Pre-existent left atrial scarring in patients undergoing pulmonary vein antrum isolation: an independent predictor of procedural failure. *J Am Coll Cardiol.* 2005;45:285–292.

98. Pappone C, Oreto G, Rosanio S, et al. Atrial electroanatomic remodeling after circumferential radiofrequency pulmonary vein ablation: efficacy of an anatomic approach in a large cohort of patients with atrial fibrillation. *Circulation.* 2001;104:2539–2544.

99. Pappone C, Santinelli V, Manguso F, et al. Pulmonary vein denervation enhances long-term benefit after circumferential ablation for paroxysmal atrial fibrillation. *Circulation.* 2004;109:327–334.

100. Matsuo S, Lim KT, Haïssaguerre M. Ablation of chronic atrial fibrillation. *Heart Rhythm.* 2007;4:1461–1463.

101. Berruezo A, Tamborero D, Mont L, et al. Pre-procedural predictors of atrial fibrillation recurrence after circumferential pulmonary vein ablation. *Eur Heart J.* 2007;28:836–841.

102. Cappato R, Calkins H, Chen SA, et al. Worldwide survey on the methods, efficacy, and safety of catheter ablation for human atrial fibrillation. *Circulation.* 2005;111:1100–1105.

103. Packer DL, Keelan P, Munger TM, et al. Clinical presentation, investigation, and management of pulmonary vein stenosis complicating ablation for atrial fibrillation. *Circulation.* 2005;111:546–554.

104. Pappone C, Oral H, Santinelli V, et al. Atrio-esophageal fistula as a complication of percutaneous transcatheter ablation of atrial fibrillation. *Circulation.* 2004;109:2724–2726.

105. Sacher F, Monahan KH, Thomas SP, et al. Phrenic nerve injury after atrial fibrillation catheter ablation: characterization and outcome in a multicenter study. *J Am Coll Cardiol.* 2006;47:2498–2503.

106. Pappone C, Rosanio S, Augello G, et al. Mortality, morbidity, and quality of life after circumferential pulmonary vein ablation for atrial fibrillation: outcomes from a controlled nonrandomized long-term study. *J Am Coll Cardiol.* 2003;42:185–197.

107. Hsu LF, Jais P, Sanders P, et al. Catheter ablation for atrial fibrillation in congestive heart failure. *N Engl J Med.* 2004;351:2373–2383.

108. Purerfellner H, Martinek M, Aichinger J, et al. Quality of life restored to normal in patients with atrial fibrillation after pulmonary vein ostial isolation. *Am Heart J.* 2004;148:318–325.

109. Weerasooriya R, Jais P, Hocini M, et al. Effect of catheter ablation on quality of life of patients with paroxysmal atrial fibrillation. *Heart Rhythm.* 2005;2:619–623.

110. Khan MN, Jais P, Cummings J, et al. Pulmonary-vein isolation for atrial fibrillation in patients with heart failure. *N Engl J Med.* 2008;359:1778–1785.

111. Oral H, Chugh A, Ozaydin M, et al. Risk of thromboembolic events after percutaneous left atrial radiofrequency ablation of atrial fibrillation. *Circulation.* 2006;114:759–765.

112. Pappone C, Rosanio S, Oreto G, et al. Circumferential radiofrequency ablation of pulmonary vein ostia: A new anatomic approach for curing atrial fibrillation. *Circulation.* 2000;21;102:2619–2628.

113. Beukema WP, Elvan A, Sie HT, et al. Successful radiofrequency ablation in patients with previous atrial fibrillation results in a significant decrease in left atrial size. *Circulation.* 2005;112:2089–2095.

114. Bertaglia E, Stabile G, Senatore G, et al. Long-term outcome of right and left atrial radiofrequency ablation in patients with persistent atrial fibrillation. *Pacing Clin Electrophysiol.* 2006;29:153–158.

115. Estner HL, Hessling G, Ndrepepa G, et al. Electrogram-guided substrate ablation with or without pulmonary vein isolation in patients with persistent atrial fibrillation. *Europace.* 2008;10:1281–1287.

116. Haïssaguerre M, Sanders P, Hocini M, et al. Catheter ablation of long-lasting persistent atrial fibrillation: critical structures for termination. *J Cardiovasc Electrophysiol.* 2005;16:1125–1137

117. Estner HL, Hessling G, Ndrepepa G, et al. Acute effects and long-term outcome of pulmonary vein isolation in combination with electrogram-guided substrate ablation for persistent atrial fibrillation. *Am J Cardiol.* 2008;101:332–337.

Catheter Ablation of Atrioventricular Nodal Reentrant Tachycardia and the Atrioventricular Junction

19

Ablation of Atrioventricular Nodal Reentrant Tachycardia and Variants

Mario D. Gonzalez, Javier E. Banchs, and Jaime Rivera

Key Points

Mechanism of atrioventricular nodal reentrant tachycardia (AVNRT) is reentry involving fast and slow atrioventricular (AV) nodal pathways.

The typical slow-fast form of AVNRT is diagnosed by the presence of a long atrium–His bundle (AH) interval (>180 milliseconds) during tachycardia, with the earliest retrograde atrial activation localized at the level of the superior part of the triangle of Koch, just behind the tendon of Todaro (fast pathway or anterior approach to the AV node).

The fast-slow variant has a short AH interval during tachycardia (<180 milliseconds), and early retrograde atrial activation is localized near the coronary sinus (CS) ostium or in the proximal portion of the CS.

The slow-slow variant has a long AH interval (>180 milliseconds), with early retrograde atrial activation near the coronary sinus (CS) ostium or in the proximal portion of the CS similar to the fast-slow form of AVNRT.

The left-sided variant is similar to the slow-fast type, but slow pathway conduction cannot be eliminated from the right atrium or proximal CS.

The ablation target for all variants is the antegrade or retrograde slow pathway.

Catheter navigation systems are useful to label sites of interest. Electroanatomic mapping systems are optional, and cryoablation may be used for selected cases.

The acute success rate is almost 100%, with a 1% to 2% rate of recurrence. The rate of complications (AV block) is 0.5% or less.

Atrioventricular nodal reentrant tachycardia (AVRNT) is the most common form of regular supraventricular tachycardia.[1] It occurs more frequently in women than in men, and the initial episode of tachycardia tends to occur at an older age than in patients with atrioventricular reentrant tachycardia.[2] Although AVNRT can have a benign course, it can also result in disabling symptoms, especially in elderly patients. Patients frequently complain of regular rapid pounding in the neck due to almost simultaneous atrial and ventricular contractions.[3] A review of 500 consecutive patients studied in our laboratory revealed a mean age of 47 ± 15 years (range, 16 to 87 years); 367 (73%) of these patients were females. Twenty-two patients (4.4%) presented with syncope. In 11 (2.2%), sustained AVNRT was induced during an electrophysiology study performed to investigate the cause of syncope. Syncope did not recur after elimination of the arrhythmia.

Catheter ablation eliminates AVNRT in most patients with a low risk for complications.[4] Therefore, it can be offered as a first-line therapy to symptomatic patients and to those who cannot tolerate or do not wish to take antiarrhythmic agents.[5] In addition, patients with high-risk occupations may undergo catheter ablation as first-line therapy. This chapter focuses on the electrophysiology diagnosis and ablation of AVNRT and its variants. All forms of atrioventricular (AV) nodal reentry can be treated by a combined anatomic and electrogram-guided approach, to guide a safe and successful ablation.

Anatomy of the Atrioventricular Node and Its Inputs

The anatomy of the AV node and its relationship with nearby atrial structures and with the His bundle were described in great detail by Tawara.[6] The AV node is located in the AV septum. It is in contact with both the right and the left atria. The AV node is not insulated from the surrounding myocardium as it occurs with the His bundle or the right bundle branch.[7,8] Right-sided and left-sided inputs[9] provide activation to the AV node proceeding from both atria. Histologically, the AV node is a discrete structure that can be traced in consecutive sections. It is constituted by specialized myocardium with characteristic immunohistochemistry expressing HCN_4, which is the major isoform of the funny channel.[10] The compact AV node is located at the apex of the triangle of Koch. This triangle is bounded by the tendon of Todaro posteriorly, the ostium of the coronary sinus (CS) inferiorly, and the septal leaflet of the tricuspid valve anteriorly.[11] However, AV nodal tissue extends well beyond the compact AV node. AV nodal conduction is modulated by autonomic regulation. The right coronary artery provides the AV nodal artery in 90% of patients and may run in the subendocardium close to the CS ostium, which may explain the rare instances of AV nodal block during radiofrequency (RF) ablation in the area of the slow pathway, despite considerable distance from the compact AV node.[12]

Pathophysiology

The fundamental studies of a century ago by Gaskell,[13] His,[14] and Tawara[15] form the basis for the present understanding of the anatomy and physiology of the AV node. Mines, in 1913,[16] was the first to describe the existence of two regions in the specialized conduction system with different conduction and recovery properties. Moe and associates[17] later demonstrated the existence of two AV nodal pathways underlying AVNRT. The fast AV nodal pathway (β pathway) was found to have a longer refractory period than the slow AV nodal pathway (α pathway). These different electrophysiologic properties facilitate the onset and maintenance of AVNRT. Mendez and colleagues[18] found that the two AV nodal pathways located in the upper portion of the AV node in the rabbit communicated with a final "lower common pathway." Denes and associates[19] were the first to document the presence of dual AV nodal pathways in patients with and without AVNRT. The initial reported prevalence (10%) of dual AV nodal pathways[20] is low compared with present-day findings, probably because electrophysiology studies were initially performed without

sedation and therefore under a predominant adrenergic tone. Now under sedation, dual AV nodal pathways are found in most patients, even in those without AVNRT.[21,22] Dual AV nodal pathways can be uncovered using single atrial extrastimuli of increasing prematurity (Fig. 19-1) or during decremental atrial stimulation A 50-millisecond "jump" in the atrium–His bundle (AH) interval following a premature atrial extrastimulus is considered the hallmark of dual AV nodal physiology. Nevertheless, the lack of a jump does not rule out the existence of two distinct AV nodal pathways. In this regard, a "continuous" AV nodal conduction curve is observed in a subgroup of individuals with inducible AVNRT.[23]

Dual AV nodal physiology is a normal behavior of the human AV node. The response of the AV node to premature stimulation and to different cycle lengths indicates the presence of two or more populations of AV nodal or perinodal cells with different refractoriness and conduction times. As mentioned previously, the presence of dual AV nodal physiology in itself does not imply the presence of AVNRT. A common misconception is to look for dual AV nodal physiology when AVNRT is suspected and to search for another arrhythmia when a jump is not observed. This simplistic approach can prevent identification of the correct mechanism of the arrhythmia. Consistent with these observations, we have found similar incidences of dual AV nodal physiology in patients with and without AVNRT. A jump of 50 milliseconds or longer was present in 83% (417 of 500) of patients with AVNRT and in 77% (385 of 500) of patients without AVNRT (studied for other reasons); this difference was not statistically significant. The magnitude of the jump, however, was greater in patients with AVNRT (93 ± 7 versus 61 ± 7 milliseconds, $P < .05$). If dual AV nodal pathways are present in most individuals with or without AVNRT, what is required to induce AVNRT? One explanation may be the fact the slow AV nodal pathways is "slower" in patients with AVNRT, as

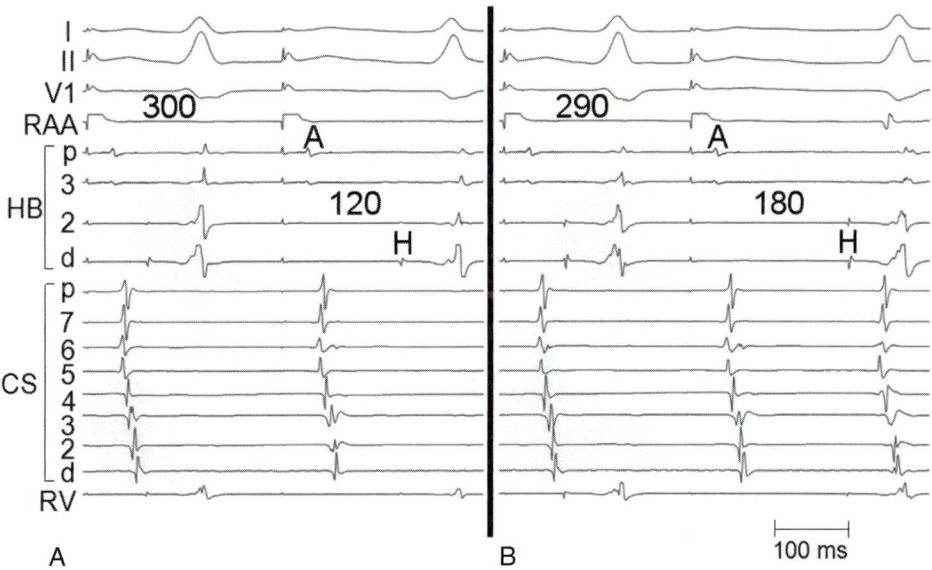

FIGURE 19-1. Demonstration of dual atrioventricular (AV) nodal pathways. Single extrastimuli of progressively shorter coupling intervals were delivered from the right atrial appendage (RAA) at a basic drive of 600 msec. A "jump" or sudden increase of the atrium–His bundle interval from 120 msec (**A**) to 180 msec (**B**) occurs after shortening of the atrial extrastimulus from 300 to 290 msec. The atrial extrastimulus in **B** conducts through the slow AV nodal pathway, followed by retrograde conduction through the fast AV nodal pathway to activate the atrium (echo beat). A, atrial electrogram; CS, coronary sinus; d, distal; H, His recording; HB, His bundle; p, proximal; RAA, right atrial appendage; RV, right ventricle.

reflected by a greater jump in those with clinical arrhythmia. This may represent an increase of collagen with age, which is supported by experimental studies that facilitate the induction of AVNRT by creating lesions that prevent antegrade activation by the superior approach to the AV node in dogs.[24] A longer conduction time over the antegrade slow pathway allows recovery of excitability of the retrograde limb (fast or slow AV nodal pathway). Anatomic differences may be important because a larger CS ostium is observed in most patients with AVNRT (Fig. 19-2) and may allow for greater conduction time over the slow pathway.[25,26] The frequency of premature atrial or ventricular beats and the length of the excitable gap also modulate the frequency and duration of AVNRT. Finally, the coexistence of AVNRT with other arrhythmias, as well as occurrence of familial forms of AVNRT, suggests the possibility of an underlying abnormality.[27–29]

Disagreement still exists regarding the nature and location of the slow and fast AV nodal pathways. One possibility is that these pathways represent longitudinal dissociation of conduction within the AV node itself. The other option is that they represent different inputs to the AV node. Before the advent of surgical and catheter ablation, the slow and fast AV nodal pathways were believed to be part of the AV node, representing regions with different electrophysiologic properties (i.e., longitudinal dissociation). In fact, several experimental and clinical observations supported an intranodal location of these AV nodal pathways and the reentrant circuit supporting AVNRT.[30–33] In some patients with AVNRT, atrial activation close to the AV node can be dissociated from the reentrant circuit without interruption of the tachycardia (Fig. 19-3).[33,34] This observation suggests that reentry confined to the AV node can sustain AVNRT without atrial involvement. Different degrees of ventriculoatrial (VA) block during AVNRT occur in the upper common pathway, allowing continuation of the tachycardia without retrograde atrial activation. In a similar fashion, the His-Purkinje system and the ventricles are not part of the reentrant circuit. This is demonstrated by episodes of 2:1 AV block with persistence of AVNRT (Fig. 19-4). Block can occur either proximal or distal to His bundle activation. This block is functional and occurs in tachycardias with short cycle lengths, which find the His-Purkinje system refractory.

Earliest atrial activation during retrograde AV nodal conduction can occur in the upper or lower portion of the triangle of Koch, depending on whether the fast or the slow AV nodal pathway is activated.[35] These observations and the results of surgical and catheter ablation of the anterior (superior) or posterior (inferior) approaches to the AV node[36–41] led to the conclusions that the fast and slow AV nodal pathways have an extranodal component and that the atrium is required to sustain AVNRT. However, the portion of the atrium that is involved in the reentrant circuit remains elusive.

The original description of the AV node, made by Tawara in 1906,[15] included posterior extensions of the AV node reaching both the mitral and tricuspid annuli. These

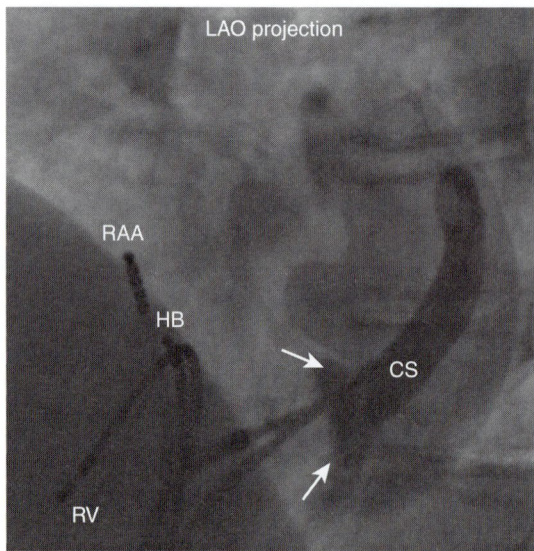

FIGURE 19-2. Coronary sinus angiogram in a patient with slow-fast atrioventricular nodal reentrant tachycardia (AVNRT). Radiograph in the left anterior oblique (LAO) projection of the mapping catheters and angiogram of the coronary sinus performed with a pigtail catheter introduced through a preshaped long sheath. *Arrows* show the borders of the coronary sinus ostium. A larger coronary sinus ostium has been suggested as the anatomic substrate for greater conduction time in the slow pathway of patients with AVNRT. Multipolar catheters are positioned in the coronary sinus (CS), right atrial appendage (RAA), His bundle (HB), and right ventricle (RV).

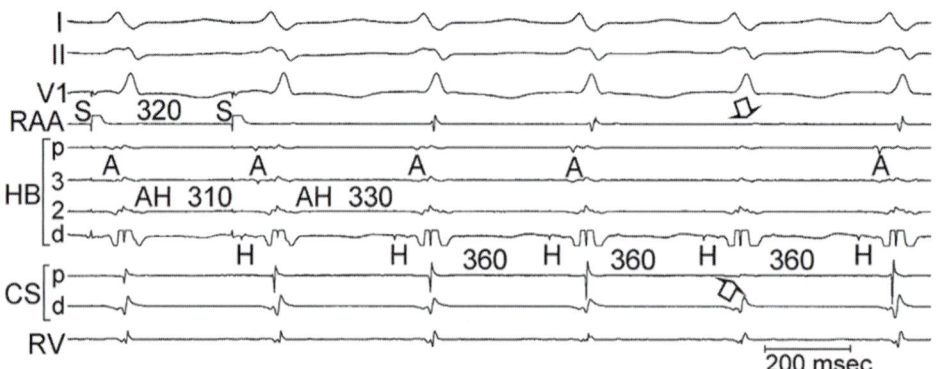

FIGURE 19-3. Induction of sustained slow-fast atrioventricular nodal reentrant tachycardia (AVNRT). Rapid atrial pacing at a cycle length of 320 msec results in sustained AVNRT following a critical prolongation of the AH interval (330 msec). The cycle length of the tachycardia was 360 msec. The third tachycardia complex fails to conduct to the atrium (*arrows*) without perturbation of the tachycardia. A, atrial electrogram; CS, coronary sinus; d, distal; H, His recording; HB, His bundle; p, proximal; RAA, right atrial appendage; RV, right ventricle. (*From Gonzalez MD, Contreras L, Cardona F, et al. V-A block during atrioventricular nodal reentrant tachycardia: reentry confined to the AV node. Pacing Clin Electrophysiol. 26:775-778, 2003. With permission.*)

observations were later confirmed by Becker, Inoue, and Anderson[42,43] (Fig. 19-5). More recently, a left atrial input to the AV node, proceeding from the mitral annulus, was demonstrated in humans.[9] This left atrial input to the AV node represents the electrophysiologic counterpart of the leftward extension of the AV node. Therefore, in addition to the right-sided superior (anterior) and inferior (posterior) inputs to the AV node, the mitral annulus provides an independent input for activation proceeding from the left atrium[9] (Fig. 19-5) These inputs probably participate in the various forms of AVNRT by providing entrance and exit sites in a reentry that involves the atrium,[44] or they may represent exit points from an "intranodal" circuit sustaining AVNRT.[33] Ventriculoatrial conduction over the slow pathway has been shown to result in earliest atrial activation on the left side of the interatrial septum, which is abolished with ablation of the slow pathway in the right atrium.[45] Consistent with the clinical observation of "intranodal" reentry,[33,34,46,47] different forms of AVNRT can be contained within the transitional cells of the posterior AV nodal input in a rabbit heart,[48] owing to functional dissociation of cellular activation.[49] Figure 19-6 depicts possible reentrant circuits that are either contained in the compact AV node or involve the right- and left-sided inputs. As can be observed, there are multiple possible reentrant loops. Identifying the reentrant mechanism in a given patient can be difficult even with entrainment maneuvers.

Diagnosis

Three main forms of AVNRT are observed: slow-fast, slow-slow, and fast-slow AVNRT. In a single patient, one, two, or all three forms may be present at different times during the electrophysiology study. There is no electrophysiologic finding that alone is diagnostic of AVNRT; the diagnosis is made on the weight of typical features and the exclusion of atrial tachycardias, junctional tachycardia, and septal accessory AV pathways using entrainment maneuvers (Table 19-1). Electrophysiologic variables of different forms of AV nodal reentry are given in Table 19-2.

An initial careful baseline electrophysiologic study is required before any ablation procedure. This is especially relevant for AVNRT because other supraventricular or ventricular arrhythmias may mimic this arrhythmia or coexist. The presence of a concealed accessory AV pathway should be ruled out before induction of the tachycardia by performing parahisian and differential ventricular pacing.

The baseline study will demonstrate dual AV nodal physiology in about 85% of patients with AVNRT,[19,20,22,23,35] but dual AV nodal physiology can also be observed in patients without AVNRT. Conversely, the absence of verifiable dual AV nodal physiology does not rule out AVNRT. The diagnostic criteria for dual AV nodal physiology are listed in Table 19-3. Prolongation of the AH interval to more than180 milliseconds during

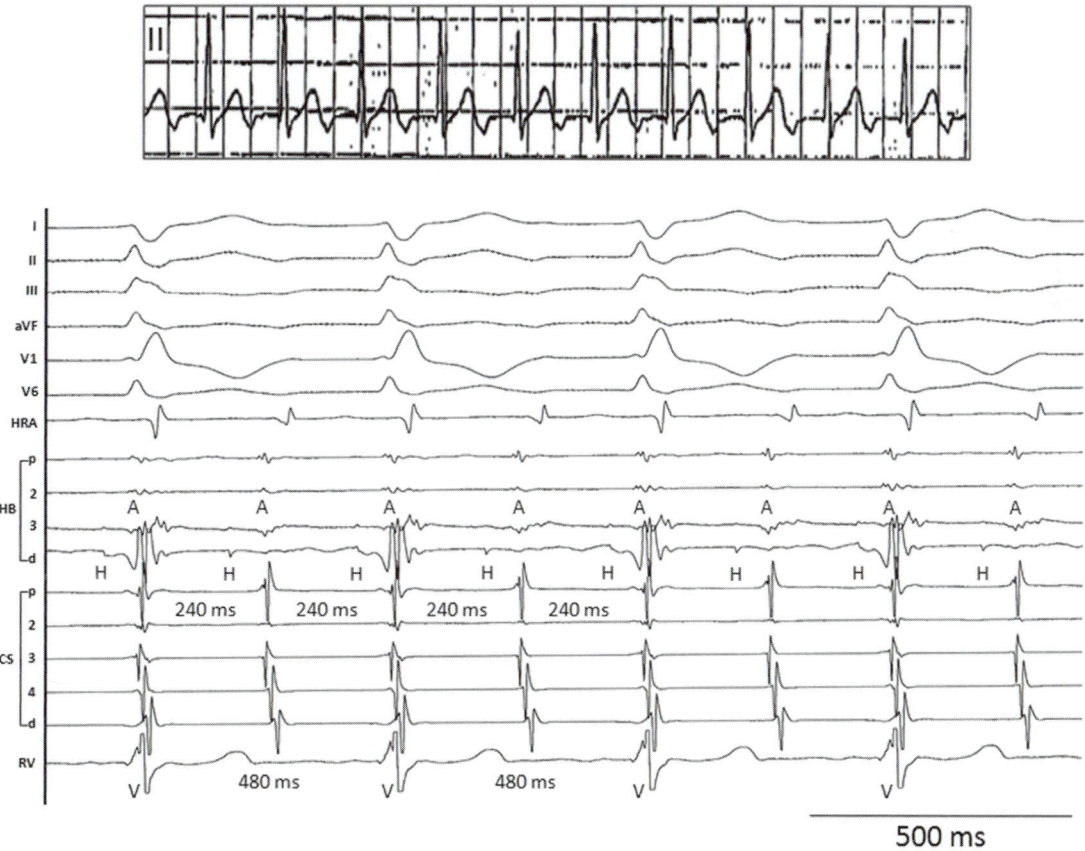

FIGURE 19-4. Slow-fast atrioventricular nodal reentrant tachycardia (AVNRT) with 2:1 conduction to the ventricles. At the *top*, a rhythm strip with the characteristic electrocardiographic manifestation of AVNRT with 2:1 atrial-to-ventricular conduction is shown. Negative P waves in inferior leads during tachycardia are the nonconducted atrial depolarizations. These P waves are located equidistant between QRS complexes. The ventricular cycle length in tachycardia doubles the atrial cycle length. Functional block during AVNRT (cycle length, 240 msec) occurs distal to His bundle activation (H) as shown in the *lower panel*. Because ventricular activation occurs almost simultaneously with retrograde atrial activation, the only visible P waves are the nonconducted ones. A, atrial electrogram; CS, coronary sinus; d, distal; H, His recording; HB, His bundle; HRA, high right atrium; p, proximal; RV, right ventricle.

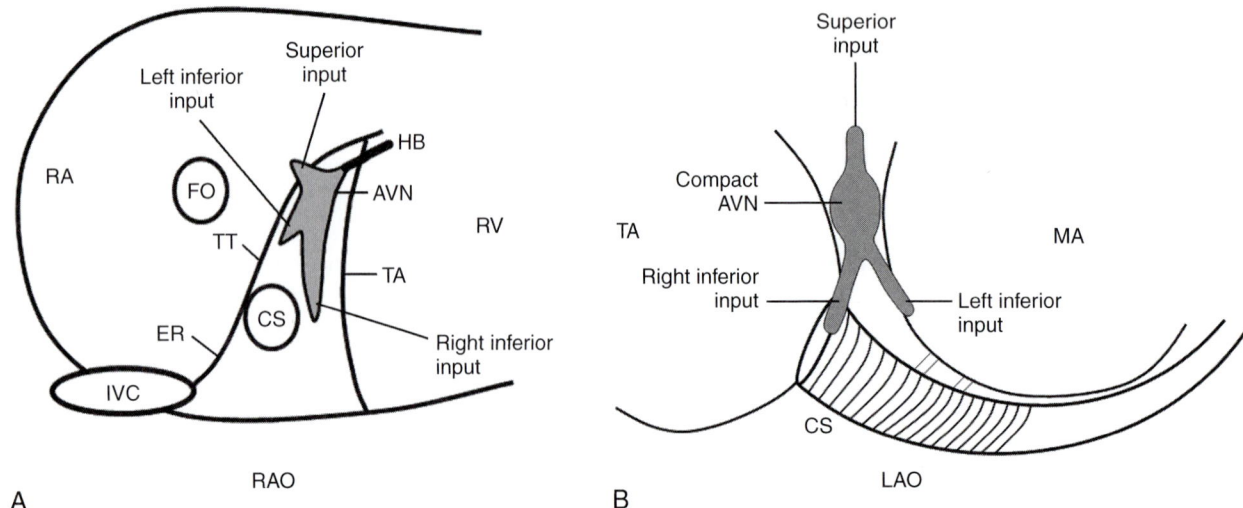

FIGURE 19-5. A, Schematic representation of atrioventricular (AV) node inside the triangle of Koch as viewed from the right anterior oblique projection (RAO). The boundaries of the triangle of Koch are defined by the tendon of Todaro (TT), the tricuspid annulus (TA), and the ostium of the coronary sinus (CS). The superior, left inferior, and right inferior inputs are shown. ER, eustachian ridge; FO, fossa ovalis; IVC, inferior vena cava; RA, right atrium; RV, right ventricle. **B,** Schematic representation of AV node (AVN) as viewed from the left anterior oblique projection (LAO). The AVN is shown above the coronary sinus (CS) along with the mitral annulus (MA) and the tricuspid annulus (TA). The superior extension ("anterior" in the old anatomic nomenclature) is in contact with both atria. The right inferior input is in contact with the coronary sinus. The left inferior input is in contact with the mitral annulus. *(Modified from Gonzalez MD, Contreras LJ, Cardona F, et al. Demonstration of a left atrial input to the atrioventricular node in humans.* Circulation. *2002;106:2930-2934. With permission.)*

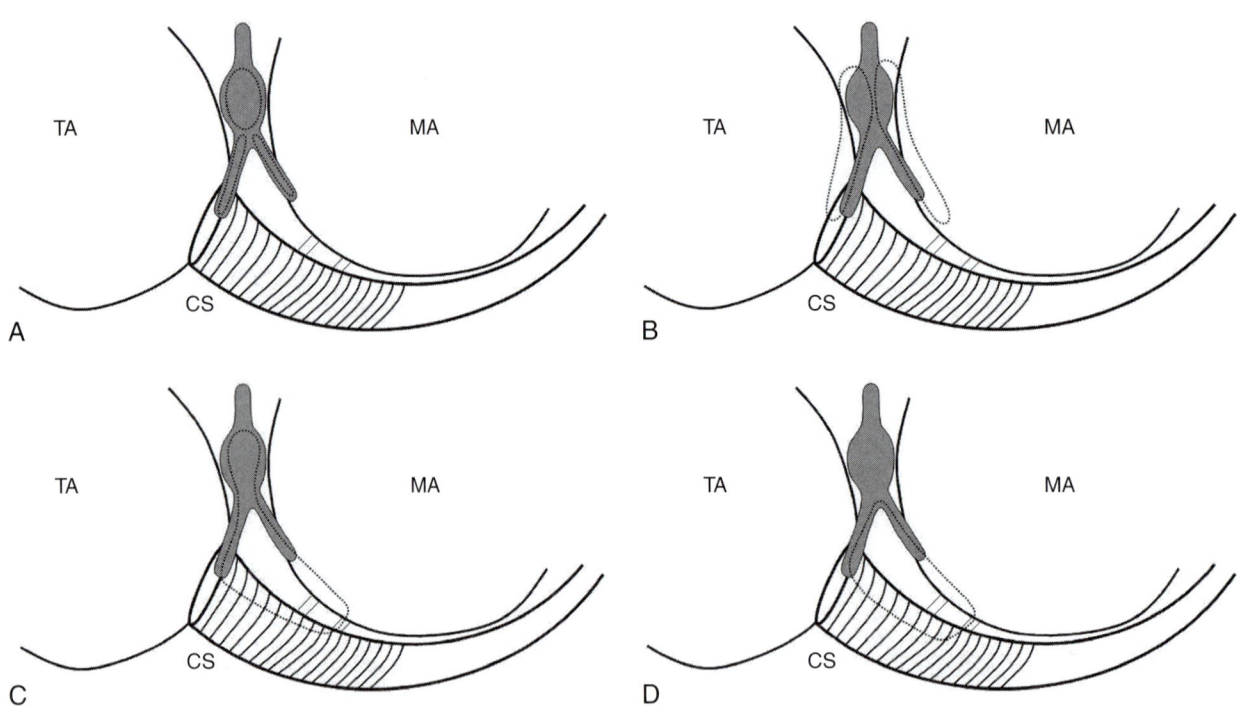

FIGURE 19-6. Hypothetical reentrant circuits underlying different forms of atrioventricular nodal reentrant tachycardia (AVNRT). **A,** Reentry *(broken lines)* confined to different segments of the atrioventricular (AV) node without participation of the atria. **B,** Reentry involving atrial tissue and different segments of the compact AV node and its inputs. **C,** Reentry involving the musculature of the coronary sinus connecting both inferior inputs and the compact AV node. This circuit has been proposed to describe slow-fast AV nodal reentry. **D,** Reentry similar to that in **C** without involvement of the compact AV node. This circuit has been proposed to describe slow-slow and fast-slow AV nodal reentry. Within a given reentrant circuit, opposite wavefronts will give rise to different forms of AVNRT. CS, coronary sinus; MA, mitral annulus; TA, tricuspid annulus.

decremental atrial pacing is usually indicative of conduction over the slow pathway[1,19,50] This frequently manifests as a paced PR interval greater than the PP interval such that the paced atrial depolarization conducts not to the next QRS but to the second QRS following the pacing stimulus (Fig. 19-7). During atrial extrastimulus testing, dual AV nodal physiology is typically manifested by a jump of 50 milliseconds or longer in the A2H2 interval following a shortening in the A1A2 interval by 10 milliseconds (Fig. 19-1). When two atrial extrastimuli are delivered, a jump from fast to slow pathway conduction is defined as an increase in the A3H3 interval

TABLE 19-1

DIAGNOSTIC CRITERIA OF ATRIOVENTRICULAR NODAL REENTRANT TACHYCARDIA AND VARIANTS

Slow-Fast

Dual AV nodal physiology in most (85%) cases

Long AH interval (>180 msec) during tachycardia

Initiation tachycardia dependent on critical AH interval during antegrade slow pathway conduction

Earliest retrograde atrial activation in tachycardia posterior to the tendon of Todaro, posterior and to the left of the His bundle near apex of triangle of Koch

Ventricular postpacing interval > 115 msec longer than TCL

VA interval during ventricular pacing at TCL minus VA interval during tachycardia > 85 msec

Late ventricular extrastimuli that advance His bundle activation also advance retrograde atrial activation and reset the tachycardia

Exclude atrial tachycardia and reciprocating tachycardia by appropriate maneuvers

Slow-Slow

Same as for slow-fast variant except for early retrograde atrial activation near the CS ostium*

Initiation dependent on critical HA interval during retrograde slow pathway conduction

At identical cycle length, the HA interval during ventricular pacing is usually longer than that observed during tachycardia (lower common pathway)

Fast-Slow

Short AH interval during tachycardia (<180 msec)

Inverted P waves in inferior leads during long RP tachycardia

Initiation dependent on critical HA interval during retrograde slow pathway conduction

Early retrograde atrial activation near the CS ostium or in the proximal portion of the CS*

At identical cycle length, the HA interval during ventricular pacing is usually longer than that observed during tachycardia (lower common pathway)

AH interval during atrial pacing at TCL > 40 msec longer than AH interval in tachycardia

Exclude atrial tachycardia and reciprocating tachycardia by appropriate maneuvers

Left-Sided

Same as for slow-fast variant except for the following:

- Inability to eliminate 1:1 slow pathway conduction from right atrium or CS

- Short HA interval (<15 msec) may be present

- Double response to atrial extrastimulus may be present

*The sequence of CS activation may simulate the presence of a posteroseptal or left-sided accessory pathway.
AH, atrium–His bundle; AV, atrioventricular; CS, coronary sinus; HA, His bundle–atrium; TCL, tachycardia cycle length.

TABLE 19-2

ELECTROPHYSIOLOGIC VARIABLES OF DIFFERENT FORMS OF ATRIOVENTRICULAR NODAL REENTRANT TACHYCARDIA

Variable	Slow-Fast (Range)	Slow-Slow (Range)	Fast-Slow (Range)
TCL (msec)	361 ± 59 (235-660)	411 ± 62 (320-565)	342 ± 61 (250-440)
AH (msec)	312 ± 61 (190-545)	282 ± 71 (185-470)	90 ± 39 (35-160)
HA (msec)	45 ± 11 (25-145)	141± 32 (90-210)	245 ± 62 (125-405)
Site of earliest retrograde atrial activation	Posterior and to the left of the catheter recording His bundle activation	At the CS ostium or in the CS up to 1.1 ± 0.5 cm from the ostium	At the CS ostium or in the CS up to 1.5 ± 0.7cm from the ostium

AH, atrium–His interval; CS, coronary sinus; HA, His atrium interval; TCL, tachycardia cycle length.

of 50 milliseconds or more in response to a decrement of 10 milliseconds in the A2A3 interval (A1A2 being constant).[50] The induction of AV nodal echo beats is an indication of longitudinal dissociation of the AV node, that is, dual AV nodal physiology. The diagnosis of retrograde dual AV nodal physiology is made based on jumps but is also dependent on changes of earliest atrial activation site (Table 19-3).[35] Retrograde His bundle–atrial (HA) interval jumps, and retrograde slow, antegrade fast AV nodal echo beats may be seen. In addition,

a change in the site of earliest retrograde atrial activation from near the His bundle area to the proximal CS region indicates a transition from retrograde fast pathway to retrograde slow pathway conduction.

Induction of AVNRT is dependent on achieving a critical AH interval[23] for typical slow-fast AVNRT; this requires exclusive antegrade slow pathway conduction, which can be achieved by atrial extrastimulus testing or atrial burst pacing near the Wenckebach cycle length. If antegrade slow pathway conduction cannot be achieved because short

TABLE 19-3

FEATURES OF DUAL ATRIOVENTRICULAR NODAL PHYSIOLOGY AND SLOW PATHWAY CONDUCTION

Dual AV Nodal Physiology

>50 msec increase in A2H2 interval with ≤10 msec decrease in A1A2 interval

>50 msec increase in AH interval with 10 msec decrease in atrial pacing rate

Abrupt change in slope of AV nodal conduction curve without "jump" (children especially)

Double response (two ventricular responses to a single atrial activation due to simultaneous fast and slow pathway conduction)

Slow Pathway Conduction

AH interval > 180 msec

Stable PR interval > paced PP interval in absence of isoproterenol

Stable VA interval > RR interval with ventricular pacing (retrograde slow pathway)

Earliest retrograde atrial activation near coronary sinus ostium (exclude accessory pathway)

A1A2, coupling interval of a single atrial extrastimulus after a basic atrial pacing drive ; AH, atrium–His bundle interval; A2H2, AH interval following the atrial extrastimulus; AV, atrioventricular; VA, ventricular-atrial interval.

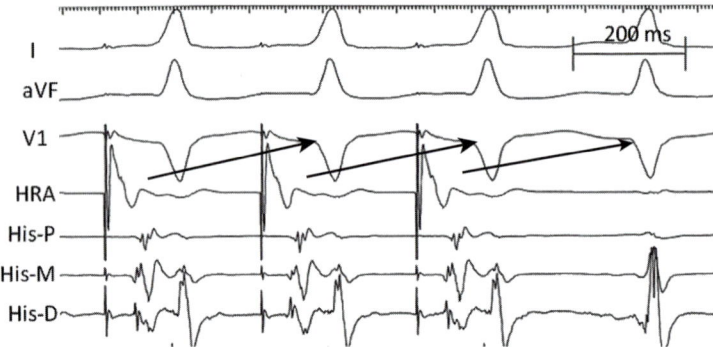

FIGURE 19-7. Antegrade slow pathway conduction during atrial pacing at 280 msec. The PR interval is 340 msec and therefore exceeds the PP interval. The stimulus conducts, not to the following QRS, but to the second QRS as indicated by the *arrows*. D, distal; HRA, high right atrium; M, mid; P, proximal.

antegrade fast pathway refractoriness, S3 stimulation, burst atrial pacing, or ventricular stimulation with or without isoproterenol may be required. If retrograde fast pathway conduction is absent during ventricular pacing (VA block or earliest retrograde atrial activation at proximal CS) or by lack of echoes or AVNRT following antegrade slow pathway conduction, isoproterenol infusion should be given.[51] Retrograde block over the fast AV nodal pathway may be due to mechanical trauma of the fast pathway by the catheter recording His bundle activity, which can be minimized by advancing the catheter to the ventricle.

Slow-Fast Variant

The typical form, or slow-fast variant, occurred in 414 (83%) of 500 patients studied at our institution. Slow-fast AVNRT can be associated with other forms of AVNRT. For example, 3.5% of patients also had slow-slow AVNRT, 2% had fast-slow AVNRT, and in 1%, the three forms coexisted in the same patient.

The electrocardiogram obtained during tachycardia can suggest the diagnosis when the retrograde P wave is superimposed on the terminal portion of the QRS, giving rise to a pseudo right bundle branch block pattern (Fig. 19-8). The tachycardia cycle length (TCL) averages 361 ± 59 milliseconds (range, 235 to 660 milliseconds). The antegrade limb of the tachycardia is the slow AV nodal

pathway, with an AH interval longer than 180 milliseconds (range, 190 to 545 milliseconds; mean, 312 ± 61 milliseconds; Table 19-2). A short VA (measured from the surface QRS to the earliest intracardiac atrial electrogram) time of less than 60 milliseconds excludes reciprocating tachycardias using a concealed accessory pathway.[23] However, atrial tachycardias with 1:1 AV conduction over the slow AV nodal pathway can have a short VA time, simulating AVNRT. The VA relationship during atrial tachycardia may change over time depending on the autonomic tone. Induction of slow-fast AVNRT is usually accomplished by atrial extrastimuli or rapid atrial stimulation. Adrenergic stimulation (isoproterenol, 1 to 4 μg/minute) may be needed. Inducibility of AVNRT sometimes occurs only after the infusion of isoproterenol has been discontinued. Occasionally, atropine, 1 to 2 mg, with or without catecholamine infusion is necessary for AVNRT induction. Regardless of the maneuver used, induction of slow-fast AVNRT from the atrium requires antegrade block over the fast AV nodal pathway, with antegrade conduction over the slow AV nodal pathway allowing retrograde conduction over the fast AV nodal pathway. Less commonly, ventricular stimulation can also induce slow-fast AVNRT. Local atrial activation near the exit site of the fast AV nodal pathway (superior aspect of the triangle of Koch) can be recorded using closely spaced electrodes (Fig. 19-9). The site of earliest retrograde atrial activation is critical to differentiate slow-fast from slow-slow AVNRT because the

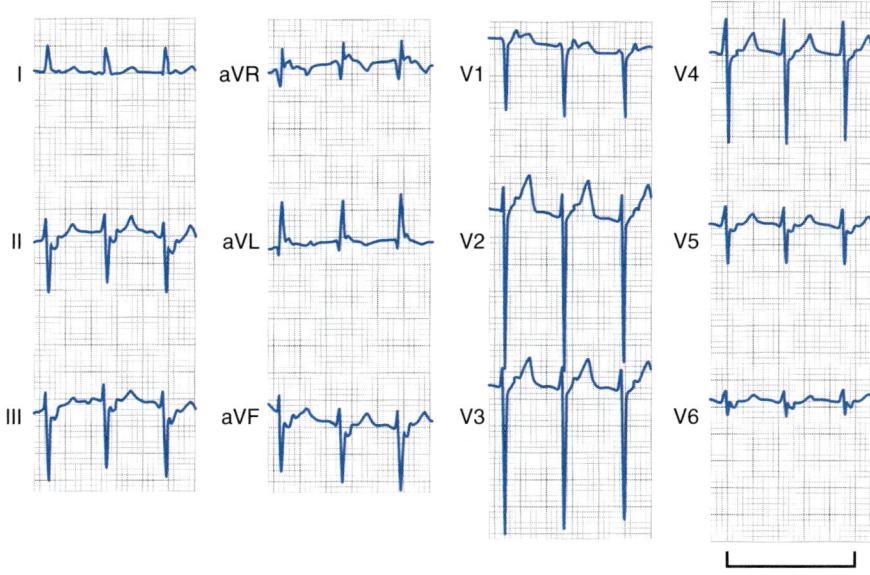

FIGURE 19-8. Electrocardiogram during slow-fast atrioventricular nodal reentrant tachycardia. This tracing was obtained in a 76-year-old man with palpitations and syncope. Retrograde P waves at the end of the QRS complex in V₁ give rise to a pseudo right bundle branch block pattern. The QRS also shows left ventricular hypertrophy and a left anterior hemiblock unrelated to the tachycardia.

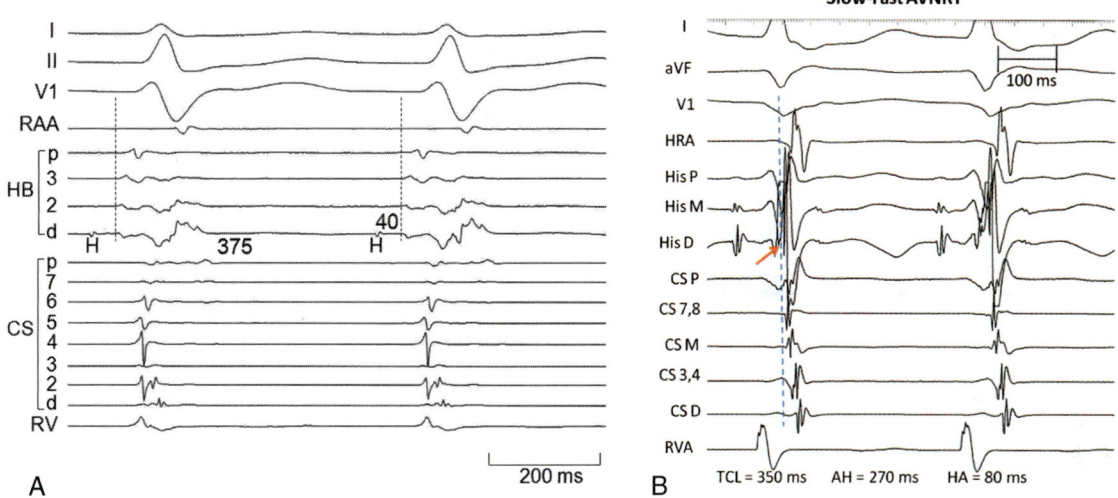

FIGURE 19-9. Two examples of slow-fast AV nodal reentry. **A,** Atrial activation precedes ventricular activation during slow-fast atrioventricular nodal reentrant tachycardia. Using close bipolar electrodes, earliest atrial activation (*dotted lines*) recorded close to the proximal portion of the His bundle precedes ventricular activation. In the absence of these recordings atrial activation would appear to be simultaneous to ventricular activation. CS, coronary sinus; d, distal; H, His recording; HB, His bundle; p, proximal; RAA, right atrial appendage; RV, right ventricle. **B,** Intracardiac electrograms recorded during slow-fast AV nodal reentry. The earliest atrial activity is recorded on the His catheter and is approximated by the vertical line. Atrial activation in the coronary sinus (CS) is concentric. The tachycardia cycle length (TCL) is 350 ms, AH interval 270 ms and HA interval 80 ms. D, distal; HRA, high right atrium; M, mid; P, proximal; RVA, right ventricular apex.

HA intervals can overlap in these two forms of tachycardia. In our population, the HA interval in the slow-fast form was 45 ± 11 milliseconds (range, 25 to 145 milliseconds). A contemporary conceptualization of the reentry circuit for slow-fast AVNRT is shown in Figure 19-6C. In this model, retrograde atrial activation through the fast pathway activates both the left and right sides of the atrial septum. The wavefront of right atrial activation fails to penetrate into the triangle of Koch because of block along the eustachian ridge.[22] The left atrial wavefront, however, activates the CS myocardium and propagates to the CS ostium and inferior triangle of Koch between the ostium and the tricuspid valve. The wavefront then ascends the atrial septum in the triangle of Koch to activate the fast pathway and complete the circuit.[22] In this conceptualization, the right infe-

rior extension comprises the anterograde slow pathway, and the fibers crossing the superior tendon of Todaro comprise the retrograde fast pathway.[22] Ablation within the CS or left atrium is necessary when the left inferior extension or left atrial myocardium provides the critical portion to the reentry circuit rather than the right inferior extension.

Although slow-fast AVNRT usually demonstrates early retrograde atrial activation posterior to the site recording His bundle activation (so-called concentric atrial activation), about 6% of patients demonstrate early retrograde atrial activation in the CS (so-called eccentric atrial activation) because of muscular connections between the left atrium and the CS (Fig. 19-10A).[52] The response after ventricular overdrive pacing is an additional maneuver to support the diagnosis of AVNRT.

During ventricular pacing with atrial entrainment, the VA interval is more than 85 milliseconds longer than the corresponding VA interval during tachycardia.[53,54] Upon cessation of ventricular pacing with tachycardia continuation, a V-A-V response is noted.[55,56] In addition, the difference between the ventricular postpacing interval (PPI) and TCL is more than 115 milliseconds.[54] Correction of the PPI may be needed to account for rate-

related prolongation of the return AH interval ($\Delta = [PPI - (AH\ return - AH\ supraventricular\ tachycardia) - TCL]$) (Fig. 19-10B).[57] The HA interval is typically stable during tachycardia and after pacing maneuvers.

To some extent, it is possible to dissociate both the atrium and the ventricle from the tachycardia. However, atrial or ventricular preexcitation will eventually advance AVNRT if His bundle activation is altered. AV block, either distal

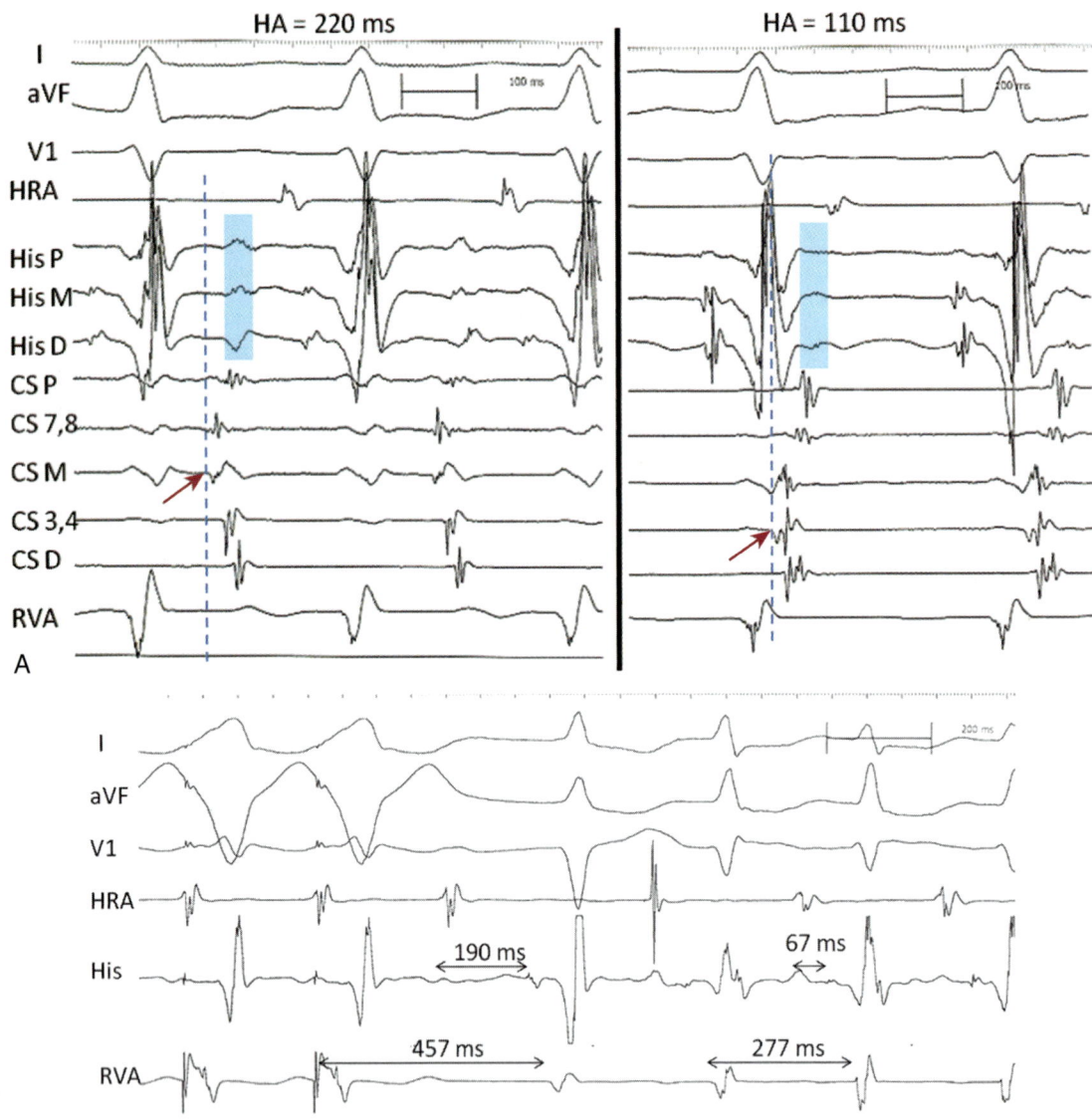

Uncorrected: PPI (457 ms) − TCL (277 ms) = 180 ms

B   **Corrected**: PPI (457 ms) − TCL (277 ms) − [AH_{PPI} (190 ms) − AH_{SVT} (67 ms)] = 57 ms

FIGURE 19-10. A, Eccentric retrograde atrial activation in the coronary sinus during atrioventricular (AV) nodal reentrant tachycardia. *Left,* The earliest atrial activity occurs at the mid-coronary sinus (CS M, *vertical line and arrow*). The His bundle–atrial (HA) interval is long at 220 msec. *Right,* In the same patient, the HA interval is shorter (110 msec) in AV nodal reentry, but the atrial activation remains earliest in the mid- (CS M) or mid-distal (CS 3,4) coronary sinus. The *shaded blue areas* highlight the timing of the atrial activation on the His catheter for clarity. D, distal; HRA, high right atrium; RVA, right ventricular apex. **B,** Correction of ventricular postpacing interval (PPI) for atrium–His bundle (AH) interval prolongation in the return cycle. Overdrive ventricular pacing that captures the atrium is terminated with continuation of a narrow complex tachycardia. The ventricular postpacing interval is long compared with the tachycardia cycle length (TCL) (difference > 115 msec) consistent with AV nodal reentry. The AH interval in the return cycle is prolonged (190 msec) compared with that in tachycardia (67 msec) because of concealed or decremental conduction in the AV node. After correction for this AH prolongation, the difference between the postpacing interval and the tachycardia cycle length is < 115 msec (57 msec), consistent with AV reciprocating tachycardia. The patient underwent successful ablation of a concealed posteroseptal pathway. CS, coronary sinus; D, distal; HRA, high right atrium; M, mid; RVA, right ventricular apex; SVT, supraventricular tachycardia.

to His or between the His and lower common pathway, is sometimes seen at the onset of tachycardia. Late ventricular extrastimuli introduced during His refractoriness will not perturb AVNRT, but those that are able to advance retrograde His bundle activation will preexcite the atrium and entrain the tachycardia.

Slow-Slow Variant

Slow-slow AVNRT occurred in 49 (10%) of our 500 patients with AVNRT. In this form of reentry, a slow AV nodal pathway is used as the antegrade limb, and another slow AV nodal pathway as the retrograde limb (Fig. 19-11).

Reentry using both the right and left inferior AV nodal inputs has been proposed.[22] The electrocardiogram during tachycardia may show characteristic negative P waves in inferior and precordial leads, typical of earliest retrograde atrial activation in the proximal CS (Fig. 19-11).[58] This tachycardia can be induced by atrial or ventricular stimulation and frequently requires administration of isoproterenol. As previously mentioned, although the HA interval is usually longer than that recorded during slow-fast AVNRT, an overlap in the HA intervals between these two forms of AVNRT is frequently observed (Table 19-2).[22] In our patients, the ranges of HA during slow-slow and slow-fast AVNRT were 90 to 210 milliseconds and 25 to 145

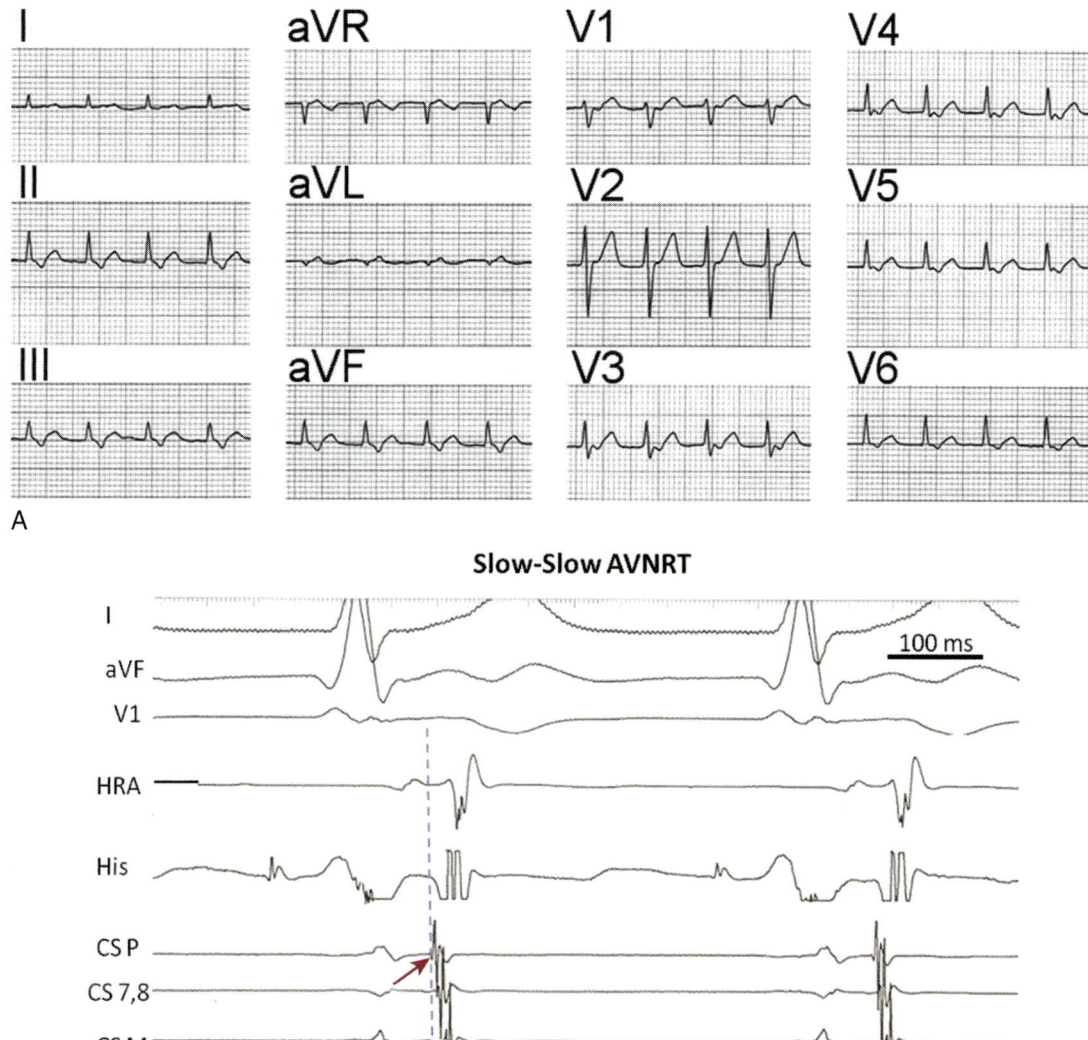

FIGURE 19-11. Slow-slow AV nodal reentry. **A,** Surface electrocardiogram showing slow-slow atrioventricular (AV) nodal reentry with the P wave in the ST segment. The P wave is inverted in the inferior leads. **B,** Intracardiac electrograms recorded during slow-slow AV nodal reentry. Note that the earliest atrial activation (*vertical line and arrow*) occurs at the proximal coronary sinus (CS P). The tachycardia cycle length (TCL) is 480 msec, the atrium–His bundle interval is 290 msec, and the His bundle–atrial (HA) interval is 190 msec. CS, coronary sinus; D, distal; HRA, high right atrium; M, mid; RVA, right ventricular apex.

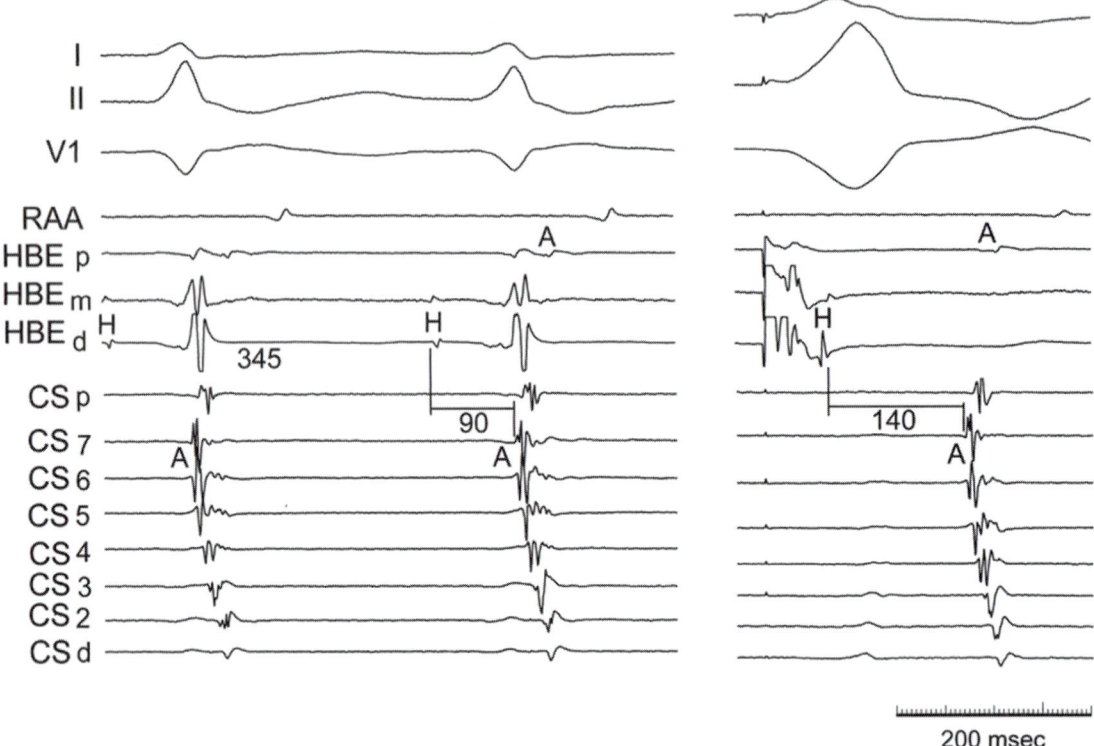

FIGURE 19-12. Demonstration of a lower common pathway in atrioventricular (AV) nodal reentrant tachycardia using a retrograde slow AV nodal pathway. *Left,* The His bundle–atrial (HA) interval during tachycardia measured to the earliest atrial activation site in the proximal coronary sinus (CS 7) is 90 msec. *Right,* During ventricular stimulation at the tachycardia cycle length (345 msec), the HA interval is 140 msec, consistent with a common lower pathway distal to the reentrant circuit supporting the tachycardia. CS, coronary sinus; D, distal; HBE, His bundle electrogram; RAA, right atrial appendage; P, proximal. *(From Curtis AB, Gonzalez MD. Supraventricular tachycardia. In Naccarelli GV, Curtis AB, Goldschlager NF (eds):* Electrophysiology Self-Assessment Program. *Bethesda, MD: American College of Cardiology; 2000. With permission.)*

milliseconds, respectively (Table 19-2). The earliest site of retrograde atrial activation was found in the right atrium near the anterior edge of the CS ostium or just inside the CS (mean distance from the ostium, 1.5 ± 0.5 cm) (Fig. 19-11). *The earliest site of retrograde atrial activation near the CS ostium is what characterizes slow-slow AVNRT, and not the HA interval.* In our series, the TCL was 411 ± 62 milliseconds; the AH interval was 282 ± 71 milliseconds; the HA interval was 141 ± 32 milliseconds (range, 90 to 210 milliseconds); and the shortest HA interval (measured at the earliest atrial activation site during tachycardia) was 85 ± 43 milliseconds (Table 19-2). Short HA intervals may also occur and are typically attributed to long conduction times in the lower common pathway, almost offsetting the longer HA times. Multiple slow pathways are often demonstrable with atrial extrastimulus testing.[59] Neither the antegrade or retrograde fast pathway is necessary for this reentrant circuit and therefore may be absent.

Characteristic of the slow-slow form of AVNRT is the presence of a lower common pathway.[60] In other words, there is a portion of the AV node that is distal to, and not part of, the reentrant circuit that sustains the tachycardia. The presence of a lower common pathway is demonstrated by comparing the HA interval during tachycardia to the earliest atrial activation site, with the HA interval observed during ventricular pacing at the same cycle length as the tachycardia. In patients with slow-slow AVNRT, the HA interval during ventricular pacing (measured from the end

of the His bundle deflection) is longer than that recorded during tachycardia (Fig. 19-12).

As in the slow-fast form, preexcitation of the atrium during slow-slow AVNRT only follows ventricular extra-stimuli that advance retrograde His bundle activation (Fig. 19-13). However, because of the presence of a lower common pathway, retrograde His bundle activation needs to be advanced more than 15 milliseconds before retrograde atrial activation is also advanced.[60] In contrast, during AV reentrant tachycardia, late ventricular extrastimuli can advance retrograde atrial activation even when retrograde His bundle activation is not altered, as long as ventricular activation near the earliest atrial activation site is advanced. An atrial tachycardia with 1:1 AV conduction can be differentiated from AVNRT by comparing the sequence of atrial activation during tachycardia with that observed during ventricular pacing at a cycle length identical to that of the tachycardia. An atrial tachycardia has a different sequence of atrial activation than that observed during ventricular pacing with 1:1 VA conduction and may demonstrate a V-A-A-V response after ventricular pacing.[55] In patients with AVNRT and long retrograde conduction times, a pseudo V-A-A-V response may occur, suggesting the wrong diagnosis of atrial tachycardia (Fig. 19-14). This happens when the retrograde VA interval exceeds the paced RR interval and atrial activation precedes ventricular activation during tachycardia.

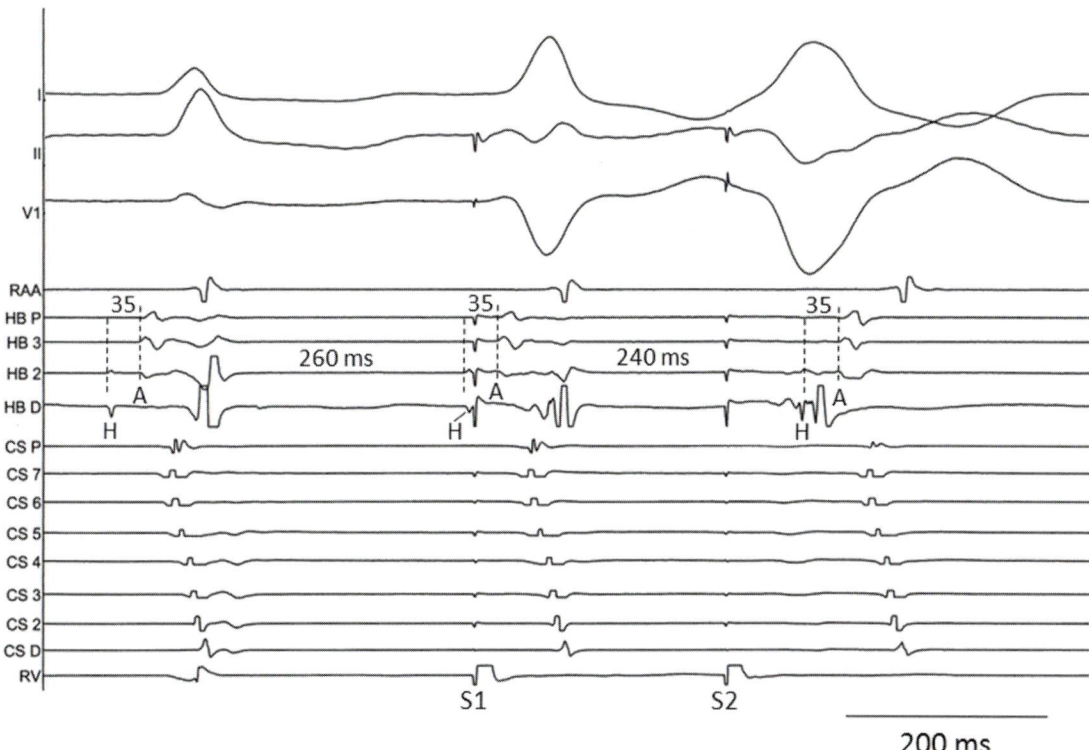

FIGURE 19-13. Entrainment of slow-fast atrioventricular nodal reentrant tachycardia (AVNRT) using double ventricular extrastimuli. S1 "peels back" the refractory period of the right ventricle, which in turn allows S2 to capture the right ventricle and advances retrograde His bundle activation. This maneuver is frequently required in AVNRT with short cycle lengths in which the ventricular effective refractory period is reached before His bundle activation can be advanced. Note that S2 advances both retrograde His bundle and atrial activations with constant His bundle–atrial (HA) intervals (35 msec), consistent with absence of lower common pathway. The sequence of atrial activation following S2 is identical to that observed during tachycardia.

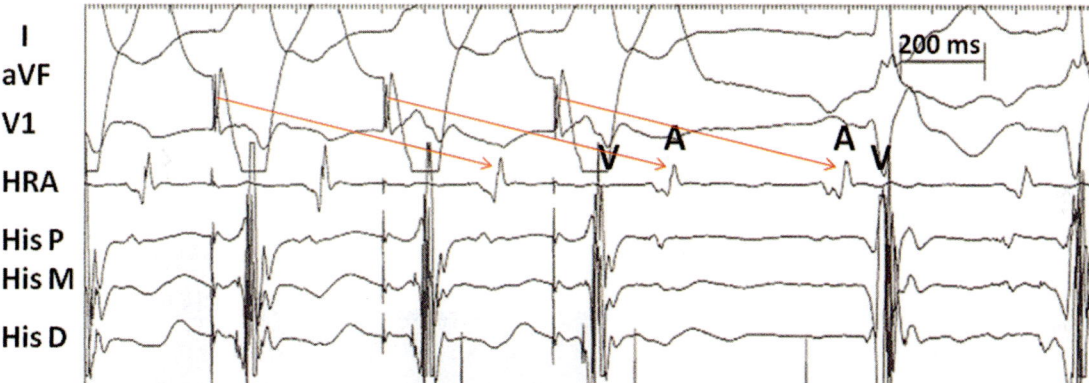

FIGURE 19-14. Pseudo V-A-A-V response to the termination of ventricular overdrive pacing during atrioventricular nodal reentry. Because of very long retrograde conduction times, the atrial electrogram during ventricular pacing is associated, not with the preceding ventricular complex, but with two complexes before (*arrows*). This pattern may be confused with the response of atrial tachycardia to ventricular overdrive pacing. A, atrial electrogram; D, distal; HRA, high right atrium; M, mid; V, ventricular electrogram.

Fast-Slow Variant

The fast-slow form of AVNRT occurred in 37 (7%) of our 500 patients with AVNRT. Similar to slow-slow AVNRT, the complete reentry circuit is not fully understood. In fast-slow AVNRT, it is assumed that the fast AV nodal pathway is used as the antegrade limb and one or more slow AV nodal pathways as the retrograde limb, with the assumption that this arrhythmia is the reversal of the typical slow-fast circuit. However, this simplified concept has been challenged by the concept that fast-slow reentry may represent reentry within the right and left inferior AV nodal inputs but in a direction opposite to that of slow-

slow AVNRT.[22] The electrocardiogram during tachycardia may show a PR interval that is shorter than the RP interval (long RP tachycardia) (Fig. 19-15A). The AH interval is less than 180 milliseconds, with P waves inverted in inferior leads (Table 19-2). The HA interval is longer than the AH interval because of retrograde conduction over the slow AV nodal pathway.

Similar to the slow-slow form, fast-slow AVNRT can be induced by atrial or ventricular stimulation, frequently during administration of isoproterenol. In some patients, AVNRT is induced only by ventricular stimulation.[61] In addition, the presence of a lower common pathway results

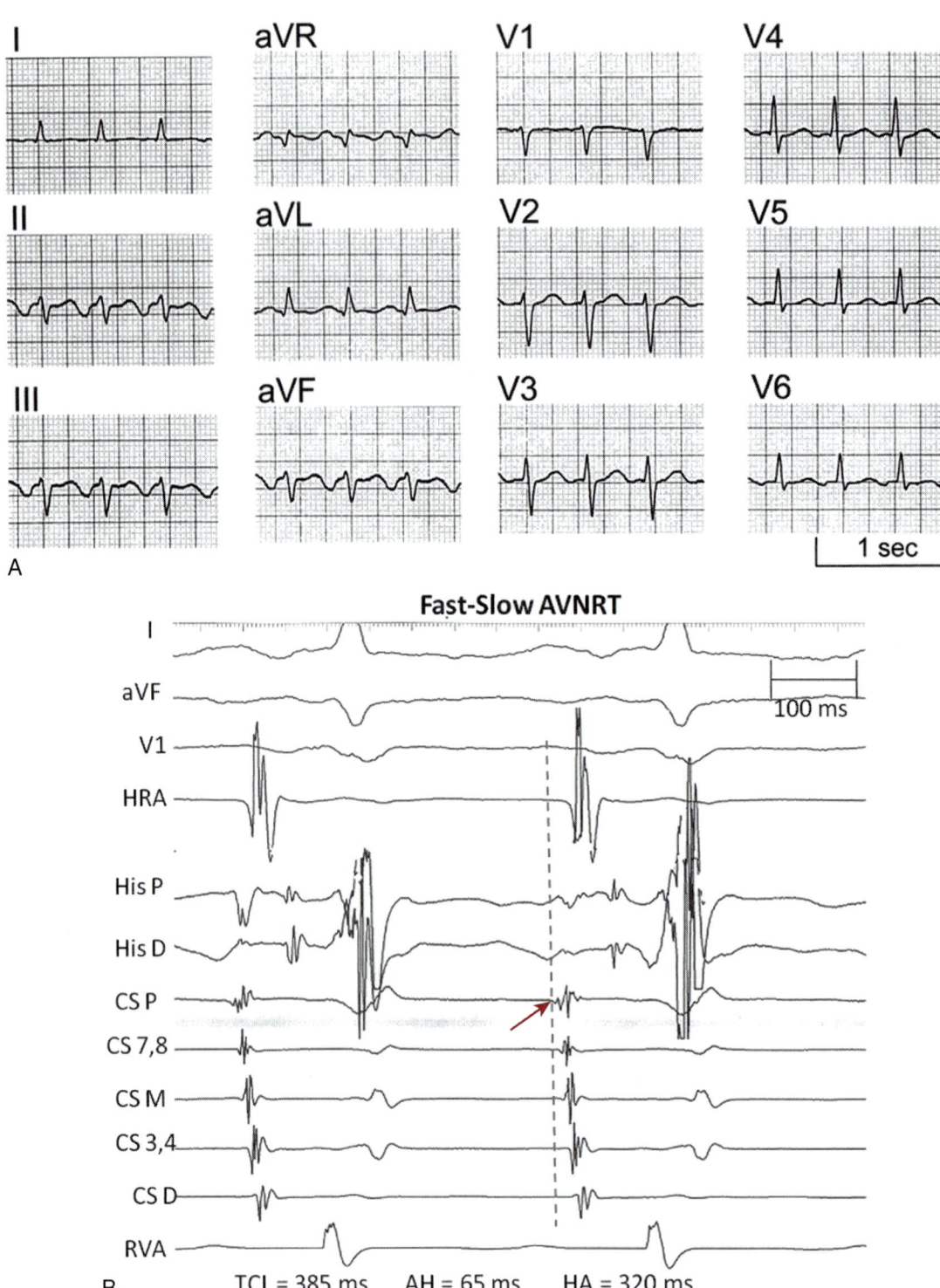

FIGURE 19-15. **A,** Electrocardiogram during fast-slow atrioventricular (AV) nodal reentrant tachycardia. Negative P waves in inferior and precordial leads are recorded before the QRS complexes with a PR shorter than the RP interval, giving rise to a long RP tachycardia pattern. **B,** Intracardiac electrograms recorded during fast-slow AV nodal reentry. Note that the earliest atrial activation (*vertical line and arrow*) occurs at the proximal coronary sinus (CS P). The tachycardia cycle length is 385 msec, the atrium–His bundle (AH) interval is 65 msec, and the His bundle–atrial (HA) interval is 320 msec. CS, coronary sinus; HRA, high right atrium; RVA, right ventricular apex; TCL, tachycardia cycle length.

in an HA interval during tachycardia that is shorter than that observed during ventricular stimulation.[60] Earliest retrograde atrial activation is close to the CS ostium (Fig. 19-15B).[58] With forms of AV nodal reentry that have long RP intervals, the AH interval during atrial pacing at the TCL exceeds the AH interval in tachycardia by greater than 40 milliseconds.[62] For AV reciprocating tachycardias,

the difference in the values of these intervals is 20 to 40 milliseconds, and for atrial tachycardias, it is less than 20 milliseconds.[62]

Left-Sided Variant

The left-sided variant occurs in up to 1.5% of patients undergoing ablation for AVNRT.[22,63] There are no

TABLE 19-4

DIFFERENTIAL DIAGNOSIS: ATRIOVENTRICULAR NODAL REENTRY, ORTHODROMIC RECIPROCATING TACHYCARDIA, AND ATRIAL TACHYCARDIA*

Maneuver	PS ORT	AVNRT	AT
Parahisian pacing	No change in V-A with loss of His capture	Increased V-A with loss of His capture	Increased V-A with loss of His capture
Late ventricular extrastimulus delivered during tachycardia	Advance atrial activation if ventricular electrogram close to location of accessory pathway is also advanced	Advances atrial activation only if retrograde His bundle activation is advanced	Unable to advance atrial activation unless His is advanced
Δ Ventricular PPI and TCL and V-A-A-V response	<115 msec unless decremental conduction, V-A-A-V response may occur with decrementally conducting APs	>115 msec, V-A-A-V response may occur with fast-slow or slow-slow AVNRT	V-A-A-V response
Δ VA during ventricular pacing at TCL and VA during tachycardia	<85 msec	>85 msec	Variable; VA conduction may be absent
VA pacing ventricular base vs. pacing ventricular apex	VA shorter pacing base	VA shorter pacing apex	VA shorter pacing apex
Retrograde V-A conduction	Nondecremental except in slowly conducting APs (e.g., PJRT)	Decremental	Decremental
Atrial and ventricular pacing at TCL	1:1 conduction present	Wenckebach conduction may occur	1:1 antegrade conduction present; VA block may be present
V-A dissociation during tachycardia	Not possible	Possible	Possible
VA interval in tachycardia	>60 msec	Typically, <60-70 msec	May be longer or shorter than 60 msec
HA interval in tachycardia	Fixed	May be variable	Variable, especially first postventricular pacing return cycle

*This table assumes that there is a single arrhythmia mechanism and no bystander or multiple accessory atrio-ventricular pathways.
Δ, difference between; AP, accessory pathway; AT, atrial tachycardia; AVNRT, atrioventricular nodal reentrant tachycardia; HA, His bundle–atrium; ORT, orthodromic reciprocating tachycardia; PS, postero-septal; V-A, paced ventricular electrogram to atrial electrogram; PPI, postpacing interval; TCL, tachycardia cycle length; VA, ventricular-atrial interval.

pathognomonic surface or intracardiac electrocardiographic findings for the left-sided AVNRT variant. Similarly, there are no clinical characteristics differentiating between these patients and those with more common forms of AVNRT.[63] The activation pattern is usually that of slow-fast AVNRT. The diagnosis is confirmed by electrophysiologic findings consistent with AVNRT but with successful slow pathway ablation from the left atrium after failure of right atrial ablation. The presence of a short HA interval (≤15 milliseconds) and the occurrence of antegrade double response to atrial pacing are sometimes noted in patients with this AVNRT variant.[22] The AH intervals and TCLs are shorter in the left-sided variant than in "right-sided" slow-fast AVNRT.[63]

Differential Diagnosis

The diagnosis of AVNRT requires exclusion of alternative mechanisms. These include AV reentry using a retrograde accessory pathway, atrial tachycardia, and junctional tachycardia (Table 19-4). Orthodromic reciprocating tachycardia can be excluded when the VA time is less than 60 milliseconds, which is common in slow-fast AVNRT.[23] Exception to this rule is a slowly conducting accessory AV pathway in which the A follows not the preceding V but the previous one. Another exception is an atrial tachycardia with 1:1

antegrade conduction in which the A occurs immediately after the previous V. During reentrant tachycardia, a critical maneuver to diagnose an accessory pathway participating as the retrograde limb is the entrainment technique. Whenever atrial activation is advanced without a change in the atrial activation sequence following a premature ventricular extrastimulus during His bundle refractoriness, a retrograde accessory pathway participating in the tachycardia is reliably diagnosed. If there is a change in the atrial activation sequence, an innocent bystander accessory pathway must be suspected. In response to ventricular overdrive pacing, orthodromic reciprocating tachycardia also produces a V-A-V response; however, the differences in VA times between pacing and tachycardia are less than 85 milliseconds, and the PPI-TCL difference is less than 115 milliseconds.[54] A long return AH interval may invalidate this maneuver unless the correction is applied (see earlier).

In sinus rhythm, parahisian pacing can identify retrograde conduction over the AV node and over anteroseptal and mid-septal accessory pathways.[64] Parahisian pacing may fail to demonstrate retrograde conduction over accessory AV pathways located at other sites. VA times determined during pacing in sinus rhythm from the base and apex of the right ventricle can help to identify the presence of an accessory pathway. With this maneuver, pacing from the base of the right ventricle will produce a shorter

VA time than apical ventricular pacing in the presence of an accessory pathway. In contrast, the VA times are shorter when pacing from the right ventricular apex when retrograde conduction occurs through the AV node.

Atrial tachycardias that originate in perinodal structures are not uncommon. Thus, atrial activation sequence may be identical to that of slow-fast AVNRT. An atrial tachycardia can be diagnosed when there is variability in the HA interval during tachycardia. Ventricular pacing at a rate faster than the rate of the tachycardia typically accelerates the atrial rate to that of the pacing rate with concealed entrainment. After abrupt termination of the pacing train, the next beat of AVNRT typically occurs at a cycle length somewhat longer than that of the tachycardia owing to the presence of decremental slow pathway conduction. However, the next beat typically has the same HA interval as during spontaneous tachycardia. In contrast, the postpacing HA interval for atrial tachycardias is typically different from that in tachycardia. The presence of a V-A-A-V sequence of activation following rapid ventricular pacing suggests (but does not prove) an atrial tachycardia as the mechanism. However, it should be recognized that slow-slow and fast-slow AVNRTs are usually associated with this same response during transient entrainment when the VA interval exceeds the ventricular pacing cycle length (see Chapter 11 and Fig. 19-14). Atrial tachycardia has a V-A-A-His-V response, however, whereas AVNRT may show a V-A-His-A-V response.[65] In addition, the permanent form of junctional reciprocating tachycardia (PJRT) with a decrementally conducting retrograde accessory pathway usually has the same response (V-A-A-V) to rapid ventricular pacing. The clear distinction between AVNRT and PJRT is made by the response to premature ventricular stimuli. Fast-slow AVNRT is not affected by appropriately timed ventricular extrastimuli unless retrograde His bundle activation is advanced, whereas during PJRT, the atrial activation may be either advanced or delayed when the V but not the His is advanced. For long RP tachycardias, comparing the AH intervals between tachycardia and atrial pacing at the TCL can differentiate among AVNRTs (difference, >40 milliseconds), atrial tachycardia (difference, <20 milliseconds), and reciprocating tachycardias (difference, >20 but <40 milliseconds).[62]

Differentiation of an accelerated junctional rhythm from slow-fast AVNRT may be difficult.[66,67] Both tachycardias have a short and constant HA conduction interval with earliest retrograde atrial activation near the apex of the triangle of Koch (fast pathway region, behind the tendon of Todaro). An automatic junctional tachycardia can be differentiated from AVNRT by the response to premature atrial contractions (PACs) introduced during or before AV junctional refractoriness (Fig. 19-16).[66] A PAC introduced during AV junctional refractoriness cannot penetrate to the automatic focus and therefore cannot alter the tachycardia. In contrast, a junctional refractory PAC may advance the following beat of tachycardia by conduction in the slow pathway in AVNRT. PACs introduced before AV junctional refractoriness may advance the immediately following beat and resend an automatic tachycardia but must terminate AVNRT because of collision of the antegrade PAC wavefront and retrograde tachycardia wavefronts in the fast pathway.

Atrioventricular Nodal Reentry and Atypical Presentations

Irregular AVNRT that can be misdiagnosed as atrial fibrillation on surface electrocardiograms is an uncommon presentation of this arrhythmia. Alternating conduction over two slow AV nodal pathways with different conduction times can give rise to alternating short-long cycles during tachycardia.[59,68] Also, double-response tachycardia can occur with each sinus beat conducting over both the fast and slow pathways to produce an apparently irregular cycle length, which may be confused with atrial fibrillation. Similarly, intermittent functional block distal or proximal to the His bundle can give origin to periods of AVNRT with 1:1 AV relationship alternating with 2:1 AVNRT (Fig. 19-4). The electrocardiogram during tachycardia could be mistaken for an atrial tachycardia.[69] The distinctive characteristic of 2:1 AVNRT is the location of the nonconducted P wave centered between the preceding and following QRS (Fig. 19-4). Older individuals with underlying AV nodal disease can present with a symptomatic AV nodal reentrant arrhythmia but with a rate below 100 beats/minute. Despite a lower rate than that required to make a diagnosis of tachycardia, the mechanism of this arrhythmia is identical to that observed in younger patients with AVNRT. These older patients tend to be quite symptomatic despite the relatively slow rate, probably owing to almost simultaneous atrial and ventricular contraction. Recently, Vijavaraman and associates described a series of six patients undergoing catheter ablation for symptomatic slow AV nodal reentry. Patients were older (age, 71-83 years) with a prolonged PR interval (262 ± 54 milliseconds).[70] All patients underwent slow pathway ablation. The AV Wenckebach cycle length prolonged from 522 ± 90 milliseconds at baseline to 666 ± 48 milliseconds after ablation. Only one patient required a permanent pacemaker due to an AV Wenckebach cycle length of 710 milliseconds after ablation. The arrhythmia rate is slower, likely because of underlying AV nodal disease—thus, their risk for AV block after ablation is probably higher than for others with AVNRT.

Atrioventricular Nodal Reentry and Other Arrhythmias

Patients presenting with clinical arrhythmias other than AVNRT can have easily inducible AVNRT in the electrophysiology laboratory. In 31 (6%) of 500 patients, in addition to AVNRT, we induced AV reentrant tachycardia using an accessory AV pathway. A focal atrial tachycardia was present in 36 (7%) of 500 patients and originated from the following sites: crista terminalis ($n = 22$), CS ostium ($n = 3$), fast AV nodal pathway region ($n = 5$), and mitral annulus–aorta junction ($n = 6$).[71]

Atrial fibrillation is often associated with AVNRT. In a study of 629 patients undergoing atrial fibrillation ablation, 27 (4.3%) had inducible AVNRT.[72] These patients were younger than those without AVNRT, and ablation limited to AVNRT was associated with reduction of clinical recurrences of atrial fibrillation. Similar results were reported by Katritsis and colleagues.[73] Among 409 patients with atrial fibrillation, AVNRT was inducible in 7 (1.7%),

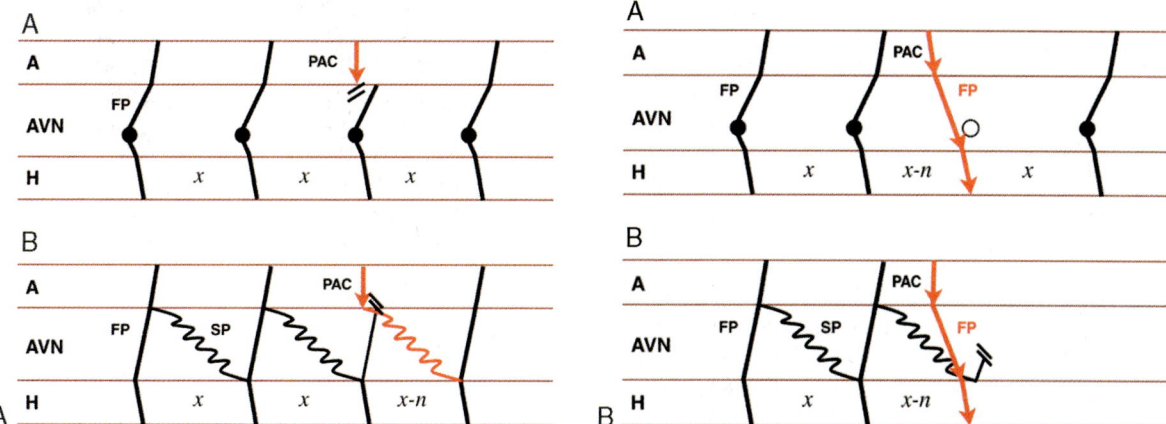

FIGURE 19-16. Atrial extrastimulus testing to differentiate AV nodal reentry from an automatic junctional tachycardia. **Panel A,** Response to premature atrial complex (PAC) delivered when the AV junction is refractory (local atrial activation from PAC occurs at or after His activation). **A,** Response in junctional tachycardia. A PAC delivered at a time the junctional focus has already depolarized the atrioventricular node (AVN) and is unable to influence the immediate or the next junction beat. *Solid circles* represent junction focus; *black lines* show conduction through AVN, His (H), and atrium (A). **B,** Response in atrioventricular node reentry tachycardia (AVNRT). A similarly timed PAC cannot influence the immediate next beat but can influence the following (*x-n*) beat of AVNRT by conduction through the slow pathway. *Black lines* show conduction through AVN, H, and A, and *red lines* show PAC and its response. Although this figure shows advancement of the next beat (*x-n*), delay of the next beat or termination of tachycardia are also specific to AVNRT. *Orange arrow* indicates PAC. FP, fast atrioventricular node pathway; SP, slow atrioventricular node pathway; *x* and *x-n*, H-H intervals. **Panel B,** Response to PACs delivered prior to AV junctional refractoriness. **A,** Response in junctional tachycardia. The open circle represents the anticipated junctional tachycardia beat timing if no PAC were delivered. An early PAC advances the immediate junctional tachycardia beat and His timing by atrioventricular (AV) nodal fast pathway activation, and junctional tachycardia continue. **B,** Response in AVNRT. An early PAC may advance the immediate His by activation of the AV nodal fast pathway. However, that makes the fast pathway refractory and unavailable for retrograde conduction, terminating the AVNRT circuit. *Orange arrow* indicates PAC and its response. A, atrium; FP, fast atrioventricular node pathway; H, His; SP, slow atrioventricular node pathway; *x* and *x-n*, H-H intervals. *(From Padanilam BJ, Manfredi JA, Steinberg LA, et al. Differentiating junctional tachycardia and atrioventricular node re-entry tachycardia based on response to atrial extrastimulus pacing. J Am Coll Cardiol. 2008;52:1711-1717. With permission.)*

and the ablation was limited to the AVNRT in 5 (1.2%), with lower recurrence of atrial fibrillation. Among patients with paroxysmal atrial fibrillation, those with no identifiable pulmonary vein triggers appear more likely to have AVNRT (11%) than those with pulmonary vein triggers (2%).[74] It has also been reported that ablation of the slow pathway decreases vulnerability to pacing-induced atrial fibrillation in patients presenting with AVNRT. In 21% to 25% of patients with idiopathic ventricular tachycardia, AVNRT is also inducible, which is not the case in patients with ventricular tachycardia associated with structural heart disease.[27,28] A comprehensive electrophysiology study is necessary during the evaluation of patients with atrial and ventricular arrhythmias to assess for inducibility of AVNRT and, as in the case of atrial fibrillation, its potential role as the trigger of the clinical arrhythmia.

Ablation

Slow-Fast Variant

Elimination of 1:1 conduction over the slow pathway is the target for ablation in all forms of AVNRT.[38,39,41,75] Once slow pathway conduction can be reproducibly demonstrated, and the diagnosis of AVNRT is confirmed, the ablation catheter is positioned along the tricuspid annulus immediately anterior to the CS ostium (Fig. 19-17).[76-78] The right anterior oblique view is especially useful for positioning catheters because it displays Koch's triangle en face. The angle of the left anterior oblique view should be adjusted so that the His catheter is perpendicular to the fluoroscopic plane. The initial target zone for slow pathway ablation is the isthmus of tissue between the tricuspid valve annulus and ostium of the

CS (Fig. 19-18A).[38,39,41,75] This area corresponds to the rightward inferior AV nodal extension described pathologically and is targeted by an anatomic and electrogram-guided approach.[39,43,75] The targets for slow pathway ablation are given in Table 19-5.

Anatomic Approach

The anatomic approach targets the area near the tricuspid annulus just outside the CS os in the inferior paraseptal region or within the proximal segment of the CS. These locations contain the musculature that is in continuity with the right and left atrial extensions of the AV node.[75] Positioning of the catheters is best performed during sinus rhythm because the atrial and ventricular electrogram components are more easily discerned. The ablation catheter should have a distal electrode 4 mm in length. The length of the deflecting segment of the ablation catheter that has proved most effective has ranged from 2.0 to 3.0 inches (D-F curves). The use of a long sheath with slight distal septal angulation (e.g., Daig SR0, St. Jude Medical, St. Paul, MN) often enhances catheter reach and stability. When using a sheath, it is important to keep the curves of the sheath and catheter coaxial. The ablation catheter is advanced into the right ventricle, moved inferiorly and medially so that it lies anterior to the ostium of the CS, and then withdrawn toward the tricuspid annulus until the distal pair of electrodes records a small atrial deflection and a large ventricular deflection (Fig. 19-18B and C). Clockwise torque will move the sheath and catheter toward the septum. The atrial electrogram at successful sites may show multiple components (Fig. 19-18B and C). The A/V ratio recorded from the distal electrode pair in sinus rhythm may range from about 1:10 to 1:3.

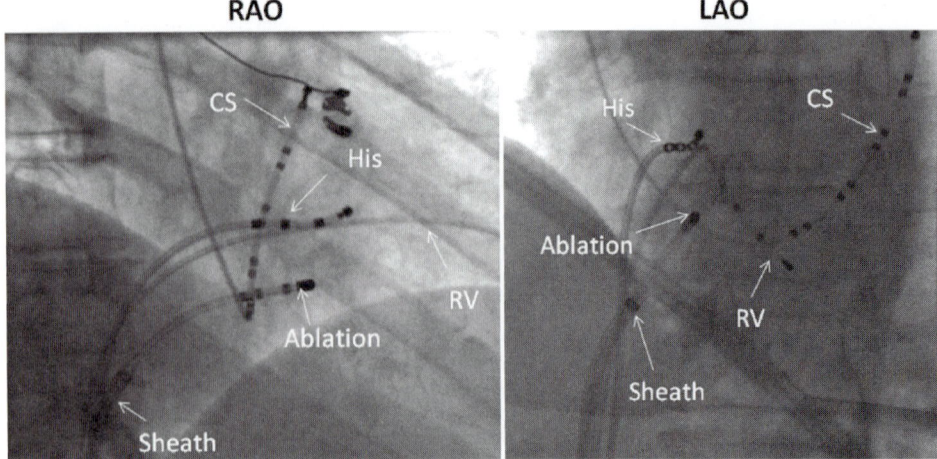

FIGURE 19-17. Catheter position for radiofrequency slow pathway ablation. The tip of the ablation catheter is between the coronary sinus (CS) os and the tricuspid valve in the right anterior oblique (RAO) view. In the left anterior oblique (LAO) view, the tip of the ablation catheter is just posterior (septal) to the His catheter at the level of the coronary sinus os. Note the angled sheath supporting the ablation catheter. RV, right ventricle.

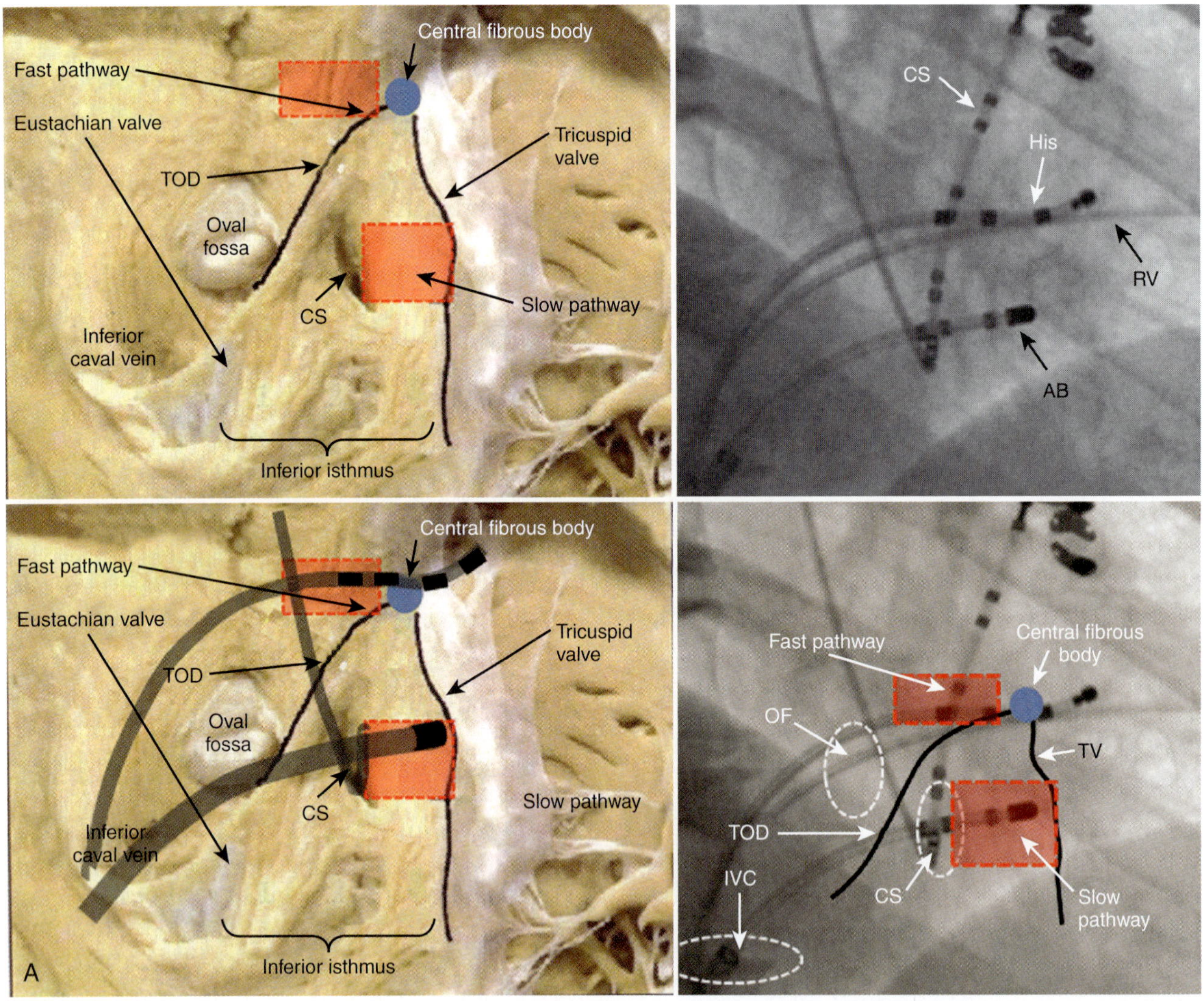

FIGURE 19-18. A, Right anterior oblique (RAO) view of the cardiac anatomy surrounding the triangle of Koch (*upper left*) and catheter positions for ablation of the slow pathway as shown in Figure 19-17 (*upper right*). The *lower panels* are annotated versions of the *upper figures*. In the *lower right*, the catheter positions are superimposed on the cardiac anatomy, showing the ablation catheter tip for slow pathway ablation in the area between the coronary sinus (CS) os and the tricuspid valve (TV). The areas for slow and fast pathway ablation are shaded in *red*. In the *lower right panel*, the salient cardiac anatomic features are superimposed on the RAO fluoroscopic view of the catheter positions. AB, ablation catheter; His, His catheter; IVC, inferior vena cava; OF, oval fossa; RV, right ventricular catheter; TOD, tendon of Todaro.

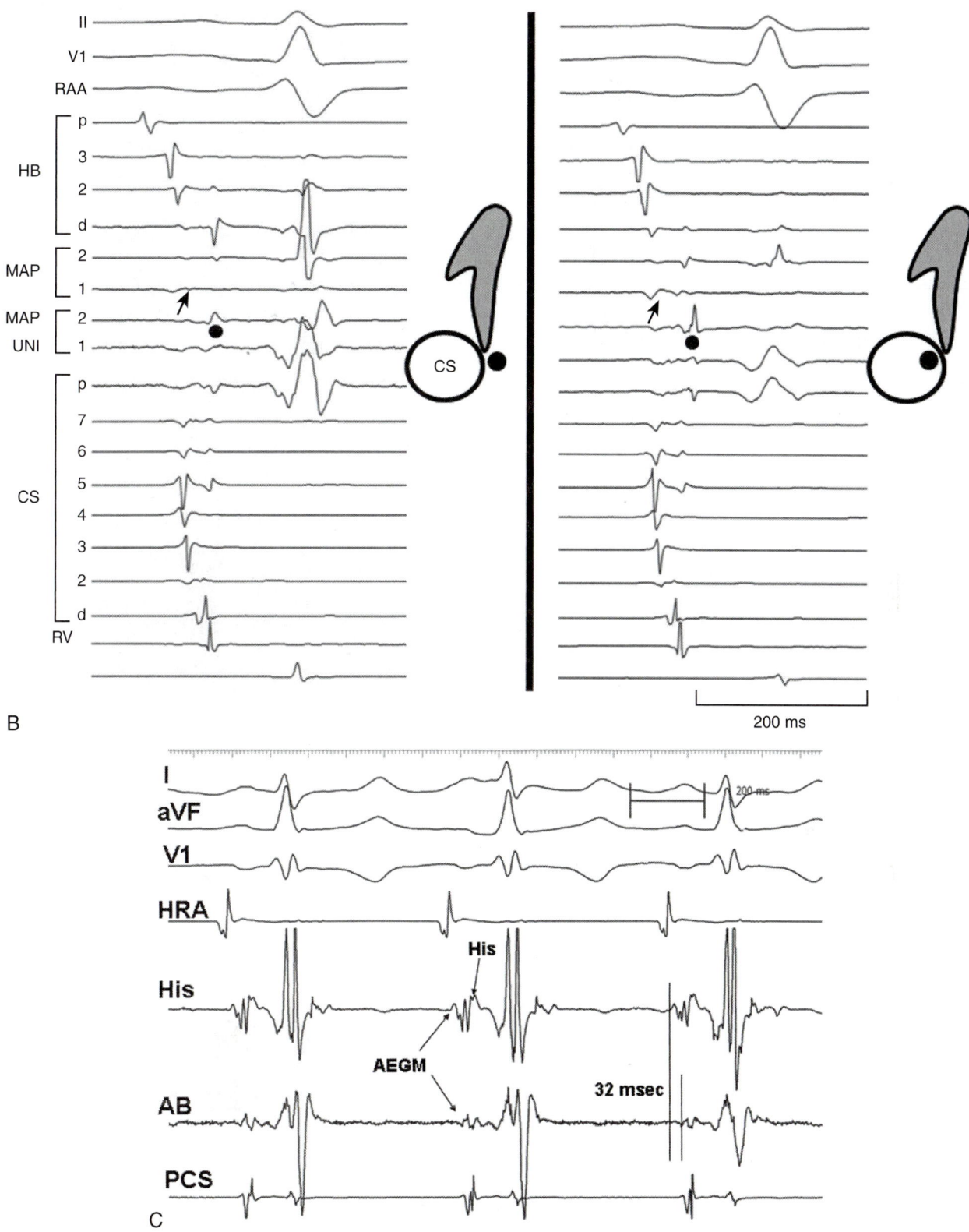

FIGURE 19-18, cont'd B, Electrograms recorded near the coronary sinus ostium and the rightward posterior (inferior) extension of the atrioventricular (AV) node. Bipolar and unipolar (UNI) recordings obtained from the mapping catheter (MAP) just before ablation of the slow AV nodal pathway. Late activation potentials (*dots*) believed to represent slow pathway activation and following local atrial activation (*arrows*) are recorded in front of the anterior edge of the coronary sinus ostium (CS, *left panel*) and just inside the coronary sinus (*right panel*). HB, His bundle; RAA, right atrial appendage; RV, right ventricle. **C,** Intracardiac electrogram at site of successful slow pathway ablation by the anatomic approach. The atrial electrogram (AEGM) on the ablation catheter (AB) is fractionated and has a 1:8 amplitude ratio compared with the ventricular electrogram. The difference in time of onset from the atrial component of the His electrogram to the onset of the atrial component of the ablation electrogram (*vertical lines*) is 32 msec. HRA, high right atrium; PCS, proximal coronary sinus. (**A,** *Adapted from Anderson et al. Heart Rhythm Society on line publication. With permission.*)

TABLE 19-5
TARGETS FOR SLOW PATHWAY ABLATION
Anatomic Guidance
Tissue between CS ostium and tricuspid annulus at the level of CS ostium (rightward inferior input)
Proximal CS musculature (connection with leftward inferior input via LA-CS connections)
Increased risk for AV block: area triangle of Koch, superior to the CS ostium A/V ratio = 1:10 to 1:3
Electrogram Guidance
Slow pathway activation potentials
Earliest retrograde atrial activation near CS (slow-slow and fast-slow AVNRT only)

A/V, atrial-to-ventricular; AV, atrioventricular; AVNRT, atrioventricular nodal reentrant tachycardia; CS, coronary sinus; LA, left atrium.

The most common site for effective ablation of slow pathway conduction is immediately anterior to or at the edge of the CS ostium.[22,75,79] Antegrade 1:1 conduction over the slow AV nodal pathway is eliminated in this area in about 95% of patients with AVNRT. Elimination of slow pathway conduction may sometimes require that the catheter be repositioned along the tricuspid annulus inferior to the CS ostium (Figs. 19-19 and 19-20). In some patients, elimination of 1:1 slow pathway conduction requires application of RF energy in the proximal portion of the CS. Moving the ablation site more cephalad is associated with an increased risk for AV block (Figs. 19-19 and 19-20).

In some patients, despite ablation near the region of the rightward inferior extension, AVNRT remains inducible. This may be due to primary or alternate slow pathway conduction over the leftward inferior extension.[22] This may be particularly true for the ablation of slow-slow AVNRT that may manifest as slow-fast or fast-slow after ablation between the tricuspid valve and CS. In these cases, ablation at a site up to 20 mm inside the CS (targeting the connection with the leftward inferior extension) may be necessary to prevent reinduction of AVNRT.[22] If the operator feels that it is necessary to ablate sites more cephalad, he or she may consider cryoablation during AVNRT because this may be associated with a lower incidence of AV nodal block.[80,81] The risk for AV block is largely related to how superiorly RF energy is applied in the Koch triangle (Fig. 19-20). For patients who are very risk averse, RF current should not be applied to sites more cephalad than the superior edge of the CS ostium.

Electrogram-Guided Approach

Two electrophysiologic approaches were described by Haïssaguerre[39] and Jackman.[41] These approaches, although they use different activation potentials, both reduce the number of RF current applications by identifying critical components of the reentrant circuit. Jackman described a sharp late potential following a low-amplitude atrial potential near the CS ostium during sinus rhythm and suggested that this potential represents the atrial connection of the slow AV nodal pathway.[41] Consistent with this concept, during retrograde slow AV nodal conduction, the sequence is inverted, and the sharp potential precedes the atrial electrogram.

This potential is usually recorded anterior or just inside the CS ostium (Fig. 19-18B). The slow potential described by Haïssaguerre is usually recorded at sites slightly superior to the site where the potential described by Jackman is observed.[39] The Haïssaguerre potential becomes delayed and of lower amplitude at rapid rates of stimulation, consistent with AV nodal properties. The locations where these two potentials can be recorded frequently overlap.[82,83] The targets for slow pathway ablation are given in Table 19-5. These potentials may represent activation of transitional cells as they approach the AV node or activation of the rightward inferior extension of the AV node.[6,43,83] In addition, these potentials are present in individuals with and without AVNRT.[83] In a randomized trial of the electrogram-guided and anatomic approaches, there were no differences in total procedure time (121 ± 57 versus 110 ± 57 minutes), fluoroscopy time (6 ± 3 versus 7 ± 3 minutes), number of RF lesions (4 ± 3 versus 4 ± 3), success rates (100% for both approaches), or recurrence rates (1.4% for both approaches).[84]

Application of Radiofrequency Current. RF current is delivered from the distal 4-mm-tip electrode of the mapping-ablation catheter toward a pair of dispersive electrode pads placed over the posterior thorax. Larger-tip or irrigated electrodes are not necessary because of the superficial location of AV nodal tissue. Impedance is carefully monitored, and RF energy is halted for any sudden drop or rise in impedance or any evidence of AV or VA block. Catheter position is continuously monitored by fluoroscopy or real-time three-dimensional catheter localization. It is advisable to initially use low power (20 to 30 W) to test for unwanted effects such as prolongation of the AH interval. After 15 seconds, the power can be gradually increased up to 50 W, with a target temperature of 55° to 60°C for 30 to 60 seconds. Energy is limited to 20 to 30 W in the proximal CS. During RF delivery, the impedance is continuously monitored because a drop in impedance is a better indicator of tissue temperature than is the tip electrode temperature. A few lesions are usually sufficient to eliminate AVNRT induction. During catheter ablation of the slow AV nodal pathway, a junctional rhythm is induced (Fig. 19-21).[85–88] Although a junctional rhythm is not specific for eliminating AVNRT, it is more commonly elicited at successful than at unsuccessful sites. During RF current delivery, we closely monitor the AH interval during sinus rhythm and retrograde conduction during junctional beats. Energy delivery must be rapidly interrupted if a junctional beat fails to conduct retrogradely through the fast AV nodal pathway to the atrium (Fig. 19-21) because this may reflect damage to the compact AV node. In rare cases, successful ablation of slow AV nodal pathway conduction can be achieved in the absence of junctional beats during RF energy application.[89] More frequently, however, successful ablation is heralded by a junctional rhythm that gradually subsides during ablation.[85] After each RF current application, programmed atrial stimulation, rapid atrial pacing, or both are performed to determine the presence or absence of slow pathway conduction or inducible AVNRT. If these characteristics remain, the catheter is repositioned, and RF current is applied at a different position. In a study involving 387 patients with AVNRT and 385 successful ablations out of 692 RF applications, the sensitivity and specificity of junctional rhythm as a sign of

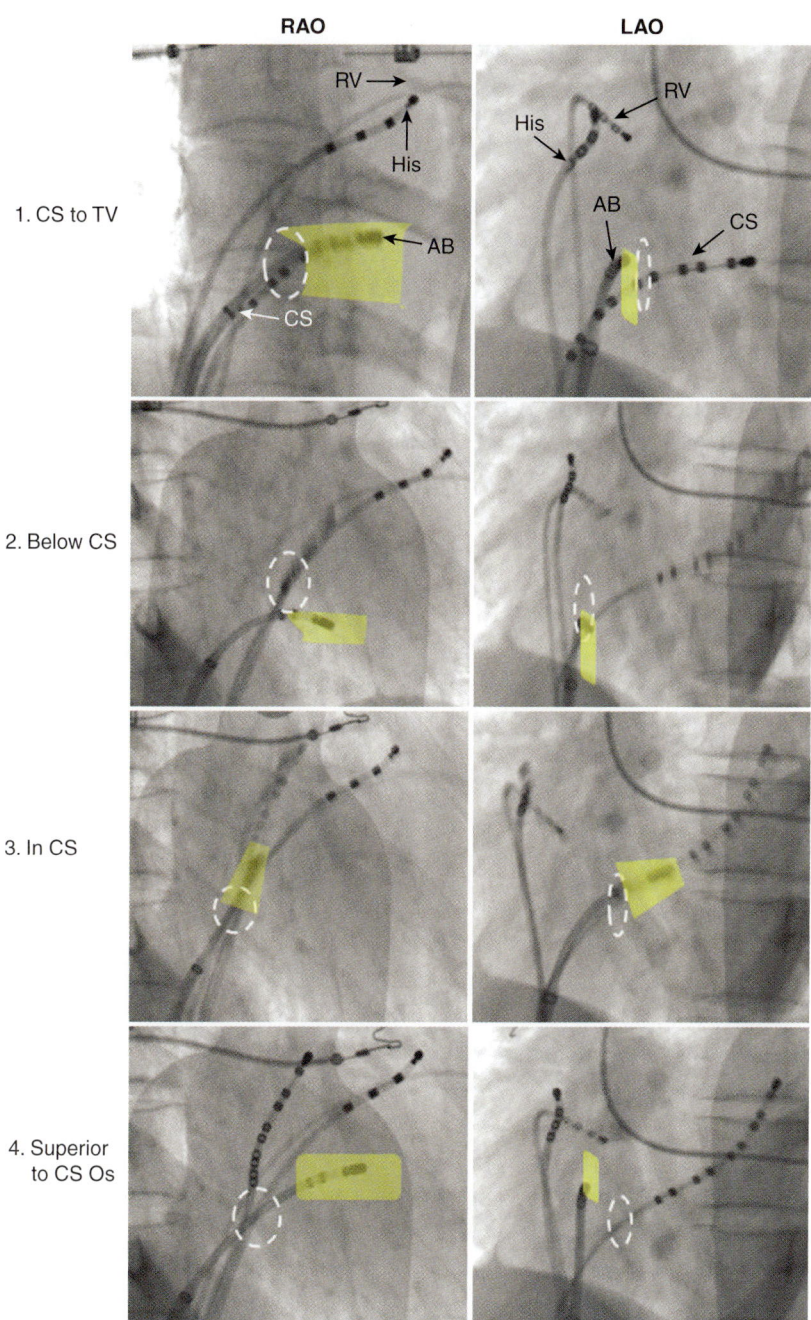

RAO

LAO

1. CS to TV

2. Below CS

3. In CS

4. Superior to CS Os

FIGURE 19-19. Progression of ablation sites (*shaded yellow areas*) for slow pathway ablation. Left panels show RAO views, right panels show LAO views. 1. The first ablation attempts are directed at the area between the coronary sinus (CS) os (*dashed circle*) and the tricuspid valve no more superiorly than the roof of the CS. 2. The second area for ablation is between the CS and tricuspid valve (TV) but inferior to the CS os. 3. The third area is the proximal CS. 4. The last area for ablation is more superiorly on the septum above the level of the CS os. The risk for atrioventricular block is increased with ablation superior to the CS os. AB, ablation catheter; His, His catheter; RV, right ventricle.

success were 99.5% and 79.1%, with a positive-predictive value of 55.5%.[79] In another study, junctional ectopy was seen more frequently (100% versus 65%) and for a longer duration (7.1 ± 7.1 versus 5.0 ± 7.0 seconds) during successful versus unsuccessful RF applications.[86]

Because the absence of junctional ectopy during RF ablation corresponds to an ineffective ablation site, it is our practice to terminate the application of RF current at a given site if an accelerated junctional rhythm is not observed within 10 to 15 seconds of reaching target power.

Although retrograde block of junctional rhythm should always be considered a potential marker of AV nodal injury, there are situations in which retrograde block occurs without AV nodal damage. Retrograde block may be anticipated with the ablation of slow-slow AVNRT in the absence of

retrograde fast pathway conduction. Also, rapid junctional rhythm at cycle lengths shorter than the 1:1 conduction rate of the fast pathway can manifest functional retrograde block. In many cases, the ERP of the fast pathway actually shortens after slow pathway ablation.[75]

Cryoablation

Cryoablation has been introduced to reduce the risk for AV block during catheter ablation of AVNRT. The 6-mm-tip catheter has proved more effective than the original 4-mm-tip catheter (Table 19-6). Rarely, an 8-mm-tip catheter is needed to create larger or deeper lesions and to reduce recurrences. The catheter positions for slow

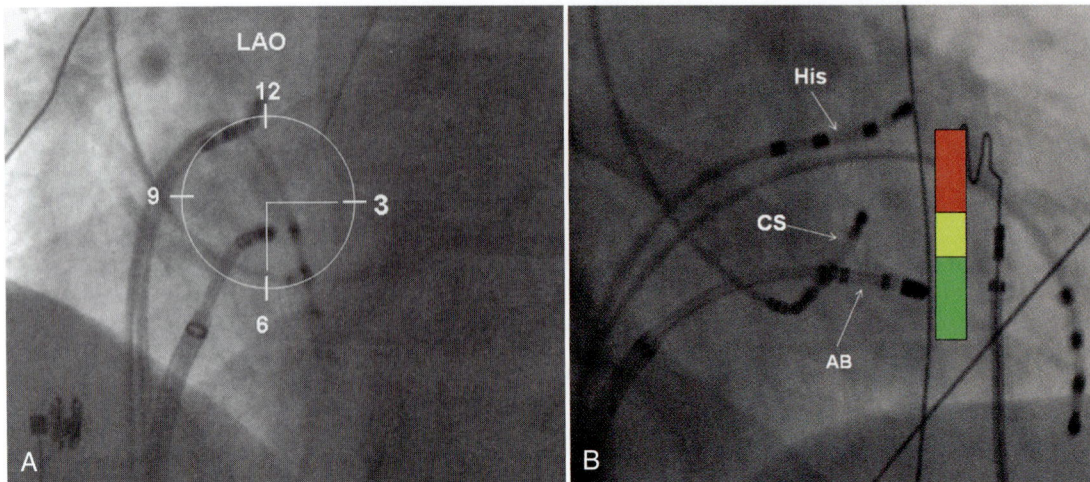

FIGURE 19-20. Limits of anatomic sites for slow pathway ablation. **A,** In the left anterior oblique (LAO) view, acceptable areas for ablation are slightly septal to the His catheter and generally between 3 and 6 o'clock, with the His catheter representing 12 o'clock and the roof of the CS 6 o'clock. **B,** Right anterior oblique view of ablation catheter (AB) at the level of the coronary sinus (CS) os near the tricuspid annulus. The estimated boundaries of the triangle of Koch are delineated by the *broken lines*. The *green marker* indicates the caudal to cranial limits with the lowest incidence of heart block. This area corresponds to sites inferior to the CS os to the superior margin (roof) of the CS os. The area in *red*, beginning near the mid-point between the CS os and the His recording, represents a high risk for atrioventricular block. The area in *yellow*, beginning at the roof of the CS, is intermediate risk for heart block.

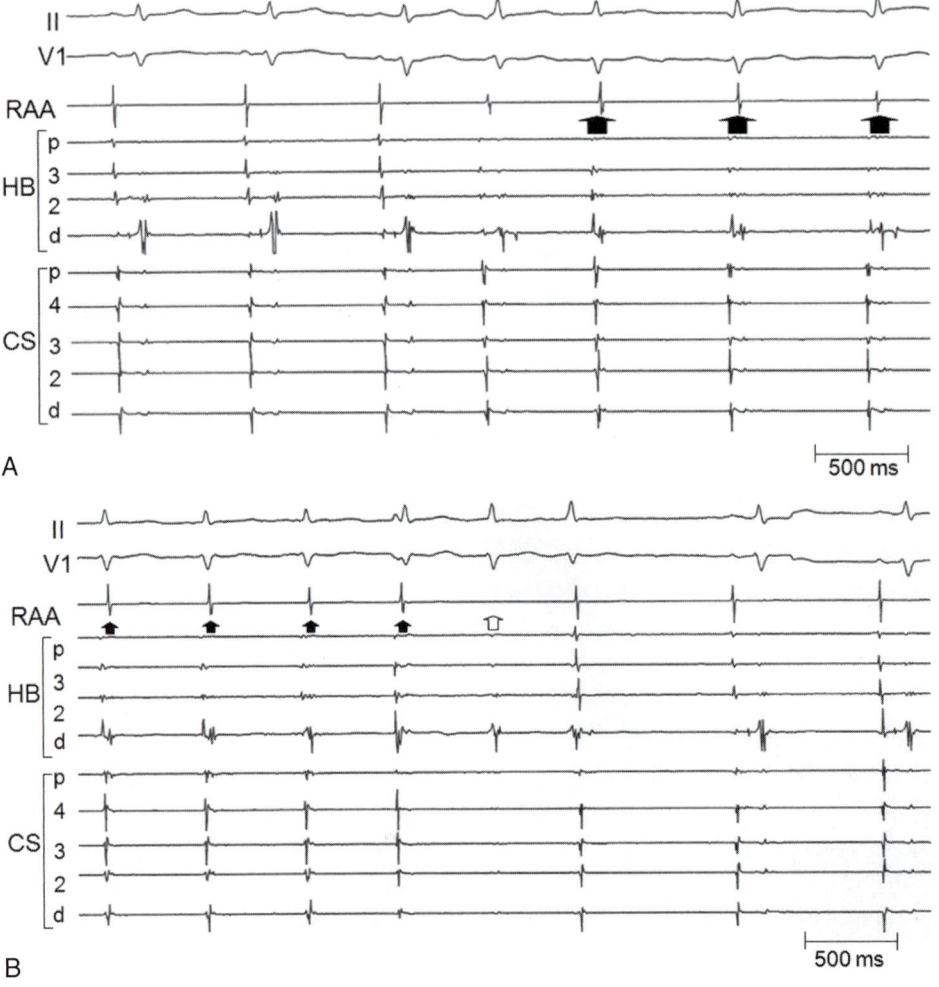

FIGURE 19-21. A, Induction of a junctional rhythm during radiofrequency application between the tricuspid annulus and the ostium of the coronary sinus (CS). One-to-one retrograde conduction over the fast atrioventricular (AV) nodal pathway (*arrows*) implies preserved normal AV nodal function during energy delivery. **B,** Retrograde block over the fast AV nodal pathway during radiofrequency application. One-to-one retrograde conduction over the fast AV nodal pathway during catheter ablation (*filled arrows*) is followed by sudden retrograde block manifested by absence of atrial activation (*open arrow*). Rapid discontinuation of energy application resulted in preservation of AV nodal conduction. HB, His bundle; RAA, right atrial appendage.

TABLE 19-6

PUBLISHED STUDIES COMPARING CRYOABLATION FOR ATRIOVENTRICULAR NODAL REENTRANT TACHYCARDIA USING THE 4- VERSUS 6-MM-TIP CATHETER

Study	No. of Patients with AVNRT	Follow-Up (mo)	APS 4 mm (%)	Rec 4 mm (%)	APS 6mm (%)	Rec 6 mm (%)	P value (Rec)
Khairy et al, 2007[98]	185	7.5	92	15	95	3	NS
Rivard et al, 2008[132]	289	5.1	91	16	90	8	0.03
Sandilands et al, 2008[99]	160	18	92	17	94	7	0.01
Chanani et al, 2008[100]	154	2.5	93	18	98	9	NS

APS, acute procedural success; AVNRT, atrioventricular nodal reentrant tachycardia; *P* values relate to recurrence rates compared with radiofrequency ablation; NS, not significant; Rec, recurrence.

pathway cryoablation are similar to those for RF energy, except with cryoablation that the successful sites are often more superior toward the compact AV node than with RF ablation (Fig. 19-22). It is not unusual that the cryoablation catheter must be positioned midway between the CS and the catheter recording His bundle activation, a position considered aggressive for RF ablation. Importantly, no junctional rhythm is produced during cryoablation. Fortunately, catheter stability during cryoablation (afforded by ice adherence to the tissue) allows for different strategies to monitor for successful ablation. In sinus rhythm or with atrial pacing, the catheter is positioned, and cryoablation is begun. The catheter quickly becomes adherent to the tissue by ice formation over the electrode. This is heralded by the loss of electrograms from the distal electrode. At this point, atrial pacing is begun to demonstrate slow pathway conduction either by repeated extrastimulus testing or by atrial pacing at a cycle length just above the one associated with Wenckebach periodicity. If slow pathway conduction is eliminated within 20 to 30 seconds, the ablation is continued for a full 4 minutes at −75°C or below.

Alternatively, cryomapping can be performed initially by reducing the electrode temperature to −30°C and monitoring for slow pathway block.[81] This allows for more rapidly reversible effects, but the superficial tissue cooling with cryomapping may provide false-negative findings; that is, cooling at lower temperatures may be successful at sites of cryomapping failure. Either cryomapping or cryoablation may be initiated during AVNRT with very little chance of catheter movement because of adherence to the tissue. Fluoroscopy is not needed to check the position of the catheter once tissue adhesion has occurred, significantly shortening fluoroscopy time.[90–92]

During cryoablation, the conduction properties of the fast and slow AV nodal pathways are continuously checked using atrial stimulation. Continuous monitoring of the AH interval is important because the lesion becomes larger than indicated by cryomapping or early in the stages of therapeutic ablation.[81,93–97] It has been suggested to pace the atrium at cycle lengths 10 to 20 milliseconds longer than the Wenckebach cycle length during cryoablation. A useful maneuver is to pace the atrium at cycle lengths 10 to 20 milliseconds longer than the Wenckebach cycle length during cryoablation to identify incipient damage to the AV node. (Mark A Wood, MD, personal communication;

Fig. 19-22). Some authors have advocated complete elimination of all slow pathway function to reduce the likelihood of recurrences after cryoablation. If high-grade block occurs, if there is dramatic prolongation of the Wenckebach cycle length (by about 100 milliseconds), or if Wenckebach block occurs at cycle lengths longer than 500 milliseconds, ablation is discontinued. Termination of AVNRT during tissue cooling, abolition of 1:1 AV conduction over the slow AV nodal pathway, and inability to reinduce AVNRT are markers of success. It is useful to reassess the status of slow pathway function and AVNRT inducibility 30 to 45 minutes after the final cryoablation lesion because acute recovery is more common than with RF ablation. Some authors have advocated complete elimination of all slow pathway function to reduce the likelihood of recurrences after cryoablation.

The choice between cryoablation and RF ablation needs to be determined on an individual basis. Patients with previous ablation near the fast AV nodal pathway region and those with a short distance between the compact AV node and the roof of the CS ostium may benefit from cryoablation because they are at higher risk for AV block. Another subgroup of high-risk patients includes those with a prolonged AH interval in the basal state. Several studies have compared the advantages and disadvantages of the two different energy sources. Available clinical data have demonstrated the effectiveness and safety of cryoablation in the treatment of AVNRT (85% to 99% acute success rate with no incidence of permanent complete heart block). Overall, recurrences have been shown to be more frequent with cryoablation (2.8% to 28%) than with conventional RF ablation. More recently, the 6-mm-tip catheter has proved more effective than the original 4-mm-tip catheter.[90,93,98–100] Table 19-7 summarizes the results of several studies that analyzed the results and recurrences of cryoablation.

Slow-Slow and Fast-Slow Variants

Ablation for slow-slow and fast-slow AVNRT targets the slow AV nodal pathway that is used for retrograde conduction. This pathway is frequently different from the slow AV nodal pathway associated with antegrade conduction.

Ablation is directed at the site of the earliest retrograde atrial activation, which is most frequently located between the tricuspid annulus and CS ostium in fast-slow AVNRT and

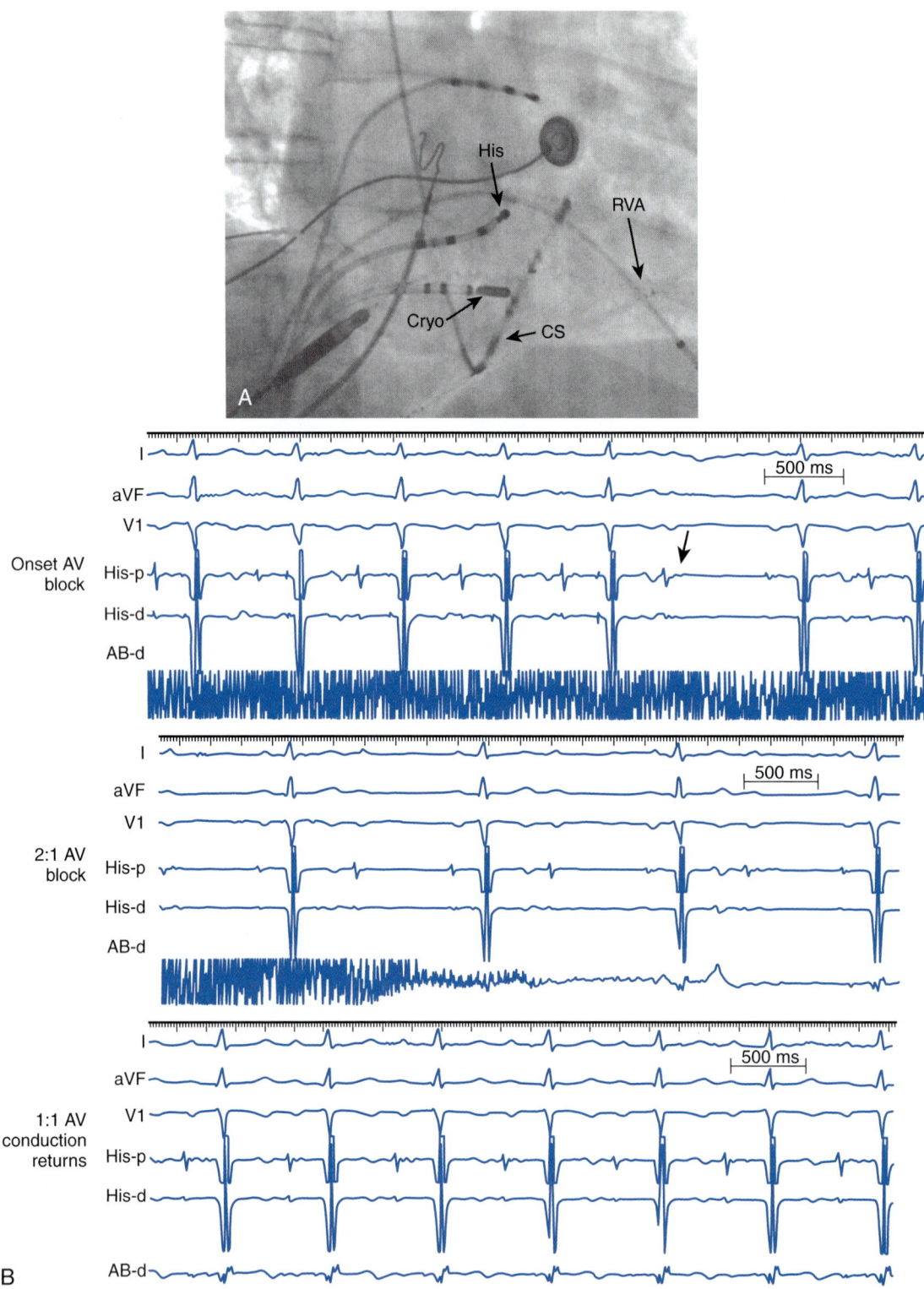

FIGURE 19-22. A, Right anterior oblique view of cryoablation catheter (Cryo) position for slow pathway ablation. The ablation tip is about halfway between the estimated location of the coronary sinus (CS) os and the His recording. Energy delivery at more inferior sites failed to terminate slow-fast atrioventricular (AV) nodal reentry in this patient. Although this site would be considered at high risk for producing AV block with radiofrequency energy, the need for cryoablation at this superior a location is not unusual. In this patient, ablation here resulted in slow pathway elimination without altering antegrade AV conduction. RVA, right ventricular apex. **B,** Transient AV block during slow pathway cryoablation. *Top,* Tachycardia was terminated by the cryoenergy; however, during the ongoing ablation, there is slight atrium–His bundle (AH) interval prolongation followed by AV block (*arrow*). *Middle,* Cryoablation is immediately discontinued, as evidenced by the return of the electrograms on the distal ablation electrodes (AB-d) as the ice investing the electrode melts. There is 2:1 AV block on termination of the ablation. *Bottom,* One minute after termination of cryoablation, 1:1 AV conduction resumes. The patient had no adverse effects from the ablation procedure, and AV nodal reentry was no longer inducible. d, distal; p, proximal.

TABLE 19-7

PUBLISHED CLINICAL STUDIES ON CRYOABLATION FOR ATRIOVENTRICULAR NODAL REENTRANT TACHYCARDIA

Study	No. of Subjects	Follow-Up (mo)	Acute Success with Cryoablation (%)	Recurrence with Cryoablation (%)	Cryoablation Catheter Tip (mm)	Acute Success with RF (%)	Recurrence with RF (%)	P Value for Cryoablation vs. RF Recurrence
Zrenner et al, 2004[133]	200	8.1	97	8	4	98	1	0.03
Friedman et al, 2004[134]	103	6	91	6	4	—	—	—
Kimman et al, 2004[95]	63	13 ± 7	93	10	4	91	9	NS
Collins et al, 2006[135]	117	12	98	8	4	100	2	NS
Jensen-Urstad et al, 2006[81]	75	12.7	99	5	6	—	—	—
Papez et al, 2006[94]	53	8.1 ± 7.0	96	12	4	96	6	NS
Gaita et al, 2006[97]	87	27 ± 13	96	10	4	—	—	N/A
Gupta et al, 2006[136]	71	2.2 ± 0.4	85	20	4	97	6	0.01
De Sisti et al, 2007[93]	69	18 ± 9	87	28	6	—	—	—
Avari et al, 2008[91]	80	10.7	97	3	6	95	2	NS
Bastani et al, 2009[137]	312	22.4 ± 12.7	99	5.8	6	—	—	—
Opel et al, 2010[138]	272	Median, 2-3 mo	93	11	6	95	3	0.02
Chan et al, 2009[92]	80	13.6	98	9	6	95	1	NS

N/A, not applicable; NS, not significant; RF, radiofrequency.

along the anterior aspect of the proximal CS in slow-slow AVNRT (Fig. 19-23).[101] For slow-slow AVNRT, it is recommended to eliminate both antegrade and retrograde slow pathway conduction to prevent recurrences of fast-slow and slow-fast AVNRT.[22] Mapping and ablation can be performed during tachycardia or during ventricular pacing to eliminate 1:1 retrograde slow AV nodal pathway conduction in patients with slow-slow or fast-slow AVNRT. Because retrograde fast pathway conduction is often poor in the setting of slow-slow AVNRT, retrograde slow pathway function can often be targeted at the site of earliest retrograde atrial activation during ventricular pacing. This site is frequently found on the anterior aspect of the proximal CS. Antegrade slow pathway is ablated as described previously for slow-fast AVNRT.

Initially, mapping is performed in the lower portion of the triangle of Koch, between the CS ostium and the tricuspid annulus, followed by mapping in the proximal portion of the CS. The site of earliest retrograde atrial activation is targeted for ablation. If ablation is performed in the proximal CS, low voltage (20 W) is initially used. The energy output is progressively increased while the impedance is monitored. Successful ablation results in elimination of retrograde conduction over the slow AV nodal pathway (Fig. 19-23).

Patients with slow-slow or fast-slow AVNRT frequently lack retrograde conduction over the fast AV nodal pathway. Therefore, during RF current application, junctional beats may have no retrograde conduction to the atrium, preventing assessment of AV nodal function during delivery of energy. In these patients, we deliver short applications of RF energy and evaluate AV nodal conduction between applications. Alternatively, overdrive atrial pacing may allow continuous monitoring of antegrade AV conduction during ablation.

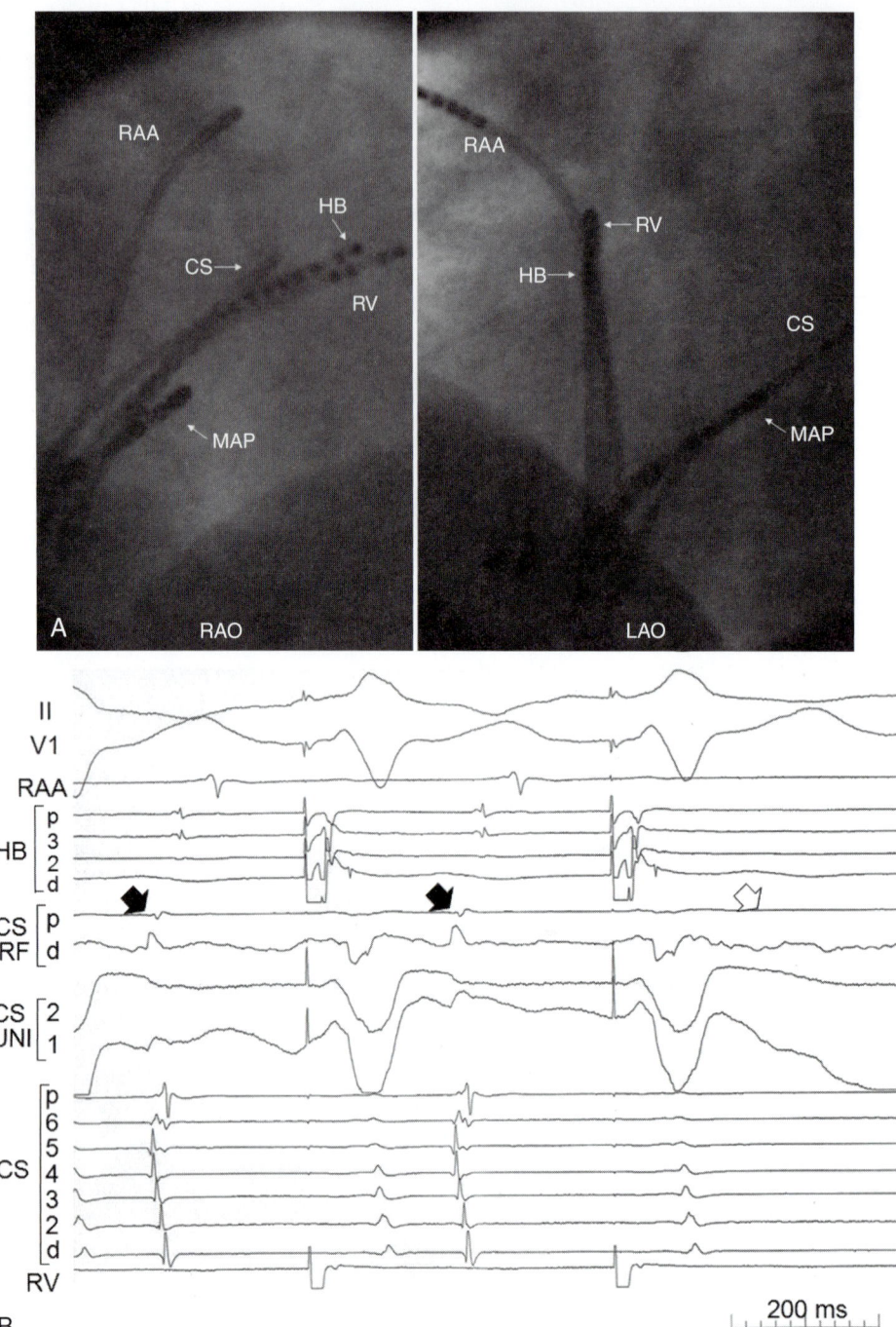

FIGURE 19-23. A, Site of earliest retrograde atrial activation during ventricular pacing in a patient with slow-slow atrioventricular nodal reentrant tachycardia. Radiographs in the right anterior oblique (RAO) and left anterior oblique (LAO) projections show the position of the mapping catheter (MAP) inside the proximal portion of the coronary sinus, about 1.5 cm from the ostium. Multipolar catheters are positioned in the coronary sinus (CS), right atrial appendage (RAA), His bundle (HB), and right ventricle (RV). **B,** Retrograde block of slow atrioventricular (AV) nodal pathway conduction during radiofrequency current ablation. During delivery of radiofrequency current through a catheter in the proximal coronary sinus (CS RF), the first two ventricular paced complexes are followed by retrograde conduction through the slow AV nodal pathway (*filled arrows*). Retrograde block over the slow AV nodal pathway is observed following the third ventricular paced complex (*open arrow*). CS, coronary sinus; d, distal; H, His recording; HB, His bundle; p, proximal; RAA, right atrial appendage; RV, right ventricle; UNI, unipolar.

Left-Sided Variant

Rarely, extensive ablation from the right atrium and CS fails to eliminate slow pathway function. In these patients, the left posterior extension of the AV node may form the slow pathway, and the slow pathway is eliminated by ablation at the posterior mitral annulus (Fig. 19-24).[63,102–104] At these sites, the tachycardia is usually reset by left atrial extrastimuli, indicating proximity to the reentrant circuit. At successful left-sided ablation sites, junctional rhythm is observed, as with ablation of "conventional" slow-fast AVNRT. Successful ablation sites are along the inferior paraseptal aspect of the mitral annulus but can be mid-septal in the left atrium.[63] These sites can be reached from the transseptal or retrograde aortic approaches. The A/V ratio is 1:10 to 1:2 at successful sites, and the average number of left-sided lesions was 9.9 ± 2.0 in one report.[63] Junctional rhythm is induced at successful left-sided ablation sites, as with right-sided slow pathway ablation.

End Points for Ablation

Before ablation, it is necessary to establish end points to be followed for ablation success. Tachycardia inducibility and 1:1 conduction over the slow AV nodal pathway are clear end points. Ablation is considered successful if the tachycardia cannot be reinduced, even during administration of isoproterenol, and 1:1 conduction over the slow AV nodal pathway is eliminated (Table 19-8).[22,75,79] Elimination of 1:1 conduction over the slow AV nodal pathway may be used as surrogate end point in cases of unreliable inducibility at baseline. Not uncommonly, AH interval jumps and slow-fast AV nodal echo beats may still be inducible after successful ablation. These echo beats are most likely the result of conduction over a different slow AV nodal pathway than the one required to sustain AVNRT. *Thus, residual AH jumps with or without single echo beats in the absence of tachycardia inducibility are an end point for ablation.*[105-107] It is important to test for noninducibility in the presence of isoproterenol after ablation even if this agent was not necessary for induction at baseline. Discontinuous AV nodal physiology can be initially demonstrated with programmed atrial stimulation in only 85% of patients in whom this arrhythmia is inducible. By careful documentation of the baseline AV node function curve, even patients with continuous AV conduction patterns can be shown to have loss of the "tail" of the curve, shortening of the maximal achievable AH interval, and prolongation of the 1:1 conduction cycle length, indicating successful slow pathway modification.[108]

Preventing Atrioventricular Block During Catheter Ablation

AV block from slow pathway ablation may occur because of direct injury to the compact AV node or fast pathway, especially if it is inferiorly displaced as an anatomic variant. In addition, damage to the AV nodal artery or preexisting fast pathway dysfunction (intrinsic or from previous ablation) may be unrecognized before slow pathway ablation. In our experience, AV block occurred in 1 (0.2%) of 500 patients during RF current delivered between the mid-portion of the CS ostium and the tricuspid annulus. In this 74-year-old man, a rapid junctional rhythm was induced, associated with retrograde VA block; despite rapid termination of energy application, the patient developed permanent AV block requiring pacemaker implantation. Delayed AV block has been documented despite preserved AV conduction at the end of the procedure.[109,110] Delayed AV block is usually confined to those patients with transient AV block during ablation.

Several strategies have been suggested to minimize the risk for ablation-induced AV block (Table 19-9). The most important method is close attention to retrograde conduction during RF ablation and immediate discontinuation in the event of any VA block. Delivery of RF energy during atrial pacing faster than the junctional rhythm rate allows for continuous assessment of antegrade conduction in cases

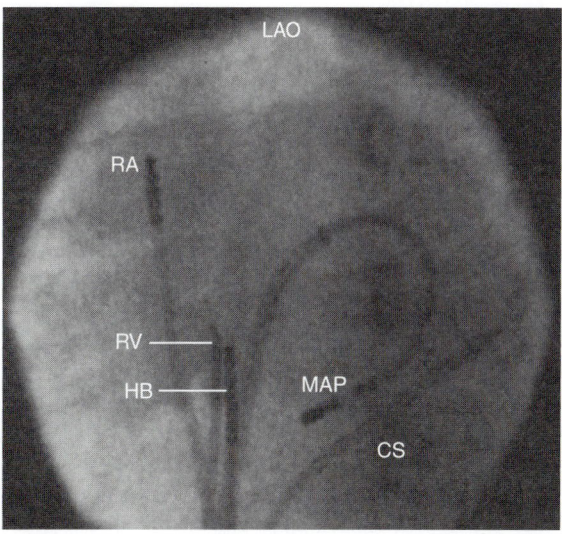

FIGURE 19-24. Catheter position at site of successful ablation in a patient with the left-sided variant of slow-fast AV nodal reentry. Intracardiac tracings and diagnostic maneuvers were consistent with slow-fast AV nodal reentry, but all attempts at ablation of slow pathway conduction from the right atrium and proximal coronary sinus were unsuccessful. Left anterior oblique (LAO) projection. The mapping catheter was introduced into the left atrium through a preformed sheath following transseptal puncture. The catheter was positioned parallel to the mitral annulus with its tip at the inferior paraseptal region. At this ablation site, junctional rhythm occurred, slow pathway function was eliminated, and tachycardia was rendered noninducible. CS, coronary sinus catheter; HB, His bundle catheter; MAP, mapping/ablation catheter; RA, right atrial catheter; RV, right ventricular catheter.

TABLE 19-8
END POINTS FOR RADIOFREQUENCY DELIVERY
Tachycardia rendered noninducible with and without isoproterenol challenge
Elimination or modification of slow pathway function
• Elimination of atrium–His bundle (AH) interval jumps
• Elimination of 1:1 antegrade conduction over the slow atrioventricular (AV) nodal pathway
• Retrograde ventricular-atrial block through the slow AV nodal pathway (fast-slow and slow-slow)
AH interval jump with single echoes only (previously inducible)
Fast pathway injury
PR interval prolongation (persistent)
Transient antegrade AV block after radiofrequency (caution warranted for further ablation)

of doubt. Rapid junctional rhythm (cycle length, <350 milliseconds) has been described as an indicator of impending AV block.[87] AV block is unlikely at sites at or below the middle level of the CS os. The risk for block increases with more superior ablation sites. AV block can occur at more inferior sites or even within the CS. Damage to the AV nodal artery may explain the occurrence of AV block even when applications are delivered far from the compact AV node.[111] Care should be taken to exclude an isorhythmic association of sinus rhythm with a junctional rhythm and VA block.

Sites with time intervals of less than 20 milliseconds between the atrial electrogram on the His bundle recording and the atrial electrogram on the ablation catheter have been

TABLE 19-9

PREVENTING ATRIOVENTRICULAR BLOCK

Method	Description	Comment
Ablation sites *below* triangle of Koch	Inferior to level of CS roof	Standard practice
Monitor retrograde junctional conduction	Discontinue RF for loss of 1:1 retrograde conduction	Standard practice
Monitor for rapid junctional rhythm[87]	Discontinue RF for junctional rhythm < 350 msec	Not prospectively tested
Δ A-A timing His and ablation recordings[112]	Difference timing between AEGM His and AEGM ablation site > 20 msec	Not prospectively tested
Pace mapping triangle of Koch[113]	Identify site on septum producing shortest stimulus to His time and avoid ablation there	Not prospectively tested
Overdrive atrial pacing	Pace atrium faster than junctional rate to monitor antegrade conduction	Not prospectively tested
Gradual power titration[114]	Start at 5 W and increase power by 5 W every 5 sec until junctional rhythm, then increase power by 10 W for total RF 120 sec	Not prospectively tested
Cryoablation	6 or 4 mm tip	Extremely low incidence of AV block

Δ, Difference; A-A, atrial-atrial interval; AEGM, atrial electrogram; AV, atrioventricular; CS, coronary sinus; RF, radiofrequency.

associated with increased risk for AV block.[112] Also, pace-mapping of the triangle of Koch to locate the site of the antegrade fast pathway may reduce the risk for AV block.[113] This practice assumes that the pacing site producing the shortest stimulus to the His electrogram interval represents the site of fast pathway insertion. Pacing is performed at low, mid, and high septal sites. In 10% of patients, the shortest interval is "displaced" into the middle or low septal locations. Ablation is directed as far as possible from mid-septal fast pathway sites. In this report, ablation was not performed at low septal sites showing the shortest stimulus to His interval.[113] The absence of antegrade fast pathway conduction before antegrade slow pathway ablation may result in AV block. The status of fast pathway conduction should be assessed before ablation, particularly in patients with long baseline PR intervals (see later). Prolongation of the AH interval during ablation is an indication of ante-grade fast pathway injury. Gradual energy titration starting with low energy levels is advised.[114] Cryoablation poses the lowest risk for persistent AV block, which at the time of this writing has not been reported in the literature.

Efficacy of Atrioventricular Nodal Modification

The acute success rate for slow pathway ablation for AVNRT is 97% to 100% in large series (Table 19-10). Randomized trials have shown equivalent outcomes using the anatomic and electrogram-guided approaches, although the electrogram-guided approach may have a lower incidence of residual slow pathway function.[84] Postprocedure recurrences of AVNRT are reported in 0.7% to 5.2% of patients. Some studies report that residual slow pathway function is a predictor of recurrence; however, this finding is not consistent.[105–107, 115–118] It is now widely accepted that any incremental benefit of more extensive ablation to eliminate all slow pathway function is offset by a higher risk for inducing AV block.[105] Slow-slow AVNRT may be associated with higher recurrence rates,

often of a different form of AVNRT. The absence of junctional tachycardia during RF application and younger age are associated with higher recurrence rates.[116]

Fast Pathway Ablation

The indications for ablation of retrograde fast pathway conduction are limited to those patients with slow-fast AVNRT in whom antegrade fast pathway function is absent or severely impaired before ablation. In most patients with prolonged preablation PR intervals, slow pathway modification remains effective and carries a low incidence of heart block.[119–124] In patients with complete absence of antegrade fast pathway function, however, slow pathway ablation may result in complete heart block. In this situation, ablation of the retrograde fast pathway function may be attempted (Fig. 19-25).[119] The fast pathway is targeted by positioning the ablation catheter to record a large His electrogram and then withdrawing the catheter toward the atrium to record a large atrial and smaller ventricular electrogram and the smallest His deflection recordable (<0.1 mV)[125,126] Attempts at targeting retrograde fast pathway only may be refined by mapping the site of earliest retrograde atrial activation in this area during AVNRT or ventricular pacing.[119] RF energy is delivered at the target site starting at low energy levels (5 to 10 W). RF delivery is interrupted with an increase in the PR interval or after showing noninducibility of AV nodal reentry.[126]

Ablation of Atrioventricular Nodal Reentry in Patients with Impaired Atrioventricular Conduction

About 3% of patients undergoing ablation for AVNRT have PR prolongation at baseline.[119–124] Patients with delayed conduction or prolonged refractoriness of the fast AV nodal pathway have an increased risk for AV block after ablation of the slow AV nodal pathway. However, several reports have documented a lack of detrimental effect of catheter ablation in such patients despite preexisting abnormal AV conduction (Table 19-11).[119–124] The lack of effect of slow AV nodal

TABLE 19-10

CONTEMPORARY RESULTS FOR RADIOFREQUENCY SLOW PATHWAY ABLATION

Study	No. of Patients	Approach	Acute Success (%)	Recurrence Rate (%)	AV Block (%)	Complication Rate (%)	Comments
Gonzalez (unpublished data)	500	Combined anatomic and electrogram guided	100	1.5	0.2	0.2, AV block; 0.4, pulmonary embolism	
Topilski et al, 2006[128]	901	Anatomic	97	2.8	3.4 transient AV block; 0.8 permanent AV block (pacemaker)	4, AV block (2 with pericardial effusion)	2 catheter (single diagnostic and ablation) approach used in 65% of patients
Kihel et al, 2006[129]	276	Combined anatomic and electrogram guided	99.6	0.7	0	1.8, pericardial effusion and pulmonary embolus	Same results <75 and >75 years old
Rostock et al, 2005[130]	578	? Anatomic	100	2.5	0.7 all PPM	Only AV block reported	Same results <75 and >75 years old
McElderry & Kay, 2006[79]	2333	Anatomic	99	1.7	0.2	0.5, AV block (3 with pericardial tamponade)	3 AV block in last 2283 patients
Estner et al, 2005[116]	506	Combined anatomic and electrogram guided	98.8	5.2	3, with 1.4 PPM	Only AV block	Younger age only risk for recurrence
Efremidis et al, 2009[84]	228	Randomized to anatomic or electrogram guided	100, both approaches	1.7, both approaches	0.9 AV block, both approaches	Only AV block	Prospective randomized trial

AV, atrioventricular; PPM, permanent pacemaker.

pathway ablation despite an abnormal fast AV nodal pathway may be explained by several factors. One possibility is that, in these patients, the left atrial (mitral annulus) input preserves AV nodal conduction despite damage to the right-sided inputs.[9] Another possibility is that, before ablation, conduction through the posterior inputs (slow AV nodal pathway) prolongs the refractory period of the anterior input (fast AV nodal pathway) because of concealed retrograde conduction of the fast pathway, the so-called linking phenomenon.[127] Nevertheless, acute AV block may occur in up to 33% of patients without evidence of dual AV nodal physiology at baseline.[119] Late AV block has been documented in 12% of patients with baseline PR prolongation.[122] It has been suggested that patients with evidence of only antegrade slow pathway conduction at baseline undergo an attempt at selective retrograde fast pathway ablation (see earlier).[119] This approach was associated with persistent intraprocedural AV block in 1 of 10 patients; however, there was no late AV block reported. In contrast, slow pathway ablation was associated with a 3% incidence of acute AV block but a 36% incidence of late AV block in patients with dual AV nodal physiology at baseline.[119] Of note, all patients progressing to late AV block had complete ablation of slow pathway function. Patients with PR prolongation before ablation should be considered at increased risk for acute or late AV block. The clinical circumstances should justify this risk, and the patient should be informed accordingly.

Complications

Complications are relatively uncommon during ablation for AVNRT (Table 19-10). Heart block represents the greatest risk and is reported to occur in 0% to 3.4% of patients (Table 19-10). The risk for requiring permanent pacemaker implantation is less than 1% in these same series. The risk for acute heart block is increased in those with absent antegrade fast pathway function, ablation superior to the CS os, greater numbers of delivered RF lesions, and junctional rhythm with retrograde block. Late heart block is greatest in patients with transient AV block during the procedure and in those with baseline PR prolongation who undergo complete slow pathway ablation. Vascular injury and pericardial tamponade may occur infrequently.

Troubleshooting the Difficult Case

As previously stated, before proceeding to ablation, the operator should be confident of the diagnosis of AVNRT. This requires eliminating as a possibility orthodromic reentrant tachycardia and atrial tachycardia with 1:1 AV conduction. Most cases of AVNRT can be successfully eliminated by delivering RF energy between the tricuspid valve annulus and the CS ostium. Securing good catheter contact is extremely important to modify conduction over

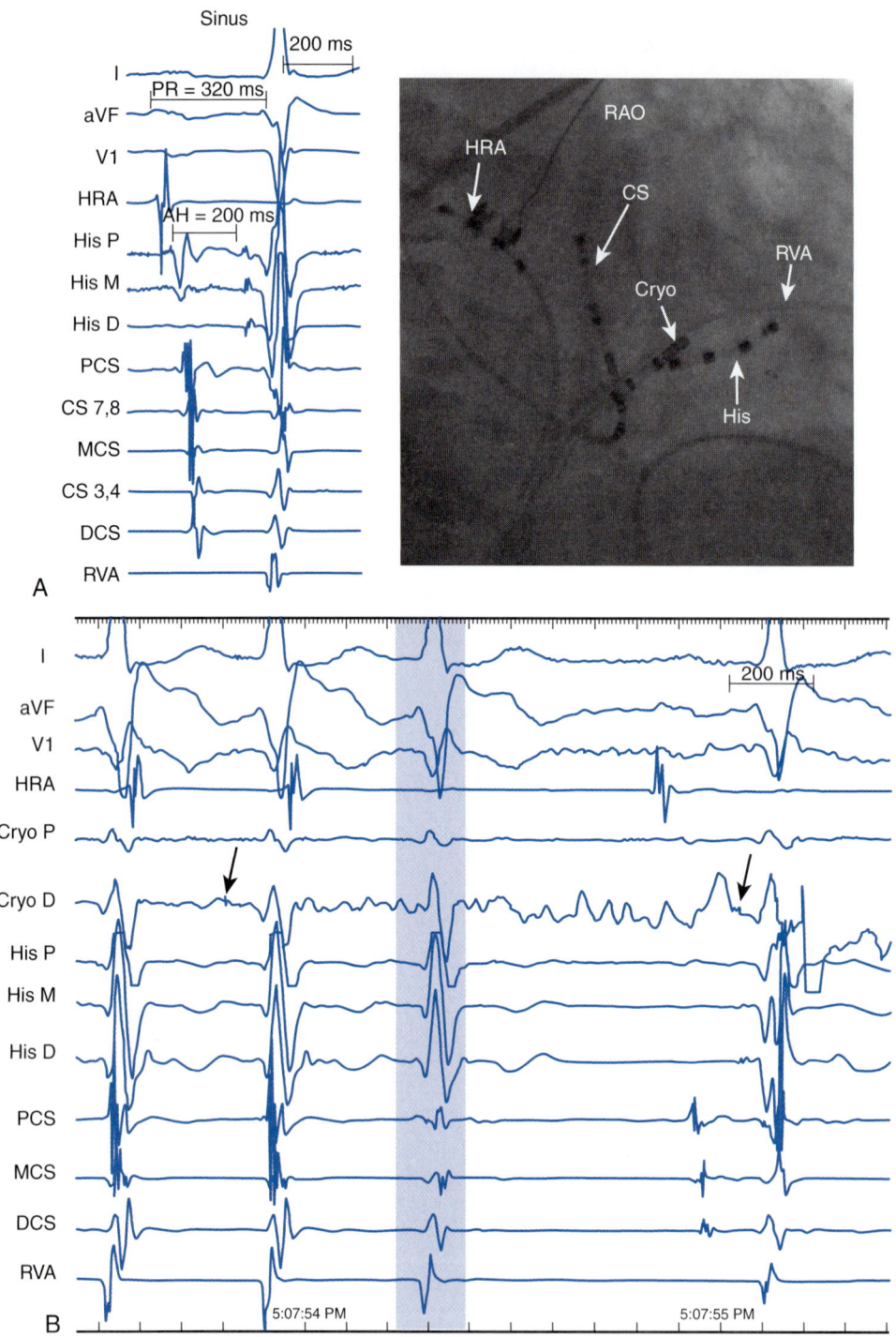

FIGURE 19-25. Retrograde fast pathway ablation with cryoenergy in an elderly patient with slow-fast atrioventricular (AV) nodal reentry and prolonged PR interval at baseline. **A,** The surface and intracardiac recordings are shown in the *left panel*. The PR interval is 320 msec, with an atrium–His bundle (AH) interval of 200 msec, suggestive of slow pathway conduction. No dual antegrade AV nodal physiology could be demonstrated. The *right panel* shows a 4-mm-tip cryoablation catheter (Cryo) positioned in the fast pathway area in a right anterior oblique (RAO) view. CS, coronary sinus; D, distal; HRA, high right atrium; M, mid; P, proximal; RA, right ventricular apex. **B,** Intracardiac recordings during cryoablation at the catheter position shown in **A**. During slow-fast AV nodal reentry, there is tachycardia termination with failure of retrograde fast pathway conduction in the third cardiac cycle (*blue highlight*). The next cycle consists of a sinus beat with AV conduction times as at baseline. The *arrows* show the His potential when discernible through the ablation catheter ice artifact. AV nodal reentry was noninducible, and antegrade AV conduction was unchanged. Cryo, cryoablation catheter; CS, coronary sinus; D, distal; His, His bundle catheter; HRA, high right atrium; M, mid; P, proximal; RVA, right ventricular apex.

the slow AV nodal pathway. When ablation at these sites is unsuccessful, alternative sites of ablation should be considered. Ablation within the proximal CS can be particularly beneficial when application of RF current in the usual position between the tricuspid annulus and the CS ostium does not result in an accelerated junctional rhythm. Only

after failing to eliminate slow pathway conduction at these sites do we consider ablation in the inferior portion of the mitral annulus and more rarely higher in the triangle of Koch. Ablation above the superior edge of the CS ostium is associated with an increased risk for AV block (Table 19-12). Induction of AV nodal reentry is infrequently a

TABLE 19-11

ABLATION FOR ATRIOVENTRICULAR NODAL REENTRANT TACHYCARDIA WITH PRE-EXISTING PR PROLONGATION

Study	No. of Subjects	Ablation Approach	Baseline PR Interval (msec)	Acute AVB (%)	Late AVB	Comments
Reithmman et al, 2006[119]	43	Retrograde FP ablation without DANP ($n = 10$)	289 ± 66	10	0 (61 ± 39 mo)	3 sudden deaths late after SP ablation as well
		SP ablation with DANP ($n = 33$)	239 ± 31	33	12 (37 ± 25 mo)	
Sra et al, 1994[121]	7	SP	210-290	0	0 (20 ± 6 mo)	PR and WBCL unchanged
Natale et al, 1997[123]	7	SP	230-300	0	0 (3 mo)	Anterior ablation sites required
Pasquie et al, 2006[120]	10	SP	222 ± 15	20, transient AVB (<5 min)	0 (39 ± 21 mo)	In 1 patient, PR increased from 220 to 320 msec
Basta et al, 1997[124]	18	SP	FP ERP > 500 msec baseline	22, transient AVB (<5 min)	0 (18 ± 11 mo)	Only 2 patients with FP function before ablation
Li et al, 2001[122]	18	SP	235 ± 28	0	33	Late heart block more common after complete SP ablation
Reithmann et al, 1998[131]	5	Retrograde FP	53	0	0	PR increased to 276 $\pm$ 48

AVB, atrioventricular block; DANP, dual AV nodal physiology; ERP, effective refractory period ; FP, fast pathway; WBCL, Wenckebach cycle length.

TABLE 19-12

TROUBLESHOOTING THE DIFFICULT CASE

Problem	Causes	Solution
Difficult to induce AVNRT	Retrograde fast AV nodal pathway block due to catheter manipulation	Avoid catheter contact with the fast AV nodal region
	Increased vagal tone due to sedation	Administer isoproterenol and/or atropine
	Similar fast and slow pathway refractoriness	Atrial burst pacing, programmed atrial and ventricular stimulation, isoproterenol, atropine
Poor catheter stability	Prominent eustachian ridge	Use long sheath with septal angulation, apply clockwise torque, create compound angle sheath anteriorly and catheter posteriorly
Prolonged AH interval before ablation	Absence or prolonged conduction over fast pathway	Ablate retrograde fast pathway (slow-fast variant), cryoablation of slow pathway (reversible), advise patient of risk for AV block
No junctional rhythm during ablation	Poor catheter contact	Use long/adjustable/angled sheath or long-reach catheter, assess for slow pathway function (possible ablation without junctional rhythm)
	Unusual slow pathway location	Ablate below CS, in proximal CS, above CS (risk for AV block) or left atrium
Change to different form of AVNRT	Multiple slow pathways	May require ablation of retrograde slow pathway function, ablate both rightward and leftward inferior extensions
VA block during junctional rhythm	Ablation near compact AV node, AV nodal artery, or anomalous fast pathway location	Ablate inferiorly, start very low energy or use cryoablation, map ablation stimulus to His time or His AEGM to ablation AEGM times
	Slow-slow variant (absent retrograde fast pathway function)	Confirm variant, ablation during atrial pacing
Nonspecific end points	Poorly inducible tachycardia	Assess for modification of slow pathway function, AV nodal conduction curves after junctional rhythm
	Absence of dual AV nodal physiology	Monitor for junctional rhythm and inducibility, assess for alteration AV and VA conduction properties

AEGM, atrium electrogram; AH, atrium–His bundle; AV, atrioventricular; AVNRT, atrioventricular nodal reentry tachycardia; CS, coronary sinus; VA, ventricular-atrial.

problem. AV nodal reentry is usually greatly influenced by autonomic tone. Reduced sedation, hyperventilation, isoproterenol, and atropine may facilitate induction. Catheter stability is sometimes problematic but is usually remedied by the use of a long sheath with slight septal angulation. The use of a catheter with adequate "reach" adds to catheter stability. At times, a large eustachian ridge may prevent the ablation catheter from achieving a septal position. In this case, turning the angled sheath anteriorly and then directing the catheter posteriorly allows the catheter to negotiate around the obstacle. If no junctional rhythm is apparent with RF ablation between the tricuspid annulus and the CS ostium, mapping of the proximal CS may identify slow pathway potentials and provide successful ablation. As noted earlier, patients with absent or poor antegrade fast pathway function are at risk for heart block after slow pathway ablation. The status of the antegrade fast pathway should be documented before ablation. If fast pathway function is poor and the decision is to proceed with ablation, AV conduction must be closely monitored during ablation. Cryoablation is probably safer than RF ablation in these patients. A summary of common problems encountered during ablation of AVNRT and possible solutions is given in Table 19-12.

References

1. Wu D, Denes P, Amat-Y-Leon F, et al. Clinical, electrocardiographic and electrophysiologic observations in patients with paroxysmal supraventricular tachycardia. *Am J Cardiol.* 1978;41:1045–1051.
2. Porter MJ, Morton JB, Denman R, et al. Influence of age and gender on the mechanism of supraventricular tachycardia. *Heart Rhythm.* 2004;1:393–396.
3. Gursoy S, Steurer G, Brugada J, et al. Brief report: the hemodynamic mechanism of pounding in the neck in atrioventricular nodal reentrant tachycardia. *N Engl J Med.* 1992;327:772–774.
4. Morady F. Catheter ablation of supraventricular arrhythmias: state of the art. *Pacing Clin Electrophysiol.* 2004;27:125–142.
5. Blomstrom-Lundqvist C, Scheinman MM, Aliot EM, et al. ACC/AHA/ESC guidelines for the management of patients with supraventricular arrhythmias: executive summary. *J Am Coll Cardiol.* 2003;42:1493–1531.
6. Tawara S. *The Conduction System in the Mammalian Heart: An Anatomico-histological Study of the Atrioventricular Bundle and the Purkinje Fibers.* Jena, Germany: Verlag Von Gustav Fischer; 1906:3–7.
7. Aschoff L. Referay uber die Herzstorungen in ihren Beziehungen zu den spezifischen Muskelsystem des Herzens. *Verh Dtsch Pathol Ges.* 1910;14:3–35.
8. Monckeberg JG. Beitrage zur normalen und pathologischen Anatomie des Herzens. *Verh Dtsch Pathol Ges.* 1910;14:64–71.
9. Gonzalez MD, Contreras LJ, Cardona F, et al. Demonstration of a left atrial input to the atrioventricular node in humans. *Circulation.* 2002;106:2930–2934.
10. Yanni J, Boyett MR, Anderson RH, Dobrzynski H. The extent of the specialized atrioventricular ring tissues. *Heart Rhythm.* 2009;6:672–680.
11. Bharati S. Anatomic-morphologic relations between AV nodal structure and function in the normal and diseased heart. In: Mazgalev TN, Tchou PJ, eds. *Atrial AV Nodal Physiology: A View from the Millennium.* Futura: Armonk, NY; 2000:25–28.
12. Arid JM, Armstrong O, Rogez JM, et al. Arterial vascularisation of the atrioventricular node. *Surg Radiol Anat.* 2000;22:93–96.
13. Gaskell WH. On the innervation of the heart, with especial reference to the heart of the tortoise. *J Physiol.* 1883;4:43–127.
14. His W Jr. Die Thätigkeit des embryonalen Herzens und deren Bedeutung für die Lehre von der Herzbewegung beim Erwachsenen. *Arb Med Klin Leipzig.* 1893;1:14–49.
15. Tawara S. *The Conduction System in the Mammalian Heart: An Anatomico-histological Study of the Atrioventricular Bundle and the Purkinje Fibers.* Jena, Germany: Verlag Von Gustav Fischer; 1906.
16. Mines GR. On dynamic equilibrium of the heart. *J Physiol.* 1913;46:349–382.
17. Moe GK, Preston JB, Burlington H. Physiologic evidence for a dual A-V transmission system. *Circ Res.* 1956;4:357–375.
18. Mendez C, Moe GK. Demonstration of a dual AV nodal conduction system in the isolated rabbit heart. *Circ Res.* 1966;19:378–393.
19. Denes P, Wu D, Dhingra RC, et al. Demonstration of dual A-V nodal pathways in patients with paroxysmal supraventricular tachycardia. *Circulation.* 1973;48:549–555.
20. Denes P, Wu D, Dhingra R, et al. Dual atrioventricular nodal pathways: a common electrophysiological response. *Br Heart J.* 1975;37:1069–1076.
21. Hazlitt HA, Beckman KJ, McClelland JH, et al. Prevalence of slow AV nodal pathway potentials in patients without AV nodal reentrant tachycardia [abstract]. *J Am Coll Cardiol.* 1993;21:281A.
22. Lockwood D, Otomo K, Wang Z, et al. Electrophysiologic characteristics of atrioventricular nodal reentrant tachycardia: implications for the reentrant circuits. In: Zipes DP, Jalife J, eds. *Cardiac Electrophysiology: From Cell to Bedside.* Philadelphia: Saunders; 2004:537–557.
23. Josephson ME. Supraventricular tachycardias. In: *Clinical Cardiac Electrophysiology.* 4th ed. Philadelphia: Wolters Kluwer/Lippincott Williams & Wilkins; 2008:175–284.
24. Lo HM, Lin FY, Cheng JJ, Tseng YZ. Anatomic substrate of the experimentally created atrioventricular node re-entrant tachycardia in the dog. *Int J Cardiol.* 1995;51:273–284.
25. Okumura Y, Watanabe I, Yamada T, et al. Comparison of coronary sinus morphology in patients with and without atrioventricular nodal reentrant tachycardia by intracardiac echocardiography. *J Cardiovasc Electrophysiol.* 2004;15:269–273.
26. Ong MG, Lee PC, Tai CT, et al. Coronary sinus morphology in different types of supraventricular tachycardias. *J Interv Card Electrophysiol.* 2006;15:21–26.
27. Topilski I, Glick A, Viskin S, Belhassen B. Frequency of spontaneous and inducible atrioventricular nodal reentry tachycardia in patients with idiopathic outflow tract ventricular arrhythmias. *Pacing Clin Electrophysiol.* 2006;29:21–28.
28. Wylie JV Jr, Milliez P, Germano JJ, et al. Atrioventricular nodal reentrant tachycardia associated with idiopathic ventricular tachycardia: clinical and electrophysiologic characteristics. *J Electrocardiol.* 2007;40:94–99.
29. Hayes JJ, Sharma PP, Smith PN, Vidaillet HJ. Familial atrioventricular nodal reentry tachycardia. *Pacing Clin Electrophysiol.* 2004;27:73–76.
30. Mignone RJ, Wallace AG. Ventricular echoes: evidence for dissociation of conduction and reentry within the AV node. *Circ Res.* 1996;19:638–649.
31. Josephson ME, Kastor JA. Paroxysmal supraventricular tachycardia: is the atrium a necessary link? *Circulation.* 1976;54:430–435.
32. Loh P, de Bakker JMT, Hocini M, et al. Reentrant pathway during ventricular echoes is confined to the atrioventricular node: high-resolution mapping and dissection of the triangle of Koch in isolated, perfused canine heart. *Circulation.* 1999;100:1346–1353.
33. Gonzalez MD, Contreras L, Cardona F, et al. V-A block during atrioventricular nodal reentrant tachycardia: reentry confined to the AV node. *Pacing Clin Electrophysiol.* 2003;26:775–778.
34. Morihisa K, Yamabe H, Uemura T, et al. Analysis of atrioventricular nodal reentrant tachycardia with variable ventriculoatrial block: characteristics of the upper common pathway. *Pacing Clin Electrophysiol.* 2009;32:484–493.
35. Sung RJ, Waxman HL, Saksena S, et al. Sequence of retrograde atrial activation in patients with dual atrioventricular nodal pathways. *Circulation.* 1981;64:1059–1067.
36. Haïssaguerre M, Warin JF, Lemetayer P, et al. Closed chest ablation of retrograde conduction in patients with atrioventricular nodal reentrant tachycardia. *N Engl J Med.* 1989;320:426–433.
37. Epstein LM, Scheinman MM, Langberg JJ, et al. Percutaneous catheter modification of the atrioventricular node: a potential cure for atrioventricular nodal reentrant tachycardia. *Circulation.* 1989;80:757–768.
38. Jazayeri MH, Hempe SL, Sra JS, et al. Selective transcatheter ablation of the fast and slow pathways using radiofrequency energy in patients with atrioventricular nodal reentrant tachycardia. *Circulation.* 1992;85:1318–1328.
39. Haïssaguerre M, Gaita F, Fisher B, et al. Elimination of atrioventricular nodal reentrant tachycardia using discrete slow potentials to guide application of radiofrequency energy. *Circulation.* 1992;85:2162–2175.
40. Ross DL, Johnson DC, Denniss AR, et al. Curative surgery of atrioventricular junctional ("AV nodal") reentrant tachycardia. *J Am Coll Cardiol.* 1985;6:1383–1392.
41. Jackman WM, Beckman KJ, McClelland JH, et al. Treatment of supraventricular tachycardia due to atrioventricular nodal reentry by radiofrequency catheter ablation of slow pathway conduction. *N Engl J Med.* 1992;327:313–318.
42. Becker AE, Anderson RH. Morphology of the human atrioventricular junctional area. In: Wellens HJJ, Lie KI, Janse MJ, eds. *The Conduction System of the Heart: Structure, Function, and Clinical Implications.* Leiden, Germany: HE Stenfert Kroese BV; 1976:263–286.
43. Inoue S, Becker AE. Posterior extensions of the human compact atrioventricular node: a neglected anatomic feature of potential clinical significance. *Circulation.* 1998;97:188–193.
44. Yamabe H, Shimasaki Y, Honda O, et al. Demonstration of the exact anatomic tachycardia circuit in the fast-slow atrioventricular nodal tachycardia. *Circulation.* 2001;104:1268–1273.
45. Katritsis DG, Ellenbogen KA, Becker AE, Camm AJ. Retrograde slow pathway conduction in patients with atrioventricular nodal re-entrant tachycardia. *Europace.* 2007;9:458–465.
46. Kose S, Amasyali B, Aytemir K, et al. Ventriculatrial block during atrioventricular nodal reentrant tachycardia suggesting existence of an upper common pathway. *Int Heart J.* 2005;46:333–338.
47. Otomo K, Okamura H, Noda T, et al. Unique electrophysiologic characteristics of atrioventricular nodal reentrant tachycardia with different ventriculoatrial block patterns: effects of slow pathway ablation and insights into the location of the reentrant circuit. *Heart Rhythm.* 2006;3:544–554.
48. Patterson E, Scherlag BJ. Longitudinal dissociation within the posterior AV nodal input of the rabbit. *Circulation.* 1999;99:143–155.

49. Gonzalez MD, Scherlag BJ, Mabo P, Lazzara R. Functional dissociation of cellular activation as a mechanism of Mobitz type II atrioventricular block. *Circulation.* 1993;87:1389–1398.

50. Kuo C-T, Lin K-H, Cheng N-J, et al. Characterization of atrioventricular nodal reentry with continuous atrioventricular node conduction curve by double atrial extrastimulation. *Circulation.* 1999;99:659–665.

51. Yu W-C, Chen S-A, Chiang C-E, et al. Effects of isoproterenol in facilitation induction of slow-fast atrioventricular nodal reentrant tachycardia. *Am J Cardiol.* 1996;78:1299–1302.

52. Hwang C, Martin D, Goodman J, et al. Atypical atrioventricular node reciprocating tachycardia masquerading as tachycardia using a left-sided accessory pathway. *J Am Coll Cardiol.* 1997;30:218–225.

53. Miller JM, Rosenthal ME, Gottlieb CD, et al. Usefulness of the ΔHA interval to accurately distinguish atrio-ventricular nodal reentry from orthodromic septal bypass tract tachycardias. *Am J Cardiol.* 1991;68:1037–1044.

54. Michaud GF, Tada H, Chough S, et al. Differentiation of atypical atrioventricular node re-entrant tachycardia from orthodromic reciprocating tachycardia using a septal accessory pathway by the response to ventricular pacing. *J Am Coll Cardiol.* 2001;38:1163–1167.

55. Knight BP, Zivin A, Souza J, et al. A technique for the rapid diagnosis of atrial tachycardia in the electrophysiology laboratory. *J Am Coll Cardiol.* 1999;33:775–778.

56. Knight BP, Ebinger M, Oral H, et al. Diagnostic value of tachycardia features and pacing maneuvers during paroxysmal supraventricular tachycardia. *J Am Coll Cardiol.* 2000;36:574–582.

57. Gonzalez-Torrecilla E, Arenal A, Atienza F, et al. First postpacing interval after tachycardia entrainment with correction for atrioventricular node delay: a simple maneuver for differential diagnosis of atrioventricular nodal reentrant tachycardias versus orthodromic reciprocating tachycardias. *Heart Rhythm.* 2006;3:674–679.

58. Waldo AL, Maclean AH, Karp RB, et al. Sequence of retrograde atrial activation of the human heart: correlation with P wave polarity. *Br Heart J.* 1977;39:634–640.

59. Tai CT, Chen SA, Chiang CE, et al. Multiple anterograde atrioventricular node pathways in patients with atrioventricular node reentrant tachycardia. *J Am Coll Cardiol.* 1996;28:725–731.

60. Heidbuchel H, Jackman WM. Characterization of subforms of AV nodal reentrant tachycardia. *Europace.* 2004;4:316–329.

61. Lee PC, Hwang B, Tai CT, et al. The electrophysiological characteristics in patients with ventricular stimulation inducible fast-slow form atrioventricular nodal reentrant tachycardia. *Pacing Clin Electrophysiol.* 2006;29:1105–1111.

62. Man KC, Niebauer M, Daoud E, et al. Comparison of atrial-His intervals during tachycardia and atrial pacing in patients with long RP tachycardia. *J Cardiovasc Electrophysiol.* 1995;6:700–710.

63. Kilic A, Amasyali B, Kose S, et al. Atrioventricular nodal reentrant tachycardia ablated from left atrial septum: clinical and electrophysiological characteristics and long-term follow-up results as compared to conventional right-sided ablation. *Int Heart J.* 2005;46:1023–1031.

64. Hirao K, Otomo K, Wang X, et al. Para-Hisian pacing: a new method for differentiating retrograde conduction over an accessory AV pathway from conduction over the AV node. *Circulation.* 1996;94:1027–1035.

65. Vijayaraman P, Lee BP, Kalahasty G, et al. Reanalysis of the "pseudo A-A-V" response to ventricular entrainment of supraventricular tachycardia: importance of His-bundle timing. *J Cardiovasc Electrophysiol.* 2006;17:25–28.

66. Padanilam BJ, Manfredi JA, Steinberg LA, et al. Differentiating junctional tachycardia and atrioventricular node re-entry tachycardia based on response to atrial extrastimulus pacing. *J Am Coll Cardiol.* 2008;52:1711–1717.

67. Srivathsan K, Gami AS, Barrett R, et al. Differentiating atrioventricular nodal reentrant tachycardia from junctional tachycardia: novel application of the delta H-A interval. *J Cardiovasc Electrophysiol.* 2008;19:1–6.

68. Otomo K, Nagata Y, Uno K, et al. Irregular atypical atrioventricular nodal reentrant tachycardia: incidence, electrophysiological characteristics, and effects of slow pathway ablation. *Heart Rhythm.* 2007;4:1507–1522.

69. Dixit S, Callans DJ, Gerstenfeld EP, Marchlinski FE. Reentrant and nonreentrant forms of atrioventricular nodal tachycardia mimicking atrial fibrillation. *J Cardiovasc Electrophysiol.* 2006;17:312–316.

70. Vijayaraman P, Alaeddini J, Storm R, et al. Slow atrioventricular nodal reentrant arrhythmias: clinical recognition, electrophysiological characteristics, and response to radiofrequency ablation. *J Cardiovasc Electrophysiol.* 2007;18:950–953.

71. Gonzalez MD, Contreras LJ, Jongbloed MRM, et al. Left atrial tachycardia originating from the mitral annulus-aorta junction. *Circulation.* 2004;110:3187–3192.

72. Sauer WH, Alonso C, Zado E, et al. Atrioventricular nodal reentrant tachycardia in patients referred for atrial fibrillation ablation: response to ablation that incorporates slow-pathway modification. *Circulation.* 2006;114:191–195.

73. Katritsis DG, Giazitzoglou E, Wood MA, et al. Inducible supraventricular tachycardias in patients referred for catheter ablation of atrial fibrillation. *Europace.* 2007;9:785–789.

74. Chang SL, Tai CT, Lin YJ, et al. Electrophysiological characteristics and catheter ablation in patients with paroxysmal supraventricular tachycardia and paroxysmal atrial fibrillation. *J Cardiovasc Electrophysiol.* 2008;19:367–373.

75. Kay GN, Epstein AE, Dailey SM, Plumb VJ. Selective radiofrequency ablation of the slow pathway for the treatment of atrioventricular nodal reentrant tachycardia: evidence for involvement of perinodal myocardium within the reentrant circuit. *Circulation.* 1992;85:1675–1688.

76. Moulton K, Miller B, Scott J, Woods WT. Radiofrequency ablation for AV nodal reentry: a technique for rapid transaction of the slow AV nodal pathway. *Pacing Clin Electrophysiol.* 1993;16:760–768.

77. Wathen M, Natale A, Wolfe K, et al. An anatomically guided approach to atrioventricular node slow pathway ablation. *Am J Cardiol.* 1992;70:886–889.

78. Wu D, Yeh S-J, Wang C-C, et al. A simple technique for selective radiofrequency ablation of the slow pathway in atrioventricular node reentrant tachycardia. *J Am Coll Cardiol.* 1993;21:1612–1621.

79. McElderry HT, Kay GN. Ablation of atrioventricular nodal reentry by the anatomic approach. In: Huang SKS, Wood MA, eds. *Catheter Ablation of Cardiac Arrhythmias.* Philadelphia: Saunders; 2006:325–346.

80. Skanes AC, Dubuc M, Klein GJ, et al. Cryothermal ablation of the slow pathway for the elimination of atrioventricular nodal reentrant tachycardia. *Circulation.* 2000;102:2856–2860.

81. Jensen-Urstad M, Tabrizi F, Kennebäck G, et al. High success rate with cryo-mapping and cryoablation of atrioventricular nodal reentry tachycardia. *Pacing Clin Electrophysiol.* 2006;29:487–489.

82. McGuire MA, Bourke JP, Robotin MC, et al. High resolution mapping of Koch's triangle using sixty electrodes in humans with atrioventricular junctional ("AV nodal") reentrant tachycardia. *Circulation.* 1993;88:2315–2328.

83. de Bakker JMT, Coronel L, McGuire MA, et al. Slow potentials in the atrioventricular junctional area of patients operated for atrioventricular nodal tachycardias and in isolated porcine hearts. *J Am Coll Cardiol.* 1994;23:709–715.

84. Efremidis M, Sideris A, Letsas KP, et al. Potential-guided versus anatomic-guided approach for slow pathway ablation of the common type atrioventricular nodal reentry tachycardia: a randomized study. *Acta Cardiol.* 2009;64:477–483.

85. Wagshal AB, Crystal E, Katz A. Patterns of accelerated junctional rhythm during slow pathway catheter ablation for atrioventricular nodal tachycardia: temperature dependence, prognostic value, and insights into the nature of the slow pathway. *J Cardiovasc Electrophysiol.* 2000;11:244–254.

86. McGavigan AD, Rae AP, Cobbe SM, Rankin AC. Junctional rhythm: a suitable surrogate endpoint in catheter ablation of atrioventricular nodal reentry tachycardia? *Pacing Clin Electrophysiol.* 2005;28:1052–1054.

87. Thakur RK, Klein GJ, Yee R. Junctional tachycardia: a useful marker during radiofrequency ablation for AV node reentrant tachycardia. *J Am Coll Cardiol.* 1993;22:1706–1710.

88. Jentzer J, Goyal R, Williamson B, et al. Analysis of junctional ectopy during radiofrequency ablation of the slow pathway in patients with atrioventricular node reentrant tachycardia. *Circulation.* 1994;90:2820–2826.

89. Hsieh MH, Chen SA, Tai CT, et al. Absence of junctional rhythm during successful slow-pathway ablation in patients with atrioventricular nodal reentrant tachycardia. *Circulation.* 1998;98:2296–2300.

90. Dubuc M, Guerra PG, Novak P, et al. Cryoablation outcomes for AV nodal reentrant tachycardia comparing 4-mm versus 6-mm electrode-tip catheters. *Heart Rhythm.* 2008;5:230–234.

91. Avari JN, Jay KS, Rhee EK. Experience and results during transition from radiofrequency ablation to cryoablation for treatment of pediatric atrioventricular nodal reentrant tachycardia. *Pacing Clin Electrophysiol.* 2008;31:454–460.

92. Chan NY, Mok NS, Lau CL, et al. Treatment of atrioventricular nodal reentrant tachycardia by cryoablation with a 6 mm-tip catheter vs. radiofrequency ablation. *Europace.* 2009;11:1065–1070.

93. De Sisti A, Tonet J, Barakett N, et al. Transvenous cryo-ablation of the slow pathway for the treatment of atrioventricular nodal re-entrant tachycardia: a single-centre initial experience study. *Europace.* 2007;9:401–406.

94. Papez AL, Al-Ahdab M, Dick M 2nd, Fischbach PS. Transcatheter cryotherapy for the treatment of supraventricular tachyarrhythmias in children: a single center experience. *J Interv Card Electrophysiol.* 2006;15:191–196.

95. Kimman GP, Theuns DA, Szili-Torok T, et al. CRAVT: A prospective, randomized study comparing transvenous cryothermal and radiofrequency ablation in atrioventricular nodal re-entrant tachycardia. *Eur Heart J.* 2004;25:2232–2237.

96. Kriebel T, Broistedt C, Kroll M, et al. Efficacy and safety of cryoenergy in the ablation of atrioventricular reentrant tachycardia substrates in children and adolescents. *J Cardiovasc Electrophysiol.* 2005;16:960–966.

97. Gaita F, Montefusco A, Riccardi R, et al. Acute and long-term outcome of transvenous cryothermal catheter ablation of supraventricular arrhythmias involving the perinodal region. *J Cardiovasc Med.* 2006;7:785–792.

98. Khairy P, Novak PG, Guerra PG, et al. Cryothermal slow pathway modification for atrioventricular nodal reentrant tachycardia. *Europace.* 2007;9:909–914.

99. Sandilands A, Boreham P, Pitts-Crick J, Cripps T. Impact of cryoablation catheter size on success rates in the treatment of atrioventricular nodal re-entry tachycardia in 160 patients with long-term follow-up. *Europace.* 2008;10:683–686.

100. Chanani NK, Chiesa NA, Dubin AM, et al. Cryoablation for atrioventricular nodal reentrant tachycardia in young patients: predictors of recurrence. *Pacing Clin Electrophysiol.* 2008;31:1152–1159.

101. Wang Z, Otomo K, Shah N, et al. Slow/slow and fast/slow atrioventricular nodal reentrant tachycardia use anatomically separate retrograde slow pathways [abstract]. *Circulation.* 1999;100:I-65.

102. Jais P, Haïssaguerre M, Shah DC, et al. Successful radiofrequency ablation of a slow atrioventricular nodal pathway on the left posterior atrial septum. *Pacing Clin Electrophysiol.* 1999;22:525–527.

103. Altemose GT, Scott LR, Miller JM. Atrioventricular nodal reentrant tachycardia requiring ablation on the mitral annulus. *J Cardiovasc Electrophysiol.* 2000;11:1281–1284.

104. Sorbera C, Cohen M, Wolf P, et al. Atrioventricular nodal reentry tachycardia: slow pathway ablation using the transseptal approach. *Pacing Clin Electrophysiol.* 2000;23:1343–1349.

105. Lindsay BD, Chung MK, Gamache MC, et al. Therapeutic end points for the treatment of atrioventricular node reentrant tachycardia by catheter-guided radiofrequency current. *J Am Coll Cardiol.* 1993;22:733–740.

106. Hummel JD, Strickberger SA, Williamson BD, et al. Effect of residual slow pathway function on the time course of recurrences of atrioventricular nodal reentrant tachycardia after radiofrequency ablation of the slow pathway. *Am J Cardiol.* 1995;75:628–630.

107. Manolis AS, Wang PJ, Estes NA 3rd. Radiofrequency ablation of slow pathway in patients with atrioventricular nodal reentrant tachycardia: do arrhythmia recurrences correlate with persistent slow pathway conduction or site of successful ablation? *Circulation.* 1994;90:2815–2819.

108. Sheahan RG, Klein GJ, Yee R, et al. Atrioventricular node reentry with "smooth" AV node function curves: a different arrhythmia substrate? *Circulation.* 1996;93:969–972.

109. Gaita F, Riccardi R, Calo L. Importance and implications of the occurrence of AV block following radiofrequency ablation. *Heart.* 1998;79:534–535.

110. Elhag O, Miller HC. Atrioventricular block occurring several months after radiofrequency ablation for the treatment of atrioventricular nodal reentrant tachycardia: a report of two cases. *Heart.* 1998;79:616–618.

111. Lin JL, Huang SK, Lai LP, et al. Distal end of the atrioventricular nodal artery predicts the risk of atrioventricular block during slow pathway catheter ablation of atrioventricular nodal re-entrant tachycardia. *Heart.* 2000;83:543–550.

112. Hintringer F, Hartikainen J, Davies W, et al. Prediction of atrioventricular block during radiofrequency ablation of the slow pathway of the atrioventricular node. *Circulation.* 1995;92:3490–3496.

113. Delise P, Sitta N, Bonso A, et al. Pace mapping of Koch's triangle reduces risk of atrioventricular block during ablation of atrioventricular nodal reentrant tachycardia. *J Cardiovasc Electrophysiol.* 2005;16:30–35.

114. Bortone A, Boveda S, Jandaud S, et al. Gradual power titration using radiofrequency energy: a safe method for slow-pathway ablation in the setting of atrioventricular nodal re-entrant tachycardia. *Europace.* 2009;11:178–183.

115. Tebbenjohanns J, Pfeiffer D, Schumacher B, et al. Impact of local atrial electrogram in AV nodal reentrant tachycardia: ablation versus modification of the slow pathway. *J Cardiovasc Electrophysiol.* 1995;6:245–251.

116. Estner HL, Ndrepepa G, Dong J, et al. Acute and long-term results of slow pathway ablation in patients with atrioventricular nodal reentrant tachycardia: an analysis of the predictive factors for arrhythmia recurrence. *Pacing Clin Electrophysiol.* 2005;28:102–110.

117. Baker JH, Plumb VJ, Epstein AE, Kay GN. Predictors of recurrent atrioventricular nodal reentry after selective slow pathway ablation. *Am J Cardiol.* 1994;73:765–769.

118. Chen S-A, Wu T-J, Chiang C-E, et al. Recurrent tachycardia after selective ablation of slow pathway in patients with atrioventricular nodal reentrant tachycardia. *Am J Cardiol.* 1995;6:131–137.

119. Reithmann C, Remp T, Oversohl N, Steinbeck G. Ablation for atrioventricular nodal reentrant tachycardia with a prolonged PR interval during sinus rhythm: the risk of delayed higher-degree atrioventricular block. *J Cardiovasc Electrophysiol.* 2006;17:973–979.

120. Pasquie JL, Scalzi J, Macia JC, et al. Long-term safety and efficacy of slow pathway ablation in patients with atrioventricular nodal re-entrant tachycardia and pre-existing prolonged PR interval. *Europace.* 2006;8:129–133.

121. Sra JS, Jazayeri MR, Blanck Z, et al. Slow pathway ablation in patients with atrioventricular node reentrant tachycardia and a prolonged PR interval. *J Am Coll Cardiol.* 1994;24:1064–1068.

122. Li Y-G, Gronefeld G, Manchura C, Hohnloser SH. Risk of development of delayed atrioventricular block after slow pathway modification in patients with atrioventricular nodal reentrant tachycardia and a pre-existing prolonged PR interval. *Eur Heart J.* 2001;22:89–95.

123. Natale A, Grenfield RA, Geiger MJ, et al. Safety of slow pathway ablation in patients with long PR interval: further evidence of fast and slow pathway interaction. *Pacing Clin Electrophysiol.* 1997;20:1698–1703.

124. Basta MN, Krahn AD, Klein GJ, et al. Safety of slow pathway ablation in patients with atrioventricular nodal reentrant tachycardia and a long fast pathway effective refractory period. *Am J Cardiol.* 1997;80:155–159.

125. Lee MA, Morady F, Kadish A, et al. Catheter modification of the atrioventricular junction with radiofrequency energy for control of atrioventricular nodal reentrant tachycardia. *Circulation.* 1991;83:827–835.

126. Langberg JJ, Kim YN, Goyal R, et al. Conversion of typical to "atypical" atrioventricular nodal reentrant tachycardia after radiofrequency catheter modification of the atrioventricular junction. *Am J Cardiol.* 1992;69:503–508.

127. Gonzalez MD, Greenspon AJ, Kidwell GA. Linking in accessory pathways: functional loss of antegrade pre-excitation. *Circulation.* 1991;83:1221–1231.

128. Topilski I, Rogowski O, Glick A, et al. Radiofrequency ablation of atrioventricular nodal reentry tachycardia: a 14 year experience with 901 patients at the Tel Aviv Sourasky Medical Center. *Israeli Med J.* 2006;8:455–459.

129. Kihel J, Da Costa A, Kihel A, et al. Long-term efficacy and safety of radiofrequency ablation in elderly patients with atrioventricular nodal re-entrant tachycardia. *Europace.* 2006;8:416–420.

130. Rostock T, Risius T, Ventura R, et al. Efficacy and safety of radiofrequency catheter ablation of atrioventricular nodal reentrant tachycardia in the elderly. *J Cardiovasc Electrophysiol.* 2005;16:608–610.

131. Reithmann C, Hoffmann E, Grünewald A, et al. Fast pathway ablation in patients with common atrioventricular nodal reentrant tachycardia and prolonged PR interval during sinus rhythm. *Eur Heart J.* 1998;19:929–935.

132. Rivard L, Dubuc M, Guerra PG, et al. Cryoablation outcomes for AV nodal reentrant tachycardia comparing 4-mm versus 6-mm electrode-tip catheters. *Heart Rhythm.* 2008;5:230–234.

133. Zrenner B, Dong J, Schreieck J, et al. Transvenous cryoablation versus radiofrequency ablation of the slow pathway for the treatment of atrioventricular nodal re-entrant tachycardia: a prospective randomized pilot study. *Eur Heart J.* 2004;25:2226–2231.

134. Friedman PL, Dubuc M, Green MS, et al. Catheter cryoablation of supraventricular tachycardia: results of the multicenter prospective "frosty" trial. *Heart Rhythm.* 2004;1:129–138.

135. Collins KK, Dubin AM, Chiesa NA, et al. Cryoablation versus radiofrequency ablation for treatment of pediatric atrioventricular nodal reentrant tachycardia: initial experience with 4-mm cryocatheter. *Heart Rhythm.* 2006;3:564–570.

136. Gupta D, Al-Lamee RK, Earley MJ, et al. Cryoablation compared with radiofrequency ablation for atrioventricular nodal re-entrant tachycardia: analysis of factors contributing to acute and follow-up outcome. *Europace.* 2006;8:1022–1026.

137. Bastani H, Schwieler J, Insulander P, et al. Acute and long-term outcome of cryoablation therapy of typical atrioventricular nodal reentrant tachycardia. *Europace.* 2009;11:1077–1082.

138. Opel A, Murray S, Kamath N, et al. Cryoablation versus radiofrequency ablation for treatment of atrioventricular nodal reentry tachycardia: cryoablation with 6-mm-tip catheters is still less effective than radiofrequency ablation. *Heart Rhythm.* 2010;7:340–343.

20
Atrioventricular Junction Ablation and Modification for Heart Rate Control of Atrial Fibrillation

Lynne Hung, Ling-Ping Lai, and Shoei K. Stephen Huang

Key Points

The mechanism of atrial fibrillation is multiple wavelets or rotors in the atria with rapid ventricular response through the atrioventricular junction.

Mapping uses a combined anatomy- and electrogram-guided approach.

The right-sided approach target is just proximal to or below the His bundle electrode position or at the proximal His position. The left-sided approach target is just below the aortic valve at the septal site where a His potential can be recorded.

Use of preformed sheaths may be helpful, and irrigated-tipped ablation catheter is sometimes necessary.

Sources of difficulties include inability to record the His potential and failure of the right-sided approach.

Atrial fibrillation (AF) is a common tachyarrhythmia in humans.[1,2] It is responsible for low cardiac output, symptoms of palpitations, and systemic thromboembolic events. For the treatment of AF, rhythm control and rate control strategies are both widely used. Restoration and maintenance of sinus rhythm are sometimes difficult; however, randomized clinical trials have demonstrated no benefit of rhythm control over rate control strategies.[3,4] The traditional way of achieving ventricular rate control is the use of atrioventricular (AV) nodal blocking agents including β-blockers, calcium channel blockers, and digitalis. With the advent of catheter ablation techniques, AV junction ablation has evolved as an important and effective means to achieve ventricular rate control in patients refractory

to medical management. This chapter describes the techniques of radiofrequency (RF) catheter ablation for ventricular rate control in patients with AF.

Complete Atrioventricular Junction Ablation

Complete AV junction ablation provides an effective way to control the ventricular rate during AF. However, a permanent pacemaker must be implanted to provide adequate heart rate because the junctional escape rhythm after ablation is typically slow and unreliable.[5] Initially, this technique was used in patients with tachycardia-bradycardia syndrome, who also need a pacemaker. Its indication was later extended to those with drug-refractory, poorly controlled, rapid ventricular rates from atrial arrhythmias. This technique has also been used in patients with AF and a normal ventricular rate.[6] Early works on AV junction ablation were achieved by direct current (DC) shock.[5,6] Today, RF energy has completely replaced DC shock as the energy source for catheter ablation of the AV junction.[7–30] Cryoablation of the AV node has also been reported.[31] However, it has not gained popularity because RF energy is widely available and highly effective and there has been no demonstrable advantage to cryoablation for this application.

Before AV junction ablation is performed, appropriate ventricular backup pacing must be ensured. This can be achieved by either placing a temporary electrode catheter at the right ventricular apex or implanting a permanent pacemaker before the ablation procedure. By implanting the device weeks before the ablation procedure, the problems associated with postimplantation pacemaker system malfunction are avoided. For patients with a permanent pacemaker implanted before ablation, care should be taken to ensure effective pacing during ablation because interaction between RF energy and the pacemaker may occur. The skin patch should be placed as far away as possible from the pacemaker. The pacemaker should be set to VVI or VOO mode at 40 to 50 beats/minute before ablation.

Ventricular asystole or extreme bradycardia may occur during RF energy application because of destruction of the AV junction and inhibition of the permanent pacemaker by RF energy. Turning off the ablation power supply restores pacemaker activity. Further ablation can be performed with the pacemaker in the VOO mode. After ablation, permanent pacemakers should be interrogated to assess for alterations in pacemaker programming or changes in pacing or sensing thresholds. The pacemaker is often set at a high rate to reduce the risk for sudden cardiac death after AV junction ablation (discussed later).

Mapping and Ablation

For the ablation procedure, an approach from the right side is usually tried first.[10] The anatomy of the AV node and conduction system is reviewed in Chapters 6 and 19. The procedure can be performed under the guidance of fluoroscopy and electrograms. A 4-mm-tip RF ablation catheter is typically placed through a sheath in the femoral vein. However, access to the AV node can also be done with the sheath placed in the subclavian vein at the time of pacemaker implant.[32] In this method, two sheaths are placed in the subclavian vein. A right ventricular pacemaker lead placement is done through one of the sheaths. An ablation catheter is inserted through the other sheath. Once the AV node is successfully ablated, the ablation catheter is removed, and an atrial pacemaker lead can be inserted, if necessary.

To ablate the AV node, the ablation catheter is positioned at the compact node region, which is located at the atrial mid-septal region, just proximal and inferior to the His bundle catheter position, under fluoroscopy (Fig. 20-1). Ablation of the AV conduction system as proximally as possible increases the chance that an escape rhythm will emerge. Typically, it is not the size of the His, but its relationship to atrial and ventricular electrogram. A large His with equally sized atrial and ventricular signals (Fig. 20-2) is not as desirable as an atrial-to-ventricular electrogram ratio (A/V ratio) greater than 1:2.

Ideally, the ablation is guided by mapping very proximal His bundle recordings. The ablation catheter is positioned to record the maximal His potential. Although it is often

tempting to ablate at the site of maximal His recording, ablation at this site often produces right bundle branch block only. The catheter is then withdrawn toward the atrium to record an A/V ratio of 1:1 or 1:2 and a small His electrogram, usually less than 0.15 mV in amplitude. The catheter tip may need to be deflected slightly inferiorly to follow the course of the AV conduction system. Some advocate use of unipolar ablation electrograms to recognize the most proximal His recording. Here, the His potential shows an entirely negative (QS) morphology, reflecting the entire His activation proceeding away from the electrode. During AF, mapping may be complicated by variable atrial electrogram amplitudes and obfuscation of the His electrogram by the continuous atrial activity (Fig. 20-3). However, the failure to record the His often predicts failure to AV junctional ablation on the right side.[33] Cardioversion to sinus rhythm may allow better demonstration of the His potential.

With standard 4-mm-tip ablation electrodes, RF is delivered for 60 seconds at 50 to 60 W with target temperatures of 55° to 65°C. One study showed that a temperature range of 60° ± 7°C was required to achieve permanent AV nodal block, whereas at lower temperature, accelerated junctional rhythm is seen. Successful ablation sites usually produce accelerated junctional rhythm within 5 seconds and complete AV nodal block within 30 seconds (Fig. 20-4).[34] The use of preformed sheaths with a slight septal angulation and large-curve catheters may improve the stability of the catheter at the desired position. It is

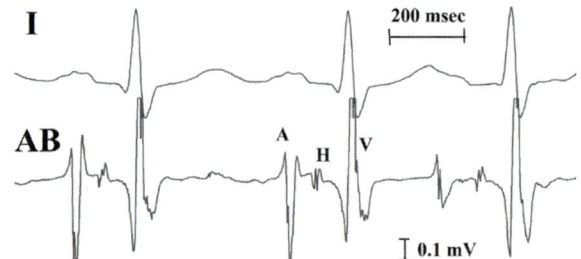

FIGURE 20-2. Surface electrocardiographic leads and electrograms from the distal ablation catheter (AB) showing an atrial (A)–to–ventricular (V) electrogram ratio of 1:1.5 and a small His potential (H) with amplitude of 0.12 mV.

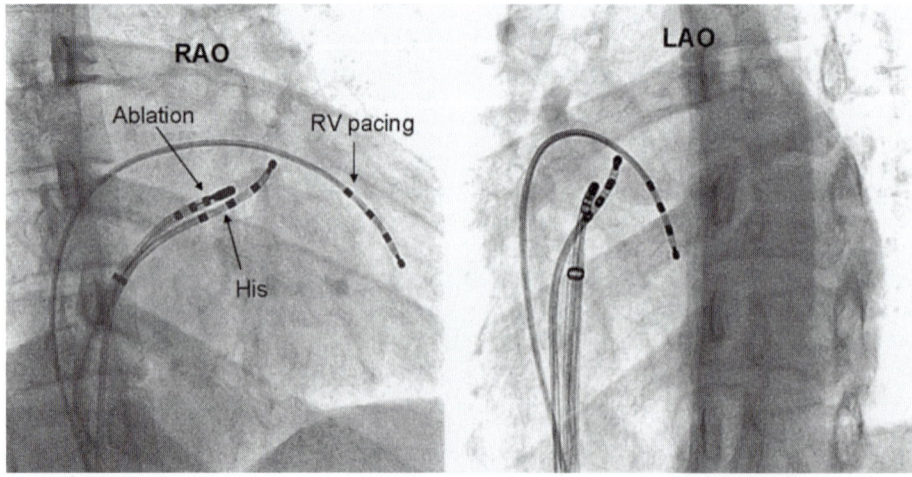

FIGURE 20-1. Standard right-sided approach for ablation of the atrioventricular junction. Right anterior oblique (RAO) and left anterior oblique (LAO) fluoroscopic views showing the ablation catheter aligned with the proximal His catheter (His) along the septum. RV, right ventricle.

highly advisable to carefully map and ensure catheter stability to avoid delivering ineffective lesions. Multiple ineffective deliveries may produce tissue edema and swelling that then obscure the His recording and distance the ablation catheter from the target tissue. During energy application, effective AV junction ablation is usually marked by accelerated junctional rhythm followed by slowing of the ventricular response and emergence of a paced ventricular rhythm.

A left-sided approach is used if the approach from the right side of the heart is undesirable or unsuccessful,[10,11] which occurs in about 5% of patients. The ablation catheter enters the left ventricle from the retrograde transaortic approach. The left-sided portion of the His bundle emerges on the septum just below the aortic valve (Fig. 20-5). It is helpful to maintain a catheter in the His position in the right side of the heart as an anatomic reference while mapping the left side of the septum. After the aortic valve is

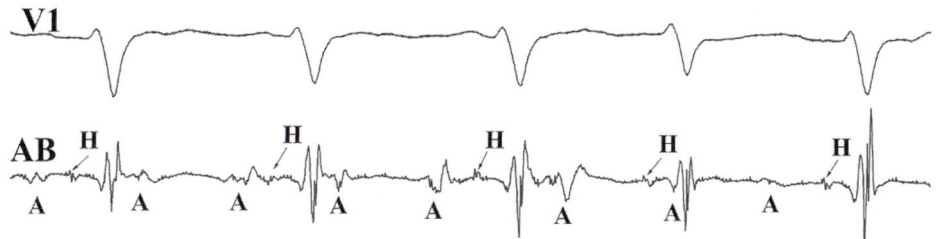

FIGURE 20-3. Mapping of the His bundle in atrial fibrillation. The irregular atrial electrograms (A) may obscure the His recording (H). In addition, variation in the amplitude of A complicates estimation of the atrial-to-ventricular electrogram ratio. AB, ablation catheter.

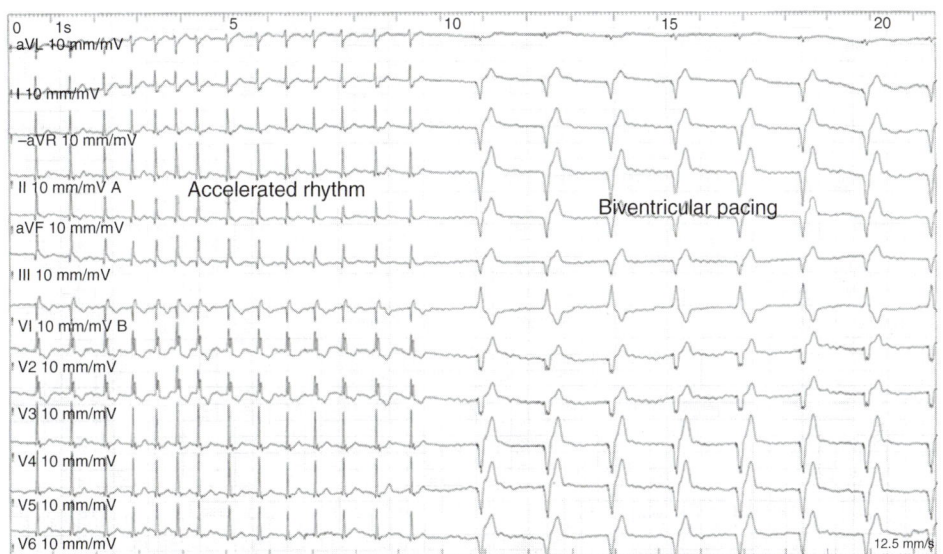

FIGURE 20-4. Successful ablation usually occurs with junctional escape rhythm within 5 seconds of radiofrequency delivery, and complete heart block is seen within 30 seconds. Note the biventricular pacing after heart block.

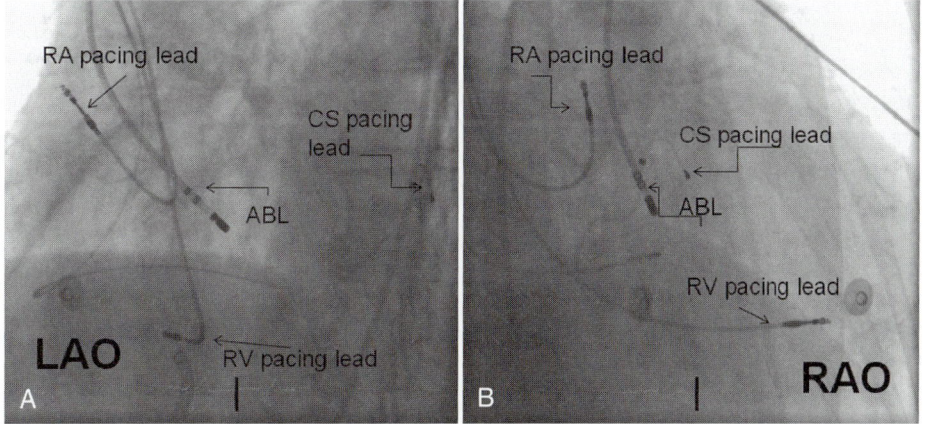

FIGURE 20-5. Atrioventricular junction ablation with a left-sided approach in patient with device. Left anterior oblique (LAO) (A) and right anterior oblique (RAO) (B) fluoroscopic images of catheter position during ablation. The ablation catheter (ABL) was just below the aortic valve. This patient already has a biventricular device, and no other catheter, except the ablation catheter, is required. The ablation catheter can record the atrium–His-ventricular electrogram. CS, coronary sinus; His, His catheter; RA, right atrium; RV, right ventricle.

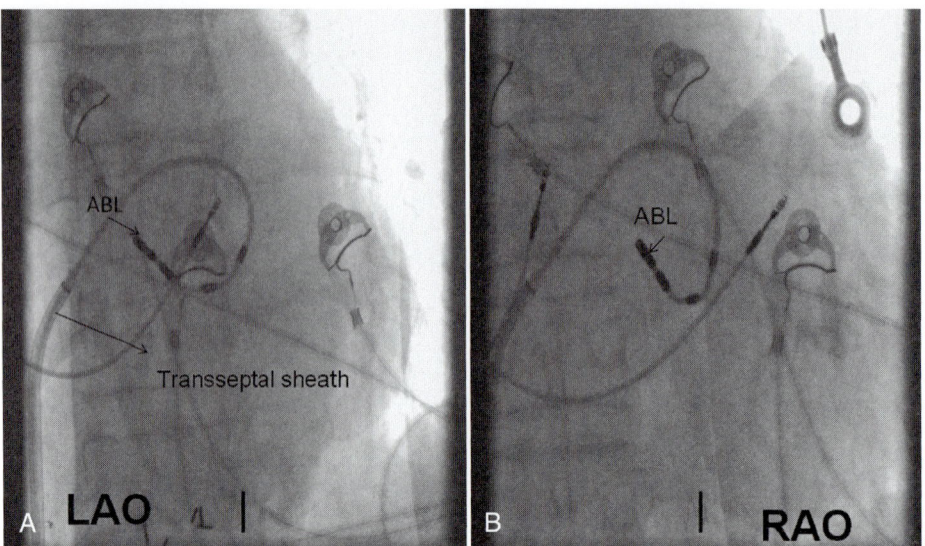

FIGURE 20-6. Transseptal access for left-sided approach. Left anterior oblique (LAO) (**A**) and right anterior oblique (RAO) (**B**) projections show looping of the magnetic navigation Stereotaxis catheter (Biosense Webster, Diamond Bar, CA) to access the atrioventricular node for ablation. ABL, ablation catheter.

crossed with a tight curve on the ablation catheter, the curve can be maintained on the catheter while it is rotated toward the septum and withdrawn to the aortic valve. Alternatively, the ablation catheter can be straightened and directed toward the inferior apical septum, then withdrawn toward the His bundle until the His potential is recorded beneath the noncoronary aortic cusp. A His electrogram is recorded at the site of ablation. The His potential must be differentiated from the left bundle branch recording. In older patients with aortic disease or peripheral arterial disease, the AV node can be approached through a transseptal puncture from the right atrium. The ablation catheter is directed to the left ventricle and placed under the aortic valve (Fig. 20-6).

The left-sided His activation should occur essentially at the same time as the right-sided His. The left bundle branch is typically recorded 1 to 1.5 cm inferior to the optimal His bundle recording site. The left bundle branch recording is identified by a potential-to-ventricular electrogram interval of 20 milliseconds or less and an A/V ratio of 1:10 or less. Electrogram recordings and catheter positions for the left conduction system are discussed in Chapter 27 and 29. In rare circumstances in which standard right-sided and left-sided approaches are both unsuccessful, energy delivery in the noncoronary or right aortic cusp where the His bundle potential is recorded may lead to complete AV block.[12]

In patients with preexisting *complete* bundle branch block, ablation of the contralateral bundle branch results in complete heart block. Mapping and ablation of the bundle branches are described in Chapter 29. Complete heart block may also result from ablation of both fast and slow pathway inputs to the AV node (Fig. 20-7). The targets for ablation are listed in Table 20-1.

For patients with chronically elevated ventricular rates, abrupt normalization of the heart rate by ablation and pacing may produce repolarization abnormalities and fatal polymorphic ventricular tachycardia.[27–30]

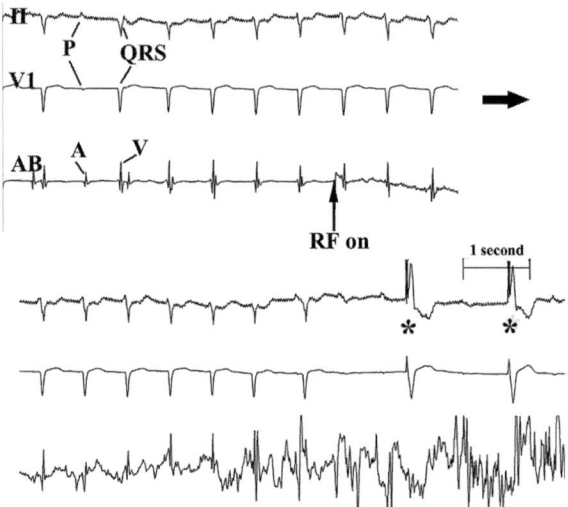

FIGURE 20-7. Induction of complete heart block by ablation of the fast and slow pathway atrioventricular (AV) nodal inputs. Electrocardiographic leads II and V_1 and the ablation (AB) electrograms are shown in this continuous tracing. A clear His recording could not be obtained in this patient. This recording was made after attempts at ablation of the proximal His bundle by anatomic guidance resulted only in fast pathway ablation and a very long PR interval of 600 msec. At the start of the tracing, there is a blocked P wave in sinus rhythm, revealing the very long PR interval. With radiofrequency energy delivery to the slow pathway region (RF on), there is the development of complete AV block and a ventricular paced rhythm (*). A, atrial electrogram; P, P wave; QRS, QRS interval; RF, radiofrequency energy; V, ventricular electrogram.

This phenomenon resulted in a significant incidence of sudden death after AV junctional ablation before it was appreciated in the early experience. Currently, the risk for postprocedure polymorphic ventricular arrhythmias has been essentially eliminated by programming the permanent pacemaker lower rate limit to 80 to 90 beats/minute immediately after ablation. The lower rate limit is then reduced by 10 beats/minute each month until the desired lower rate limit is achieved.

TABLE 20-1

TARGETS FOR ABLATION

Distal AV Node–Proximal His Junction (Right-Sided Approach)

Small His electrogram (≤0.15 mV)

A/V ratio 1:1 or ≥1:2

QS morphology to unipolar His recording

Left-Sided His Bundle

H-V interval >30-40 msec

A/V ratio about 1:5 to 1:10

Site <1-1.5 cm below aortic valve, on the septum

Compact AV Node

Site proximal and slightly inferior to His catheter in the triangle of Koch

Mid-septal, posteroseptal for AV node modification and more anterior approach for permanent AV block

A/V ratio 1:1 or ≥1:2

Bundle Branches

Right Bundle Branch

Absent or minimal atrial electrogram

BB-V interval <30-35 msec

Left Bundle Branch

A/V ratio ≤1:10

BB-V interval ≤20 msec

Site about 1-1.5 cm below aortic valve, on the septum

AV, atrioventricular; A/V ratio, atrial-to-ventricular electrogram ratio; BB, bundle branch; BB-V ratio, bundle branch–to-ventricular; H-V, His-to-ventricular.

Outcomes

The overall success rate for AV junction ablation is essentially 100% in recent reports.[13–20] A recurrence of AV conduction occurs in about 5% of patients. Brignole and colleagues[13] performed a multicenter, randomized study in 43 patients to compare AV junction and pharmacologic treatment in patients with symptomatic AF. The report showed that AV junction ablation with pacemaker implantation was superior in controlling symptoms related to palpitations, dyspnea, and exercise intolerance in a 6-month follow-up period. The improvement in quality of life was also greater in the ablation group. Similar results were shown in another, uncontrolled but larger series of 107 patients.[14] In the latter series, not only did the quality of life improve, but also the number of doctor visits, hospital admissions, and episodes of heart failure were all significantly decreased. Therefore, the medical costs were substantially reduced. With regular R-R intervals, the cardiac output and overall cardiac performance, as well as exercise capacity, can be improved.[15,16] A reduction of left ventricular dimension and increased contractility have also been shown 6 months after ablation.[17] For those with tachycardia-related cardiomyopathy, a recovery of left ventricular size and function has been reported.[18,19]

A meta-analysis of clinical outcomes after AV junctional ablation and pacing in 1181 patients reported in 21 studies demonstrated improvements in quality of life, ejection fraction, and exercise time.[20] Symptoms and health care use were decreased. Total mortality in this study was 6% at 1 year, and in long-term follow-up, it was similar to that in the general population with AF.[21]

Recent studies suggest that biventricular pacing is better than right ventricular pacing after AV junction ablation for AF, especially in patients with left ventricular dysfunction.[35–38] The patients with biventricular pacing appear to have improved functional capacity and an increase in left ventricular ejection fraction.[39] According to the 2008 ACC/AHA/HRS guideline, biventricular pacing is a class IIA indication for patients who are pacemaker dependent with New York Heart Association functional class III or IV.[40]

Complications directly related to the ablation procedure are rare, especially with right-sided procedures. The risk for postablation polymorphic ventricular arrhythmias has largely been eliminated by programming the pacemaker lower rate limit to 80 to 90 beats/minute after the procedure. Alterations in pacemaker function are common during RF delivery and include inhibition, asynchronous pacing, and induction of pacemaker-mediated tachycardia.[25,29] Interference may be enhanced in unipolar pacing systems. Problems persisting after termination of RF delivery are uncommon but include persistent reset mode requiring reprogramming, elevation of pacing or sensing thresholds, and direct damage to pacemaker leads.[25] For these reasons, permanent pacemakers should be thoroughly evaluated both before and after ablation.

Troubleshooting the Difficult Case

AV junctional ablation is usually a simple and straightforward procedure. It is perhaps this fact that compounds the operator's frustration when a case becomes difficult. The most common problem encountered is the inability to record a clear His potential. This may result from an intramyocardial course of the His bundle or from obfuscation of the His by scar or fibrosis (e.g., from prior surgery). In this instance, localization of the His bundle may be facilitated by use of a separate multipolar mapping catheter. A systematic search of the septum inferiorly and superiorly at variable extents into the ventricle often reveals its location. Pacing from the distal ablation electrodes at high output may identify areas of QRS narrowing, identifying His capture. The continuous atrial activity of AF may obscure the proximal His recording. By cardioversion, even if brief, the His may become apparent. The inability to record the His is a frequent problem after delivery of multiple ineffective lesions to the target area. The resulting edema and tissue swelling may physically distance the ablation catheter from the target tissue. This problem is best avoided by careful mapping and selective RF delivery only to favorable sites with stable catheter positions. If the His cannot be identified by any means, anatomically based lesions may be attempted from the right side of the heart before left-sided ablation is attempted. In this instance, the use of irrigated-tip or large-tip catheters may compensate for the absence of precise mapping. A line of lesions on the

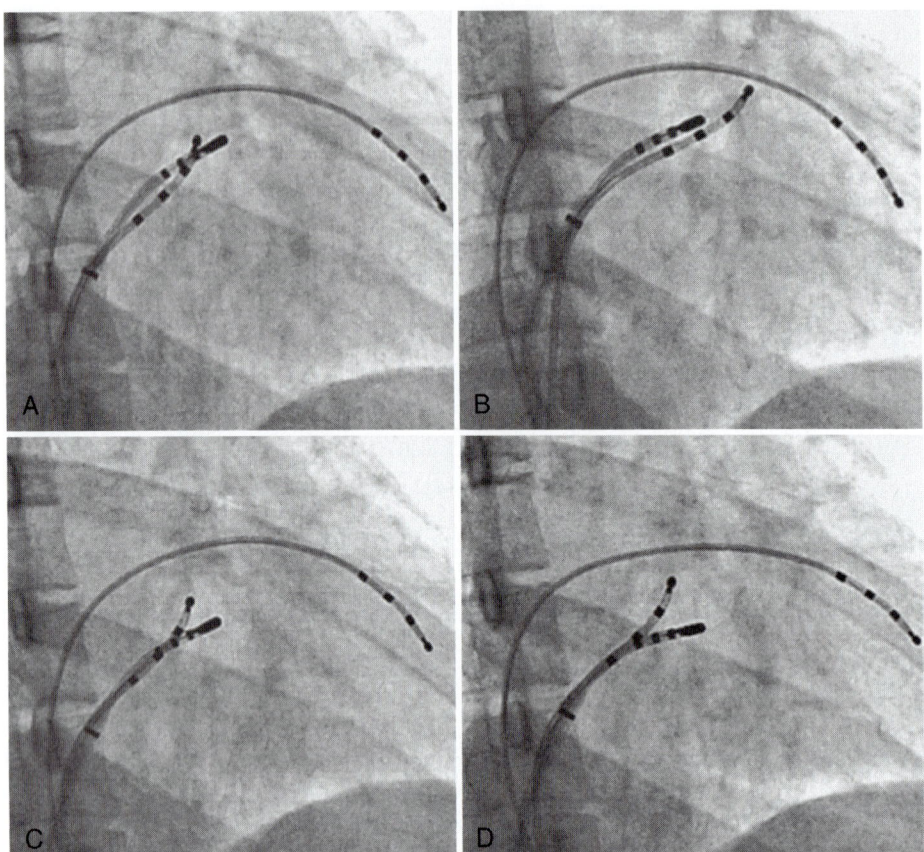

FIGURE 20-8. Right anterior oblique views of ablation catheter positions to create a linear lesion perpendicular to the estimated course of the His bundle when the His bundle cannot be recorded. From **A** through **D**, the ablation catheter is moved superiorly to inferiorly, with the His catheter as reference. Complete heart block was achieved at the site in **D**.

septum perpendicular to the course of the His bundle may be effective (Fig. 20-8).

Despite clear His recordings, RF lesions may fail to induce heart block. This typically results from unstable catheter positions or poor tissue contact. The use of long preformed sheaths with septal angulation can be helpful, especially in the setting of enlarged cardiac chambers. The use of irrigated-tip or large-tip catheters coupled with high-output generators is sometimes necessary. If heart block cannot be achieved from the right ventricle, the left ventricular approach should be tried. If this also fails to target the compact AV node, individual bundle branches or AV nodal inputs are possible.

Loss of ventricular pacing may interrupt an otherwise successful lesion delivery. For patients with permanent pacemakers, reprogramming to VOO mode is usually corrective. Pacemakers should be interrogated fully before ablation, to assess thresholds and battery status. If near elective replacement indicators, reversion to magnet noise or reset mode may result in loss of capture. Rarely, damage to pacing leads or to the electrode-tissue interface can result in more lasting problems. Loss of pacing from temporary pacing leads is usually the result of lead dislodgment. If the ablation catheter is preset for pacing from the distal electrodes, the catheter can readily be advanced into the ventricle for pacing if the other systems fail. Common

problems related to AV junctional ablation and their solutions are listed in Table 20-2.

Atrioventricular Junction Modification

AV junction modification without causing complete AV block can also be achieved by catheter ablation but is now rarely used in clinical practice. It has been reported that selective ablation of the slow pathway of the AV node results in an increase in AV refractoriness and therefore decreases the ventricular rate.[41–48] In practice, the technique is similar to that used for treating AV nodal reentrant tachycardia. Ablation is begun in the slow pathway region of the low posteroseptal right atrium during AF. It is delivered at sites with A/V ratios of 1:2 to 1:4. While the ventricular response is monitored, lesions are delivered in incremental steps superiorly toward the midseptal area. Ablation is not given at sites in which a His potential is recorded or that exceed 0.02 mV.[47] The end point is reduction of the ventricular response to less than 100 beats/minute, and ideally to between 60 and 80 beats/minute. At this point, an isoproterenol or atropine challenge may be administered and ablation continued until the heart rate is less than 120 beats/minute during the pharmacologic stress.[45] The

TABLE 20-2

TROUBLESHOOTING THE DIFFICULT CASE

Problem	Cause	Solution
Inability to record His potential	Intramyocardial course or His obscured by scar or fibrosis	Mapping with multipolar catheter Pace-map from ablation catheter for His capture (QRS narrowing) Create anatomically based linear lesion perpendicular to His Ablate from left ventricle Target compact AV node or AV nodal inputs
	Acute tissue edema from ineffective RF lesions His obscured by atrial activity in AF	Careful initial mapping and catheter instability to limit ineffective lesions Cardiovert and reinitiate AF after ablation
Ineffective RF delivery	Poor tissue contact	Use preformed sheath; change catheter reach, curve, or stiffness Overdrive ventricular pacing to reduce cardiac motion Ablate from left ventricle
	Intramyocardial course, insufficient lesion size	Use irrigated RF or large-tip catheter with high-output generator Ablate from left ventricle Ablate right and left bundle branches separately
Loss of pacing during ablation	Pacemaker inhibition from EMI Pacemaker reset mode Displacement of temporary pacemaker wire	Program VOO or asynchronous pacing Check battery status before ablation Careful catheter manipulation; use screw in temporary pacemaker wire, temporary pacing from ablation catheter advanced into right ventricle

AF, atrial fibrillation; AV, atrioventricular; EMI, electromagnetic interference; RF, radiofrequency energy.

patient should be monitored for 24 to 72 hours after the procedure for recurrences of rapid ventricular rates (which are not uncommon), excessively slow rates, and AV block or polymorphic ventricular arrhythmias. AV junction modification leads to satisfactory ventricular rate control in 25% to 85% of patients.[41–50]

Complications of the procedure include AV block necessitating permanent pacing in as many as 21% of patients.[50] The onset of complete AV block may be delayed for days after the procedure.[47] The occurrence of transient high-grade AV block during the ablation procedure may identify those at risk for late heart block.[47] The occurrence of repolarization abnormalities with polymorphic ventricular tachycardia has also been documented after AV nodal modification without pacemaker implantation.[47]

This technique has been largely abandoned because of the high incidence of AV block and polymorphic ventricular arrhythmias, both of which may occur days after the procedure.[47] These problems are overcome by the presence of a permanent pacemaker, the avoidance of which is the primary benefit of AV junctional modification. In addition, there have been consistent benefits to complete AV junctional ablation and pacing in the literature, with no reported superiority of the AV nodal modification approach.[20,49]

References

1. Kannel WB, Abbott RD, Savage DD, et al. Epidemiologic features of atrial fibrillation. *N Engl J Med.* 1982;306:1018–1022.
2. Alpert JS, Petersen P, Godtfredsen J. Atrial fibrillation: natural history, complications and management. *Annu Rev Med.* 1988;39:41–52.
3. Van Gelder IC, Hagens VE, Bosker HA, et al. Rate Control versus Electrical Cardioversion for Persistent Atrial Fibrillation Study Group. A comparison of rate control and rhythm control in patients with recurrent persistent atrial fibrillation. *N Engl J Med.* 2002;347:1834–1840.
4. Wyse DG, Waldo AL, DiMarco JP, et al. Atrial Fibrillation Follow-up Investigation of Rhythm Management (AFFIRM) Investigators. A comparison of rate control and rhythm control in patients with atrial fibrillation. *N Engl J Med.* 2002;347:1825–1833.
5. Curtis AB, Kutalek SP, Prior M, et al. Prevalence and characteristics of escape rhythms after radiofrequency ablation of the atrioventricular junction: results from the registry for AV junction ablation and pacing in atrial fibrillation. Ablate and Pace Trial Investigators. *Am Heart J.* 2000;139:122–125.
6. Natale A, Zimerman L, Tomassoni G, et al. Impact on ventricular function and quality of life of transcatheter ablation of the atrioventricular junction in chronic atrial fibrillation with a normal ventricular response. *Am J Cardiol.* 1996;78:1431–1433.
7. Evans T, Scheinman M, Zipes D, et al. The percutaneous cardiac mapping and ablation registry: final summary of results. *Pacing Clin Electrophysiol.* 1988;11:1621–1626.
8. Evans T, Scheinman M, Bardy G, et al. Predictors of in-hospital mortality after direct current catheter ablation of atrioventricular junction: results of a prospective, international, multicenter study. *Circulation.* 1991;84:1924–1937.
9. Simantirakis EN, Vardakis KE, Kochiadakis GE, et al. Left ventricular mechanics during right ventricular apical or left ventricular-based pacing in patients with chronic atrial fibrillation after atrioventricular junction ablation. *J Am Coll Cardiol.* 2004;43:1013–1018.
10. Sousa O, Gursoy S, Simonis F, et al. Right-sided versus left-sided radiofrequency ablation of the His bundle. *Pacing Clin Electrophysiol.* 1992;15:1454–1459.
11. Sousa J, El-Atassi R, Rosenheck S, et al. Radiofrequency catheter ablation of the atrioventricular junction from the left ventricle. *Circulation.* 1991;84:567–571.
12. Cuello C, Huang SKS, Wagshal AB, et al. Radiofrequency catheter ablation of the atrioventricular junction by a supravalvular non-coronary aortic cusp approach. *Pacing Clin Electrophysiol.* 1994;17:1182–1185.
13. Brignole M, Gianfranchi L, Menozzi C, et al. Assessment of atrioventricular junction ablation and DDDR mode-switching pacemaker versus pharmacological treatment in patients with severely symptomatic paroxysmal atrial fibrillation: a randomized controlled study. *Circulation.* 1997;96:2617–2624.
14. Fitzpatrick AP, Kourouyan HD, Siu A, et al. Quality of life and outcomes after radiofrequency His-bundle catheter ablation and permanent pacemaker implantation: impact of treatment in paroxysmal and established atrial fibrillation. *Am Heart J.* 1996;131:499–507.
15. Buys EM, Hemel NM, Kelder JC, et al. Exercise capacity after his bundle ablation and rate response ventricular pacing for drug refractory chronic atrial fibrillation. *Heart.* 1997;77:238–241.
16. Rodriguez LM, Smeets JL, Xie B, et al. Improvement in left ventricular function by ablation of atrioventricular nodal conduction in selected patients with lone atrial fibrillation. *Am J Cardiol.* 1993;72:1137–1141.
17. Brignole M, Menozzi C, Gianfranchi L, et al. Assessment of atrioventricular junction ablation and VVIR pacemaker versus pharmacological treatment in patients with heart failure and chronic atrial fibrillation: a randomized, controlled study. *Circulation.* 1998;98:953–960.

18. Redfield MM, Kay GN, Jenkins LS, et al. Tachycardia-related cardiomyopathy: a common cause of ventricular dysfunction in patients with atrial fibrillation referred for atrioventricular ablation. *Mayo Clin Proc.* 2000;75:790–795.

19. Lemery R, Brugada P, Cheriex E, Wellens HJ. Reversibility of tachycardia-induced left ventricular dysfunction after closed-chest catheter ablation of the atrioventricular junction for intractable atrial fibrillation. *Am J Cardiol.* 1987;60:1406–1408.

20. Wood MA, Brown-Mahoney C, Kay GN, Ellenbogen KA. Clinical outcomes after ablation and pacing therapy for atrial fibrillation: a meta-analysis. *Circulation.* 2000;101:1138–1144.

21. Ozcan C, Jahangir A, Friedman PA, et al. Long-term survival after ablation of the atrioventricular node and implantation of a permanent pacemaker in patients with atrial fibrillation. *N Engl J Med.* 2001;344:1043–1051.

22. Willems R, Wyse DG, Gillis AM, Atrial Pacing Periablation for Paroxysmal Atrial Fibrillation (PA3) Study Investigators. Total atrioventricular nodal ablation increases atrial fibrillation burden in patients with paroxysmal atrial fibrillation despite continuation of antiarrhythmic drug therapy. *J Cardiovasc Electrophysiol.* 2003;14:1296–1301.

23. Gianfranchi L, Brignole M, Menozzi C, et al. Progression of permanent atrial fibrillation after atrioventricular junction ablation and dual-chamber pacemaker implantation in patients with paroxysmal atrial tachyarrhythmias. *Am J Cardiol.* 1998;81:351–354.

24. Wood MA, Curtis AB, Takle-Newhouse TA, et al. Survival of DDD pacing mode after atrioventricular junction ablation and pacing for refractory atrial fibrillation. *Am Heart J.* 1999;137:682–685.

25. Buurke MC, Kopp DE, Alberts M, et al. Effects of radiofrequency current on previously implanted pacemaker and defibrillator lead systems. *J Electrocardiol.* 2001;34(suppl):143–148.

26. Gillis AM, Connolly SJ, Lacombe P, et al. Randomized crossover comparison of DDDR versus VDD pacing after atrioventricular junction ablation for prevention of atrial fibrillation. The Atrial Pacing Periablation for Paroxysmal Atrial Fibrillation (PA3) Study Investigators. *Circulation.* 2000;102:736–741.

27. Darpo B, Walfridsson H, Aunes M, et al. Incidence of sudden death after radiofrequency ablation of the atrioventricular junction for atrial fibrillation. *Am J Cardiol.* 1997;80:1174–1177.

28. Ozcan C, Jahangir A, Friedman PA, et al. Sudden death after radiofrequency ablation of the atrioventricular node in patients with atrial fibrillation. *J Am Coll Cardiol.* 2002;40:105–110.

29. Sadoul N, Blankoff I, de Chillou C, et al. Effects of radiofrequency catheter ablation on patients with permanent pacemakers. *J Interv Card Electrophysiol.* 1997;1:227–233.

30. Geelen P, Brugada J, Andries E, et al. Ventricular fibrillation and sudden death after radiofrequency ablation of the atrioventricular junction for atrial fibrillation. *Pacing Clin Electrophysiol.* 1997;20:343–348.

31. Dubuc M, Khairy P, Rodriguez-Santiago A, et al. Catheter cryoablation of the atrioventricular node in patients with atrial fibrillation: a novel technology for ablation of cardiac arrhythmias. *J Cardiovasc Electrophysiol.* 2001;12:439–444.

32. Issa ZF. An approach to ablate and pace: AV junction ablation and pacemaker implantation performed concurrently from the same venous access site. *Pacing Clin Electrophysiol.* 2007;30:1116–1120.

33. Abe H, Bhandari AK, Lerman R, et al. A low amplitude His-bundle potential predicts failure of the right-sided approach for atrioventricular junction ablation. *Jpn Circ J.* 2000;64:257–261.

34. Nath S, DiMarco JP, Mounsey JP, et al. Correlation of temperature and pathophysiological effect during radiofrequency catheter ablation of the AV junction. *Circulation.* 1995;92:1188–1192.

35. Touboul P. Atrioventricular nodal ablation and pacemaker implantation in patients with atrial fibrillation. *Am J Cardiol.* 1999;83:241D–245D.

36. Occhetta E, Bortnik M, Dell'era G, et al. Evaluation of pacemaker dependence in patients on ablate and pace therapy for atrial fibrillation. *Europace.* 2007;9:1119–1123.

37. Doshi RN, Daound EG, Fellows C, et al. Left ventricular-based cardiac stimulation post AV nodal ablation evaluation (the PAVE study). *J Cardiovasc Electrophysiol.* 2005;16:1160–1165.

38. Brignole M, Gianfranchi L, Menozzi C, et al. Assessment of atrioventricular junction ablation and DDDR mode-switching pacemaker versus pharmacological treatment in patients with severely symptomatic paroxysmal atrial fibrillation: a randomized controlled study. *Circulation.* 1998;98:953–960.

39. Valls-Bertault V, Fatemi M, Gilard M, et al. Assessment of upgrading to biventricular pacing in patients with right ventricular pacing and congestive heart failure after atrioventricular junctional ablation for chronic atrial fibrillation. *Europace.* 2004;6:438–443.

40. Epstein AE, DiMarco JP, Ellenbogen KA, et al. ACC/AHA/HRS 2008 Guidelines for device-based therapy of cardiac rhythm abnormalities: executive summary. *J Am Coll Cardiol.* 2008;51:2085–2105.

41. Tebbenjohanns J, Schumacher B, Korte T, et al. Bimodal RR interval distribution in chronic atrial fibrillation: impact of dual atrioventricular nodal physiology on long-term rate control after catheter ablation of the posterior atrionodal input. *J Cardiovasc Electrophysiol.* 2000;11:497–503.

42. Blanck Z, Dhala AA, Sra J, et al. Characterization of atrioventricular nodal behavior and ventricular response during atrial fibrillation before and after a selective slow-pathway ablation. *Circulation.* 1995;91:1086–1094.

43. Della Bella P, Carbucicchio C, Tondo C, et al. Modulation of atrioventricular conduction by ablation of the "slow" atrioventricular node pathway in patients with drug-refractory atrial fibrillation or flutter. *J Am Coll Cardiol.* 1995;25:39–46.

44. Menozzi C, Brignole M, Gianfranchi L, et al. Radiofrequency catheter ablation and modulation of atrioventricular conduction in patients with atrial fibrillation. *Pacing Clin Electrophysiol.* 1994;17:2143–2149.

45. Feld G. Radiofrequency catheter ablation versus modification of the AV node for control of rapid ventricular response in atrial fibrillation. *J Cardiovasc Electrophysiol.* 1995;6:217–228.

46. Canby RC, Roman CA, Kessler DJ, et al. Selective radiofrequency ablation of the "slow" atrioventricular nodal pathway for control of the ventricular response to atrial fibrillation. *Am J Cardiol.* 1996;77:1358–1361.

47. Morady F, Hasse C, Strickberger A, et al. Long-term follow-up after radiofrequency modification of the atrioventricular node in patients with atrial fibrillation. *J Am Coll Cardiol.* 1997;27:113–121.

48. Fleck RP, Chen PS, Boyce K, et al. Radiofrequency modification of atrioventricular conduction by selective ablation of the low posterior septal right atrium in a patient with atrial fibrillation and a rapid ventricular response. *Pacing Clin Electrophysiol.* 1993;16:377–381.

49. Proclemer A, Della Bella P, Tondo C, et al. Radiofrequency ablation of atrioventricular junction and pacemaker implantation versus modulation of atrioventricular conduction in drug refractory atrial fibrillation. *Am J Cardiol.* 1999;83:1437–1442.

50. Williamson BD, Ching Man K, Daoud E, et al. Radiofrequency catheter modification of atrioventricular conduction to control the ventricular rate during atrial fibrillation. *N Engl J Med.* 1993;331:910–917.

Catheter Ablation of Accessory Atrioventricular Connections

21
Ablation of Free Wall Accessory Pathways

Mark A. Wood

Key Points

The atrioventricular annulus is mapped for atrial or ventricular accessory pathway (AP) insertion sites or the AP itself.

Ablation targets include the earliest site of atrial or ventricular activation by the AP, sites of AP potentials, and sites of electrogram polarity reversal (left free wall APs).

Special equipment includes preformed sheaths (especially for the transseptal approach) and multielectrode halo mapping catheters (right free wall). Catheter navigation systems are useful, and electroanatomic mapping is optional.

Sources of difficulty are misdiagnosis of atrioventricular nodal reentry with eccentric atrial activation or atrial tachycardia as orthodromic reciprocating tachycardia, catheter stability (especially with right free wall APs), and epicardial APs.

Free wall locations are the most common positions for accessory pathways (APs) in clinical practice. Right and left free wall APs account for 10% to 20% and 50% to 60% of all APs, respectively.[1] These pathway locations each present distinct challenges to the electrophysiologist. Left free wall APs are amenable to ablation and have the highest success rates and lowest incidences of recurrence. The left heart location is less accessible, however, necessitating arterial or transseptal approaches. In contrast, right free wall APs are readily approached from simple venous access but have the lowest success rates and highest incidences of recurrence.

Anatomy

The anatomy of the tricuspid annulus is different from that of the mitral annulus.[2-4] The hinge of the mitral atrioventricular (AV) annulus is a well-formed and distinct cord of fibrous tissue around the annulus (Fig. 21-1A). This accretion of fibrous tissue is interposed between the atrial and ventricular

myocardia. On the ventricular side of the mitral annulus, basal cords of ventricular myocardium may descend in a curtain-like fashion from the mitral hinge to insert into the trabeculations on the ventricular wall. These cords may limit catheter mobility beneath the valve during attempts at left free wall AP ablations. In the limited human histologic descriptions of left free wall APs, the atrial connection is usually discrete and near the annulus.[2,3] The pathways then skirt the annulus on its epicardial aspect and may cross at variable depths within the epicardial fat pad (Fig. 21-1B). The ventricular insertion usually branches into multiple connections with the ventricle that may be displaced away from the annulus, toward the apex.[2,3] The histologically determined length of an AP is typically 5 to 10 mm, with a maximal diameter of 0.1 to 7 mm.[5] The left-sided epicardial AV groove is shallow but contains the left circumflex artery near the annulus and the coronary sinus (CS) more remote from the annulus. Although the CS is useful for quickly mapping the mitral valve area, it runs an average of 10 to 14 mm on the atrial side of the true annulus.[6] This separation from the annulus is more pronounced in the proximal 20 mm of the CS. Therefore, during catheter mapping, the CS location and electrograms are best regarded as gross estimates of the true AP location on the annulus. The anterior limit of the left free wall is anatomically well demarcated by the aortic-mitral valve continuity, which rarely contains AP connections. The exact location of this continuity is difficult to recognize by fluoroscopy alone. The posterior limit of the left free wall is anatomically continuous with the posteroseptal area and is arbitrarily defined on fluoroscopy.

In contrast to the mitral annulus, the tricuspid valve annulus is less well formed and frequently discontinuous.[2,3] The right atrial and right ventricular myocardia tend to overlap or fold over one another as they insert on the tricuspid annulus (Fig. 21-1B). Right free wall APs may cross discontinuities in the less distinct fibrous annulus or skirt the epicardial aspect of the annulus, as do left free wall APs.[2,3] The less developed tricuspid annulus and acute angulation of the tricuspid leaflets toward the ventricle make catheter positions along the right free wall unstable. Fluoroscopic definition of the right free wall is difficult because there are no clear landmarks for guidance.

Because of the association of Ebstein anomaly with right-sided APs, the anatomy of this condition merits special consideration.[7] In this disorder, the tricuspid valve leaflets are

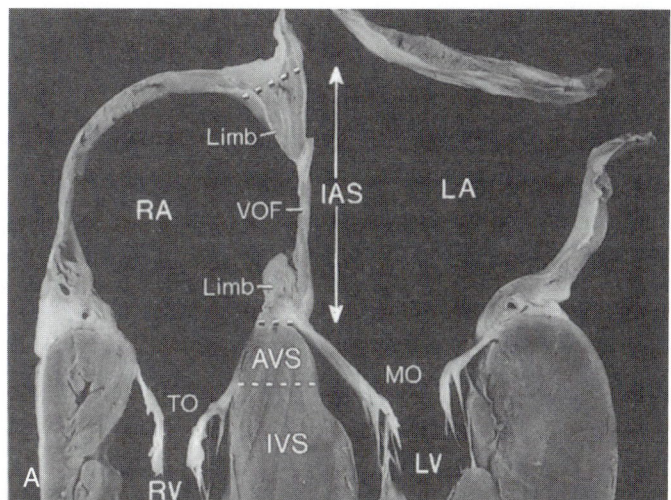

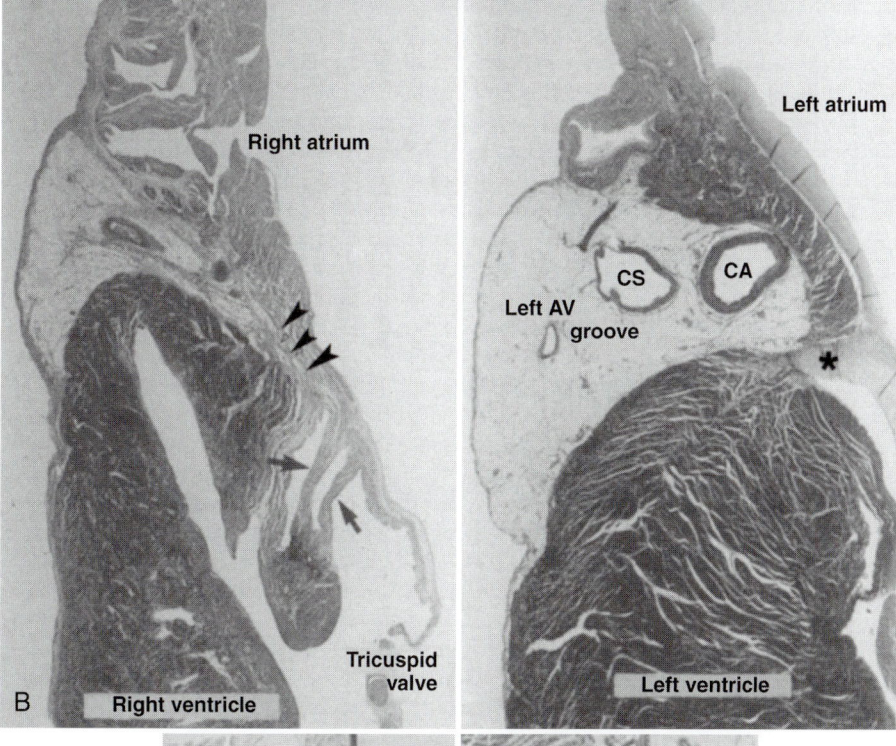

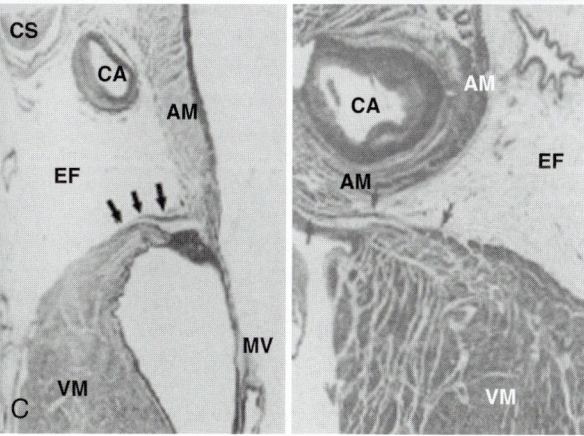

FIGURE 21-1. A, Gross histologic section demonstrating a cross section of the AV valves along the free walls. Note the more apical position of the tricuspid valve (TO) compared with the mitral valve (MO). AVS, atrioventricular septum; IAS, interatrial septum; IVS, interventricular septum; LA, left atrium; limb, limbus; LV, left ventricle; RA, right atrium; RV, right ventricle; VOF, foramen ovale. **B,** Histologic sections of the tricuspid (*left panel*) and mitral valve (*right panel*) annuli through the free walls. Along the tricuspid annulus, the atrial and ventricular myocardia fold over one another, separated by a poorly defined fibrous component (*arrowheads*). The *arrows* show two cords supporting the base of the valve leaflet. In the *right panel*, the distinct fibrous component to the mitral annulus creates a well-formed hinge (*asterisk*) for the mitral valve and separates the atrial and ventricular myocardia. Note the relation of the circumflex coronary artery (CA) and coronary sinus (CS) to the mitral annulus. AV, atrioventricular. **C,** Histologic sections of the mitral annulus in patients with a left posterior accessory pathway (*left panel*) and a left lateral accessory pathway (*right panel*). In each case, the accessory pathways (*arrows*) cross in the epicardial fat pad (EF) on the epicardial aspect of the annulus fibrosus. Note the distant location of the coronary sinus (CS) to the accessory pathway in the *left panel*. In the *right panel*, atrial myocardium (AM) encircles the circumflex coronary artery (CA). MV, mitral valve; VM, ventricular myocardium. (**A,** *From Classification and terminology of cardiovascular abnormalities. In Emmanouilides GC, Riemenschneider TA, Allen HD,* Moss and Adams' Heart Disease in Infants, Children, and Adolescents: Including the Fetus and Young Adult. *Baltimore, Williams & Williams, 1995:115.* **B,** *From Ho SY, Anderson RH. Anatomy of accessory pathways. In Farre J, Moro C [eds]:* Ten Years of Radiofrequency Catheter Ablation. *Armonk, NY: Futura; 1998:149-163.* **C,** *From Becker A, Anderson R, Durrer D, et al. The anatomic substrates of Wolff-Parkinson-White syndrome: a clinico-pathologic correlation in seven patients.* Circulation. *1978;57:870-879. With permission.)*

tethered to the ventricular wall for variable distances from the annulus. This contributes to catheter instability during mapping of the tricuspid annulus. Although not anatomically displaced, the true tricuspid annulus may be poorly developed, with extensive discontinuities of the fibrous architecture.[3] Electrograms recorded from the annulus in Ebstein anomaly may be of low amplitude and fragmented owing to the disorganized tissue.[8] This fragmentation adds to the difficulty in mapping the tricuspid annulus in this condition. APs in Ebstein anomaly are often multiple and may skirt the epicardial aspect of the annulus or pass subendocardially through gaps in the fibrous annulus.[2,3]

A complete description of free wall accessory AV connections must also include those resulting from connections of the ventricle to the CS musculature, the ligament of Marshall, and the atrial appendage. Mahaim-type atriofascicular connections are described in Chapter 24. The venous wall of the CS is surrounded by a continuous sleeve of atrial myocardium that extends for 25 to 51 mm from the CS ostium.[9] This muscle is continuous with the right atrial myocardium proximally but is usually separated from the left atrium by adipose tissue. This separation may be bridged by strands of striated muscle, however, producing electrical continuity between the CS musculature and the left atrium (Fig. 21-2). These connections,

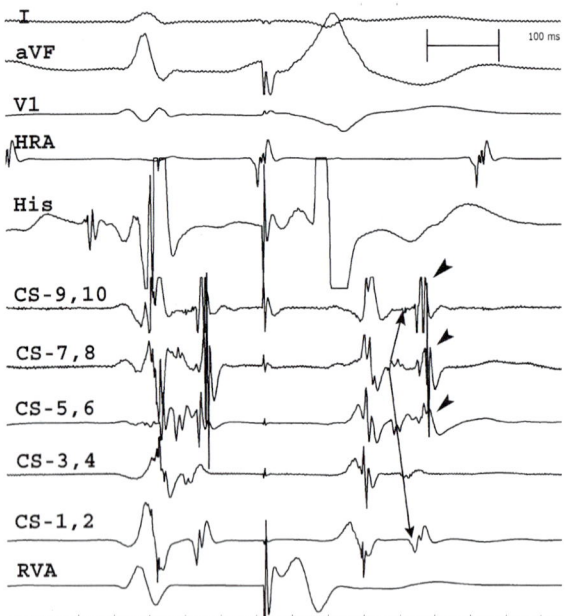

FIGURE 21-2. Coronary sinus (CS) potentials recorded during mapping of left lateral accessory pathway. The first complex represents orthodromic reciprocating tachycardia with earliest atrial activation at CS 7,8. The second complex is a premature ventricular stimulus that reverses the sequence of ventricular activation along the CS. This separates the atrial and ventricular potentials without altering the atrial activation sequence. After the ventricular electrogram on the CS tracings, there are low-amplitude, low-frequency far-field atrial potentials (*arrows*). After the atrial potentials on CS 5,6 through CS 9,10, there are high-amplitude, high-frequency CS musculature potentials (*arrowheads*) that are activated in a proximal-to-distal sequence. This is interpreted as activation of the proximal CS atrium by the accessory pathway with atrial conduction proximally to the point of connection to the CS musculature. The CS musculature then conducts proximally to distally along a portion of the CS catheter. CS 9,10, proximal CS; CS 1,2, distal CS; HRA, high right atrium; RVA, right ventricular apex.

which can be broad and very extensive, are reported in up to 80% of hearts in autopsy series.[9] Electrical continuity of the CS musculature with the ventricle is less common, but it may provide the substrate for reciprocating tachycardias.[10] Ventricular connections may result from CS musculature extensions over the middle cardiac vein, posterior cardiac vein, or AV groove branch of the distal left circumflex artery. Ventricular connections with the CS are described in 3% to 6% of hearts at autopsy.[10] Sun and associates[10] reported that 36% of patients (most with previously failed ablation) who had left posterior or left posteroseptal AV connections actually used the CS musculature as the intermediary between the atrium and ventricle in reciprocating tachycardias.

The ligament of Marshall is a vestigial fold of pericardium that carries the vein of Marshall from its origin as a branch of the distal CS to its termination near the left superior pulmonary vein. This structure may also contain bundles of muscle fibers that are continuous with the CS musculature. These fibers may end blindly, or they may insert directly into the left atrial musculature at the inferior interatrial pathway.[11] With proximal connections between the CS musculature and the ventricle, the ligament of Marshall can support AV reciprocating tachycardia.[11]

Another unusual form of AV connection is a direct epicardial muscular continuity between the atrial appendage and the ventricle.[12-14] Several reports of connections between the right atrial appendage and ventricle are available, whereas left-sided connections appear even more rare.[14] The developmental basis for these connections is unknown. Because of epicardial ventricular insertions more than 1 cm apical to the annulus and atrial origins within the atrial appendage, endocardial mapping of the annulus for conventional APs is perplexing.[12,13] For left-sided connections, mapping of the anterior coronary venous branches may demonstrate the earliest ventricular activation.[14] At surgical division of one such right-sided connection, a broad band of myocardium under the epicardial fat pad was noted from the base of the atrial appendage to the base of the right ventricle.[12] Case reports describe successful catheter ablation of these connections from the right atrial appendage.[13]

Pathophysiology

Diagnosis

As with APs at other locations, free wall APs may participate in reciprocating tachycardias or undergo bystander activation during tachycardias mechanistically unrelated to the presence of the AP. Free wall APs have been associated with specific electrophysiologic characteristics.[15] Compared with septal and left free wall locations, right free wall APs are less likely to demonstrate retrograde conduction, to participate in reciprocating tachycardias, and to be associated with inducible atrial fibrillation.[15] Pathways in the right free wall may be more likely to demonstrate decremental antegrade conduction than those in other locations. Compared with right free wall pathways, left free wall APs are more likely to demonstrate decremental retrograde conduction and have longer retrograde refractory periods.[15]

Surface electrocardiogram (ECG) localization of manifest free wall APs is imperfect and becomes less accurate if minimal preexcitation is present (QRS <120 milliseconds).[16] ECG algorithms for AP localization are most accurate for the diagnosis of left free wall APs compared with all other locations, achieving at least 90% sensitivity and almost 100% specificity.[16–20] In using any localization algorithm, one must be aware of the portion of the QRS complex on which the algorithm is based. Some algorithms use only the first 20 to 60 milliseconds of the delta wave, whereas others are based on the morphology or polarity of the entire QRS complex.[18–21] Provided that significant preexcitation is present, all left free wall APs should demonstrate a positive delta wave in V_1, with the R wave greater than the S wave (R > S) in lead V_1 or V_2 at the latest (Fig. 21-3). A negative delta wave in lead I, aVL, or V_6 is pathognomonic of a left lateral pathway. As the pathway location moves from posterior to lateral to anterior, the delta waves in the inferior leads, especially aVF and III, change from negative to isoelectric to positive in polarity.

As opposed to left free wall APs, the ECG diagnosis of right free wall APs is the least accurate and least consistent among algorithms,[16–18,20] with a sensitivity of 80% to 90% and a specificity of 90% to 100%. Confusion may arise in the interpretation of a positive delta wave in V_1 as indicating a left-sided AP (Fig. 21-4). This finding is diagnostic of a left free wall AP only if R > S; a positive delta wave with R < S in V_1 is consistent with a right free wall AP or a minimally preexcited left free wall AP. A negative delta wave in V_1 is consistent with a septal AP. Therefore, most algorithms identify right free wall APs by a positive initial delta wave in V_1 but a late transition to R > S in the precordial leads at V_3 or later, coupled with leftward orientation to the initial delta wave, such as delta wave positivity in lead I or aVL.[18–20] As the pathway location moves from the right superior free wall to the right middle and right inferior free wall, the delta wave in inferior leads aVF and II changes from positive to isoelectric to negative.[18–20] A useful algorithm for AP localization that is based on the initial 20 milliseconds of the delta wave is shown in Figure 21-5.

The location of the AP can also be inferred from the surface ECG by the polarity of the retrograde P waves during orthodromic reciprocating tachycardia (ORT).[22,23] A negative P wave in lead I is highly suggestive of a left free wall location, with a 95% positive-predictive value.[23] A negative P wave in lead V_1 is highly suggestive of a right-sided AP. The presence of a positive retrograde P wave in lead I suggests a right free wall AP with a positive-predictive value of 99%.[23] For either right or left free wall APs, the presence of negative P waves in all three inferior leads indicates an inferior location, whereas positive P waves in these leads indicate a superior location. Isoelectric or biphasic P waves in any of the inferior leads suggest a middle free wall location.[22]

At electrophysiologic testing, the hallmark of any ORT is the demonstration of obligatory 1:1 atrial and ventricular activation for persistence of the tachycardia (Table 21-1).[24] The diagnosis of ORT using a free wall AP also requires an eccentric atrial activation sequence earliest along the right or left atrial free wall. Coupled with such an eccentric atrial activation sequence, ORT is highly suggested by demonstration of the shortest QRS-to-atrium time greater than or equal to 60 milliseconds, constant ventricle-to-atrium times despite changes in the tachycardia cycle length, and the ability to advance atrial activation by a premature ventricular stimulus delivered during His bundle refractoriness.[24] The last finding indicates the presence of an AP but does not prove participation in the tachycardia. A preexcitation index greater than 70 milliseconds is consistent with a left lateral AP.[25] The preexcitation index is the difference between the tachycardia cycle length and the longest coupling interval of a right ventricular apical premature stimulus that advances the atrium.[25] *Diagnostic* of a free wall pathway is prolongation of the QRS-to-atrium (or His-to-atrium) time during reciprocating tachycardia (and usually of the tachycardia cycle length as well) by 35 to 40 milliseconds or longer with ipsilateral bundle branch block.[24,26] Left anterior fascicular block also prolongs the QRS-to-atrium time in patients with left free wall APs.[26] Coupled with an eccentric atrial activation sequence, the ability to reproducibly terminate the tachycardia with a premature ventricular stimulus delivered during His bundle refractoriness also proves an ORT. Parahisian pacing techniques consistently indicate the presence of retrograde conduction over right free wall APs.[27] The response of left

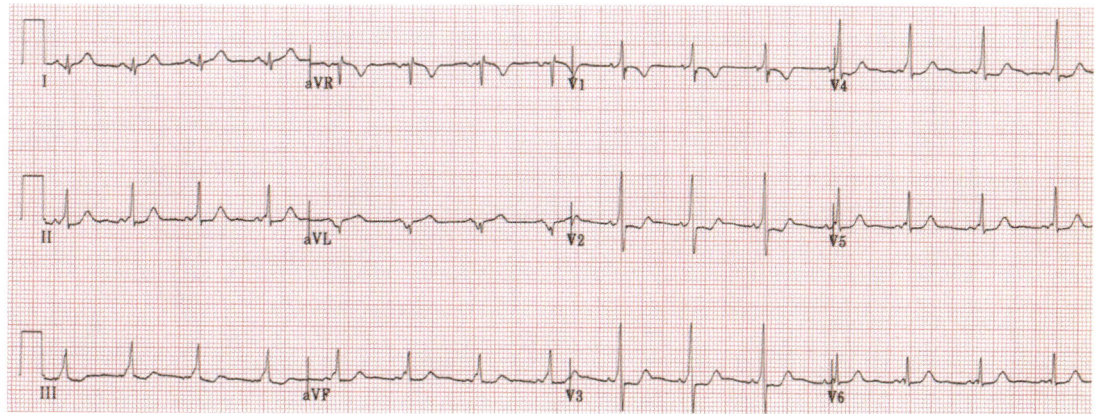

FIGURE 21-3. Twelve-lead electrocardiogram in sinus rhythm from a patient with a manifest left lateral accessory pathway. The positive delta wave in V_1 with R > S wave indicates a left free wall location. The negative delta waves in leads I and aVL are pathognomonic of a left free wall position. The positive delta waves in leads II, III, and aVF suggest a position anterolateral on the annulus.

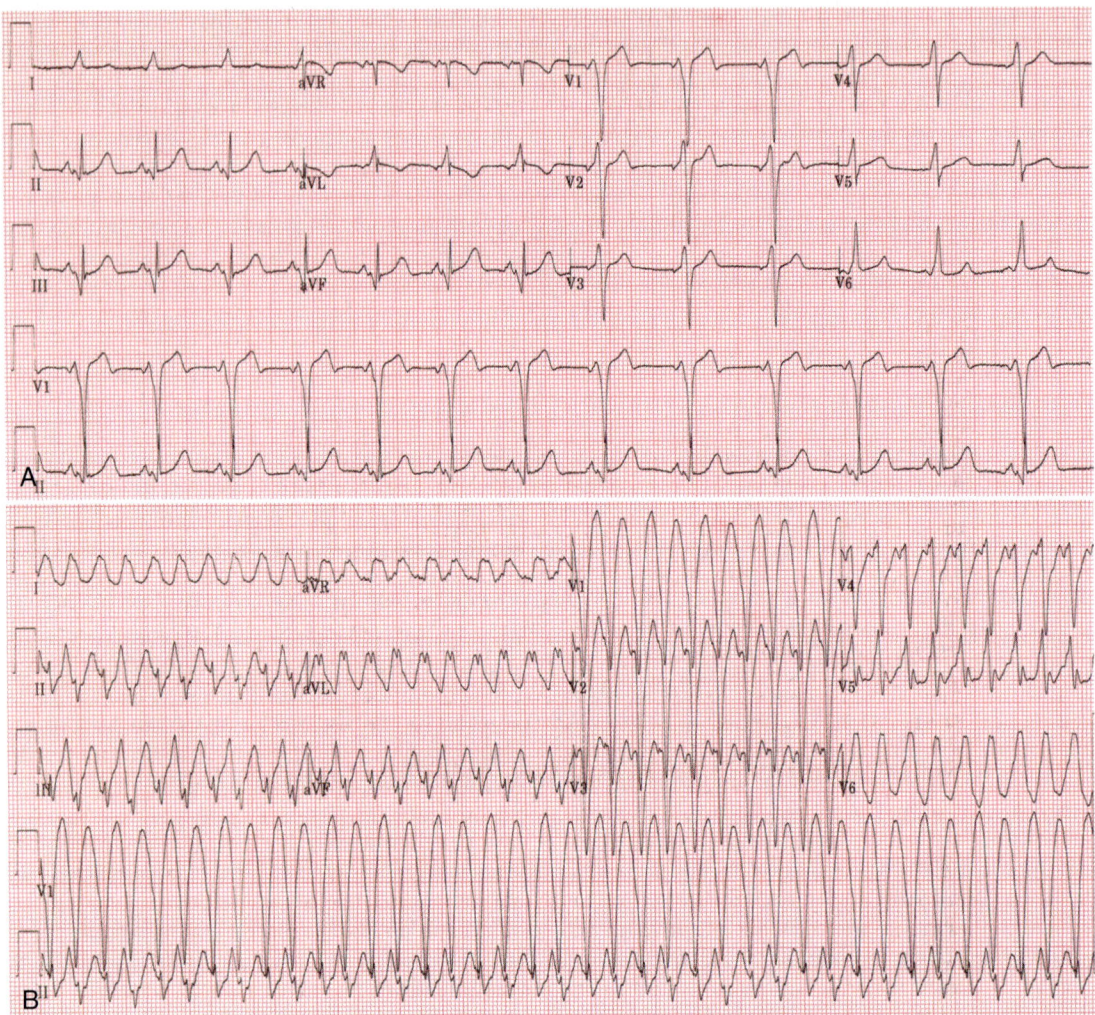

FIGURE 21-4. A, Twelve-lead electrocardiogram (ECG) in sinus rhythm from a patient with a manifest right free wall accessory pathway. The delta wave is positive in lead V_1; however, the transition to R > S wave in the precordial leads does not occur until V_5, indicating a right free wall location. The delta waves are negative in leads II, III, and aVF, indicating a position inferiorly on the right ventricular free wall. **B,** ECG from the same patient during antidromic reciprocating tachycardia using the right free wall pathway. The QRS complex is fully preexcited.

FIGURE 21-5. Algorithm for accessory pathway localization by surface electrocardiogram (ECG). This algorithm is based on the polarity of the first 20 msec of the delta wave. Left free wall pathways are readily identified by an isoelectric or negative delta wave in lead I or an R > S wave in V_1. Note that with right free wall pathways, the initial component of the delta wave is positive in V_1 but with R < S wave. Right free wall pathways are identified by a late transition to R > S usually in V_3 or later. LAL, left anterolateral; LL, left lateral; LP, left posterior; LPL, left posterolateral; MS, mid-septal; PSMA, posteroseptal mitral annulus; PSTA, posteroseptal tricuspid annulus; RA, right anterior; RAL, right anterolateral; RL, right lateral. *(From Arruda MS, McClelland J, Wang X, et al. Development and validation of an ECG algorithm for identifying accessory pathway ablation site in Wolff-Parkinson-White syndrome.* J Cardiovasc Electrophysiol. *1998;9:2–12. With permission.)*

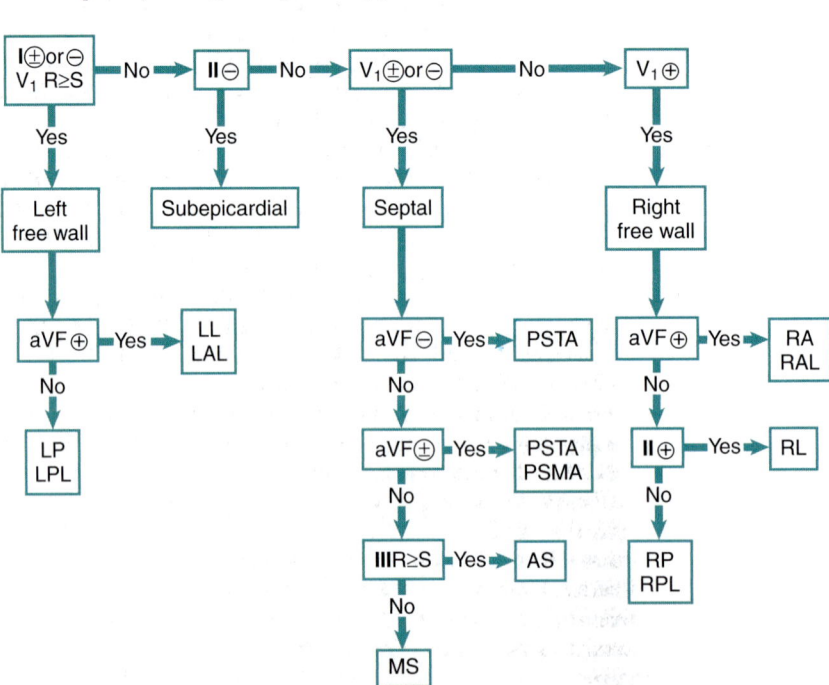

TABLE 21-1

DIAGNOSTIC CRITERIA

Orthodromic Tachycardia

Obligatory 1:1 AV relationship with earliest atrial activation on AV free wall

Shortest V-to-A time ≥60 msec

Constant V-to-A conduction times despite TCL variations

Advance atrial activation during His refractoriness (proves pathway presence but not participation in tachycardia)

Preexcitation index >70 msec (left lateral AP)

Ipsilateral bundle branch block prolongs His- (or V-) to-A time (and usually TCL) by ≥35 msec*

Reproducible tachycardia termination by premature ventricular stimuli during His refractoriness without conduction to atrium†

Antidromic Tachycardia

Obligatory 1:1 AV relationship with earliest ventricular activation on free wall

QRS morphology in tachycardia consistent with maximal preexcitation

Tachycardia QRS morphology reproduced by atrial pacing near pathway insertion

Each limb of tachycardia circuit supports conduction at TCL

Advance ventricular activation by atrial extrastimuli near insertion with advancement of subsequent His and atrial activation†

Changes in V-to-His interval precede changes in TCL

Exclusion of ventricular tachycardia and bystander participation, especially AV nodal reentry (His-to-A time in tachycardia ≤70 msec consistent with AV nodal reentry)

* Proves free wall AP-mediated tachycardia.
† Proves AP-mediated tachycardia.
A, atrium; AP, accessory pathway; AV, atrioventricular; His, bundle of His; TCL, tachycardia cycle length; V, ventricle

free wall APs to parahisian pacing is more complex. In about 25% of cases of left free wall APs, parahisian pacing is consistent with retrograde conduction over only the AV node. His capture may lead to a paradoxical shortening of the ventricle-to-atrium times, with left lateral APs due to the more rapid activation of the left free wall through the His-Purkinje system than occurs with septal ventricular capture alone.

The diagnostic features of antidromic reciprocating tachycardia are given in Table 21-1. Preexcited reciprocating tachycardias may use the AV node or a second AP as the retrograde limb. There are no surface ECG features that are diagnostic of antidromic tachycardia, but the diagnosis is excluded by demonstration of other than a 1:1 atrial-to-ventricular relationship.

Differential Diagnosis

ORTs using free wall APs must be differentiated from atrial tachycardias arising from near the AV valve annuli or, rarely, from the CS musculature.[28] Differentiation between atrial tachycardia and ORT is best accomplished by dissociating the ventricles from the tachycardia. The demonstration of a V-A-A-V response after termination of ventricular pacing that *entrains* the atrium excludes an ORT and confirms an atrial tachycardia.[29] The ability to

initiate the tachycardia with ventricular pacing, initiation with a critical AV or ventriculoatrial (VA) interval, and advancement of the same atrium activation sequence with premature ventricular stimuli during His refractoriness are all consistent with an ORT rather than AV nodal reentry.[24]

About 6% of cases of AV nodal reentry are associated with an eccentric atrial activation sequence that is earliest in the posterior or distal CS, with even the shortest VA times being longer than 60 milliseconds (Fig. 21-6).[30] This pattern is easily confused with ORT using a left-sided concealed AP, both at electrophysiologic testing and on the surface ECG, because the retrograde P wave during AV nodal reentrant tachycardia (AVNRT) is negative in leads I and aVL and positive in V_1. The eccentric atrial activation sequence is usually demonstrated with ventricular pacing as well. The keys to the diagnosis of AVNRT with eccentric atrial activation are (1) demonstration of dual AV nodal physiology, (2) ability to also induce "typical" AV nodal reentry with concentric atrial activation or variable patterns of retrograde atrial activation in most patients, (3) absence of retrograde VA conduction without isoproterenol, (4) inability to advance the atrium with premature ventricular stimuli during His refractoriness (may require left ventricular pacing), (5) demonstration of only decremental retrograde VA conduction, and (6) ability to dissociate the atrium and ventricle from the tachycardia.[30] Standard slow pathway ablation in the posteroseptal right atrium eliminates the tachycardia in these cases.

The differential diagnosis of an antidromic tachycardia includes ventricular tachycardia and bystander AP participation. Ventricular tachycardia should be diagnosed by the dissociation of the atrium from the tachycardia or a variable His-to-atrium timing relationship without alteration of the tachycardia cycle length. Antidromic tachycardia is diagnosed by demonstrating an obligatory 1:1 atrium-to-ventricle relationship during tachycardia, reproduction of tachycardia QRS morphology by atrial pacing at the presumed AP insertion site, and advancement of the ventricular *and* subsequent atrial activation by a premature atrial stimulus near the AP site (Table 21-1).[24]

Bystander participation of the AP is best recognized by dissociation of AP conduction from the tachycardia. The demonstration of a His-to-atrium interval of 70 milliseconds or less indicates AV nodal reentry with bystander AP rather than an antidromic reciprocating tachycardia.[24]

Mapping

The most widely used approaches to mapping of free wall APs rely on identification of the earliest ventricular activation during antegrade AP conduction and earliest retrograde atrial activation during ORT (Table 21-2). However, mapping based on electrogram morphology rather than timing can be performed in some situations. Both unipolar and bipolar recordings are helpful. Unipolar recordings from the electrode tip provide information on local activation through electrogram timing and morphology. Bipolar recordings from the distal electrode pair reflect timing and more clearly demonstrate the electrogram components and AP potentials.

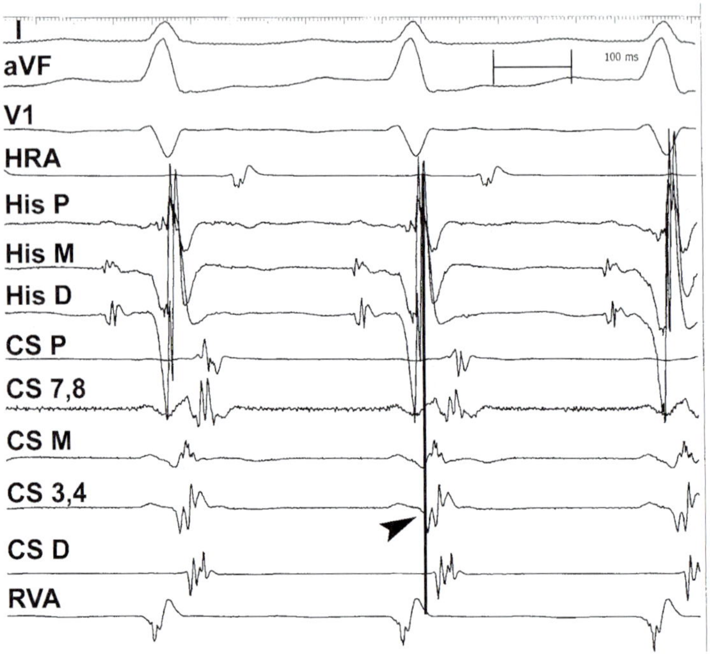

FIGURE 21-6. Eccentric retrograde atrial activation during atrioventricular (AV) nodal reentrant tachycardia. The first cardiac cycle is annotated, with ventricle-to-atrium (V-A) activation times indicated by *vertical lines*. The earliest atrial activation occurs in the next most distal bipole (*arrowhead*, CS 3,4) in the coronary sinus (CS). The tachycardia was rendered noninducible by slow pathway ablation. The V-A times are short for reciprocating tachycardia in this example but can be long with the eccentric activation sequence in AV node reentry as well. D, distal; HRA, high right atrium; M, mid; P, proximal; RVA, right ventricular apex.

TABLE 21-2

TARGET SITES

Left Free Wall

Presumed AP potential

Delta-VEGM ≤0 msec (antegrade conduction)

VEGM-AEGM ≤40 msec (retrograde conduction)

AEGM-VEGM ≤40 msec (antegrade conduction)

AEGM amplitude >0.4 mV

QRS-AEGM interval ≤70 msec (retrograde conduction)

Isoelectric VEGM-AEGM interval ≤5 msec (retrograde conduction)

Site of AEGM polarity reversal (in tachycardia)

Right Free Wall

Presumed AP potential

Delta-VEGM ≤ −10 msec

AEGM amplitude >1 mV

AEGM-VEGM ≤40 msec (antegrade conduction)

QRS-AEGM interval ≤70 msec (retrograde conduction)

Isoelectric VEGM-AEGM interval ≤5 msec (retrograde conduction)

AEGM, atrial electrogram; AP, accessory pathway; Delta, delta wave onset; QRS, QRS onset; VEGM, ventricular electrogram.

Left Free Wall Accessory Pathways

Mapping of left free wall APs is facilitated by multielectrode recordings from a CS catheter; however, the anatomic distance from the true mitral annulus limits the accuracy of CS mapping alone to identify target sites for ablation (Fig. 21-7). Left free wall APs can be ablated without the use of CS catheters (single catheter technique); however, the CS catheter is standard, along with right atrial, His, and right ventricular catheters.[31,32] Mapping and ablation may be performed by the transaor-

tic (retrograde) approach or the transseptal approach. The transaortic approach is directed at sites beneath the mitral annulus and therefore targets the AP ventricular insertion. For the transaortic approach, the catheter is always prolapsed across the aortic valve to prevent perforation of the leaflets or entry into the coronary arteries. The catheter most readily crosses the aortic valve, with the J curvature of the deflected catheter tip opening to the right of the fluoroscopy screen (anteriorly) in the right anterior oblique view. After entering the left ventricular cavity, the J curvature is maintained on the catheter tip, and the catheter is rotated in a counterclockwise direction to turn the catheter tip posteriorly toward the annulus (Fig. 21-8). The catheter then can be opened slightly to engage a subannular position, or it can be withdrawn to cross over the annulus into the left atrium. The catheter tip is either moved incrementally in steps beneath the annulus or made to slide along the mitral annulus for mapping before being dropped down beneath the annulus for energy delivery (Fig. 21-8). It is often difficult to achieve stable catheter positions for the far lateral and anterior mitral annulus with the transaortic approach.

The transseptal approach is primarily directed at mapping the atrial side of the annulus or the mitral annulus itself. As opposed to the transaortic approach, in which the ablation electrode is perpendicular to and beneath the annulus, the transseptal approach is directed at positions on or above the annulus, with the electrodes parallel to the annulus (Fig. 21-9).[1,34] After passing through the atrial septum, the catheter is directed laterally with a large sweeping curve, to direct the tip back toward the atrial septum. With the aid of preformed sheaths, the catheter tip is made to slide along the annulus by advancing and withdrawing the catheter (Fig. 21-9). Anterior mitral valve positions are readily reached with the transseptal approach (Fig. 21-10). Although catheter mobility is greater, catheter stability may be more problematic than with the transaortic approach.

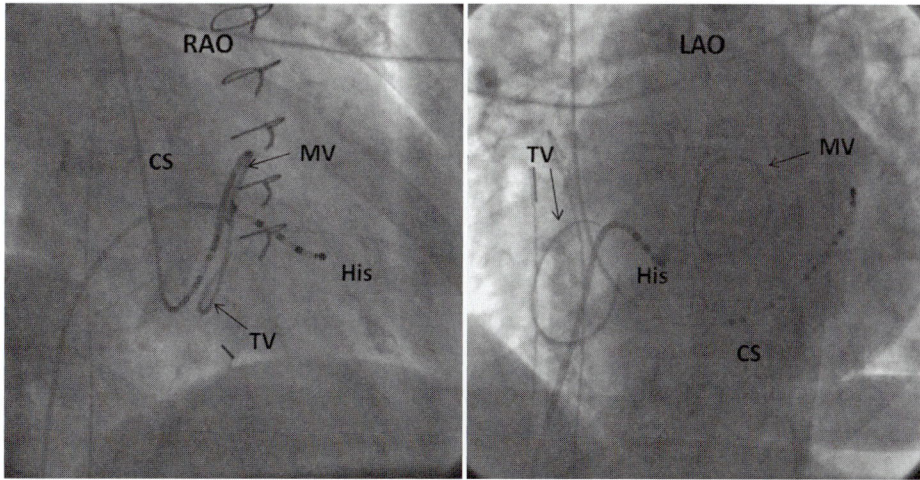

FIGURE 21-7. Fluoroscopic position of tricuspid (TV) and mitral (MV) valve annuli as defined by valvuloplasty rings. Note the separation of the mitral valve annulus from the coronary sinus catheter (CS) in the left anterior oblique (LAO) view. RAO, right anterior oblique.

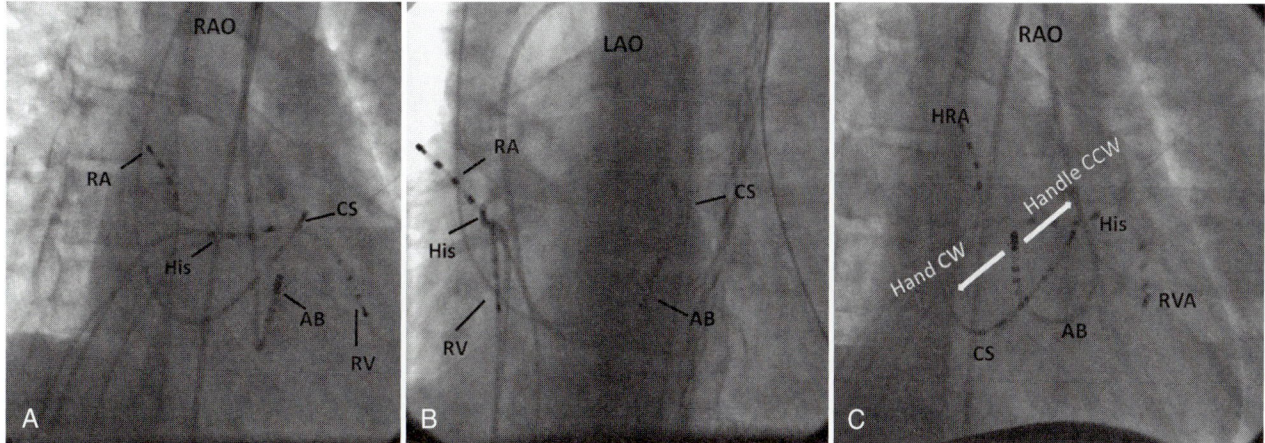

FIGURE 21-8. Catheter positions in right anterior oblique (RAO) (**A**) and left anterior oblique (LAO) (**B**) views for ablation of left free wall accessory pathway by the retrograde transaortic approach. **C,** Catheter-tip motion in response to torque on the handle once in mapping position. AB, ablation catheter; CCW, counterclockwise; CW, clockwise; CS, coronary sinus catheter; His, His bundle catheter; RA, right atrial catheter; RV, right ventricular catheter.

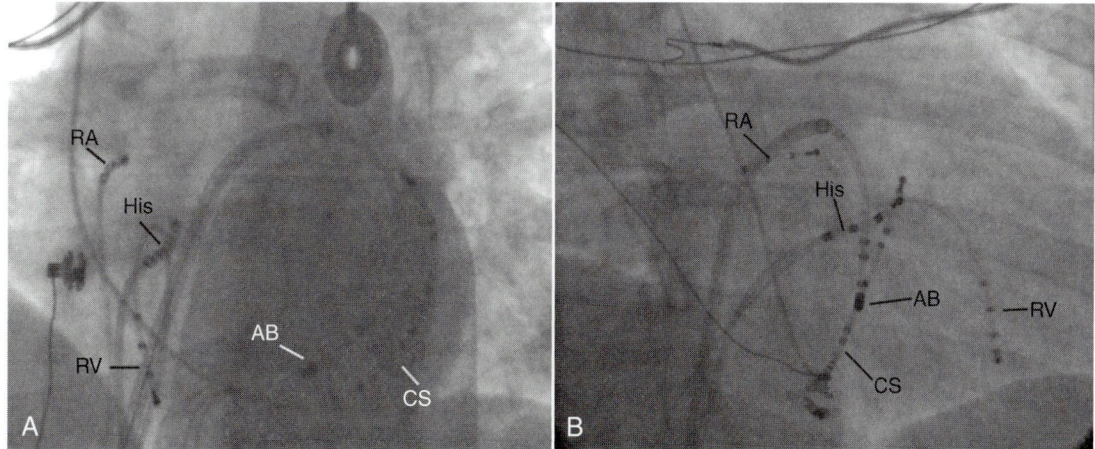

FIGURE 21-9. Catheter positions for transseptal approach to ablation of left free wall accessory pathway. **A,** Left anterior oblique view showing the preformed transseptal sheath (Daig SL2 Swartz Sheath) crossing the foramen ovale and used to position the ablation catheter (AB) along the proximal mitral annulus. From this position, the ablation catheter can be easily advanced to move proximally on the annulus and withdrawn to move distally. **B,** Right anterior oblique view of catheter positions. The ablation catheter has been moved slightly more distally. Note that the tip of the ablation catheter is slightly on the ventricular side of the coronary sinus catheter (CS). His, His bundle catheter; RA, right atrial catheter; RV, right ventricular apical catheter.

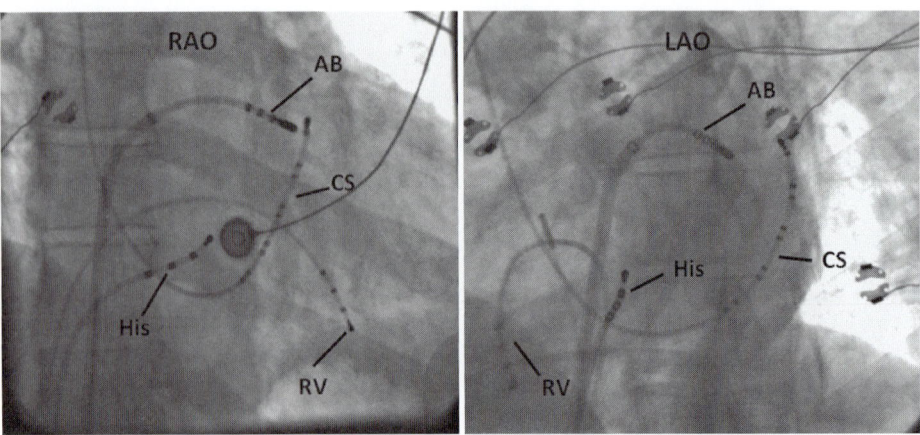

FIGURE 21-10. Transseptal approach to ablation of a left anterior accessory pathway. Turning the sheath and catheter in a counterclockwise direction allows advancing the tip into the left ventricle. By advancing the sheath, the superior aspect of the annulus is reached. The ablation catheter is then straightened and withdrawn to map the annulus. AB, ablation catheter; CS, coronary sinus catheter; His, His bundle catheter; LAO, left anterior oblique; RAO, right anterior oblique; RV, right ventricular apical catheter.

The decision regarding use of the transaortic or transseptal approach is based on physician familiarity and certain patient characteristics. Because the two approaches are complementary, it is best for the physician to be familiar with both techniques. The transseptal approach is favored in the presence of peripheral vascular disease, aortic valve disease or prosthesis, or small ventricular chambers. In children weighing less than 30 kg, the transaortic approach may be associated with frequent valve trauma.[33] The transseptal approach provides better access to far lateral and anterolateral AP locations. The transseptal approach may be contraindicated in the presence of distorted cardiac anatomy such as congenital heart disease, pneumonectomy, kyphoscoliosis, or severe dilation of the aorta or right atrium.

The characteristics of electrograms at successful ablation sites have been studied extensively for left free wall APs.[34–39] Most of these data are derived from early experience with ablation by the transaortic approach and have not been reproduced for the transseptal approach. Five electrogram characteristics have been described as useful in predicting successful ablation sites when mapping antegrade AP activation by the transaortic approach: (1) delta-to-ventricle (V) interval, (2) atrial electrogram amplitude, (3) electrogram stability, (4) local AV electrogram interval, and (5) presence of a presumed AP potential. The delta-to-V interval should be measured from the onset of the delta wave to the peak or intrinsicoid deflection of bipolar mapping electrograms.[36,37,40] For unipolar electrograms, the maximal negative dV/dt reflects local ventricular activation.[40] The absence of a QS morphology in the unipolar electrogram indicates a site with a less than 10% chance of ablation success.[40] Pacing from near the AP insertion accentuates the degree of preexcitation. For left free wall APs, a delta-to-V time of less than or equal to 0 milliseconds is usually recorded at successful ablation sites, with average intervals of only –2 to –10 milliseconds (Fig. 21-11).[35,37,41]

The atrial electrogram amplitude at successful sites should be greater than 0.4 to 1 mV, or the atrial-to-ventricular (A/V) ratio should be greater than 0.1 by the transaortic approach. The small atrial electrogram amplitude indicates the subannular position of the catheter. The absence of any atrial electrogram suggests a position

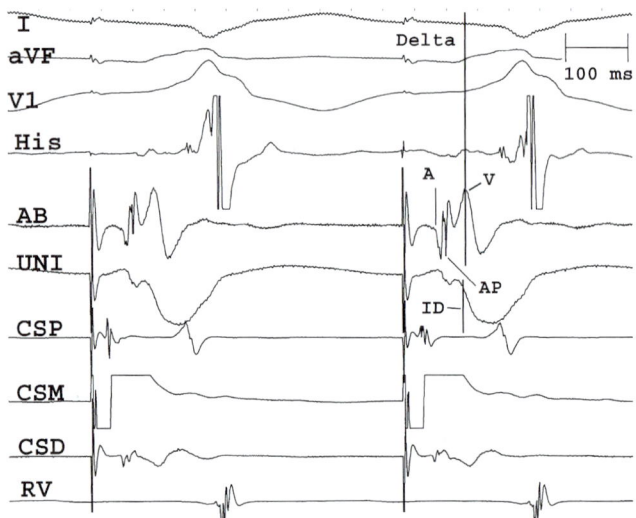

FIGURE 21-11. Mapping antegrade left free wall accessory pathway (AP) activation during pacing from the middle coronary sinus (CSM). The onset of the delta wave (Delta) is marked by the *vertical line* on the surface electrocardiographic leads (*top three tracings*). On the bipolar distal ablation electrodes (AB), the onset of the local atrial electrogram (A) and local ventricular electrogram (V) are marked. The local atrium-to-ventricle (A-V) interval is 25 msec, and the peak of the local bipolar ventricular electrogram coincides with delta wave onset (Delta-V = 0). The intrinsicoid deflection (ID) of the unipolar electrogram (UNI) precedes delta wave onset by about 5 msec. The unipolar ventricular ablation electrogram is entirely negative (QS morphology) and fuses with the atrial electrogram. A discrete high-frequency electrogram between the atrial and ventricular components represents a possible AP potential. CSD, distal coronary sinus; CSP, proximal coronary sinus; RV, right ventricle.

too far from the annulus. For transseptal mapping, an A/V ratio equal to 1 is sought along the mitral annulus.[32] Greater and lesser ratios indicate atrial and ventricular displacement of the catheter, respectively. Electrogram stability is defined as less than 10% change in the atrial and ventricular electrogram amplitudes or A/V ratio over 5 to 10 cardiac cycles.[35,37,39]

The transaortic approach usually provides good catheter stability because the catheter is "wedged" beneath the mitral valve. For the transseptal approach, stability can be assessed by consistent electrogram amplitudes, catheter motion concordant with the CS catheter, and, when on the atrial side of the annulus, consistent "PR" segment elevation on the unipolar electrogram.[13] The last finding also indicates sufficient catheter contact with the atrial myocardium. Local AV intervals of 40 milliseconds or less should be sought, with average intervals of 25 to 50 milliseconds reported for successful ablation sites (Fig. 21-11).[38,39] The AV intervals for left free wall APs are longer than for other AP locations, and the times at successful sites overlap with those at unsuccessful sites. The local AV times alone, therefore, have limited specificity in identifying successful ablation sites for left-sided APs.

Finally, the recording of a presumed AP potential has been used to define appropriate ablation sites. The ability to record AP potentials may be influenced by the catheter approach used to map the annulus. Presumed AP potentials are defined as discrete, high-frequency potentials that occur between the atrial and ventricular electrograms and at least 10 milliseconds before the onset of the delta wave (Fig. 21-11).[34-36,38,42] The amplitude of AP potentials ranges from 0.5 to 1 mV.[35] The validation of a signal as a true AP potential is a tedious process and is not practical in the clinical setting. It is probably for this reason that "AP potentials" are reported at 35% to 94% of successful ablation sites and at up to 72% of unsuccessful sites.[35,36,38,42,43] The recording of larger AP potentials in the CS than along the mitral annulus suggests the presence of an epicardial AP.[44]

For mapping of retrograde AP conduction during ORT or ventricular pacing, electrogram characteristics reported to identify successful sites include catheter stability, presence of a presumed AP potential, continuous electrical activity, and the local VA interval.[34,35,39] These data are derived largely from studies of ablation from the transaortic approach. Catheter stability is defined the same as for mapping of antegrade conduction. The presence of a presumed AP potential is reported at only 37% to 67% of successful ablation sites during retrograde AP conduction mapping.[34,35,39] It is possible that AP potentials are obscured by the large ventricular electrogram with the transaortic approach. The QRS onset-to–local atrial electrogram (QRS-A) interval is usually about 70 milliseconds in the absence of a left ventricular conduction delay (Fig. 21-12).[34,35] The local VA interval at successful ablation sites is typically 25 to 50 milliseconds.[34,35,39] At very short VA intervals, the atrial electrogram may be inscribed on the terminal portion of the ventricular electrogram. Continuous electrical activity (<5 milliseconds isoelectric interval between V and A electrograms) and the "pseudo-disappearance" of the atrial electrogram into the ventricular electrogram are manifestations of extremely short VA times.[34,37] One group has reported successful ablation by pace-mapping beneath the mitral annulus with the ablation catheter and measuring the stimulus-to-atrial times recorded on the CS catheter.[45] The site producing the shortest stimulus-to-atrial interval should be at the ventricular insertion of the AP. The average stimulus-to-atrial interval at successful sites was 46 ± 15 milliseconds.[45]

The predictive accuracy of any single electrogram characteristic for identifying a successful ablation site rarely exceeds 30%. The electrogram must satisfy three or four criteria to achieve 60% to 80% predictive values.[37,42] Multivariate predictors of successful ablation sites are given in Table 21-3.

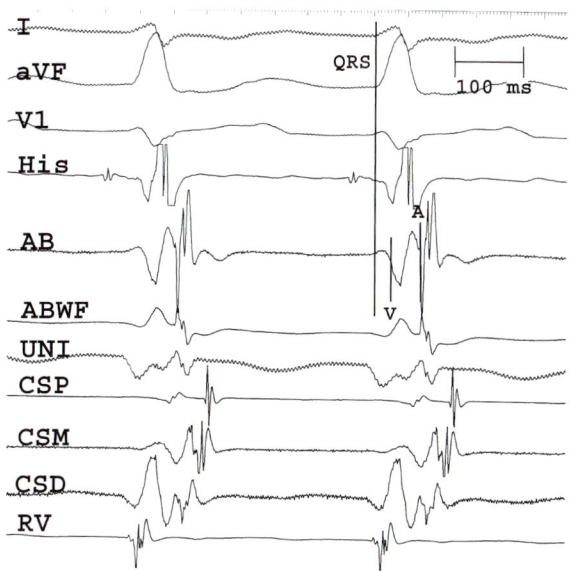

FIGURE 21-12. Electrograms from successful ablation site during mapping of retrograde accessory pathway (AP) conduction in orthodromic reciprocating tachycardia. The distal coronary sinus is earliest on this catheter. The QRS onset (QRS) to local atrial electrogram (A) interval on the ablation catheter is 68 msec and is shown by the *vertical lines*. The local ventricular (V) to atrial interval on the ablation electrodes is 40 msec. Note the isoelectric morphology of the atrial component of the electrogram on the wide filtered ablation electrogram (ABWF), representing the atrial insertion point of the AP (see text). AB, ablation catheter; CSD, distal coronary sinus; CSM, middle coronary sinus; CSP, proximal coronary sinus; His, His bundle catheter; RV, right ventricle; UNI, unipolar electrogram.

One problem with mapping retrograde atrial activation times is the difficulty in discriminating between atrial and ventricular components of the electrograms. This problem may be addressed in several ways. One method is to compare the electrogram recorded on the ablation catheter while simultaneously pacing the atrium and the ventricle with the electrogram recorded during ventricular pacing alone (Fig. 21-13).[46]

Another approach to unmasking distinct components of antegrade and retrograde electrograms exploits the oblique course of AP conduction across the AV annulus.[47] For left free wall APs, the ventricular insertion is usually more proximal in the CS than the atrial insertion.[47,48] When the ventricular insertion of the AP is activated by a wavefront conducting in the same direction as the oblique AP propagation, the VA intervals recorded on mapping electrodes are short and may overlap (Figs. 21-14 and 21-15). By reversing the direction of wavefront activation, the local VA intervals may be prolonged if conduction over the AP "backtracks" past ventricular sites previously activated. The same separation of components of antegrade-conducted electrograms is possible by reversing the direction of activation of the atrial AP insertion. For left lateral APs, pacing of the basal posteroseptal right ventricle provides counterclockwise activation of the ventricular insertion (from the left anterior oblique perspective), whereas pacing of the high right ventricular outflow tract near the pulmonic valve provides clockwise activation of the ventricular insertion. Because the ventricular AP insertion tends to be more proximal along the CS than the atrial insertion, the VA intervals are typically prolonged by clockwise activation with right ventricular outflow tract pacing. A change in

MULTIVARIATE PREDICTORS OF SUCCESSFUL LEFT FREE WALL ABLATION SITES BY THE TRANSAORTIC APPROACH

Study	AP Potential	EGM Stability	Delta-V Interval (msec)	A Amplitude	Local AV Interval (msec)	Local VA Interval (msec)	Best Positive-Predictive Value (%)
Hindrick et al, 1955[36]	+	—	Value not specified	—	—	—	70
Bashir et al, 1993[37]	+	—	10	—	—	—	20-25
Chen et al, 1992[35]	+	<10% change in EGM amplitude	0	A >1 mV	—	—	62
Cappato et al,1994[38]	+	—	≤0	A/V ratio ≥0.1	≤40	—	87
Xie et al, 1996[39]	+	—	0	—	30	≤30	67
Villacastin et al, 1996[34]	+	—	—	—	—	Pseudo-disappearance	59

A, atrial electrogram; AP, accessory pathway; AV, atrium-to-ventricle; Delta, delta wave onset; EGM, electrogram; V, ventricular electrogram; VA, ventricle-to-atrium; –, not reported.

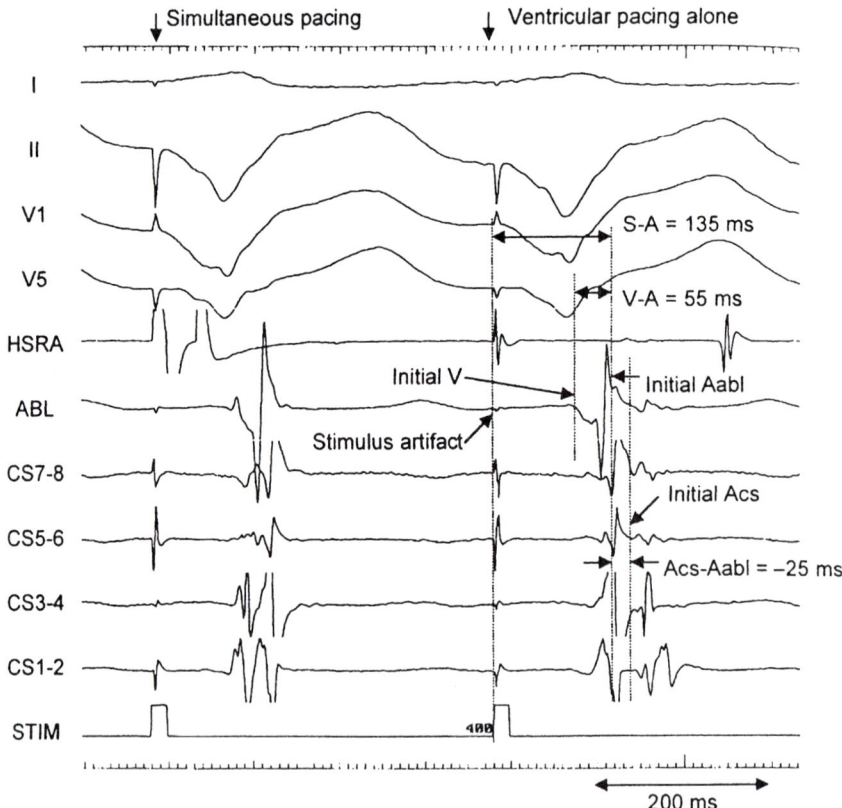

FIGURE 21-13. Use of simultaneous atrial and ventricular pacing to discriminate components of mapping electrograms in a patient with left-sided accessory pathway. The penultimate beat of the drive train comprises simultaneous atrial and ventricular pacing (labeled). The atrial electrogram is advanced relative to the ventricular electrogram and precedes it. No electrical activity follows the ventricular activation in this beat. The last beat of the drive comprises only ventricular pacing. Retrograde conduction over the accessory pathway is evident by atrial activation now following the ventricular electrograms. By comparing the electrograms from the two cardiac cycles the atrial and ventricular components of the electrograms are more apparent. Aabl, onset local retrograde atrial electrogram on the ablation catheter; ABL, ablation; Acs, onset local atrial electrogram recorded on the coronary sinus; CS1-2, distal coronary sinus; CS7-8, proximal coronary sinus; HRSA, high septal right atrium; S-A, interval between stimulus artifact (Stim) and local atrial electrogram; V-A, interval between local ventricular and atrial electrograms. *(From Nakao K, Seto S, Iliev II, et al. Simultaneous atrial and ventricular pacing to facilitate mapping of concealed left-sided accessory pathways. Pacing Clin Electrophysiol. 2002;25:922-928. With permission.)*

local VA times of greater than 15milliseconds is considered to represent a significant change in the activation wavefront. For reversing atrial activation wavefronts of left free wall APs, CS pacing proximal and distal to the site of earliest retrograde atrial activity is used. For antegrade mapping, pacing distal to the atrial insertion should provide a counterclockwise activation wavefront and the longest AV intervals. The target sites are AP potentials or just to the

side of the earliest site of atrial or ventricular activation predicted to be the mid-AP site by changes in the local electrogram times. Note that this technique does not target the sites of the shortest AV or VA times.

A useful technique for ablation of left free wall pathways from the transseptal approach is to identify the point of atrial electrogram polarity reversal when mapping the annulus.[49] This vectorial technique obviates the need to measure VA

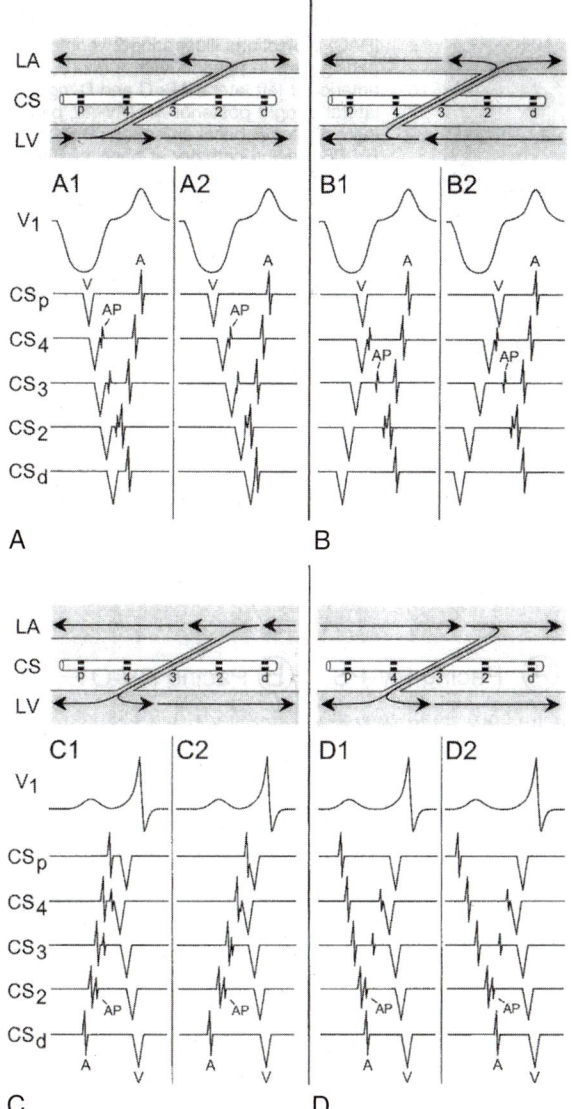

FIGURE 21-14. Activation of oblique accessory pathways. Schematic of antegrade and retrograde activation of an oblique left free wall accessory pathway (AP) from opposing directions. **A** and **B** demonstrate activation of the ventricular insertion from the proximal-to-distal and distal-to-proximal directions, respectively. **C** and **D** represent activation of the atrial insertion from the distal-to-proximal and proximal-to-distal directions, respectively. Note the separation of the components of the electrograms when the AP is activated from the direction opposite to the direction of conduction over the pathway. A, atrial potential; CS, coronary sinus; d, distal; LA, left atrium; LV, left ventricle; p, proximal; V, ventricular potential. *(From Kenichiro O, Gonzalez M, Beckman K, et al. Reversing the direction of paced ventricular and atrial wavefronts reveals an oblique course in accessory AV pathways and improves localization for catheter ablation. Circulation. 2001;104:550-556. With permission.)*

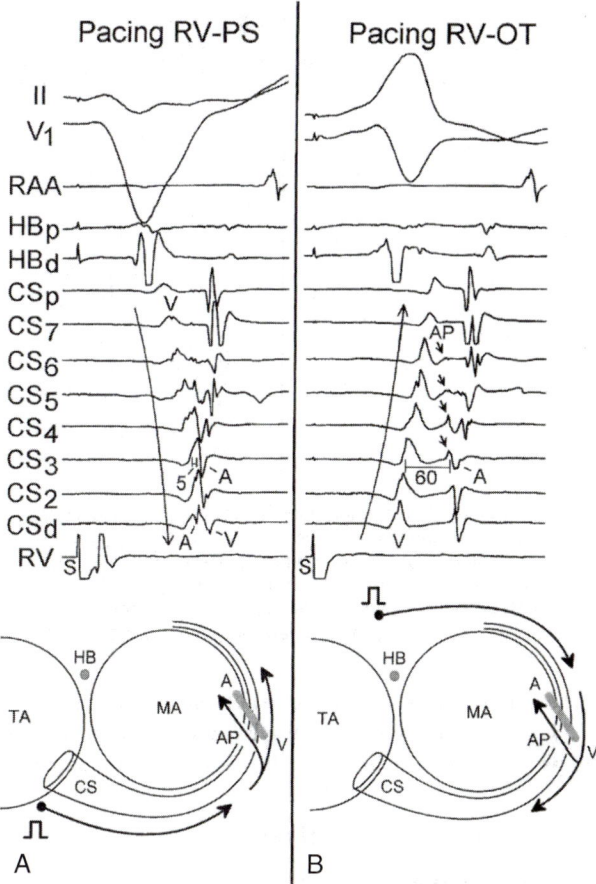

FIGURE 21-15. Reversing the direction of activation of the ventricular insertion in a patient with a left lateral accessory pathway (AP). The schematics show the presumed pathway orientation and wavefront propagation. When activated from proximal to distal by right ventricular posteroseptal (RV-PS) pacing (**A**), the coronary sinus (CS) electrograms overlap considerably. When activated from distal to proximal by right ventricular outflow tract (RV-OT) pacing (**B**), there is greater separation of the electrogram components and definition of an AP potential. HB, his bundle; MA, mitral annulus; RAA, right atrial appendage; S, stimulus artifact; TA, tricuspid annulus. *(From Kenichiro O, Gonzalez M, Beckman K, et al. Reversing the direction of paced ventricular and atrial wavefronts reveals an oblique course in accessory AV pathways and improves localization for catheter ablation. Circulation. 2001;104: 550-556. With permission.)*

intervals. Through transseptal access, the ablation electrode bipole is oriented parallel to the axis of the annulus. Wide-bandpass electrogram filtering is set to 0.5 to 500 Hz to accentuate the directional characteristics of the electrogram polarity. The bipole is then moved proximally and distally, parallel to the annulus, during ORT, and the polarity of the atrial electrogram is noted. With the tip electrode negative and the proximal electrode positive, the atrial electrogram will be predominantly negative at catheter positions on the annulus proximal to the atrial insertion (Fig. 21-16). At positions distal to the atrial insertion, the direction of the atrial activation wavefront is reversed relative to the bipole, and the atrial electrogram is predominantly positive. The point at which the atrial electrogram becomes isoelectric marks the atrial insertion and the site for ablation. The positive-predictive value of electrogram reversal for identifying the successful ablation site is 75%.[49] To be effective, this technique requires that the mapping bipole remain parallel with the axis of atrial activation on the annulus.

Right Free Wall Accessory Pathways

Mapping and ablation of right free wall APs is more difficult than for left-sided APs because of the absence of a venous structure paralleling the tricuspid annulus and because of catheter instability. To facilitate rapid localization of right free wall APs, it is often useful to employ a circular multielectrode halo catheter positioned near the

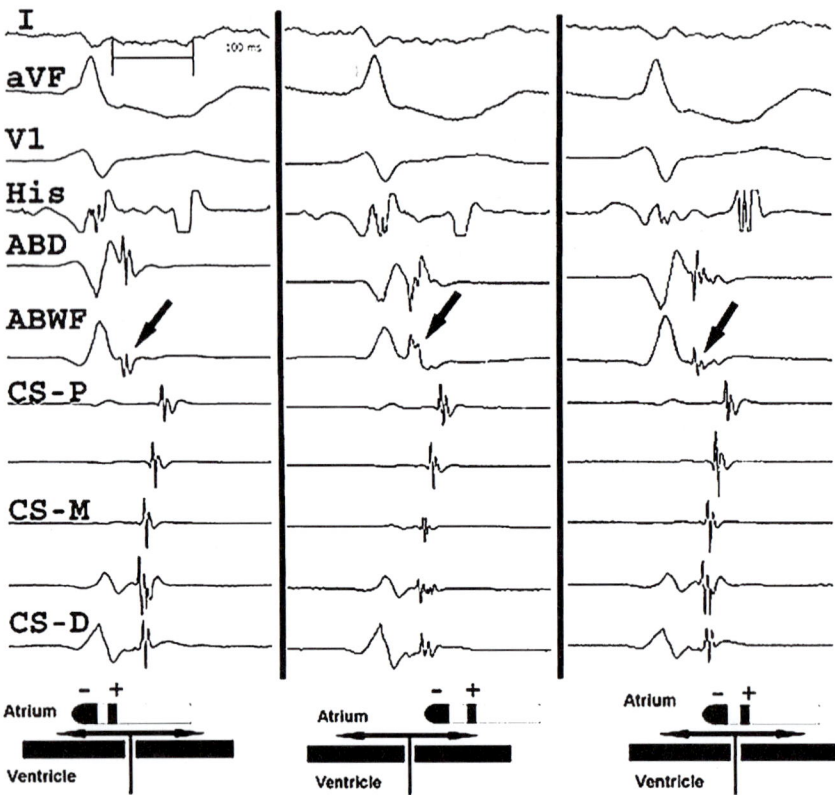

FIGURE 21-16. Atrial electrogram polarity reversal during mapping of orthodromic reciprocating tachycardia using a left free wall accessory pathway. *Left,* During reciprocating tachycardia, the distal bipolar ablation electrograms are displayed with standard (ABD) filtering at 30-500 Hz and wide filtering (ABWF) at 0.5-500 Hz. In this panel, the electrode is parallel to the annulus and proximal to the site of atrial accessory pathway (AP) insertion. The atrial component of the ABWF electrogram (*arrow*) is negative. *Middle,* The distal electrode pair has been moved distal to the site of the AP insertion, represented by the positive atrial component to the ABWF electrogram. *Right,* When the electrode pair is directly over the atrial insertion of the AP, the atrial component to the ABWF electrogram is isoelectric as the wavefront spreads away from the electrode pair in two opposing directions. The schematics at the *bottom* of the tracings illustrate the relation of the electrodes to the atrial insertion site. CS, coronary sinus; D, distal; M, mid; P, proximal.

tricuspid annulus (Fig. 21-17). Use of this catheter or, rarely, of 2-French (2F) mapping catheters positioned in the right coronary artery represents the closest equivalent to a CS mapping for the right side of the heart.[8] Catheter mapping from the subclavian or right internal jugular approach is sometimes more productive than from the femoral approach. As for transseptal access to the left side of the heart, the use of preformed sheaths to direct the ablation catheter to specific locations on the tricuspid annulus is helpful. The sheaths allow for placement of the mapping catheter parallel to the annulus for mapping, as with the transseptal approach to left APs (Fig. 21-17).

Because of the relative infrequency of right free wall APs, multivariate analyses of electrogram characteristics specific to this site that predict successful ablation are not available. Presumably, the stability and AP criteria defined for left APs are applicable. For ablation along the tricuspid annulus, a 1:1 A/V ratio is usually sought.[41,50] Most series have also used retrograde local VA times of 40 milliseconds or less as a criterion for radiofrequency (RF) delivery. The timing of local ventricular activation before delta wave onset is usually earlier than for left APs (Fig. 21-18). Haïssaguerre and colleagues[41,50] found that the local ventricle preceded delta wave onset by 18 ± 10 milliseconds for right APs and 2 ± 6 milliseconds for left APs at successful sites. The average local AV time was 28 ± 7 milliseconds for right-sided APs. In children, the local AV times were 11 to 26 milliseconds, with delta-to-V electrogram intervals of –28 to –52

milliseconds at sites of successful right free wall AP ablation in five patients.[51] If it is difficult to discriminate the components of the local electrograms, reversal of the activating wavefronts may be useful, as described earlier.[47] For right free wall APs, opposing ventricular wavefronts are produced by pacing the right ventricle near the annulus, anterior and posterior to the site of earliest retrograde AP conduction. Opposing atrial activation is produced by pacing on either side of the presumed atrial insertion.

For both right and left free wall pathways, it is my opinion that computerized *mapping* of electrical activation is optional. This is because there are usually relatively few points of electrical interest. Electroanatomic mapping systems have been shown to dramatically reduce fluoroscopic exposure to pediatric patients, however.[51] The catheter *navigation* capabilities of computerized systems are very helpful because they allow the operator to precisely return to sites of interest (Fig. 21-19).

Ablation

Before ablation energy delivery, it is essential to obtain the most stable catheter position possible. Catheter dislodgment before completion of the ablation lesion may transiently suppress AP function, allowing future recovery. Catheter stability is enhanced by the use of preformed sheaths and catheters with sufficient curvature or reach to

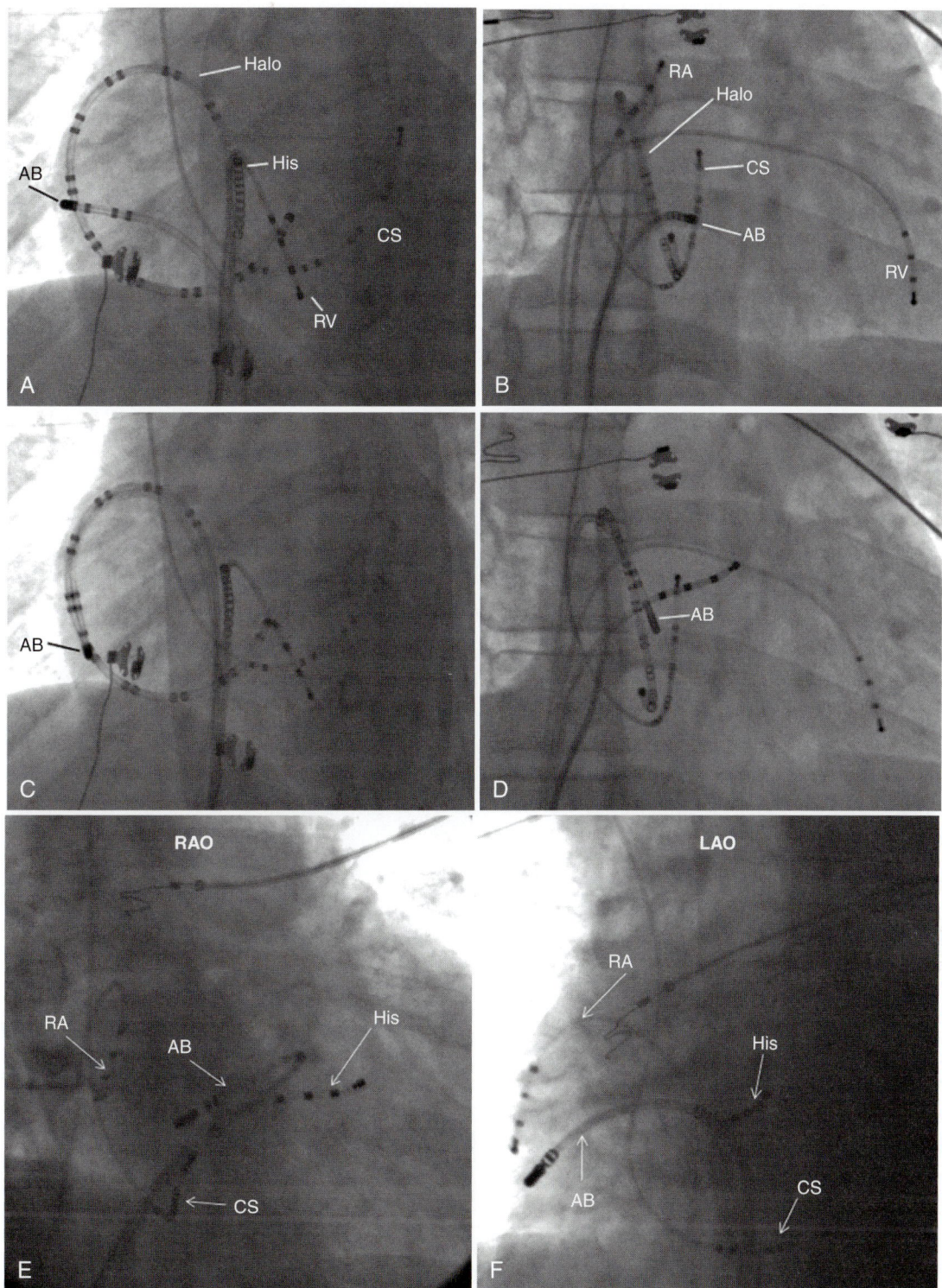

FIGURE 21-17. Catheter positions for ablation of a right free wall accessory pathway. **A,** Left anterior oblique (LAO) 40-degree view showing the 20-electrode halo catheter parallel to the tricuspid annulus and the ablation (AB) catheter near electrodes 11 and 12 along the free wall. The His, right ventricular apical (RV), and coronary sinus (CS) catheters are shown. **B,** Right anterior oblique (RAO) 30-degree view of the same catheter positions as in **A,** except that the His bundle catheter is replaced by a right atrial (RA) catheter. Note that the ablation catheter tip is to the ventricular side of the halo catheter. **C,** LAO 40-degree view with the ablation catheter now placed parallel to the tricuspid annulus. **D,** RAO 30-degree view of catheter positions in **C. E** and **F,** Ablation of right free wall accessory pathway with ablation catheter (AB) positioned under the tricuspid annulus. A Daig SR3 sheath is used to direct the catheter into the ventricle and under the annulus. In this patient, catheter positions on the atrial aspect of the annulus were unstable or unsuccessful. The accessory pathway was ablated at this site. An irrigated catheter was needed because of excessive temperatures with low energy deliveries with a standard catheter.

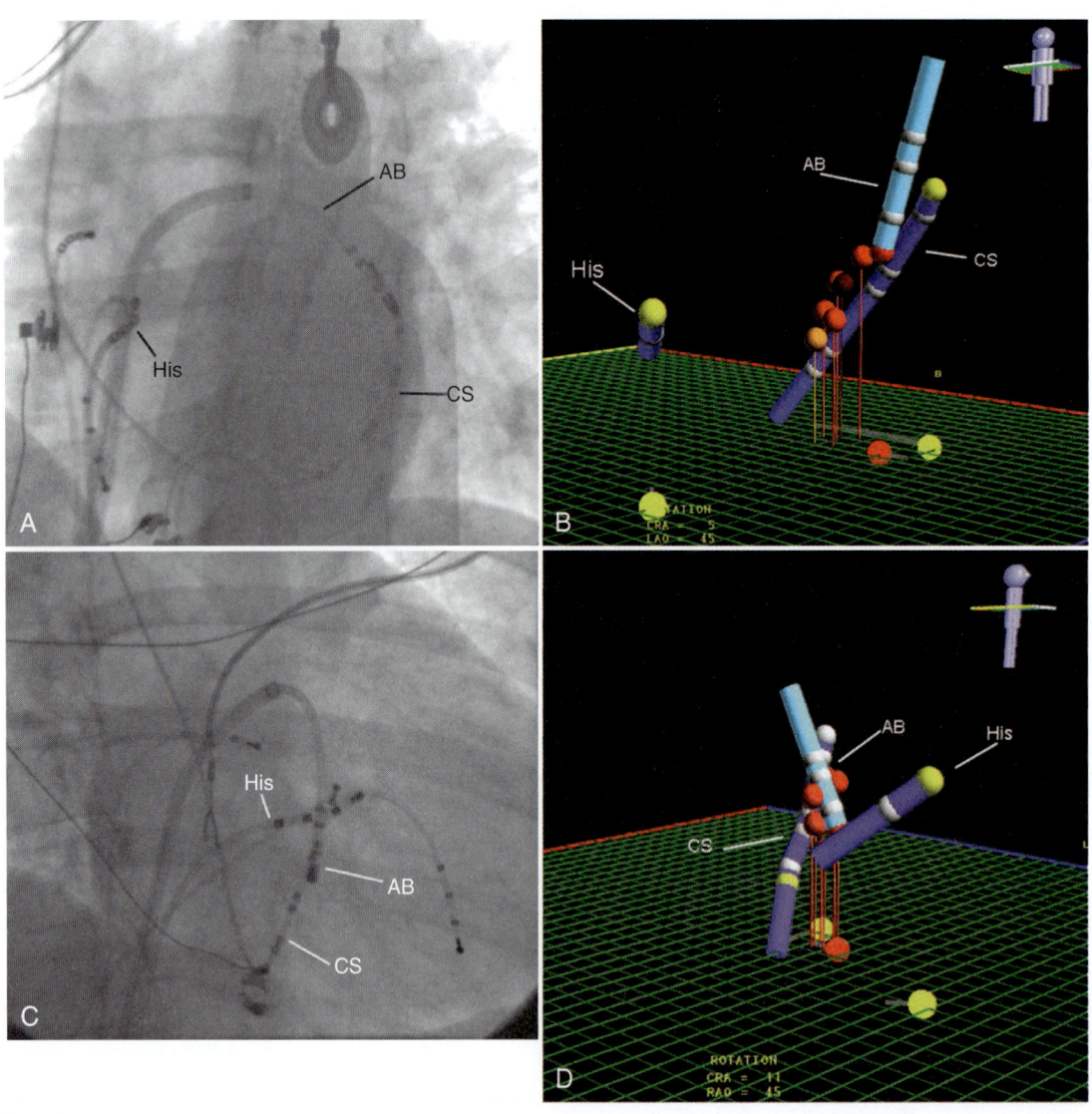

FIGURE 21-18. Electrograms from the site of successful ablation of a right free wall accessory pathway. *Left,* On the distal ablation bipole (AB), there is continuous electrical activity with the local ventricular electrogram (V) preceding the delta wave (Delta) onset by 25 msec. The local atrial (A)–to–ventricular (V) electrogram interval is 38 msec. The unipolar distal ablation electrogram (UNI) has a QS morphology. *Right,* After ablation, the ablation electrogram shows prolongation of the AV times, but the morphology of the local atrial electrogram is unchanged. DCS, distal coronary sinus; MCS, middle coronary sinus; PCS, proximal coronary sinus; RVA, right ventricular apex.

FIGURE 21-19. Use of a nonfluoroscopic catheter navigation system for ablation of a left free wall accessory pathway. **A,** Left anterior oblique (LAO) fluoroscopic view of the ablation catheter (AB) in the far lateral free wall near coronary sinus (CS) electrodes 3 and 4. **B,** Comparable LAO representation of the ablation catheter, His bundle catheter, and distal six CS electrodes in the nonfluoroscopic navigation system. The *red spheres* indicate sites of radiofrequency delivery, with the *dark red marker* being the successful site. **C,** Right anterior oblique (RAO) fluoroscopic view of catheter positions as in **A. D,** RAO nonfluoroscopic navigation system view comparable to **C.** In both **C** and **D,** the ablation catheter is seen slightly on the ventricular side of the coronary sinus catheter.

TABLE 21-4

CATHETER ABLATION OF LEFT FREE WALL ACCESSORY PATHWAYS FROM WITHIN THE CORONARY SINUS

Study	Energy Type	No. of Patients	Maximal Power	Target Temperature	Duration (sec)	Success (No./Total)	Complications
Wang et al, 1992[56]	RF	5	Not reported	Power control	—	5/5 (100%)	Not reported
Haïssaguerre et al, 1992[57]	RF	7	30 W	Power control	60	6/7 (85%)	CS mural thrombus (2 patients)
Giorgberidze et al, 1995[58]	RF	5	Not reported	Power control	—	3/5 (60%)	None
Langberg et al, 1993[59]	RF	2	28 ± 9W	Power control	—	2/2 (100%)	Not reported
Cappato et al, 1993[60]	RF	6	Not reported	Power control	—	6/6 (100%)	None
Yamane et al, 2000[55]	Irrigated RF	7	30 W maximum	50°C	60	7/7 (100%)	Stenosis of cardiac veins (2 patients)
Gaita et al, 2002[61]	Cryoablation	1	NA	−75°C	240	1/1 (100%)	None

CS, coronary sinus; NA, not applicable; RF, radiofrequency; —, not reported.

access the target site. Cardiac motion can be minimized during ablation by discontinuing the use of isoproterenol and by rapid ventricular pacing at rates of 120 beats/minute or greater. With ventricular pacing to entrain reciprocating tachycardias, the ablation catheter is less subject to dislodgment on termination of the arrhythmia. Adequate sedation should be established before RF delivery because the patient may move in response to pain. Marking of the catheter site with computerized navigation systems or by fluoroscopy may allow return to successful sites despite catheter dislodgment (Fig. 21-19). Standard 4-mm-tip RF catheters are usually adequate for free wall APs.

The target temperatures for right and left free wall APs is typically 60° to 65°C.[52] Favorable ablation sites should not be abandoned until temperatures higher than 50° to 55°C are achieved. For impedance monitoring, a 5- to 10-ohm decrease in impedance usually signifies tissue heating. The energy needed to reach the target temperature varies with catheter location. Low blood flow positions beneath the mitral or tricuspid annulus may require little energy because of the absence of convective cooling. Loss of AP function should occur within 1 to 6 seconds after RF energy delivery.[53] Longer times to success may be associated with higher recurrence rates. Endocardial cryoablation is effective for free wall AP ablation and offers the advantage of complete catheter stability due to adherence to the tissue during ablation.[54] Large-tip (6 or 8 mm) cryoablation catheters should be used to minimize the likelihood of AP recurrence. After successful ablation, thorough electrophysiologic testing should be undertaken to document the complete elimination of AP function and to exclude other mechanisms of tachycardias.

For resistant APs, irrigated catheters may prove successful by delivering greater energies.[55] For irrigated systems, target maximal temperatures of 50°C with 50 W maximal power may safely eliminate 94% of APs after failed conventional RF delivery.[55] Use of passively cooled large-tip catheters with high-output generators may also result in larger lesions.

Epicardial left free wall APs may require ablation from within the CS (Table 21-4).[44,55-61] Epicardial APs account for 4% of all left free wall APs and 10% of failed ablations.[44] Before CS ablation, CS angiography may be used to delineate the anatomy, exclude diverticulum, and assess possible damage to the CS from the ablation. Also, coronary angiography may be performed to determine the proximity of the ablation site to the left circumflex artery. Much published experience included non–temperature-controlled ablation in a small series of patients (Table 21-4). Mural thrombus in the CS was reported in one series.[57] For temperature-controlled RF within the CS, target temperatures of 60°C with power limits of 20 to 30W have been used.[55] For resistant epicardial APs, irrigated RF ablation within the CS may be effective. For irrigated catheters, the target temperature is 50°C with maximal power of 20 to 30 W delivered for 60 seconds at effective sites.[55] No complications were reported in small series of patients, and irrigated RF may be the preferred RF modality within the CS. Cryoablation in the CS has been used effectively and may carry a lower risk for injury to the circumflex coronary artery than RF ablation.[61] Right and left epicardial APs may also be ablated by direct epicardial mapping achieved by percutaneous pericardial access (Fig. 21-20).[62]

The use of robotic and magnetic navigation systems for free wall AP ablation may theoretically improve catheter stability (Fig. 21-21) and maneuverability, but superiority to manual ablation has not been demonstrated.

Clinical Results

Left Free Wall Accessory Pathways

The rates of success for left free wall AP ablation are the highest of any AP location and are typically greater than 90% (Table 21-5).[32,49,63-76] In the largest reported single-center series, 96% of 388 patients with left free wall APs were successfully ablated by the transseptal approach.[63] The recurrence rates for left free wall APs are the lowest

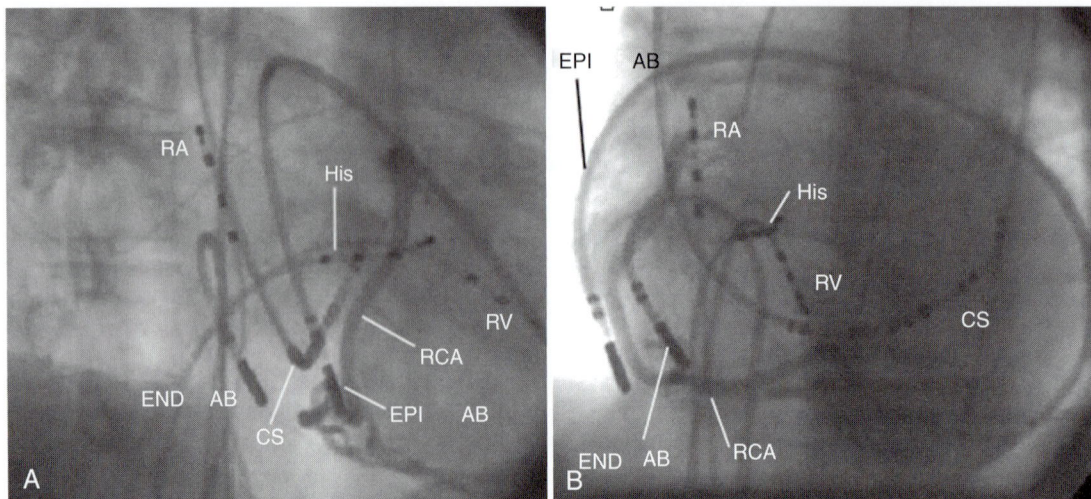

FIGURE 21-20. Percutaneous epicardial catheter approach to ablation of an epicardial right inferior free wall pathway. **A,** In this right anterior oblique view, the epicardial ablation catheter (EPI AB) enters the pericardial space from subxiphoid access and encircles the heart from posterior to anterior to reach the site of successful ablation. Attempts at ablation from the endocardial catheter (END AB) failed. The right coronary artery (RCA) is visualized by angiography and is very near the epicardial ablation catheter. **B,** Same catheter positions shown in left anterior oblique view. His, His bundle catheter; RA, right atrial catheter; RV, right ventricular catheter. (Courtesy of Dr. K. Shivkumar.)

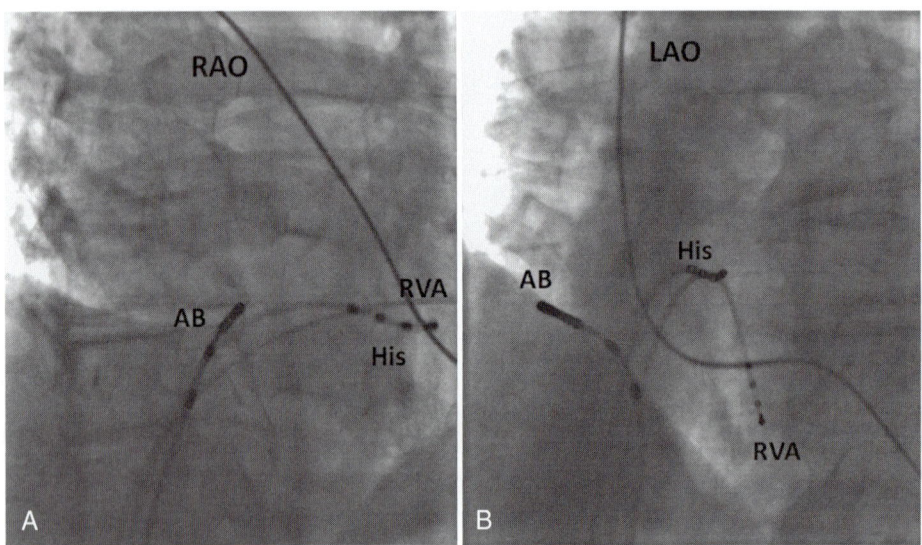

FIGURE 21-21. A and **B,** Stereotaxis magnetic ablation catheter (AB) navigation for ablation of a right free wall pathway. The catheter is very stable along the middle free wall tricuspid annulus despite the absence of a preformed sheath. His, His bundle catheter; RVA, right ventricular apex.

of any location, at 2% to 5%.[32,49,63–65] Recurrences are more likely with concealed APs, delivery of transiently effective pulses, or need for more than five lesions for acute success.[53,66–68] The success rates for ablation by the transaortic and transseptal approaches appear to be similar in direct comparisons (Table 21-6).[69–76] These studies usually report similar total procedure times, fluoroscopy times, and rates of crossover to the other approach. Overall, complication rates appear to be similar, but some studies have found a trend toward a higher rate of complications with the transaortic approach.[71,73] In comparative trials, there are no features that predict the success of one approach or the other.[70] Because the techniques are complementary, it is to the operator's advantage to be familiar with both, allowing crossover should one approach fail. Because arterial access is required for the retrograde transaortic approach, vascular complications may be more common with this technique.[71,73] The success rates for ablation of concealed left

APs by the transaortic approach are lower in some reports, possibly because of the smaller atrial electrograms recorded with this approach.

The success rates for right free wall AP ablation are the lowest of any AP location, averaging about 90% but ranging from 66% to 100% (Table 21-7).[32,41,51,66,77,78] In the largest series of 92 patients with right free wall APs, the success rate was 90%.[77] The lower success rate is attributed in general to greater catheter instability for right free wall locations. The recurrence rates are higher for right free wall APs than for other locations, ranging from 9% to 16.7% (Table 21-7).[32,41,66,77,78] The right free wall location is a predictor of recurrence in some studies.[77] The success rates are lower still for patients with Ebstein anomaly. In the largest reported series of 100 such patients, 52 had right free wall APs.[79] The initial success rate for these pathways was 79%, with a 32% recurrence rate. In another report of 21 patients with Ebstein anomaly, only 76% of patients had

TABLE 21-5

RESULTS OF TRANSSEPTAL ABLATION FOR LEFT FREE WALL ACCESSORY PATHWAYS

Study	No. of Patients	Success (%)	Compli-cations (%)	Recurrence (%)	Cross-over (%)*	Fluoro-scopy Time (min)	Procedure Time (hr)	Comments
De Ponti et al, 1998[63]	388	96	1.2	1.2	2	—	—	Complication rate includes ablation of atrial tachycardias
Swartz et al, 1993[32]	76	97	2	2	0	63 ± 47	4.9 ± 2.2	Complication rate includes other pathway locations
Fisher & Swartz, 1992[49]	26	100	0	0	0	25 ± 10.5	2.8 ± 0.9	Vectorial 3D mapping
Yip et al, 1997[64]	49	92	4	4	4	22.5 ± 15.2	1.7 ± 0.05	Preformed transseptal sheaths
Manolis et al, 1995[65]	31	100	0	3	0	76 ± 48	5.4 ± 1.9	"W sign" used for mapping

3D, three-dimensional.
* Crossover to transaortic approach.

elimination of all right-sided APs.[8] In these patients, acute success was predicted by a body surface area less than or equal to 1.7 m², a mild degree of tricuspid regurgitation, and mild severity of Ebstein anomaly.[79] Only body surface area predicted long-term success, however.

Complications

The complication rate for the transaortic approach to left-sided APs ranges from 0% to 8% and is typically less than 4%.[32,49,63-65,69–76] Half of all complications are vascular related because of arterial access and include hematomas, dissections, pseudoaneurysms, and AV fistulas.[80,81] Almost unique to the transaortic approach is damage to the aortic or mitral valve. Aortic valve damage occurs in up to 30% of pediatric patients undergoing a retrograde ablation technique.[33] Aortic leaflet perforation and catheter entrapment in the mitral valve apparatus have been reported.[82,83] The latter may require transesophageal echocardiography to direct the extraction, and surgical removal has been necessary. By removing the CS catheter, the mitral annulus may be relaxed, facilitating catheter removal. Dissection or thrombosis of the left main coronary artery has resulted from catheter trauma or energy delivery in the artery.[84] There is a 2% risk for thromboembolic events due to thrombus formation on the catheter, despite anticoagulation or dislodgment of aortic debris.[85] A 1.5% risk for tamponade, stroke, pericardial effusion, or cardiac perforation is reported for ablations at all locations. The risk for complications is higher for patients older than 65 years of age.[86]

The reported incidences of complications with the transseptal approach are 0% to 6% in adults and 0% to 25% in pediatric series.[32,49,63–65,74,87,88] The transseptal approach greatly reduces the incidence of vascular complications but introduces potential complications from atrial septal puncture. In large series of transseptal procedures performed in the catheterization laboratory, the incidence of major complications related to access was 1.3% and included tampon-

ade (1.2%), embolization (0.08%), and death (0.08%).[89] Thermal injury to the circumflex artery is also possible.

There are limited reports of ablation within the CS. To date, only mural thrombus or venous branch stenosis has been reported.[57] There remain the risks for perforation, catheter adhesion, and coronary artery injury, however.

Complications from right free wall AP ablation are rare and are less common than for other AP locations.[32,41,66,78,90] Cardiac perforation may rarely occur, as may pulmonary embolism. Stenosis of a marginal right coronary artery branch was reported in a child with Ebstein anomaly.[91] Mapping of the right coronary artery can lead to arterial injury or thrombosis.

Troubleshooting the Difficult Case

The most common causes of failed AP ablations are inability to access the target site (25% of cases), catheter instability (23%), mapping errors due to oblique AP orientation (11%), epicardial AP (8%), and recurrent atrial fibrillation (3%).[92] These problems and possible solutions are listed in Table 21-8. Misdiagnosis of the arrhythmia mechanism is more common for left than for right free wall APs. For left free wall APs, the diagnosis of ORT may be mimicked by AV nodal reentry with eccentric atrial activation or by atrial tachycardias arising from the CS musculature or the ligament of Marshall.[11,28,30] These arrhythmias can be recognized by the presence of decremental retrograde conduction only and by the ability to dissociate the ventricle from the tachycardia. It should be noted that, during retrograde AV nodal conduction in patients without APs, the far lateral to anterolateral CS is frequently activated in a distal-to-proximal sequence.[93] This results from rapid conduction over Bachmann bundle and may

TABLE 21-6

COMPARISON OF TRANSAORTIC AND TRANSSEPTAL ABLATION PROCEDURES

Study	Approach	No. of Patients	Success (%)	Recurrence (%)	Complications (%)	Crossover (%)*	Procedure Time (Range)	Fluoroscopy Time (Range) (min)	Comments
Deshpande et al, 1994[69]	TA	42	95	—	4.7	4.7	244 ± 82 min	51 ± 22	—
	TS	58	75	—	3.4	24	268 ± 8 8min	53 ± 22	—
Lesh et al, 1993[70]	TA	89	85	—	6.7	12	220 ± 13 min	44 ± 4	—
	TS	33	85	—	6.1	12	205 ± 13 min	45 ± 5	—
Natale et al, 1992[71]	TA	49	88	4	4	6	—	42 ± 29	—
	TS	31	100	0	0	0	—	34 ± 18	—
Saul et al, 1993[72]	TA	50	40	—	—	14	3.3 (2-9.5) hr*	52 (18-259)	Pediatric patients
	TS	13	100	—	—	0	4.3 (2-6) hr*	58 (14-197)	
Manolis et al, 1994[73]	TA	50	87	11	8	10	7.1 ± 2.4 hr*	121 ± 81*	—
	TS	23	96	4	0	17	5.5 ± 2.1 hr*	81 ± 57	
Vora et al, 1994[74]	TA	13	100	16	8	0	—	38 ± 30*	Nonrandomized pediatric patients
	TS	36	100	0	3	0	—	61 ± 45	
Ma et al, 1995[75]	TA	50	100	0	0	4	77 ± 20 min	12 ± 7	Randomized study (abstract)
	TS	50	96	0	0	0	81 ± 19 min	13 ± 8	
Montenero et al, 1996[76]	TA	10	100	—	—	—	—	45 ± 10	Pediatric patients
	TS	18	100	—	—	—	—	23 ± 1	
Katritsis et al, 2001[96]	TA	23	87	4	0	13	156 ± 58 min†	37 ± 25†	Single catheter for both approaches
	TS	21	90	5	0	5	119 ± 39 min	22 ± 21	

TA, transaortic approach; TS, transseptal approach; —, not reported.
* Crossover to other approach.
† P < .05 transaortic versus transseptal.

be confused with retrograde conduction over an AP. Parahisian pacing maneuvers validate the presence of retrograde right free wall AP conduction with consistency, but left free wall APs may be missed.[27]

Difficulties with mapping may occur if no favorable ablation sites are found. If both antegrade and retrograde AP conduction are present, it may be useful to map conduction in the opposite direction to that which is problematic (i.e., map retrograde conduction if antegrade mapping fails).[92]

Most APs have an oblique course, and the atrial and ventricular insertions can be several centimeters apart. If no early antegrade or retrograde sites are found for left free wall APs in the CS, direct mapping of the mitral annulus should be performed because the CS is usually anatomically removed from the course of the AP. It is possible to place multielectrode halo catheters along the mitral annulus through transseptal access for difficult cases. Altering of the direction of AP antegrade or retrograde activation may make the

TABLE 21-7

SUCCESS RATES FOR RIGHT FREE WALL ACCESSORY PATHWAYS*

Study	No. of Patients	Acute Success (%)	Recurrence (%)	Comments
Calkins et al, 1999[77]	92	90	14	Power-controlled ablation
Swartz et al, 1993[32]	12	67	16.7	Power-controlled ablation
Jackman et al, 1991[78]	14	100	9	Power-controlled ablation
Lesh et al, 1992[66]	21[†]	80	11.8	Power-controlled ablation
Haïssaguerre et al, 1994[41]	32	93.7	11	—
Drago et al, 2002[51]	21	95	0	Pediatric series with electroanatomic mapping

* Non–Ebstein's anomaly series.
† No. of accessory pathways.

TABLE 21-8

TROUBLESHOOTING THE DIFFICULT CASE

Problem	Causes	Solution
Misdiagnosis	Atrioventricular nodal reentry with eccentric atrial activation	Demonstrate only decremental retrograde conduction, dissociate atrium and/or ventricle from tachycardia
	Atrial tachycardia near atrioventricular annulus or from CS musculature	Dissociate ventricle from tachycardia
No early or favorable target sites	Poor catheter mobility	Use preformed sheaths or halo catheter, change catheter reach or stiffness
	CS distant from mitral annulus	Map mitral annulus directly
	Unable to discriminate component electrograms	Map AP conduction in opposite direction, change approach of mapping catheter (e.g., transaortic to transseptal), reverse direction of AP activation wavefront, map electrogram polarity reversal, simultaneous pacing
	Long AP conduction times	Map electrogram polarity reversal or shortest times with electroanatomic mapping system
	Epicardial AP location	Map CS and venous branches, map right coronary artery, epicardial mapping by pericardial access, map atrial appendages or ventricle apical to atrioventricular annulus
	Ligament of Marshall connection	Map left atrium anterior to left superior pulmonary vein
	Ebstein anomaly	Simultaneous atrial and ventricular pacing or atrial or ventricular premature stimuli to separate fractionated electrograms, map right coronary artery, use computerized mapping system
Unsuccessful energy delivery	Poor catheter stability and/or contact	Use preformed sheaths, change catheter curvature, reach, or stiffness; change catheter approach to ablation site (e.g., femoral to subclavian for right-sided AP); for 1 rapid pacing during ablation, use cryoablation
	Low temperatures with radiofrequency ablation	Improve catheter contact; use high-output generator and large-tip catheter
	Low current delivery with radiofrequency ablation	Lower system impedance (additional skin patches); use irrigated or cooled radiofrequency catheter; use cryoablation
	Epicardial AP	Ablation in CS or tributary with cryoablation or cooled radiofrequency; percutaneous epicardial ablation
	Wrong location	Continued mapping, map polarity reversal, map AP conduction in alternate direction, map for epicardial AP, consider unusual AP location

AP, accessory pathway; AV, atrioventricular; CS, coronary sinus.

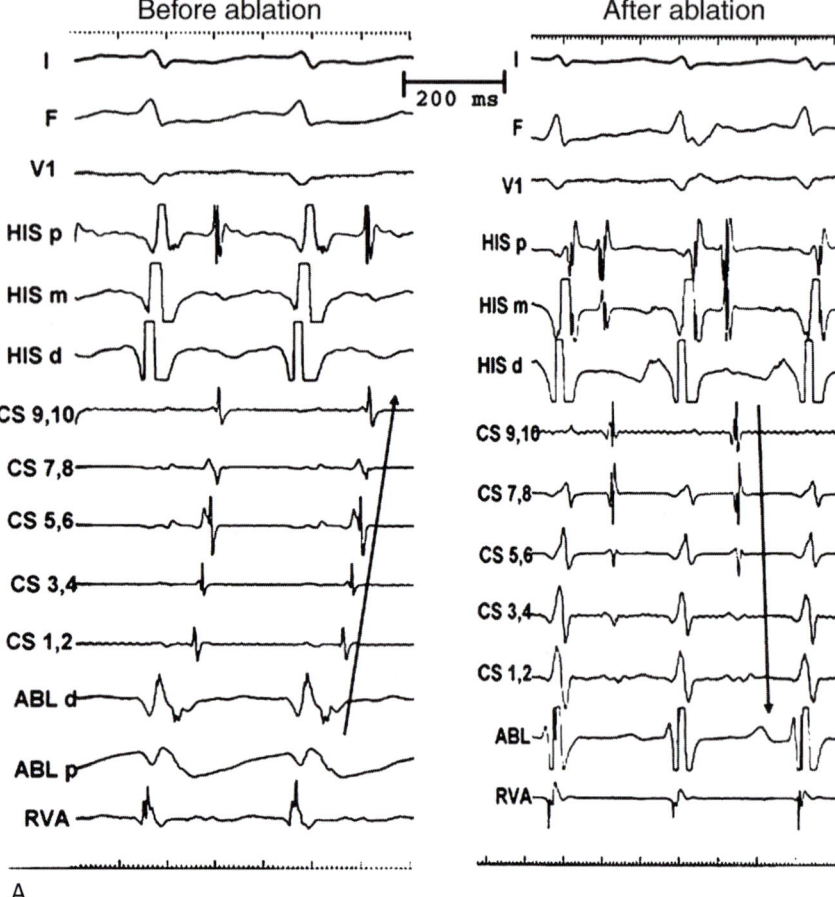

FIGURE 21-22. Intra-atrial conduction block after radiofrequency energy delivery for left lateral accessory pathway (AP). **A,** Electrograms and surface electrocardiogram (ECG) tracings in orthodromic reciprocating tachycardia with earliest atrial activation in the distal coronary sinus (CS 1,2). After ablation, the tachycardia cycle length is unchanged at 310 msec, but ventricle-to-atrium (VA) times are prolonged and the atrial activation is earliest in the proximal His electrogram (HIS p). The CS is now activated from proximal (CS 9,10) to distal. ABL d, ablation distal; ABL p, ablation proximal; I, F, V$_1$, surface ECG leads; RVA, right ventricle.

electrogram components more apparent and reveal AP potentials.[47] This approach can be used for right free wall APs as well. Changing the approach of the mapping catheter to access sites of interest may be needed. For left APs, changing from transaortic to transseptal mapping, or vice versa, may be helpful. For right-sided APs, changing from the femoral to a subclavian or internal jugular approach can be tried. If the AP demonstrates slow antegrade or retrograde conduction, the usual timing criteria used to identify successful ablation sites may not be applicable. In such cases, the earliest activation sites should be sought. Mapping of electrogram polarity reversal is particularly helpful in this situation because this technique is independent of electrogram timing.[49] The use of 2F multielectrode catheters to map the CS branches or the right coronary artery can be tried.[94] For complex cases, the use of electroanatomic mapping systems can be valuable. The occurrence of frequent atrial fibrillation may preclude mapping, especially for retrograde-only APs. In such cases, small incremental doses of ibutilide (0.1 mg to maximum of 1 to 2 mg) may prevent atrial arrhythmias without altering AP conduction.

Poor catheter mobility and stability are the most common reasons for failed AP ablations.[92] Catheter stability can be enhanced by using preformed sheaths, or different catheter curvatures and shaft stiffness, or by changing the approach to the ablation site (e.g., transaortic to transseptal). Slower pacing or the use of cryothermic energy may also stabilize the catheter during ablation. The use of robotic catheter navigation systems may enhance catheter stability (Fig. 21-21).

RF ablation may also fail because of the inability to deliver sufficient current or to achieve satisfactory temperatures at the target site. If low current delivery is a problem, cooled ablation electrodes can be used.[55] If satisfactory temperatures cannot be reached despite full energy delivery, poor catheter contact is likely.

The inability to ablate an AP from endocardial approaches suggests an epicardial location.[44] Further attempts at endocardial ablation slightly away from the annulus may occasionally be successful for pathways inserting off the annulus. Left free wall epicardial APs may be recognized by earliest activation times or large AP potentials recorded in the CS or in a venous tributary. Coronary muscular connections to the ventricle are typically mapped to the proximal middle cardiac vein or a posterior venous branch.[10] Ablation within the CS or venous branch may be necessary. For these applications, cryoablation provides the greatest safety, followed by irrigated-tip RF ablation and, finally, noncooled RF ablation. Epicardial mapping and ablation through percutaneous pericardial access provides another approach to epicardial AV connections.[63,95]

Intra-atrial conduction block without alteration of AP conduction after ablation delivery may occur in 6.9% of attempts at left free wall AP ablation.[96] In this situation, the resulting abrupt change or reversal of the retrograde atrial activation sequence may be misinterpreted as the appearance of a new arrhythmia (Fig. 21-22). Careful mapping along the CS distal to the ablation site will reveal persistent sites of early atrial activation.

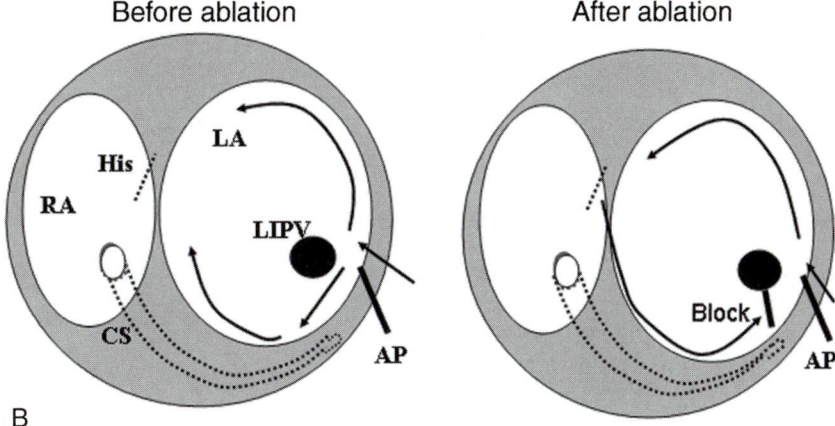

Before ablation

After ablation

B

FIGURE 21-22, cont'd. B, Schematic illustration of the reentry circuits before and after ablation. Before ablation, there is left atrial activation radiating proximally and distally from the AP insertion (*arrows*). After ablation, intra-atrial block results in left atrial activation only distally from the AP insertion. The wavefront crosses over the roof of the left atrium to the atrial septum and then conducts proximal to distal in the CS. The ablation catheter recorded a VA time of 40 msec distal to the site of block, and the tachycardia was terminated with ablation to this site. His, His bundle; LA, left atrium; LIPV, left inferior pulmonary vein; RA, right atrium.

References

1. Yee R, Klein GJ, Prystowsky E. The Wolff-Parkinson-White syndrome and related variants. In: Zipes D, ed. *Cardiac Electrophysiology: From Cell to Bedside.* 3rd ed. Philadelphia: WB Saunders; 2000:845–861.
2. Becker AE, Anderson RH. The Wolff-Parkinson-White syndrome and its anatomical substrates. *Anat Rec.* 1981;201:169–177.
3. Becker A, Anderson R, Durrer D, et al. The anatomical substrates of Wolff-Parkinson-White syndrome: a clinical correlation in seven patients. *Circulation.* 1978;57:870–879.
4. Anderson R, Ho S. Anatomy of the atrioventricular junctions with regard to ventricular preexcitation. *Pacing Clin Electrophysiol.* 1997;20: 2072–2076.
5. Klein G, Hackel D, Gallagher J. Anatomic substrate of impaired conduction over an accessory atrioventricular pathway in the Wolff-Parkinson-White syndrome. *Circulation.* 1980;61:1249–1256.
6. Shinbane J, Lesh M, Stevenson W, et al. Anatomic and electrophysiologic relation between the coronary sinus and mitral annulus: implications for ablation of left-sided accessory pathways. *Am Heart J.* 1998;135:93–98.
7. Ho SY, Goltz D, McCarthy K, et al. The atrioventricular junctions in Ebstein malformation. *Heart.* 2000;83:444–449.
8. Cappato RI, Schluter M, Weiss C, et al. Radiofrequency current catheter ablation of accessory atrioventricular pathways in Ebstein's anomaly. *Circulation.* 1996;94:376–383.
9. Chauvin M, Shah D, Haïssaguerre M, et al. The anatomic basis of connections between the coronary sinus musculature and the left atrium in humans. *Circulation.* 2000;101:647–652.
10. Sun Y, Arruda M, Otomo K, et al. Coronary sinus-ventricular accessory connections producing posteroseptal and left posterior accessory pathways: incidence and electrophysiological identification. *Circulation.* 2002;106:1362–1367.
11. Hwang C, Peter C, Chen P. Radiofrequency ablation of accessory pathways guided by the location of the ligament of Marshall. *J Cardiovasc Electrophysiol.* 2003;14:616–620.
12. Milstein S, Dunnigan A, Tang C, et al. Right atrial appendage to right ventricle accessory atrioventricular connection: a case report. *Pacing Clin Electrophysiol.* 1997;20:1877–1880.
13. Goya M, Takahashi A, Nakagawa H, et al. A case of catheter ablation of necessary atrioventricular connection between the right atrial appendage and right ventricle guided by a three-dimensional electroanatomic mapping system. *J Cardiovasc Electrophysiol.* 1999;10:1112–1118.
14. Arruda M, McClelland J, Beckman K, et al. Atrial appendage-ventricular connections: a new variant of preexcitation. *Circulation.* 1994;90:I–126.
15. De Chillou C, Rodriguez L, Schlapfer J, et al. Clinical characteristics and electrophysiologic properties of atrioventricular accessory pathways: Importance of the accessory pathway location. *J Am Coll Cardiol.* 1992;20:666–671.
16. Katsouras C, Greakas G, Goudevenos J, et al. Localization of accessory pathways by the electrocardiogram: which is the degree of accordance of three algorithms in use? *Pacing Clin Electrophysiol.* 2004;27:189–193.
17. Teo W, Klein G, Guiraudon G, et al. Predictive accuracy of electrophysiologic localization of accessory pathways. *J Am Coll Cardiol.* 1991;18:527–532.
18. Arruda M, McClelland J, Wang X, et al. Development and validation of an ECG algorithm for identifying accessory pathway ablation site in Wolff-Parkinson-White syndrome. *J Cardiovasc Electrophysiol.* 1998;9:2–12.
19. Chiang C, Chen S, Teo W, et al. An accurate stepwise electrocardiographic algorithm for localization of accessory pathways in patients with Wolff-Parkinson-White syndrome from a comprehensive analysis of delta waves and r/s ratio during sinus rhythm. *Am J Cardiol.* 1995;76:40–46.
20. Boersma L, Garcia-Moran E, Mont L, et al. Accessory pathway localization by QRS polarity in children with Wolff-Parkinson-White syndrome. *J Cardiovasc Electrophysiol.* 2002;13:1222–1226.

21. Xie B, Heald S, Bashir Y, et al. Localization of accessory pathways from the 12-lead electrocardiogram using a new algorithm. *Am J Cardiol.* 1994;74:161–165.
22. Chen S, Tai C. Ablation of atrioventricular accessory pathways: current technique-state of the art. *Pacing Clin Electrophysiol.* 2001;24:1795–1809.
23. Fitzgerald DM, Hawthorne HR, Crossley GH, et al. P wave morphology during atrial pacing along the atrioventricular ring: ECG localization of the site of origin of retrograde atrial activation. *J Electrocardiol.* 1996;29:1–10.
24. Josephson M. Preexcitation syndromes. In: Josephson M, ed. *Clinical Cardiac Electrophysiology: Techniques and Interpretations.* 3rd ed. Philadelphia: Lippincott Williams & Wilkins; 2002:322–424.
25. Miles WM, Yee R, Klein GJ, et al. The preexcitation index: an aid in determining the mechanism of supraventricular tachycardia and localizing accessory pathways. *Circulation.* 1986;74:493–500.
26. Yang Y, Cheng J, Glatter K, et al. Quantitative effects of functional bundle branch block in patients with atrioventricular reentrant tachycardia. *Am J Cardiol.* 2000;85:826–831.
27. Hirao K, Otomo K, Wang X, et al. Para-Hisian pacing: a new method for differentiating retrograde conduction over an accessory AV pathway from conduction over the AV node. *Circulation.* 1996;94:1027–1035.
28. Pavin D, Boulmier D, Daubert J, et al. Permanent left atrial tachycardia: radiofrequency catheter ablation through the coronary sinus. *J Cardiovasc Electrophysiol.* 2002;13:395–398.
29. Knight BP, Zivin A, Souza J, et al. A technique for the rapid diagnosis of atrial tachycardia in the electrophysiology laboratory. *J Am Coll Cardiol.* 1999;33:775–781.
30. Hwang C, Martin D, Goodman J, et al. Atypical atrioventricular node reciprocating tachycardia masquerading as tachycardia using a left-sided accessory pathway. *J Am Coll Cardiol.* 1997;30:218–225.
31. Kuck K-H, Schluter M. Single-catheter approach to radiofrequency current ablation of left-sided accessory pathways in patients with Wolff-Parkinson-White syndrome. *Circulation.* 1991;84:2366–2375.
32. Swartz F, Tracy CM, Fletcher RD. Radiofrequency endocardial catheter ablation of accessory atrioventricular pathway atrial insertion sites. *Circulation.* 1993;87:487–499.
33. Minich LL, Snider AR, Dick M. Doppler detection of valvular regurgitation after radiofrequency ablation of accessory connections. *Am J Cardiol.* 1992;70:116–117.
34. Villacastin J, Almendral J, Medina O, et al. "Pseudodisappearance" of atrial electrogram during orthodromic tachycardia: new criteria for successful ablation of concealed left-sided accessory pathways. *J Am Coll Cardiol.* 1996;27:853–859.
35. Chen X, Borggrefe M, Shenasa M, et al. Characteristics of local electrogram predicting successful transcatheter radiofrequency ablation of left-sided accessory pathways. *J Am Coll Cardiol.* 1992;20:656–665.
36. Hindricks G, Kottkamp H, Chen X, et al. Localization and radiofrequency catheter ablation of left-sided accessory pathways during atrial fibrillation. *J Am Coll Cardiol.* 1995;25:444–451.
37. Bashir Y, Heald SC, Katritsis D, et al. Radiofrequency ablation of accessory atrioventricular pathways: predictive value of local electrogram characteristics for the identification of successful target sites. *Br Heart J.* 1993;69:315–321.
38. Cappato R, Schlüter M, Mont L, Kuck K-H. Anatomic, electrical and mechanical factors affecting bipolar endocardial electrogram: impact on catheter ablation of manifest left free-wall accessory pathways. *Circulation.* 1994;90: 884–894.
39. Xie B, Heald SC, Camm AJ, et al. Successful radiofrequency ablation of accessory pathways with the first energy delivery: the anatomic and electrical characteristics. *Eur Heart J.* 1996;17:1072–1079.

40. Barlow MA, Klein GJ, Simpson CS, et al. Unipolar electrogram characteristics predictive of successful radiofrequency catheter ablation of accessory pathways. *J Cardiovasc Electrophysiol.* 2000;11:146–154.

41. Haïssaguerre M, Gaita F, Marcus FI, et al. Radiofrequency catheter ablation of accessory pathways: a contemporary review. *J Cardiovasc Electrophysiol.* 1994;5:532–552.

42. Calkins H, Kim Y-N, Schmaltz S, et al. Electrogram criteria for identification of appropriate target sites for radiofrequency catheter ablation of accessory atrioventricular connections. *Circulation.* 1992;85:565–573.

43. Jackman WM, Friday KJ, Fitzgerald DM, et al. Localization of left free-wall and posteroseptal accessory atrioventricular pathways by direct recordings of accessory pathway activation. *Pacing Clin Electrophysiol.* 1989;12:204–214.

44. Langberg JJ, Man KC, Vorperian VR, et al. Recognition and catheter ablation of subepicardial accessory pathways. *J Am Coll Cardiol.* 1993;22:1100–1104.

45. Yamabe H, Shimasaki Y, Honda O, et al. Localization of the ventricular insertion site of concealed left-sided accessory pathways using ventricular pace mapping. *Pacing Clin Electrophysiol.* 2002;25:940–950.

46. Nakao K, Seto S, Iliev II, et al. Simultaneous atrial and ventricular pacing to facilitate mapping of concealed left-sided accessory pathways. *Pacing Clin Electrophysiol.* 2002;25:922–928.

47. Otomo K, Gonzalez M, Beckman K, et al. Reversing the direction of paced ventricular and atrial wavefronts reveals an oblique course in accessory AV pathways and improves localization for catheter ablation. *Circulation.* 2001;104:550–556.

48. Tai C-T, Chen S-A, Chiang C-E, et al. Identification of fiber orientation in left free-wall accessory pathways: Implications for radiofrequency ablation. *J Interv Cardiac Electrophysiol.* 1997;1:235–241.

49. Fisher WG, Swartz JF. Three dimensional electrogram mapping improves ablation of left-sided accessory pathways. *Pacing Clin Electrophysiol.* 1992;15:2344–2356.

50. Haïssaguerre M, Fischer B, Warin J-F, et al. Electrogram patterns predictive of successful radiofrequency catheter ablation of accessory pathways. *Pacing Clin Electrophysiol.* 1992;15:2138–2145.

51. Drago F, Silvetti M, Di Pino A, et al. Exclusion of fluoroscopy during ablation treatment of right accessory pathway in children. *J Cardiovasc Electrophysiol.* 2002;13:778–782.

52. Langberg JJ, Calkins H, El-Atassi R, et al. Temperature monitoring during radiofrequency ablation of accessory pathways. *Circulation.* 1992;86:1469–1474.

53. Twidale N, Wang Z, Beckman KJ, et al. Factors associated with recurrences of accessory pathway conduction after radiofrequency catheter ablation. *Pacing Clin Electrophysiol.* 1991;14:2042–2048.

54. Rodriguez L, Geller J, Tse H, et al. Acute results of transvenous cryoablation of supraventricular tachycardia (atrial fibrillation, atrial flutter, Wolff-Parkinson-White syndrome, atrioventricular nodal reentry tachycardia). *J Cardiovasc Electrophysiol.* 2002;13:1082–1089.

55. Yamane T, Jais P, Shah D, et al. Efficacy and safety of an irrigated-tip catheter for the ablation of accessory pathways resistant to conventional radiofrequency ablation. *Circulation.* 2000;102:2565–2568.

56. Wang X, McCelland J, Beckman K, et al. Left free-wall accessory pathway ablation from the coronary sinus: unique coronary sinus electrogram pattern. *Circulation.* 1992;86:I–586.

57. Haïssaguerre M, Gaita F, Fischer B, et al. Radiofrequency catheter ablation of left lateral accessory pathways via the coronary sinus. *Circulation.* 1992;86:1464–1468.

58. Giorgberidze I, Saksena S, Krol RB, Mathew P. Efficacy and safety of radiofrequency catheter ablation of left-sided accessory pathways through the coronary sinus. *Am J Cardiol.* 1995;76:359–365.

59. Langberg JJ, Man KC, Vorperian VR, et al. Recognition and catheter ablation of subepicardial accessory pathways. *J Am Coll Cardiol.* 1993;22:1100–1104.

60. Cappato R, Weiss C, Brown E, et al. Catheter ablation of manifest accessory pathways related to the coronary sinus. *New Trends Arrhythmias.* 1993;9:421.

61. Gaita F, Paperini L, Riccardi R, et al. Cryothermic ablation within the coronary sinus of an epicardial posterolateral pathway. *J Cardiovasc Electrophysiol.* 2002;13:1160–1163.

62. Schweikert RA, Saliba WI, Tommassoni G, et al. Percutaneous pericardial instrumentation for endo-epicardial mapping of previously failed ablations. *Circulation.* 2003;108:1329–1335.

63. De Ponti R, Zardini M, Storti C, et al. Trans-septal catheterization for radiofrequency catheter ablation of cardiac arrhythmias. *Eur Heart J.* 1998;19:943–950.

64. Yip ASB, Chow W-H, Yung T-C, et al. Radiofrequency catheter ablation of left-sided accessory pathways using a transeptal technique and specialized long intravascular sheaths. *Jpn Heart J.* 1997;38:643–650.

65. Manolis AS, Wang PJ, Estes NAM. Radiofrequency ablation of atrial insertion of left-sided accessory pathways guided by the "W sign". *J Cardiovasc Electrophysiol.* 1995;6:1068–1076.

66. Lesh MD, Van Hare GF, Schamp DJ, et al. Curative percutaneous catheter ablation using radiofrequency energy for accessory pathways in all locations: results in 100 consecutive patients. *J Am Coll Cardiol.* 2004;19:1303–1309.

67. Chen X, Borggrefe M, Hindricks G, et al. Radiofrequency ablation of accessory pathways: characteristics of transiently and permanently effective pulses. *Pacing Clin Electrophysiol.* 1992;15:1122–1130.

68. Langberg JJ, Calkins H, Kim Y-N, et al. Recurrence of conduction in accessory atrioventricular connections after initially successful radiofrequency catheter ablation. *J Am Coll Cardiol.* 1992;19:1588–1592.

69. Deshpande SS, Bremmer S, Sra JS, et al. Ablation of left free-wall accessory pathways using radiofrequency energy at the atrial insertion site: transseptal versus transaortic approach. *J Cardiovasc Electrophysiol.* 1994;5:219–231.

70. Lesh MD, Van Hare GF, Scheinman MM, et al. Comparison of the retrograde and transeptal methods for ablation of left free-wall accessory pathways. *J Am Coll Cardiol.* 1993;22:542–549.

71. Natale A, Wathen M, Yee R, et al. Atrial and ventricular approaches for radiofrequency catheter ablation of left-sided accessory pathways. *Am J Cardiol.* 1992;70:114–116.

72. Saul JP, Hulse JE, De W, et al. Catheter ablation of accessory atrioventricular pathways in young patients: use of long vascular sheaths, the transeptal approach and a retrograde left posterior parallel approach. *J Am Coll Cardiol.* 1993;21:571–583.

73. Manolis AS, Wang PJ, Estes NAM. Radiofrequency ablation of left-sided accessory pathways: transaortic versus transseptal approach. *Am Heart J.* 1994;128:896–902.

74. Vora AM, McMahon S, Jazayeri MR, Dhala A. Ablation of atrial insertion sites of left-sided accessory pathways in children: efficacy and safety of transeptal versus transaortic approach. *Pediatr Cardiol.* 1997;18:332–338.

75. Ma C, Dong J, Yang X, et al. A randomized comparison between retrograde and transseptal approach for radiofrequency ablation of left-sided accessory pathways. *Pacing Clin Electrophysiol.* 1995;18:479.

76. Montenero AS, Drago F, Crea F, et al. Ablazione transcatetere con radiofrequenza delle tachicardie sopraventricolari in eta pediatrica: risultati immediati e di un follow-up a medio termine. *G Ital Cardiol.* 1996;26:31–40.

77. Calkins H, Yong P, Miller J, et al. Catheter ablation of accessory pathways, atrioventricular nodal reentrant tachycardia, and the atrioventricular junction: final results of a prospective, multicenter clinical trial. *Circulation.* 1999;99:262–270.

78. Jackman WM, Wang X, Friday KJ, et al. Catheter ablation of accessory atrioventricular pathways (Wolff-Parkinson-White syndrome) by radiofrequency current. *N Engl J Med.* 1991;324:1605–1611.

79. Reich J, Auld D, Hulse E, et al. The Pediatric Radiofrequency Ablation Registry's experience with Ebstein's anomaly. *J Cardiovasc Electrophysiol.* 1998;9:1370–1377.

80. Greene TO, Huang SKS, Wagshal AB, et al. Cardiovascular complications after radiofrequency catheter ablation of supraventricular tachyarrhythmias. *Am J Cardiol.* 1994;74:615–617.

81. Chen S-A, Chiang C-E, Tai C-T, et al. Complications of diagnostic electrophysiologic studies and radiofrequency catheter ablation in patients with tachyarrhythmias: an eight-year survey of 3,966 consecutive procedures in a tertiary referral center. *Am J Cardiol.* 1996;77:41–46.

82. Conti JB, Geiser E, Curtis AB. Catheter entrapment in the mitral valve apparatus during radiofrequency ablation. *Pacing Clin Electrophysiol.* 1994;17:1681–1685.

83. Seifert MJ, Morady F, Calkins H, et al. Aortic leaflet perforation during radiofrequency ablation. *Pacing Clin Electrophysiol.* 1991;14:1582–1585.

84. Kosinoki DJ, Grubb BP, Burket MW, et al. Occlusion of the left main coronary artery during radiofrequency ablation for the Wolff-Parkinson-White syndrome. *Eur JCPE.* 1993;1:63–66.

85. Epstein MR, Knapp LD, Martindill M, et al. Embolic complications associated with radiofrequency catheter ablation. *Am J Cardiol.* 1996;77:655–658.

86. Hindricks G. The multicentre European radiofrequency survey (MERFS): complications of radiofrequency catheter ablation of arrhythmias. *Eur Heart J.* 1993;14:1644–1653.

87. Dick M, O'Conner BK, Serwer GA, et al. Use of radiofrequency current to ablate accessory connections in children. *Circulation.* 1991;84:2318–2324.

88. Benito F, Sanchez C. Radiofrequency catheter ablation of accessory pathways in infants. *Heart.* 1997;78:160–162.

89. Roelke M, Smith AJC, Palacios IF. The technique and safety of transeptal left heart catheterization: the Massachusetts General Hospital experience with 1,279 procedures. *Cathet Cardiovasc Diagn.* 1994;32:332–339.

90. Calkins H, Langberg J, Sousa J, et al. Radiofrequency catheter ablation of accessory atrioventricular connections in 250 patients. *Circulation.* 1992;19:1303–1309.

91. Bertram H, Bokenkamp R, Peuster M, et al. Coronary artery stenosis after radiofrequency catheter ablation of accessory atrioventricular pathways in children with Ebstein's malformation. *Circulation.* 2001;103:538–543.

92. Morady F, Strickberger SA, Man KC, et al. Reasons for prolonged or failed attempt at radiofrequency catheter ablation of accessory pathways. *J Am Coll Cardiol.* 1996;27:683–689.

93. Suzuki F, Tosaka T, Ashikawa H, et al. Earlier activation of the distal than the proximal site of the coronary sinus may represent retrograde conduction through AV node: significance of recording of far distal coronary sinus. *Pacing Clin Electrophysiol.* 1996;19:331–341.

94. Cappato R, Schluter M, Weiss C, et al. Mapping of the coronary sinus and great cardiac vein using a 2-French electrode catheter and a right femoral approach. *J Cardiovasc Electrophysiol.* 1997;8:371–376.

95. Valderrabano M, Cesario DA, Sen J, et al. Percutaneous epicardial mapping during ablation of difficult accessory pathways as an alternative to cardiac surgery. *Heart Rhythm.* 2004;3:311–316.

96. Luria DM, Nemec J, Etheridge SP, et al. Intra-atrial conduction block along the mitral annulus during accessory pathway ablation: evidence for a left atrial "isthmus." *J Cardiovasc Electrophysiol.*. 2001;12:744–749.

22
Ablation of Posteroseptal Accessory Pathways

Mark A. Wood

Key Points

> Mapping of posteroseptal accessory pathways (APs) may involve the inferior right and left paraseptal atrioventricular (AV) annuli, proximal coronary sinus (CS), middle cardiac vein, posterior cardiac vein, and coronary venous diverticula.
>
> Ablation targets are the accessory pathway potentials, the earliest atrial or ventricular activation by AP conduction for endocardial APs, and the CS muscular extension potentials and ventricular insertions for epicardial accessory AV connections.
>
> Angiographic catheters for injection of the CS and possibly the right coronary artery may be needed, as may preformed sheaths and apparatus for transseptal access. Irrigated radiofrequency ablation or cryoablation systems and catheter location and navigation systems may be helpful.
>
> Sources of difficulty include complex anatomy, possibly requiring right- and left-sided mapping, epicardial connections involving the coronary venous system and diverticula, and injury to the right coronary artery or AV nodal artery from ablation.

Posteroseptal accessory pathways (APs) are the second most common location for accessory connections and account for 25% to 30% of APs in most series.[1-4] Surgically, these connections are the most difficult to transect, owing to the complex anatomy of the posteroseptal region.[5,6] In the electrophysiology laboratory, ablation of these connections is associated with longer procedure times, greater fluoroscopic exposure, and more radiofrequency (RF) lesions than any other location.[7,8] Nevertheless, these pathways are ablated with catheter-based techniques, with a very

high degree of success despite the potential complexity of mapping in this area.[3,4,7-11]

Anatomy

The term *posteroseptal* is inaccurate because this region is inferior to the true atrial septum according to attitudinally based nomenclature.[12-15] The term *inferoparaseptal* would be more anatomically correct; however, the posteroseptal terminology is ingrained in the literature and will be used in this chapter.

The anatomy of the posteroseptal region is more complex than for any other AP location. This area includes the pyramidal space, which represents the confluence of all four cardiac chambers and the coronary sinus (CS) in their closest proximity (Fig. 22-1).[12-15] The superior boundary of the pyramidal space is the central fibrous body. The anterior aspect is the ventricular septum, and the posterior walls are formed by the convergence of the left and right atria. The tricuspid valve annulus is displaced apically 5 to 10 mm in relation to the mitral annulus (Fig. 21-1A in Chapter 21). In this gap between the mitral and tricuspid annuli lies the right atrium–left ventricular sulcus. Here is the junction between the inferomedial right atrium and the posterosuperior process of the left ventricle. The right atrium in this area is separated from the left ventricle by only a thin sheet of fibrous tissue that may be readily crossed by accessory connections (Fig. 22-2).[12-15] The ostium of the CS abuts the superior margin of the right atrial–left ventricular sulcus and the paraseptal mitral annulus in the pyramidal space. This proximity may allow for the ablation of APs from the proximal CS in many cases. In anatomic series, the distance from the CS ostium (os) to the left margin of the posteroseptal space is 2.3 ± 0.4 cm.[12] Thus, the left boundary of the posteroseptal space is often defined as extending 2 cm from the CS os. The topography of the right posteroseptal space from the right atrial perspective includes the inferior portion of the triangle of Koch and the area around the ostium of the CS (Fig. 22-2).[15]

APs in this region can take a variety of courses (Fig. 22-3). From the surgical literature, most of these connections are believed to be right atrial–to–left ventricular pathways skirting the atrioventricular (AV) annulus.[2,5,6,10,16] The course of

383

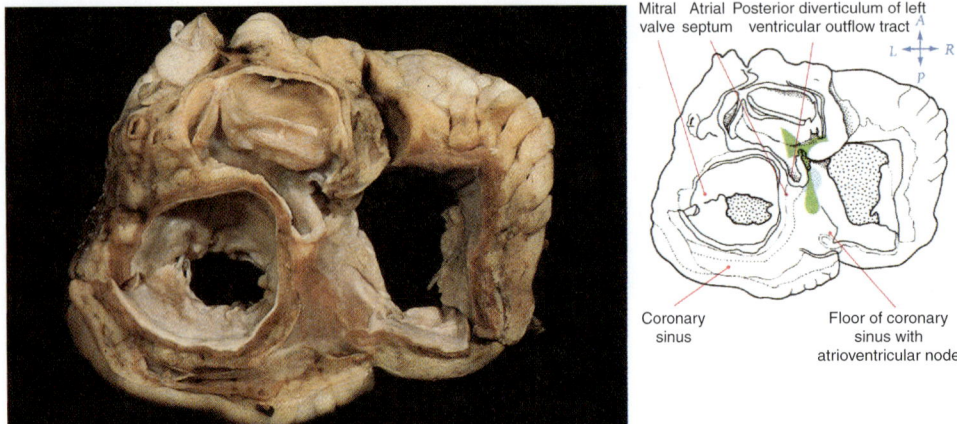

FIGURE 22-1. Anatomy of pyramidal space and posteroseptal regions in the human heart. This short-axis view is cut through the level of the coronary sinus (labeled). The position of the atrioventricular node and conduction axis is illustrated in the schematic. Note the fat-filled pyramidal space formed between the mitral and tricuspid annuli and above the floor of the coronary sinus. *(From Wilcox BR, Anderson RH [eds]:* Surgical Anatomy of the Heart. *Edinburgh: Churchill Livingstone; 1985:4-5. With permission.)*

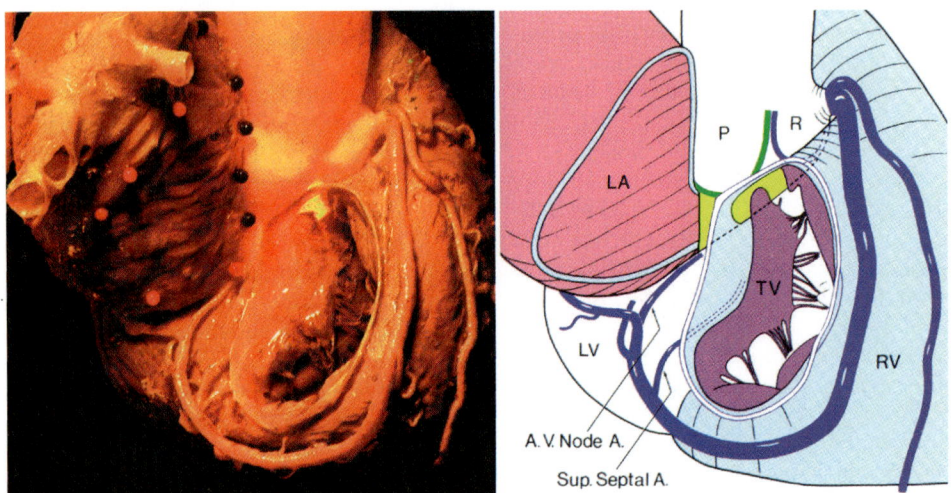

FIGURE 22-2. View of the pyramidal space and right endocardial posteroseptal region from the perspective of the right atrium. The atrioventricular nodal artery is seen in the pyramidal space and may be vulnerable to injury from ablation in the posteroseptal region. In the schematic representation of the heart, the left ventricle is *white,* and the right ventricle is *blue.* Note the region of the right atrium *(cut away)* above the tricuspid valve that is in apposition with the superior-posterior portion of the left ventricle. This area may give rise to right atrial–to–left ventricular accessory pathways. A, artery; LA, left atrium; LV, left ventricle; P, posterior aortic cusp; R, right aortic cusp; RV, right ventricle; Sup., superior; TV, tricuspid valve; V, ventricle. *(From McAlpine WA.* Heart and Coronary Arteries. *New York: Springer-Verlag; 1975:160-162. With permission.)*

such connections can be explained by the interface of the inferior medial right atrium with the posterosuperior process of the left ventricle in this region (Fig. 22-2). AP connections may also run from the paraseptal left atrium to left ventricle and from the paraseptal right atrium to right ventricle (Fig. 22-3).[7] In up to 20% of posteroseptal connections, the AV circuit results from CS musculature connections between the ventricle and left atrium (Fig. 22-4).[16] Of these connections, 70% are associated with normal CS anatomy. In the normal human heart, a sleeve of myocardial tissue that is continuous with the right atrial myocardium invests the proximal portion of the CS. In 2% to 3% of autopsy specimens, this myocardium forms extensions over the middle or posterior cardiac veins to the epicardial aspect of the left ventricle.[16] If the CS muscular coat also

has electrical connection to the left ventricle, the circuit for an epicardial accessory AV connection is present.[17] The anatomy of this region of the heart can be explored interactively on the Visible Human Server (http://visiblehuman.epfl.ch/intapplet.php).

In 21% of patients with CS muscular extensions to the left ventricle, the connection occurs in association with a CS diverticulum.[16] These venous anomalies arise within the proximal 1.5 cm of the CS and before the middle cardiac vein in most cases; however, they can arise from the middle or posterior cardiac veins themselves (Fig. 22-5). The body of the diverticulum is typically within the epicardial layers of the posterior-superior process of the left ventricle.[2] The walls of a CS diverticulum contain ventricular musculature and are often seen to contract on angiography.[16]

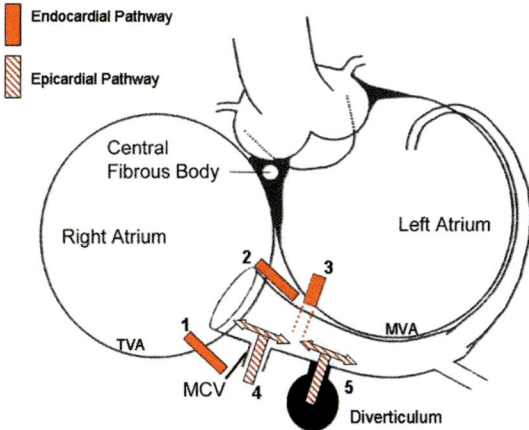

FIGURE 22-3. Schematic showing possible courses of accessory atrioventricular connections in the posteroseptal region. A short-axis view of the heart is shown. MCV, middle cardiac vein; MVA, mitral valve annulus; TVA, tricuspid valve annulus; 1, right atrial–to–right ventricular connection (or septal summit) crossing tricuspid annulus; 2, right atrial–to–left ventricular connection inserting in the posterior superior process of the left ventricle; 3, left atrial–to–left ventricular connection crossing the mitral annulus; 4, coronary sinus muscular extension to left ventricle over the middle (or posterior) cardiac vein; 5, coronary sinus muscular connection to diverticulum that contains muscular fibers in continuity with the left ventricle. Note that connections 4 and 5 are epicardial and connect to the atria by the coronary sinus musculature.

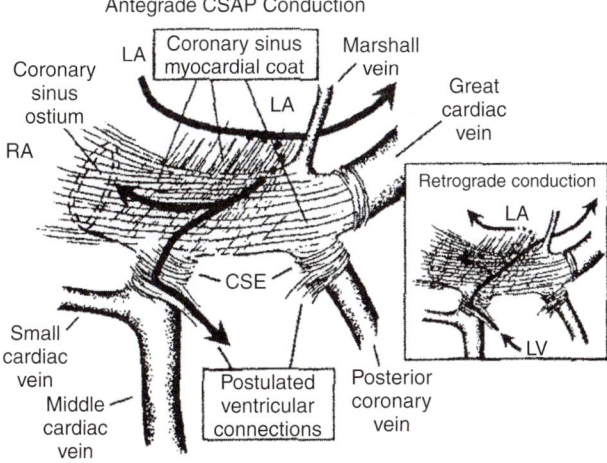

FIGURE 22-4. Schematic for possible anatomic basis of connections between the coronary sinus musculature and left ventricular myocardium (LV). The coronary sinus musculature may form extensions (CSE) over the proximal portions of the middle and posterior cardiac veins. If connections between the coronary sinus musculature and the left (LA) or right (RA) atrial myocardium exist as well, the substrate for reciprocating tachycardias is formed. CSAP, coronary sinus accessory pathway. *(From Sun Y, Arruda M, Otomo K, et al. Coronary sinus–ventricular accessory connections producing posteroseptal and left posterior accessory pathways: incidence and electrophysiologic identification. Circulation. 2002;106:1362-1367. With permission.)*

This musculature is in continuity with the epicardial left ventricle and with the CS musculature at the mouth of the diverticulum to form the reentry circuit. CS diverticula are reported in up to 9% of all patients presenting for ablation; if present in patients with evidence of a posteroseptal AP, they are usually the site of the connection.[16,18,19] CS muscular extensions forming accessory AV connections may be associated with coronary venous anomalies other than diverticula.[16]

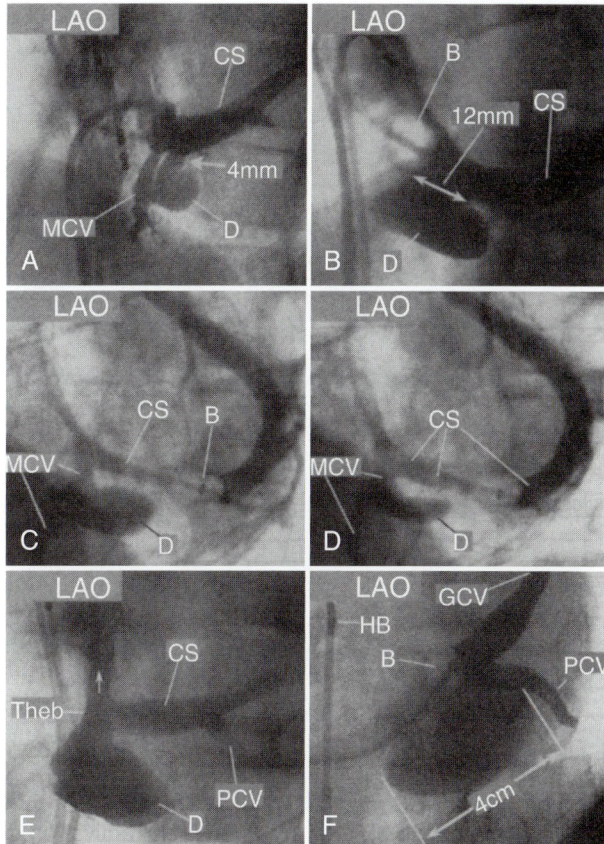

FIGURE 22-5. Coronary sinus (CS) diverticulum (D) visualized by occlusive venography. Dimensions of the anomalies are shown. In **A, B,** and **E,** the diverticula arise from the coronary sinus. In **C** and **D,** the diverticula arise from the middle cardiac vein (MCV). In **F,** the diverticulum arises near the posterior cardiac vein (PCV). GCV, great cardiac vein; LAO, left anterior oblique; Theb, Thebesian value. *(From Sun Y, Arruda M, Otomo K, et al. Coronary sinus–ventricular accessory connections producing posteroseptal and left posterior accessory pathways: incidence and electrophysiologic identification. Circulation. 2002;106:1362-1367. With permission.)*

Pathophysiology

As with any AP connection, posteroseptal connections may participate in reciprocating tachycardia or be activated as a bystander. The pathways associated with permanent junctional reciprocating tachycardia (PJRT) are most commonly found in the posteroseptal location but can rarely be found in free wall locations as well.[10,11] These connections are usually concealed and exhibit slow and decremental retrograde conduction properties that result in incessant reciprocating tachycardia.[10,11]

Diagnosis and Differential Diagnosis

On the surface electrocardiogram (ECG), the distinction between right and left posteroseptal APs has been made based on the presumed site of ventricular insertion. This classification of the surface ECG features has limited ability to predict the site of successful ablation as right- or left-sided, however.[7,9,20,21] For those pathways considered to be right-sided, the delta wave in lead V_1 is negative to

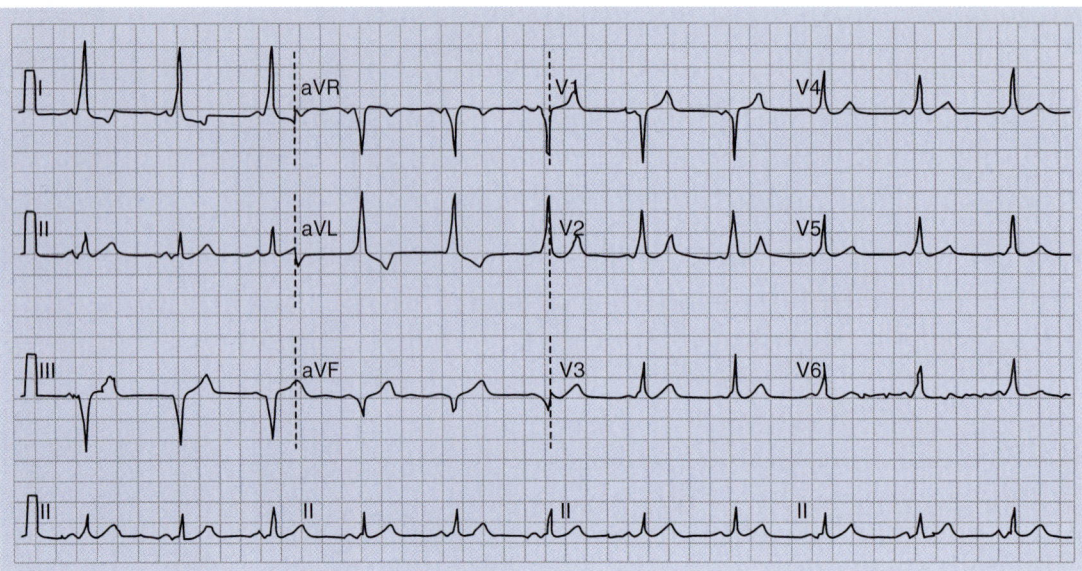

FIGURE 22-6. Surface electrocardiogram from a patient with a manifest right posteroseptal accessory pathway. Note the negative delta wave in lead V_1 and abrupt transition to R > S in lead V_2. In addition, the delta waves are negative in leads III and aVF but upright in lead II. This pathway was ablated along the posteroseptal tricuspid annulus.

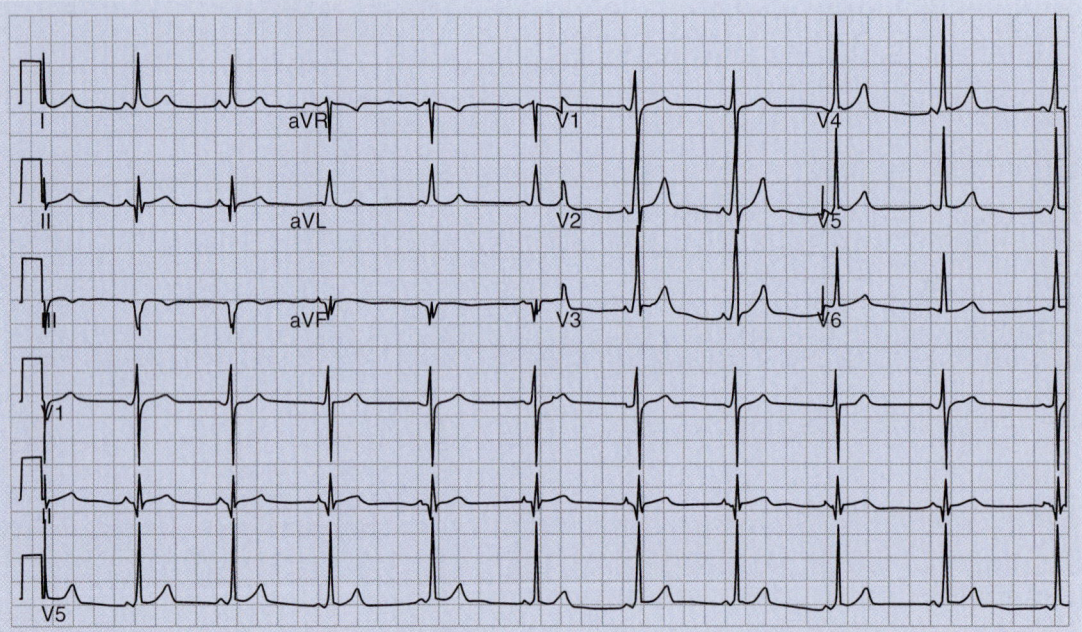

FIGURE 22-7. Surface electrocardiogram consistent with a left posteroseptal accessory pathway. The delta wave is positive in V_1 and the transition to R > S is in V_2. The delta waves are negative in leads II, III, and aVF. This pathway was ablated 1cm within the coronary sinus.

isoelectric, with abrupt transition to R > S in lead V_2 (75% of cases) or V_3 (Fig. 22-6). The delta waves are deeply negative in lead III and usually in aVF as well. Those pathways classified as left posteroseptal in location have a more variable ECG presentation, with the delta wave positive or isoelectric in V_1 and sometimes with R > S in V_1 (Fig. 22-7). Lead III is negative, but lead aVF is less commonly negative. In either case, a negative delta wave in lead II was previously thought to be sensitive for indicating an epicardial posteroseptal connection, but larger studies

demonstrated this to not be the case.[16] During orthodromic reciprocating tachycardia (ORT), the P-wave morphology on surface ECG commonly is negative in II, III, and aVF; positive in aVR and aVL; and biphasic or isoelectric in V_1. These features do not allow discrimination of right- and left-sided APs based on P-wave morphology.[22] Of interest, with loss of preexcitation during reciprocating tachycardia or after ablation, prominent T-wave inversion is often noted, with posteroseptal pathways believed to reflect a cardiac memory phenomenon.[23]

TABLE 22-1

DIAGNOSTIC CRITERIA FOR POSTEROSEPTAL ACCESSORY PATHWAY CONNECTIONS

Type of Connection	Criteria
Posteroseptal AP	Features of AP traversing pyramidal space or inserting along (1) tricuspid annulus near CS ostium; (2) proximal CS, its ostium or tributary vessels; or (3) inferior paraseptal mitral annulus VA interval prolongation 10-30 msec during ORT with ipsilateral bundle branch block
CS muscular extension—antegrade*	Rapid downstroke in unfiltered unipolar endocardial VEGM >15 msec later than onset of far-field ventricular potential at site >1 cm apical to tricuspid and mitral annuli Ventricular activation from MCV, PCV, or CS diverticulum precedes endocardial ventricular activation High-frequency potential (similar to AP potential) from CS muscular extension recorded from MCV, PCV, or CS diverticulum before ventricular activation CS muscular extension potential can be dissociated from local atrial and ventricular activity by programmed stimulation
CS muscular extension—retrograde*	Earliest high-frequency potential (similar to AP potential) recorded from MCV, PCV, or CS diverticulum CS muscular extension potential followed by activation of CS muscular coat near the orifice of the vein CS muscular potentials propagate leftward, activating left atrium before right atrium (in absence of prior ablation) CS muscular extension potential can be dissociated from local atrial and ventricular activation
PJRT	Tachycardia present >12 hr/day ORT with typically concealed, slow decrementally conducting AP (>50 msec increase in VA time with tachycardia or pacing), usually in posteroseptal region Exclude fast-slow AVNRT and low septal atrial tachycardia

AP, accessory pathway; AVNRT, atrioventricular nodal reentrant tachycardia; CS, coronary sinus; MCV, middle cardiac vein; ORT, orthodromic reciprocating tachycardia; PCV, posterior cardiac vein; PJRT, permanent junctional reciprocating tachycardia; VA, ventricular-to-atrial; VEGM, ventricular electrogram.
* From Sun Y, Arruda M, Otomo K, et al. Coronary sinus-ventricular accessory connections producing posteroseptal and left posterior accessory pathways. *Circulation.* 2002;106:1362-1367.

PJRT manifests with a distinctive ECG pattern, however. This long-RP tachycardia is present for more than 12 hours per day and typically has large inverted P waves in leads II, III, and aVF.[10,11]

Based on intracardiac recordings, posteroseptal pathways are diagnosed by the demonstration of antegrade or retrograde AP conduction, or both, with pathway insertion in the inferior right or left paraseptal region, in the proximal 2 cm of the CS, including the ostium and its tributaries (Table 22-1).[8,9,19] The diagnosis of CS musculature-to-ventricular connections is based on demonstrating earlier epicardial than endocardial antegrade ventricular activation, earliest retrograde activation of CS musculature with subsequent atrial activation, and AP-like potentials representing activation of the CS muscular connections (Figs. 22-8 and 22-9; Table 22-1).[16] Reciprocating tachycardias using posteroseptal APs must be differentiated from AV nodal reentry with an eccentric atrial activation sequence and from slow-slow AV nodal reentry with long ventriculoatrial (VA) intervals and earliest atrial activation near the CS os.[24] The differential diagnosis is best accomplished by timed ventricular stimulation during His refractoriness during tachycardia. The diagnosis of reciprocating tachycardia is made by the ability to terminate the tachycardia by premature ventricular complexes that do not conduct to the AV node or atrium and is supported by the ability to advance atrial activation during His refractoriness. The use of parahisian pacing, response of ventricular postpacing interval, comparison of His bundle–to-atrial interval during supraventricular tachycardia, and ventricular pacing at the same cycle length are also important methods of making the differential diagnosis (Table 22-2).[25]

PJRT is diagnosed by demonstrating a slowly and decrementally conducting AP participating in incessant ORT (Table 22-1). About 80% of these pathways are located in the posteroseptal region, and they demonstrate antegrade conduction in the minority of patients.[10,11] PJRT using a posteroseptal AP must be differentiated from the fast-slow (atypical) form of AV nodal reentry and from atrial tachycardia. In PJRT, the atrial activation may be advanced or delayed or the tachycardia terminated without conduction to the atria by premature ventricular stimuli during His refractoriness. In addition, the atrial-to–His bundle (AH) interval during atrial pacing at the tachycardia cycle length is within 20 to 40 milliseconds of the AH interval in tachycardia in PJRT. In atypical AV nodal reentry, the difference in AH intervals is greater than 40 milliseconds. A true V-A-A-V response to the termination of ventricular pacing with tachycardia entrainments indicates an atrial tachycardia rather than an ORT.

Mapping

The potential locations for posteroseptal APs are many, and the anatomy of this region is complex (Fig. 22-3). For these reasons, it is best to adopt a systematic approach to mapping in this area.[2,7] Regardless of the surface ECG manifestations as right- or left-sided, most of these connections can be ablated from a right endocardial approach along the inferior paraseptal tricuspid annulus or in the proximal CS (Fig. 22-10; **Videos 22-1 and 22-2**).[2,7–9] Features that suggest successful ablation from the right endocardial approach include a negative delta wave in V_1, a difference in VA time between the His recording and the earliest CS recording of less than 25 milliseconds (validated for concealed APs), and the presence of a long-RP tachycardia (Table 22-3).[2,7,9] The finding of fragmented or double potentials at the site of earliest (exclusively) retrograde AP conduction in the CS is common for posteroseptal pathways.[26–34] The finding of a sharp, near-field (CS muscular) electrogram followed by a blunt, far-field (atrial) electrogram at this site suggests a right-sided

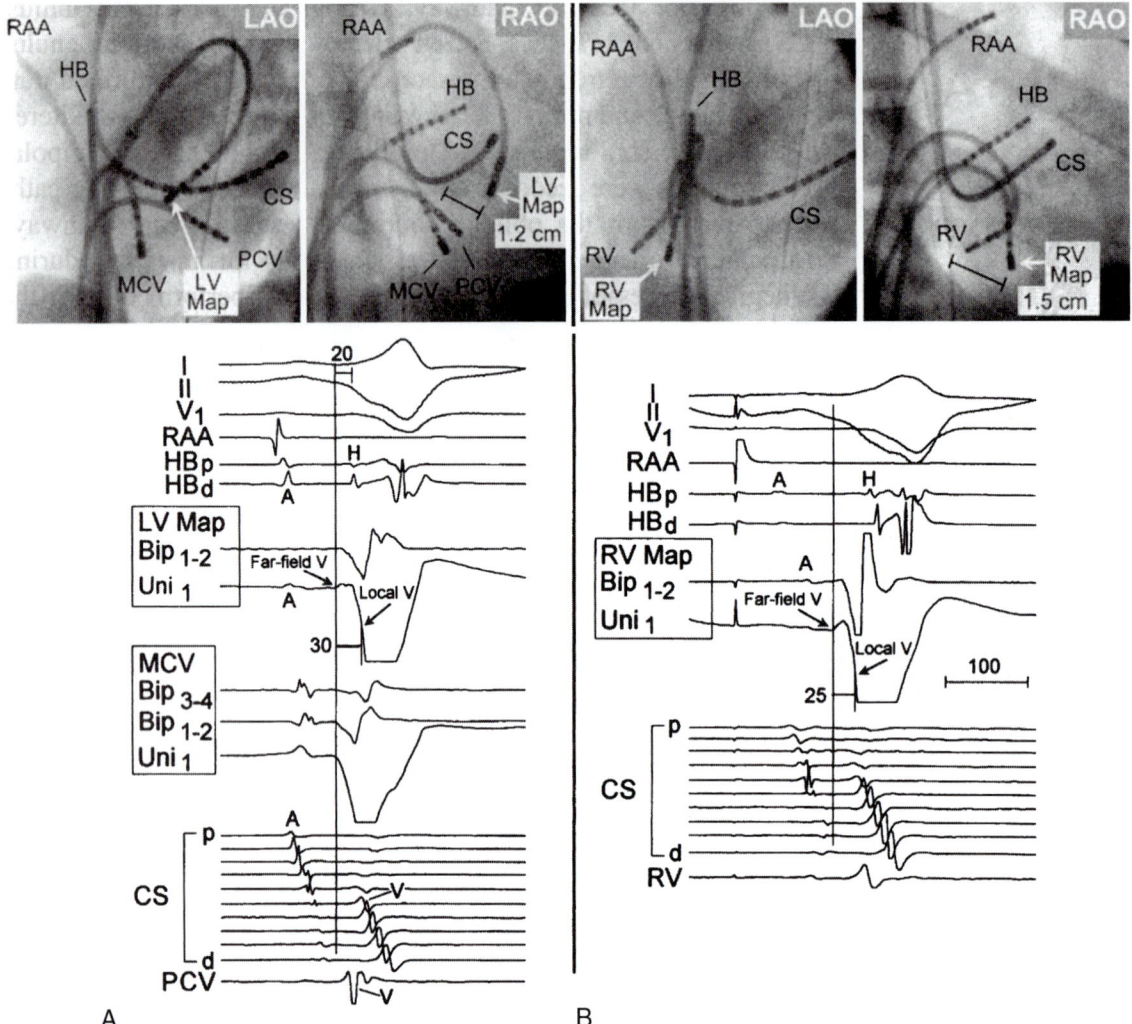

FIGURE 22-8. Intracardiac recordings from a patient with coronary sinus muscular extensions in the middle cardiac vein (MCV). **A,** The earliest ventricular activation from the left ventricular endocardium (LV Map) is far-field (*vertical line*) and 20 msec before the delta wave onset. The local ventricular activation (local V) is 30 msec after the far-field potential. The earliest ventricular activation is recorded from a catheter deep in the MCV. Bip, bipolar recording; Uni, unipolar recording. The catheter positions are shown. **B,** The earliest endocardial right ventricular recording (local V) occurs 25 msec after a far-field ventricular potential with the catheter 1.5 cm from the posteroseptal tricuspid annulus. A, atrial electrogram; CS, coronary sinus; d, distal; H, His recording; HB, His bundle; I, II, V₁, surface electrocardiogram leads; LAO, left anterior oblique; LV, left ventricle; p, proximal; PCV, posterior cardiac vein; RAA, right atrial appendage; RAO, right anterior oblique; RV, right ventricle; V, ventricular electrogram. *(From Sun Y, Arruda M, Otomo K, et al. Coronary sinus–ventricular accessory connections producing posteroseptal and left posterior accessory pathways: incidence and electrophysiologic identification. Circulation. 2002;106:1362-1367. With permission.)*

endocardial or an epicardial (coronary venous system) AP location (Fig. 22-11).

There are also features that predict the need for left endocardial ablation. If present, these findings may justify primary left-sided mapping or an early transition to left endocardial mapping. Features associated with successful ablation from the left endocardial approach are earliest retrograde atrial activation in the middle CS, a difference in VA time between the His electrogram and the earliest CS atrial electrogram of greater than 25 milliseconds (validated for concealed APs), an increase in the VA time of 10 to 30 milliseconds with left bundle branch block, R > S in V₁, and earliest retrograde atrial activation recorded greater than 15 mm from the CS ostium (Table 22-3).[7,9] In addition, a CS electrogram morphology at the site of earliest retrograde atrial activation demonstrating a blunt, far-field (atrial) component preceding the sharp, near-field (CS musculature) component

suggests the need for left-sided endocardial ablation (Fig. 22-11).[34] Use of a systematic mapping strategy may reduce procedure and fluoroscopic times through the elimination of unnecessary right-sided mapping (Fig. 22-12).[7]

Some authors have suggested assessing the response of the VA interval during ORT to the development of bundle branch block as a means of predicting the need for right- or left-sided ablation.[2,7–9] If the VA interval is prolonged by less than 10 milliseconds with ipsilateral bundle branch block, the AP is likely to be truly septal in location. Similarly, increases in the VA time of greater than 35 milliseconds suggest a free wall location. If the VA interval increases by 10 to 30 milliseconds with right or left bundle branch block, the pathway is considered to have, respectively, a right or left ventricular insertion. The site of insertion then indicates the approach to ablation as right or left endocardial. Despite the electrophysiologic rationale

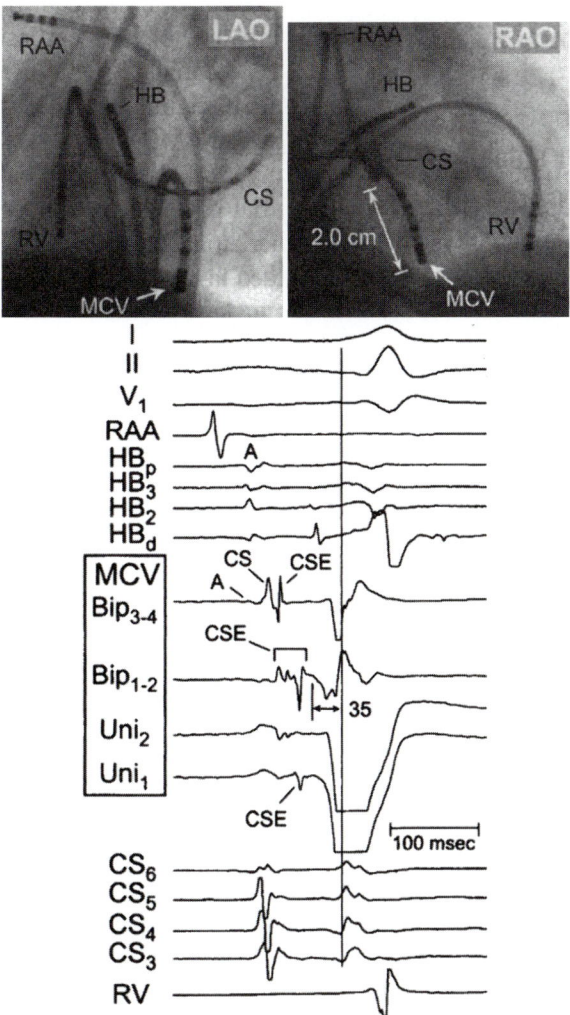

FIGURE 22-9. Recordings of antegrade coronary sinus muscular extension potentials (CSE). The CSE recordings are made from the mapping catheter 2 cm deep into the middle cardiac vein. Analogous to an accessory pathway potential, the CSE potentials are interposed between the atrial and ventricular electrograms and precede delta wave onset. A, atrial electrogram; CS, coronary sinus; d, distal; H, His recording; HB, His bundle; I, II, V₁, surface electrocardiogram leads; LAO, left anterior oblique; LV, left ventricle; p, proximal; PCV, posterior cardiac vein; RAA, right atrial appendage; RAO, right anterior oblique; RV, right ventricle. *(From Sun Y, Arruda M, Otomo K, et al. Coronary sinus–ventricular accessory connections producing posteroseptal and left posterior accessory pathways: incidence and electrophysiologic identification. Circulation. 2002;106:1362-1367. With permission.)*

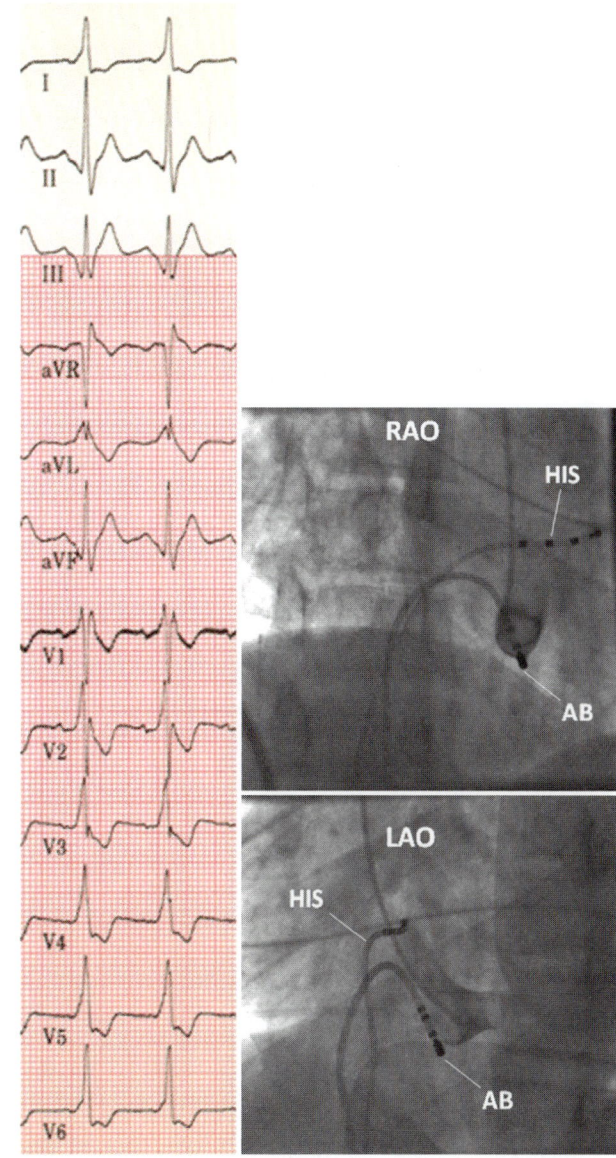

FIGURE 22-10. Ablation of a right posteroseptal accessory pathway (AP) at the coronary sinus (CS) os. CS contrast injection delineates the proximal CS anatomy in RAO and LAO views. This ablation catheter position eliminated AP conduction despite the surface electrocardiogram *(left panel)* showing a positive delta wave in V₁. AB, ablation catheter; HIS, His bundle catheter.

TABLE 22-2		
DIFFERENTIATING POSTEROSEPTAL ORTHODROMIC RECIPROCATING TACHYCARDIA FROM ATRIOVENTRICULAR NODAL REENTRANT TACHYCARDIA		
Maneuver	**Posteroseptal ORT**	**AVNRT**
Parahisian pacing	No change in Stim-A with loss of His capture	Increased Stim-A with loss of His capture
PVC during His refractoriness	Advances (or delays) atrial activation or terminates tachycardia without conduction to atrium	Unable to advance atrial activation Terminates tachycardia only with conduction to atrium
Difference between ventricular PPI and TCL	<115 msec	>115 msec
Difference between VA during ventricular pacing at TCL and VA during tachycardia	<85 msec	>85 msec
VA pacing at ventricular base vs pacing at ventricular apex	VA shorter with pacing of base	VA shorter with pacing of apex

AVNRT, atrioventricular nodal reentrant tachycardia; ORT, orthodromic reciprocating tachycardia; PPI, postpacing interval; PVC, premature ventricular complex; Stim-A, ventricular stimulus–to–atrial electrogram interval; TCL, tachycardia cycle length; VA, ventricular-to-atrial interval.

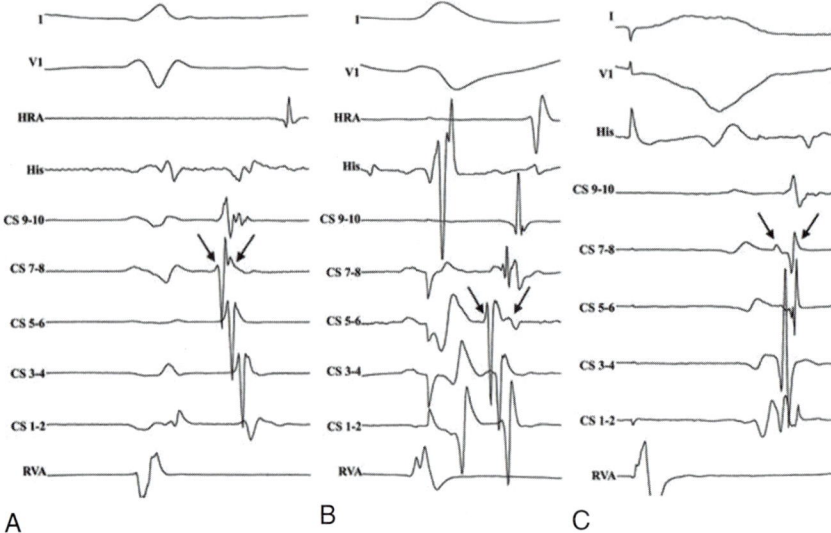

A   B   C

FIGURE 22-11. Use of double potentials on coronary sinus electrograms to predict site of successful ablation. The site of earliest retrograde coronary sinus (CS) activation during exclusive accessory pathway conduction is examined. **A,** A larger sharp, near-field electrogram (*arrow*) believed to represent activation of the CS musculature precedes the smaller, blunt, far-field electrogram (*arrow*) component representing activation of atrial myocardium. This electrogram was recorded in a patient with a right endocardial accessory pathway (AP). **B,** This sharp/blunt electrogram pattern (*arrows*) was recorded from a patient with an epicardial AP. **C,** This blunt/sharp electrogram pattern (*arrows*) was recorded from a patient with a left endocardial AP. HRA, high right atrium; RVA, right ventricular apex. *(From Pap R, Traykov VB, Makai A, et al. Ablation of posteroseptal and left posterior accessory pathways guided by left atrium-coronary musculature activation sequence.* J Cardiovasc Electrophysiol. *2008;19:653-658. With permission.)*

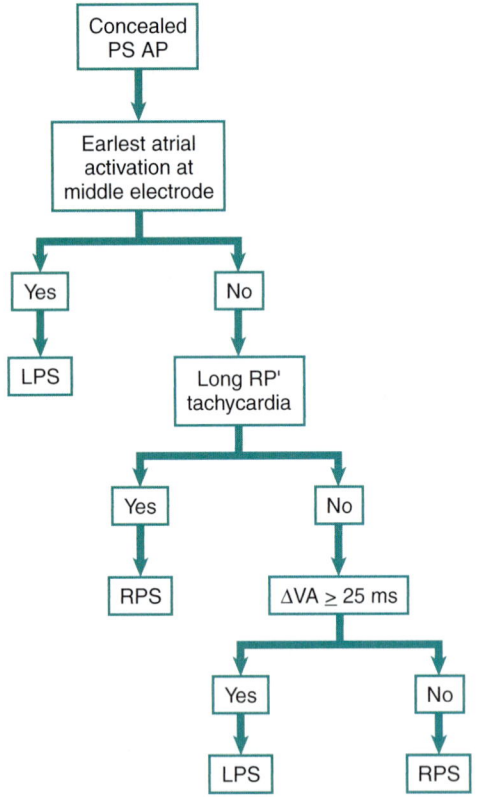

FIGURE 22-12. Algorithm for identifying the need for left endocardial ablation of concealed posteroseptal (PS) accessory pathways (AP). ΔVA, difference in ventricular-to-atrial conduction time between the His bundle recording and the earliest site in the coronary sinus; L, left; R, right. *(From Chiang CE, Chen S, Tai C, et al. Prediction of successful ablation on concealed posteroseptal accessory pathways by a novel algorithm using baseline electrophysiological parameters.* Circulation. *1996;93: 982-991. With permission.)*

TABLE 22-3	
PREDICTORS OF ABLATION SITE	
Right Side Favored	**Left Side Favored**
Difference between VA at His and earliest VA in CS <25 msec	Difference between VA at His and earliest VA in CS >25 msec
Long-RP tachycardia	Earliest retrograde atrial activation in ORT at middle CS
Negative delta wave in V_1*	R > S wave in V_1
Earliest VA <15 mm from CS os	Earliest VA >15 mm from CS os
Sharp/blunt CS EGM at earliest retrograde site[†]	Blunt/sharp CS EGM at earliest retrograde site

* From Haïssaguerre M, Gaita F, Marcus FI, Clementy J. Radiofrequency catheter ablation of accessory pathways: a contemporary review. *J Cardiovasc Electrophysiol.* 1994;5:533-552.
[†] Pap R, Traykov VB, Makai A, et al. Ablation of posteroseptal and left posterior accessory pathways guided by left atrium - coronary musculature activation sequence. *J Cardiovasc Electrophysiol.* 2008;19:653-658.
CS, coronary sinus; EGM, electrogram; ORT, orthodromic reciprocating tachycardia; VA, ventricular-to-atrial interval.

for this finding, it is frequently inaccurate in predicting the site of successful ablation.[9]

If endocardial mapping fails, attention should turn to the coronary venous system.[16] Features that suggest an epicardial accessory AV connection using CS musculature include the presence of a CS diverticulum, a negative delta wave in lead II, a steep positive delta wave in aVR, and a deep S wave in V_6 (Table 22-4).[26] The combination of a steep positive delta wave in aVR and R < S in V_6 provides a 91% positive-predictive value for ablation within the CS or middle cardiac vein. A negative delta wave in lead II alone has a 50% positive-predictive value.[26] A CS electrogram at the site of earliest retrograde AP conduction with sharp

TABLE 22-4

PREDICTORS OF EPICARDIAL POSTEROSEPTAL ATRIOVENTRICULAR CONNECTION

Finding	Sensitivity (%)	Specificity (%)	PPV (%)
Steep negative delta wave in lead II*	87	79	50
Steep positive delta wave in lead aVR*	61	98	88
Deep S wave in lead V$_6$*	70	87	57
Presence of CS diverticulum	NA	NA	NA
Sharp/blunt CS EGM at earliest retrograde site†	100	47	NA

* From Takahashi A, Shah D, Jais P, et al. Specific electrocardiographic features of manifest coronary vein posteroseptal accessory pathways. *J Cardiovasc Electrophysiol.* 1998;9:1015-1025.
† Estimated from Pap R, Traykov VB, Makai A, et al. Ablation of posteroseptal and left posterior accessory pathways guided by left atrium-coronary musculature activation sequence. *J Cardiovasc Electrophysiol.* 2008;19:653-658.
CS, coronary sinus; NA, not assessed; PPV, positive-predictive value.

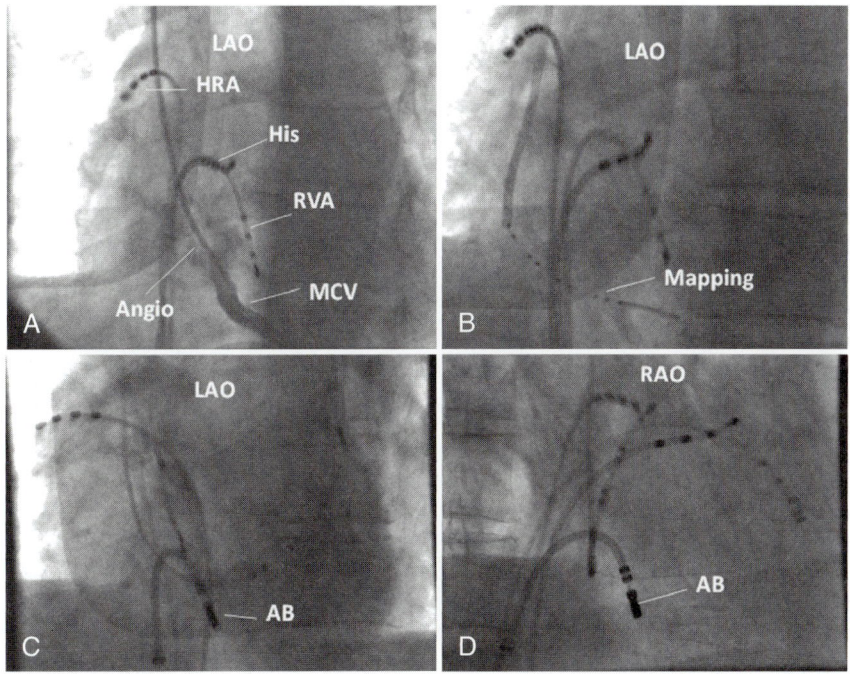

FIGURE 22-13. Use of 2-French multipolar catheter to map the middle cardiac vein (MCV) from the right internal jugular venous approach. **A,** MCV venogram is performed with angiographic (Angio) catheter in left anterior oblique (LAO) view. **B,** The mapping catheter is passed through the angiographic guide. Very early retrograde electrical activity was recorded during orthodromic tachycardia from the proximal MCV. **C** and **D,** LAO and right anterior oblique (RAO) views of the irrigated catheter at the site of successful ablation in the MCV. AB, ablation catheter; His, His bundle catheter; HRA, high right atrium; RVA, right ventricular apex.

(CS musculature) followed by blunt (atrial) components is suggestive of either an epicardial coronary sinus musculature AP or a right endocardial AP (Fig. 22-11).[34] With these findings or failure of tricuspid annular mapping, attention should turn quickly to detailed CS angiography and thorough mapping of the proximal CS, middle and posterior cardiac veins, and any diverticulum visualized. Retrograde CS angiography can be performed with an 8-French guiding sheath introduced from the femoral, internal jugular, or subclavian vein approaches.[16]

A technique for occlusive venography has been described and is preferred by experienced centers, however.[16] A steerable, balloon-tipped, lumen catheter (Vueport, Cardima, Fremont, CA) is introduced into the body of the CS or great cardiac vein. After the balloon is gently inflated, 5 to 15 mL of contrast medium is slowly injected to fill the distal CS. With continued injection, the entire venous system is filled through collaterals, and the catheter can be slowly withdrawn to enhance retrograde filling of the proximal structures (Fig. 22-5).[16] The coronary venous system can also be visualized by injection of the left coronary artery. CS muscular connections are present in up to 21% of all patients with posteroseptal connections and in up to 47% of patients with previously failed ablation in this region.[16] CS mapping is facilitated in some cases by catheter manipulation from the right internal jugular or by left subclavian vein approaches (Fig. 22-13). These connections most commonly occur in the middle cardiac vein (82%), followed by the posterior cardiac vein (11%), both veins (5%), and the floor of the CS between these two veins (2%).[16] The connections are recorded 5 to 20 mm deep into the veins.[16] The features that are diagnostic of accessory connections using coronary muscular connections with the left ventricle are given in Table 22-1.

TABLE 22-5

TARGETS FOR ABLATION

AP potentials

Local AV or VA ≤40 msec

Right-sided V-to-delta interval >15 msec

Left-sided V-to-delta interval > 0 msec

Ventricular insertion for epicardial connections

AP, accessory pathway; AV, atrial-to-ventricular interval; VA, ventricular-to-atrial interval; onset of delta-to-V, delta wave to local ventricular.

Conventional electrogram criteria for selecting right-sided ablation sites apply: local AV and VA times of 40 milliseconds or less and local ventricular activation greater than 15 milliseconds before delta wave onset (Table 22-5).[1,3,4,9] For mitral annular mapping, the earliest ventricular activation before delta onset is typically later than for right-sided APs. Some authors describe a high frequency of fractionated atrial electrograms at the site of successful mapping of retrograde conduction.[9] Many authors have stressed the frequency and benefit of recording AP potentials from accessory connections in this area.[4,9,15,16] The demonstration of AP potentials may be enhanced by reversing the direction of atrial or ventricular activation at the AP insertion sites.[27] For epicardial connections, the activity of the CS muscular connections can be recorded, analogous to conventional AP connections (Fig. 22-9).[16] The site of successful ablation is in the posteroseptal tricuspid annulus in 35% to 65%, proximal CS in 31% to 33%, mitral annulus in 4% to 23%, and CS diverticula in 9% to 21% of patients.[2–4,7,9] PJRT is targeted at the site of shortest VA time and by mapping for negative unipolar atrial electrograms.[10,11] The AP is located in the posteroseptal right atrium or proximal CS in 76% of cases, is in a mid-septal location in 12%, and is right or left posterior or lateral in the remainder.[11]

Ablation

For ablation along the tricuspid or mitral annulus, conventional RF ablation with 4-mm-tip catheters is usually sufficient (Fig. 22-14; see Fig. 22-11).[3,4,7–10] Standard RF ablation can also be delivered in the proximal 1 cm of the CS. The left endocardium can be approached by retrograde transaortic or transseptal techniques (Fig. 22-15; see Fig. 22-14). For ablation more distally in the CS or in venous tributaries or diverticulum, greater care is necessary (Figs. 22-8 and 22-9). In these cases, conventional RF may be associated with high electrode temperatures due to venous occlusion and lack of cooling. The result may be low power delivery and limited lesion size or coagulum formation with catheter adherence to the venous wall. For these situations, the use of an irrigated catheter system may allow for greater power delivery with a lower risk for coagulum formation. Cryoablation may be an alternative with a low potential for vascular injury.[28]

Finally, for ablation within the CS and its proximal tributaries, the proximity of the ablation site to the right coronary artery must be considered. Based on angiography, sites greater than 2 mm away from the right coronary artery may

be treated with irrigated RF limited to 12 to 15 W. For sites less than 2 mm from the right coronary artery, RF energy carries a significant risk for arterial damage, and cryoablation is the modality of choice.

Not uncommonly, ablation of the atrial insertion of posteroseptal AP connections alters the retrograde activation sequence without eliminating reciprocating tachycardia. Although this situation may represent multiple APs, it is believed in many instances to result from multiple CS-atrial connections. In such cases, targeting the single ventricular insertion site may be more efficient.

Despite the complex nature of posteroseptal APs, the success rate for ablation is high, at 93% to 98%.[1,3,4,7–11,22] Complications are common to any ablation procedure for right and left endocardial approaches. Ablation within the CS, its branches, or diverticula carries the risk for venous perforation and tamponade[29] or venous occlusion.[29] Damage to the right coronary artery is also possible.[30] Rarely, heart block has resulted from posteroseptal ablation, possibly from damage to the AV nodal artery. Recurrence rates are reported to be about 12% but range from 6% to 50%.[31–33]

Troubleshooting the Difficult Case

Sources of difficulty most frequently arise from the complex and extensive mapping required to localize APs in this region (Table 22-6). This problem can be minimized by adhering to a systematic approach to mapping. In general, mapping begins in the right endocardium unless there are signs that strongly suggest the need for a left endocardial approach (Table 22-3). From the right endocardium, the proximal CS is mapped, and venography is performed if no attractive sites are identified. If the venography is unrevealing for diverticula or other anomalies, the left endocardium is mapped by a transaortic or transseptal technique. If one approach fails, switching to the other may be useful. It may be necessary to compare the AV and VA conduction times recorded from the right and left sides to direct more detailed mapping at the site of the shorter time. Because of slow and decremental conduction of some APs in this area, conventional criteria for identifying favorable ablation sites based on short AV and VA times may not apply. In this instance, careful cataloguing of the conduction times at all sites may identify the shortest as the best site for ablation. Alternatively, AP potentials can be sought, aided by reversal of the activation wavefront for the atrial and ventricular insertions. Careful CS venography should be performed early in the difficult case because the presence of a venous anomaly usually identifies the site of the accessory connection. Changing retrograde atrial activation with ablation of CS muscular connections can cause confusion. In this instance, targeting the ventricular insertion may be more efficient. Ablation within the CS tributary branches and diverticula may lead to excessive electrode temperatures with conventional RF catheters. The use of irrigated RF at low power settings may be required. Cryoablation is an attractive alternative to RF for ablation in the venous branches, especially when ablating near the right coronary artery. Ablation in the venous branches should be preceded by right coronary angiography to evaluate this risk.

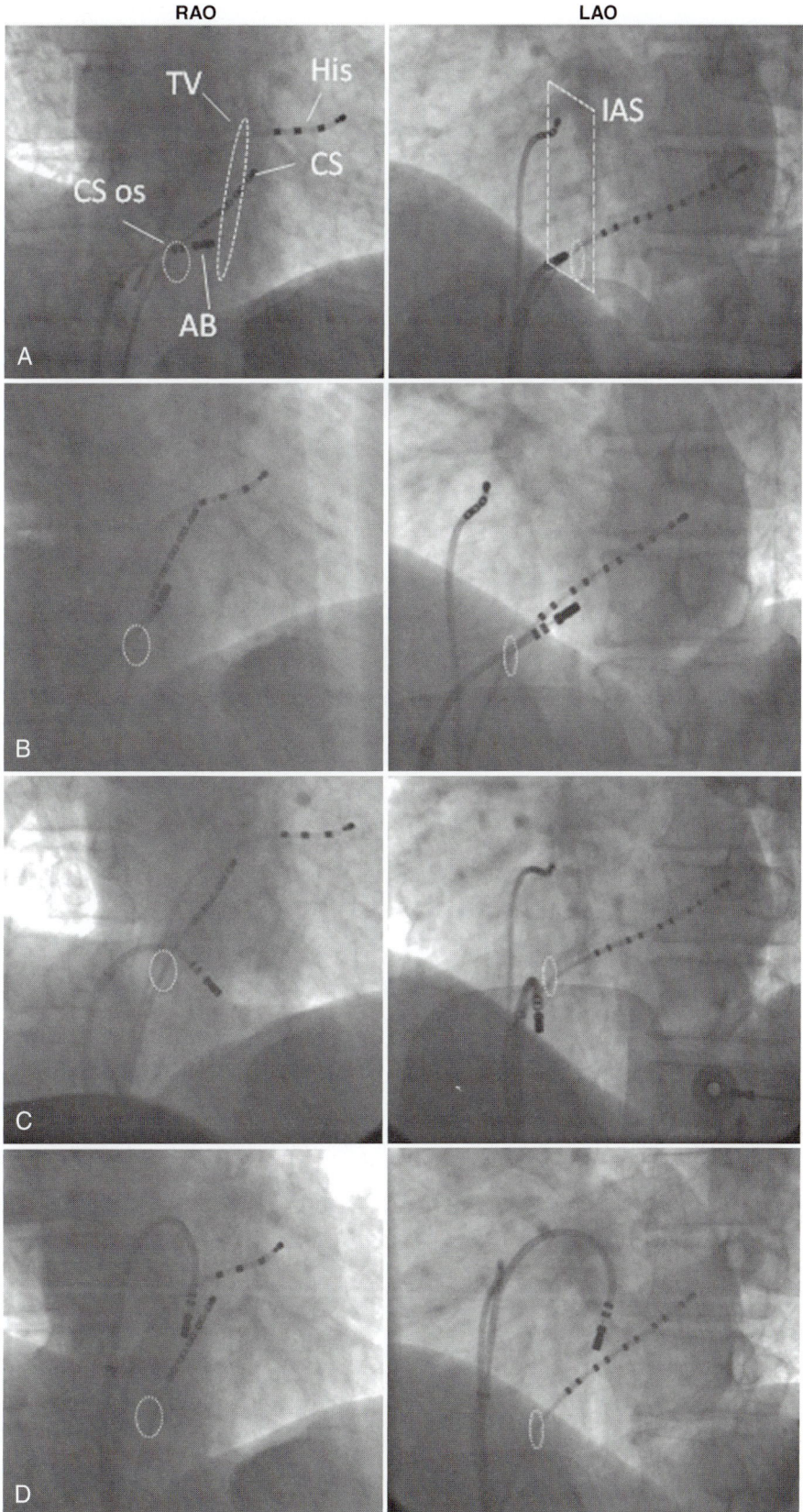

FIGURE 22-14. Examples of ablation catheter (AB) positions for posteroseptal accessory pathways (AP). Right anterior oblique (RAO) views are shown on the left, and left anterior oblique (LAO) views on the right. **A,** Right-sided AP just superior to the coronary sinus (CS) os. The estimated positions of the CS os, tricuspid valve (TV), and intra-atrial septum (IAS) are shown. **B,** Ablation within the proximal CS. **C,** Ablation inferior to the CS os between the CS and TV. **D,** Transseptal approach to a left posteroseptal AP.

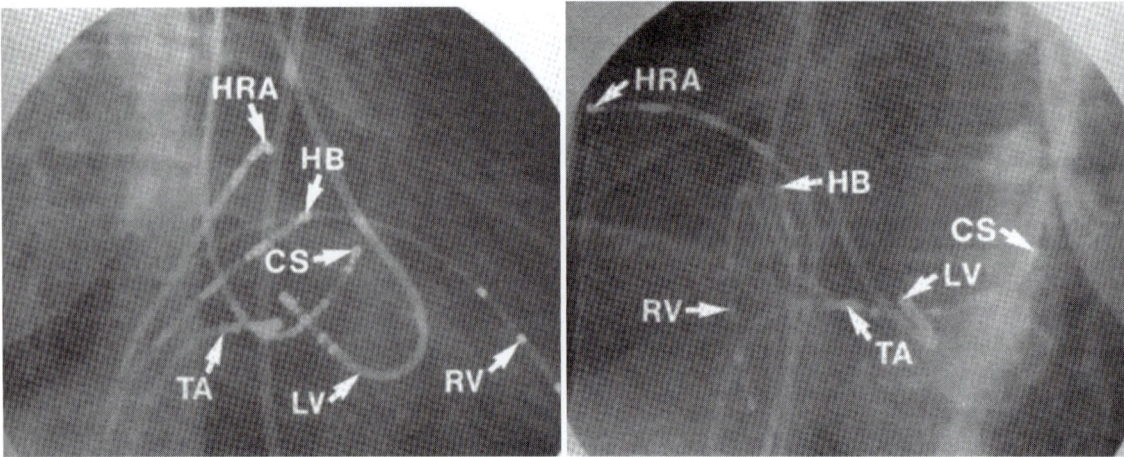

FIGURE 22-15. Right anterior oblique (RAO) (*top*) and left anterior oblique (LAO) (*bottom*) fluoroscopic views of catheter positions for mapping the left and right posteroseptal regions. The left ventricle (LV) catheter is introduced by the retrograde transaortic approach. The right ventricle (RV) catheter is simultaneously positioned at the coronary sinus ostium. CS, coronary sinus; HB, His bundle; HRA, high right atrium; TA, tricuspid annulus. *(From Jazayeri MR, Deshpande S, Dhala A, et al. Transcatheter mapping and radiofrequency ablation of cardiac arrhythmias.* Curr Probl Cardiol. *1994;6:285–396. With permission.)*

TABLE 22-6		
TROUBLESHOOTING THE DIFFICULT CASE		
Problem	**Cause**	**Solution**
No early sites	Incomplete mapping	Map proximal CS and tributaries; CS venogram for venous anomalies; map left heart, map from right internal jugular or subclavian approach
	Oblique AP course	Reverse direction of activation of AP to separate electrogram components and map AP potentials
	Epicardial AV connection	Map proximal CS tributaries, perform CS venography
	Slow and/or decremental AP conduction	Map shortest of prolonged conduction times or map AP potentials
Changing retrograde activation with ablation	Broad band atrial insertion or multiple CS musculature to atrial connections	Target ventricular insertion especially within CS venous system
Low power delivery	Low blood flow location	Use irrigated RF
	RF in CS tributary or diverticulum	Use irrigated RF; or, if near right coronary artery use (<2 mm), use cryoablation
Epicardial connection near right coronary artery	Epicardial connection in proximal CS venous system	Use cryoablation

AP, accessory pathway; AV, atrioventricular; CS, coronary sinus; RF, radiofrequency.

References

1. Calkins H, Kim Y-N, Schmaltz S, et al. Electrogram criteria for identification of appropriate target sites for radiofrequency catheter ablation of accessory atrioventricular connections. *Circulation*. 1992;85:565–573.
2. Jazayeri MR, Deshpande S, Dhala A, et al. Transcatheter mapping and radiofrequency ablation of cardiac arrhythmias. *Cardiology*. 1994;19:285–296.
3. Calkins H, Yong P, Miller J, et al. Catheter ablation of accessory pathways, atrioventricular nodal reentrant tachycardia, and the atrioventricular junction: final results of a prospective, multicenter clinical trial. *Circulation*. 1999;99:262–270.
4. Jackman WM, Wang X, Friday KJ, et al. Catheter ablation of accessory atrioventricular pathways (Wolff-Parkinson-White syndrome) by radiofrequency current. *N Engl J Med*. 1991;324:1605–1611.
5. Sealy WC, Gallagher JJ. The surgical approach to the septal area of the heart based on the experiences with forty-five patients with Kent bundles. *J Thorac Cardiovasc Surg*. 1980;79:542–551.
6. Sealy WC, Mikat EM. Anatomical problems with identification and interruption of posterior septal Kent bundles. *Ann Thorac Surg*. 1983;36:584–595.
7. Chiang C, Chen S, Tai C, et al. Prediction of successful ablation site of concealed posteroseptal accessory pathways by a novel algorithm using baseline electrophysiological parameters. *Circulation*. 1996;93:982–991.
8. Dhala AA, Deshpande SS, Bremner S, et al. Transcatheter ablation of posteroseptal accessory pathways using a venous approach and radiofrequency energy. *Circulation*. 1994;90:1799–1810.
9. Haïssaguerre M, Gaita F, Marcus FI, Clementy J. Radiofrequency catheter ablation of accessory pathways: a contemporary review. *J Cardiovasc Electrophysiol*. 1994;5:533–552.
10. Haïssaguerre M, Montserrat P, Warin JF, et al. Catheter ablation of left posteroseptal accessory pathways and of long RP tachycardias with a right endocardial approach. *Eur Heart J*. 1991;12:845–859.
11. Gaita F, Haïssaguerre M, Giustetto C, et al. Catheter ablation of permanent junctional reciprocating tachycardia with radiofrequency current. *J Am Coll Cardiol*. 1995;25:648–654.
12. Davis LM, Byth K, Ellis P, et al. Dimensions of the human posterior septal space and coronary sinus. *Am J Cardiol*. 1991;68:621–625.
13. Hood MA, Cox JL, Lindsay BD, et al. Improved detection of accessory pathways that bridge posterior septal and left posterior regions in the Wolff-Parkinson-White syndrome. *Am J Cardiol*. 1992;70:205–210.
14. McAlpine WA. *Heart and Coronary Arteries: An Anatomical Atlas for Clinical and Surgical Treatment*. New York: Springer-Verlag; 1975.
15. Sánchez-Quintana D, Ho SY, Cabrera JA, et al. Topographic anatomy of the inferior pyramidal space: relevance to radiofrequency catheter ablation. *J Cardiovasc Electrophysiol*. 2001;12:210–217.
16. Sun Y, Arruda M, Otomo K, et al. Coronary sinus-ventricular accessory connections producing posteroseptal and left posterior accessory pathways. *Circulation*. 2002;106:1362–1367.
17. Kasai A, Anselme F, Saoudi N. Myocardial connections between left atrial myocardium and coronary sinus musculature in man. *J Cardiovasc Electrophysiol*. 2001;12:981–985.

18. Chiang CE, Chen SA, Yang CR, et al. Major coronary sinus abnormalities: identification of occurrence and significance in radiofrequency ablation of supraventricular tachycardia. *Am Heart J.* 1994;127:1279–1289.
19. Weiss C, Cappato R, Schluter M, et al. Anomalies of the coronary venous system in patients with and without accessory pathways [abstract]. *J Am Coll Cardiol.* 1995;25:18A.
20. Chiang CE, Chen SA, Teo WS, et al. An accurate stepwise electrocardiographic algorithm for localization of accessory pathways in patients with Wolff-Parkinson-White syndrome from a comprehensive analysis of delta waves and R/S ratio during sinus rhythm. *Am J Cardiol.* 1995;76:40–46.
21. Arruda M, McClelland J, Wang X, et al. Development and validation of an ECG algorithm for identifying accessory pathway ablation site in Wolff-Parkinson-White syndrome. *J Cardiovasc Electrophysiol.* 1998;9:2–12.
22. Chen S-A, Tai C-T. Ablation of atrioventricular accessory pathways: current technique-state of the art. *Pacing Clin Electrophysiol.* 2001;24:1795–1809.
23. Wood MA, DiMarco JP, Haines DE. Electrocardiographic abnormalities following radiofrequency catheter ablation of accessory bypass tracts in Wolff-Parkinson-White syndrome. *Am J Cardiol.* 1992;70:200–204.
24. Hwang C, Martin D, Goodman J, et al. Atypical atrioventricular node reciprocating tachycardia masquerading as tachycardia using a left-sided accessory pathway. *J Am Coll Cardiol.* 1997;30:218–225.
25. Miller JM, Rosenthal ME, Gottlieb CD, et al. Usefulness of the DHA interval to accurately distinguish atrio-ventricular nodal reentry from orthodromic septal bypass tract tachycardias. *Am J Cardiol.* 1991;68:1037–1044.
26. Takahashi A, Shah D, Jais P, et al. Specific electrocardiographic features of manifest coronary vein posteroseptal accessory pathways. *J Cardiovasc Electrophysiol.* 1998;9:1015–1025.
27. Otomo K, Gonzalez M, Beckman K, et al. Reversing the direction of paced ventricular and atrial wavefronts reveals an oblique course in accessory AV pathways and improves localization for catheter ablation. *Circulation.* 2001;104:550–556.
28. Gaita F, Paperini L, Riccardi R, et al. Cryothermic ablation within the coronary sinus of an epicardial posterolateral pathway. *J Cardiovasc Electrophysiol.* 2002;13:1160–1163.
29. Wang X, Jackman WM, McClelland J, et al. Sites of successful radiofrequency ablation of posteroseptal accessory pathways [abstract]. *Pacing Clin Electrophysiol.* 1992;15:535.
30. Duong T, Hui P, Mailhot J. Acute right coronary artery occlusion in an adult patient after radiofrequency catheter ablation of a posteroseptal accessory pathway. *J Invasive Cardiol.* 2004;16:657–659.
31. Chen SA, Chiang CE, Tsang WP, et al. Recurrent conduction in accessory pathway and possible new arrhythmias after radiofrequency catheter ablation. *Am Heart J.* 1993;125:381–387.
32. Yee R, Klein GJ, Guiraudon GM. The Wolff-Parkinson-White syndrome. In: Zipes DP, Jalife J, eds. *Cardiac Electrophysiology: From Cell to Bedside.* Philadelphia: WB Saunders; 1995:1199–1214.
33. Calkins H, Prystowski E, Carlson M, et al. Temperature monitoring during radiofrequency catheter ablation procedures using closed loop control. *Circulation.* 1994;90:1279–1286.
34. Pap R, Traykov VB, Makai A, et al. Ablation of posteroseptal and left posterior accessory pathways guided by left atrium-coronary musculature activation sequence. *J Cardiovasc Electrophysiol.* 2008;19:653–658.

Video

Video 22-1. Proximal coronary sinus (CS) venogram in the LAO view showing relation ablation catheter at the inferior boarder of the CS os. A His catheter is also in position.

Video 22-2. Proximal coronary sinus (CS) venogram in RAO projection showing relation ablation catheter at the inferior boarder of the CS os. A His catheter is also in position.

23

Catheter Ablation of Superoparaseptal ("Anteroseptal") and Mid-Septal Accessory Pathways

John M. Miller, Mithilesh K. Das, Anil V. Yadav, and Deepak Bhakta

Key Points

Diagnosis of superoparaseptal ("anteroseptal") and mid-septal accessory pathways (APs) is made on the basis of an electrocardiographic pattern (if overt preexcitation is present) and evidence of mid-septal and anteroseptal AP insertions.

Orthodromic supraventricular tachycardia using a mid-septal AP must be differentiated from atrioventricular (AV) nodal reentry and septal or parahisian atrial tachycardias.

Mapping of superoparaseptal APs is done to locate the site with the earliest anterograde ventricular activation near or anterior to the His bundle recording, the earliest anterograde ventricular activation–to–delta wave interval (15 to 40 msec pre-delta), and earliest retrograde atrial activation in the region of the His bundle recording. Recording a discrete AP potential is very helpful but not always achievable.

Mapping of mid-septal APs is done to locate the site of the earliest anterograde ventricular activation between the coronary sinus (CS) ostium and the His recording location, the earliest anterograde ventricular activation–to–delta wave interval (15 to 25 msec pre-delta), and the earliest retrograde atrial activation between the CS ostium and the His recording location. Left mid-septal connections are rare.

The ablation target is the site of earliest anterograde ventricular activation or retrograde atrial activation on the AV annulus. Recording the AP potential can verify the correct target.

The use of preformed vascular sheaths may be helpful; catheter navigation systems are often useful to "tag" sites of interest, and cryoablation may be useful. Cooled radiofrequency ablation is rarely needed and is possibly contraindicated.

Sources of difficulty include lack of catheter stability, proximity to normal conduction system with risk for heart block, catheter-induced mechanical block of pathway conduction, and accelerated junctional rhythm (narrow QRS) during ablation mistaken for elimination of preexcitation.

Atrioventricular (AV) accessory pathways (APs) are thin fibers, usually composed of typical myocardial cells that allow electrical communication between atrium and ventricle extrinsic to the normal AV node–His bundle axis. The clinical expression of these pathways ranges from simply causing an abnormal electrocardiogram to forming an integral component of a macro-reentrant circuit incorporating atrial and ventricular myocardium, AV node and His bundle, and the AP (AV reciprocating supraventricular tachycardia [SVT]) to functioning as an alternative pathway for transmission of rapid atrial tachyarrhythmias such as flutter and fibrillation to the ventricles. Symptoms may range from none to occasional mild palpitations to severe palpitations accompanied by dyspnea, chest discomfort, lightheadedness, and even syncope or cardiac arrest from rapidly conducted atrial fibrillation.

Since its introduction in the late 1980s, catheter ablation of APs has become a relatively routine matter in most electrophysiology laboratories. However, ablation of pathways in the so-called anterior and mid-septal locations remains a challenge for even experienced operators because of the proximity of these pathways to the normal cardiac conduction system (AV node and His bundle). Inadvertent injury to these structures resulting in the need for permanent pacing, especially in a young patient, is a serious adverse outcome. Fortunately, techniques have been developed to decrease the likelihood of this complication. This chapter discusses the relevant anatomy of these pathways and the use of these techniques.

Anatomy and Nomenclature

Current nomenclature of septal pathways is undergoing modification. A reexamination of the anatomy of the AV junctions has suggested that the terminology used in the original descriptions of AP locations was anatomically inaccurate and, in some cases, frankly misleading. Most electrophysiology trainees have had the experience of asking, "Why is my attending telling me to move the catheter *anteriorly* when I see it moving toward the head?" A reclassification of cardiac electrophysiologic anatomy has been developed to try to correct these antiquated but ingrained terms.[1] In addition, a more complete understanding of the anatomy of the atrial and ventricular septa has resulted in a "shrinking" of the atrial septum: most trainees conceive of the atrial septum as a relatively large disk comprising the intersection of two spheres compressed together. In fact, the true muscular atrial septum is much smaller, consisting of a relatively thin rim of atrial tissue surrounding the fossa ovalis.[2-4] This has implications for how precisely one must position a needle and catheter to safely puncture the septum for left atrial access and also for evaluation and ablation of the pathways under consideration in this chapter.

In the old vernacular, "anteroseptal" pathways were regarded as being located in the apex of the triangle of Koch, connecting the atrial and ventricular septa in the region of the His bundle. In the anatomically accurate nomenclature, these pathways are more properly regarded as *superoparaseptal* because there is no atrial septum in the region anterior to the His recording location (atrial walls are separated here by the aortic root) (Fig. 23-1). These connections are thus right free wall, paraseptal pathways. Posteriorly, pathways in the region of the ostium of the coronary sinus (CS), which previously were called "posteroseptal," are in fact *posterior paraseptal*, because the CS itself is, by definition, entirely posterior to the atrial septum. Pathways located between these two boundaries of the septum have been called "mid-septal" or "intermediate septal," but, because they are the only truly septal interconnections, they may simply be called *septal*. Further complicating the situation is the fact that the AV valves are not isoplanar; the tricuspid valve is slightly inferiorly displaced relative to the mitral valve such that a portion of the medial right atrium is juxtaposed to subaortic left ventricular muscle, rather than right ventricle.

In the discussion that follows, we will consider that superoparaseptal ("anteroseptal") APs are located in the apex of the triangle of Koch at a site from which a small His potential can usually be recorded. True septal or midseptal APs are located in the floor of the triangle of Koch, between the His recording location and the anterior portion of the CS ostium.

Diagnosis and Differential Diagnosis

Superoparaseptal Accessory Pathways

Superoparaseptal APs comprise 6% to 7% of all APs in most large series. About 80% of these APs exhibit anterograde conduction, and 20% are retrograde-only conducting ("concealed"); only about 5% conduct exclusively in the anterograde direction. Because these pathways connect the right atrial and right ventricular paraseptal free

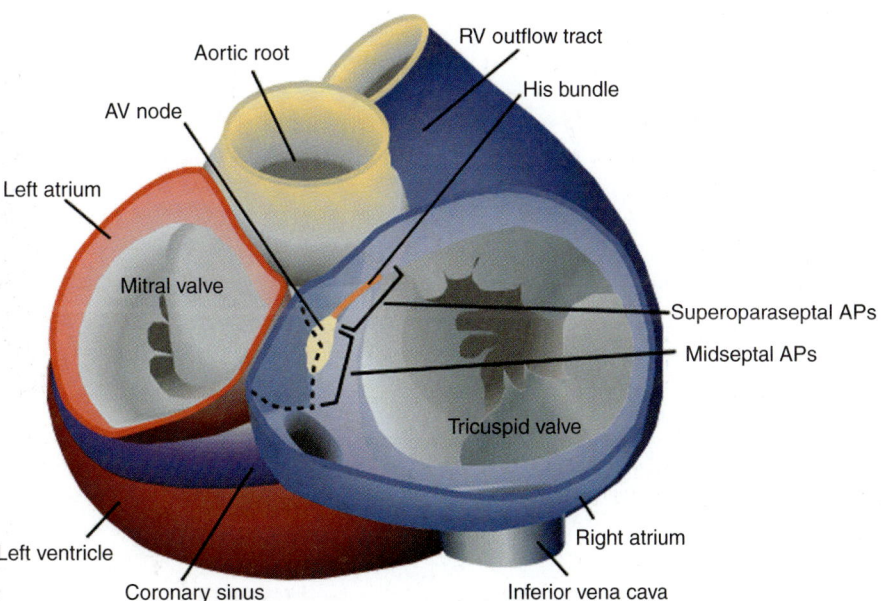

FIGURE 23-1. View of atrioventricular (AV) groove from above with most of the atrial muscle removed; the right atrial rim has been rendered semitransparent to reveal structures beneath. Note the small dimensions of the actual atrial septum (*dashed line*). True septal ("mid-septal") pathways have an atrial insertion on the right or left side in this region, in which the AV node resides. Pathways in the region of the His bundle, previously called anteroseptal, in fact have free wall and not septal atrial insertions (hence "superoparaseptal" pathways). APs, accessory pathways.

walls in a region that is cephalad, or superior, as well as anterior, to most of the rest of the ventricular mass, an anterograde conducting pathway manifests positive delta waves in the inferior leads (II, III, and aVF) and the lateral precordial leads (V_3 through V_6); negative delta waves are present in lead V_1 and often in lead V_2 (Fig. 23-2). Leads I and aVL have positive delta waves (negative in aVR). During orthodromic SVT, the P wave is typically situated in the early portion of the ST segment; although retrograde, it usually positive in the inferior leads because much of the atrial mass is located caudad from the atrial insertion (Fig. 23-3).

Mid-Septal Accessory Pathways

Mid-septal pathways account for 5% or less of all APs in most series. About 85% of mid-septal APs show anterograde conduction (15% are retrograde only), with only about 4% conducting anterograde only. These APs connect atrium and ventricle in a complex region that can give rise to slightly different delta wave polarities in different individuals. A typical preexcitation pattern has predominantly positive delta waves in leads I, II, aVL, and V_2 through V_6, with leads III and aVF usually having predominantly

negative delta waves and aVR and V_1 having isoelectric delta waves. Variations in this pattern, especially in the inferior leads and in V_2, have been reported. During SVT, because of the more posterior location of the pathway's atrial insertion (near the compact AV node), the P wave is usually inverted in the inferior leads. Multiple APs are present in up to 25% of patients with mid-septal APs.

Electrophysiologic Testing

The electrophysiologic diagnosis of SVT incorporating a superoparaseptal or mid-septal pathway is usually relatively straightforward (Table 23-1); however, the atrial activation sequence during SVT may resemble that of normal AV nodal output (unlike the situation with left or right free wall APs, in which the atrial activation sequence during SVT is eccentric). This similarity of atrial activation can provide a diagnostic challenge in some cases. Standard diagnostic techniques, including introduction of ventricular premature extrastimuli during His refractoriness in an episode of SVT, should be used to define the tachycardia mechanism. In some cases, such as when the ventricular-to-atrial interval is very short or SVT is nonsustained or noninducible, other techniques must be used to establish

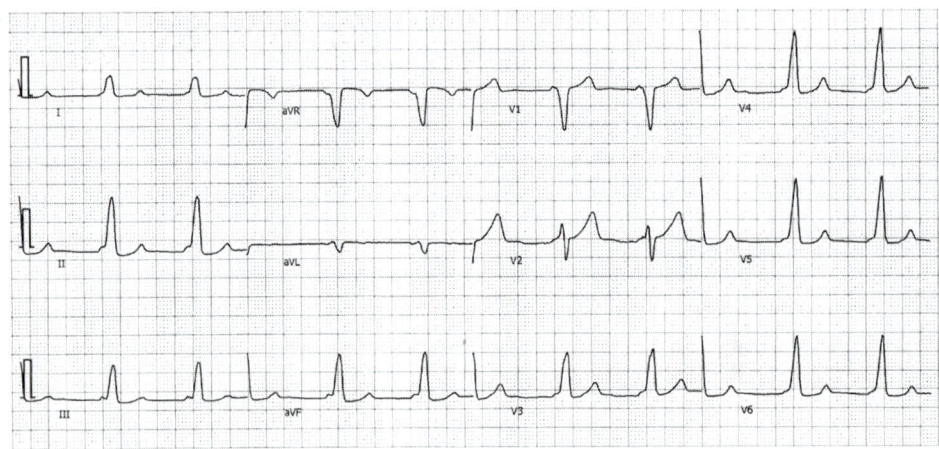

FIGURE 23-2. Electrocardiogram of superoparaseptal accessory pathways with anterograde conduction, showing a very short PR segment and positive delta waves in I, II, III, aVF, and lateral precordial leads.

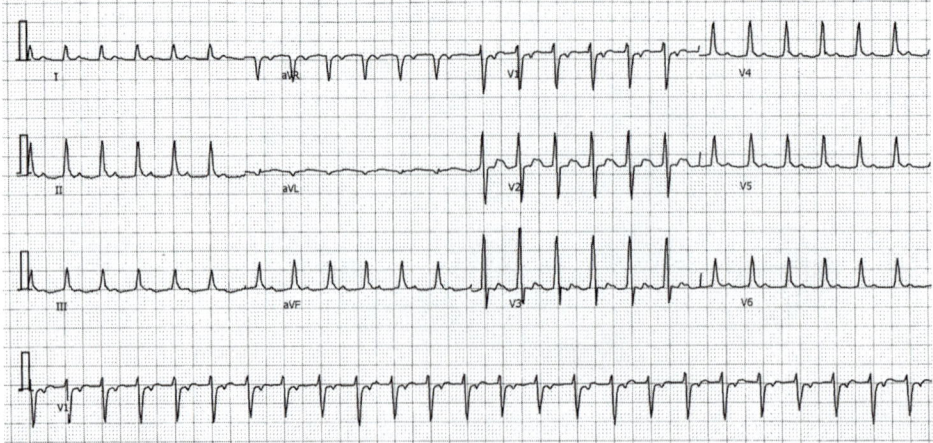

FIGURE 23-3. Electrocardiogram of supraventricular tachycardia incorporating a retrograde-conducting superoparaseptal accessory pathway. Note the positive P waves in the inferior leads with negative P-wave polarity in leads aVR and V_1.

the presence of an AP. These include parahisian pacing, differential site ventricular pacing, comparison of His bundle–to-atrial (HA) intervals, and entrainment of SVT.

Pacing from a location near the His bundle (parahisian pacing) can distinguish retrograde conduction over an AP from that over the AV node, as follows: at low pacing outputs, ventricular capture occurs, whereas at higher outputs, the His bundle and proximal right bundle branch are captured with the adjacent ventricular myocardium, resulting in a narrower QRS. If an AP in the regions under consideration is present, the stimulus-to-atrial interval will be identical regardless of whether the His is captured because these APs typically conduct more rapidly than the AV node. If there is no AP, the stimulus-to-atrial interval is longer with ventricular-only capture than when the His is captured because, with ventricular pacing, the impulse must travel some distance using relatively slow myocyte-myocyte conduction before it encounters elements of the His-Purkinje network to begin activating it retrogradely. With His capture, the impulse need only traverse the AV node to activate the atrium (Fig. 23-4).[5] This technique can be used to assess whether the AP has been successfully ablated (Fig. 23-5).

Using a principle similar to that of parahisian pacing, comparison of the stimulus-to-atrial intervals observed with right ventricular apical versus basal stimulation can demonstrate the presence of an AP. The apex, although physically more distant from the atrium than the ventricular base, is nonetheless electrically closer because of the proximity of the distal right bundle branch to the pacing site. Entry into the rapidly conducting His-Purkinje system allows a shorter stimulus-to-atrial interval during pacing from the apex than from the base. From the base, the impulse must again travel relatively slowly over some distance through ventricular myocardium before it engages the His-Purkinje system (Fig. 23-6). Fixed-rate

pacing or extrastimuli during SVT can be used.[6] This technique can also be used to confirm successful AP ablation.

Comparison of the HA intervals observed during SVT and during ventricular pacing at the SVT cycle length can distinguish AV nodal reentry from septal pathway–dependent orthodromic SVT. The HA interval during AV nodal reentry should be the same as, or slightly shorter than, the interval during ventricular pacing. The His bundle and atrium are activated in parallel during SVT but in series during pacing.[7] However, the HA during orthodromic reciprocating tachycardia should be much longer than that during ventricular pacing because the His bundle and atrium are activated in series during SVT but in parallel during pacing (the opposite of the situation in AV nodal reentry).[7]

Similarly, overdrive right ventricular apical pacing at a cycle length slightly faster than that of SVT (entrainment of SVT) can distinguish atypical AV nodal reentry from orthodromic SVT using a septal AP. If AV nodal reentry is present, the stimulus-to-atrial interval during ventricular pacing will exceed the QRS-to-atrial interval by more than 85 milliseconds, and the ventricular postpacing interval will exceed the SVT cycle length by more than 115 milliseconds. In orthodromic SVT using a septal AP, these intervals are less than the cutoff values noted. This distinction occurs because the pacing site is remote from the SVT circuit in AV nodal reentry but near or within it in orthodromic SVT.[8] Although this criterion was meant for and tested in long-RP tachycardias, we have not seen it give misleading results in more typical septal pathways. Atrial tachycardias can be differentiated from septal orthodromic SVT by the presence of a V-A-A-V response to ventricular overdrive pacing, the ability to dissociate the ventricle from the tachycardia, and a variable HA interval during tachycardia.

TABLE 23-1

DIAGNOSTIC CRITERIA

Technique	Criteria
Surface ECG: Sinus Rhythm (in Presence of Preexcitation)	
Superoparaseptal APs	Delta waves predominantly positive in leads I, II, III, aVL, aVF, and V_3 through V_6; negative in aVR and V_1, and often in V_2
Mid-septal APs	Delta waves predominantly positive in I, II, aVL, and V_2 through V_6; negative in III and aVF; negative or isoelectric in aVR and V_1
Surface ECG: Orthodromic SVT	
	P waves (in early ST segment); may be positive in inferior leads (superoparaseptal APs)
Intracardiac Recordings and Electrophysiology	
	Premature ventricular extrastimulus during His refractoriness can advance atrial activation or terminate tachycardia without causing atrial activation
	ΔHA interval (SVT versus ventricular pacing) to distinguish orthodromic SVT from AV nodal reentry
	Mid-septal pathways may exhibit "decremental" conduction properties (anterograde or retrograde)
	Parahisian or differential site ventricular pacing useful to prove existence of pathway, confirm its ablation (if normal retrograde AV node/His conduction intact)
Superoparaseptal APs	Earliest anterograde ventricular activation at or anterior to His recording location
	Earliest retrograde atrial activation in His bundle recording
	Small (<0.1 mV) His deflection in ablation recording
	Sensitivity to mechanical block by catheter manipulation
Mid-septal APs	Earliest anterograde ventricular and retrograde atrial activation between His and coronary sinus ostium

AP, accessory pathway; AV, atrioventricular; ECG, electrocardiogram; ΔHA, difference in His-to-atrial interval; SVT, supraventricular tachycardia.

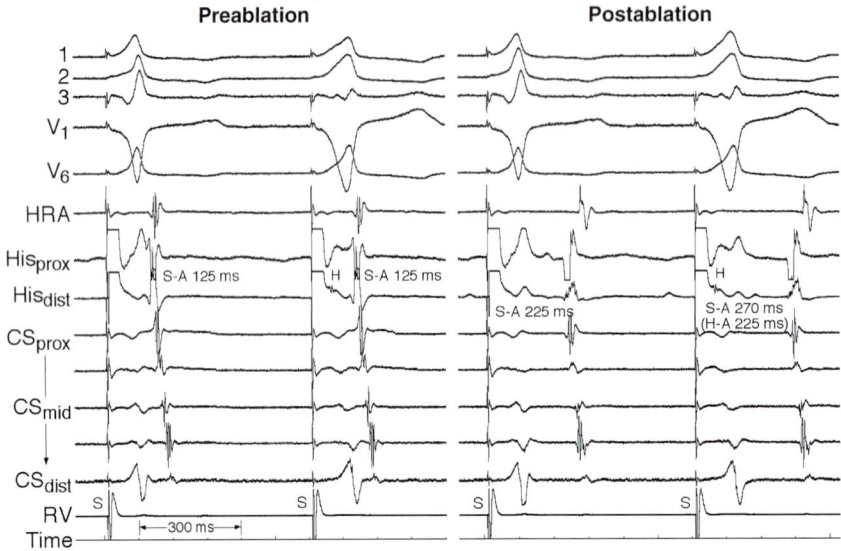

FIGURE 23-4. Parahisian pacing. In this and subsequent figures, surface leads I, II, III, V₁, and V₆ are shown with intracardiac recordings from high right atrium (HRA), His bundle proximal (prox) and distal (dist) electrode pairs, coronary sinus (CS), right ventricle (RV) near the His recording location; S denotes stimulus artifact, H the His deflection. Parahisian pacing is shown before (*left panel*) and after (*right panel*) ablation. On each panel, the first complex shows His and ventricular capture, the second ventricular capture only. Before ablation, the stimulus-atrial (S-A) interval is the same regardless of whether His capture occurs because the accessory pathway is the preferred path of conduction. In the complex on the *right*, the apparent H-A interval is shorter than the S-A interval during His capture, indicating that atrial activation is occurring independent of AV nodal conduction. After successful ablation, retrograde conduction requires His activation; the S-A interval is longer than before ablation and increases further in the absence of His capture (complex on the right) because with pure ventricular pacing, it takes longer to get to the His bundle. Once the His is activated as shown, the H-A time is the same as the S-A time during His capture.

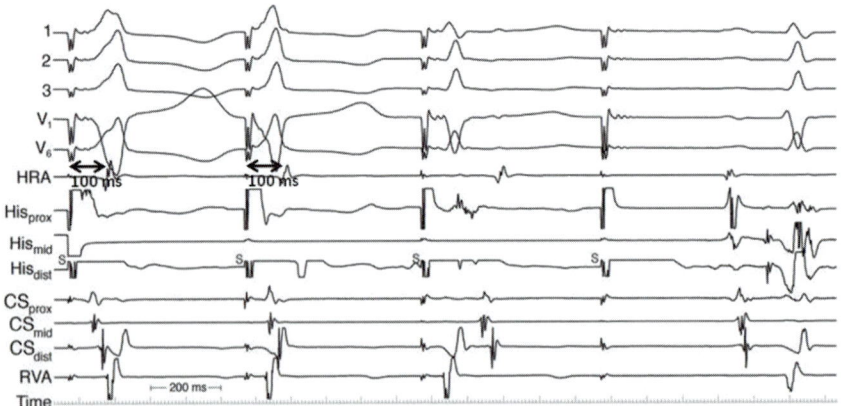

FIGURE 23-5. Parahisian pacing revealing presence of pathway after apparently successful radiofrequency application. Four stimuli from the His region result in (*left to right*) ventricular capture, His and ventricular capture, pure His capture, and no capture. The two complexes on the left have identical S-A intervals (100 msec), indicating lack of dependence on His conduction for atrial activation (i.e., accessory pathway present). A sinus complex at the *right* confirms the pure His capture complex, which has a longer S-A interval than either of the first two complexes, confirming persistence of the pathway. CS, coronary sinus; HRA, high right atrium; RVA, right ventricular apex.

Mid-septal APs occasionally present additional nuances. In some cases, these pathways have demonstrated so-called decremental conduction properties (cycle length–dependent prolongation of conduction intervals). Especially in the absence of overt preexcitation, this feature could cause confusion by suggesting conduction only through the AV node, rather than the presence of an AP.[9]

Mapping and Ablation Techniques

Superoparaseptal Accessory Pathways

Ablation of APs in the region of the His bundle may be successfully and safely accomplished using the same techniques employed for APs in other locations (Table 23-2). In the presence of preexcitation, the ventricular insertion site can be targeted by searching for the earliest site of ventricular activation during sinus rhythm; atrial pacing usually is not necessary to attain maximal preexcitation because the ventricular insertion of the AP is relatively close to the sinus node. Electrogram characteristics at successful ablation sites include (1) a ventricular activation time that precedes the surface electrocardiogram delta wave onset by 15 to 40 milliseconds; (2) a sharp QS deflection on the unipolar electrogram of the ablation electrode; (3) a sharp AP potential; and (4) an almost continuous recording incorporating atrial-AP-ventricular components (Fig. 23-7). Differentiation of atrial from ventricular components of a complex recording can usually

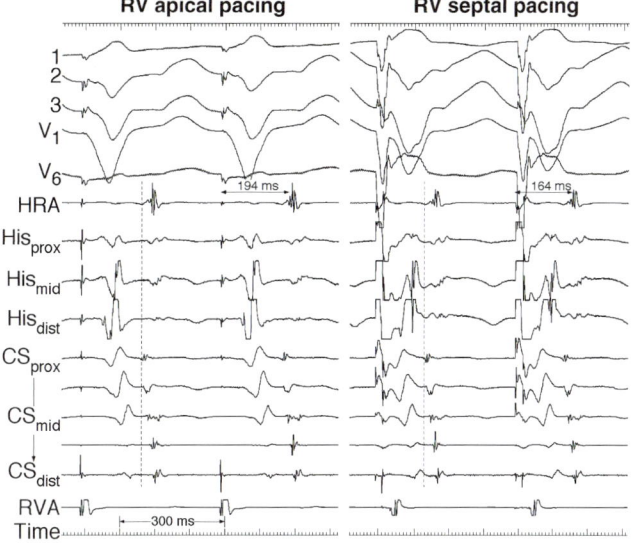

FIGURE 23-6. Differential site pacing. *Dashed lines* denote onset of atrial activation. On the *left panel*, right ventricular (RV) apical pacing yields a stimulus–high right atrium (HRA) time of 194 msec, whereas RV basal pacing yields a stimulus-HRA interval of 164 msec, indicating the presence of an extranodal. Abl, ablation catheter; CS, coronary sinus; RVA, right ventricular apex.

TABLE 23-2		
TARGET SITES FOR ABLATION		
Superoparaseptal	*Ventricular insertion site (in presence of preexcitation):* Ventricular activation time that precedes surface ECG delta wave onset by 15-40 msec Sharp QS deflection on the unipolar electrogram of the ablation electrode Presence of a sharp AP potential between atrial and ventricular electrograms Nearly continuous recording with atrial-AP-ventricular components preceding delta wave onset Small (<0.1 mV) His deflection may be present (may be obscured by ventricular electrogram) *Atrial insertion site (in presence of retrograde conduction):* Earliest atrial electrogram Presence of a sharp AP potential between atrial and ventricular electrograms Small (<0.1 mV) His deflection may be present		
Mid-septal	*Ventricular insertion site (in presence of preexcitation):* Ventricular activation time that precedes the surface ECG delta wave onset by 15-40 msec Sharp QS deflection on the unipolar electrogram of the ablation electrode Presence of a sharp AP potential between ventricular and atrial electrograms preceding delta wave onset Nearly continuous recording with atrial-AP-ventricular components *Atrial insertion site (in presence of retrograde conduction):* Earliest atrial electrogram Presence of a sharp AP potential between ventricular and atrial electrograms		

AP, accessory pathway; ECG, electrocardiogram.

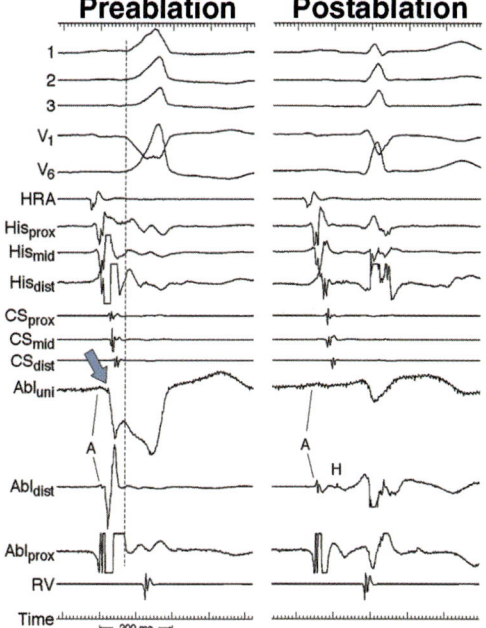

FIGURE 23-7. Site of superoparaseptal accessory pathway ablation. The *dashed line* indicates the onset of the delta wave. Note the sharp negative deflection in the unipolar electrogram (*arrow*) with a diminutive atrial electrogram that is clearly evident as such only post ablation. Note also the His potential (H) in the post-ablation recording. A, atrial electrogram; Abl, ablation catheter; CS, coronary sinus; HRA, high right atrium; RV, right ventricle; uni, unipolar electrogram.

be accomplished by introducing atrial extrastimuli or burst pacing that blocks in the AP. Pre-delta wave activation times are longer (i.e., earlier) in right-sided than in left-sided APs in general, and especially so with superoparaseptal APs.[10] The site with the longest (earliest) pre-delta time should be sought. (For example, even if the pre-delta time in the first site sampled is 15 milliseconds, ablation should not be performed there until multiple other nearby sites have been sampled, none of which has a longer interval.) Fluoroscopically, this can be very close to the His bundle recording site (Fig. 23-8). It is important to distinguish the AP potential from the His recording; repeated bursts of pacing or premature stimuli will usually accomplish this (Fig. 23-9).

During orthodromic SVT, the site with the earliest atrial electrogram activation, often with an AP potential, is the target. It is important to distinguish between the site with the *shortest ventricular-to-atrial interval* and the site with the *earliest atrial activation time;* they are often the same site, but if they are not, the site with the earliest atrial activation time is preferred. The ventricular and atrial electrograms may be almost fused during SVT or ventricular pacing; introduction of premature ventricular extrastim-

uli during either pacing or SVT may separate the electrogram components, allowing the operator to correctly assess the timing of atrial activation as well as relative electrogram amplitudes. Also during SVT, the amplitude of the His bundle electrogram in the ablation recording can be assessed. The AP can be safely ablated if the His deflection is less than 0.2 mV in amplitude, although there is probably less chance of injury if it is smaller still.

Ordinarily, one should ablate on the ventricular aspect of the annulus if this site is stable; atrial sites (ratio of atrial to ventricular electrogram amplitudes, >0.4) may yield successful ablation but with a slightly higher risk for injury to the normal conduction system. A long vascular sheath may help stabilize the position of the catheter tip regardless of whether an atrial or a ventricular site is chosen. Some operators prefer to ablate with a catheter introduced from

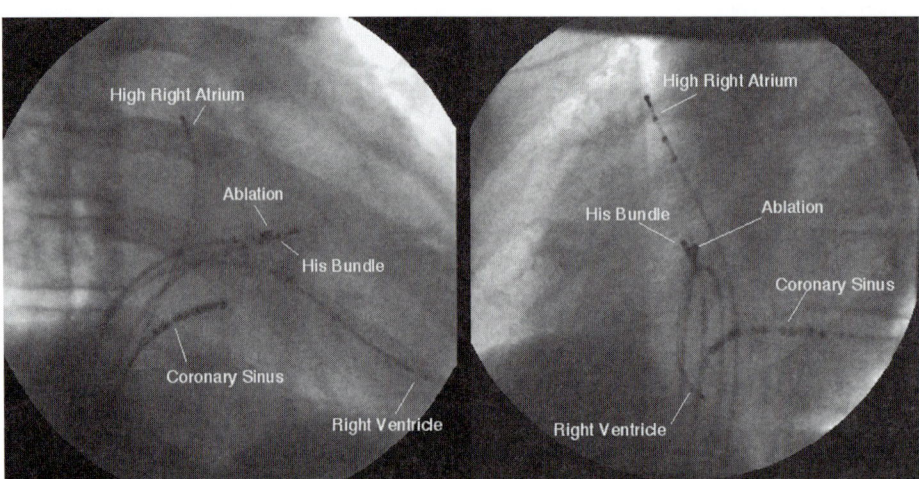

FIGURE 23-8. Fluoroscopic images of superoparaseptal accessory pathway ablation site. Catheters and views as labeled; note the near-superimposition of the ablation catheter and His recording electrodes. Ablation at this site was successful without injury to the His bundle.

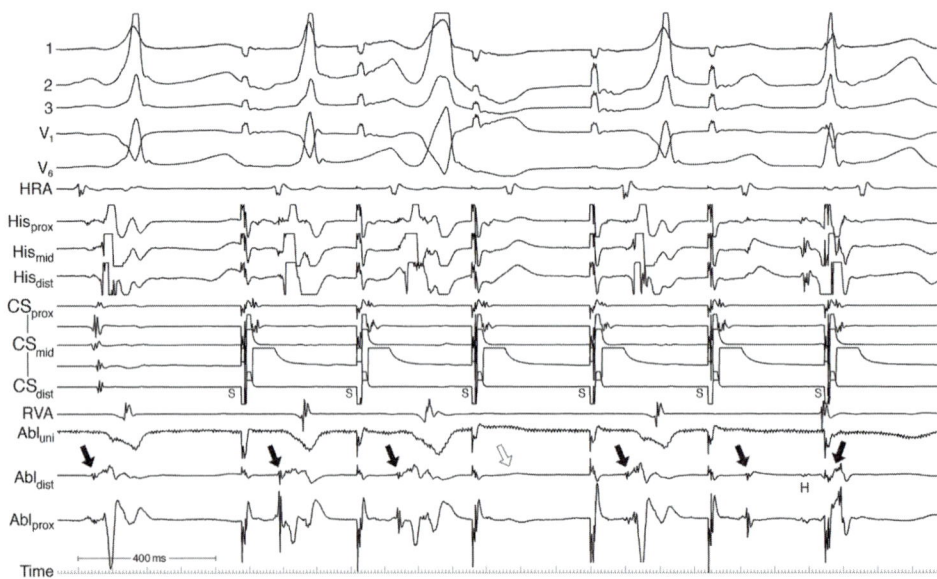

FIGURE 23-9. Proof of accessory pathway (AP) potential recording. *Filled arrows* indicate AP potential, *open arrows* its absence. A sinus rhythm complex is followed by a burst of pacing from the coronary sinus, resulting in conduction over the AP after the first two stimuli but not the third stimulus, that captures atrium but blocks in the AP (hence no AP potential; this proves the potential was not atrial in origin.). The fourth stimulus is like the first, but the fifth stimulus blocks distal to the AP (thus, it is not ventricular in origin). A small His potential (H) is seen in the ablation recording, indicating the proximity to the normal conduction system (as well as that the AP potential is not the His spike). Abl, ablation catheter; CS, coronary sinus; HRA, high right atrium; RVA, right ventricular apex; uni, unipolar electrogram.

the internal jugular vein approach, either positioning the catheter tip on the atrial aspect or advancing it slightly across and beneath the tricuspid annulus to ablate from the ventricular aspect.

It is worth spending extra time to fine-tune the ablation site, ensuring both the best possible timing and the morphology of the ablation electrogram as well as catheter-tip stability. Delivering as few ablation applications as possible (and, consequently, doing as little damage as possible) is an important goal when ablating in the vicinity of the AV node and His bundle. Mapping systems that can "tag" or track the location of mapping or ablation sites may be useful in guiding the operator either toward more favorable sites or away from sites that are less attractive. If the best ablation site is very close to the His bundle recording site, the His recording catheter can occasionally be advanced slightly into the ventricle, leaving the insulated portion of the catheter as a potential physical barrier overlying the His bundle.

Once a site has been chosen for ablation, radiofrequency (RF) energy delivery should begin at relatively low power (30 W) and low temperature (50° to 60°C) settings but with firm catheter contact. Poor contact may result in only minimal damage but with edema formation that then distorts electrograms and may lead to an increased physical barrier to subsequent effective energy delivery. If preexcitation is present, ablation may be attempted during sinus rhythm or during atrial pacing. Unsuccessful energy applications should be stopped after no more than 15 seconds; continued energy delivery at such sites is unlikely to be beneficial but may have already caused damage to the AV node or His bundle that cannot be discerned as long as preexcitation persists. It is useful to try to ensure that normal AV node–His conduction is still intact after one or two failed ablation energy deliveries. Use of higher energies, or of large-tip catheters capable of causing more extensive damage, has practically no role in ablation of these APs; the cause of ablation failure in these APs is almost always incorrect localization or poor contact, and not inadequacy of a standard-sized RF lesion.

For nonseptal concealed APs, ablation is usually performed during ventricular pacing so that loss of AP conduction can be readily monitored. However, use of this method for ablation of pathways in the vicinity of the AV node and His bundle could result in inadvertent damage to these structures that would not be evident until after cessation of pacing (when it may be too late). Alternative methods for ablation of concealed APs in this region include ablation during sinus rhythm, during SVT, and during atrial-entrained SVT.

Ablation during sinus rhythm has the advantage of allowing monitoring for either PR prolongation or accelerated junctional rhythm, indicating damage to the normal conduction system and prompting cessation of energy delivery. However, AP ablation success cannot be assessed until ventricular pacing is performed after cessation of RF delivery.

Ablation during SVT allows monitoring of both normal conduction and ablation success (SVT terminates in retrograde limb). However, the sudden change in heart rate associated with successful ablation and cessation of SVT can lead to ablation catheter displacement and incomplete ablation. With ablation during atrial-entrained SVT, atrial pacing is performed slightly faster than the SVT cycle length while ablation energy is delivered. When the AP conduction is ablated, SVT terminates, but the heart rate does not change; therefore, the likelihood of catheter movement is

decreased, and complete ablation is facilitated. Because this method allows monitoring of efficacy (AP ablation) and safety (normal AV conduction) and addresses the problem of catheter movement, it is preferred.

Cryomapping and ablation have been introduced as techniques to avoid unwanted damage to the AV node and His bundle.[11,12] With cryomapping, the catheter tip is first cooled to 0°C at potential ablation sites; if AP conduction is lost without damage to the normal conduction elements, the catheter-tip temperature can be decreased to –80°C for cryoablation. Cold-induced attenuation of normal pathway conduction may be hard to appreciate because preexcitation is near-maximal in sinus rhythm or with right atrial pacing; instead, if CS pacing results in a greater degree of normal conduction (less preexcitation), application of cold to the AV node or His bundle will result in an increase in preexcitation. Such areas should be noted as sites at which ablation definitely should not be performed.

Troubleshooting the Difficult Case

Successful ablation of superoparaseptal APs poses particular challenges (Table 23-3). These APs are by definition close enough to the His bundle that a small His potential is usually recorded in the ablation signal (or sometimes first becomes evident after successful ablation). Inadvertent damage to the His bundle or the AV node is the primary hazard in ablating these APs. Additional potential difficulties include AP sensitivity to catheter trauma and accelerated junctional rhythm during RF energy delivery.

These pathways are often very superficial (toward the endocardial surface), and catheter trauma results in transient block of pathway conduction in one or both directions in up to 38% of cases (Fig. 23-10).[13] If this occurs, and the catheter has moved ("grazed" the pathway as it was passing by), one can only wait and hope that pathway conduction resumes. This may take up to 30 minutes. Isoproterenol has been used by some to try to facilitate resumption of conduction; although this has been reported to be successful, the additional waiting time may have been responsible for return of AP conduction, rather than the medication, and there are no controlled studies of isoproterenol in this setting. If the catheter tip is still at the site at which trauma interrupted AP conduction, one can proceed with ablation despite lack of return of conduction after a reasonable waiting period (10 to 15 minutes). Use of mapping systems that allow tagging of sites on a three-dimensional rendering of the heart may be helpful in this regard, but only if sites with acceptable electrogram characteristics were designated as such before catheter-mediated loss of AP conduction. If catheter-induced AP block occurs and one is uncertain as to whether the catheter is still at the site that caused mechanical block, it may be appropriate to move the catheter well away from the site (i.e., its continued presence may be causing ongoing mechanical block). In this situation, tagging of the site with a mapping system can be very helpful: if conduction returns after the catheter is moved away, the mapping reference facilitates replacement of the tip back to the same site.

Accelerated junctional rhythm during RF energy delivery (Fig. 23-11) occurs in up to 5% of patients[14] and results

TABLE 23-3

TROUBLESHOOTING THE DIFFICULT CASE

Problem	Causes	Possible Solutions
Pathway block during mapping	Catheter trauma of superficially located pathway	Careful catheter manipulation If catheter remains in the same location that caused block, wait up to 1 hr for recovery
Accelerated junctional rhythm	Heating of AV node	Stop RF application immediately; reposition catheter
Right bundle branch block during RF application	Catheter positioned too distally	Reposition catheter
Unable to successfully ablate at earliest site of RA activation in SVT	Poor catheter contact	Vascular sheath; alter approach (switch to SVC or femoral vein)
	Incorrect location on right side Left-sided atrial or ventricular pathway insertion	Continue mapping Map LA/LV septum; LVOT; noncoronary sinus of Valsalva
Large His potential in best ablation recording	True parahisian pathway	Use cryomapping to test sites before ablation Advance His catheter so that insulated shaft "shields" His bundle from ablation energy

AV, atrioventricular; LA, left atrium; LV, left ventricle; LVOT, left ventricular outflow tract; RA, right atrium; RF, radiofrequency; SVC, superior vena cava; SVT, supraventricular tachycardia.

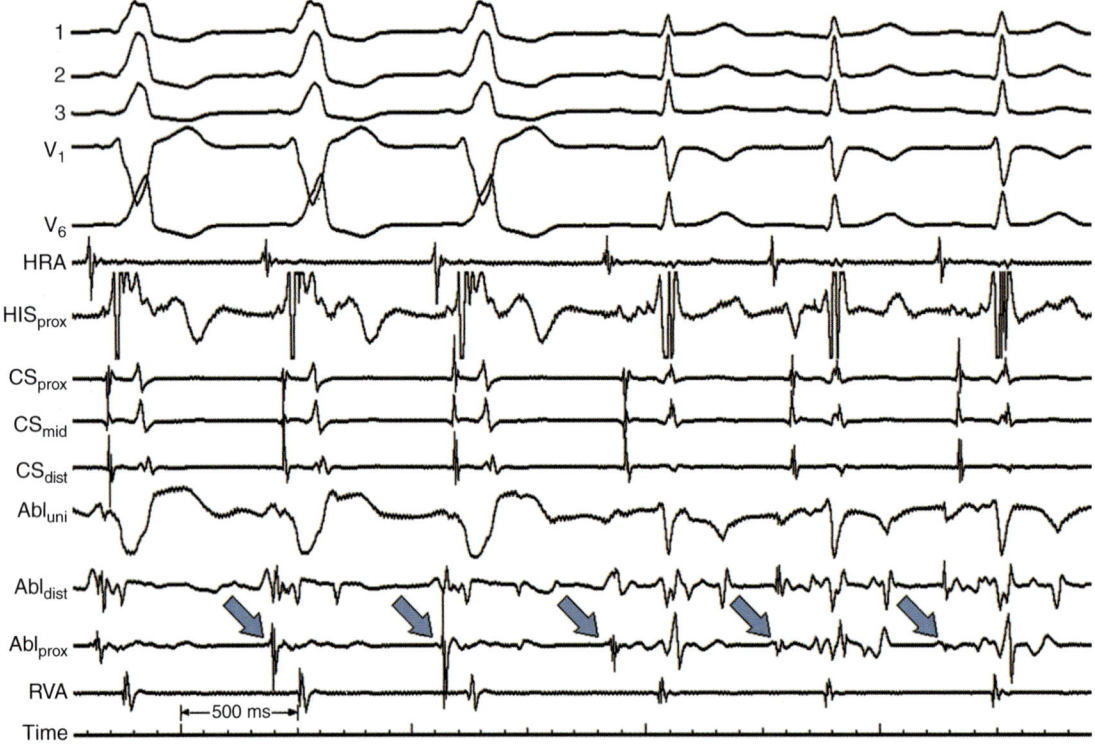

FIGURE 23-10. Mechanical block in superoparaseptal accessory pathway due to catheter manipulation. The first three beats show preexcitation; the last three do not, owing to catheter trauma. *Diagonal arrows* show a changing atrial electrogram in the ablation recording, indicating unstable catheter position. Abl, ablation catheter; CS, coronary sinus; HRA, high right atrium; RVA, right ventricular apex.

from heating of the His bundle. Accelerated junctional rhythm typically results in a narrow QRS complex on the electrocardiogram, a finding that may erroneously suggest that the AP has been successfully ablated and that energy delivery should continue. In fact, this is exactly the wrong thing to do because the His bundle may be undergoing destruction. The operator has only seconds to discontinue RF energy delivery before the His bundle is destroyed. If energy delivery continues, progressive acceleration of the junctional discharge rate may occur, as during intentional His bundle ablation. This can provide an important

warning to the operator if the danger has not already been appreciated. Fortunately, the His bundle is contained within a fibrous sheath that is somewhat protective against inadvertent ablation. Of note, cryoablation does not result in accelerated junctional rhythm; however, absence of this rhythm during cryoablation should not be interpreted as lack of risk for damaging the normal conduction system.

Parahisian pathways represent a subgroup of the superoparaseptal pathways that are more closely related to the His bundle (His deflection, >0.1 mV).[15] Despite this proximity to the His, these APs can still be ablated successfully without

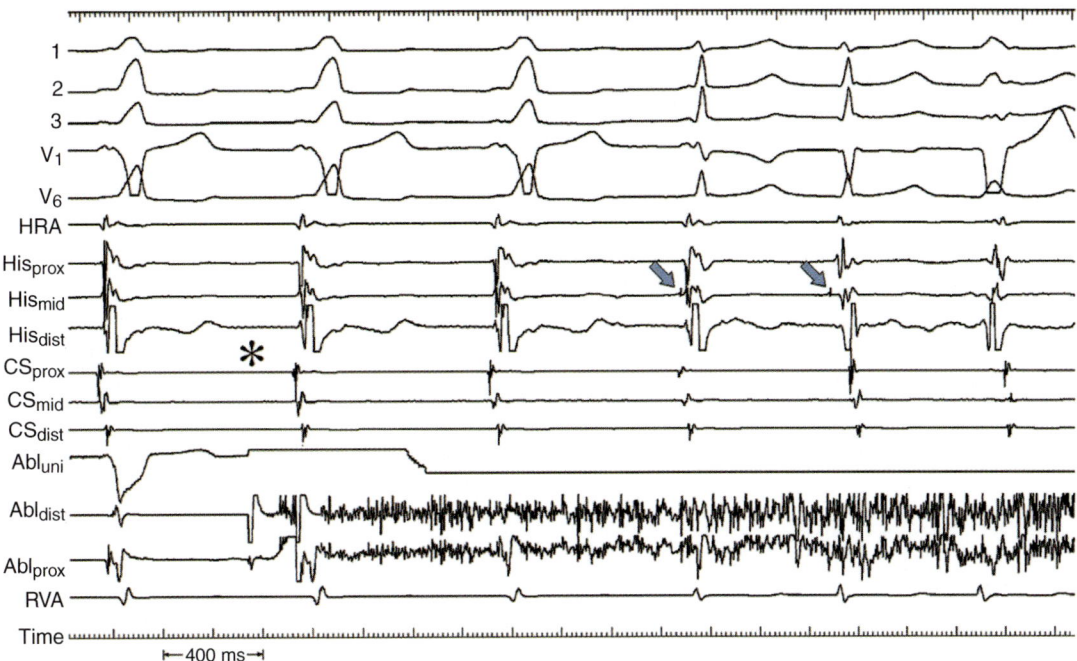

FIGURE 23-11. Accelerated junctional rhythm during ablation attempt (superoparaseptal accessory pathway [AP]). Radiofrequency (RF) delivery is begun at the *asterisk*; the next two preexcited beats are followed by two narrow QRS complexes, but not due to AP ablation. Instead, these are accelerated junctional complexes caused by heating of the His bundle (*arrows*). RF application was stopped just after the end of the recording. The AP was eventually ablated with preservation of normal atrioventricular conduction. Abl, ablation catheter; CS, coronary sinus; HRA, high right atrium; RVA, right ventricular apex.

incurring His bundle injury, perhaps because of the insulating effect of the fibrous sheath surrounding the His bundle. Some authors have observed inappropriate sinus tachycardia shortly after ablation of APs in this location, presumably due to alteration of parasympathetic tone caused by the ablation.[16] This is self-limited and requires no treatment.

Rare cases have been reported in which superoparaseptal APs could be ablated only at sites other than the expected apex of the triangle of Koch. These sites have included the left ventricular outflow tract[17] and the noncoronary sinus of Valsalva.[18] If several attempts at ablation in the expected right ventricular region have failed to interrupt AP conduction, one should evaluate other, less common ventricular insertion sites such as these.

Using the techniques described, superoparaseptal pathways can be successfully ablated in more than 95% of patients, with about 1% risk for heart block or other significant complications. Right bundle branch block occurs in up to 10% of cases.[14] Cryoablation has been less successful on long-term follow-up than RF ablation (up to 20% recurrence after hospital discharge)[11,12]; whether this is due to an inherent inferiority of cryoablation or simply less familiarity with the technique is not clear. Assessment of successful ablation includes standard techniques (i.e., lack of preexcitation at rest or with decremental atrial pacing, lack of any retrograde conduction, or conduction only over the AV node with cycle length–dependent prolongation of conduction time). Parahisian pacing and differential-site right ventricular pacing can also be used (see earlier discussion).

Mid-Septal Accessory Pathways

The principles of ablation of mid-septal APs are similar to those for superoparaseptal APs (Fig. 23-12). Care should

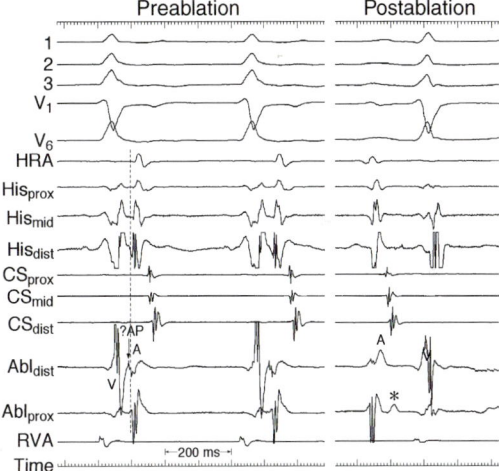

FIGURE 23-12. Site of mid-septal accessory pathway (AP) ablation. The *left panel* shows supraventricular tachycardia incorporating a retrograde-conducting mid-septal pathway with earliest atrial activation in the distal ablation (Abl$_{dist}$) recording followed by the His region. The Abl$_{dist}$ also shows a possible AP potential between ventricular and atrial components (*small arrow*). After ablation, the ablation recordings do not show a His potential, but a deflection similar to some so-called slow atrioventricular nodal pathway recordings is seen (*asterisk*). CS, coronary sinus; HRA, high right atrium; RVA, right ventricular apex.

be taken to ablate on the ventricular side of the annulus to avoid AV nodal damage (Fig. 23-13). Mid-septal APs are successfully ablated in about 98% of cases, with about a 1% risk for complete AV block, although transient AV block may occur in up to 5% of patients. Junctional rhythm during RF delivery is seen in up to 50% of cases.[14]

Occasionally, ablation of mid-septal APs is not successful after several RF applications on the tricuspid annulus.

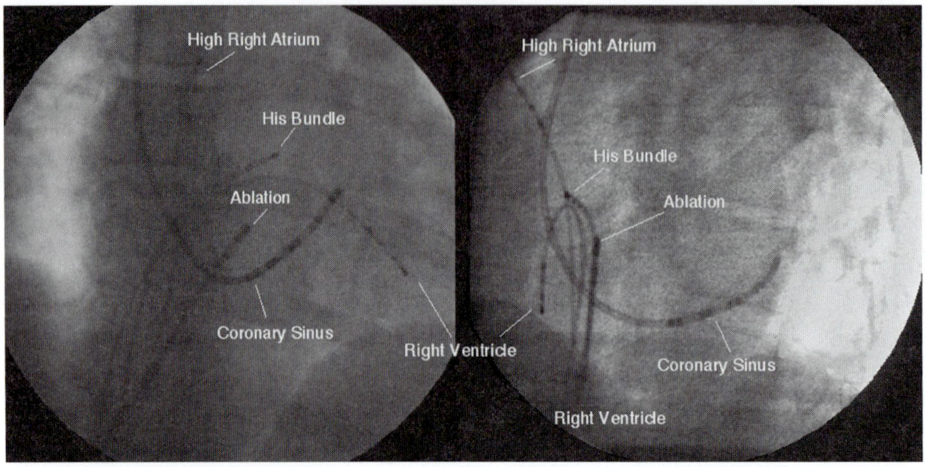

FIGURE 23-13. Fluoroscopic images of mid-septal accessory pathway ablation site. Catheters and views as labeled. The ablation catheter is situated between the coronary sinus ostium and His recording electrodes, in the region of the compact atrioventricular (AV) node. Ablation at this site was successful without damaging the AV node.

In most cases, this is due to poor site selection or poor electrode-endocardial contact at an appropriate site. In some cases, ablation can be successful only if it is performed from the left side of the septum. Clues to the presence of a left mid-septal AP are absence of sites with pre-delta wave intervals in excess of 10 milliseconds if preexcitation is present, absence of an AP potential at all sites on the tricuspid annulus, and relatively long local ventricular-to-atrial intervals (>60 milliseconds) on the tricuspid annulus. Left-sided ablation may be performed using the retrograde aortic or the transseptal approach. The surface electrocardiogram preexcitation pattern is not specific enough to suggest the necessity of a left-sided approach.[14]

APs in both superoparaseptal and mid-septal regions can be safely and successfully ablated using only two electrode catheters (an ablation catheter and a right ventricular catheter for assessing retrograde conduction).[19] Most operators prefer to use additional catheters for fluoroscopic (coronary sinus) and electrical (His bundle) reference.

Recurrence of AP conduction after apparently successful ablation occurs in up to 15% of right-sided APs, including superoparaseptal and mid-septal APs.[20] Poor catheter stability is the most common cause (suboptimal ablation due to poor contact), although in the case of APs near the AV node and His bundle, operator timidity (unwillingness to deliver adequate energy to the area for fear of causing heart block) may be responsible for incomplete ablation. Common problems encountered in the ablation of septal pathways and their solutions are listed in Table 23-3.

Conclusion

Ablation of APs in the region of the normal conduction system presents special challenges to the electrophysiologist. Although differentiation of AP-related SVTs from atrial tachycardias and AV nodal reentry can sometimes be difficult, the major challenge remains avoidance of damage to the AV node and His bundle that would require permanent pacing. Fortunately, this complication can usually be avoided by careful attention to catheter positioning and monitoring of normal AV conduction.

References

1. Cosio FG, Anderson RH, Kuck KH, et al. ESCWGA/NASPE/P experts consensus statement. Living anatomy of the atrioventricular junctions: a guide to electrophysiologic mapping. Working Group of Arrhythmias of the European Society of Cardiology. North American Society of Pacing and Electrophysiology. J Cardiovasc Electrophysiol. 1999;10:1162–1170.
2. Anderson RH, Brown NA. The anatomy of the heart revisited. Anat Rec. 1996;246:1–7.
3. Anderson RH, Brown NA, Webb S. Development and structure of the atrial septum. Heart. 2002;88:104–110.
4. Anderson RH, Webb S, Brown NA, et al. Development of the heart. 2. Septation of the atriums and ventricles. Heart. 2003;89:949–958.
5. Hirao K, Otomo K, Wang X, et al. Para-Hisian pacing: a new method for differentiating retrograde conduction over an accessory AV pathway from conduction over the AV node. Circulation. 1996;94:1027–1035.
6. Goldberger J, Wang Y, Scheinman M. Stimulation of the summit of the right ventricular aspect of the ventricular septum during orthodromic atrioventricular reentrant tachycardia. Am J Cardiol. 1992;70:78–85.
7. Miller JM, Rosenthal ME, Gottlieb CD, et al. Usefulness of the delta HA interval to accurately distinguish atrioventricular nodal reentry from orthodromic septal bypass tract tachycardias. Am J Cardiol. 1991;68:1037–1044.
8. Michaud GF, Tada H, Chough S, et al. Differentiation of atypical atrioventricular node re-entrant tachycardia from orthodromic reciprocating tachycardia using a septal accessory pathway by the response to ventricular pacing. J Am Coll Cardiol. 2001;38:1163–1167.
9. Coppess MA, Altemose GT, Jayachandran JV, et al. Unusual features of intermediate septal bypass tracts. J Cardiovasc Electrophysiol. 2000;11:730–735.
10. Xie B, Heald SC, Camm AJ, et al. Characteristics of bipolar electrograms during anterograde mapping: the importance of accessory atrioventricular pathway location. Am Heart J. 1996;131:720–723.
11. Gaita F, Haïssaguerre M, Giustetto C, et al. Safety and efficacy of cryoablation of accessory pathways adjacent to the normal conduction system. J Cardiovasc Electrophysiol. 2003;14:825–829.
12. Wong T, Markides V, Peters NS, Davies DW. Clinical usefulness of cryomapping for ablation of tachycardias involving perinodal tissue. J Interv Card Electrophysiol. 2004;10:153–158.
13. Belhassen B, Viskin S, Fish R, et al. Catheter-induced mechanical trauma to accessory pathways during radiofrequency ablation: incidence, predictors and clinical implications. J Am Coll Cardiol. 1999;33:767–774.
14. Kuck KH, Ouyang F, Goya M, Boczor S. Ablation of anteroseptal and midseptal accessory pathways. In: Zipes DP, Haïssaguerre M, eds. Catheter Ablation of Arrhythmias. 2nd ed. Armonk, NY: Futura; 2002:305–320.
15. Haïssaguerre M, Marcus F, Poquet F, et al. Electrocardiographic characteristics and catheter ablation of parahisian accessory pathways. Circulation. 1994;90:1124–1128.
16. Pappone C, Stabile G, Oreto G, et al. Inappropriate sinus tachycardia after radiofrequency ablation of para-Hisian accessory pathways. J Cardiovasc Electrophysiol. 1997;8:1357–1365.

17. Miyauchi Y, Kobayashi Y, Morita N, et al. Successful radiofrequency catheter ablation of an anteroseptal (superoparaseptal) atrioventricular accessory pathway from the left ventricular outflow tract. *Pacing Clin Electrophysiol.* 2004;27:668–670.
18. Tada H, Naito S, Nogami A, Taniguchi K. Successful catheter ablation of an anteroseptal accessory pathway from the noncoronary sinus of Valsalva. *J Cardiovasc Electrophysiol.* 2003;14:544–546.
19. Brugada J, Puigfel M, Mont L, et al. Radiofrequency ablation of anteroseptal, para-Hisian, and mid-septal accessory pathways using a simplified femoral approach. *Pacing Clin Electrophysiol.* 1998;21:735–741.
20. Twidale N, Wang XZ, Beckman KJ, et al. Factors associated with recurrence of accessory pathway conduction after radiofrequency catheter ablation. *Pacing Clin Electrophysiol.* 1991;14:2042–2048.

24
Ablation of Atriofascicular "Mahaim Fiber" Accessory Pathways and Variants

Henry Chen, Amin Al-Ahmad, Henry H. Hsia, Mintu Turakhia, Paul C. Zei, and Paul J. Wang

Key Points

Mapping of the atriofascicular (Mahaim fiber) accessory pathways is directed at identification of the atrial insertion site on tricuspid annulus. This site is identified by discrete accessory pathway potential.

Ablation targets include the atrial or ventricular pathway insertion on the tricuspid annulus or distally in right ventricle (more difficult).

Special equipment includes mapping and ablation catheters and a long sheath; computerized mapping is optional.

Sources of difficulty are ablation of distal ventricular insertion site, catheter instability during mapping, and accessory pathway sensitivity to mechanical trauma.

An evolution in the understanding of a unique type of accessory pathway that demonstrates slow, decremental, and exclusively antegrade conduction, originally termed *Mahaim fiber*, has occurred over several decades of histopathologic, electrophysiologic, and surgical observations. In 1938, Mahaim and colleagues originally described pathologic findings of discrete accessory conductive pathways connecting the atrioventricular (AV) node and the ventricle.[1,2] Later observations of a unique preexcitation tachycardia syndrome that demonstrated nodal-like slow and decremental conduction led to the speculation that the fibers described by Mahaim were responsible.[3,4] Although these observations fit the behavior of nodoventricular and nodofascicular connections, the most common etiology for these unusual preexcitation patterns is now recognized to be atriofascicular accessory pathways.[4–12] The term Mahaim

fiber has evolved a variety of meanings. For some, the true Mahaim fiber is the nodofascicular or nodoventricular connection faithful to the original pathologic description. Over time, the term became a generic description for any pathway with slow decremental conduction properties. These properties may now be better described as *Mahaim physiology* without implicating specific anatomic connections. Current use, although varied, tends to use Mahaim fiber to describe the most common pathway associated with decremental properties, the atriofascicular pathway. In this chapter, we favor the unambiguous term *atriofascicular pathway* over the term Mahaim fiber.

Atriofascicular Pathway Anatomy

Our current concepts of the pathways have been shaped by modern surgical and electrophysiologic data. The proximal insertion of the pathway is at the atrial margin of the free wall tricuspid annulus and the distal insertion either at the right bundle branch (RBB) (atriofascicular) or directly into ventricular myocardium (AV) (Figs. 24-1 to 24-3).[6–8,10–17] Most of the atriofascicular pathways are on the right side of the heart, although there have been rare cases reported of left-sided pathways.[18–20] In addition, there is a report of a decrementally conducting AV accessory pathway at the mitral annulus–aorta junction.[21] The atrial component of the pathway (usually located at or near the lateral, anterolateral, or posterolateral tricuspid annulus) has AV nodal-like properties and is responsible for the decremental conduction properties of the pathway.[10]

The atrial insertion connects to a long fiber, similar to the RBB, that inserts distally into the apical ventricular myocardium or travels along the right ventricular endocardial surface to insert into the RBB.[10] The long pathways often have wide distal insertion, which can be up to 0.5 to 2 cm in diameter.[13]

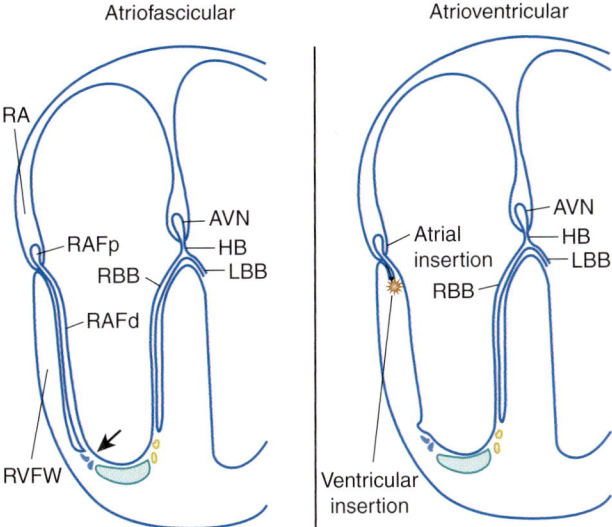

FIGURE 24-1. Schematic representation of Mahaim pathways demonstrating atrioventricular connections (short and long) as well as atriofascicular connection. Note the distal arborization of long accessory tracts. AVN, atrioventricular node; HB, His bundle; LBB, left bundle branch; RA, right atrium; RAFp, right atriofascicular proximal insertion; RBB, right bundle branch; RVFW, right ventricular free wall. *(Adapted from Jackman WM, et al. Ablation of right atriofascicular (Mahaim) accessory pathways. In: Zipes DE, ed. Catheter Ablation of Cardiac Arrhythmias. Armonk, NY: Futura; 1994:187-210. With permission.)*

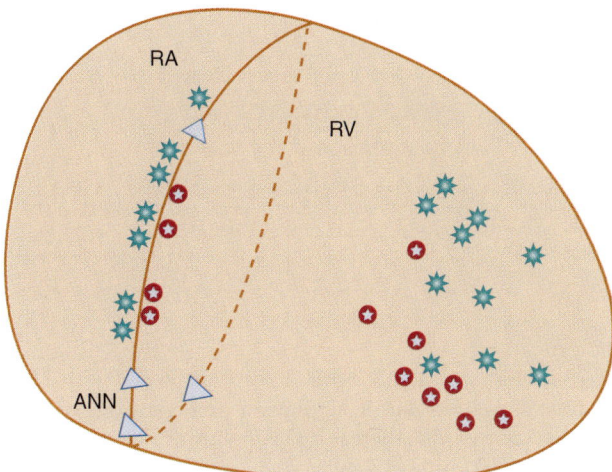

FIGURE 24-2. Pathway insertion sites (in 21 patients). In the right anterior oblique perspective, the tricuspid annulus is depicted by the *brown line* and the *dotted brown line* (septal aspect), the atriofascicular pathway insertions are represented by the *blue stars*, the long atrioventricular pathway insertions are represented by the *white stars on red background*, and the short atrioventricular pathway insertions are represented by the *triangles*. ANN, annulus; RA, right atrium; RV, right ventricle. *(From Haïssaguerre M, Warin JF, Le Metayer P, et al. Characteristics of the ventricular insertion sites of accessory pathways with anterograde decremental conduction properties. Circulation. 1995;91:1077-1085. With permission.)*

Pathophysiology

Atriofascicular accessory pathways are characterized by specific electrophysiologic properties that must be appreciated to understand the manifestations of these connections. During sinus rhythm, they demonstrate only minimal preexcitation. These accessory pathways conduct only in the antegrade direction and exhibit long baseline conduction time, decremental conduction, Wenckebach behavior,

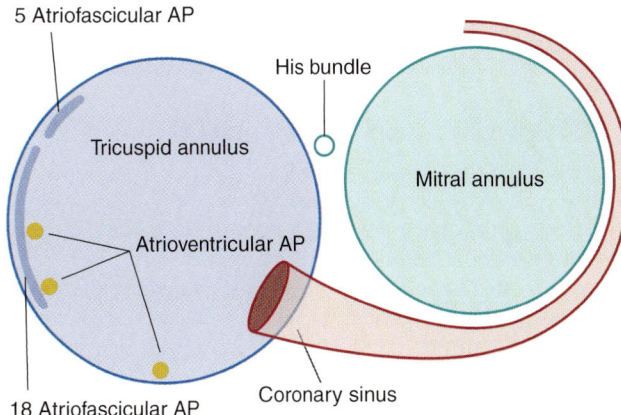

FIGURE 24-3. Schematic representation in vertical perspective of tricuspid annulus insertion sites in 26 patients. Twenty-three patients were found to have atriofascicular accessory pathways (AP), and three were found to have atrioventricular accessory pathways. *(From McClelland JH, Wang X, Beckman KJ, et al. Radiofrequency catheter ablation of right atriofascicular [Mahaim] accessory pathways guided by accessory pathway activation potentials. Circulation. 1994;89:2655-2666. With permission.)*

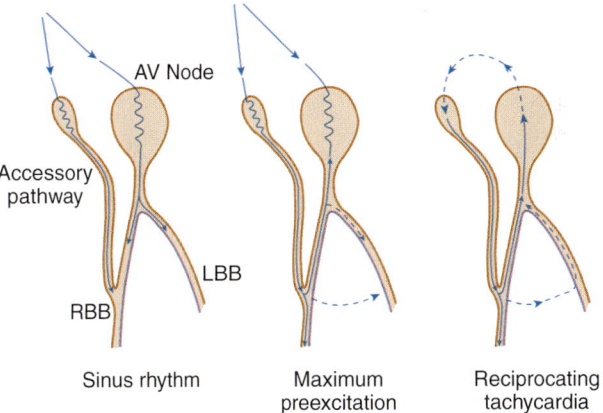

FIGURE 24-4. Mechanism of tachycardia. In sinus rhythm, the atrial signal may travel down the accessory pathway as well as the atrioventricular (AV) node. During maximal preexcitation, or antidromic reciprocating tachycardia, the signal travels antegrade down the accessory pathway. It then retrogradely activates the bundle of His and then the AVN. LBB, left bundle branch; RBB, right bundle branch. *(From Leitch JW, Klein GJ, Yee R. New concepts on nodoventricular accessory pathways. J Cardiovasc Electrophysiol. 1990;1:220-230. With permission.)*

and transient conduction block with adenosine.[10,22,23] With very rare exceptions, these pathways are right-sided. A summary of nine series of patients (99 total) demonstrated no patients with left-sided atriofascicular accessory pathways.[10-15,24-26] The anatomy of the atriofascicular connection has been described as a duplication of the AV nodal and fascicular conduction system. The proximal atrial insertion is the site of conduction delay in the pathway. As a parallel circuit with the AV nodal system, the pathway forms the basis for AV reentry. Because of the universal absence of retrograde conduction in these pathways, they directly participate in antidromic reciprocating tachycardia only. During tachycardia, conduction travels antegrade down the accessory pathway, to the RBB (typically), and retrograde back up to the His bundle, AV node, and then atrium (Fig. 24-4).[12] Atriofascicular pathways sometimes occur with other accessory pathways, which can serve as the retrograde limb in the reentrant circuit. AV node reentrant tachycardia may be present, with the atriofascicular accessory pathways serving a "bystander" role.[12,16,27,28]

Diagnosis and Differential Diagnosis

Patients with Mahaim-type accessory pathways can be young with or without cardiac structural abnormality. There have been reported associations with Ebstein anomaly of the tricuspid valve[29,30] as well as dual AV nodal pathways and coexistent accessory pathways.[22,31,32] Familial occurrence of Mahaim-type accessory pathways has been reported.[33] Among all accessory pathways, atriofascicular pathways are relatively uncommon, accounting for up to 2% to 3%.[11,22,32] The actual incidence may be greater owing to potential underreporting because the surface electrocardiogram during sinus rhythm may appear normal without evident preexcitation.

Electrocardiographic Characteristics

In sinus rhythm, there is typically little or no preexcitation (Table 24-1; Fig. 24-5). Minimal ventricular preexcitation may be suggested by the absence of septal Q waves in leads I, aVL, V_5, and V_6 or the presence of an rS QRS complex in lead III.[34-36] During preexcitation or antidromic tachycardia, the QRS axis is between 0 and –75 degrees, QRS width is 0.15 seconds or less, QRS transition occurs after V_4, and cycle length is between 220 and 450 milliseconds.[36] This QRS morphology is that of typical or atypical left bundle branch (LBB) block depending on the proximity of pathway insertion to the RBB.[36]

Electrophysiologic Findings

Atrial pacing with decreasing cycle lengths prolongs the PR interval (decremental conduction) and widens the QRS duration (preexcitation) (Fig. 24-6; Table 24-1). The His bundle–ventricular (HV) interval shortens, and the atrial–delta wave (A-delta) interval prolongs.[12] Progressively faster pacing can cause prolongation of the PR and QRS intervals up to a point of maximal preexcitation, beyond which AV block occurs. Often, preexcited tachycardia can be induced when a critical pacing interval is reached or when pacing is stopped abruptly.

Because these pathways are usually located along the tricuspid annulus, right atrial pacing commonly produces greater preexcitation than pacing from the coronary sinus.

Similar to rapid atrial pacing, delivery of early atrial extrastimuli can cause prolongation of the PR and QRS intervals. Even shorter coupling intervals will ultimately lead to a point of maximal preexcitation and then ultimately AV block. If conduction then goes exclusively antegrade down the accessory pathway, antidromic tachycardia can be initiated. This impulse travels down the accessory pathway, enters the distal RBB (or LBB in the setting of RBB block) either directly or after activation of intervening myocardium, activates the ventricle, then travels retrograde in the His system and AV node to the atrium to complete the circuit (Fig. 24-7). There is progressive prolongation of conduction to eventual block with injection of adenosine.

During preexcitation or antidromic tachycardia, the earliest ventricular activation is seen at the right ventricular

TABLE 24-1

DIAGNOSTIC CRITERIA FOR ATRIOFASCICULAR ACCESSORY PATHWAYS

Electrocardiography

LBBB morphology

QRS interval ≤150 msec (commonly)

Axis between 0 and –75 degrees

Late R > S wave transition at V_4 or V_5

Electrophysiologic Study

AP conduct only in antegrade direction

AP exhibits slow, decremental conduction proximal to AP potential with fixed AP-to-V interval

AP conduction block with adenosine

Prolongation of PR and AH intervals associated with shortening HV interval in response to atrial pacing/extrastimuli

Earliest ventricular activation during preexcitation at RV apex

In Tachycardia

Features of antidromic reciprocating tachycardia with ability to advance V and subsequent A activation with PAC during AV nodal refractoriness

Short VH interval (<50 msec)

Earliest ventricular activation and short postpacing interval in RV apex

RBB activation before His (in absence of RBBB)

Increased VA and VH with RBBB without change in preexcitation

VH in SVT < VH with RV pacing

HA in SVT = HA with RV pacing

A, atrium; AP, accessory pathway; HA, His bundle–to-atrial interval; LBBB, left bundle branch block; PAC, premature atrial extrastimulus; RBB(B), right bundle branch (block); RV, right ventricular; SVT, supraventricular tachycardia; V, ventricle; VA, ventricular-to-atrial interval; VH, ventricular-to–His bundle interval.

apical catheter, with activation at or before the QRS onset (Figs. 24-7 and 24-8). RBB activation precedes the His bundle activation during significant preexcitation. In antidromic tachycardia, there is typically short HV and ventriculoatrial (VA) intervals (retrograde atrial activation begins near the end of the QRS); however, these intervals may be prolonged in the setting of retrograde RBB block.

Introduction of an atrial extrastimulus, usually from the lateral right atrium, during tachycardia can prove both the presence of the atriofascicular pathway and its participation in the reentrant circuit. Atrial extrastimuli are delivered late to prevent the premature extrastimulus from conducting down the AV node.[6] The atrial extrasystole should be delivered late enough to first observe the retrograde atrial activation at the atrial septum or coronary sinus ostium before the paced atrial beat.[10] The presence of an atriofascicular pathway is suggested if this atrial extrasystole during AV nodal refractoriness preexcites the ventricle. If it advances the subsequent atrial signal that follows the QRS, then the participation of the pathway in the reentrant circuit is also demonstrated. Mere presence of the accessory pathway without involvement in the reentrant tachycardia may occur in cases of other pathways (e.g., AV node reentrant tachycardia), in which the accessory pathway acts as a bystander.

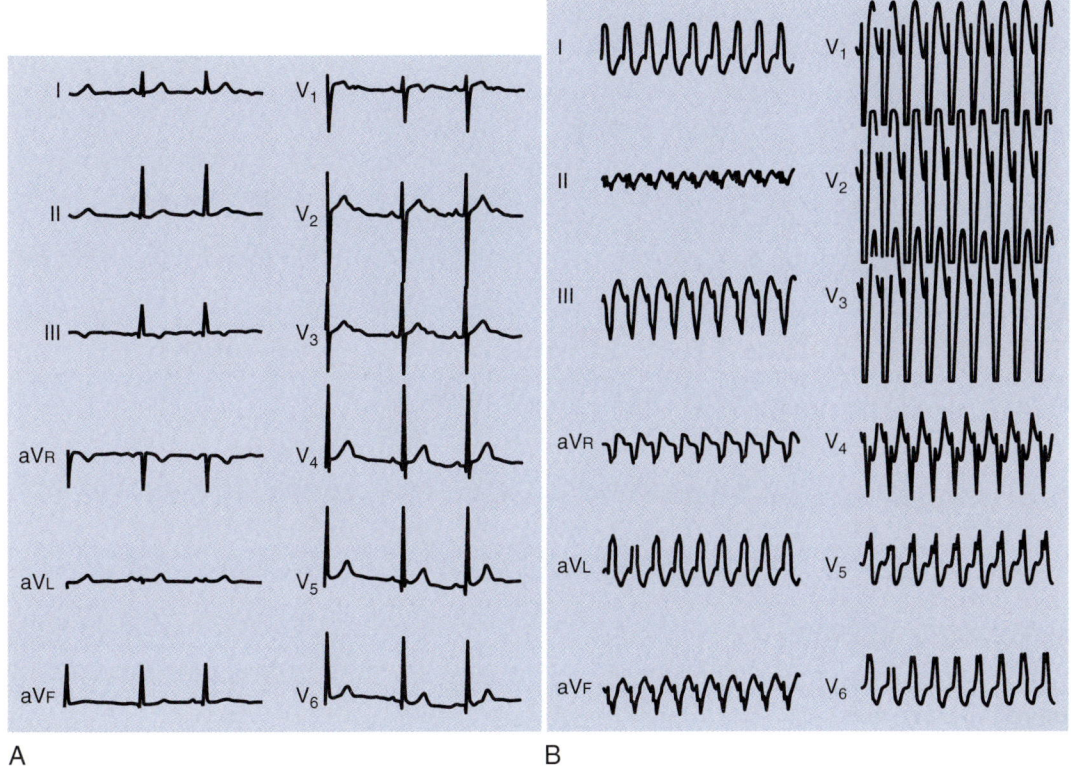

FIGURE 24-5. Surface electrocardiogram of a patient with Mahaim accessory pathway. **A,** Sinus rhythm. No preexcitation is observed. **B,** Reciprocating tachycardia, in which left bundle branch morphology is seen. *(From Okishige K, Goseki Y, Itoh A, et al. New electrophysiologic features and catheter ablation of atrioventricular and atriofascicular accessory pathways: evidence of decremental conduction and the anatomic structure of the Mahaim pathway. J Cardiovasc Electrophysiol. 1998;9:22-33. With permission.)*

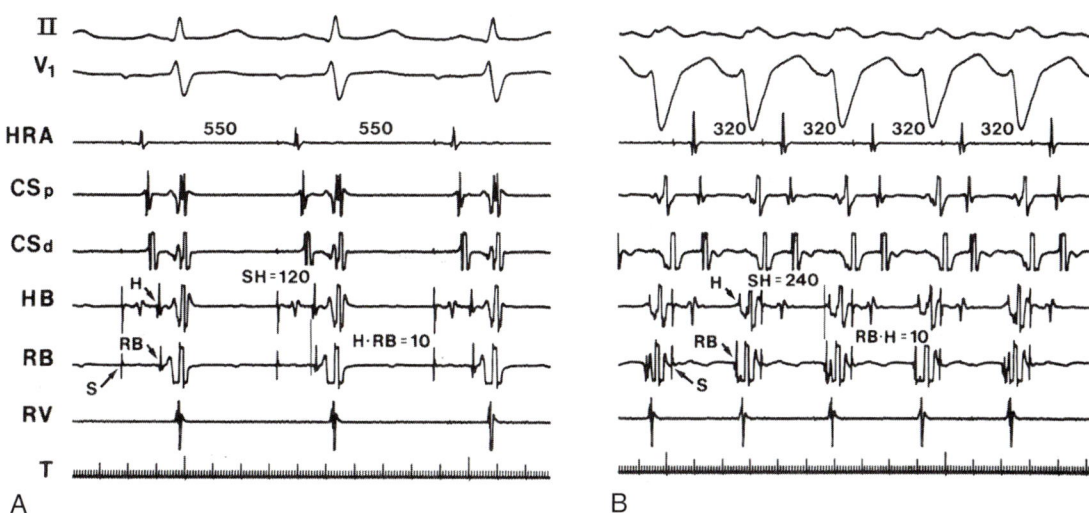

FIGURE 24-6. Atrial pacing. **A,** Atrial pacing at cycle length of 550 msec demonstrates no preexcitation in the QRS morphology, and antegrade conduction through the right bundle is suggested by the His–right bundle interval. **B,** when the atrial pacing cycle length is shortened to 320 msec, there is maximal preexcitation with widened QRS morphology, and the sequence of His and right bundle activations is reversed. Intracardiac leads are high right atrium (HRA), proximal and distal coronary sinus (CSp and CSd, respectively), His bundle (HB), right bundle branch (RB), and right ventricular apex (RV). Surface electrocardiogram leads are II and V1. *(From Tchou P, Lehmann MH, Jazayeri M, Akhtar M. Atriofascicular connection or a nodoventricular Mahaim fiber? Electrophysiologic elucidation of the pathway and associated reentrant circuit. Circulation. 1988;77:837-848. With permission.)*

Intracardiac Recordings

The criteria to diagnose an atriofascicular pathway by intracardiac recordings are given in Table 24-1. There should be evidence of an antegrade-only, slow, decrementally conducting AP with atrial insertion along the tricuspid annulus (usually) and ventricular insertion in the distal right bundle. For AV pathways, the insertion is usually the right ventricular free wall near the annulus. The atriofascicular pathway demonstrates decremental conduction between the atrial insertion and the AP potential as well as a fixed AP-to-ventricular interval.

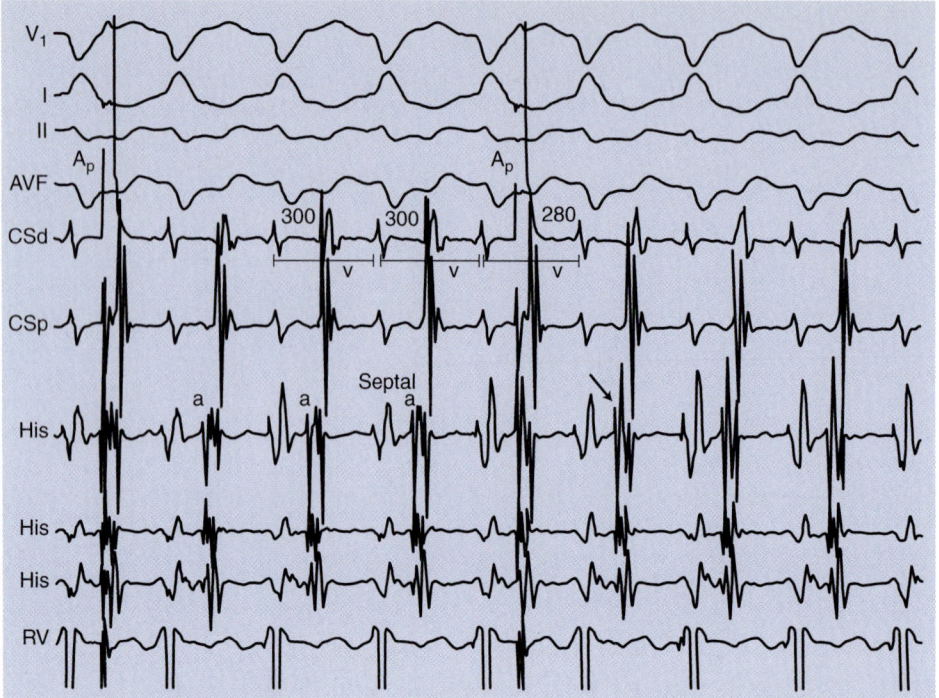

FIGURE 24-7. Introduction of atrial extrastimulus during tachycardia, timed after deflection of septal atrial electrogram. Advancement of the following QRS complex (with identical preexcited morphology) *and* retrograde atrial activation *(arrow)* are displayed. Such findings demonstrate the participation of the Mahaim accessory pathway in the tachycardia circuit rather than atrioventricular nodal reentry. Surface electrocardiogram leads include V₁, I, II, and aVF. Intracardiac recordings are from the coronary sinus distal and proximal (CSd and CSp), His bundle, and right ventricular apex (RV). Septal atrial electrogram is marked with "a," and ventricular electrogram is noted with "v." *(From Grogin HR, Lee RJ, Kwasman M, et al. Radiofrequency catheter ablation of atriofascicular and nodoventricular Mahaim tracts.* Circulation. *1994;90:272–281. With permission.)*

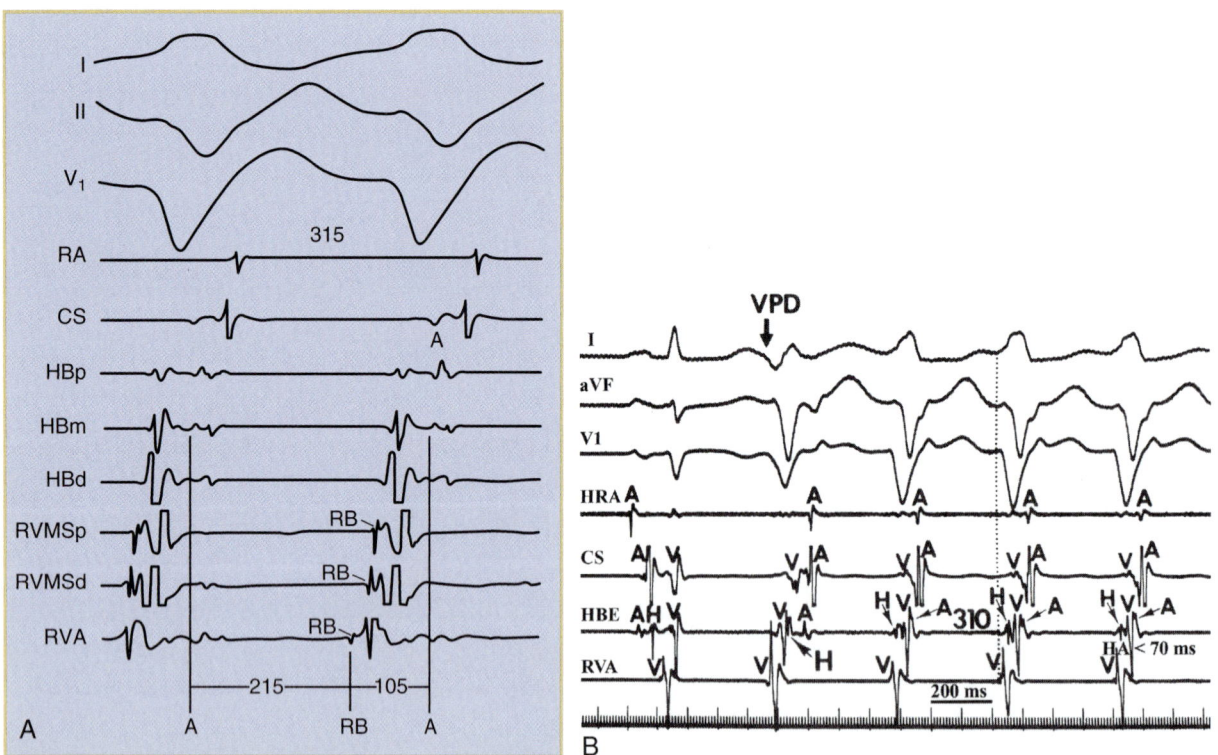

FIGURE 24-8. A, Intracardiac electrogram of patient in reciprocating tachycardia, demonstrating typical features: left bundle branch morphology, ventricular activation preceded by retrograde activation of right bundle branch (RB), early retrograde activation of the His bundle causing short ventriculoatrial interval, and long accessory pathway conduction time causing long atrioventricular interval. CS, coronary sinus; d, distal; HB, His bundle; m, middle; p, proximal; RA, right atrium; RVA, right ventricular apex; RVMSd, right ventricular midseptum distal; RMVSp, right ventricular midseptum proximal. **B,** Bystander Mahaim conduction during atrioventricular (AV) nodal reentry. After one beat of sinus rhythm, a premature ventricular contraction (VPD) is delivered *(arrow)*, inducing AV nodal reentry. The cycle length is 310 msec. The *dotted line* demarcates the QRS onset. The preexcited tachycardia shows a His bundle–atrial (HA) interval after the VPD, which represents the HA interval that would be expected in antidromic tachycardia. The short HA interval in tachycardia is consistent with AV nodal reentry and bystander Mahaim preexcitation. A, atrial electrogram; CS, coronary sinus; HRA, high right atrium; RVA, right ventricular apex; V, ventricular electrogram. *(A, From McClelland JH, Wang X, Beckman KJ, et al. Radiofrequency catheter ablation of right atriofascicular [Mahaim] accessory pathways guided by accessory pathway activation potentials.* Circulation. *1994;89:2655–2666; B, from Josephson ME. Clinical cardiac electrophysiology. In: Techniques and Interpretations, 3/e. Philadelphia: Lippincott Williams & Wilkins, 2002:322–424. Writh permission)*

During antidromic reciprocating tachycardia, an atriofascicular connection should demonstrate the following: (1) short ventricular-to–His bundle (VH) interval (in absence of RBB block); (2) earliest ventricular activation near the right ventricular apex, with short postpacing intervals from this location; (3) retrograde activation of the RBB before His bundle activation (in absence RBB block); (4) increased VA interval and tachycardia cycle length with RBB block; (5) VH interval in tachycardia shorter than the VH interval with right ventricular pacing; (6) a His bundle–to-atrial (HA) interval in tachycardia equal to the HA interval with right ventricular pacing; and (7) ability to advance ventricular and subsequent atrial activation by a premature atrial stimulus delivered during AV nodal refractoriness.[32] The effects of RBB block in tachycardia are to prolong the VA and VH intervals in tachycardia and also to produce antegrade right bundle activation after His depolarization. This latter finding results from transmyocardial conduction to the left ventricle, LBB, His bundle, and then the right bundle. RBB block produces no change in the pattern of preexcitation.

The AV connection should meet criteria for antidromic reciprocating tachycardia, but, compared with the atriofascicular connections, it demonstrates earliest ventricular activation near the tricuspid annulus, wider preexcited QRS complexes, and longer VH intervals (37 ± 9 milliseconds for AV versus 16 ± 5 milliseconds for atriofascicular) (Fig. 24-9).[37]

Differential Diagnosis

The differential diagnosis of atriofascicular connections includes ventricular tachycardia, LBB block aberrancy, bystander participation, and nodoventricular or nodofascicular connections (Table 24-2). Ventricular tachycardia

should be excluded by the demonstration of obligatory 1:1 atrial and ventricular activation for perpetuation of the tachycardia and by the ability to reset the ventricle and subsequent atrial activation by a premature atrial stimulus delivered during AV nodal refractoriness. Bundle branch reentry with LBB block morphology has an HV interval greater than the HV interval in sinus rhythm and His activation before RBB activation. Supraventricular tachycardia with LBB block aberrancy is proved by recording a normal or prolonged HV interval with antegrade His activation during tachycardia. Bystander participation can be demonstrated by dissociating conduction over the AP from continuation of the tachycardia. AV nodal reentry is not an uncommon finding associated with atriofascicular pathways. AVNRT with bystander pathway activation is suggested by continuation of tachycardia at the same cycle length with block in AP, HA interval in tachycardia shorter than during RV pacing, HA interval in tachycardia of less than 70 msec, His activation before or on time with right bundle activation in absence of RBB block, fusion of the QRS complex, and a VH interval in tachycardia shorter than with right ventricular pacing, which in turn is shorter than the HV interval.[37,38] QRS fusion during tachycardia should not occur during antidromic tachycardia but may be seen during bystander participation.

The exclusion of nodoventricular and nodofascicular connections is also necessary. These rare connections arise from the AV node to insert into the right ventricular myocardium and distal RBB, respectively (see later). These connections may manifest with narrow- or wide-complex tachycardia and AV dissociation. Narrow-complex tachycardia results from retrograde conduction in the AP to the AV node, with the His-Purkinje system forming the antegrade limb. During antidromic tachycardia, the VH interval

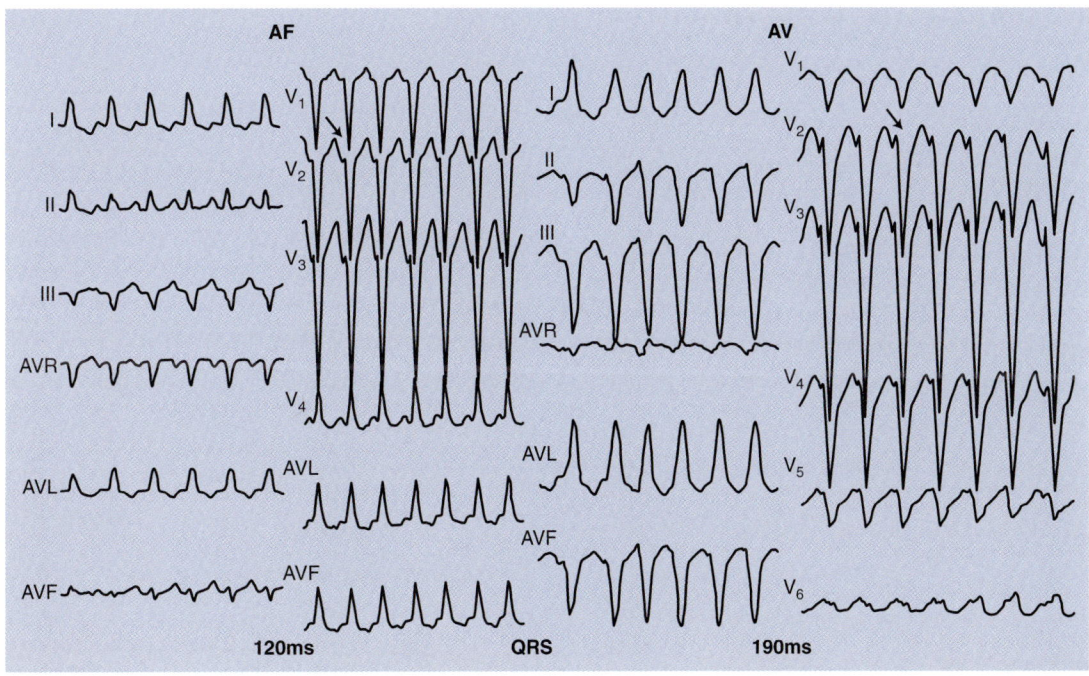

FIGURE 24-9. Surface electrocardiograms of patients with atriofascicular (AF) accessory pathway (*left*) and atrioventricular (AV) accessory pathway (*right*). The QRS duration is longer, and the initial R wave in the anterior leads (*arrow*) is broader in the electrocardiogram of the atrioventricular accessory pathway. (*From Haïssaguerre M, Warin JF, Le Metayer P, et al. Characteristics of the ventricular insertion sites of accessory pathways with anterograde decremental conduction properties. Circulation. 1995;91:1077-1085.*)

TABLE 24-2

DIFFERENTIAL ELECTROPHYSIOLOGIC FINDINGS FOR LEFT BUNDLE BRANCH BLOCK TACHYCARDIAS

Connection/ Arrhythmia	Proximal Insertion	Distal Insertion	HV with Decremental Atrial Pacing	VH in Tachycardia	Effect of RAFW PAC in Tachycardia	AV Dissociation in Tachycardia	HA in Tachycardia*	QRS Fusion from Atrial Activation during Tachycardia†	Sequence of His and RBB in Tachycardia*
Atriofascicular	RA free wall	Distal RBB	Decreases, then fixed	Short† and <VH with RV pacing	V and subsequent A advance when septal A refractory	Not possible	= HA with RV pacing	Not possible	RBB before His
Decremental atrioventricular	RA free wall	RV near TVA or mid RV	Decreases, then fixed	Intermediate§ and >VH with RV pacing	A and subsequent V advanced when septal A refractory	Not possible	= HA with RV pacing	Not possible	RBB before His
Typical atrioventricular (antidromic tach)	RA near TVA	RV near TVA	Decreases	Intermediate§ and >VH with RV pacing	V and subsequent A advanced if near atrial insertion	Not possible	= HA with RV pacing	Not possible	Usually RBB before His
Nodoventricular	AV node	Ventricular myocardium	Decreases, then fixed	>VH with RV pacing	V advanced if septal A advanced	Possible	= HA with RV pacing	Not possible	RBB before His
Nodofascicular	AV node	Distal RBB	Decreases, then fixed	Short† and <VH with RV pacing	V advanced if septal A advanced	Possible	= HA with RV pacing	Not possible	RBB before His
RV fascicular VT	RV fascicular system	RV fascicular system	Normal	Short	V advanced only if His/RBB advanced	Possible	= HA with RV pacing	Possible	RBB before His
Fasciculoventricular	His or RBB	RV myocardium	Short and fixed	Bystander only	Bystander only	Bystander only	Bystander only	Bystander only	His before RBB
Intra-myocardial VT	RV or V septum	RV or V septum	Normal or prolonged	Usually intermediate§ or long	V advanced only if septal A and His advanced	Common	= HA with RV pacing	Possible	Typically RBB before His
BBR	Usually RBB antegrade	Myocardium and LBB retrograde	Usually fixed and prolonged	HV in tach ≥HV in sinus rhythm	V advanced only if septal A and His advanced	Common	= HA with RV pacing	Not possible	Typically His before RBB with H-RBB interval ≤H-RBB interval in sinus rhythm
AVNRT with bystander atriofascicular	RA free wall	Distal RBB	Decreases then fixed	<70 msec and/ or <VH with RV pacing	Usually no effect	Possible	<HA with RV pacing	Possible	His before or on time with RBB
SVT LBBB aberrancy	Variable depending on mechanism	Variable depending on mechanism	Fixed or prolonged	HV fixed	Variable depending on mechanism	Depends on mechanism	Depends on mechanism	Not possible	His before RBB

* Assumes no RBBB.
† Assumes absence of second accessory pathway.
‡ VH < 50 msec.
§ VH = 50-80 msec.

A, atrium; AV, atrioventricular; AVNRT, atrioventricular nodal reentrant tachycardia; BBR, bundle branch reentry; HA, His-to-atrial tachycardia; His, His bundle; HV, His-to-ventricular interval; His, His-to-atrial interval; LBB(B), left bundle branch (block); PAC, premature atrial contraction; RBB(B), right bundle branch (block); RA, right atrium; RAFW, right atrial free wall; RV, right ventricle; SVT, supraventricular tachycardia; tach, tachycardia; TVA, tricuspid valve annulus; V, ventricle; VH, ventricle-to-His interval; VT, ventricular tachycardia.

may be short (<50 milliseconds for nodofascicular) or intermediate (50 to 80 milliseconds for nodoventricular) in the absence of RBB block.[37] These tachycardias should not be advanced by premature atrial stimulation during AV nodal refractoriness (above the level of the AP insertion) and are advanced only if the septal atrial activation is advanced.

Mapping

Techniques for mapping and ablating these pathways have been derived from their unique properties. Because these accessory pathways conduct only in an anterograde direction without much preexcitation in sinus rhythm, mapping is usually performed during antidromic AV tachycardia, atrial pacing, or atrial extrastimuli.

1. *Identification of the site of discrete Mahaim potential at the tricuspid annulus.* This technique is the most commonly used.[10,13,15,28,38,39] By scanning the tricuspid annulus at the right atrial free wall with the catheter tip, one looks for the localization of the presence of accessory pathway or Kent potentials.[10,12,14] Distinct atrial, accessory pathway, and ventricular potentials can be found at the atrial insertion site. The Mahaim potential represents the atrial insertion site (Fig. 24-10) and provides the best site for ablation of these accessory pathways.[39–41]

2. *Atrial pace-mapping at the tricuspid annulus.* Localizing the point that produces the shortest stimulus-to-preexcitation

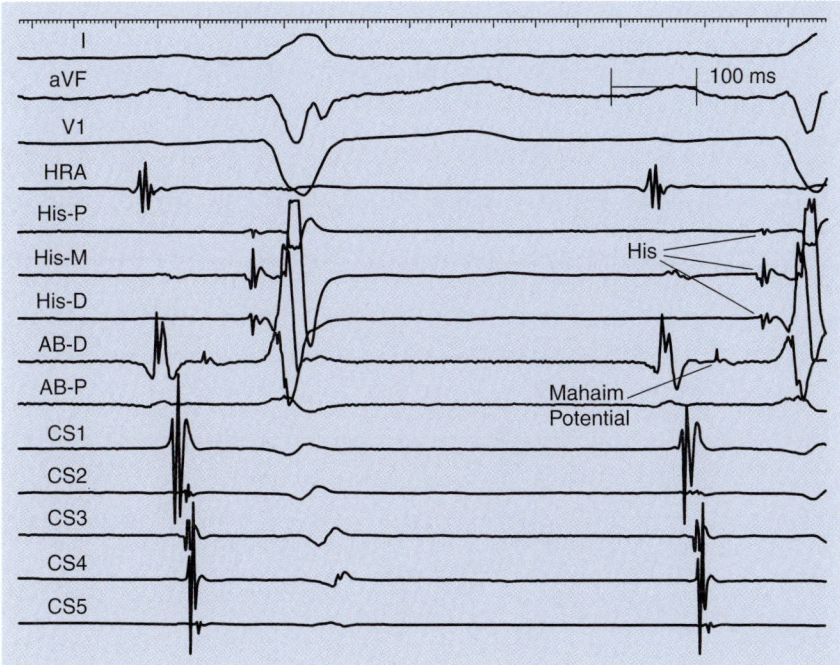

A

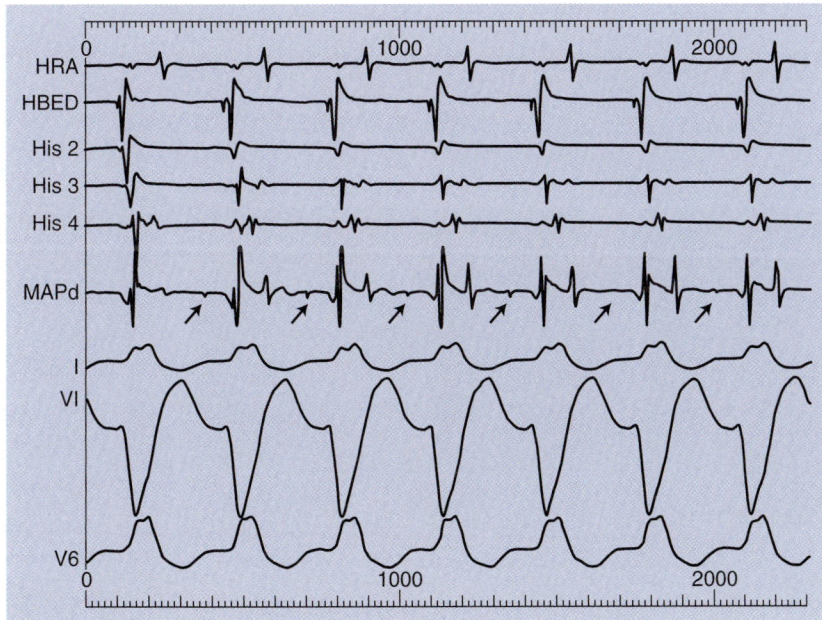

Speed: 100 mm/s

B

FIGURE 24-10. Mahaim potential. **A,** Sinus rhythm. The distal His catheter demonstrates His large potentials, and the posterior tricuspid annulus recording (AB-D) has a discrete Mahaim potential, which occurs slightly earlier than the His bundle potential. **B,** Tachycardia with Mahaim potentials (arrows). Note that both the Mahaim potentials and the His bundle activation precede the surface QRS deflection. The Mahaim potential and the His bundle potential on the HBED electrode precede ventricular activation. Note that in tachycardia, but not in sinus rhythm, the ventricular activation and onset of QRS precede retrograde His bundle activation. Surface electrocardiogram leads are I, aVL, V_1, and V_6. Intracardiac signals are from the high right atrium (HRA), distal His bundle (HBED), middle His bundle (His 2 and 3), proximal His bundle (His 4), and right ventricular apex (MAPd). *(From Heald SC, Davies DW, Ward DE, et al. Radiofrequency catheter ablation of Mahaim tachycardia by targeting Mahaim potentials at the tricuspid annulus. Br Heart J. 1995;73:250-257. With permission.)*

(delta wave) interval with atrial pacing can be used in an effort to identify the atrial insertion site. The major limitations of this method are the technical difficulty of positioning the catheter and distinguishing sites of similar S-delta intervals.[14]

3. *Introducing an atrial extrastimulus.* Similar to atrial pace-mapping, localization of the spot from which a late premature atrial extrastimulus delivered during preexcited tachycardia results in the greatest advancement of the next QRS can be used to locate the atrial insertion site. This technique involves introducing a late premature atrial extrastimulus at different spots to identify the one that provides the greatest advancement of the next QRS complex with fixed coupling interval or the site from which the longest coupled atrial extrastimulus during tachycardia causes resetting of the cycle (Fig. 24-11).[15] This method has also been found to be technically difficult and time-consuming[11,15,42]

4. *Activation mapping of the ventricle.* The ventricular insertion site, especially when at the level of the tricuspid annulus, can be localized with this method.[13,41,42] For more distally inserting accessory pathways, mapping for the earliest ventricular activation is difficult. These pathways tend to arborize widely into the ventricular tissue, causing difficulty to completely ablate the ventricular insertion.[13] Often, this results in a change in the preexcitation electrogram rather than abolition. Nonetheless, there are few reports of successful ablation at the ventricular insertion of the accessory pathways.[41,43]

5. *Mechanical disruption of conduction.* These accessory pathways have particular sensitivity to mechanical trauma compared with other accessory pathways.[11,14,24] Cappato and colleagues have demonstrated that merely applying pressure to the accessory pathway with the catheter tip easily induces conduction block (Figs. 24-12 and 24-13).[11] This phenomenon can be

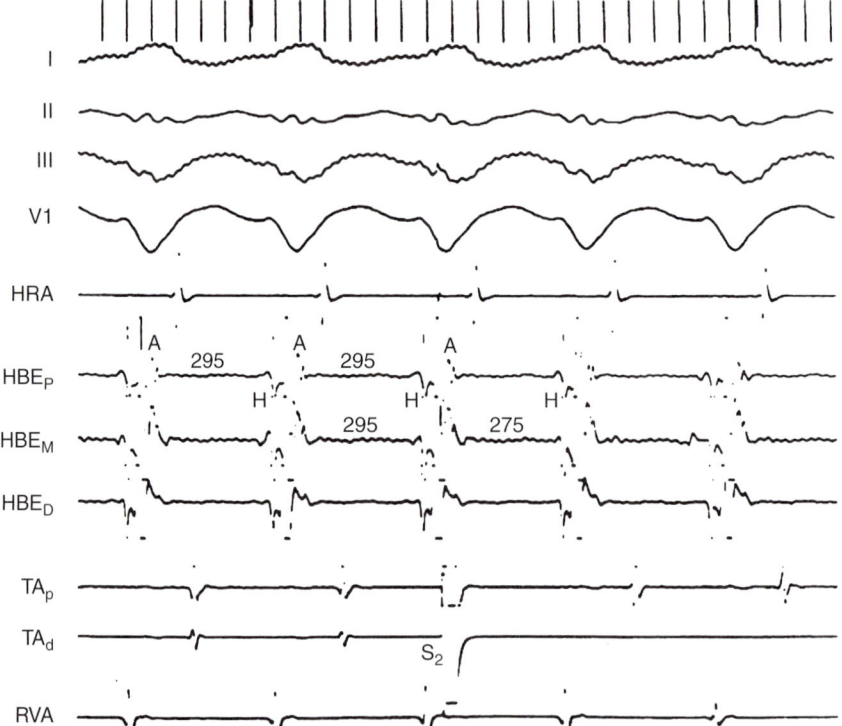

FIGURE 24-11. Locating atrial insertion site using atrial extrastimulus. After an atrial extrastimulus (S₂) is delivered in a right lateral location during tachycardia, there is atrial–His bundle (AH) interval shortening in the recording from the proximal His bundle electrogram (HBE$_P$) as the His signal is advanced 20 msec while the preceding atrial electrogram is not. This finding implies that the proximal insertion of the accessory pathway is located in a different area than the atrial insertion of the atrioventricular node. This stimulus location also identified the site at which the latest atrial extrastimulus advanced the His deflection but not the atrial signal in the His bundle recording, implicating that catheter location as the atrial insertion of the accessory pathway. Surface electrocardiogram leads are I, II, III, and V₁. Intracardiac recordings are from the high right atrium (HRA), proximal His bundle (HBE$_P$), middle His bundle (HBE$_M$), distal His bundle (HBE$_D$), and proximal and distal tricuspid annulus (TA$_P$ and TA$_d$, respectively). *(Adapted from Klein LS, Hackett K, Zipes DP, et al. Radiofrequency catheter ablation of Mahaim fibers at the tricuspid annulus. Circulation. 1993;87:738-747. With permission.)*

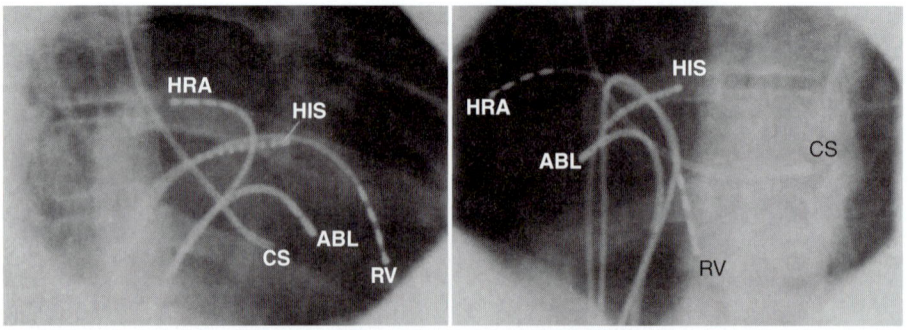

FIGURE 24-12. Catheter placement. The ablation catheter (ABL) is placed with the tip at the atrial insertion of the accessory pathway, positioned in the posterolateral region of the tricuspid annulus. Mapping catheters include quadripolar catheters in the high right atrium (HRA) and in the right ventricular apex (RV), a decapolar catheter at the bundle of His (HIS), and a 12-polar catheter in the coronary sinus (CS). The *top panel* displays 30 degrees in right anterior oblique view, and the *bottom panel* displays 30 degrees in left anterior oblique view. *(From Cappato R, Schluter M, Weib C, et al. Catheter-induced mechanical conduction block of right-sided accessory fibers with Mahaim-type preexcitation to guide radiofrequency ablation. Circulation. 1994;90:282-290. With permission.)*

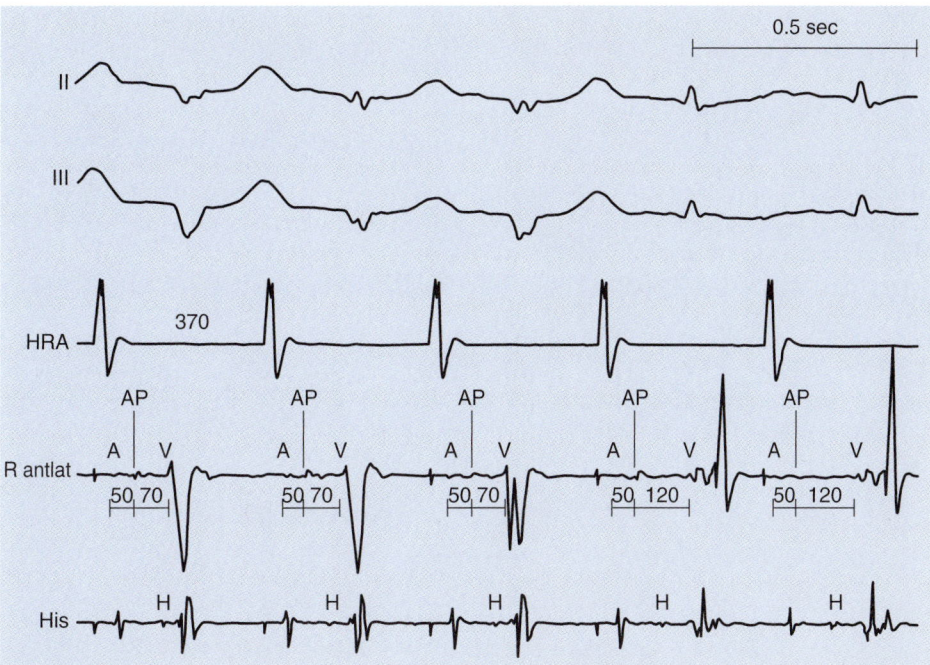

FIGURE 24-13. Mechanical disruption. During pacing at the high right atrium, preexcitation is lost (last two beats) after manipulation of the mapping catheter in the anterolateral tricuspid annulus, demonstrating mechanically-induced block in the accessory pathway. In addition, the mapping catheter continues to record accessory pathway potential (AP), localizing site of antegrade conduction block at the subannular level of the atrial input. While the A-AP interval stays constant, the AP-V interval lengthens 50 msec after the onset of mechanical disruption of the accessory pathway conduction. Surface electrocardiogram leads are II and III. Intracardiac recordings are from high right atrium (HRA), mapping catheter in right anterolateral tricuspid annulus (R antlat), and bundle of His. *(From Cappato R, Schluter M, Weib C, et al. Catheter-induced mechanical conduction block of right-sided accessory fibers with Mahaim-type preexcitation to guide radiofrequency ablation. Circulation. 1994;90:282-290. With permission.)*

used to help identify the location of the accessory pathway. The catheter tip is positioned along the tricuspid annulus and has gentle pressure exerted and brought along the tricuspid annular groove. After induction of mechanical block (sudden loss of preexcitation or prolongation of the AV interval, suggesting location of tricuspid annular crossing), one waits for the return of the preexcitation (can be sometimes up to hours) and chooses that spot for ablation.[11,44] There are several criticisms to this technique. Namely, there is a significant amount of waiting time for the return of the preexcitation after block was induced, and if the catheter has moved after block, the spot cannot be found again until the conduction recurs. Electroanatomic mapping may help with this problem.

Ablation

Although practice variations exist, typically a femoral vein approach is used with a 7-French, 4-mm electrode, deflectable-tip catheter for mapping and ablation. Long, curved-tip sheaths may provide greater catheter stability and may help position the catheter tip at different places along the tricuspid annulus. For mapping the ventricle, the catheter can cross the tricuspid annulus and be situated below the tricuspid valve. Mapping is then performed in the left anterior oblique view, with the tricuspid annulus in the center. Mapping techniques discussed earlier are then performed (during tachycardia or with pacing).

TABLE 24-3
TARGET SITES FOR ATRIOFASCICULAR PATHWAY ABLATION
Atrial Aspect of Tricuspid Annulus
Site of Mahaim potential
Site of shortest stimulus-to-preexcitation (delta wave)
Site of greatest advancement of subsequent QRS complex after introduction of late premature atrial extrastimulus
Ventricular Insertion Site
Site identified by activation mapping

Most commonly, ablation is performed at the atrial insertion using mapping of discrete Mahaim pathways (Tables 24-3 and 24-4). Loss of preexcitation during ablation is usually observed (Fig. 24-14).

Usually, these accessory pathways are right-sided, traveling along the free wall tricuspid annulus to the ventricular myocardium or more commonly to the RBB fascicle (there have been isolated reports of decrementally conducting left-sided accessory pathways). Although most successful ablations are in the lateral or anterolateral tricuspid annulus (80% reported), there have been rare cases of right atrial posterior or posteroseptal atrial insertions.[19]

Although there may be practice variations, the target temperature for ablation is usually 60° to 70°C, delivered for 10 to 15 seconds while evaluating for termination of

TABLE 24-4

STUDIES OF MAPPING AND ABLATION FOR ATRIOFASCICULAR ACCESSORY PATHWAYS

Study	No. of Patients	Mapping Method	Mapping Outcome	Ablation Method	Ablation Outcome	Follow-Up	Complications
Tchou et al, 1988[6]	1	Atrial and ventricular pacing, delivery of AES	Late AES during tachycardia preexcited ventricle while unable to conduct through AVN, thus demonstrating right atrial component of AP independent of AVN				
Haïssaguerre et al, 1990[42]	3	V pace-mapping for ventricular insertion		DC energy to ventricular insertion	100% success	12, 14, and 16 mo: no recurrence	Subclavian vein thrombosis (2 pts) pulmonary embolism (1 pt)
Klein et al, 1993[15]	4	Atrial extrastimuli during SVT Stimulus-to-delta wave	Atriofascicular (3 pts), atrioventricular (1 pt)	RFE to posterior and lateral TA	100% success	8 mo: no recurrent tachycardia	None
Grogin et al, 1994[12]	6	Discrete MP	Atriofascicular AP (4 pts), nodoventricular AP (2 pts)	AFP: RFE to atrial side of TA (2 pts), to ventricular side of TA (1 pt), to distal ventricular insertion (1 pt) Nodoventricular pathways: RFE to mid-septal region	100% success	Not reported	Not reported
Cappato et al, 1994[11]	11	Mechanical block at subannular TA in 8 pts (2 pts in atrial fibrillation)	Successful ablation in all 8 pts at subannular TA; failures: 1 pt who had ablation at ventricular insertion, 1 pt who had ablation at supra-annular TA; in 1 pt, mechanical block was not achieved but ablated at subannular TA in SVT	RFE applied to site identified by mechanical block during atrial pacing (6 pts) or in atrial fibrillation (2 pts)	In 5/6 pts who had ablation in A pacing, recurrence of preexcitation in 12 hr; additional ablation the next day, overall conduction eliminated in 9 of 11 pts (82%)	9.5 ± 2.3 mo, preexcitation recurred in 1 pt	Not reported
McClelland et al, 1994[10]	23	Discrete MP	22 pts had single, discrete high-frequency AP potential at TA	RFE applied to site recording AP potential (TA in 19 pts and RV free wall in 3 pts)	100% success (22 pts)	18 ± 13 mo: no tachycardia recurrence (all) EPS at 3.8 ± 1.7 mo (9 pts) had no AP conduction	Small thrombus in superior vena cava (catheter-induced trauma)
Li et al, 1994[25]	4	Discrete MP			100% success		
Heald et al, 1995[24]	21	Discrete MP		RFE to site identified by MP at ventricular aspect of TA; or if no MP, then site found by stimulus-to–delta wave mapping	18 (90%)	9 mo: 1 recurrence (5%)	None

Study	N	Mapping criteria	Details	Ablation	Success	Follow-up	Complications
Haissaguerre et al, 1995[13]	21	Discrete MP	17 patients w/long APs (10 with AFP, 7 with AVP) and 4 with short AVP	RFE to distal or to TA sites in long AP and RFE to TA in short AP patients	100% success	12 mo: no recurrence	Not reported
Brugada et al, 1995[39]	4	Discrete MP		RFE to TA	100% success	5 mo: no recurrence	None
Okishige et al, 1998[14]	7	Proximal site: discrete MP along TA Distal site: earliest bipolar ventricular activation relative to preexcitation signal	7 pts with AFP or AVP, 6 pts with discrete MP observed	RFE to atrial or ventricular aspect of TA, localized to MP site or to site detected by S-delta mapping.	100% success	19 mo: no recurrence of AP conduction	None
Bohora et al, 2008[37]	15	(1) M potential with constant M potential–to–ventricular electrogram interval during atrial pacing; (2) stimulus–to–delta wave; (3) mechanical trauma	Right lateral tricuspid annulus (13 pts), 6:30 position (1 pt); 5-o'clock position (1 pt)	RFE	14 pts RF ablation: 13 pts had loss of AP conduction and 1 pt had partial loss Ablation not performed in 1 pt owing to proximity to AV node	1 pt had tachycardia recurrence	None

AES, atrial extrastimulus; AFP, atriofascicular pathway; AP, accessory pathway; AV, atrioventricular; AVN, atrioventricular node; AVP, atrioventricular pathway; MP, Mahaim potential; pt, patient; RF, radiofrequency; RFE, radiofrequency energy; SVT, supraventricular tachycardia; TA, tricuspid annulus;

accessory pathway conduction or tachycardia. If either occurs, radiofrequency ablation is continued for a total of 30 to 60 seconds, and the patient is monitored thereafter for recurrence. If the tachycardia or AP conduction does not terminate, alternate ablation sites are selected.[45]

During radiofrequency ablation of Mahaim-type accessory pathways, an irregular rhythm often occurs, reflecting automaticity of the accessory pathway due to heating.[46] Failed ablation lesions, in contrast, do not result in accelerated tachycardias from the accessory pathway.[47]

Catheter ablation of these pathways appears to be safe and highly successful with little recurrence. Success rates of ablation of tricuspid annulus discrete potentials has been quite high.[11,44] Overall ablation success rates are about 90% to 95% with about a 5% recurrence rate.[10-15,24,25,45,48]

Troubleshooting the Difficult Case

Although the mapping techniques generally offer a high probability of successful localization, and ablation is generally quite successful, there are specific difficulties that may arise (Table 24-5).

In some cases, it may be difficult to record a Mahaim potential. Because ventricular activation at the tricuspid annulus is not usually the earliest, it is generally difficult to map ventricular activation at that location. Alternative methods such as identifying the shortest S-delta or bump mapping may be necessary.

Catheter movement, particularly during a change in rhythm during ablation, may interfere with successful

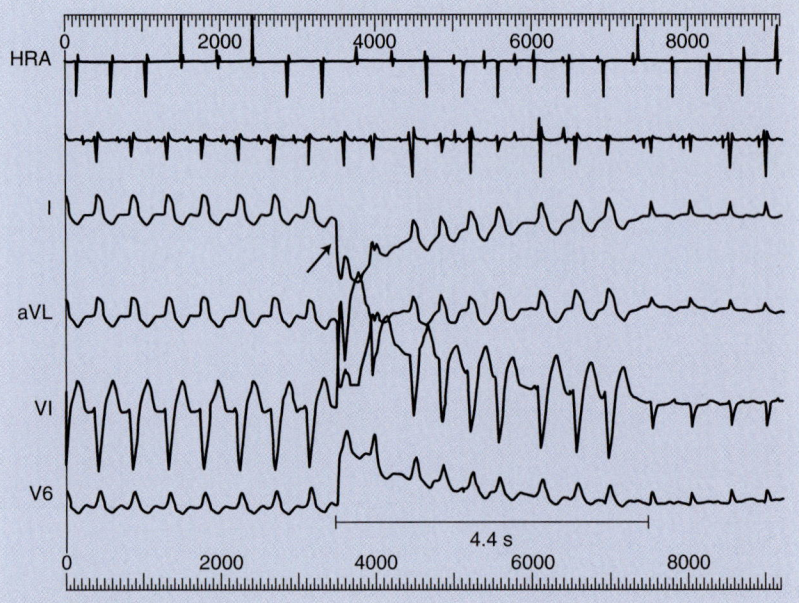

Speed: 25 mm/s

A

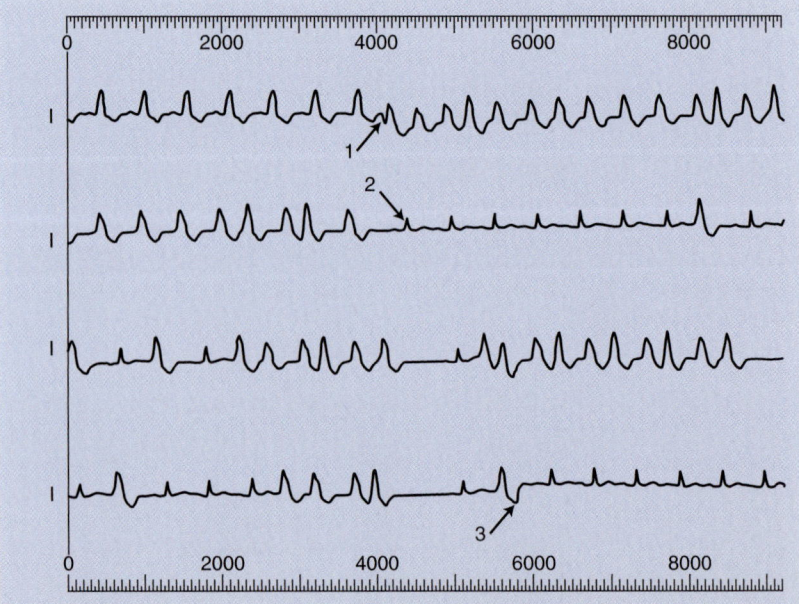

Speed: 25 mm/s

B

FIGURE 24-14. Radiofrequency energy ablation. **A,** Intracardiac recordings from the high right atrium and distal His bundle as well as surface recordings from leads I, aVL, V₁, and V₆. After 4.4 seconds of energy delivery, there is block of Mahaim pathway conduction and resultant normalization of surface QRS complex. **B,** A continuous recording from surface electrocardiogram lead I. Typical pattern of stuttering block is demonstrated during energy application. The onset of radiofrequency energy (1) is followed by initial block in Mahaim during energy application after 9.5 seconds (2). Ectopic activity from the Mahaim pathway was observed until the end of the first 30 seconds of energy application (3). *(From Heald SC, Davies DW, Ward DE, et al. Radiofrequency catheter ablation of Mahaim tachycardia by targeting Mahaim potentials at the tricuspid annulus. Br Heart J. 1995;73:250-257. With permission.)*

ablation. Catheter stability can be increased with use of long, curved-tip sheaths.

Finally, these pathways are very sensitive to mechanical trauma.[11,44] If a catheter bumps into it, there may be pause of accessory pathway activity, which can be from minutes to hours. Thus, the ability to relocate the accessory pathway is confounded by the time it takes to recover. Three-dimensional mapping[49,50] and noncontact mapping[51] may be used to mark the position of the catheter when accessory pathway conduction is lost after bumping and to anatomically guide ablation of the accessory pathway.

Other Accessory Pathway Variants

A list of accessory pathway variants is given in Table 24-6 and illustrated in Figure 24-15. If atriofascicular pathways are considered uncommon, other pathway variants are very rare. These pathways must be recognized, however, to treat the rare patient with these structures and to avoid unnecessary treatment for purely bystander pathways (fasciculoventricular).

TABLE 24-5

TROUBLESHOOTING THE DIFFICULT CASE

Problem	Causes	Solution
Inability to identify insertion site at TA for ablation	Absence of retrograde conduction precludes localizing spot of earliest retrograde atrial activation. Pathways with ventricular insertion distal to TA cannot be localized by evaluating for earliest ventricular activation at the TA.	Map during antidromic AVRT or atrial pacing Map for the area that provides shortest atrioventricular interval
Poor catheter stability	Sudden change in rhythm and heart rate Poor catheter contact	Use long sheath Use electroanatomic mapping to relocalize catheter tip to previous location
Transient conduction block during mapping or ablation	High sensitivity to mechanical trauma, such as bumping catheter into accessory pathway	Use electroanatomic mapping Wait until reappearance of AP activity (may take minutes to hours)

AP, accessory pathway; AVRT, atrioventricular tachycardia; TA, tricuspid annulus.

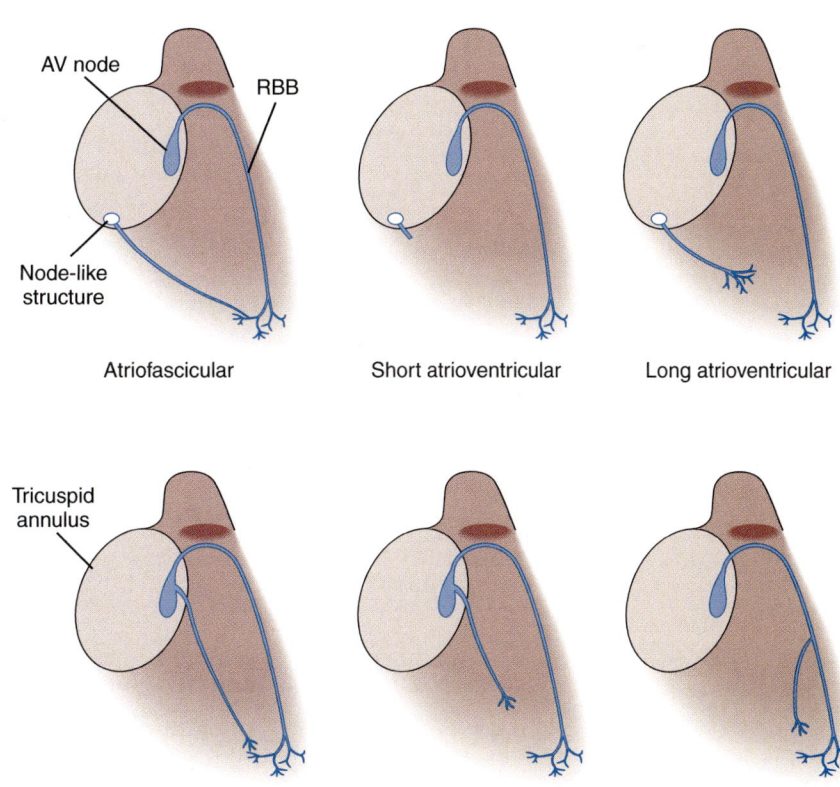

FIGURE 24-15. Anatomic courses of accessory pathway variants. AV, atrioventricular; RBB, right bundle branch. *(From Sternick EB, Wellens HJJ. Historical notes and classification of variants of ventricular preexcitation. In: Variants of Ventricular Preexcitation. Malden, MA: Blackwell Futura; 2006:1-6. With permission.)*

Decrementally Conducting Atrioventricular Pathways

Decremental conduction is defined as cycle length–dependent prolongation in conduction through the accessory pathway by 30 milliseconds or longer.[52] One type of decremental pathway is the short decremental AV connections.[52] These connections share features of typical Mahaim atriofascicular physiology and anatomy except that the ventricular insertion in the former occurs near the tricuspid annulus or in the middle right ventricle.[52] Current conceptions are that these pathways consist of the proximal accessory AV node but without the long distal portion to the right ventricular apex. Instead, these fibers insert into the right ventricle near the tricuspid valve or middle free wall. These fibers lack retrograde accessory pathway conduction and may show block with adenosine but differ from typical Mahaim atriofascicular connections in showing greater overt preexcitation, having no reversal of the His-RBB activation in sinus rhythm (due to insertion remote from the RBB), and being less likely to participate in reciprocating tachcyardias.[52] These connections are ablated near the tricuspid annulus analogous to typical Mahaim connections.[24]

Decrementally conducting "conventional" AV accessory pathways without AV nodal-like behavior have also been described. The physiology of these connections is exemplified in the setting of permanent junctional reciprocating tachycardia. Decremental conduction may result from circuitous pathway geometry, impedance mismatch along the pathway, previous ablation attempts, or unrecognized insertion into the AV node.[53] These connections typically demonstrate decremental conduction in one direction across the AV annulus but fail to conduct in the opposite direction. These pathways may be found in the left or right heart but predominate on the right.

Nodofascicular and Nodoventricular Accessory Pathways

Nodoventricular and nodofascicular fibers are the accessory connections originally described histologically by Mahaim.[1] The proximal insertion for these connections is into the AV node, with variable degrees of physiologic conduction delay occurring above and below the site of pathway insertion. The nodofascicular connection inserts distally into the His bundle, RBB, or rarely left bundle system (the left posterior fascicle has been reported).[54] For nodoventricular fibers, the distal connection is into the septal ventricular myocardium near the tricuspid annulus. The pathways tend to show either antegrade- or retrograde-only conduction. Bidirectional conduction over these accessory pathways appears extremely rare.[29] The diagnostic criteria are given in Table 24-6. Antidromic tachycardias involving the accessory pathway are much more common than orthodromic reentry (Fig. 24-16). AV dissociation may occur during tachycardia because of proximal pathway insertion into the

TABLE 24-6		
ACCESSORY PATHWAY VARIANTS		
Pathway Variant	**Diagnostic Features**	**Ablation Targets**
Atriofascicular (Mahaim)	See Table 24-1	See Table 24-1
Decrementally conducting atrioventricular	Cycle length–dependent prolongation in conduction time through AP to ≥30 msec	
• Short/intermediate Mahaim	Decremental conduction with AV nodal behavior and insertion near TV or mid RV	Mahaim potential or site of earliest ventricular activation
• Decremental antegrade atrioventricular	Decremental conduction without AV nodal behavior	Site of earliest ventricular activation during preexcitation
• Decremental concealed atrioventricular	Decremental conduction without AV nodal behavior	Site of earliest retrograde atrial activation during ORT
Nodoventricular	Prolongation of PR and AH intervals associated with shortening HV interval in response to atrial pacing/extra stimuli LBBB preexcitation pattern Retrograde conduction over AV node* Preexcitation linked to activation of AV node/septal atrium AV dissociation possible during reciprocation tachycardia Tachycardia not advanced with PAC during AVN/septal atrial refractoriness Loss of preexcitation with His pacing	Earliest ventricular activation
Nodofascicular	Prolongation of PR and AH intervals associated with shortening HV interval in response to atrial pacing/extra stimuli LBBB preexcitation pattern Retrograde conduction over AV node* Preexcitation linked to activation of AV node/septal atrium AV dissociation possible during reciprocation tachycardia Tachycardia not advanced with PAC during AVN/septal atrial refractoriness	Possibly earliest ventricular activation but same limitations as atriofascicular, parahisian, or mid-septal TV
Fasciculoventricular	HV interval <35 msec Fixed degree of preexcitation at all atrial cycle lengths Continued preexcitation during His bundle pacing	Not indicated for ablation

* Assumes absence of other accessory AV connections.

AH, atrial-to-His; AP, accessory pathway; AVN, atrioventricular node; HV, His-to-ventricular; LBBB, left bundle branch block; ORT, orthodromic reciprocating tachycardia, PAC, premature atrial stimulus; TV, tricuspid valve.

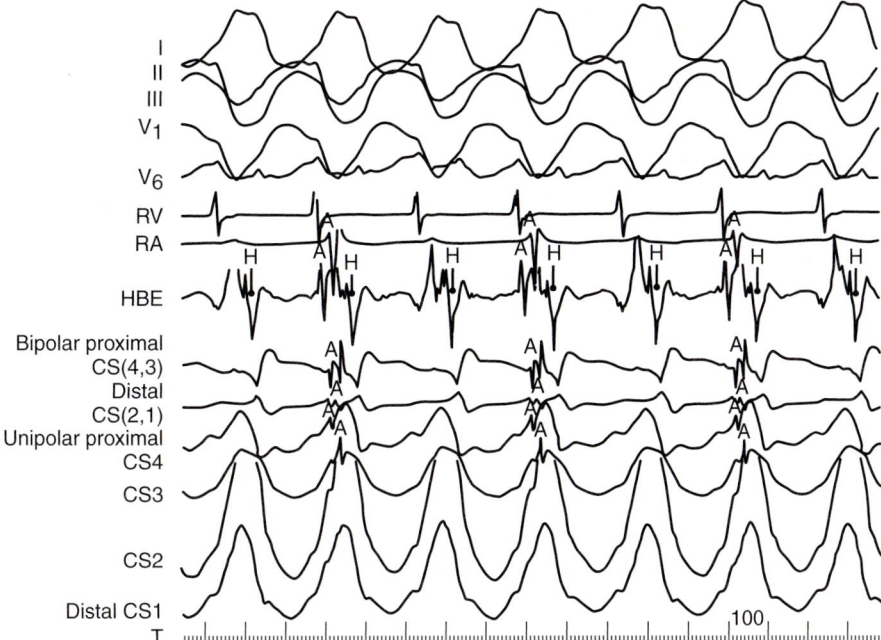

FIGURE 24-16. Surface and intracardiac recordings during reciprocating tachycardia in a patient with a nodoventricular accessory pathway. The pathway serves as the antegrade limb, and the His-Purkinje system is the retrograde limb. Left bundle branch block morphology is present on surface electrocardiogram. A sharp His bundle deflection (H) is shown late in the QRS with a ventricular–His bundle (VH) interval of 100 msec. Note the 2:1 retrograde conduction to the atrium (A). CS, coronary sinus; HBE, His bundle electrogram; RA, right atrium; RV, right ventricle. *(From Gallagher JJ, Smith WM, Kasell JH. Role of Mahaim fibers in cardiac arrhythmias in man. Circulation. 1981;64:176-189. With permission.)*

distal AV node. Distal insertion above the His bifurcation or in the proximal bundle branch may allow for transient infrahisian block to occur during tachycardia and render the tachycardia cycle length unperturbed by bundle branch blocks. These variant pathways frequently occur in association with dual AV nodal physiology and typical AV pathways. Thus, bystander activation is common.[54] There are limited reports detailing ablation of nodoventricular and nodofascicular connections. Because of the origin from the AV node, attempts to ablate the proximal insertion may carry a significant risk for AV block. Ablation of fast or slow AV nodal pathways theoretically could result in heart block but spare the tachycardia circuit itself. Ablation should target the distal insertion site if possible. These sites may be identified by recording accessory pathway potentials, sites of earliest ventricular activation (nodoventricular), or sites at which extrastimuli during tachycardia and His refractoriness produce the greatest degree of His-His interval decrement.[54] For nodofascicular fibers, the earliest ventricular activation is near the apex, and as with typical Mahaim atriofascicular connections, ablation at this site may not be successful. Most reports indicate successful ablation sites along the middle right ventricular septum. There are limited data on the use of cryoablation for these connections, but this modality may be safer than radiofrequency.[55] There are rare reports of ablation of a nodo-His connection at the level of the tricuspid valve in the low septal right atrium.[56,57]

Fasciculoventricular Accessory Pathways

Fasciculoventricular connections arise from the His bundle or bundle branches to insert into the ventricular septum. Both right- and left-sided connections have been reported.[58] Although these connections do not participate directly in any reentrant circuits, they are associated with

other arrhythmogenic accessory pathways as bystander participants. These circuits must be recognized to avoid unnecessary ablation, especially if misdiagnosed as a mid-septal AV pathway. The HV interval is less than 35 milliseconds. The hallmark finding is a fixed degree of preexcitation with all atrial cycle lengths. The continued presence of preexcitation during pure His pacing is pathognomonic. These pathways have not been convincingly shown to participate in a reentry circuit and do not require ablation.

References

1. Mahaim I, Winston MR. Recherches d'lanatomic comparee et du pathologic experimental sur les connexions hautes du faisceau de His-Tawara. *Cardiologia.* 1941;5:189–260.
2. Mahaim I, Benatt A. Nouvelles recherches sur les connexions superieures de la branche gauche du faisceau de His-Tawara avec cloison interventriculaire. *Cardiologia.* 1938;1:61–76.
3. Wellens HJ. The preexcitation syndrome. In: Wellens HJ, ed. *Electrical Stimulation of the Heart in the Study and Treatment of Tachycardias.* Baltimore: University Park Press; 1971:97–109.
4. Anderson RH, Becker AE, Brechenmacher C, et al. Ventricular preexcitation: a proposed nomenclature for its substrates. *Eur J Cardiol.* 1975;3:27–36.
5. Ellenbogen KA, O'Callaghan WG, Colavita PG, et al. Catheter atrioventricular junction ablation for recurrent supraventricular tachycardia with nodoventricular fibers. *Am J Cardiol.* 1985;55:1227–1229.
6. Tchou P, Lehmann MH, Jazayeri M, Akhtar M. Atriofascicular connection or a nodoventricular Mahaim fiber? Electrophysiologic elucidation of the pathway and associated reentrant circuit. *Circulation.* 1988;77:837–848.
7. Gillette PC, Garson A Jr, Cooey DA, et al. Prolonged and decremental antegrade conduction properties in right anterior atrioventricular connections: wide QRS antidromic tachycardia of left bundle block pattern without Wolff-Parkinson-White configuration in sinus rhythm. *Am Heart J.* 1982;103:66.
8. Klein GJ, Guiraudon GM, Kerr CR, et al. "Nodoventricular" accessory pathway: evidence for a distinct accessory atrioventricular pathway with atrioventricular node-like properties. *J Am Coll Cardiol.* 1988;11:1035.
9. Bhandari A, Morady F, Shen EN, et al. Catheter-induced His bundle ablation in a patient with reentrant tachycardia associated with a nodoventricular tract. *J Am Coll Cardiol.* 1984;4:611–616.
10. McClelland JH, Wang X, Beckman KJ, et al. Radiofrequency catheter ablation of right atriofascicular (Mahaim) accessory pathways guided by accessory pathway activation potentials. *Circulation.* 1994;89:2655–2666.
11. Cappato R, Schluer M, Weiss C, et al. Catheter-induced mechanical conduction block of right-sided accessory fibers with Mahaim-type preexcitation to guide radiofrequency ablation. *Circulation.* 1994;90:282–290.
12. Grogin HR, Lee RJ, Kwasman M, et al. Radiofrequency catheter ablation of atriofascicular and nodoventricular Mahaim tracts. *Circulation.* 1994;90:272–281.

13. Haïssaguerre M, Cauchemez B, Marcus F, et al. Characteristics of the ventricular insertion sites of accessory pathways with anterograde decremental conduction properties. *Circulation.* 1995;91:1077–1085.
14. Okishige K, Goseki Y, Itoh A, et al. New electrophysiologic features and catheter ablation of atrioventricular and atriofascicular accessory pathways: evidence of decremental conduction and the anatomic structure of the Mahaim pathway. *J Cardiovasc Electrophysiol.* 1998;9:22–33.
15. Klein LS, Hackett FK, Zipes DP, Miles WM. Radiofrequency catheter ablation of Mahaim fibers at the tricuspid annulus. *Circulation.* 1993;87:738–747.
16. Haïssaguerre M, Capos J, Marcus FI, et al. Involvement of a nodofascicular connection in supraventricular tachycardia with VA dissociation. *J Cardiovasc Electrophysiol.* 1994;5:854–862.
17. Prystowsky EM, Miles WM, Heger JJ, Zipes DP. Preexcitation syndromes: mechanisms and management. *Med Clin North Am.* 1984;68:831.
18. Hluchy J, Schlegelmilch P, Schickel S, et al. Radiofrequency ablation of a concealed nodoventricular Mahaim fiber guided by a discrete potential. *J Cardiovasc Electrophysiol.* 1999;10:603–610.
19. Johnson CT, Brooks C, Jaramillo J, et al. A left free-wall, decrementally conducting, atrioventricular (Mahaim) fiber: diagnosis at electrophysiological study and radiofrequency catheter ablation guided by direct recording of a Mahaim potential. *Pacing Clin Electrophysiol.* 1997;20:2486–2488.
20. Tada H, Nogami A, Naito S, et al. Left posteroseptal Mahaim fiber associated with marked longitudinal dissociation. *Pacing Clin Electrophysiol.* 1999;22:1696–1699.
21. Francia P, Pittalis M, Ali H, Cappato R. Electrophysiological study and catheter ablation of a Mahaim fibre located at the mitral annulus-aorta junction. *J Interv Card Electrophysiol.* 2008;23:153–157.
22. Ellenbogen KA, Rogers R, Old W. Pharmacological characterization of conduction over a Mahaim fiber: evidence for adenosine sensitive conduction. *Pacing Clin Electrophysiol.* 1989;12:1396–1404.
23. Betts TR. Mahaim tachycardia and intravenous adenosine. *Heart.* 2006;92:1408.
24. Heald SC, Davies DW, Ward DE, et al. Radiofrequency catheter ablation of Mahaim tachycardia by targeting Mahaim potentials at the tricuspid annulus. *Br Heart J.* 1995;73:250–257.
25. Li HG, Klein GJ, Thakur RK, Yee R. Radiofrequency ablation of decremental accessory pathways mimicking "nodoventricular" conduction. *Am J Cardiol.* 1994;74:829–833.
26. Lee PC, Kanter R, Gomez-Martin O, et al. Quantitative assessment of the recovery property of atriofascicular/atrioventricular-type Mahaim fiber. *J Cardiovasc Electrophysiol.* 2002;13:535–541.
27. Beurrier D, Brembilla-Perrot B, Bragard MF. Radiofrequency catheter ablation of a nodofascicular Mahaim tract. *Herz.* 1996;21:314–319.
28. Kottkamp H, Hindricks G, Shenasa H, et al. Variants of preexcitation—specialized atriofascicular pathways, nodofascicular pathways, and fasciculoventricular pathways: electrophysiologic findings and target sites for radiofrequency catheter ablation. *J Cardiovasc Electrophysiol.* 1996;7:916–930.
29. Davidson NC, Morton JB, Sanders P, Kalman J. Latent Mahaim fiber as a cause of antidromic reciprocating tachycardia: recognition and successful radiofrequency ablation. *J Cardiovasc Electrophysiol.* 2002;13:74–78.
30. Broadhurst P, Redfern C. Radiofrequency ablation of a "concealed" Mahaim-type accessory pathway. *Pacing Clin Electrophysiol.* 2008;30:1032–1035.
31. Gallagher JJ, Smith WM, Kasell JH, et al. Role of Mahaim fibers in cardiac arrhythmias in man. *Circulation.* 1981;64:176–189.
32. Ellenbogen KA, Ramirez NM, Packer DL, et al. Accessory nodoventricular (Mahaim) fibers: a clinical review. *Pacing Clin Electrophysiol.* 1986;9:868–884.
33. Ott P, Marcus FI. Familial Mahaim syndrome. *Ann Noninvasive Electrocardiol.* 2001;6:272–275.
34. Murdock CJ, Leitch JW, Klein GJ, et al. Epicardial mapping in patients with "nodoventricular" accessory pathways. *Am J Cardiol.* 1991;68:208–214.
35. Sternick EB, Timmermans C, Sosa E, et al. The electrocardiogram during sinus rhythm and tachycardia in patients with Mahaim fibers: the importance of an "rS" pattern in lead III. *J Am Coll Cardiol.* 2004;44:1626–1635.
36. Bardy GH, Fedor JM, German LD, et al. Surface electrocardiographic clues suggesting presence of a nodofascicular Mahaim fiber. *J Am Coll Cardiol.* 1984;3:1161–1168.
37. Bohora S, Dora SK, Namboordri S, et al. Electrophysiology study and radiofrequency catheter ablation of atriofascicular tracts with decremental properties (Mahaim fibre) at the tricuspid annulus. *Europace.* 2008;10:1428–1433.
38. Mounsey JP, Griffith MJ, McComb JM. Radiofrequency ablation of a Mahaim fiber following localization of Mahaim pathway potentials. *J Cardiovasc Electrophysiol.* 1994;5:432–437.
39. Brugada J, Martinez-Sanchez J, Kuzmicic B. Radiofrequency catheter ablation of atriofascicular accessory pathways guided by discrete electrical potentials recorded at the tricuspid annulus. *Pacing Clin Electrophysiol.* 1995;18:1388–1394.
40. Okishige K, Strickberger A, Walsh E. Catheter ablation of the atrial origin of a decrementally conducting atriofascicular accessory pathway by radiofrequency current. *J Cardiovasc Electrophysiol.* 1991;2:465–475.
41. Miller JM, Harper GR, Rothman SA, Hsia HH. Radiofrequency catheter ablation of an atriofascicular pathway during atrial fibrillation: a case report. *J Cardiovasc Electrophysiol.* 1994;5:846–853.
42. Haïssaguerre M, Warin JF, Le Metayer P, et al. Catheter ablation of Mahaim fibers with preservation of atrioventricular nodal conduction. *Circulation.* 1990;82:418–427.
43. Haïssaguerre M, Fischer B, Le Metayer P, Warin JF. Nature of the distal insertion site of Mahaim fibers as defined by catheter ablation [abstract]. *Eur Soc Cardiol.* 1993.
44. Belhassen B, Viskin S, Fish R, et al. Catheter-induced mechanical trauma to accessory pathways during radiofrequency ablation: incidence, predictors and clinical implications. *J Am Coll Cardiol.* 1999;33:767–774.
45. Tomassoni G, et al. Ablation of right free wall and atriofascicular accessory pathways. In: Singer I, ed. *Interventional Electrophysiology.* Philadelphia: Lippincott Williams & Wilkins; 2001:193–236.
46. Sternick EB, Gerken LM, Vrandecic MO, et al. Appraisal of "Mahaim" automatic tachycardia. *J Cardiovasc Electrophysiol.* 2002;13:244–249.
47. Ma FS, Ma J, Chu JM, et al. The automaticity of Mahaim fibre and its response to effective ablation. *Chinese Med J.* 2004;117:1768–1771.
48. Miller JM, Olgin JE. Catheter ablation of free-wall accessory pathways and "Mahaim" fibers. In: Zipes DF, Haïssaguerre M, eds. *Catheter Ablation of Arrhythmias.* Armonk, NY: Futura; 2002:277–303.
49. Worley S. Use of a real-time three-dimensional magnetic navigation system for radiofrequency ablation of accessory pathways. *Pacing Clin Electrophysiol.* 1998;21:1636–1645.
50. Morita N, Kobayashi Y, Katoh T, Takano T. Anatomic and electrophysiologic evaluation of a right lateral atrioventricular Mahaim fiber. *Pacing Clin Electrophysiol.* 2005;28:1138–1141.
51. Fung JW, Chan HCK, Chan WWL, et al. Ablation of the Mahaim pathway guided by noncontact mapping. *J Cardiovasc Electrophysiol.* 2002;13:1064.
52. Sternick EB, Wellens HJJ. The short AV decrementally conduction fibers. In: *Variants of Ventricular Preexcitation.* Malden, MA: Blackwell Futura; 2006:59–73.
53. Sternick EB, Wellens HJJ. Conduction disturbances in accessory pathways. In: *Variants of Ventricular Preexcitation.* Malden, MA: Blackwell Futura; 2006:103–115.
54. Sternick EB, Wellens HJJ. Nodoventricular and nodofascicular fibers. In: *Variants of Ventricular Preexcitation.* Malden, MA: Blackwell Futura; 2006:75–81.
55. Papagiannis J, Vachtsevanos L, Rammos S, Kanter R. Cryoablation of a nodoventricular Mahaim fiber. *J Interv Card Electrophysiol.* 2005;14:111–116.
56. Haïssaguerre M, Campos J, Marcus FI, et al. Involvement of a nodofascicular connection in supraventricular tachycardia with VA dissociation. *J Cardiovasc Electrophysiol.* 1994;5:854–862.
57. Okumura K, Yamabe H, Yasue H. Radiofrequency catheter ablation of concealed atrio-His bypass tract involved in paroxysmal supraventricular tachycardia. *Pacing Clin Electrophysiol.* 1994;17:1686–1690.
58. Sternick EB, Wellens HJJ. Fasciculoventricular fibers. In: *Variants of Ventricular Preexcitation.* Malden, MA: Blackwell Futura; 2006:83–102.

25

Special Problems in Ablation of Accessory Pathways

*Basilios Petrellis, Allan C. Skanes, George J. Klein,
Andrew D. Krahn, and Raymond Yee*

Key Points

The approach to the difficult accessory pathway ablation is, first, to exclude "cognitive" ablation failure by confirming the tachycardia diagnosis and reevaluating the electrograms.

Second, use a systematic approach to identify contributing technical factors, such as pathway-related factors (including location and atypical configuration) and associated cardiac structural abnormalities.

Finally, devise an appropriate strategy. This may include optimizing pathway localization, adjusting the ablation approach to improve stability and tissue contact, and changing the ablation modality (conventional versus saline-cooled radiofrequency ablation or cryoablation).

The atrioventricular (AV) groove is normally composed of fibrous tissue devoid of electrical conductive properties; this commits ventricular activation to proceed over the specialized AV conduction tissue, the His-Purkinje system. Accessory pathways (APs) are considered a remnant of incomplete separation of the atrial and ventricular myocardium by the annulus fibrosus during cardiogenesis. The resulting myocardial bridges are capable of electrical conduction that may facilitate early ventricular activation and provide the arrhythmogenic substrate for AV reentrant tachycardia.

Because of its low risk and high efficacy, catheter ablation is first-line therapy for symptomatic patients with APs.[1-5] Ablation of APs was historically achieved first by surgical dissection and subsequently by direct current energy applied through transvenous catheters. The first successful catheter ablation of an AP using radiofrequency (RF) energy was performed in 1984.[6]

Although successful pathway elimination is achieved in more than 95% of cases, primary success is occasionally elusive, resulting in lengthy procedures or multiple attempts. Furthermore, AP conduction may return after initial success. This chapter aims to outline problems that may be encountered during ablation of APs and to propose practical solutions.

General Considerations

The incidence of successful elimination and recurrence after RF catheter ablation of APs has been well documented.[2-4,7-11] Initial ablation success is highest for left-sided pathways (97%) and is lower for right-sided (88%) and septal connections (89%). Recurrence is also less frequent at left free wall locations (5%) than at the right free wall (17%) and septum (11%).

Failed RF catheter ablation of APs is most frequently related to technical difficulties or misdiagnosis (Table 25-1). Other factors include the coexistence of structural cardiac abnormalities, atypical pathway configuration, and high-risk AP locations, such as those adjacent to the AV node or within the coronary sinus (CS).

Inability to Heat

Technical considerations such as catheter instability or difficult access may give rise to poor endocardial contact, leading to insufficient energy delivery and local heat production at the ablation target. This problem is more frequently encountered with right-sided APs because of a less clearly defined anatomic groove delineating the tricuspid annulus. Poor energy delivery, indicated by a low power output of the RF generator during temperature-controlled RF ablation, may achieve the desired tip-tissue interface temperature but does not provide adequate depth of energy penetration for elimination of AP conduction. Tissue contact and catheter access to the target site are often improved by the use of long, preformed intravascular sheaths or deflectable ablation catheters of varying reach, curve, and tip size, which are designed in a variety of configurations to allow access to all locations on either the tricuspid or the mitral annulus.

Energy delivery is further enhanced by the use of passively cooled large-tip catheters or saline-irrigated (cooled-tip) catheters that infuse normal saline during RF delivery. Because interfacial heating is reduced, coagulum formation and char at the catheter tip are prevented, allowing the point

TABLE 25-1

CAUSES OF FAILED CATHETER ABLATION OF ACCESSORY PATHWAYS

Inability to Heat

Catheter instability, poor tissue contact, difficult access to target site

Pathway location beyond range of RF lesion size (e.g., epicardial location)

Misdiagnosis

Misinterpretation of electrophysiologic data

Previous ablation, low-amplitude, or distorted electrogram recordings

Incomplete electrophysiology study, inaccurate pathway localization, incomplete mapping

Multiple tachycardia mechanisms (e.g., AP with AVNRT or ectopic tachycardia, pathway-to-pathway tachycardia)

Associated Structural Cardiac Abnormalities

Ebstein anomaly

Persistent left-sided superior vena cava

Atypical Pathway Configuration

Multiple APs

Oblique APs

Epicardial APs

Atypical AP connections

High-Risk AP Location

Adjacent to the AV node: mid-septal or anteroseptal pathway (risk for inadvertent AV block)

Epicardial APs: accessible within the coronary sinus or associated with diverticulum (risk for arterial stenosis–circumflex artery or distal right coronary branches)

AP, accessory pathway; AV, atrioventricular; AVNRT, atrioventricular nodal reentrant tachycardia; RF, radiofrequency energy.

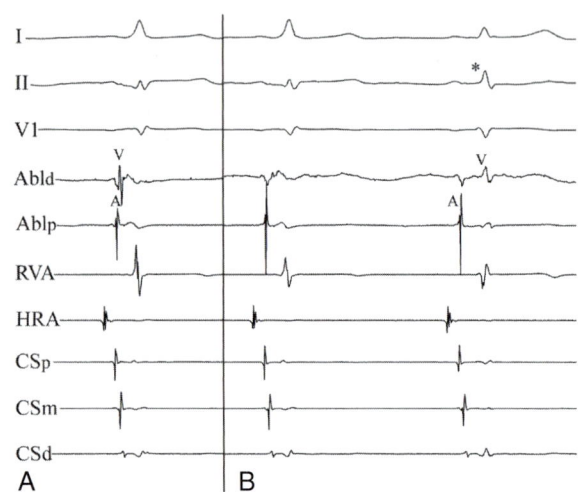

FIGURE 25-1. Misinterpretation of electrophysiologic data may lead to ablation failure. **A,** Mapping of a right posterior free wall accessory pathway during sinus rhythm. The ablation catheter (Abl) is located at the atrial aspect of the tricuspid annulus (6-o'clock position, left anterior oblique 30-degree projection). At first inspection, only an atrial electrogram appears to be recorded. Closer inspection reveals balanced atrial (A) and ventricular (V) electrograms confirming an annular catheter position. The earlier atrial electrogram is recorded proximally (Ablp) and the ventricular electrogram distally (Abld). Electrogram fusion is frequently observed with right-sided accessory pathways, and misinterpretation can result in failure to identify the successful ablation site. **B,** Radiofrequency current application at this site eliminated pathway conduction demonstrated by loss of preexcitation (*asterisk*) and separation of the previously fused A and V electrograms. CS, coronary sinus (p, proximal; m, mid; d, distal); HRA, high right atrium; RVA, right ventricular apex.

of maximal heating to be shifted into the tissue rather than focused at the tissue surface. Deeper conductive heating produces deeper tissue lesions.

Catheter stability may be compromised if ablation is performed during orthodromic AV reentrant tachycardia. Ablation during tachycardia is sometimes necessary if retrograde fusion during ventricular pacing obscures the pathway location in patients with concealed APs. Abrupt heart rate slowing on RF-induced termination of tachycardia frequently results in catheter dislodgment, preventing full-duration RF current delivery at the successful site. Entrainment of the tachycardia by ventricular pacing during ablation overcomes this potential problem.[12] While maintaining retrograde activation over the AP, entrainment prevents an abrupt change in ventricular rate, allowing a stable catheter position during pathway ablation for continued RF energy delivery despite tachycardia termination.

Misdiagnosis

Misinterpretation of electrophysiologic data, by failure or inability to recognize atrial or ventricular activation sequence or AP potentials, prohibits accurate pathway localization. Appropriate interpretation of data may be precluded by factors attributable to the AP, such as overlapping electrograms, which are often seen with multiple and right free wall pathways (Fig. 25-1), or distorted low-amplitude

electrograms at the site of RF lesions in patients with a previously unsuccessful ablation attempt.

Incomplete mapping may prevent accurate localization, a point of particular relevance to posteroseptal APs. If thorough mapping at the posteroseptal region on the right fails to identify a successful ablation site, careful mapping of the CS and the left posteroseptal region is essential. In the event that an epicardial pathway is suspected, CS angiography may identify a coexistent CS diverticulum or aneurysm.

A complete initial electrophysiology study is necessary to exclude an unrecognized or unexpected tachycardia mechanism, because APs, atrioventricular nodal reentrant tachycardia (AVNRT), and ectopic tachycardias infrequently coexist. Furthermore, successful AP ablation may lead to the emergence of a latent AP, causing symptom recurrence and need for a repeat procedure. A repeat diagnostic study after presumed successful pathway ablation is strongly recommended to exclude this possibility.

A number of published series have identified factors associated with difficult or failed ablation and recurrence of AP conduction. In a retrospective analysis, Morady and associates[13] identified six factors contributing to a failed or prolonged ablation session. In the failure group, the proportion of APs located at the right free wall was significantly greater than in the overall group (29% versus 16%), with right anterolateral and right posterolateral locations specifically overrepresented.

Of the six factors identified, problems related to catheter manipulation and inaccurate pathway localization accounted for most cases (48% and 26%, respectively). Other contributing factors included the presence of an epicardial pathway (5%), recurrent atrial fibrillation

FIGURE 25-2. Demonstration of an accessory pathway (AP) potential using a nonfluoroscopic mapping system. The electrogram was recorded at the right anterolateral atrioventricular (AV) ring adjacent to the *blue tag*. Ablation lesions that eliminated AP conduction along with sites of lesion expansion are seen as *red tags*. In difficult cases, nonfluoroscopic mapping systems catalogue sites of interest. RVA, right ventricular apex.

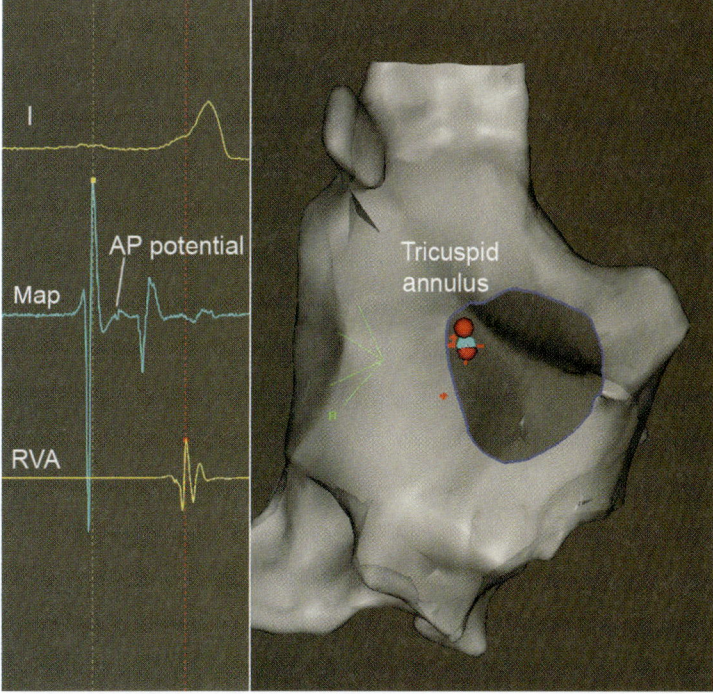

interfering with mapping (3%), unusual AP anatomy (1.5%), and procedure-related vascular complications (3%) preventing an ablation attempt.

Problems Related to Catheter Manipulation

Inability to guide the ablation catheter to the endocardial target, catheter instability, or inadequate tissue contact, or a combination of these, contributed to failed or prolonged ablation in 48% of Morady's patients.[13] Successful pathway elimination was achieved in some cases by a change in the ablation approach. Specifically, for left-sided pathways, a retrograde aortic approach was switched to a transseptal approach; for pathways located on the right, an inferior vena cava approach was switched to a superior vena cava approach. In other cases, the use of a long guiding sheath, multiple operators, or ablation catheters of varying distal configurations during tip deflection proved successful.

Inaccurate Pathway Localization

Inaccurate pathway localization may lead to RF energy application at inappropriate sites, a problem that was encountered in two circumstances.[13] The first occurred when the surface electrocardiogram (ECG) suggested right posteroseptal preexcitation but subsequent successful ablation was achieved at the left posteroseptal region. In the second type, failure was observed during ablation of unrecognized oblique APs caused by disparate atrial and ventricular insertions at the AV junction. As a result, ventricular insertion sites did not correspond to the site of earliest retrograde atrial activation during ventricular pacing or orthodromic tachycardia. Similarly, atrial insertion sites were not identified by the earliest anterograde ventricular activation during preexcitation. Success was ultimately achieved by identifying the atrial or ventricular insertion sites on their corresponding side of the annulus or by ablating a midportion of the pathway itself, as identified by AP potentials.

Other Factors

Epicardial APs were identified in a small number of patients in whom successful elimination was achieved by application of RF energy within the CS after failure at the corresponding endocardial site.[13] In these patients, prominent AP potentials recorded within the CS were absent or of small amplitude at the endocardial surface. An unusual AP course was identified in one patient, in whom the ventricular insertion was at the anterior wall of the right ventricle, 2 cm from the tricuspid annulus. Delivery of RF current at this site eliminated pathway conduction and confirmed its atypical ventricular insertion.

Similar findings were reported by Xie and colleagues.[14] Primary ablation failure was observed in 10% of patients and was associated with catheter instability, epicardial pathway course, and a right-sided location, particularly in midseptal and anteroseptal positions. Recurrence was seen in 6% during a mean follow-up period of 20 months and was predicted by a right free wall location, time to conduction block after onset of RF current greater than 12 seconds, poor ablation electrogram stability, and inability to deliver the desired temperature despite maximal power output, a reflection of poor electrode-tissue contact.

Twidale and coworkers[15] reported recurrence in 8% of patients during a mean follow-up period of 8.5 months. Again, recurrence was more frequent with anteroseptal, right free wall, and posteroseptal connections (12% to 14%), and concealed pathways recurred more frequently (16%) than manifest pathways (5.5%). In addition to the time to conduction block from onset of RF, a strong predictor for pathway recurrence was failure to record an AP potential at the ablation site, with the difference attributable to less accurate pathway localization (Fig. 25-2).

Specific Challenges

Ablation of Epicardial Accessory Pathways

Coronary Sinus and Epicardial Accessory Pathways

The CS originates at its ostium within the right atrium and extends distally to the valve of Vieussens, where it receives the great cardiac vein. Other major tributaries include the left obtuse marginal vein, the posterior left ventricular vein (PCV), the middle cardiac vein (MCV), and the right coronary vein, also known as the small cardiac vein (Fig. 25-3).[16]

The CS provides a conduit for catheter access, permitting mapping of left-sided APs adjacent to the mitral annulus and of posteroseptal (paraseptal) APs traversing the inferior pyramidal space. Moreover, it provides a means of access to epicardial areas of the myocardium for potential ablation of epicardial pathways.

A myocardial coat around the CS is present in all individuals.[17,18] It is composed of bands of muscle arising from the right and left atrial walls[19] and extends in most cases to, and occasionally beyond, the great cardiac vein. Electrical continuity therefore exists between both atria and this muscular sleeve.[20] The tributaries of the CS are usually devoid of a myocardial coat. Nonetheless, sleeve-like muscular extensions covering the proximal portions of the MCV and PCV are present in 3% and 2% of hearts, respectively,[17] potentially serving as connections between the ventricle and the CS and completing a CS-AP connection (Fig. 25-4).

The association of CS diverticula with posteroseptal and left posterolateral APs is well documented.[21–24] Myocardial fibers found within diverticula frequently connect the ventricle with the CS musculature. Other anatomic anomalies, such as fusiform or bulbous enlargement of the CS tributaries, have also been reported to be associated with such connections.

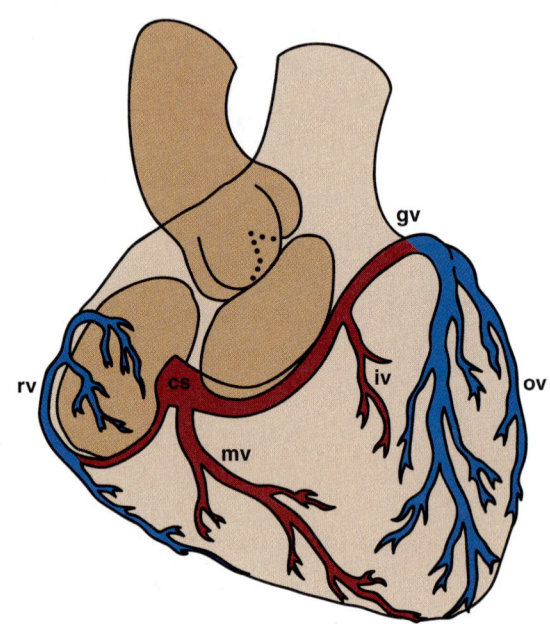

FIGURE 25-3. Schematic representation of the coronary venous system. cs, Coronary sinus; gv, great cardiac vein; iv, inferior left cardiac vein; mv, middle cardiac vein; ov, obtuse left cardiac vein; rv, right cardiac vein.

Antegrade CSAP conduction

Coronary sinus Myocardial coat

LA

LA

Coronary sinus ostium

Marshall vein

Great cardiac vein

RA

Retrograde conduction

LA

CSE

LV

Small cardiac vein

Posterior coronary vein

Postulated ventricular connections

Middle cardiac vein

FIGURE 25-4. Schematic for possible anatomic basis of connections between the coronary sinus musculature and left ventricular myocardium (LV). The coronary sinus musculature may form extensions (CSE) over the proximal portions of the middle and posterior cardiac veins. If connections between the coronary sinus musculature and the left (LA) or right (RA) atrial myocardium exist as well, the substrate for reciprocating tachycardias is formed. CSAP, coronary sinus accessory pathway. *(From Sun Y, Arruda M, Otomo K, et al. Coronary sinus–ventricular accessory connections producing posteroseptal and left posterior accessory pathways: incidence and electrophysiological identification. Circulation. 2002;106:1362–1367. With permission.)*

Sun and associates[25] identified a CS AP in 36% of 480 patients with posteroseptal or left posterior APs. During antegrade AP conduction, the presence of a CS AP was established by the recording of ventricular activation at the MCV, PCV, or neck of a CS diverticulum earlier than endocardial ventricular activation. At the same site, a high-frequency potential was recorded before the earliest recorded far-field ventricular potential. This high-frequency potential, analogous to an AP potential, was generated by the muscular extension of the CS myocardial coat, which formed a connection to the epicardial surface of the ventricle.

Retrograde angiography in patients with CS AP demonstrated a CS diverticulum in only 21% of cases, most frequently extending from the CS and the MCV. Fusiform or bulbous venous enlargement was identified in 9% of patients, but CS anatomy was normal in the remaining 70%, suggesting that most CS APs occur without a diverticulum or other venous anomaly.

Because of their epicardial location, successful ablation of these APs is accomplished only by RF current delivered within the CS or by direct percutaneous catheter access to the pericardial space. Specific ECG features have been described to identify manifest pathways requiring such an approach.[26] A negative delta wave in lead II predicts a successful ablation site within the CS or MCV with a sensitivity of 87%, but with a relatively low specificity (79%) and positive predictive value (50%). However, a steep positive delta wave in lead aVR and a deep S wave in lead V_6 (R < S) yields high specificity and positive-predictive values, 99% and 91%, respectively, for a successful ablation site within the CS. These ECG findings, along with a difficult or previously failed ablation attempt, suggest that contrast definition of the coronary venous anatomy and subsequent detailed mapping may prove helpful in identification of a successful epicardial ablation target.

RF ablation within the coronary venous system has been shown to be successful and safe for the elimination of epicardial APs (Fig. 25-5).[27-35] Reports of CS injury after RF catheter ablation are infrequent, possibly because of the lack of clinical sequelae and symptoms of CS stenosis. Nevertheless, RF current delivery within the vein has been associated with endoluminal thrombosis, stenosis, perforation leading to pericardial tamponade, and damage to adjacent structures. The proximity of the right coronary artery and its AV nodal branch with the proximal MCV, and crossover points of the left anterior descending and left circumflex arteries with the great cardiac vein, represent potential sites of susceptibility for coronary artery spasm or myocardial infarction during RF ablation.[36-38] Selective coronary angiography to delineate the relation of a prospective ablation site to the coronary arteries is prudent before RF current application within the CS. Luminal patency may also be reassessed after ablation. Irrigated RF ablation may be safer in this situation than noncooled RF, owing to the lower incidence of impedance rises and coagulum formation. Cryoablation may be the modality of choice for these cases.

Cryothermal ablation within the CS has been successfully employed to eliminate epicardial posterolateral APs.[39] Cryolesions are associated with less endothelial disruption and thrombus formation than RF lesions. Furthermore, the safety of cryothermal ablation adjacent to the coronary arteries has been demonstrated by extensive surgical experience[40] and by recent catheter-based studies using animal models.[41,42] A percutaneous epicardial approach using RF energy has also been successfully employed for elimination of posteroseptal APs associated with CS diverticula after multiple failed transvenous ablation attempts.[43,44]

Atrial Appendage-to-Ventricular Accessory Pathways

Most reported epicardial APs occur adjacent to a CS diverticulum, the MCV, or the great cardiac vein.[45] The atrial appendage-to-ventricular pathway is a recognized variant of AP connections that is characterized by an epicardial course connecting the atrial appendage and the ventricular base, most frequently on the right side. RF energy at endocardial sites may be ineffective, resulting in failure of ablation or recurrence of pathway conduction.

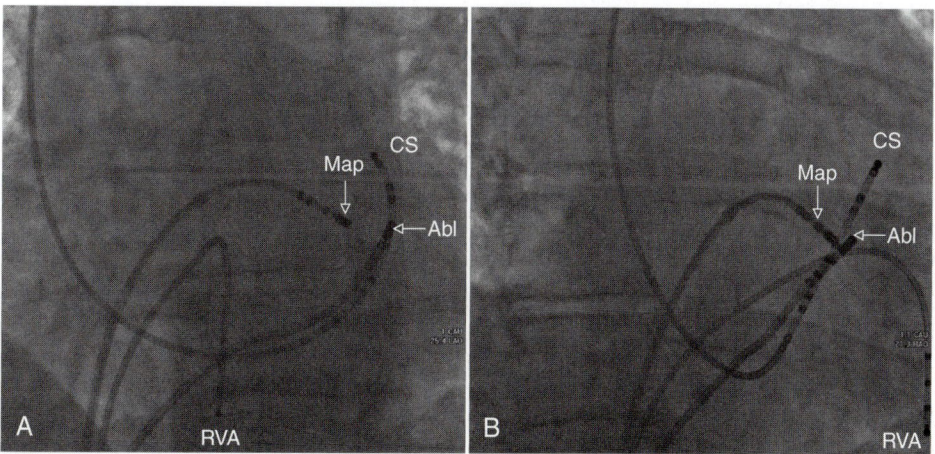

FIGURE 25-5. Radiofrequency (RF) ablation within the coronary sinus, fluoroscopic images in left anterior oblique (**A**) and anteroposterior (**B**) projections. Endocardial RF current delivered adjacent to the mitral annulus (Map), where local myocardial activation was optimum, failed to eliminate accessory pathway conduction. An ablation catheter (Abl) positioned within the coronary sinus identified a discrete accessory pathway potential. Low-power (15 W) RF current delivery at this site resulted in permanent pathway elimination within seconds of application. Abl, coronary sinus ablation catheter; CS, coronary sinus; Map, endocardial ablation catheter; RVA, right ventricular apex.

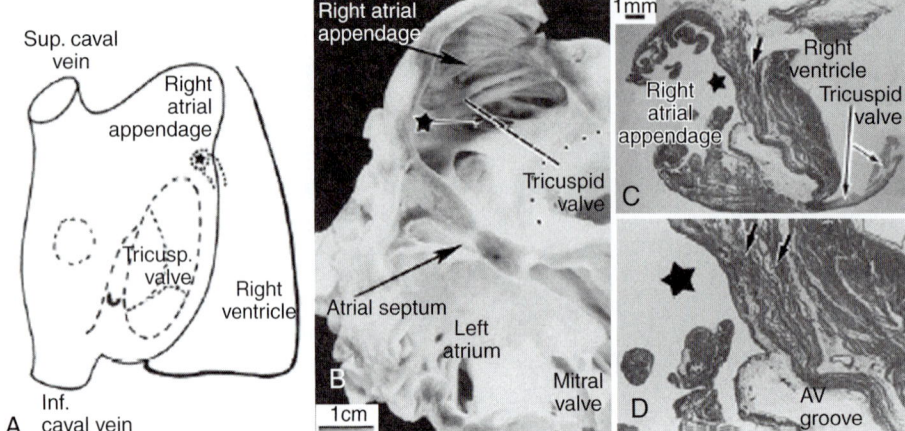

FIGURE 25-6. A, Diagram showing the location of an accessory connection joining the floor of the right atrial appendage (*star*) to the supraventricular crest. **B,** The heart is sectioned in a plane to show the four cardiac chambers from a posterior perspective. The *broken line* marks the level of the histologic sections shown in panels **C** and **D**. Note the distance between the pouch (*star and arrow*) and the hinge of the tricuspid valve (*dotted line*). **C,** This section through the atrioventricular (AV) junction shows the pouch (*star*) overlying the superior wall of the right ventricle and the band of accessory tissue (*arrow*). **D,** This magnification of the pouch reveals the muscular band (*arrows*) from the wall of the pouch to the ventricular myocardium. *(From Heaven DJ, Till JA, Ho SY. Sudden death in a child with an unusual accessory connection. Europace. With permission.)*

The first histologic documentation of this pathway type was at autopsy after the sudden death of a pediatric patient with known Wolff-Parkinson-White syndrome.[46] A bandlike muscular structure extending from the underside of the right atrial appendage to the right ventricle was identified during dissection of the right AV groove (Fig. 25-6). Internally, this structure corresponded to a pouch with a muscular wall that coursed through the epicardial fat and ultimately continued into the ventricular myocardium about 5 mm from the annular insertion of the tricuspid valve.

Features suggestive of this pathway variant include (1) a preexcitation pattern indicative of a right anterior or right anterolateral pathway; (2) retrograde atrial activation recorded earlier in the right atrial appendage than at the tricuspid annulus; (3) a relatively long ventriculoatrial (VA) conduction time during tachycardia, consistent with a long epicardial AP course and earliest ventricular activation recorded more than 1 cm apical to the tricuspid annulus; (4) failed or transient loss of pathway conduction with RF delivery at the tricuspid annulus; and (5) the need for high-energy delivery within the appendage to achieve permanent pathway elimination.

Arruda and colleagues[47] reported three bidirectional APs, each with an atrial insertion at the atrial appendage, representing fewer than 0.5% of cases in their series of 646 patients undergoing catheter ablation for the Wolff-Parkinson-White syndrome. After unsuccessful RF catheter ablation, pathway conduction was eliminated in two patients by surgical separation of the atrial appendage from the ventricle at a site distant to the annulus, on the left side in one patient and on the right in the other. RF current eliminated conduction in the third patient when delivered to the tip of the right atrial appendage. Similarly, Milstein and associates[48] observed a bridge of tissue crossing from the base of the right atrial appendage into the fat pad overlying the base of the right ventricle at least 10 mm distal to the tricuspid annulus at surgery. Transection of this tissue resulted in loss of preexcitation.

Successful RF catheter ablation was also reported by Soejima and associates[49]; however, application of RF current within the appendage was limited by frequent impedance rises when a 4-mm-tip electrode ablation catheter was used. High-energy delivery and elimination of impedance rise was achieved by substitution of an 8-mm large-tip ablation catheter. Similar advantages are afforded by saline-irrigated catheters.

Nonfluoroscopic three-dimensional mapping has also facilitated catheter ablation.[50] In our laboratory, this approach was used in a patient with three prior unsuccessful ablation attempts. The baseline 12-lead ECG was suggestive of a right-sided AP (Fig. 25-7). At electrophysiology study, earliest atrial activation occurred within the right atrial appendage during orthodromic reentrant tachycardia and ventricular pacing (Fig. 25-8). Initial ablation attempts were made using a 4-mm-tip electrode ablation catheter, but successful pathway elimination within the right atrial appendage was achieved with a saline-irrigated catheter. Adding complexity to a technically challenging case was the presence of a broad pathway insertion or muscle "band" that acted like multiple discrete APs. This feature had undeniably contributed to the failure of previous attempts. Electroanatomic mapping proved invaluable by allowing remapping of earliest retrograde atrial activation after ablation of successive pathway "strands."

Epicardial elimination of an atrial appendage–to-ventricular pathway was reported in a patient who had undergone multiple unsuccessful endocardial attempts.[51] Transcutaneous instrumentation through a subxiphoid puncture permitted insertion of a 7-French (7F) deflectable catheter into the epicardial space. Epicardial mapping using a three-dimensional electroanatomic mapping system assisted localization of the earliest atrial activation and an AP potential at the anterior aspect of the heart. Delivery of low-power RF current at 20 W permanently eliminated pathway conduction without recurrence.

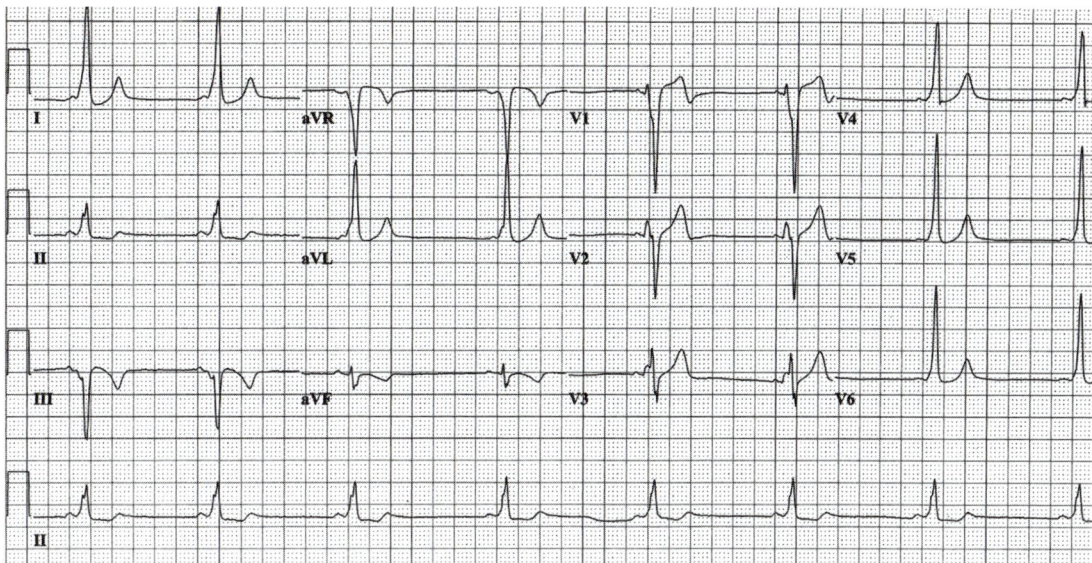

FIGURE 25-7. The 12-lead electrocardiogram during sinus rhythm was suggestive of a right-sided accessory pathway.

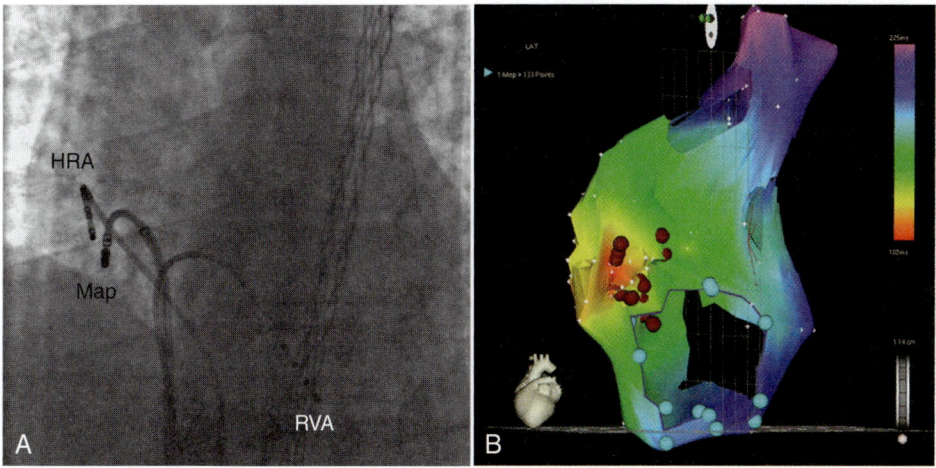

FIGURE 25-8. A, The mapping catheter identifies the site of successful pathway elimination within the right atrial appendage (left anterior oblique [LAO] projection). Elimination of conduction was achieved using a saline-irrigated ablation catheter allowing higher energy delivery producing a larger, deeper lesion. **B,** Electroanatomic right atrial activation map constructed during right ventricular pacing (LAO projection). Earliest retrograde atrial activation was localized to the right atrial appendage (*red area*). *Brown markers* indicate ablation sites. *Light blue markers* outline the tricuspid annulus. HRA, high right atrium; Map, ablation catheter; RVA, right ventricular apex.

Ablation of Accessory Pathways Associated with Structural Cardiac Abnormalities

APs are commonly associated with a variety of structural heart disorders, including Ebstein anomaly, a persistent left superior vena cava, hypertrophic cardiomyopathy, and L-transposition of the great vessels. Ebstein anomaly, although rare, is the most common congenital heart disease associated with the Wolff-Parkinson-White syndrome.[52]

Ebstein Anomaly

Ebstein anomaly is characterized by apical displacement of the tricuspid valve into the right ventricle, with atrialization of the area of right ventricle between the true tricuspid annulus and the anomalous attachments of the septal and posterior leaflets. The atrialized right ventricle is thinned and dilated, and the remainder of the ventricular chamber is diminished in size. Associated cardiac anomalies include a patent foramen ovale, atrial and ventricular septal defects, and right ventricular outflow tract obstruction.

About 20% to 30% of patients with Ebstein anomaly experience AV reciprocating tachycardia,[53,54] and the presence of preexcitation with atrial tachyarrhythmias is associated with sudden cardiac death. Right bundle branch block pattern is typically present because of posteroseptal conduction delay, and its absence should raise suspicion of the presence of an AP.

Accessory AV connections associated with Ebstein anomaly are usually right-sided and located along the dysplastic portion of the tricuspid annulus,[54] where abnormal endocardial electrograms are frequently recorded.[53] These connections, along with difficulty localizing the true AV groove fluoroscopically, the presence of multiple AV connections in up to 50% of patients,[52,54,55] and the presence of significant tricuspid regurgitation, hinder precise pathway localization and impair catheter stability and tissue contact. These factors ultimately account for the lower reported rates of success compared with catheter ablation of pathways not associated with this malformation. RF catheter ablation is not limited by previous surgical intervention because successful pathway elimination has been achieved in patients presenting with cardiac arrhythmias after tricuspid valve replacement.[56,57]

Cappato and coworkers[55] reported their experience of RF catheter ablation in 21 patients with symptomatic AV reciprocating tachycardia and Ebstein anomaly. Of the 34 APs identified, all were right-sided, with most located in the posteroseptal (9), posterior (10), and posterolateral (10) positions. Normal endocardial electrograms were recorded at all sites along the tricuspid annulus with successful abolition of all APs in 10 patients. In the remaining 11 patients, continuous fragmented electrical activity with multiple spikes was recorded along the surface of the atrialized ventricle in the posteroseptal and posterolateral regions, permitting conventional endocardial AP localization in only 1 patient. In all other patients, epicardial mapping through the right coronary artery was attempted. Selective right coronary angiography was performed to assess vessel size and an anatomic course confined to the AV groove. An over-the-wire system was used to advance a 2F multipolar catheter to map AP potentials and earliest anterograde ventricular or retrograde atrial activation during slow withdrawal of the catheter. The intracardiac mapping catheter was then positioned at the endocardial site that best matched the anatomic location and electrogram configuration recorded by the epicardial electrode pair, and RF energy was delivered. With this approach, APs were eliminated in 5 patients but did not assist pathway localization or could not be performed because of an adverse vessel course in the remaining patients.

Overall, Cappato and coworkers[55] reported successful AP ablation in 76% of patients, compared with their experience of 95% success for right-sided pathways in the absence of Ebstein anomaly. Factors identified that contributed to lower success included (1) abnormal and ill-defined tricuspid annulus anatomy with resultant catheter instability and poor tissue contact, and (2) recording of fractionated activation potentials at the atrialized ventricle, impairing the ability to identify AP potentials and the site of earliest antegrade ventricular and retrograde atrial activation.

In another reported series of five patients,[58] the importance of localization of the "electrical" AV ring, where balanced atrial and ventricular electrograms were recorded, was emphasized. The inferiorly displaced anatomic annulus was initially mapped and found to be devoid of balanced electrograms with short AV intervals or AP potentials. Repositioning of the ablation catheter at the true annulus, guided anatomically by insertion of a guidewire into the right coronary artery, identified electrograms in which successful RF pathway elimination was achieved in each patient. All the AV connections were located in the right posterior and posterolateral region.

Reich and colleagues[59] reported their pediatric experience of RF ablation in Ebstein anomaly, which included 59 patients with AP-mediated arrhythmias. Multiple APs occurred in 33% of the patients, and the pathways were right-sided in 96%. Acute success was achieved for 79% of right free wall pathways and 89% of right septal pathways. The reported rate of complications was low and included one patient who required permanent pacemaker implantation because of the development of complete heart block. Coronary artery occlusion after AP ablation has been reported in two pediatric patients with Ebstein anomaly.[60]

Electroanatomic mapping techniques may facilitate pathway localization after failed conventional mapping.[61] Construction of a right atrial activation map permits demarcation of the "electrical" AV junction, where balanced atrial and ventricular electrograms are recorded at the endocardium. This approach is analogous to use of the right coronary artery as an anatomic landmark but eliminates the need for coronary arterial instrumentation and its associated risks.

Persistent Left Superior Vena Cava

Failure of involution of the left cardinal vein during embryologic development results in a persistent left superior vena cava (LSVC). It is the most common systemic venous anomaly, occurring with an incidence of 0.5% in the general population[62] and in 4% of patients with congenital heart disease.[63] Associated cardiac anomalies include atrial septal defect, tetralogy of Fallot, AV canal defect, and partial anomalous pulmonary venous connection.[64]

In its pure form, the LSVC enters the left atrium between the appendage and the left pulmonary veins, providing direct transvenous access to the left side of the heart. Rarely, it is accompanied by complete absence of the right superior vena cava, permitting right heart access only by the femoral approach. Alternatively, an anastomosis with the CS results in an LSVC-to-CS fistula that acts as a conduit for systemic venous return to the right atrium. The CS in this instance is significantly dilated owing to increased blood flow. Infrequently, atresia of the CS ostium results in absence of a connection to the right atrium; consequently, coronary venous blood is directed systemically, to the left subclavian vein.

CS anomalies frequently coexist with AV APs,[65,66] occurring more frequently in patients with AP-mediated tachycardia (4.7%) than in patients with AVNRT (0.6%). Such abnormalities include vertical CS angulation, hypoplasia, narrowing, and persistent LSVC-to-CS fistula. Furthermore, CS abnormalities are anatomically related to the location of the APs and frequently preclude CS catheterization.

Although echocardiographic examination may demonstrate CS dilation, the presence of an LSVC-to-CS fistula is usually first discovered during CS instrumentation at electrophysiology study. When advanced, a left subclavian venous catheter travels in an anomalous inferior course in the left chest to the posterior aspect of the heart. Alternatively, passage of the catheter from the CS to the left subclavian vein is observed when the catheter is introduced through a femoral or right jugular vein approach (Fig. 25-9). The inability to advance the catheter into the CS should raise suspicion of associated atresia of the CS ostium.

Although asymptomatic, the presence of an LSVC-to-CS fistula may complicate catheter ablation of left-sided pathways. The cavernous nature of the vessel may

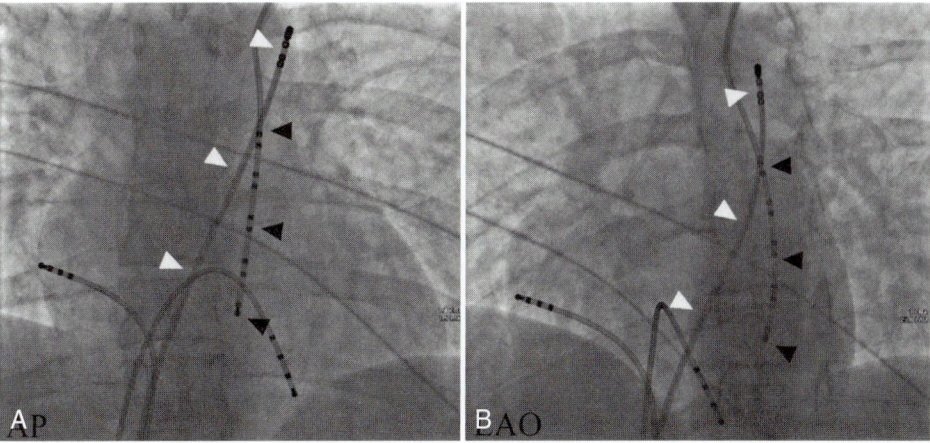

FIGURE 25-9. Fluoroscopic images of a persistent left superior vena cava and associated coronary sinus fistula in the anteroposterior (**A**) and left anterior oblique (**B**) projections. An anomalous inferior course in the left chest to the posterior aspect of the heart is identified as a decapolar mapping catheter is advanced from the left subclavian vein (*black arrowheads*). A deflectable catheter advanced through the ostium into the coronary sinus from the inferior vena cava (*white arrowheads*) confirms the presence of a fistulous connection. The cavernous nature of the coronary sinus is suggested by the distance separating the catheters, indicated by *arrows*. Unsuccessful passage of a guidewire from the right subclavian vein to the right atrium confirmed associated absence of a right superior vena cava.

prohibit precise pathway localization because of excessive motion and poor electrode contact of the CS mapping catheter. Alternatively, the CS may be located at a site distant to the mitral annulus. Successful pathway ablation requires a modified approach.[67–71] Ultimately, if the CS cannot be used to guide ablation, a single-catheter technique with careful mapping of the mitral annulus is obligatory.

Ablation of Pathways with Atypical Configuration
Multiple Accessory Pathways
The reported incidence of multiple APs is 3% to 15%.[52,72–80] APs have been defined as multiple when they are separated at the AV junction by 1 to 3 cm based on an approximation of distance during catheter mapping; however, it is difficult to differentiate multiple pathways from those with broad atrial or ventricular insertions or an oblique course. Multiple pathways are typically located unilaterally and are most frequently two in number. Clinical variables associated with their presence include Ebstein anomaly[52,73,77–80] and a history of preexcited reciprocating tachycardia.[52,78,80] Several reports also suggest a higher incidence in patients with right free wall and posteroseptal AV connections,[52,74,77–79] possibly related to the presence of multiple discontinuities in the tricuspid annulus fibrosus.[81,82]

Notable electrophysiologic properties distinguish patients with multiple APs from those with a single pathway. Multiple pathways provide the substrate for complex reentrant circuits, potentially resulting in multiple atrial wavefronts and the development of atrial fibrillation during reciprocating tachycardia. In addition, shorter AP effective refractory periods and measured R-R intervals during atrial fibrillation (<250 milliseconds) are a reflection of superior AP conduction in these patients. The combination of enhanced pathway conduction with more frequent occurrence of atrial fibrillation potentially increases the risk for deterioration into ventricular fibrillation and sudden cardiac death.[78–80,83,84]

Multiple APs are identified during the electrophysiologic study by (1) the occurrence of different patterns of preexcitation during atrial pacing or atrial fibrillation with different delta wave morphologic and ventricular activation patterns; (2) different sites of atrial activation during right ventricular pacing or orthodromic reciprocating tachycardia; (3) preexcited tachycardia using a second pathway as the retrograde limb of the circuit; (4) mismatch between the atrial and ventricular ends of the AP as assessed by comparing antidromic and orthodromic reciprocating tachycardia (mismatch distance, >1 cm); and (5) change from orthodromic to antidromic reciprocating tachycardia, or vice versa.[72,78] Some pathways cannot be identified during the baseline study and become evident only during RF ablation after successful interruption of the dominant pathway.

Several published series have demonstrated safe and efficacious elimination of multiple pathways with success rates of 86% to 98%.[74–76,78] Many reports have shown rates of success equivalent to those in patients possessing a single pathway, but others have not.[75,77,79] Predictably, however, procedure duration, radiation exposure time, and number of ablation pulses have been significantly greater.[74,75,76,79] A higher rate of recurrent pathway conduction is also reported, ranging from 8% to 12%.[74,75,77–79]

From a practical standpoint, failure to recognize the existence of multiple pathways may result in primary ablation failure or recurrent tachycardia. A multipolar CS mapping catheter imparts detailed information on VA timing in addition to atrial and ventricular activation at multiple sites along the mitral annulus. This is invaluable during ablation of left-sided pathways, which are most frequently located at the posterior and lateral regions of the AV junction, within reach of the CS catheter. Therefore, subtle activation changes during ablation are easily recognizable (Fig. 25-10). Mapping of the tricuspid annulus with a multielectrode catheter is less convenient but can be achieved with a multipolar halo catheter positioned near the tricuspid annulus. Brief current applications in the presence of multiple pathways may be erroneously considered ineffective

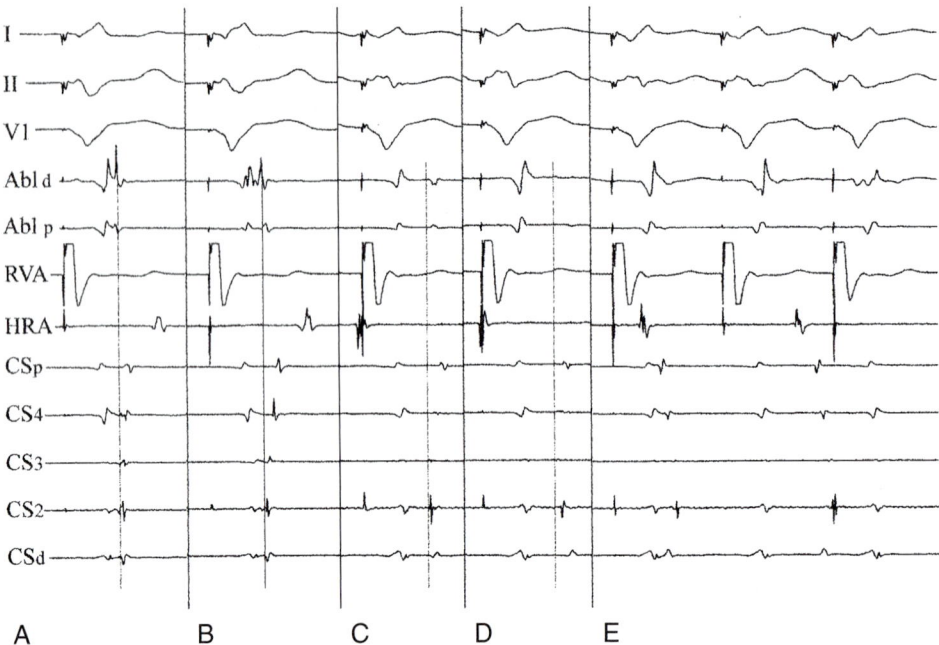

FIGURE 25-10. Radiofrequency ablation of multiple concealed accessory pathways. The ablation catheter is positioned adjacent the mitral annulus at the site of earliest recorded retrograde atrial activation (*vertical dashed lines*) during right ventricular pacing. Panels **A** to **D** demonstrate the intracardiac recordings preceding each current application. With successive pathway elimination, subtle changes in local ventriculoatrial (VA) interval and retrograde atrial activation sequence is observed. A total of four accessory pathways were identified with separate atrial insertions along the posterolateral and lateral mitral annulus. The development of ventriculoatrial block heralded success (**E**). Abl, ablation catheter (d, distal; p, proximal); CS, coronary sinus (p, proximal; d, distal); HRA, high right atrium; RVA, right ventricular apex.

if subtle activation changes, such as prolongation of local VA timing or changes in surface delta wave morphology, are unrecognized.

To reduce primary ablation failure, the following key points must be emphasized: (1) apparent failure of current application at a site of optimal electrogram timing and morphology should raise suspicion of the presence of multiple APs; (2) commitment to a full-duration current application at such a site should be undertaken with careful scrutiny of local VA timing or delta wave morphologic changes; and (3) meticulous remapping of the AV junction should be undertaken to identify any new site of early activation or presence of an AP potential, indicative of a distinct pathway. The procedure described earlier should be repeated until elimination of all pathways is achieved. Again, the importance of careful observation during RF application in such cases cannot be overemphasized.

Despite a meticulous approach, recurrent tachycardia may occur. Recurrent tachycardia, although most commonly caused by recurrence of AP conduction, should raise the possibility of other tachycardia mechanisms. Recurrence of clinical symptoms due to AP conduction occurred in 4.2% of cases in a series of 1280 patients who underwent ablation of an AP.[85] Manifestation of a previously unrecognized pathway caused symptom recurrence in 0.7% of patients and was subsequently ablated at an anatomic site distinct from the initial target. These "dormant" pathways were usually concealed and not identified at the time of initial study, suggesting intermittent conduction. Recurrence of tachycardia may also occur because of transient interruption of conduction, either by mechanical pressure of the mapping catheter or by delivery of RF current. These findings strongly support the recommendation

for a complete diagnostic electrophysiology study with isoproterenol to confirm elimination of pathway conduction after apparently successful ablation.

Oblique Accessory Pathways

Atrioventricular APs are usually regarded as following a course perpendicular to the AV groove, producing the shortest local ventriculoatrial interval at the site of the pathway during orthodromic AV reentrant tachycardia or ventricular pacing. Appropriately, this site is considered a favorable target for AP ablation.[86,87] However, studies suggest that APs frequently follow an oblique course.[88-91]

Jackman and colleagues[88,89] identified AP potentials associated with left free wall and posteroseptal APs using a multipolar mapping catheter inserted into the CS. By mapping AP potentials along the length of the CS, an oblique course was established in 87% of left-sided pathways; the atrial insertion was identified 4 to 30 mm (median, 14 mm) proximal (posterior) to its corresponding ventricular insertion.

Oblique APs are also identified by a change of the local VA or AV interval as a result of reversing the direction of paced ventricular and atrial wavefronts.[90] Such a change in local activation was observed in 87% of patients with a single left- or right-sided AP presenting for catheter ablation. Local atrial and ventricular activation was recorded using a multipolar (20-electrode) catheter placed in the CS or positioned around the tricuspid annulus in patients with a right free wall AP. Based on the site of earliest recorded retrograde atrial activation, two ventricular pacing sites were selected on either side, to produce a clockwise and counterclockwise wavefront to the AP. Similarly, two atrial pacing

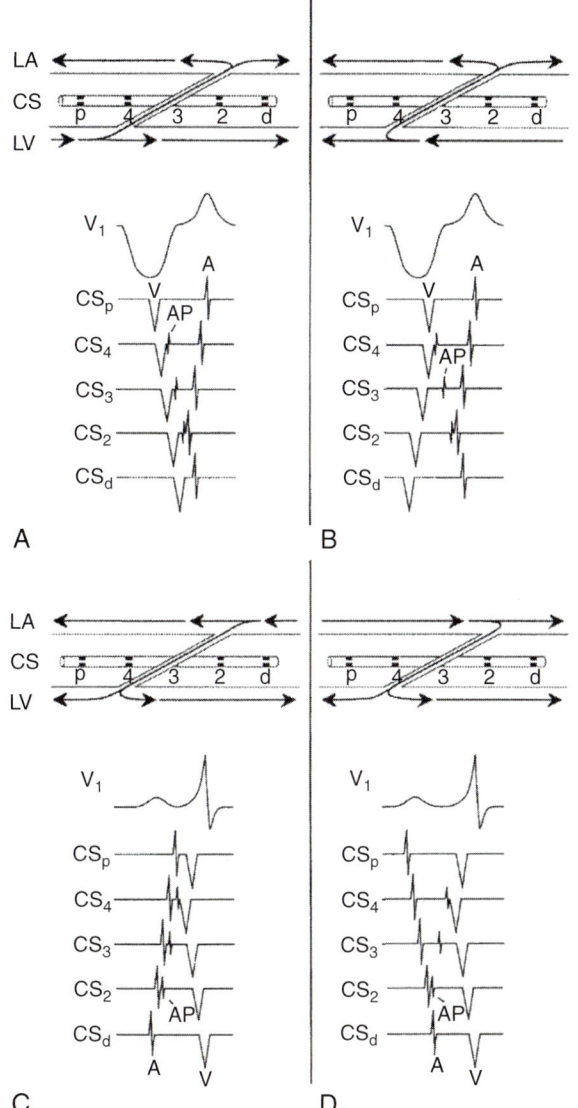

FIGURE 25-11. Activation of oblique accessory pathways. Schematic of antegrade and retrograde activation of an oblique left free wall accessory pathway (AP) from opposing directions. **A** and **B** demonstrate activation of the ventricular insertion from the proximal to distal and distal to proximal directions, respectively. **C** and **D** represent activation of the atrial insertion from the distal to proximal and proximal to distal directions, respectively. Note the separation of the components of the electrograms when the AP is activated from the direction opposite to the direction of conduction over the pathway. A, atrial potential; CS, coronary sinus; d, distal; LA, left atrium; LV, left ventricle; p, proximal; V, ventricular potential. *(From Otomo K, Gonzalez MD, Beckman KJ, et al. Reversing the direction of paced ventricular and atrial wavefronts reveals an oblique course in the accessory AV pathways and improves localization for catheter ablation. Circulation. 2001;104:550-556. With permission.)*

sites were selected to reverse the atrial wavefront along the annulus surrounding the site of earliest recorded antegrade ventricular activation.

A ventricular wavefront propagating from the direction of the ventricular end produced a short local-VA interval because activation along the AP proceeded to the earliest atrial activation site simultaneously with the ventricular wavefront (Fig. 25-11A, CS_2). Consequently, the ventricular potential often masked the AP potential and overlapped the atrial electrogram, masking earliest

atrial activation. Conversely, a wavefront propagating in the opposite direction resulted in a longer local-VA interval because the ventricular wavefront had to pass the site of earliest atrial activation before reaching the ventricular end of the AP (Fig. 25-11B, CS_2). This countercurrent wavefront was found to expose the AP potential and the atrial activation sequence, allowing identification of an appropriate ablation target. Similarly, atrial pacing in the direction of the atrial end resulted in a short local-AV interval (Fig. 25-11C, CS_4), and a countercurrent wavefront lengthened the local-AV interval, exposing the AP potential and ventricular activation sequence (Fig. 25-11D, CS_4).

In a study of concealed left-sided APs, Yamabe and colleagues[91] compared the ventricular insertion site with the corresponding atrial insertion, which was identified at the site of earliest recorded retrograde atrial activation within the CS. The ventricular insertion was identified at the site of shortest measured stimulus-to-atrial (Stim-A) interval during pacing delivered at mapping sites under the mitral valve leaflet. In 49% of patients, a number of observations indicated an oblique pathway course. First, the site of the shortest Stim-A interval did not coincide fluoroscopically with the site at which the earliest retrograde atrial activation was recorded. In these patients, the Stim-A interval at the shortest Stim-A site was significantly shorter than that at the corresponding ventricular side of earliest retrograde atrial activation. Second, during tachycardia, the interval between the onset of the surface QRS and the retrograde atrial electrogram (QRS-A interval) was longer at the shortest Stim-A site than at the site of earliest retrograde atrial activation. In all patients, elimination of pathway conduction was achieved by a single application of RF energy to the ventricular side of the mitral annulus at the site of the shortest identified Stim-A interval.

Successful elimination of pathway conduction can be achieved by application of RF current at or anywhere between the atrial and ventricular insertion sites, although targeting of an isolated AP potential is associated with the highest rate of ablation success (Fig. 25-12).[2,86,92] Oblique AV APs provide a challenge to ablation because of the inherent difficulties in identifying AP potentials due to obscured or overlapping electrograms and disparate myocardial insertions at the AV junction. An assumption of a perpendicular pathway course may lead to an inappropriate or suboptimal ablation site, underscoring the importance of selecting an ablation site guided by the appropriate data. Specifically, the atrial insertion site is best identified by the earliest recorded atrial activation during retrograde mapping, and the ventricular insertion site is best identified by the earliest recorded ventricular activation during antegrade mapping on the corresponding side of the annulus. Ablation here or at sites where discrete AP potentials are recorded will most likely yield success.

Atypical Accessory Pathways

Failure of RF catheter ablation may be caused by the complexity of the AP course. Pathways with an atypical course and those with connections to the His-Purkinje system are considered AP variants (Table 25-2; Fig. 25-13). The differential diagnosis of these connections is discussed in Chapter 24.

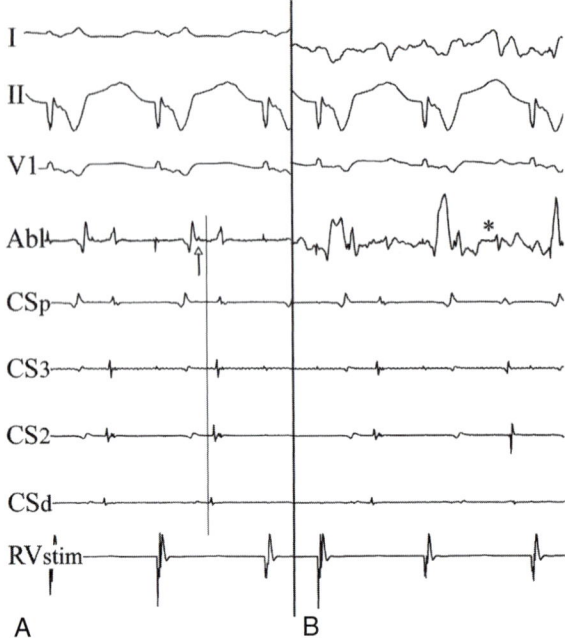

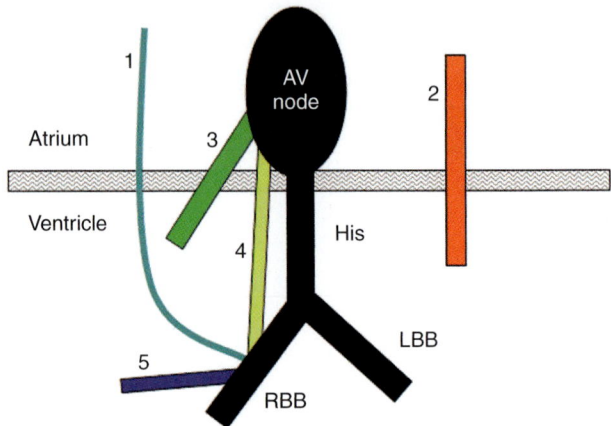

FIGURE 25-13. Schematic of variant endocardial accessory atrioventricular (AV) connections. (1) Atriofascicular pathway. (2) Atrioventricular pathway. (3) Nodoventricular pathway. (4) Nodofascicular pathway. (5) Fasciculoventricular pathway. LBB, left bundle branch; RBB, right bundle branch.

FIGURE 25-12. Intracardiac recordings during mapping and ablation of an oblique left-sided atrioventricular accessory pathway. **A,** An ablation catheter (Abl) positioned at the atrial aspect of the mitral annulus recording of retrograde activity during ventricular pacing. A discrete accessory pathway potential is recorded between the ventricular and atrial electrograms (*arrow*). Note that earliest retrograde atrial activation is recorded at the distal coronary sinus (*vertical line*), significantly earlier than recorded at the site of the ablation catheter. Atrial activation recorded at the ablation catheter coincides with activation at the proximal coronary sinus. **B,** Within seconds of radiofrequency current application at this site, permanent elimination of accessory pathway conduction occurred, indicated by a change in atrial activation sequence (*asterisk*). Following ablation, the discrete accessory pathway potential adjacent the ventricular electrogram was no longer recorded. Abl, ablation catheter; CS, coronary sinus (p, proximal; d, distal); RVstim, right ventricular apex.

TABLE 25-2
ACCESSORY PATHWAY VARIANTS
Accessory Pathways with His-Purkinje Connections
Atriofascicular
Atrium–His bundle
Nodoventricular, nodofascicular
Fasciculoventricular
Accessory Pathways with Atypical Course
Epicardial accessory pathways
Coronary sinus
Atrial appendage to ventricle
Aortomitral continuity
Other

One anatomically distinct pathway variant is an epicardial connection extending between the atrial appendage and the ventricular base.[46–48] In such cases, the AP traverses the epicardial fat from an atrial insertion at the floor of the left or right atrial appendage to the base of the ventricle, usually at a site distant to the tricuspid or mitral annulus. Endocardial RF current application at the AV junction is

either unrewarding or results in only transient elimination of pathway conduction. Mapping within the atrial appendage allows recording of retrograde atrial activation earlier than at the tricuspid annulus and may also identify the presence of an AP potential. Conventional mapping at annular locations will fail to identify an atrial or ventricular insertion site, leading to ablation failure.

Similarly, posteroseptal and left posterior APs may require ablation through the CS because of their epicardial location. Failure of RF energy at the endocardium should prompt a search within the CS for identification of high-frequency potentials, analogous to AP potentials, and atrial and ventricular activation occurring earlier than at the corresponding endocardial site. Successful elimination may be achieved by cautious application of RF current or by cryothermal ablation.

Rarely, an AP with a truly atypical course is encountered. This is best exemplified by an anteroseptal AP with a ventricular insertion at the outflow tract region, reported by our institution in 1992.[93] More than 10 years later, an anatomically identical pathway was encountered. An atypical AP, more specifically an atypical ventricular insertion site, was suggested by the surface ECG during preexcited atrial fibrillation. The preexcitation pattern did not conform to typical pathways at the AV ring but was suggestive of right ventricular outflow tract preexcitation, exhibiting left bundle branch block morphology with an inferior axis (Fig. 25-14).

In both instances, the AP course was confirmed by the standard electrophysiology study using pacing maneuvers and careful mapping to accurately identify the atrial and ventricular insertion sites. The ventricular insertion site of our most recent case was identified by earliest ventricular activation recorded at the anterior septal right ventricular outflow tract during CS pacing, where local activation preceded the surface delta wave by 10 milliseconds (Fig. 25-15). The atrial insertion was precisely localized to a site adjacent the AV node in the right anterior septum off the tricuspid annulus (1-o'clock position, left anterior oblique 30-degree projection), where the shortest stimulus-to-delta wave interval was identified (Fig. 25-16). Cryothermic mapping (reversible loss of preexcitation without AV

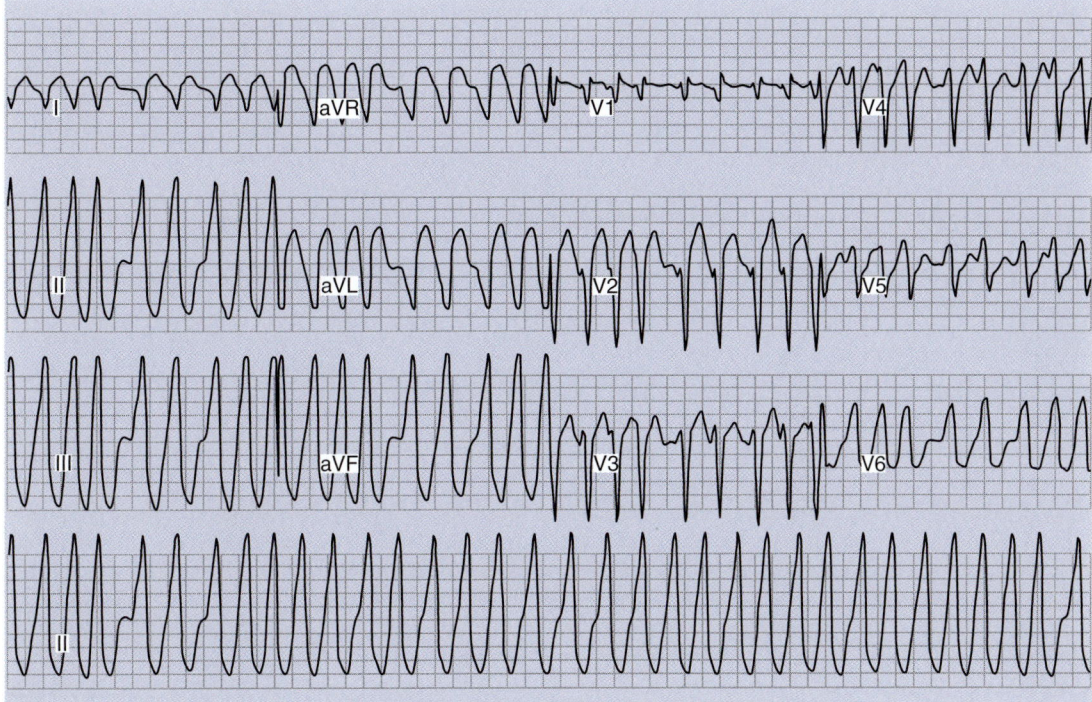

FIGURE 25-14. Twelve-lead electrogram recorded during preexcited atrial fibrillation. An unusual preexcitation pattern with precordial R-wave transition suggesting a right-sided accessory pathway but QS complexes in leads I and aVL consistent with a left lateral pathway. The left bundle branch block QRS morphology with inferior axis is suggestive of right ventricular outflow tract preexcitation.

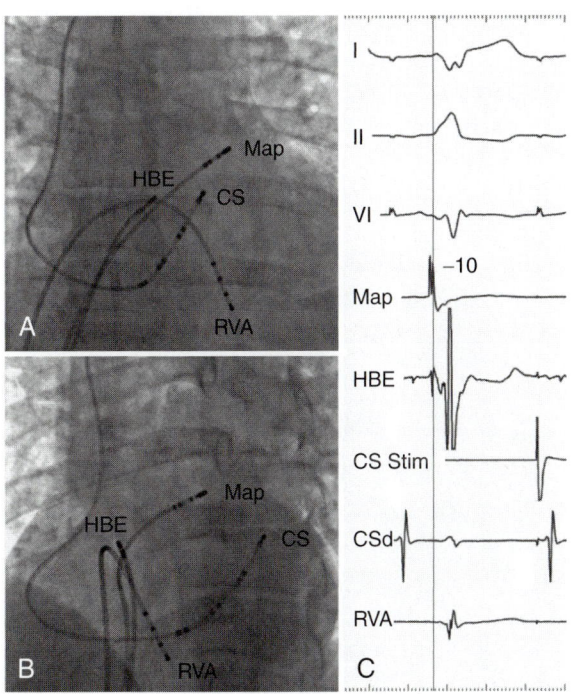

FIGURE 25-15. Ventricular insertion site of the accessory pathway in the anteroposterior (**A**) and left anterior oblique (**B**) projections identified by earliest ventricular activation during coronary sinus pacing. Intracardiac electrograms (**C**) indicate ventricular activation at the ablation catheter preceding the surface delta wave by 10 msec. CS, coronary sinus (Stim, pacing site; d, distal); HBE, His bundle electrogram; Map, ablation catheter; RVA, right ventricular apex.

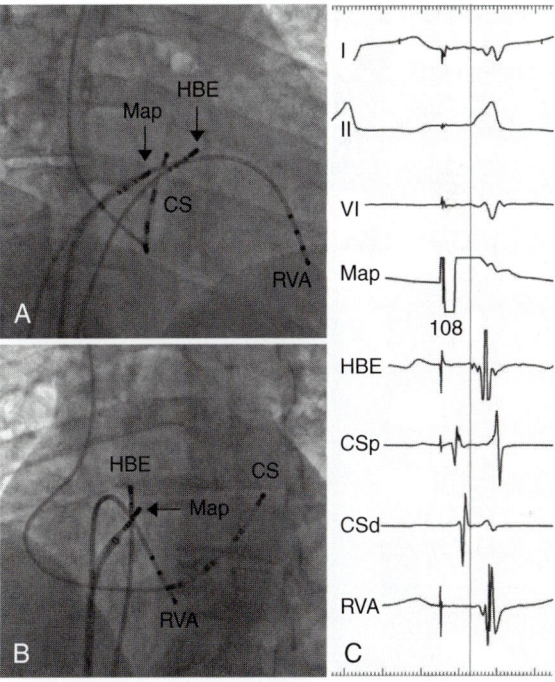

FIGURE 25-16. Atrial insertion site of the accessory pathway in the right anterior oblique (**A**) and left anterior oblique (**B**) projections identified during stimulus-to-delta pace mapping. Note the anatomic proximity of the accessory pathway to the site of the recorded His bundle electrogram. Intracardiac electrograms (**C**) indicate the shortest stimulus-to-delta interval identified (108 msec) at the site of successful elimination of accessory pathway conduction during ice mapping and radiofrequency ablation. CS, coronary sinus (p, proximal; d, distal); HBE, His bundle electrogram; Map, ablation catheter; RVA, right ventricular apex.

block) confirmed the atrial insertion site when cooled to –30°C, and RF current application at this site resulted in permanent pathway elimination.

Although uncommon, these examples illustrate the importance of a complete electrophysiology study and accurate interpretation of all available data. If endocardial mapping or ablation at the AV ring is unrewarding, consideration should be given to the presence of an atypical AP. In these instances, endocardial mapping at sites off the AV ring or within the CS may prove invaluable.

Another rare location for an accessory pathway is the aortomitral continuity (Fig. 25-17).[94] Anatomically, this junction comprises a continuous fibrous ring located between the noncoronary aortic cusp and the posterior portion of the left coronary cusp. Very rarely, muscular connections may cross this structure from the left atrium to left ventricle. The preexcitation pattern associated with these pathways usually shows positive or isoelectric delta waves in leads I and aVL, negative in V_1, and positive in the inferior leads.[94] Concealed pathways occur in this unusual position as well. The retrograde P waves during orthodromic reciprocating tachycardia are usually isoelectric or negative in leads I and aVL and positive in the inferior leads. Successful ablation has been reported through the retrograde aortic approach or transseptal approach, or within the sinus of Valsalva.

New Technologies

Saline-Cooled Radiofrequency Ablation

RF energy is typically delivered in a unipolar fashion to the myocardial surface through the electrode tip of an ablation catheter. The passage of alternating current through the tissues to a large dispersive patch applied to the patient's skin produces resistive heat at the tip-tissue interface. Conductive heating from the catheter tip through the tissue results in a thermal gradient within the adjacent myocardium. Tissue heating to more than 50°C results in irreversible myocardial tissue damage[95] and the production of permanent RF ablation lesions.

The temperature recorded at the tip-tissue interface is the most accurate predictor of RF lesion volume. As interface temperature is increased, deeper ablation lesions are produced. However, at an interface temperature of 100°C, plasma boiling and coagulum formation at the catheter tip result in a sudden impedance rise, loss of thermal conductivity, and loss of effective tissue heating.[96] Tip temperature monitoring aims to prevent excessive interfacial heating and loss of efficacy of energy delivery.

Power delivery is another important determinant of RF lesion size and is limited during conventional RF ablation by a tip-tissue interface temperature of 100°C. Greater RF energy delivery can be achieved by the use of saline-irrigated (cooled-tip) catheters. Cooling the electrode tip with infused normal saline reduces interfacial heating and shifts the point of maximal heating into the tissue rather than focusing it at the tissue surface.[97,98] As a result, deeper conductive heating occurs and produces deeper tissue lesions, an attribute essential for targets beyond the range of conventional RF lesions, such as epicardial APs. Large (8- to 10-mm) ablation electrodes provide a similar effect through passive convective cooling of the electrode by local blood flow.

Cryothermal Ablation

Cryoablation was first used as an alternative to surgical dissection of arrhythmic substrates during arrhythmia surgery in the 1970s. Evolution of cryoablation technologies has yielded catheter-based delivery systems providing a novel ablation modality and an alternative to RF energy for transvenous catheter ablation.

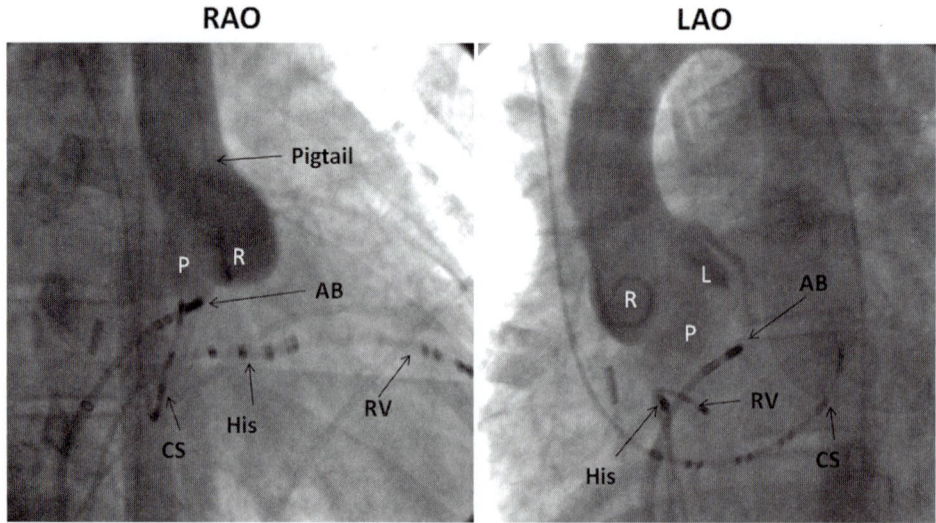

FIGURE 25-17. Catheter positions during successful ablation of a concealed accessory pathway at the aortomitral continuity. Aortogram is being performed through a pigtail catheter in the right aortic cusp (R). The ablation catheter (AB) is positioned between the left aortic cusp (L) and the posterior or noncoronary cusp (P) through transseptal access. CS, coronary sinus catheter; His, His bundle catheter; RV, right ventricular catheter. LAO, left anterior oblique; RAO, right anterior oblique.

Since its introduction, percutaneous cryoablation has been shown to be safe and effective for the treatment of supraventricular arrhythmias and atrial fibrillation.[99–102] In addition, properties unique to cryothermy offer potential advantages over RF energy in selected clinical applications.[103,104]

The clinical effects of cryothermy are achieved by cooling tissue to subzero temperatures. A cryoablation console controls the delivery of pressurized nitrous oxide gas from a storage cylinder to the tip of the ablation catheter; the gas then expands and causes cooling. The amount of heat and the speed at which it is removed allow for a permanent or transient effect in the target cells.

When tissue is cooled to −20°C, the formation of extracellular ice results in a hyperosmotic extracellular environment, forcing an outward shift of intracellular fluid. This leads to cell shrinkage, causing damage to the cell membrane and intracellular constituents. On rewarming, reversal of these effects results in cell swelling and disruption of the cell membrane. If the tissue is cooled to −40°C or lower, intracellular ice formation leads to irreversible destruction of intracellular organelles and cellular membranes, with ensuing cell death.

If cooling is limited to less extreme temperatures, the tissue effects at the cellular level are fully reversible. At temperatures between 0° and −10°C, loss of membrane transport capability and ion pump function occurs, prohibiting tissue depolarization and conduction. Reversible loss of electrophysiologic function during cooling permits testing of the functionality of a prospective ablation target before the creation of a permanent destructive lesion. This unique property of cryothermy is commonly known as *ice mapping*.

Cryothermy also affords exceptional electrode tip-tissue interface stability during mapping and ablation due to "cryoadherence." As the temperature is reduced below 0°C, progressive ice formation at the catheter tip causes its adherence to the adjacent tissue, ensuring secure contact of the tip to the target site during respiration and cardiac motion. Furthermore, cryolesions are associated with less endothelial disruption and thrombus formation than RF lesions,[105,106] and the safety of cryothermal ablation adjacent to coronary arteries has been demonstrated by extensive surgical experience and recent catheter-based studies using animal models.[41,42]

Impact of Location on Ablation of Accessory Pathways

The location of an AP may dictate the need for special consideration of the ablation approach to reduce potential complications. By definition, septal APs have an atrial insertion located within the triangle of Koch. Anteroseptal and mid-septal pathways course near the septum in close anatomic relationship to the His bundle and AV node. As a result, surgical division or RF catheter ablation is associated with an increased risk for AV block, reported to occur in up to 36% of patients.[107–109] Not infrequently, ablation of such pathways is postponed in the absence of drug-refractory symptoms or a short antegrade effective refractory period and rapidly conducted atrial fibrillation.

This difficulty notwithstanding, several studies have demonstrated effective RF interruption of these pathways with preservation of AV nodal conduction.[110–114] Conventional RF energy with step-up power titration has been successful with a low incidence of AV block.[113] Placement of a His bundle recording catheter as a reference point allows estimation of the distance between the ablation target and the AV node. Once a suitable target without a His bundle recording is identified, RF energy may be delivered, commencing at a power setting of 10 W. If pathway interruption has not occurred after 10 to 15 seconds, the power is increased by 5 W every 10 to 15 seconds, with continuous attention given to the earliest recognition of AV nodal impairment (development of atrium-to-His [AH] interval prolongation or AV block), accelerated nodal rhythm, or catheter displacement. Ablation commencing with a low power setting has been recommended by several authors to achieve the desired result while producing the smallest possible lesion.[111–113] The success of this approach and the frequently observed temporary conduction block after catheter-induced mechanical trauma suggest a superficial subendocardial location of these pathways.

An alternative and possibly safer approach for elimination of septal pathways is cryoablation. The well-established properties of cryothermy, including reversibility, small discrete lesion size, and cryoadherence, make this ablation modality particularly suitable if lesions are required adjacent to the AV node. Stability secures accurate lesion placement, and reversibility allows functional testing of the target before ablation, a combination that makes inadvertent permanent AV block an unlikely complication (Fig. 25-18). This technology intuitively offers significant advantages over RF energy in this setting.

Epicardial APs also warrant special consideration. Posteroseptal and left posterolateral pathways may be accessible only through the CS or by intrapericardial access. Application of RF current within the CS has been reported to be safe and successful; however, vascular complications, including venous thrombosis, stenosis, perforation, tamponade, and arterial injury, infrequently occur. Thorough mapping and the use of high standards in accepting suitable electrograms for ablation, including identification of AP potentials, can minimize complications by reducing the number of required RF current pulses. Risk may also be reduced by the use of lower delivered energy and temperature-guided ablation with conventional RF. Irrigated cooled-tip catheters may facilitate ablation by allowing delivery of higher energy within the confined space of the CS, preventing the impedance rises that may be observed with conventional catheters. Furthermore, selective coronary arterial angiography may reduce arterial injury by defining the anatomic relation of the ablation target to the coronary vessels.

The complications associated with RF energy delivery within the CS are all but eliminated when cryoablation is used. Cryothermy has been safely and successfully employed within the CS for elimination of posterolateral epicardial APs.[39] Preservation of the endothelial surface, less thrombus formation, and safe application adjacent to the coronary arteries are potential benefits offered by this modality compared with RF energy.

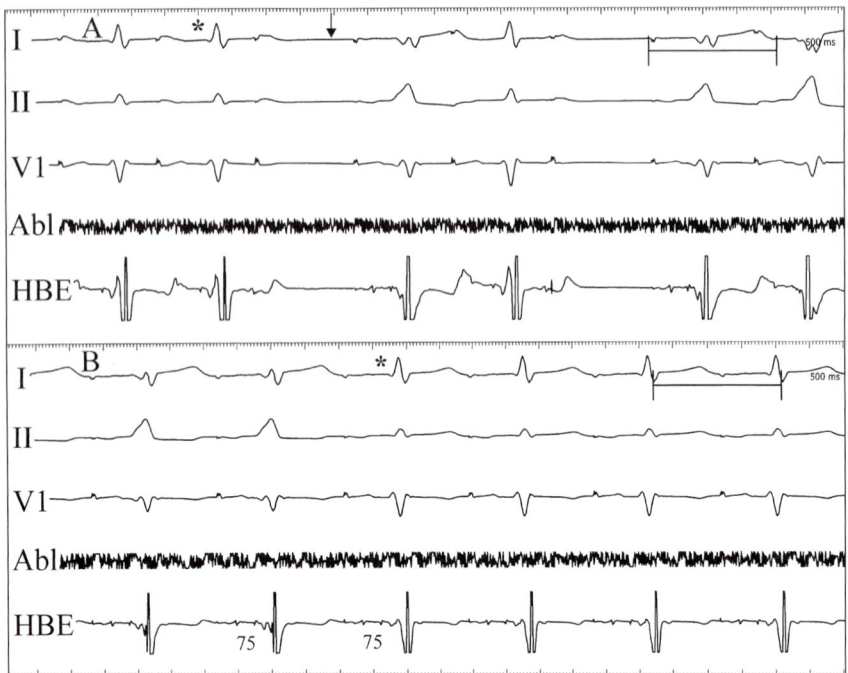

FIGURE 25-18. Cryoablation of an anteroseptal accessory pathway. **A,** During ice mapping (−30°C) at the atrial insertion site, intermittent loss of preexcitation (*asterisk*) and transient AV block (*arrow*) is observed with return of conduction at rewarming. **B,** Further ice mapping identified a site where loss of preexcitation occurred without atrioventricular block (*asterisk*) before permanent pathway elimination. Note that the atrial–His bundle interval (75 msec) remains unchanged with loss of preexcitation. Abl, ablation catheter; HBE, His bundle electrogram.

Failure to eliminate AP conduction with conventional RF often prompts substitution with a saline-irrigated catheter.[115] Ablation failure may relate to AP anatomy, such as a broad pathway insertion or an epicardial location. Conversely, suboptimal energy delivery may be contributory, as can occur with catheter instability or poor tissue contact. In these circumstances, successful ablation is often accomplished by enhanced delivery of RF energy to the tissue, which in turn produces larger and deeper endomyocardial lesions. However, the benefits of saline-irrigated RF ablation are not without risk. Higher energy delivery may permit subendocardial tissue temperature to rise above 100°C. Plasma boiling and tissue desiccation at these temperatures, frequently accompanied by an audible pop, may result in crater formation and wall rupture, particularly in thin-walled cavities such as the atria or outflow tracts. Accordingly, saline-irrigated RF ablation should be used judiciously, with power limited to 30 W[116,117] and at temperatures not exceeding 45°C,[118–120] to reduce the risk for "steam pop" and perforation.

Approach to the Patient Requiring Repeat Ablation

Primary failure or recurrent tachycardia after initial ablation success may necessitate a repeat ablation procedure. Patients may be referred from other laboratories or may undergo a subsequent attempt at the same institution. In any case, a systematic approach to identifying contributing factors and formulation of an appropriate ablation strategy are essential to improve the likelihood of success (Table 25-3).

Although the most frequent causes of primary ablation failure are technical, the contribution of "cognitive" failure must not be underestimated. Inaccurate pathway localization and tachycardia misdiagnosis are the next most common causes of failed ablation.[13] Consequently, a thorough review of all available information, including the clinical history, the 12-lead ECG during sinus rhythm and tachycardia, and findings of the initial electrophysiology study, is essential. Accompanying correspondence from the referring physician may document relevant technical information, including difficult target site access, catheter instability, or perinodal ablation.

Confirmation of the tachycardia diagnosis is the single most critical step in the management of repeat ablation. This is achieved only by completion of a full repeat diagnostic electrophysiology study. New findings, incongruent with preceding data, may provide grounds for a previously failed attempt. If the tachycardia mechanism is verified, localization of the AP and repeat ablation should be undertaken. *Importantly, maximal preexcitation during sinus rhythm and lack of tachycardia inducibility should raise suspicion of previous inadvertent AV nodal injury, particularly in the setting of anteroseptal or mid-septal APs.* Consequently, demonstration of intact AV nodal function during the baseline study is crucial because the anterograde conducting AP may represent the only electrical connection between the atrium and ventricle, and its elimination will result in complete AV block and pacemaker dependence.

Instability and difficult target site access may be overcome by the use of purpose-specific long intravascular sheaths, ablation catheters of different reach or distal configuration, an alternative ablation approach (e.g., retrograde aortic versus transseptal), or attempt by a second operator. Larger and deeper ablation lesions produced by saline-irrigated catheters may allow elimination of epicardial APs

TABLE 25-3

APPROACH TO FAILED ABLATION AT THE SITE OF AN "IDEAL" ELECTROGRAM

Reevaluate Electrogram Interpretation

Presence of far-field activity on the electrogram before the rapid deflection suggests need for more accurate pathway localization
Use a unipolar electrogram to help determine ideal timing compared with the rapid deflection of the bipolar electrogram
Possible misinterpretation of closely approximated A and V electrograms
Assess and compare local A and V activation during sinus rhythm and A or V pacing
Brush back and forth from A to V to clarify timing of A and V activation (especially at the right free wall, where A and V may be superimposed*)
Pacing maneuvers to dissociate the putative AP potential from A and V electrograms (useful in the presence of fractionated electrograms)

Instability

Remap using a long sheath or different catheter curve to improve stability
Consider an alternative approach: SVC versus IVC, retrograde aortic versus transseptal
Entrainment during AVRT to prevent dislodgment with RF termination of tachycardia
Cryoablation

Consider an Alternative Target

Posteroseptal pathways
May be left-sided or epicardial, possibly accessible through the coronary sinus
Atypical accessory pathways and nonannular AV pathways
Map at sites away from the AV annulus (e.g., appendage, outflow tract)

High-Risk Target

Ablation target adjacent to the AV node or within the coronary sinus
Consider cryothermal ablation

Unrecognized Change

Possible multiple accessory pathways
Commit to full-duration energy application if subtle changes in electrogram timing or QRS morphology are observed, then remap and repeat

Transient Elimination of AP Conduction

Time to elimination is a good indicator of ablation catheter proximity to the pathway
Instability—as above
Multiple accessory pathways
Carefully reevaluate preexcitation pattern or retrograde atrial activation sequence
"Deep" or epicardial location
Consider using a saline-irrigated catheter

* See Figure 25-1.

A, atrium; AP, accessory pathway; AV, atrioventricular; AVRT, atrioventricular reentrant tachycardia; IVC, inferior vena cava; RF, radiofrequency energy; SVC, superior vena cava; V, ventricle.

or permit delivery of RF energy within a confined space, such as the CS. In addition, cryoablation may afford a degree of safety for ablation targets in high-risk locations, such as those adjacent to the AV node or within the CS and its branches.

Fortunately, failures to eliminate AP conduction and recurrence of tachycardia after apparently successful ablation are infrequent outcomes of therapeutic intervention for AV reentrant tachycardia. In these cases, perseverance and patience usually prevail.

References

1. Hindricks G, the Multicentre European Radiofrequency Survey (MERFS). Complications of radiofrequency catheter ablation of arrhythmias: the Multicentre European Radiofrequency Survey (MERFS) of the Working Group on Arrhythmias of the European Society of Cardiology. *Eur Heart J.* 1993;14:1644–1653.
2. Jackman WM, Wang X, Friday KJ, et al. Catheter ablation of atrioventricular accessory pathways (Wolff-Parkinson-White syndrome) by radiofrequency current. *N Engl J Med.* 1991;324:1605–1611.
3. Kuck KH, Schluter M, Geiger M, et al. Radiofrequency current catheter ablation of accessory atrioventricular pathways. *Lancet.* 1991;337:1557–1561.
4. Lesh MD, Van Hare GF, Schamp DJ, et al. Curative percutaneous catheter ablation of using radiofrequency energy for accessory pathways in all locations: results in 100 consecutive patients. *J Am Coll Cardiol.* 1992;19:1303–1309.
5. Calkins H, Yong P, Miller JM, et al. Catheter ablation of accessory pathways, atrioventricular nodal reentrant tachycardia, and the atrioventricular junction: final results of a prospective, multicentre clinical trial. *Circulation.* 1999;99:262–270.
6. Borgreffe M, Budde T, Podczeck A, et al. High frequency alternating current ablation of an accessory pathway in humans. *J Am Coll Cardiol.* 1987;10:576–582.
7. Schluter M, Geiger M, Siebels J, et al. Catheter ablation using radiofrequency current to cure symptomatic patients with tachyarrhythmias related to an accessory atrioventricular accessory pathway. *Circulation.* 1991;84:1644–1661.
8. Calkins H, Langberg J, Sousa J, et al. Radiofrequency catheter ablation of accessory atrioventricular connections in 250 patients: abbreviated therapeutic approach to Wolff-Parkinson-White syndrome. *Circulation.* 1992;85:1337–1346.
9. Warin JF, Haissaguerre M, D'ivernois C, et al. Catheter ablation of accessory pathways: technique and results in 248, patients. *Pacing Clin Electrophysiol.* 1990;13:1609–1614.
10. Kay GN, Epstein AE, Dailey SM, et al. Role of radiofrequency ablation in the management of supraventricular arrhythmias: experience in 760 consecutive patients. *J Clin Electrophysiol.* 1993;4:372–389.
11. Leather RA, Leitch JW, Klein GJ, et al. Radiofrequency catheter ablation of accessory pathways: a learning experience. *Am J Cardiol.* 1991;68:1651–1655.
12. Li HG, Klein GJ, Zardini M, et al. Radiofrequency catheter ablation of accessory pathways during entrainment of AV reentrant tachycardia. *Pacing Clin Electrophysiol.* 1994;17:590–594.
13. Morady F, Strickberger SA, Man KC, et al. Reasons for prolonged or failed attempts at radiofrequency catheter ablation of accessory pathways. *J Am Coll Cardiol.* 1996;27:683–689.

14. Xie B, Heald SC, Camm AJ, et al. Radiofrequency catheter ablation of accessory atrioventricular: primary failure and recurrence of conduction. *Heart.* 1977;77:363–368.

15. Twidale N, Wang XZ, Beckman KJ, et al. Factors associated with recurrence of accessory pathway conduction after radiofrequency catheter ablation. *Pacing Clin Electrophysiol.* 1991;14:2042–2048.

16. Ho S, Sánchez-Quintana D, Becker AE. A review of the coronary venous system: a road less travelled. *Heart Rhythm.* 2004;1:107–112.

17. Lüdinghausen VM, Ohmachi N, Boot C. Myocardial coverage of the coronary sinus and related veins. *Clin Anat.* 1992;5:1–15.

18. Chauvin M, Shah DC, Haïssaguerre M, et al. The anatomic basis of connections between the coronary sinus musculature and the left atrium in humans. *Circulation.* 2000;101:647–652.

19. Ho SY, Sánchez-Quintana D, Cabrera JA, Anderson RH. Anatomy of the left atrium: implications for radiofrequency ablation of atrial fibrillation. *J Cardiovasc Electrophysiol.* 1999;10:1525–1533.

20. Antz M, Otomo K, Arruda M, et al. Electrical conduction between the right atrium and the left atrium via the musculature of the coronary sinus. *Circulation.* 1998;98:1790–1795.

21. Gerlis LM, Davies MJ, Boyle R, et al. Pre-excitation due to accessory sinoventricular connections associated with coronary aneurysms: a report of two cases. *Br Heart J.* 1985;53:314–322.

22. Segni ED, Siegal A, Katzenstein M, et al. Congenital diverticulum of the heart arising from the coronary sinus. *Br Heart J.* 1986;56:380–384.

23. Guiraudon GM, Guiraudon CM, Klein GJ, et al. The coronary sinus diverticulum: a pathologic entity associated with Wolff-Parkinson-White syndrome. *Am J Cardiol.* 1988;62:733–735.

24. Ho SY, Russell G, Roland E. Coronary venous aneurysms and accessory atrioventricular connections. *Br Heart J.* 1988;60:348–351.

25. Sun Y, Arruda M, Otomo K, et al. Coronary sinus-ventricular accessory connections producing posteroseptal and left posterior accessory pathways: incidence and electrophysiological identification. *Circulation.* 2002;106:1362–1367.

26. Takahashi A, Shah DC, Jais P, et al. Specific electrocardiographic features of manifest coronary vein posteroseptal accessory pathways. *J Cardiovasc Electrophysiol.* 1998;9:1015–1025.

27. Haïssaguerre M, Gaita F, Fischer B, et al. Radiofrequency catheter ablation of left lateral accessory pathways via the coronary sinus. *Circulation.* 1992;86:1464–1468.

28. Beukema WP, Van Dessel PF, Van Hemel NM, Kingma JH. Radiofrequency catheter ablation of accessory pathways associated with a coronary sinus diverticulum. *Eur Heart J.* 1994;15:1415–1418.

29. Villacastin J, Merino JL, Almendral J, et al. Radiofrequency ablation of a posteroseptal accessory pathway associated with coronary sinus diverticulum. *Rev Esp Cardiol.* 1995;48:638–641.

30. Kleinman D, Winters SL. Successful catheter ablation of an inferoseptal accessory pathway within the coronary sinus in a patient with a previously unsuccessful attempt at surgical interruption: coronary sinus ablation for Wolff-Parkinson-White syndrome. *J Electrocardiol.* 1996;29:55–60.

31. Takatsuki S, Mitamura H, Ieda M, Ogawa S. Accessory pathway associated with an anomalous coronary vein in a patient with Wolff-Parkinson-White syndrome. *J Cardiovasc Electrophysiol.* 2001;12:1080–1082.

32. Kusano KF, Morita H, Fujimoto Y, et al. Catheter ablation of an epicardial accessory pathway via the middle cardiac vein guided by monophasic action potential recordings. *Europace.* 2001;3:164–167.

33. Davidson NC, Cooper MJ, Ross DL. Radiofrequency catheter ablation of a posteroseptal accessory pathway with two diverticula of the coronary sinus. *Circulation.* 2001;104:240–241.

34. Lewalter T, Yang A, Schwab JO, Lüderitz B. Accessory pathway catheter ablation inside the neck of a coronary sinus diverticulum. *J Cardiovasc Electrophysiol.* 2003;14:1386.

35. Hussin A, Sanders P, Kistler PM, et al. Accessory pathway in left inferoposterior diverticulum masquerading as left posterior pathway due to conduction over coronary sinus to left atrium connection. *J Cardiovasc Electrophysiol.* 2003;14:403–406.

36. Hartzler GO, Giorgi LV, Diehl AM, Hamaker WR. Right coronary spasm complicating electrode catheter ablation of a right lateral accessory pathway. *J Am Coll Cardiol.* 1985;6:250–253.

37. Chatelain P, Zimmermann M, Weber R, et al. Acute coronary occlusion secondary to radiofrequency catheter ablation of a left lateral accessory pathway. *Eur Heart J.* 1995;16:859–861.

38. de Paola AA, Leite LR, Arfelli E. Mechanical reperfusion of acute right coronary artery occlusion after radiofrequency catheter ablation and long term follow-up angiography. *J Invasive Cardiol.* 2003;15:173–175.

39. Gaita F, Paperini L, Riccardi R, Ferraro A. Cryothermic ablation within the coronary sinus of an epicardial posterolateral accessory pathway. *J Cardiovasc Electrophysiol.* 2002;13:1160–1163.

40. Klein GJ, Harrison L, Ideker RF, et al. Reaction of the myocardium to cryosurgery: electrophysiology and arrhythmogenic potential. *Circulation.* 1979;59:364–372.

41. Skanes AC, Jones DL, Teefy P, et al. Safety and feasibility of cryothermal ablation within the mid- and distal coronary sinus. *J Cardiovasc Electrophysiol.* 2004;15:1319–1323.

42. Yagi T, Nakagawa H, Khammar GS, et al. Safety and efficacy of cryo-ablation in the canine coronary sinus [abstract]. *Circulation.* 2001;104:II-620.

43. Saad EB, Marrouche NF, Cole CR, Natale A. Simultaneous epicardial and endocardial mapping of a left-sided posteroseptal accessory pathway associated with a large coronary sinus diverticulum: successful ablation by transection of the diverticulum's neck. *Pacing Clin Electrophysiol.* 2002;25:1524–1526.

44. Sapp J, Soejima K, Couper G, Stevenson W. Electrophysiology and anatomic characterization of an epicardial accessory pathway. *J Cardiovasc Electrophysiol.* 2001;12:1411–1414.

45. Anderson RH, Ho SY. Anatomy of the atrioventricular junctions with regard to ventricular preexcitation. *Pacing Clin Electrophysiol.* 1997;20:2072–2076.

46. Heaven DJ, Till JA, Ho SY. Sudden death in a child with an unusual accessory connection. *Europace.* 2000;2:224–227.

47. Arruda M, McClelland J, Beckman K, et al. Atrial appendage-ventricular connections: a new variant of preexcitation [abstract]. *Circulation.* 1994;90:I-126.

48. Milstein S, Dunnigan A, Tang C, Pineda E. Right atrial appendage to right ventricle accessory atrioventricular pathway: a case report. *Pacing Clin Electrophysiol.* 1997;20:1877–1880.

49. Soejima K, Mitamura H, Miyazaki T, et al. Catheter ablation of accessory atrioventricular connection between right atrial appendage to right ventricle: a case report. *J Cardiovasc Electrophysiol.* 1998;9:523–528.

50. Goya M, Takahashi A, Nakagawa H, Iesaka Y. A case of catheter ablation of accessory atrioventricular connection between the right atrial appendage and right ventricle guided by a three-dimensional electroanatomic mapping system. *J Cardiovasc Electrophysiol.* 1999;10:1112–1118.

51. Lam C, Schweikert R, Kanagaratham L, Natale A. Radiofrequency ablation of a right atrial appendage-ventricular accessory pathway by transcutaneous epicardial instrumentation. *J Cardiovasc Electrophysiol.* 2000;11:1170–1173.

52. Colavita PG, Packer DL, Pressley JC, et al. Frequency, diagnosis and clinical characteristics of patients with multiple accessory atrioventricular pathways. *Am J Cardiol.* 1987;59:601–606.

53. Kastor JA, Goldreyer BN, Josephson ME, et al. Electrophysiologic characterization of Ebstein's anomaly of the tricuspid valve. *Circulation.* 1975;52:987–995.

54. Smith WM, Gallagher JJ, Kerr CR, et al. The electrophysiologic basis and management of symptomatic and recurrent tachycardia in patients with Ebstein's anomaly of the tricuspid valve. *Am J Cardiol.* 1982;49:1223–1234.

55. Cappato R, Schluter M, Weiss C, et al. Radiofrequency current catheter ablation of accessory atrioventricular pathways in Ebstein's anomaly. *Circulation.* 1996;94:376–383.

56. Kocheril AG, Rosenfeld LE. Radiofrequency ablation of an accessory pathway in a patient with corrected Ebstein's anomaly. *Pacing Clin Electrophysiol.* 1994;17:986–990.

57. Ai T, Horie M, Washizuka T, et al. Successful radiofrequency current catheter ablation of accessory atrioventricular pathway after tricuspid replacement in Ebstein's anomaly. *Jpn Circ J.* 1998;62:791–793.

58. Okishige K, Azegami K, Goseki Y, et al. Radiofrequency ablation of tachyarrhythmias in patients with Ebstein's anomaly. *Int J Cardiol.* 1997;60:171–180.

59. Reich J, Auld D, Hulse JE, et al. The pediatric radiofrequency ablation registry's experience with Ebstein's anomaly. *J Cardiovasc Electrophysiol.* 1998;9:1370–1377.

60. Bertram H, Bökenkamp R, Peuster M, et al. Coronary artery stenosis after radiofrequency catheter ablation of accessory atrioventricular pathways in children with Ebstein's malformation. *Circulation.* 2001;103:538–543.

61. Ai T, Ikeguchi S, Watanuki M, et al. Successful radiofrequency current catheter ablation of accessory atrioventricular pathway in Ebstein's anomaly using electroanatomic mapping. *Pacing Clin Electrophysiol.* 2002;25:374–375.

62. Steinberg I, Dubilier W, Lucas D. Persistence of left superior vena cava. *Dis Chest.* 1953;24:479–488.

63. Fraser RS, Dvorkin J, Rossall RE, Eidem R. Left superior vena cava: a review of associated congenital heart lesions, catheterisation data, and roentgenologic findings. *Am J Med.* 1961;31:771–776.

64. Bjerregaard P, Laursen HB. Persistent left superior vena cava. *Acta Paediatr Scand.* 1980;69:105–108.

65. Chiang CE, Chen SA, Yang CR, et al. Major coronary sinus abnormalities: identification of occurrence and significance in radiofrequency ablation of supraventricular tachycardia. *Am Heart J.* 1994;127:1279–1289.

66. Weiss C, Cappato R, Willems S, et al. Prospective evaluation of coronary sinus anatomy in patients undergoing electrophysiology study. *Clin Cardiol.* 1999;22:537–543.

67. Ma CS, Hu D, Fang Q, et al. Catheter ablation of a left-sided accessory pathway with a left superior vena cava. *Am Heart J.* 1995;130:613–615.

68. Takatsuki S, Mitamura H, Ieda M, Ogawa S. Accessory pathway associated with an anomalous coronary vein in a patient with Wolff-Parkinson-White syndrome. *J Cardiovasc Electrophysiol.* 2001;12:1080–1082.

69. Kursaklioglu H, Kose S, Barcin C, et al. Radiofrequency catheter ablation of a left lateral accessory pathway in a patient with persistent left superior vena cava. *Heart Dis.* 2002;4:162–165.

70. Chiou CW, Chen SA, Chiang CE, et al. Radiofrequency catheter ablation of paroxysmal supraventricular tachycardia in patients with congenital heart disease. *Int J Cardiol.* 1995;50:143–151.

71. O'Callaghan WG, Colavita PG, Kay GN, et al. Persistent left superior vena cava: localization of site of ectopic atrial pacemaker and associated atrioventricular accessory pathway. *Am Heart J.* 1985;111:1200–1202.

72. Gallagher JJ, Sealy WC, Kasell J, Wallace AG. Multiple accessory pathways in patients with the pre-excitation syndrome. *Circulation.* 1976;54:571–591.

73. Iwa T, Magara T, Watanabe Y, et al. Interruption of multiple accessory pathways in patients with the Wolff-Parkinson-White syndrome. *Ann Thorac Surg.* 1980;30:313–325.
74. Chen SA, Chiang CE, Chiou CW, et al. Reappraisal of radiofrequency ablation of multiple accessory pathways. *Am Heart J.* 1993;125:760–771.
75. Yeh SJ, Wang CC, Wen MS, et al. Radiofrequency ablation in multiple accessory pathways and the physiologic implications. *Am J Cardiol.* 1993;15:1174–1180.
76. Wang LX, Ding YS, Hu DY. Endocardial mapping and radiofrequency catheter ablation of multiple atrioventricular accessory pathways. *Chin Med J.* 1994;107:83–87.
77. Iturralde Torres P, Lara S, Picos Bovio E, et al. Radiofrequency ablation in multiple accessory pathways. *Arch Inst Cardiol Mex.* 1996;66:390–399.
78. Huang JL, Chen SA, Tai CT, et al. Long-term results of radiofrequency catheter ablation in patients with multiple accessory pathways. *Am J Cardiol.* 1996;78:1375–1379.
79. Iturralde P, Guevara-Valdivia M, Rodríguez-Chàvez L, et al. Radiofrequency ablation of multiple accessory pathways. *Europace.* 2002;4:273–280.
80. Weng KP, Wolff GS, Young ML. Multiple accessory pathways in paediatric patients with Wolff-Parkinson-White syndrome. *Am J Cardiol.* 2003;91:1178–1183.
81. Verduyn Lunel AA. Significance of annulus fibrosus of heart in relation to AV conduction and ventricular activation in cases of Wolff-Parkinson-White syndrome. *Br Heart J.* 1972;34:1263–1271.
82. Becker AE, Anderson RH, Durrer D, Wellens HJ. The anatomic substrates of Wolff-Parkinson-White syndrome. *Circulation.* 1978;57:870–879.
83. Klein GJ, Bashore TM, Sellers TD, et al. Ventricular fibrillation in the Wolff-Parkinson-White syndrome. *N Engl J Med.* 1979;301:1080–1085.
84. Teo WS, Klein GJ, Guiraudon GM, et al. Multiple accessory pathways in the Wolff-Parkinson-White syndrome as a risk factor for ventricular fibrillation. *Am J Cardiol.* 1991;67:889–891.
85. Schluter M, Cappato R, Ouyang F, et al. Clinical recurrences after successful accessory pathway ablation: the role of "dormant" accessory pathways. *J Cardiovasc Electrophysiol.* 1997;8:1366–1372.
86. Silka MJ, Kron J, Halperin BD, et al. Analysis of local electrogram characteristics correlated with successful radiofrequency catheter ablation of accessory atrioventricular accessory pathways. *Pacing Clin Electrophysiol.* 1992;15:1000–1007.
87. Swartz JF, Tracy CM, Fletcher RD. Radiofrequency endocardial catheter ablation of accessory atrioventricular pathway atrial insertion sites. *Circulation.* 1993;87:487–499.
88. Jackman WM, Friday KJ, Yeung-Lai-Wah JA, et al. New catheter technique for recording left free-wall accessory atrioventricular pathway activation: Identification of pathway fiber orientation. *Circulation.* 1988;78:598–611.
89. Jackman WM, Friday KJ, Fitzgerald DM, et al. Localization of left free-wall and posteroseptal accessory atrioventricular pathways by direct recording of accessory pathway activation. *Pacing Clin Electrophysiol.* 1989;12:204–214.
90. Otomo K, Gonzalez MD, Beckman KJ, et al. Reversing the direction of paced ventricular and atrial wavefronts reveals an oblique course in the accessory AV pathways and improves localization for catheter ablation. *Circulation.* 2001;104:550–556.
91. Yamabe H, Shimasaki Y, Honda O, et al. Localization of the ventricular insertion site of concealed left-sided accessory pathways using ventricular pace mapping. *Pacing Clin Electrophysiol.* 2002;25:940–950.
92. Calkins H, Kim YN, Schmaltz S, et al. Electrogram criteria for identification of appropriate target sites for radiofrequency catheter ablation of accessory atrioventricular accessory connections. *Circulation.* 1992;85:565–573.
93. Teo WS, Guiraudon G, Klein GJ, et al. A unique preexcitation pattern related to an atypical anteroseptal accessory pathway. *Pacing Clin Electrophysiol.* 1992;15:1696–1701.
94. Tada H, Naito S, Taniguchi K, Nogami A. Concealed left anterior accessory pathways: two approaches for successful ablation. *J Cardiovasc Electrophysiol.* 2003;14:204–208.
95. Haines DE. The biophysics of radiofrequency catheter ablation in the heart: the importance of temperature monitoring. *Pacing Clin Electrophysiol.* 1993;16:586–591.
96. Haines DE, Verow AF. Observations on electrode tissue interface temperature and effect on electrical impedance during radiofrequency ablation of ventricular myocardium. *Circulation.* 1990;82:1034–1038.
97. Nakagawa H, Yamanashi WS, Pitha JV, et al. Comparison of in vivo tissue temperature profile and lesion geometry for radiofrequency ablation with a saline-irrigated electrode versus temperature control in a canine thigh muscle preparation. *Circulation.* 1995;91:2264–2273.
98. Demazumder D, Mirotznik MS. Schwartzman D. Biophysics of radiofrequency ablation using an irrigated electrode. *J Interv Cardiol Electrophysiol.* 2001;5:377–389.
99. Skanes AC, Dubuc M, Klein GJ, et al. Cryothermal ablation of the slow pathway for the elimination of atrioventricular nodal reentrant tachycardia. *Circulation.* 2000;102:2856–2860.
100. Dubuc M, Khairy P, Rodriguez-Santiago A, et al. Catheter cryoablation of the atrioventricular node in patients with atrial fibrillation: A novel technology for ablation of cardiac arrhythmias. *J Cardiovasc Electrophysiol.* 2001;12:439–444.
101. Rodriguez LM, Geller C, Tse HF, et al. Acute results of transvenous cryoablation of supraventricular tachycardia (atrial fibrillation, atrial flutter, Wolff-Parkinson-White syndrome, atrioventricular nodal tachycardia). *J Cardiovasc Electrophysiol.* 2002;13:1082–1089.
102. Lanzotti ME, De Ponti R, Tritto M, et al. Successful treatment of anteroseptal accessory pathways by transvenous cryomapping and cryoablation. *Ital Heart J.* 2002;3:128–132.
103. Skanes AC, Klein GJ, Krahn AD, Yee R. Advances in energy delivery. *Coron Artery Dis.* 2003;14:15–23.
104. Skanes AC, Yee R, Krahn AD, Klein GJ. Cryoablation of atrial arrhythmias. *Card Electrophysiol Rev.* 2002;6:383–388.
105. Ayala-Paredes F, Sturmer ML, Macle L, et al. Catheter-based cryothermal versus radiofrequency ablation: Morphometric lesion characteristics [abstract]. *Pacing Clin Electrophysiol.* 2002;25:663.
106. Khairy P, Chauvet P, Lehmann J, et al. Lower incidence of thrombus formation with cryoenergy versus radiofrequency catheter ablation. *Circulation.* 2003;107:2045–2050.
107. Gallagher JJ, Selle JG, Sealy WC, et al. Intermediate septal accessory pathways (IS-AP): a subset of preexcitation at risk for complete heart block/failure during WPW surgery [abstract]. *Circulation.* 1986;74(suppl II):II–387.
108. Epstein AE, Kirklin JK, Holman WL, et al. Intermediate septal accessory pathways: electrocardiographic characteristics, electrophysiologic observations and their surgical implications. *J Am Coll Cardiol.* 1991;17:1570–1578.
109. Yeh SJ, Wang CC, Wen MS, et al. Characteristics and radiofrequency ablation therapy of intermediate septal accessory pathways. *Am J Cardiol.* 1994;73:50–56.
110. Kuck KH, Schluter M, Gursoy S. Preservation of atrioventricular nodal conduction during radiofrequency catheter ablation of midseptal accessory pathway. *Circulation.* 1992;86:1743–1752.
111. Schluter M, Kuck KH. Catheter ablation from right atrium of anteroseptal accessory pathways using radiofrequency current. *J Am Coll Cardiol.* 1992;19:663–670.
112. Haïssaguerre M, Marcus F, Poquet F, et al. Electrocardiographic characteristics and catheter ablation of para-Hisian accessory pathways. *Circulation.* 1994;90:1124–1128.
113. Tai CT, Chen SA, Chiang CE, et al. Electrocardiographic and electrophysiologic characteristics of anteroseptal, midseptal and para-Hisian accessory pathways: implication for radiofrequency catheter ablation. *Chest.* 1996;109:730–740.
114. Gatzoulis K, Apostolopoulos T, Costeas X, et al. Paraseptal accessory connections in the proximity of the atrioventricular node and the His bundle: additional observations in relation to the ablation technique in a high risk area. *Europace.* 2004;6:1–9.
115. García-García J, Almendral J, Arenal A, et al. Irrigated tip catheter ablation in right posteroseptal accessory pathways resistant to conventional ablation. *Pacing Clin Electrophysiol.* 2002;25:799–803.
116. Skrumeda LL, Mehra R. Comparison of standard and irrigated radiofrequency ablation in the canine ventricle. *J Cardiovasc Electrophysiol.* 1998;9:1196–1205.
117. Mittleman RS, Huang SKS, De Guzman WT, et al. Use of saline infusion electrode catheter for improved energy delivery and increased lesion size in radiofrequency catheter ablation. *Pacing Clin Electrophysiol.* 1995;18:1022–1027.
118. Wharton JM, Wilber DJ, Calkins H, et al. Utility of tip thermometry during radiofrequency ablation in humans using an internally perfused saline cooled catheter [abstract]. *Circulation.* 1997;96:I–318.
119. Barold HS, Jain MK, Dixon-Tulloch E, et al. What is the optimal temperature limit for the temperature-controlled cooled radiofrequency ablation? [abstract]. *Circulation.* 1998;98:I–644.
120. Barold HS, Jain MK, Dixon-Tulloch E, et al. A comparison of temperature-controlled cooled tip versus standard temperature-controlled radiofrequency ablation in left ventricular myocardium [abstract]. *Circulation.* 1998;98:I–644.

Catheter Ablation
of Ventricular Tachycardia

PART VII

26
Ablation of Ventricular Outflow Tract Tachycardias

Sanjay Dixit, David Lin, and Francis E. Marchlinski

Key Points

Mapping of ventricular outflow tract tachycardias includes the right or left ventricular outflow tract, aortic cusps, pulmonary artery, and possibly epicardial mapping.

The ablation targets are the site of earliest activation and the site of identical pace-mapping.

Electroanatomic mapping systems are often useful. Noncontact mapping may be helpful for nonsustained tachycardias. Irrigated radiofrequency ablation catheters or large-tip catheters may be needed. Coronary angiographic catheters may be needed to visualize coronary arteries.

Sources of difficulty include tachycardias that are noninducible or nonsustained, electrocardiographic localization based on electrocardiogram morphology, and ablation near the coronary arteries or His bundle.

Ventricular tachycardias (VTs) are usually observed in the setting of structural heart disease.[1,2] However, in 10% of the patients presenting with VT, the routine diagnostic modalities demonstrate no myocardial damage.[1] These arrhythmias have been called *idiopathic ventricular tachycardias* (IVTs), and they consist of various subtypes that have been defined by their clinical presentation (e.g., repetitive monomorphic tachycardias, exercise-induced sustained ventricular arrhythmias) and their underlying mechanism (e.g., adenosine-sensitive triggered arrhythmias, β-blocker–dependent automatic arrhythmias, intrafascicular or interfascicular reentrant arrhythmias).[3–5] Importantly, the mechanistically different subgroups of IVT favor certain anatomic locations within the heart and hence manifest specific electrocardiogram (ECG) patterns that help to identify their site of origin.

Outflow tract tachycardias comprise a subgroup of IVTs that are predominantly localized in and around the right and left ventricular outflow tracts (RVOT and LVOT, respectively). Lerman and colleagues[6,7] elegantly demonstrated that the mechanism underlying this group of arrhythmias appears to be triggered activity due to delayed afterdepolarizations that are determined by intracellular calcium release (load). The release of calcium is negatively affected by adenosine, which thus inhibits the afterdepolarizations and their clinical manifestations, and these arrhythmias are typically "adenosine sensitive."

In a group of 122 patients who underwent ablation of IVT at our center between January 1999 and December 2003, using the site of successful ablation or the earliest activation marked on the magnetic electroanatomic map (MEAM) as the gold standard, the site of origin was localized to the RVOT region in 88 patients (72%). Of the remaining 34 patients, 14 manifested fascicular VT, 9 had a site of origin localized to the aortic cusps or the left ventricular (LV) epicardium, and in 11, the site of origin of clinical arrhythmia was localized to the endocardium of the basal LV.[8] Therefore, most outflow tract tachycardias in our series were found to originate in the RVOT, which is in concurrence with other reports.[1,5]

This chapter describes briefly the common features of outflow tract tachycardias as a group and then focuses more specifically on the various sites of origin for illustrating the effect of anatomic location on ECG morphology. It then outlines strategies that we have used for ablation based on the site of origin in the outflow tract region.

Clinical Presentation

In general, outflow tract tachycardias manifest at a relatively early age. Lerman and associates[9] found equal distribution of the tachycardia between the two sexes. In our experience, VT originating in the RVOT shows a predilection for females (69.6%), whereas LVOT is predominantly seen in males (8 of 11 patients).[8,10]

The typical presentation of these arrhythmias consists of "salvos" of paroxysmal ventricular ectopic beats and nonsustained VT; however, sustained tachycardia is not uncommon. Most patients (48% to 80%) experience palpitations. Presyncope and lightheadedness may also be observed (28% to 50%). True syncope is infrequently seen (overall incidence, <10%), and these rhythm disorders are rarely life-threatening (there is only one case of documented fatality by cardiac arrest).[11–13] However, in a recent case series by Haïssaguerre and associates,[14] ventricular ectopic beats with morphology and intracardiac localization suggesting a site of origin in the RVOT region were shown to consistently initiate ventricular fibrillation in a selected group of patients with Brugada and long QT syndromes. Outflow tract tachycardias are typically provoked by exercise, and treadmill testing can reproduce the clinical VT in most patients.[11,15,16] The arrhythmia may occur during the acceleration of heart rate with exercise or during the recovery phase of exercise, suggesting that there is a combination of critical heart rate and endogenous catecholamine release that potentiates the rhythm disturbance.[17] Other triggers for inducing or enhancing the arrhythmia include stress, anxiety, and stimulants such as caffeine. In females, outflow tachycardias are more often observed during premenstrual and perimenopausal periods and with gestation, suggesting the role of hormonal influences. Our own experience suggests that, in female patients, a hormonal trigger for outflow tract tachycardia initiation is more common than exercise.[18]

Lack of Structural Heart Disease

In most patients presenting with these arrhythmias, cardiac function is generally well preserved. Structural heart disease has been traditionally assessed in most studies with the use of ECGs, chest radiographs, echocardiography, radionuclide imaging and stress testing, and cardiac catheterization. A more recent study using cine magnetic resonance imaging in patients with RVOT tachycardia showed evidence for right ventricular (RV) outflow abnormalities (focal wall thinning, diminished systolic wall thickening, and abnormal systolic wall motion localized to the anterior and lateral RVOT).[19] However, these findings were

not corroborated in another study using similar imaging techniques.[20] Researchers have also attempted to analyze the cardiac sympathetic innervation of ventricles in these patients using ^{123}I-metaiodobenzylguanidine scintigraphy and have inconsistently found regional deficiencies in sympathetic innervation.[21–24] Recent observational studies have shown the existence of more profound LV dysfunction in a subset of patients manifesting premature ventricular complexes (PVCs) originating from the RVOT or the basal LV region.[25,26] Importantly, in a subgroup of these patients, following successful PVC ablation, there was significant improvement in the LV function, suggesting that this was likely tachycardia-mediated cardiomyopathy. These observations obviously refute the heretofore held belief that outflow tract tachycardias are benign arrhythmias. Thus, it is worthwhile to follow patients with this condition by serial imaging studies (echocardiograms, magnetic resonance imaging studies), and if deterioration in LV dysfunction is observed, that perhaps may be a reason for a more aggressive management strategy.

Anatomy

Outflow tract tachycardia, as the name implies, originates primarily from the outflow tract of either ventricle and, in these regions, is further localized to even narrower zones. In our series, most RVOT tachycardias (≥80%) originated in the superior, septal, and anterior aspect (under the pulmonic valve),[10] whereas LVOT tachycardias were localized predominantly to the medial aspect of the basal LV (septal-parahisian region, aortomitral continuity, and superior mitral annulus), the epicardial region of the LV above the aortic valve, and the left and right aortic cusps.[8] If the outflow tract regions of both ventricles together are analyzed, as is illustrated in Figure 26-1, it becomes obvious that most of the

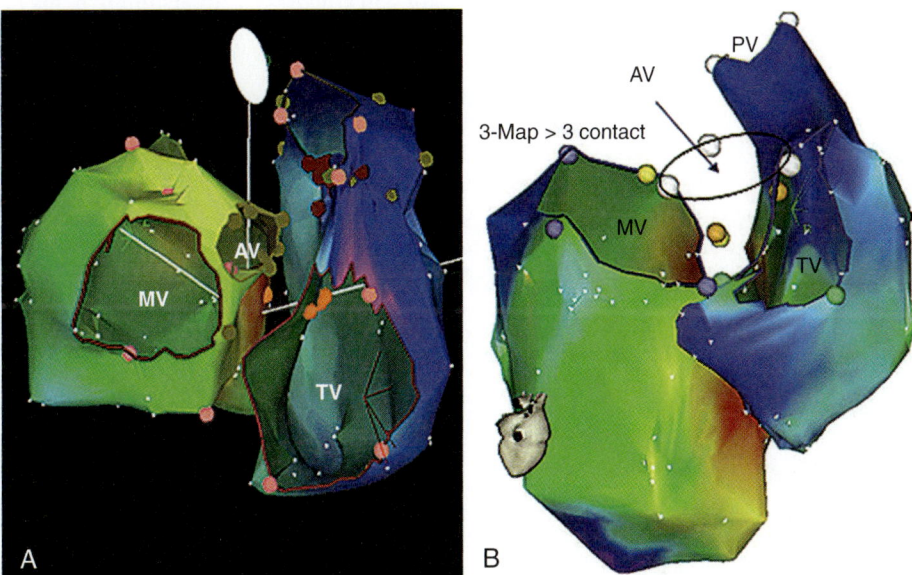

FIGURE 26-1. Anatomic relationship between the outflow tract regions of the right and left ventricles on magnetic electroanatomic mapping–generated endocardial shells. **A,** The aortic valve (AV) sits perpendicular. **B,** The aortic valve is oriented parallel to the plane of the pulmonic valve (PV). In our opinion, this change in AV orientation is age related, with the former seen more commonly in older patients as the aortic arch begins to unfold. These variations may influence the characteristics of pace maps and arrhythmias originating from aortic cusps, especially the right coronary cusp. See text for details. MV, mitral valve; TV, tricuspid valve.

outflow tract tachycardias originate from a fairly narrow anatomic zone. The relative proximity of the LVOT and RVOT areas was further reinforced by our observations in autopsied human hearts. A probe advanced from the supero-anterior and septal aspect of RVOT (under the pulmonic valve) toward the LV initially was seen to overlie the basal LV epicardium and superior aspect of the left interventricular septum (Fig. 26-2). If advanced further, the probe extended toward the aortomitral continuity and superior mitral annulus, sites from which most outflow tract tachycardias have been localized.[27] LV myocardium typically extends above the line of attachment of the right coronary cusp into the aortic sinus.[28] The noncoronary and left coronary cusps usually lack ventricular myocardial extensions; however, myocardial extensions may occur into all three cusps. Myocardial extensions occur above the pulmonic valve as well. Thus, ablation above semilunar valves may be necessary to target these myocardial extensions or because of the proximity of these sites to other cardiac structures (such as ablation of the posterior RVOT from the right coronary cusp).

This predisposition of outflow tract tachycardias (90%) to a specific region in the heart raises an interesting question with regard to the tissue characteristics, which may favor triggered activity and arrhythmogenesis in the area. We have noticed that most outflow tract VTs originate in perivalvular tissue, which may be anatomically predisposed to fiber disruption. Whether it is a normal anatomic finding seen in all people or is an exclusive developmental anomaly manifested in a selected group, not unlike bypass tracts, remains to be determined. It is, of course, possible that a subclinical process (myocarditis or pericarditis) may enhance fiber disruption or cause local autonomic changes, predisposing the tissue to triggered activity and arrhythmogenesis. Of note, a small percentage of outflow tract tachycardias can be seen in other anatomic locations, including the lateral and inferolateral aspect of the mitral annulus, the RV inflow region, the mid-ventricular septum, and the inferoapical area of the LV. In a recent report of seven patients with RVOT tachycardia,

the earliest intracardiac activation was demonstrated above the plane of the pulmonic valve. However, in most of these cases, successful ablation was still performed in the superior RVOT under the valve plane.[1,29–34.]

Diagnosis

Electrocardiographic Patterns and Anatomic Location

From the foregoing discussion, it would appear that, given the relatively narrow anatomic zone from which outflow tract tachycardias arise, these tachycardias should manifest broadly similar ECG characteristics. Nevertheless, outflow tract tachycardias in fact manifest a variety of ECG morphologies, including left or right bundle branch block patterns, diverse axes (left, inferior, right, leftward), and various patterns of precordial transition (early, late, or none). However, ECG morphologies are predictable based on anatomic location, and recognition of specific ECG features may serve as a useful tool to accurately localize the site of origin of the clinical arrhythmia. Using pace-mapping under electroanatomic mapping guidance (see later discussion), we have characterized specific ECG features from different aspects of RVOT, basal LV, and aortic cusps that have allowed us to develop algorithms that are useful in accurately localizing clinical VT originating from this region. The following sections discuss in more detail these site-specific ECG features.

Clinical Arrhythmias from Right Ventricular Outflow Tract

The RVOT region is defined superiorly by the pulmonic valve and inferiorly by the superior margin of the RV inflow tract (tricuspid valve). The interventricular septum and the RV free wall constitute its medial and lateral aspects, respectively. We have used the following protocol for constructing electroanatomic maps of this region: The

Common sites of origin of outflow tract tachycardias

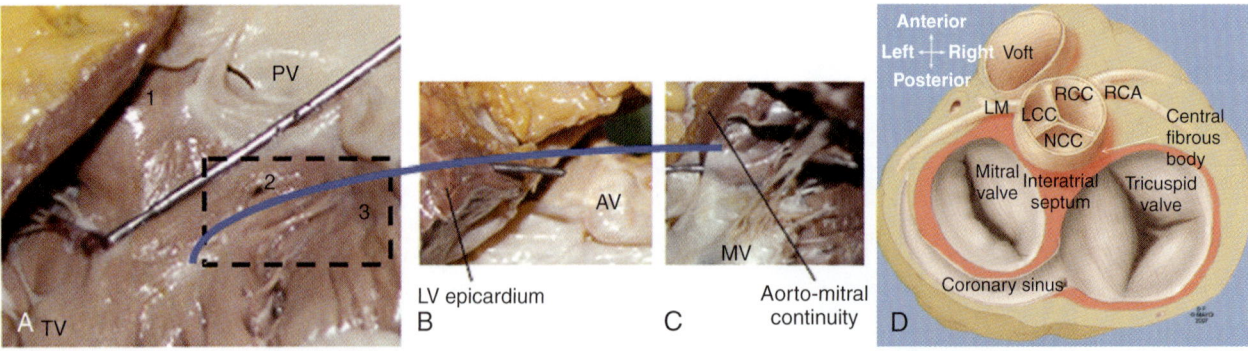

FIGURE 26-2. Right ventricular outflow tract (RVOT) (**A**), left ventricular epicardium adjacent to the anterior RVOT above the aortic valve (AV) (**B**), and aortomitral continuity and medial and superior aspect of the mitral valve (MV) (**C**). Sites in the RVOT endocardium under the pulmonic valve (PV) from posterior to anterior are labeled 1, 2, and 3. The *rectangle* represents common areas of RVOT tachycardia sites; the *blue line* illustrates the natural course of a probe advanced into the anterior RVOT (site 3), which overlies the LV epicardium and the superomedial aspect of the MV. These areas are also common sites of origin of outflow tract tachycardias, underscoring the proximity of the RVOT and basal LV. **D,** Schematic diagram of the anatomy of the outflow tracts.. The right ventricular outflow tract (Voft) is anterior and leftward of the aortic root. The anterior portion of the right coronary cusp (RCC) and left coronary cusps (LCC) underlies the RVOT. Note the close proximity of the left main coronary artery (LM) to the RVOT and the proximity of the AV conduction system (central fibrous body) to the RCC. (*Adapted from Sulieman M, Asarvatham SJ. Ablation above the semilunar valves: when, why, and how?* Heart Rhythm. *2008;5:1485-1492. With permission.*)

plane of the pulmonic valve is defined to outline the superior limit of the RVOT. The mapping catheter is advanced superiorly in the RVOT until no discrete bipolar electrograms are seen in the distal electrode pair. The catheter is then retracted until electrograms in the distal electrode pair reappear and pacing results in capture of the RVOT endocardium. This marks the level of the pulmonic valve, and at this level, three distinct points are acquired and tagged to construct the valve plane. Next, under electroanatomic mapping and fluoroscopic guidance, a detailed electroanatomic map of the entire RVOT and RV is constructed by acquiring multiple (≥75) points during sinus rhythm.

In an earlier study, based on specific ECG morphologies identified during pace mapping, we divided the septal RVOT into nine anatomic sites to facilitate the description of the catheter position (Fig. 26-3A). However, because of the predilection for clinical arrhythmias from superior RVOT, we attempted to further characterize the ECG features of pace maps from this region in 14 patients. To accomplish this, the superior-most sites in a posterior-to-anterior distribution were assigned numbers 1, 2, and 3, and their counterpart locations along the free wall of superior RVOT were also assigned numbers 1, 2, and 3 (Fig. 26-3B). The mapping catheter was positioned serially at each of these sites, which were tagged and labeled on the electroanatomic map and paced at diastolic threshold (cycle length, 400 to 500 msec) for 10 to 20 uninterrupted captured beats. A 12-lead ECG during pacing from each site was acquired. The ECG was specifically analyzed for (1) QRS amplitude and duration in all limb leads; (2) presence of "notching" of R waves in the inferior leads II, III, or aVF; (3) QRS transition pattern in the precordial leads (change from a QS/rS pattern to an RS/Rs pattern), with a change at or beyond lead V_4 defined as a late transition; and (4) QRS morphology in limb lead I. We used limb lead II as representative of all the inferior leads, to quantify the differences in R-wave amplitude and QRS duration of pace maps from septal and free wall sites.[30]

Figure 26-4 shows the pace maps from all six locations in the superior RVOT. The pace maps from septal sites manifest monophasic R waves in the inferior leads, which are taller and narrower compared with those seen in the counterpart free wall locations (Fig. 26-5A). Likewise, the duration of the R wave in lead II at septal sites is narrower than that of the R wave at free wall sites (Fig. 26-5B). The contour of the R wave in the inferior leads is also helpful in differentiating septal and free wall locations in the superior RVOT. Typically, R waves from free wall sites demonstrate characteristic "notching," which is uncommon in R waves from septal locations. Notching of the R wave was seen in 40 (95.2%) of 42 free wall sites and in only 12 (28.6%) of the 42 septal locations ($P < .05$). Another feature that can distinguish pace maps from septal and free wall sites in superior RVOT is the QRS transition pattern in the precordial leads (late versus early; Fig. 26-4). A late precordial transition was observed in 40 free wall sites (95.2%) and in only 9 septal locations (21.4 %; $P < .05$). Importantly, only 4 (9.5%) of 42 septal sites demonstrated both a late precordial transition and notching in the inferior leads, in contrast to 39 (92.9%) of 42 free wall sites ($P < .05$). We also evaluated the QRS morphology in limb lead I, during pace mapping at posterior (site 1) and anterior (site 3) locations along the septum and free wall in the RVOT (Fig. 26-4). In general, for both the free wall and septal posterior locations (site 1), the QRS in lead I manifested a positive polarity (r waves). In comparison, anterior sites (site 3) along the septum and the free wall demonstrated a negative polarity (qs pattern). Sites midway between the anterior and posterior locations (site 2) along the septum and the free wall demonstrated either a biphasic or a multiphasic QRS morphology (qr/rs pattern), or an isoelectric segment preceding the q or r wave.[35]

We also analyzed ECG morphologies of RVOT tachycardias in 28 patients and found that all arrhythmias originating from septal locations lacked notching of R waves in inferior leads. In comparison, all tachycardias originating from the free wall sites in the superior RVOT demonstrated notching. Late precordial transition was seen in 6 (85.7%) of the 7 free wall tachycardias and only 2 (9.5%) of 21 tachycardias originating from septal locations. All spontaneous arrhythmias originating from site 3 had a qs pattern in lead I with a net negative QRS polarity. In comparison, all tachycardias originating from site 1 demonstrated an R wave with a net positive QRS polarity. All of the remaining spontaneous arrhythmias (13 patients) originated from septal site 2 and demonstrated a biphasic or

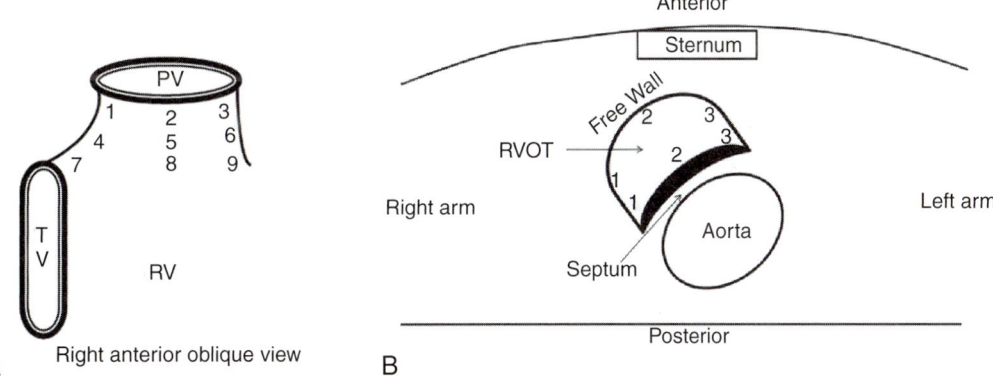

FIGURE 26-3. Schematic representation of the right ventricular outflow tract (RVOT). **A,** Locations of the nine standard mapping sites along the septal RVOT are shown in right anterior oblique projection. Sites 1 through 3 represent the first row of sites beneath the pulmonic valve. **B,** RVOT viewed from the left anterior oblique perspective. Sites 1 (most posterior) through 3 (most anterior) along the septum and free wall are shown. See text for details. RV, right ventricle; PV, pulmonic valve; TV, tricuspid valve.

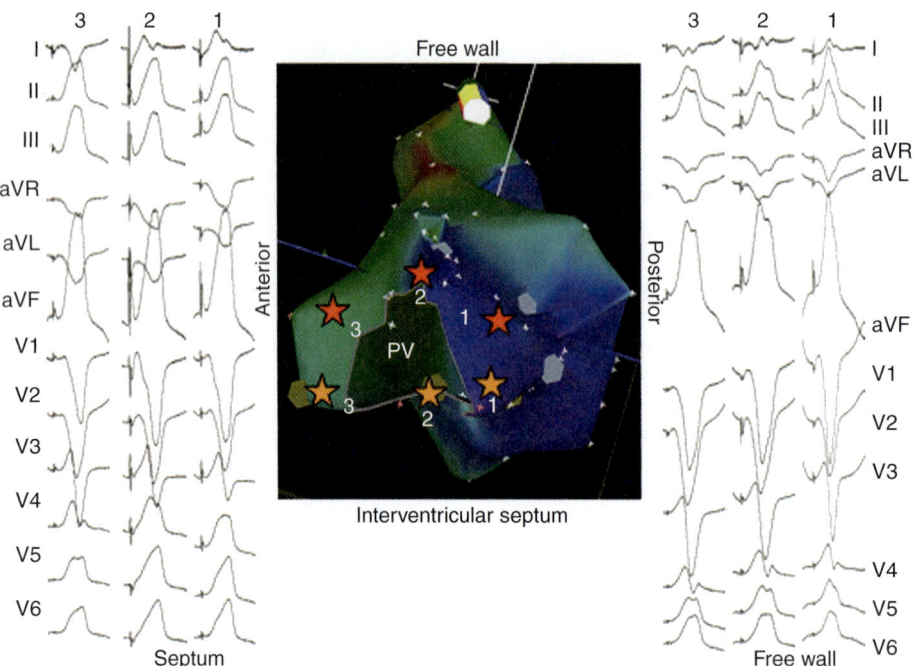

FIGURE 26-4. Twelve-lead electrocardiogram pace maps from sites 1, 2 and 3 along the septum and free wall (FW) of the right ventricular outflow tract (RVOT) showing characteristic features. Sites are labeled on the magnetic electroanatomic map (MEAM) in the center of the figure and over each pace map. The MEAM of the RVOT is shown in a coronal projection and was acquired during sinus rhythm. The three-dimensional shape of the RVOT is evident from MEAM and the cartoon in the *middle of the figure*. All pace maps show left bundle branch block morphology and inferior frontal plane axis. Differences in R waves in inferior leads (II, III, and aVF) between the FW and septal pace maps are seen (broader, shorter, and notched for the FW sites). Also, the precordial transition pattern for the FW site shows later transition (R/S ratio [1 by precordial leads V₄] compared with the septal locations. Changes in lead I when moving from more anterior and leftward, site 3 (negative QRS), to the more posterior and rightward, site 1 (positive QRS), are also shown. PV, pulmonic valve.

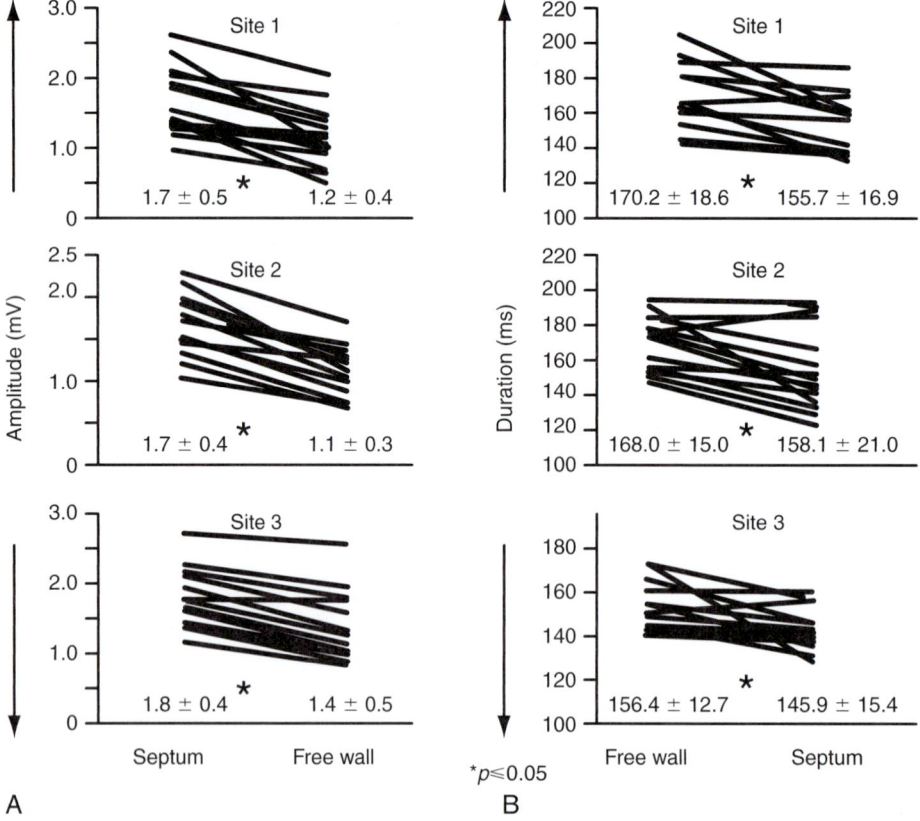

FIGURE 26-5. Comparison of QRS amplitude and width in lead II during pace mapping from septal and free wall (FW) sites. **A,** Amplitude of the R wave in limb lead II compared among sites 1, 2, and 3 along the septum and the FW. Each line represents R-wave amplitude (mV) at the same sites between the septum and the FW for each patient. The mean R-wave amplitude for the different sites are also shown. At each site, the mean R-wave amplitude in the septum was significantly greater than that in the FW. **B,** Duration of the R-wave in limb lead II compared among sites 1, 2, and 3 along the septum and the FW. Each line represents R-wave duration (msec) at the same site in the septum and the FW for each patient. The mean R-wave duration for the different sites are also shown. At each site, the mean R wave width of the FW pace maps was significantly greater than that of the septal pace maps.

multiphasic QRS morphology (10 patients) or an isoelectric segment preceding a small rs or qr (3 patients) in lead I. Table 26-1summarizes the criteria we use to localize clinical VT originating from the superior RVOT region, and Figure 26-6 shows ECG morphologies of clinical arrhythmias from various superior RVOT sites.

RVOT arising from above the pulmonic valve has been described in a series of 24 patients.[35] In these patients, VT is believed to arise from strands of myocardial tissue extending over the pulmonary artery in a fashion analogous to arrhythmogenic myocardium extending over the pulmonary veins. The tachycardias had left bundle branch block morphology with intermediate, right, or vertical frontal plane axes. Precordial transition occurred in V_2 or later. Compared with RVOT arising below the pulmonic valve, VT arising from above the valve had greater R-wave amplitude in the inferior leads. The values overlapped greatly between the two groups, however, and no ECG feature reliably separated the two patterns. The successful ablation site was 0.5 to 2.1 cm above the pulmonic valve. At the successful ablation site, a sharp presystolic electrical potential was noted in VT in most patients. In sinus rhythm, the successful ablation site not uncommonly recorded a small far-field atrial potential. Ablation was delivered with a standard 4-mm-tip radiofrequency catheter with a target temperature of 55°C for 60 to 90 seconds. All 24 patients were successfully ablated without complication or recurrence in follow-up.

Clinical Arrhythmias from Basal Left Ventricle

The basal LV constitutes ventricular myocardium bordering the mitral valve and encompasses a wide area, including septum and anterior, lateral, and inferior walls.[9,10] The

---

TABLE 26-1

ELECTROCARDIOGRAPHIC CHARACTERISTICS OF PACE MAPS FROM VARIOUS SUPERIOR RVOT SITE

Item	Septal RVOT Sites			Free Wall RVOT Sites		
	Posterior (Site 1)	Middle (Site 2)	Anterior (Site 3)	Posterior (Site 1)	Middle (Site 2)	Anterior (Site 3)
Morphology in lead I	R, Rs	rs, qrs	qs, rS	R, Rs	rs, qrs	qs, rS
Notch in inferior leads	–	–	–	+	+	+
Precordial transition	$\leq V_3$	$\leq V_3$	$\leq V_3$	$\geq V_4$	$\geq V_4$	$\geq V_4$

≤, Transition earlier than or equal to; ≥, transition later than or equal to; RVOT, right ventricular outflow tract.

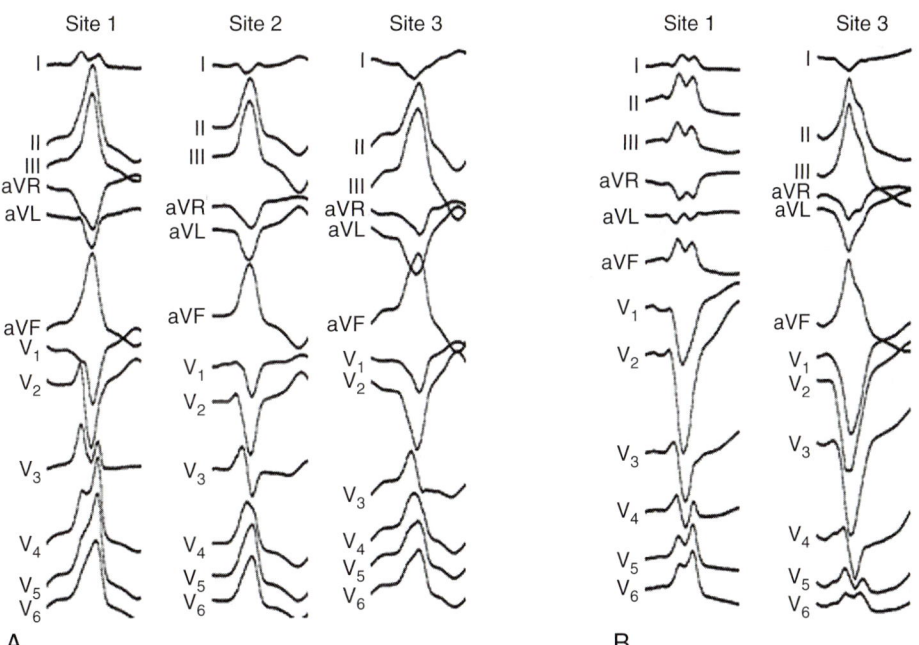

FIGURE 26-6. The unique electrocardiogram (ECG) morphologies that help in distinguishing site of origin of the clinical arrhythmia in the superior RVOT are shown. **A,** The ECG morphologies of spontaneous arrhythmias from septal sites 1, 2, and 3. **B,** The ECG morphologies of spontaneous arrhythmias from free wall (FW) sites 1 and 3. All the FW sites show notching in inferior leads and late precordial transition ($\geq V_4$). In comparison, all the septal sites lack both notching of inferior leads and late precordial transition. For both the septal and FW locations of the clinical arrhythmias, lead I helps in distinguishing anterior and leftward location (site 3; negative polarity) from posterior and leftward location (site 1; positive polarity). Site 2, which lies in between, manifests multiphasic polarity in lead I (panel **A**; see text for details).

aortic valve typically sits at the superior-most and medial aspect of this region, distorting its otherwise circular shape. To create the electroanatomic map of this region, we recommend the following protocol.

At the outset, planes of mitral and aortic valves are defined. For outlining the mitral valve, the mapping catheter is positioned in the basal LV such that the distal electrode pair records a large ventricular electrogram preceded by a smaller or equal size atrial electrogram. In this orientation, three different points (medial, lateral, and superior or inferior) are acquired to create the mitral valve plane. Next, the catheter is retracted into the aorta and then advanced down to the aortic valve, where the individual cusps (left, right, and noncoronary), as determined by distinct catheter locations on orthogonal fluoroscopy, are tagged. Intracardiac echocardiography is a useful tool to confirm accurate anatomic location of the catheter in this region (Fig. 26-7). The catheter is then readvanced into the LV, and multiple points (≥100) are acquired to create an endocardial shell. To develop ECG criteria for localizing basal LV VT, we performed pace mapping in a series of patients from four or more locations in this region, including the septal-parahisian region and the aortomitral continuity, as well as superior, superolateral, and lateral mitral annular

locations, using the pacing protocol described earlier for the RVOT. In general, pace maps from medial sites (septal-parahisian region and aortomitral continuity) show a mean QRS duration of 134 ± 28 milliseconds, initial negative forces in lead V_1 (QS or Qr complexes for septal-parahisian region and qR complexes for aortomitral continuity sites), and predominantly positive forces (R or Rs morphology) in lead I. Additionally, pace maps from the septal-parahisian region manifest an early precordial transition pattern (reversal of the ratio of Q to R waves occurring earlier than or in V_3). In comparison, pace maps from lateral basal LV sites (superolateral and lateral mitral annulus) demonstrate a mean QRS duration of 182 ± 1 milliseconds, have a right bundle branch block morphology (R or Rs, or both) in lead V_1, and are associated with a late precordial transition pattern (reversal of ratio of R to Q waves in V_5 or later) or lack of precordial transition. Also for these sites, lead I demonstrates an rS or qs morphology.[8]

Details of the pace maps from individual locations along the basal LV are shown in Figure 26-8. In general, most medial basal LV sites demonstrate the narrowest complexes, with the most positive complexes in lead I, whereas superolateral mitral annulus locations demonstrate the widest complexes, with the least positive forces in lead I. With the exception of parahisian sites, which consistently demonstrate left bundle branch block morphology and early precordial transition patterns, pace maps from all other sites in this region manifest right bundle branch block morphology. Additionally, "qR" morphology in lead V_1 is *pathognomonic* for pace maps from aortomitral continuity locations (Fig. 26-8).

Of the 122 patients who underwent ablation of IVT (both RV and LV) at our center over a 5-year period, the site of origin of clinical tachycardias in 12 patients was localized to basal LV endocardium based on MEAM-guided ablation, as follows: parahisian region (2 patients), aortomitral continuity (4 patients), superior mitral annulus (3 patients), and superolateral mitral annulus (3 patients) (Fig. 26-9). Using the previously described ECG criteria (Table 26-2), a blinded observer was able to accurately predict the site of origin of clinical tachycardia in 10 (83%) of the 12 cases, attesting to the clinical utility of our algorithm for localizing basal LV VT.

Clinical Arrhythmias from the Aortic Cusps and Surrounding Epicardium

The aortic valve, with the left and right cusps occupying positions adjacent to the left and right coronary arteries, respectively, forms the centerpiece of the heart. It is increasingly recognized that the aortic cusps and the sinus of Valsalva can also provide a site of origin of IVT.[37–40] Recognition of this fact may have important clinical implications because radiofrequency ablation inside the aortic cusps is feasible and is associated with high success rates for curing IVT originating from the region.

To determine unique ECG characteristics, we performed pace-mapping of the right coronary cusp, left coronary cusp, and noncoronary cusp in a total of 20 patients with structurally normal hearts using the same protocol as described earlier for the RVOT. The catheter position in relation to the individual aortic cusps was confirmed using one or more of the following imaging modalities:

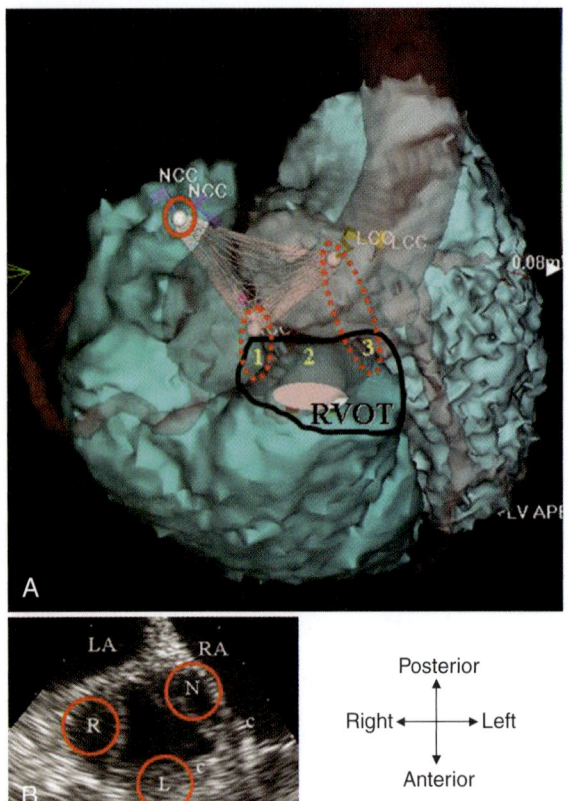

FIGURE 26-7. A, Computed tomography (CT) angiogram of the outflow tract region (coronal view) depicting the relationship between the superior right ventricular outflow tract (RVOT) and aortic cusps. The posterior septal and anterior septal RVOTs (sites 1 and 3) are in close proximity to the right and left coronary cusps (RCC and LCC), respectively. Accurate anatomic localization of the mapping catheter in the cusp region is greatly facilitated by intracardiac echocardiography (**B**), which shows the wedge-shaped right (R), left (L), and noncoronary (N) cusps. Notice how the noncoronary cusp sits between the right and the left atria (RA, LA).

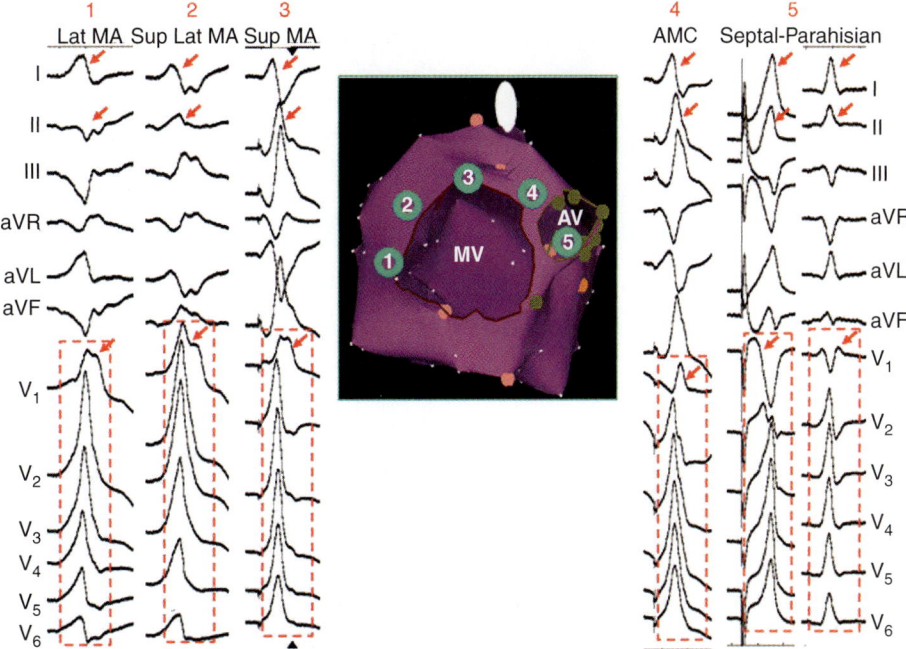

FIGURE 26-8. Representation of pace maps from various basal left ventricle (LV) locations. In a lateral-to-medial distribution, paced sites include lateral, superolateral, superior mitral annulus (Lat, Sup Lat, and Sup MA, respectively), aortomitral continuity (AMC), and septal-parahisian region (S-P). Magnetic electroanatomic map of LV in posteroanterior projection is shown in the center. QRS morphology in leads I, II, V$_1$ (*arrows*) and precordial transition pattern (*rectangles*) help in distinguishing site of origin of the pace maps. AV, aortic valve; MV, mitral valve.

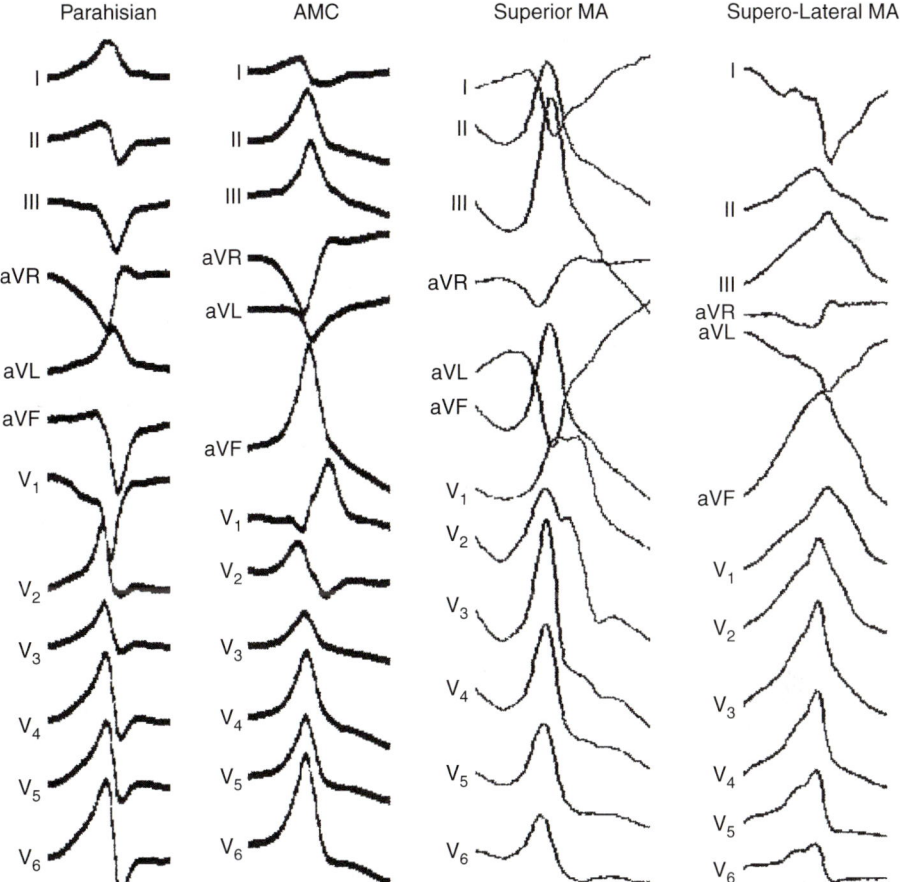

FIGURE 26-9. Typical electrocardiogram morphologies of clinical arrhythmias shown originating from basal left ventricle (LV) region that were localized based on site of successful ablation on magnetic electroanatomic mapping to the parahisian region, aortomitral continuity (AMC), superior mitral annular (MA) location, and superolateral MA location. QRS morphology in leads I and V$_1$, together with the ratio of QRS complexes in leads II/III and precordial transition pattern, can reliably distinguish medial from lateral locations in this region (see text for details).

TABLE 26-2

ELECTROCARDIOGRAPHIC CHARACTERISTICS OF PACE MAPS FROM VARIOUS BASAL LEFT VENTRICULAR SITES

Item	Septal-Parahisian	AMC	Superior MA	Superolateral MA	Lateral MA
Lead I	R or Rs	Rs or rs	rs or rS	rS or QS	rS or rs
Lead V_1	QS or Qr	qR	R or Rs	R or Rs	R or Rs
Precordial transition*	Early	None	None	None	None or late
Ratio of QRS in leads II and III	>1	≤1	≤1	≤1	>1

*Reversal of Q to R and vice versa ≤V_3 (early) and ≥V_5 (late).
AMC, aortomitral continuity; MA, mitral annulus.

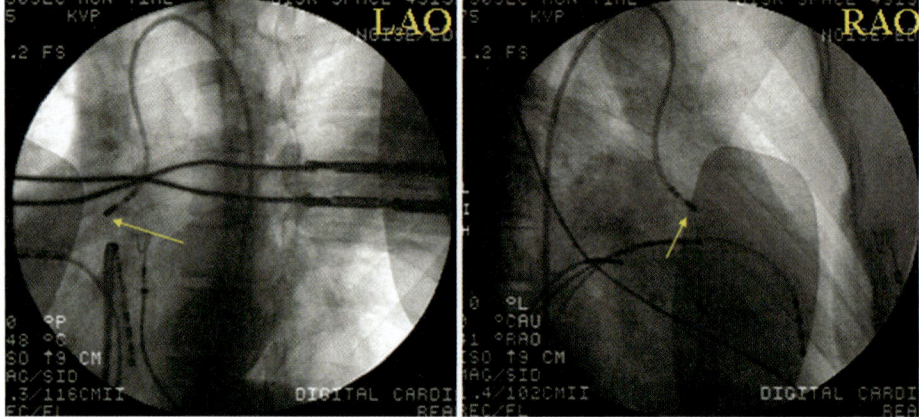

FIGURE 26-10. Typical left and right anterior oblique fluoroscopic projections (LAO and RAO, respectively) showing the mapping catheter (*yellow arrow*) by the right coronary cusp.

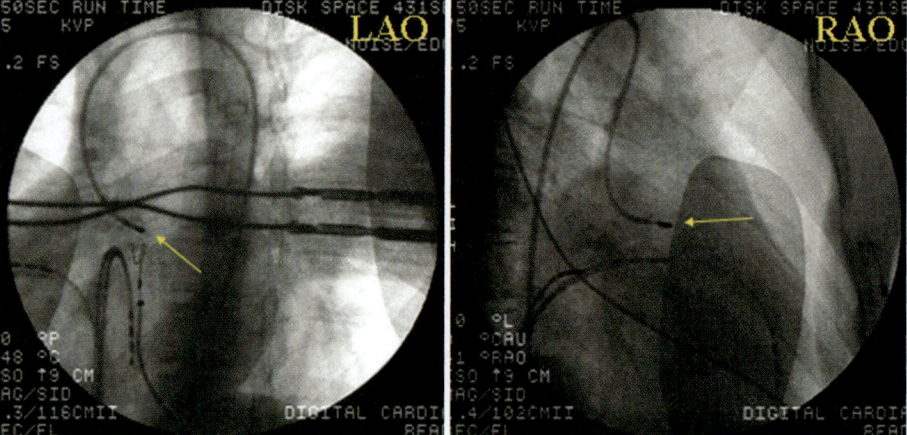

FIGURE 26-11. This figure shows the mapping catheter (*yellow arrow*) positioned at the left coronary cusp in left and right anterior oblique (LAO and RAO, respectively) fluoroscopic projections.

phased-array intracardiac ultrasound, biplane fluoroscopy, and electroanatomic mapping (Figs. 26-10 to 26-12).

Anatomic Considerations. To conceptualize the correct approach to catheter ablation in this region, it is important to understand the anatomic relations between the aortic cusps and their surrounding structures.[40,41] The pulmonic valve and adjoining RVOT region typically are located anteriorly and sit slightly superior to and rightward of the aortic valve. The posterior septal aspect of the superior RVOT typically lies adjacent to the right coronary cusp, whereas the anterior septal aspect tends to be situated at the junction of the right and left cusp or anterior to the medial aspect of the latter (Fig. 26-7).[41] Furthermore, given the frequent convex, crescent shape of the area just below the pulmonic valve, a leftward direction can also be observed when pacing at the most posterior and anterior aspects of the RVOT septum.[35]

Mapping Technique. Consistent with our previous studies, we used a standard 12-lead ECG configuration to acquire pace maps while mapping the cusp region. Using a retrograde approach through the femoral artery, we positioned a 7-French deflectable mapping catheter in

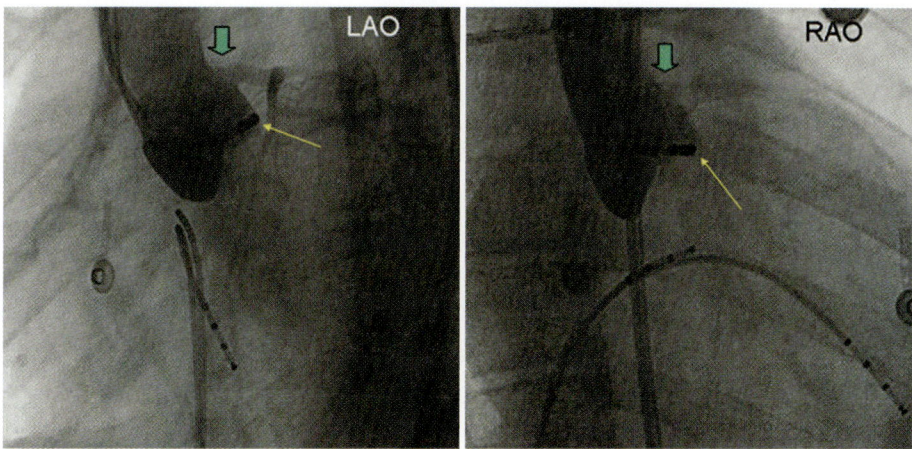

FIGURE 26-12. A representative aortogram depicting the tip of the mapping catheter (*yellow arrow*) by the left coronary cusp and its proximity to the takeoff of the left main coronary artery (*light blue arrow*). The ablation catheter tip is 4 mm, and the electrodes are spaced 5 mm apart. LAO, left anterior oblique; RAO, right anterior oblique.

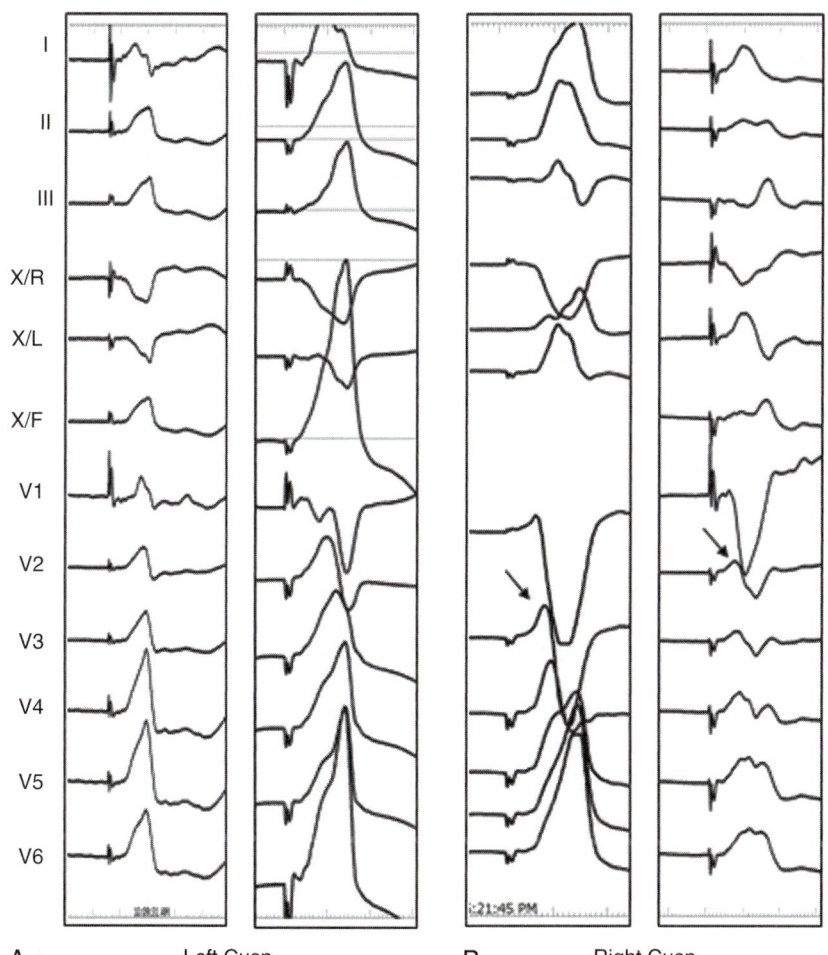

A   Left Cusp   B   Right Cusp

FIGURE 26-13. A, Two different examples of pacing from the left coronary cusp. The first example shows an M-shaped pattern in V_1, whereas it is more W shaped in the second example (*arrows*). In both cases, the overall axis is inferiorly directed, with a multiphasic QRS in V_1 and a transition by lead V_2 or earlier. **B,** Two examples of a typical pattern with pacing from the right coronary cusp. As with the left coronary cusp, the axis is inferiorly directed. However, with the right coronary cusp, the transition in the precordial leads is later ($\geq V_3$) with a left bundle branch block type pattern.

the aortic root and manipulated it toward individual valve cusps. The catheter location at each valve cusp was confirmed by various imaging modalities, as described earlier. Pacing at each site was performed as described previously, and the ECGs of pace maps were analyzed with respect to morphology, amplitude, and duration in all leads and the precordial transition pattern.

Morphology. In our series, lead V_1 was found to be the most useful in distinguishing the various sites. Left coronary cusp pacing consistently produced a multiphasic component resembling an M- or W-shaped QRS complex. Right coronary cusp pacing demonstrated a QS or QR type pattern with a predominantly negative vector in V_1 (Fig. 26-13). Pacing the noncoronary cusp universally resulted in capture of the atrium. This probably occurred because of the close proximity of the noncoronary cusp to both left and right atria.[41] The question often raised is how one can differentiate VT arising from the aortic cusps from VT arising from the RVOT region. Because of the proximity of the RVOT septum to the aortic cusps, especially the right coronary cusp, ECG features among these sites often overlap, and differences are subtle. The RVOT is anterior, superior, and leftward of the aortic valve. Ouyang and associates[39] reported that the r wave duration in V_1 and V_2 tended to be broader when VT originated from the aortic valve cusps than when it arose from the RVOT septum. Furthermore, R wave duration of longer than 50% of the total QRS duration or R/S amplitude ratio greater than 30% in V_1 or V_2 also favored an aortic cusp location.

Amplitude and Duration. In our series, evaluation of the amplitude of the R wave in inferior leads and the width of the QRS interval was inconsistent, and an absolute value of these measures could not be used to differentiate cusp pace maps. However, the QRS duration in general was wider with right coronary cusp pacing than with left coronary cusp pacing. In our experience, the mean QRS duration for pace maps from the left coronary cusp was 142 milliseconds (range, 108 to 180 milliseconds), whereas for right coronary cusp pace maps, it was 164 milliseconds (range, 141 to 241 milliseconds).[41] Because the left coronary cusp lies on the same cranial plane as the right coronary cusp, the inferior lead morphology (inferior axis) does not differ significantly between the cusps and therefore is not useful as a differentiating factor.

Precordial Transition. Analysis of the R-wave transition demonstrated that, for pace maps from left coronary cusp, precordial transition occurred in V_2 or earlier in 16 of 20 patients, whereas for right coronary cusp pace maps, the precordial transition was most commonly after V_2 (18 of 20 patients).[41] The ECG features of coronary cusp VTs are listed in Table 26-3.

Tachycardias Originating from Right and Left Coronary Cusp Commissure. Recently, in a consecutive series of patients at our center who underwent successful ablation of PVC and VT from the aortic cusp region, in 19 patients the site of origin of the tachycardia was localized to the commissure between the left and right coronary cusps.[42] This was confirmed by merging the electroanatomic shell to the geometry of the cusp region segmented from the computed tomographic angiogram as well as monitoring "live" the catheter position by intracardiac phased-array ultrasound. Unique features of tachycardias

originating from this location included QS morphology in lead V_1 with notching on the downward deflection and late potential during sinus rhythm at the site of earliest activation, which reversed during the arrhythmia.[42] Typically, these sites were found to be located higher than the actual cusps and well above the aortic root (Fig. 26-14).

Other Electrocardiographic Localization Criteria

An algorithm for the localization of outflow tract VTs by surface ECG has been published.[43] However, there may be difficulties in the universal applicability of such algorithms due to overlap in certain ECG features among VT sites, varying patient characteristics, cardiac rotation, body habitus, and so on.[43] In addition, a ratio of time to R-wave peak and total QRS duration greater than 0.54 in the precordial leads has been used as a useful indicator of an epicardial origin to outflow tract VTs.

Diagnosis by Intracardiac Recordings

The criteria for diagnosis of outflow tract VTs are given in Table 26-4. The criteria include the general features of VT and evidence of a triggered or automatic mechanism. The tachycardias are mapped to the characteristic locations described earlier.

Decision to Ablate Outflow Tract Tachycardias

The various treatment options for outflow tract tachycardia are determined mostly by the burden of the disease.[5] Because the arrhythmia is not life-threatening, electrophysiologists have the luxury of fine-tuning the treatment strategy for individual patients. If symptoms are infrequent and relatively mild, treatment is not mandated. Ablation of outflow tract tachycardias has been traditionally reserved for patients with prolonged incapacitating symptoms for whom pharmacologic treatment with β-blockers, calcium channel blockers, and class I or class III antiarrhythmics has failed.[11,15,21,36,44-47] The presence of left ventricular dysfunction due to frequent ventricular ectopy is also a strong motivation for ablation. Because the population with this arrhythmia is younger and generally healthy otherwise, and quality of life is a significant issue for them, most patients in this group at our center, when offered the choice between antiarrhythmic agents and ablation, have opted for the latter.

Mapping

The favored technique for successful ablation consists of localization of the site of origin using earliest intracardiac activation, pace-mapping, or both (Table 26-5). Careful analysis of the 12-lead ECG during tachycardia is very useful and can guide catheter localization to within 0.5 to 1 cm of the site of successful ablation.[8,10,30,31,35] Although biplane fluoroscopy permits reasonable catheter localization, use of electroanatomic mapping and the availability of intracardiac echocardiography further enhance precise

TABLE 26-3

ELECTROCARDIOGRAPHIC FEATURES OF AORTIC CUSP VENTRICULAR TACHYCARDIAS

ECG Feature	Right Coronary Cusp	Left Coronary Cusp
V_1	QS or QR predominantly negative	Multiphasic "M" or "W" configuration
Precordial transition	≥V_3	≤V_2

≤, Transition earlier than or equal to; ≥, transition later than or equal to; ECG, electrocardiogram.

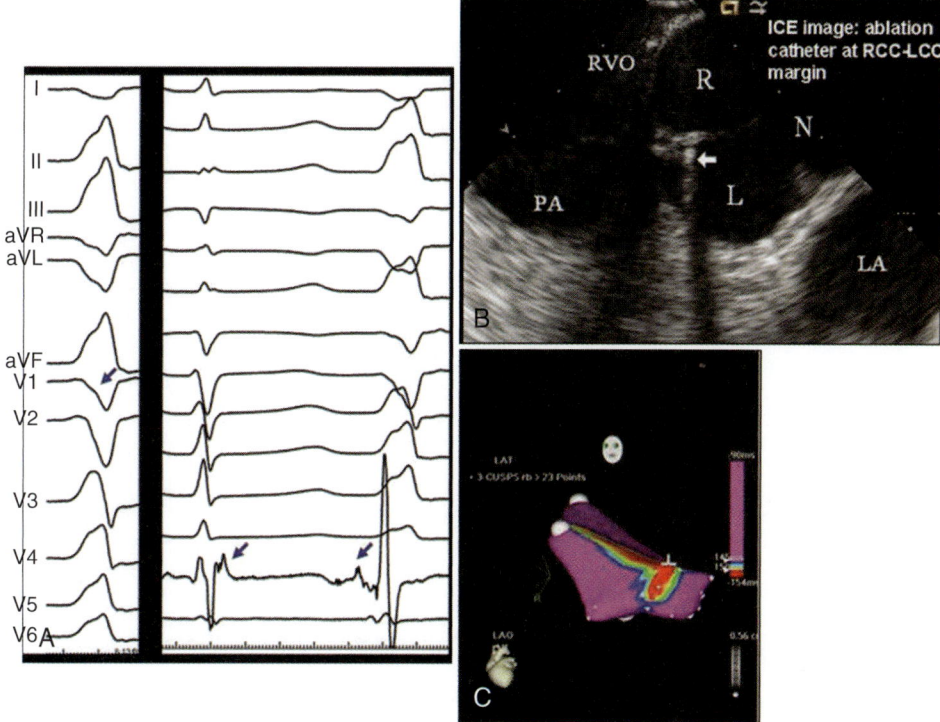

FIGURE 26-14. **A,** Typical morphology of premature ventricular complex originating from the commissure between the right and left coronary cusps. Notice QS morphology of complexes in lead V₁, with a notch seen on the down slope (*arrow*). Typically, at the site of origin of these tachycardias, a late potential is seen during sinus (*arrow*) beats that reverses during the tachycardia (*arrow*). **B,** This particular location was confirmed by visualizing catheter position on intracardiac phase array ultrasound (*arrow*). **C,** Usually, these locations were above the plane of the aortic root as seen on the electroanatomic map (*red zone*). ICE, intracardiac echocardiogram; L, left (coronary cusp); LA, left atrium; LAO, left anterior oblique; LAT, lateral projection; LCC, left coronary cusp; N, non (coronary cusp); PA, pulmonary artery; R, right (coronary cusp); RCC, right coronary cusp; RVO, right ventricular outflow tract.

<table>
<tr><td colspan="1">TABLE 26-4</td></tr>
</table>

DIAGNOSTIC CRITERIA
General features of ventricular tachycardia
Evidence of triggered or automatic mechanism (typically)
Adenosine sensitive
Noninducible by PES or initiated with burst pacing
Absence of entrainment
Earliest activation in RVOT, LVOT, AMC, or pulmonary artery

AMC, aortomitral continuity; LVOT, left ventricular outflow tract; PES, programmed electrical stimulation; RVOT, right ventricular outflow tract.

TABLE 26-5

TARGET SITES
Site of earliest ventricular activation typically >30 msec before QRS onset
Site of ≥11/12 pace map

localization by permitting three-dimensional reconstruction of intracardiac anatomy. In addition, if the endocardial shell is constructed during the tachycardia, the site of earliest activation can also be visualized.[8,10,47] We have typically used the contact electroanatomic system (Carto, Biosense Webster, Diamond Bar, CA) for mapping these

arrhythmias, but other investigators have reported comparable success rates during RVOT tachycardia ablation using noncontact electroanatomic mapping system (EnSite 3000, St. Jude Medical, St. Paul, MN). A potential advantage of the latter system is its ability to map and localize nonsustained rhythms, including isolated ventricular ectopic beats.[49]

Typically for ablation, the mapping catheter is advanced to the area of interest as suggested by the 12-lead ECG, and pace-mapping is performed at the diastolic threshold and at a rate similar to the tachycardia cycle length. The goal is to achieve an identical match (all 12 leads) between the clinical arrhythmia and the pace map, paying particular attention to subtle features such as notches in the QRS complexes in various leads. In the absence of a good match, the catheter should be repositioned with subtle movements in the area of interest. Diligent mapping is important because inability to achieve an identical match is usually associated with unsuccessful outcome. Figure 26-15 depicts the native tachycardia and an identical pace map, which was performed from the left coronary cusp. This was also the site of successful ablation.

Activation mapping can also be used to localize the site of origin.[30,31,48,50] Typically, the site of successful ablation precedes onset of QRS by about 30 milliseconds on a bipolar electrogram; if unipolar recording is performed at this location, it should have a "QS" morphology.[50] However, given the size of the catheter tip (4 to 8 mm), the site of earliest

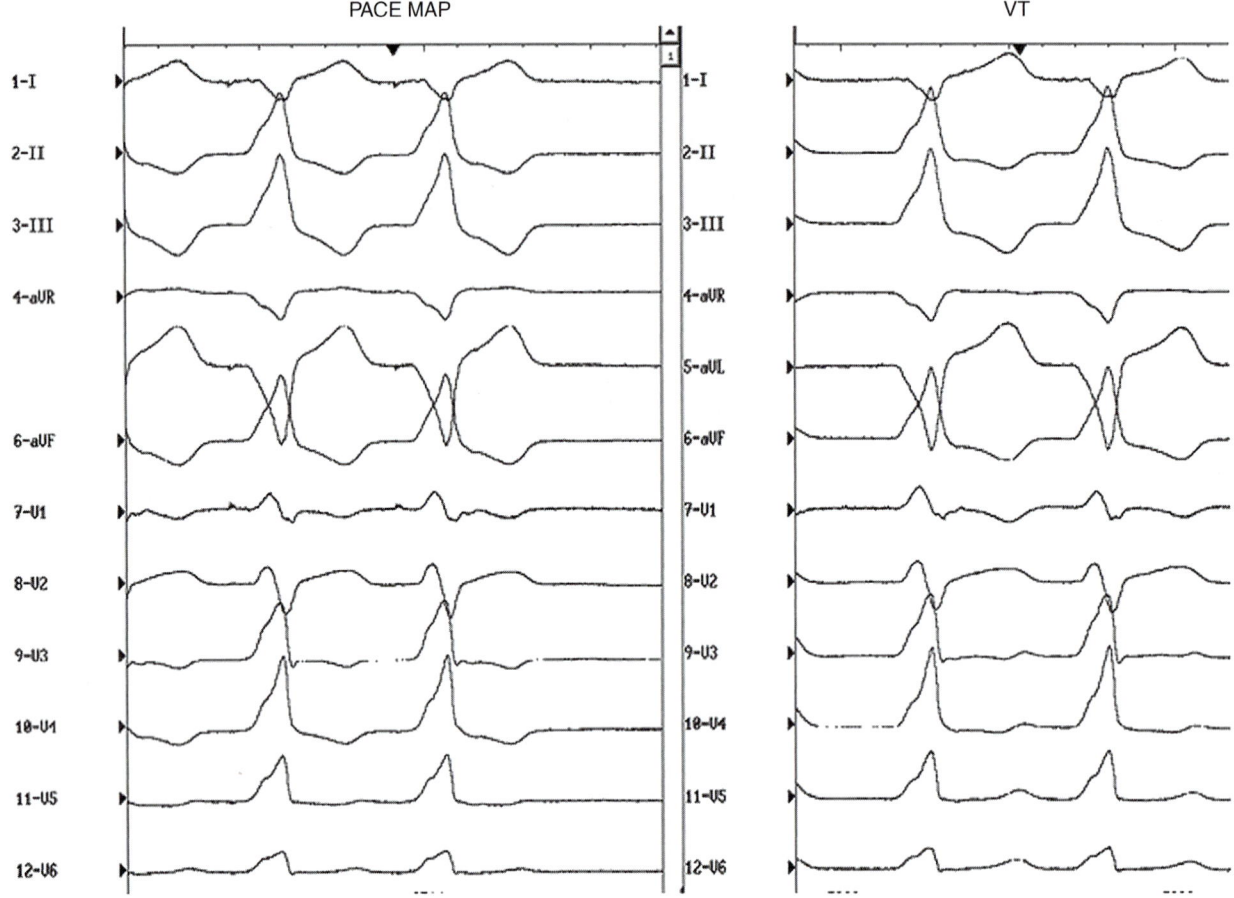

FIGURE 26-15. Clinical arrhythmia shown originating from basal left ventricle (*right panel*) and pace map (*left panel*), which was obtained from the left coronary cusp. The pace map at this site is a perfect match, and a single radiofrequency ablation from this location terminated the tachycardia. (Courtesy of Dr. Enrique Rodriguez.)

recording is not always the true site of origin and may not consistently result in successful ablation. Therefore, it is imperative to confirm an identical pace map at the site of earliest activation before ablating.[46,51]

In the event that the arrhythmia does not occur spontaneously or in response to programmed stimulation, isoproterenol is administered in incremental doses until there is an augmentation in the heart rate above baseline by about 20% to 25%. This sometimes requires doses of 10 μg/minute or higher, which in our experience are well tolerated. Because of the unpredictable nature of triggered activity, tachycardia induction may not always happen at peak heart rates; instead, it may manifest as the heart rate is slowing down after isoproterenol infusion is discontinued.[5] Aminophylline or epinephrine infusion may also enhance triggered activity and arrhythmia induction, and phenylephrine has been suggested to stimulate aortic cusp VTs (see later discussion). The triggered activity usually emanates from a narrow area (2 to 4 mm). Because of rapid conduction from the site of origin, however, a much larger area may be interpreted as having early activation unless meticulous attention is paid to electrogram analysis.[52] A large endocardial area of early ventricular activation may also represent the breakthrough point for an epicardial focus.

Ablation

Because the focus of the tachycardia is typically small in area, the site usually can be targeted using a 4-mm-tip ablation catheter in either temperature- or power-controlled mode. Our preference is temperature-control mode, with the typical settings for targeting RVOT and basal LV endocardium being 40 to 50 W, a temperature not to exceed 55°C, and a duration of up to 60 seconds.[8,10] For ablation in the aortic cusp region, we prefer to start at a lower power setting (10 to 15 W) and augment in steps of 5 to 10 W to achieve catheter-tip temperatures of 45° to 50°C, targeting an impedance drop of 5 ohms or greater.[50] It may be necessary to perform a coronary angiogram to delineate the proximity of a site of origin in the aortic cusp region to the coronary vessels. In general, delivery of radiofrequency energy within 1 cm of the coronary artery ostia should be avoided. In certain locations, such as at the anteroseptal aspect of superior RVOT or at the ventricular aspect of superolateral and lateral mitral annulus, the catheter tip may be deeply embedded in myocardium, causing poor blood flow and resulting in rapid achievement of target temperatures with low power output and minimal impedance drop. In such a scenario, switching to a larger-tip or an irrigated-tip catheter may be necessary to

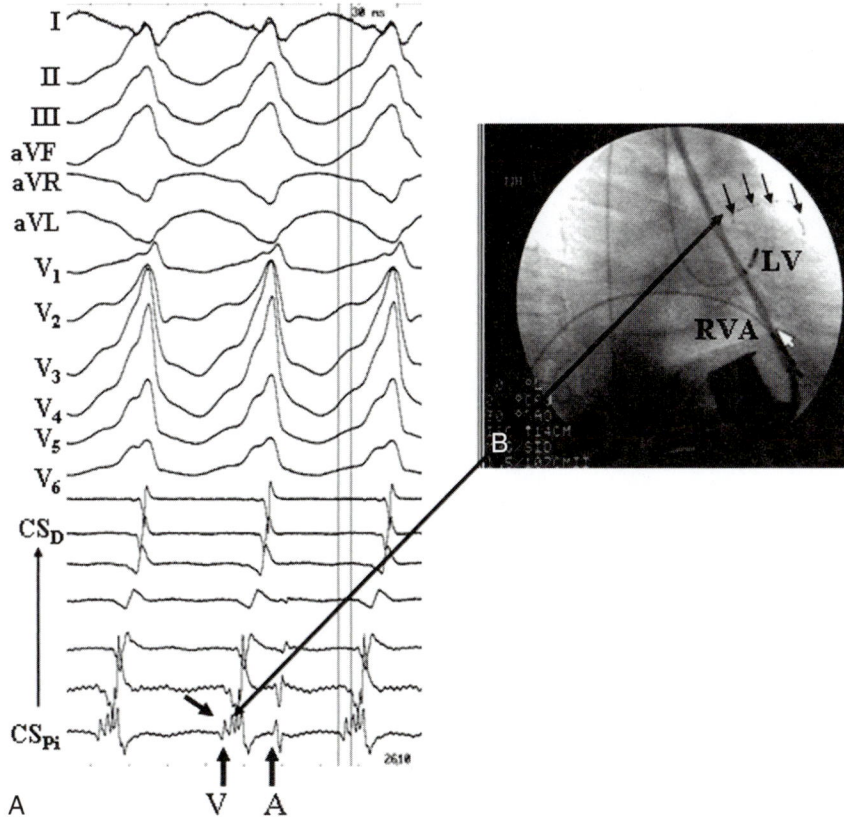

FIGURE 26-16. A, Twelve-lead ECG and recordings from the anterior branch of coronary sinus (CS) using a 2-French multielectrode mapping catheter (*arrows* on the fluoroscopic image) during tachycardia and recordings from the proximal poles of CS catheter are earliest. This was also the site for best pace mapping. **B,** Fluoroscopic image obtained in the right anterior oblique (RAO) projection. Also seen in the image are catheters at the right ventricular apex (RVA) and the left ventricle (LV) endocardium under the aortic valve. A, atrium; D, distal; Pi, proximal; V, ventricle. (Courtesy of Dr. Enrique Rodriguez.)

deliver effective energy.[50] Although it is safe to ablate from most locations in RVOT and basal LV with various catheter types, care must be exercised if the tachycardia originates close to the superior septum in the vicinity of the His bundle. In two of our initial four patients with LVOT tachycardia, a prominent His deflection was seen at the site of ideal pace maps; in both patients, ablation therapy was deferred because of the high risk for causing atrioventricular block.[10] Another area of the LVOT that requires special consideration in terms of ablation technique is the LV epicardium. It is impossible to achieve an ideal pace map for these tachycardias endocardially.[29] Options include the introduction of a low-profile, deflectable, multipolar catheter (with or without a sheath) into the branches of the coronary sinus (Fig. 26-16) or pacing from above the aortic valve in the region of the left or right coronary cusp, or both.[53] We have also used the epicardial approach for successful basal LV tachycardia ablation, following the technique described by Sosa and associates[54,55] (see Chapter 31). Because of the proximity of the epicardial coronary vessels, especially in the basal-anterior location, there are some additional risks involved with this strategy, and our practice has been to perform coronary angiography routinely before ablating in this area. Others have suggested using intravascular ultrasound.[5] Catheter visualization in some of these locations is enhanced by the use of phased-array intracardiac ultrasound, which in expert hands can accurately show the catheter-tissue interface and lesion creation in real time as well as demarcate more accurately the exact catheter location. The latter is especially important during localization and ablation of VT originating from the aortic cusp region.[50,56-58]

Clinical Outcomes and Complications

Radiofrequency ablation, if done with attention to energy settings and the coronary anatomy, is a safe treatment option with an overall success rate of 90% to 95%. In our opinion, ablation therapy may be considered first-line therapy in patients as an alternative to pursuing pharmacologic management. Some of the more common complications during RVOT and LVOT tachycardia ablations include development of complete left or right bundle branch block and aortic regurgitation.[58,59] A single case of death has been reported and on autopsy was shown to have occurred from a linear tear and hemopericardium in the RVOT.[58] There is also a report of a left main coronary artery occlusion during ablation of LVOT tachycardia originating beneath the aortic valve.[59]

Troubleshooting the Difficult Case

Common problems and potential solutions to the ablation of outflow tract VTs are listed in Table 26-6. Because of the triggered or automatic mechanism underlying most of these arrhythmias, noninducibility of the arrhythmia is a frequent obstacle. High-dose isoproterenol, hand grip exercises, and intravenous aminophylline can all be tried to facilitate tachycardia onset. Phenylephrine infusion has been described to facilitate onset of aortic cusp VTs.[60] Patience is often the key to success. Even limited amounts of ectopy may allow for pace-mapping or noncontact mapping. Noninducibility and infrequent ectopy are also problematic for defining end points for ablation. For cases with limited ectopy, "thermal mapping" of the RVOT has been described.[61] Radiofrequency energy is applied for 5 to 10 seconds to achieve tip temperatures of 45° to 50°C at sites of interest. At sites where ectopy is induced that is morphologically consistent with clinical ectopy, the radiofrequency energy is given for 30 to 60 seconds to reach tip temperatures of 50° to 60°C. The process is repeated until no further ectopy is evoked with and without isoproterenol. For RVOT especially, local conduction

TABLE 26-6

TROUBLESHOOTING THE DIFFICULT CASE

Problem	Causes	Solution
Tachycardia noninducible and rare spontaneous ectopy	Triggered or automatic mechanism	High-dose isoproterenol, and/or use aminophylline or phenylephrine (coronary cusp VTs) Pace map ectopy, thermal mapping Use noncontact mapping
Large area of earliest activation	Rapid local conduction near site of origin (usually RVOT) Origin epicardial or remote from mapping sites	Use pace mapping Careful electrogram analysis, and use unipolar electrograms Electroanatomic mapping Map epicardium or contralateral outflow tract sites
Best sites near coronary artery or His bundle	Origin in LVOT or septum	Coronary angiography before and after ablation Possibly use cryoablation
Ablation at favorable sites fails	Large area early activation (usually RVOT) Epicardial focus Incomplete mapping Insufficient lesion size	See above Map epicardium (percutaneous or by coronary veins) Reanalyze maps, expand area of mapping Use irrigated or large-tip ablation catheter

LVOT, left ventricular outflow tract; RVOT, right ventricular outflow tract; VT, ventricular tachycardia.

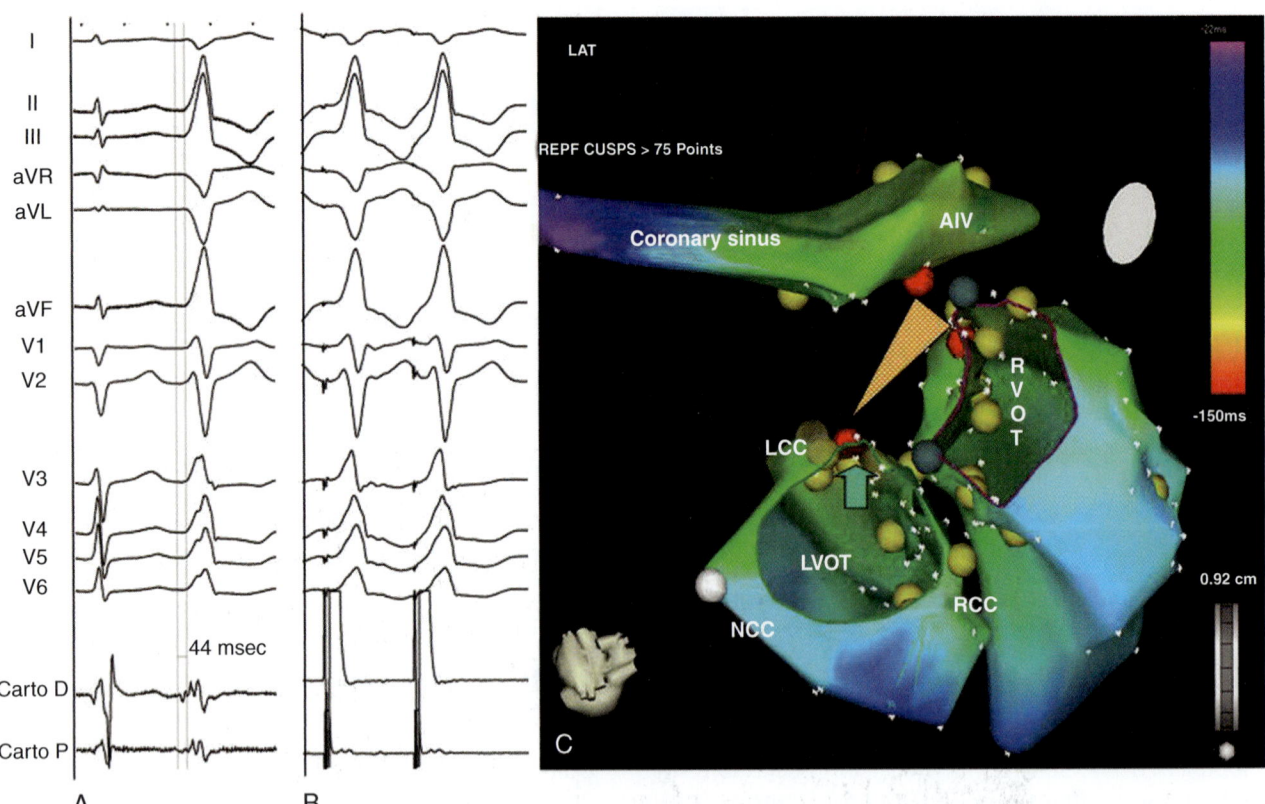

FIGURE 26-17. A, Local activation from the left coronary cusp (LCC) (pre-QRS by 44 msec) during the clinical arrhythmia (frequent monomorphic premature ventricular complexes [PVCs] with left bundle branch block morphology, inferior axis, and early precordial transition, by lead V_3). **B,** Pace map from this location, which is an excellent match of the PVC. **C,** Electroanatomic maps of the right and left ventricular outflow tracts (RVOT and LVOT, respectively) and the coronary sinus/anterior interventricular vein (AIV) that were acquired during the PVCs. Relative to the RVOT, coronary sinus, AIV, right coronary cusp (RCC), and noncoronary cusp (NCC), the LCC demonstrates the earliest activation (*arrow*). The region between the anterior septal superior RVOT, LCC, and distal coronary sinus–AIV junction (*red dots*) has been popularly nicknamed the "Bermuda Triangle." Arrhythmia foci arising from this region, depending on direction of preferential conduction, can manifest early activation and best pace maps from one or more surrounding locations and so can be frequently challenging to accurately localize.

from the focus may be very rapid, presenting a large area with early activation. Meticulous electrogram analysis and use of unipolar electrograms are essential to defining the earliest site. Sites near coronary arteries may risk injury to these vessels. Coronary angiography is recommended in such cases to define the proximity of the ablation catheter to the coronary artery. Sites near the His bundle or major fascicles may also risk injury to the conduction system. Cyroablation may offer less risk for collateral injury to these structures.

Despite appropriate target sites, ablation lesions may fail to terminate the tachycardia or prevent initiation. In the RVOT, a large area of early activation may be present, and the best site for ablation may not be easily distinguished from nearby sites. Careful electrogram analysis and pace-mapping may be remedial. An epicardial focus or a focus removed from the site of mapping may also produce favorable electrograms endocardially but be resistant to endocardial ablation. Thorough endocardial mapping and possibly mapping of the contralateral outflow tract may reveal even more favorable ablation targets. Epicardial mapping by the percutaneous approach or through the coronary sinus veins may be necessary. Frequently, in patients presenting with VT or PVC manifesting left bundle branch block morphology and inferior axis with an early precordial transition pattern (by lead V_3), extensive activation and pace-mapping in the septal RVOT, aortic cusp, and distal coronary sinus region may be required to determine the true site of origin (Fig. 26-17). Because of preferential conduction from the aortic cusps to the RVOT, pace maps in the RVOT may appear favorable for ablation yet be remote from the actual source of the ectopy. Mapping earliest ventricular activation will demonstrate significantly earlier activation in the aortic cusps in these instances.[62] Cooled ablation systems may be required to enhance energy delivery and lesion size in areas of low blood flow. Cryoablation is an option whenever there is excessive risk for collateral damage.

Conclusion

Outflow tract tachycardias are thought to be caused by adenosine-sensitive triggered activity. They are augmented by exercise and other adrenergic influences. The 12-lead ECG during the arrhythmias manifests site-specific characteristics that facilitate their localization. These arrhythmias, in general, are not life-threatening and therefore can initially be managed conservatively. However, radiofrequency ablation is a more definitive treatment option, and it can be curative in more than 90% of cases with a low risk (about 1%) for serious complications. Although it is typically reserved for patients who have failed or are intolerant to therapy with antiarrhythmic agents, ablation is an attractive initial treatment strategy in selected patients.

References

1. Lerman BB, Kenneth SM, Markovitz SM. Mechanisms of idiopathic left ventricular tachycardia. *J Cardiovasc Electrophysiol.* 1997;8:571–583.
2. Daliento L, Turrini P, Nava A, et al. Arrhythmogenic right ventricular cardiomyopathy in young versus adult patients: similarities and differences. *J Am Coll Cardiol.* 1995;25:655–664.
3. Froment R, Gallavardin L, Cahen P. Paroxysmal ventricular tachycardia: a clinical classification. *Br Heart J.* 1953;15:172.
4. Brooks R, Burgess JH. Idiopathic ventricular tachycardia: a review. *Medicine.* 1988;67:271–294.
5. Lerman BB, Stein SM, Markowitz SM, et al. Ventricular tachycardia in patients with structurally normal hearts. In: Zipes DP, Jalife J, eds. *Cardiac Electrophysiology: From Cell to Bedside.* Philadelphia: Saunders; 1999:640–656.
6. Lerman BB. Response of nonreentrant catecholamine-mediated ventricular tachycardia to endogenous adenosine and acetylcholine: evidence for myocardial receptor-mediated effects. *Circulation.* 1993;87:382–390.
7. Lerman BB, Belardinelli L, West GA, et al. Adenosine-sensitive ventricular tachycardia: evidence suggesting cyclic AMP-mediated triggered activity. *Circulation.* 1986;74:270–280.
8. Dixit S, Lin D, Zado E, Marchlinski F. Identification of distinct electrocardiographic patterns from basal left ventricle: distinguishing medial and lateral sites of origin. *Heart Rhythm.* 2004;1:S104.
9. Lerman BB, Stein KM, Markowitz SM. Idiopathic right ventricular outflow tract tachycardia: a clinical approach. *Pacing Clin Electrophysiol.* 1996;19:2120–2137.
10. Callans DJ, Menz V, Schwartzman D, et al. Repetitive monomorphic tachycardia from the left ventricular outflow tract: Electrocardiographic patterns consistent with a left ventricular site of origin. *J Am Coll Cardiol.* 1997;29:1023–1027.
11. Buxton AE, Waxman HL, Marchlinski FE, et al. Right ventricular tachycardia: clinical and electrophysiologic characteristics. *Circulation.* 1983;68:917–927.
12. Proclemer A, Ciani R, Feruglio GA. Right ventricular tachycardia with left bundle branch block and inferior axis morphology: clinical and arrhythmological characteristics in 15 patients. *Pacing Clin Electrophysiol.* 1989;12:977–988.
13. Lemery R, Brugada P, Della Bella P, et al. Non ischemic ventricular tachycardia: clinical course and long-term follow-up in patients without clinically overt heart disease. *Circulation.* 1989;79:990–999.
14. Haïssaguerre M, Extramania F, Hocini M, et al. Mapping and ablation of ventricular fibrillation associated with long QT and Brugada syndrome. *Circulation.* 2003;108:925–928.
15. Mont L, Seixas T, Brugada P, et al. Clinical and electrophysiologic characteristics of exercise-related idiopathic ventricular tachycardia. *Am J Cardiol.* 1991;68:897–900.
16. Lerman BB, Stein K, Engelstein ED, et al. Mechanism of repetitive monomorphic ventricular tachycardia. *Circulation.* 1995;92:421–429.
17. Hayashi H, Fujiki A, Tani M, et al. Role of sympathovagal balance in the initiation of idiopathic ventricular tachycardia originating from right ventricular outflow tract. *Pacing Clin Electrophysiol.* 1997;20:2371–2377.
18. Marchlinski FE, Deely MP, Zado ES. Gender specific triggers for right ventricular outflow tract tachycardias. *Am Heart J.* 2000;139:1009–1013.
19. Mehta D, Davies MJ, Ward DE, Camm AJ. Ventricular tachycardias of right ventricular origin: Markers of subclinical right ventricular disease. *Am Heart J.* 1994;127:360–366.
20. Carlson MD, White RD, Trohman RG, et al. Right ventricular outflow tract ventricular tachycardia: detection of previously unrecognized anatomic abnormalities using cine magnetic resonance imaging. *J Am Coll Cardiol.* 1994;24:720–727.
21. Markowitz SM, Litvak BL, Ramirez de Arellano EA, et al. Adenosine sensitive ventricular tachycardia: right ventricular abnormalities delineated by magnetic resonance imaging. *Circulation.* 1997;96:1192–1200.
22. Gill JS, Hunter GJ, Gane J, et al. Asymmetry of cardiac [^{123}I] meta-iodobenzylguanidine scans in patients with ventricular tachycardia and "clinically normal" heart. *Br Heart J.* 1993;59:6–13.
23. Mitrani RD, Klein LS, Miles WM, et al. Regional cardiac sympathetic denervation in patients with ventricular tachycardia in the absence of coronary artery disease. *J Am Coll Cardiol.* 1993;22:1344–1353.
24. Wichter T, Hindricks G, Lerch H, et al. Regional myocardial sympathetic dysinnervation in arrhythmogenic right ventricular cardiomyopathy: an analysis using ^{123}I-meta-iodobenzylguanidine scintigraphy. *Circulation.* 1994;89:667–683.
25. Vijgen J, Hill P, Biblo LA, Carlson MD. Tachycardia induced cardiomyopathy secondary to right ventricular outflow tract tachycardia: improvement of left ventricular systolic dysfunction after radiofrequency catheter ablation of the arrhythmia. *J Cardiovasc Electrophysiol.* 1997;8:445–450.
26. Takemoto M, Yoshimura H, Ohba Y, et al. Radiofrequency catheter ablation of premature ventricular complexes from left ventricular outflow tract improves left ventricular dilation and clinical status in patients without structural heart disease. *J Am Coll Cardiol.* 2005;45:1259–1265.
27. Bogun F, Reich S, Crawford T, et al. Radiofrequency ablation of frequent, idiopathic premature ventricular complexes: comparison with control group without intervention. *Heart Rhythm.* 2007;4:863–867.
28. Sulieman M, Asirvatham SJ. Ablation above the semilunar valves: when, why and how? Part I. *Heart Rhythm.* 2008;5:1485–1492.
29. Dixit S, Marchlinski FE. Clinical characteristics and catheter ablation of left ventricular outflow tract tachycardia. *Curr Cardiol Rep.* 2001;3:305–313.
30. Jadonath RL, Schwartzman DS, Preminger MW, et al. Utility of 12-lead electrocardiogram in localizing the origin of right ventricular outflow tract tachycardia. *Am Heart J.* 1995;130:1107–1113.
31. Movsowitz C, Schwartzman DS, Callans DJ, et al. Idiopathic right ventricular outflow tract tachycardia: Narrowing the anatomic location for successful ablation. *Am Heart J.* 1996;131:930–936.

32. Delacey WA, Nath S, Haines DE, et al. Adenosine and verapamil sensitive tachycardia originating from the left ventricle: radiofrequency catheter ablation. *Pacing Clin Electrophysiol.* 1992;15:2240–2244.

33. Sekiguchi Y, Aonuma K, Takahashi A, et al. Electrocardiographic and electrophysiologic characteristics of ventricular tachycardia originating within the pulmonary artery. *J Am Coll Cardiol.* 2005;45:887–895.

34. Lerman BB, Wesley RC, DiMarco JP, et al. Antiadrenergic effects of adenosine on His-Purkinje automaticity: evidence for accentuated antagonism. *J Clin Invest.* 1988;82:2127–2135.

35. Dixit S, Gerstenfeld EP, Callans DJ, Marchlinski FE. Electrocardiographic patterns of superior right ventricular outflow tract tachycardia: distinguishing septal and free wall sites of origin. *J Cardiovasc Electrophysiol.* 2003;13:1–7.

36. Griffith MJ, Garratt CJ, Rowland E, et al. Effects of intravenous adenosine on verapamil-sensitive "idiopathic" ventricular tachycardia. *Am J Cardiol.* 1994;73:759–764.

37. Storey J, Iwasa A, Feld G. Left ventricular outflow tract tachycardia originating from the right coronary cusp: identification of location of origin by endocardial noncontact activation mapping from the right ventricular outflow tract. *J Cardiovasc Electrophysiol.* 2002;13:1050–1053.

38. Kanagaratnam L, Tomassoni G, Schweikert R, et al. Ventricular tachycardias arising from the aortic sinus of Valsalva: an under-recognized variant of left outflow tract ventricular tachycardia. *J Am Coll Cardiol.* 2001;37:1408–1414.

39. Ouyang F, Fotuhi P, Ho SY, et al. Repetitive monomorphic ventricular tachycardia originating from the aortic sinus cusp. *J Am Coll Cardiol.* 2002;39:500–508.

40. Yacoub M, Kilner P, Birks E, Misfeld M. The aortic outflow and root: a tale of dynamism and crosstalk. *Ann Thorac Surg.* 1999;68:S37–S43.

41. Lin D, Ilkhanoff L, Gerstenfeld E, et al. Twelve lead electrocardiographic characteristics of the aortic cusp region guided by intracardiac echocardiography and electroanatomic mapping. *Heart Rhythm.* 2008;5:663–669.

42. Bala R, Garcia F, Harding J, et al. Notch in downward deflection in lead V1 defines VPDs from the right/left coronary cusp margin: anatomic and electrophysiologic observations. *Heart Rhythm.* 2008;5:PO6–PO43.

43. Ito H, Tada H, Naito S, et al. Development and validation of an ECG algorithm for identifying the optimal ablation site for idiopathic ventricular outflow tract tachycardia. *J Cardiovasc Electrophysiol.* 2003;14:1280–1286.

44. Goy JJ, Tauxe F, Fromer M, et al. Ten-years follow-up of 20 patients with idiopathic ventricular tachycardia. *Pacing Clin Electrophysiol.* 1990;13:1142–1147.

45. Gill JS, Ward D, Camm AJ. Comparison of verapamil and diltiazem in the suppression of idiopathic ventricular tachycardia. *Pacing Clin Electrophysiol.* 1992;15:2122–2125.

46. Gill JS, Mehta D, Ward DE, et al. Efficacy of flecainide, sotalol and verapamil in the treatment of right ventricular tachycardia in patients without overt cardiac abnormality. *Br Heart J.* 1992;68:392–397.

47. Wilber DJ, Baerman J, Olshansky B, et al. Adenosine-sensitive ventricular tachycardia: clinical characteristics and response to catheter ablation. *Circulation.* 1993;87:126–134.

48. Gepstein L, Hayam G, Ben-Haim SA. A novel method for nonfluoroscopic catheter-based electroanatomic mapping of the heart: In vitro and in vivo accuracy results. *Circulation.* 1997;95:1611–1622.

49. Friedman PA, Asirvatham SJ, Grice S, et al. Noncontact mapping to guide ablation of right ventricular outflow tract tachycardia. *J Am Coll Cardiol.* 2002;39:1808–1812.

50. Marchlinski FE, Lin D, Dixit S, et al. Ventricular tachycardia from the aortic cusps: localization and ablation. In: Raviele A, ed. *Cardiac Arrhythmias 2003.* Milan: Springer-Verlag Italia; 2004:357–370. Proceedings of the 8th International Workshop for Cardiac Arrhythmias, Venice 2003.

51. Coggins DL, Lee RJ, Sweeney J, et al. Radiofrequency catheter ablation as a cure for idiopathic tachycardia of both left and right ventricular origin. *J Am Coll Cardiol.* 1994;23:1333–1341.

52. Yamada T, Murakami Y, Yoshida N, et al. Preferential conduction across ventricular outflow septum in ventricular arrhythmias originating from the aortic sinus cusp. *J Am Coll Cardiol.* 2007;50:884–891.

53. Stellbrink C, Diem B, Schaurte P, et al. Transcoronary venous radiofrequency catheter ablation of ventricular tachycardia. *J Cardiovasc Electrophysiol.* 1997;8:916–921.

54. Sosa E, Scanavacca M, d'Avila A, et al. Nonsurgical transthoracic epicardial catheter ablation to treat recurrent ventricular tachycardia occurring late after myocardial infarction [see comment]. *J Am Coll Cardiol.* 2000;35:1442–1449.

55. Dixit S, Narula N, Callans DJ, Marchlinski FE. Electroanatomic mapping of human heart: epicardial fat can mimic scar. *J Cardiovasc Electrophysiol.* 2003;14:1128.

56. Ren J, Marchlinski FE, Callans DC, et al. Intracardiac Doppler echocardiographic quantification of pulmonary flow velocity: an effective technique for monitoring pulmonary vein narrowing during focal atrial fibrillation ablation. *J Cardiovasc Electrophysiol.* 2002;13:1076–1081.

57. Dixit S, Ren J-F, Callans DJ, et al. Favorable effect of pulmonic vein isolation by partial circumferential ablation on ostial flow velocity. *Heart Rhythm.* 2004;1:262–267.

58. Zhu D, Maloney JD, Simmons TE, et al. Radiofrequency catheter ablation for management of symptomatic ventricular ectopic activity. *J Am Coll Cardiol.* 1995;26:843–849.

59. Friedman PL, Stevenson WG, Bihl JA, et al. Left main coronary artery occlusion during radiofrequency catheter ablation of idiopathic outflow tract tachycardia. *Pacing Clin Electrophysiol.* 1997;20:1184.

60. Cole RC, Marrouche NF, Natale A. Evaluation and management of ventricular outflow tract tachycardia. *Card Electrophysiol Rev.* 2002;6:442–447.

61. Clyne CA, Athar H, Shah A, et al. Thermal mapping of right ventricular outflow tract tachycardia. *Pacing Clin Electrophysiol.* 2007;30:343–351.

62. Yamada T, Murakami Y, Yoshida N, et al. Preferential conduction across the ventricular outflow septum in ventricular arrhythmias originating from the aortic sinus cusp. *J Am Coll Cardiol.* 2007;50:884–891.

27
Ablation of Idiopathic Left Ventricular and Fascicular Tachycardias

Akihiko Nogami

Key Points

The mechanism of verapamil-sensitive idiopathic left ventricular tachycardia (VT) is reentry.

Diagnosis is based on demonstration of right bundle branch block and superior axis configuration (common type); right bundle branch block and inferior axis configuration (uncommon type); or a relatively narrow QRS and inferior axis configuration (rare type), together with dependence on left ventricular fascicular activation and verapamil sensitivity (termination or slowing of the tachycardia).

Ablation targets are the diastolic potential in the descending limb of the fascicular circuit or the presystolic fused Purkinje potential at the VT exit.

A multipolar electrode mapping catheter may be useful. Specialized mapping systems or irrigated ablation are rarely necessary.

The success rate of ablation is greater than 90% for the superior axis configuration (common type) and greater than 80% for the inferior axis configuration (uncommon type). The success rate for VTs with relatively narrow QRS and inferior axis configuration (rare type) is unclear.

It is difficult to distinguish verapamil-sensitive idiopathic left VT from focal verapamil-insensitive Purkinje VT by 12-lead ECG.

The mechanism of focal Purkinje VT is the abnormal automaticity from the distal Purkinje system, and the ablation target is the earliest Purkinje activation during VT.

Sustained monomorphic ventricular tachycardia (VT) is most often related to myocardial structure heart disease, including healed myocardial infarction and cardiomyopathies. However, no apparent structural abnormality is identified in about 10% of all sustained monomorphic VTs in the United States[1] and 20% of those in Japan.[2] These VTs are referred to as "idiopathic." Idiopathic VTs usually occur in specific locations and have specific QRS morphologies, whereas VTs associated with structural heart disease have a QRS morphology that tends to indicate the location of the scar. Idiopathic VT comprises multiple discrete subtypes that are best differentiated by their mechanism, QRS morphology, and site of origin. The most common idiopathic VT originates from a focus in the outflow tract of the right ventricle (see Chapter 26), and its mechanism is most likely triggered activity. In idiopathic left VT, four types of VT exist: verapamil-sensitive left fascicular VT (reentry), VT with a focal origin in the distal Purkinje system (abnormal automaticity), left ventricular outflow tract VT (triggered activity, reentry, or automaticity; see Chapter 26), and VT from the mitral annulus (triggered activity, reentry, or automaticity; see Chapter 26). This chapter focuses on the assessment and nonpharmacologic treatment of Purkinje-related VTs: verapamil-sensitive left fascicular VT and focal Purkinje VT.

Pathophysiology

Classification

Verapamil-sensitive fascicular VT is the most common form of idiopathic left VT. It was first recognized as an electrocardiographic entity in 1979 by Zipes and colleagues,[3] who identified the characteristic diagnostic triad: (1) induction with atrial pacing, (2) right bundle branch block (RBBB) and left-axis configuration, and (3) manifestation in patients without structural heart disease. In 1981, Belhassen and associates[4] were the first to demonstrate the verapamil sensitivity of the tachycardia, a fourth identifying feature. Ohe and coworkers[5] reported another type of this tachycardia, with RBBB and a right-axis deviation, in 1988. More recently, Shimoike and associates[6] described the upper septal form of this tachycardia. According to the QRS morphology, verapamil-sensitive left fascicular VT can be classified into three subgroups: (1) left posterior fascicular VT, whose QRS morphology exhibits an RBBB configuration and a superior axis (Fig. 27-1); (2) left anterior fascicular VT, whose QRS morphology exhibits an RBBB configuration and right-axis deviation (Fig. 27-2); and (3) upper septal fascicular VT, whose QRS morphology exhibits a narrow QRS configuration and normal or right-axis deviation (Fig. 27-3). Left posterior fascicular VT is common, left anterior fascicular VT is uncommon, and left upper septal fascicular VT is very rare.

Substrate and Anatomy

The anatomic basis of this tachycardia has provoked considerable interest. Some data suggest that the tachycardia may originate from a false tendon or fibromuscular band in the left ventricle.[7-9] Suwa and coworkers[8] described a

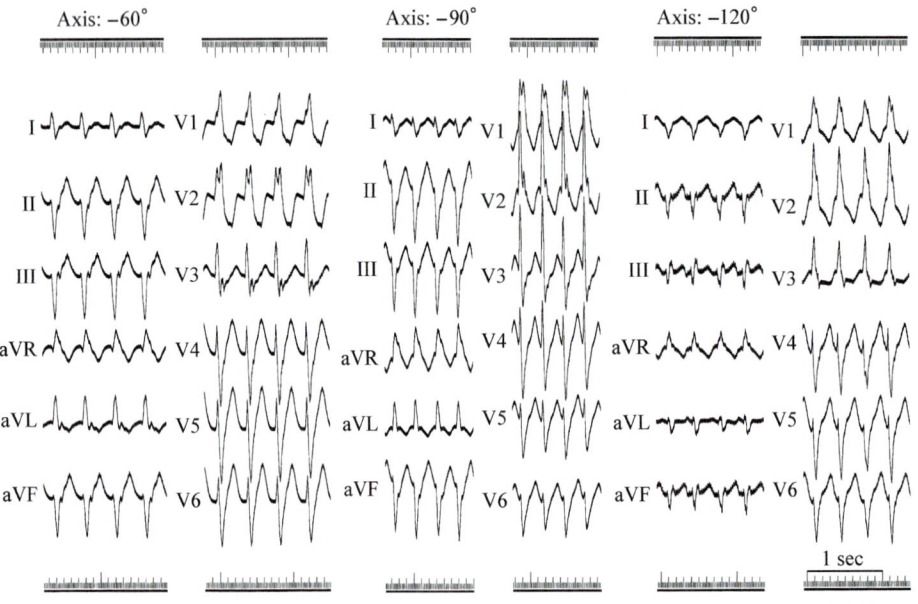

FIGURE 27-1. Twelve-lead electrocardiograms of verapamil-sensitive left posterior fascicular ventricular tachycardias (VTs). Three different VTs are shown. *(From Nogami A. Idiopathic left ventricular tachycardia: assessment and treatment. Card Electrophysiol Rev. 2002;6:448–457. With permission.)*

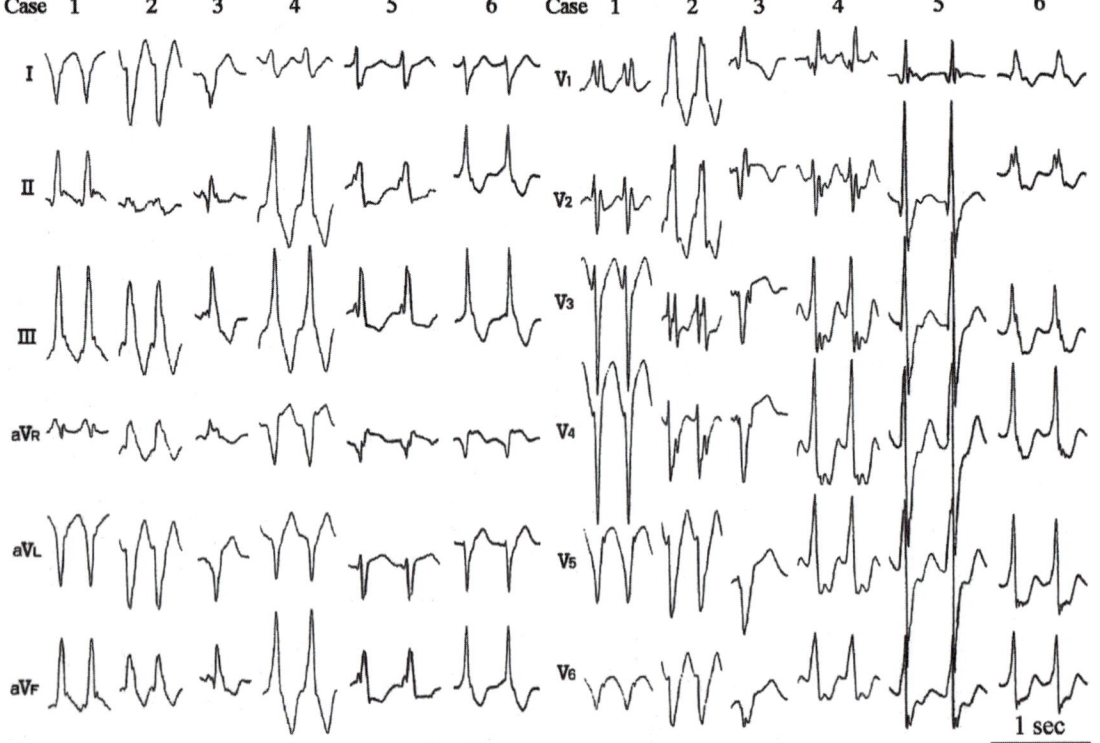

FIGURE 27-2. Twelve-lead electrocardiograms of verapamil-sensitive left anterior fascicular ventricular tachycardias in six patients. *(From Nogami A, Naito S, Tada H, et al. Verapamil-sensitive left anterior fascicular ventricular tachycardia: results of radiofrequency ablation in six patients. J Cardiovasc Electrophysiol. 1998;9:1269–1278. With permission.)*

false tendon in the left ventricle of a patient with idiopathic VT in whom the VT was eliminated by surgical resection of the tendon. Using transthoracic and transesophageal echocardiography, Thakur and colleagues[9] found false tendons extending from the posteroinferior left ventricle to the basal septum in 15 of 15 patients with idiopathic left VT but in only 5% of control patients. Maruyama and associates[10] reported a case with the recording of sequential diastolic potentials bridging the entire diastolic period and a false tendon extending from the mid-septum to the inferoapical septum. Lin and colleagues[11] found that 17 of 18 patients with idiopathic VT had this fibromuscular band but also found it in 35 of 40 control patients. They concluded that the band was a common echocardiographic finding and was not a specific arrhythmogenic substrate for this tachycardia, although they could not exclude the possibility that the band was a potential substrate of the VT. Small fibromuscular bands, trabeculae carneae, and small papillary muscles cannot be detected by echocardiography. The Purkinje networks in these small anatomic structures are important when considering the reentry circuit of verapamil-sensitive left posterior fascicular VT. This circuit is not completely defined but may comprise only fascicular tissue or fascicular tissue and ventricular myocardium.

Mechanism

The mechanism of verapamil-sensitive left VT is reentry because it can be induced, entrained, and terminated by programmed ventricle or atrial stimulation. To confirm its reentry circuit and the mechanism, my colleagues and I performed left ventricular septal mapping using an octapolar electrode catheter in 20 patients with left posterior fascicular VT[12] (Fig. 27-4). In 15 of 20 patients, two distinct potentials, P1 and P2, were recorded during the VT at the mid-septum (Fig. 27-5). Although the mid-diastolic potential (P1) was recorded earlier from the proximal rather than the distal electrodes, the fused presystolic Purkinje potential (P2) was recorded earlier from the distal electrodes. During sinus rhythm, recording at the same site demonstrated P2, which was recorded after the His bundle potential and before the onset of the QRS complex; however, the sequence of the P2 was the reverse of that seen during the VT. At the initiation of the VT by ventricular extrastimulation, retrograde conduction of the P2 was observed (Fig. 27-6). VT could be entrained from the atrium (Fig. 27-7) and from the ven-

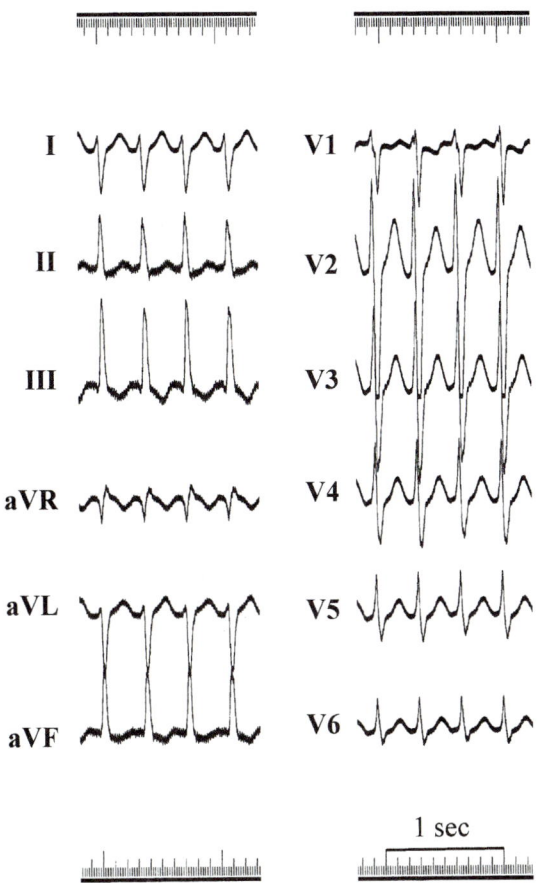

FIGURE 27-3. Twelve-lead electrocardiogram of verapamil-sensitive left upper septal ventricular tachycardia (VT). The QRS morphology during the VT was narrow (100 msec) and exhibited an R-wave transition at V₃. (*From Nogami A. Idiopathic left ventricular tachycardia: assessment and treatment.* Card Electrophysiol Rev. *2002;6:448–457. With permission.*)

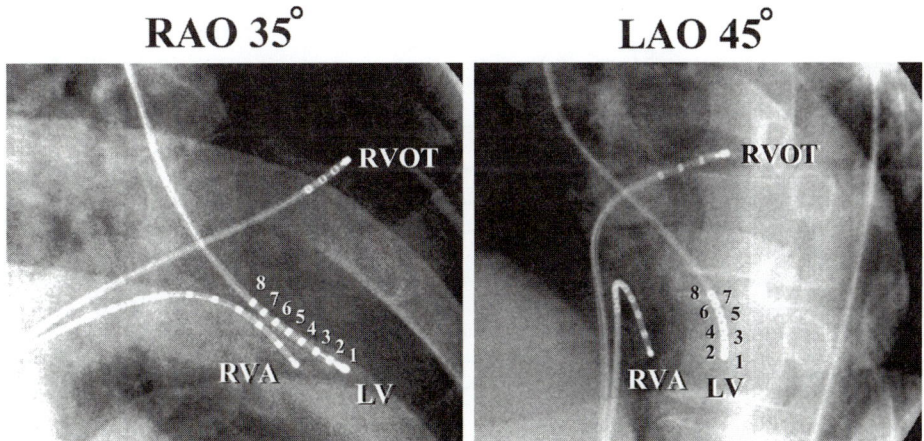

FIGURE 27-4. Representation of an octapolar electrode catheter positioned at the left ventricular septum as viewed fluoroscopically in the right anterior oblique (RAO) and left anterior oblique (LAO) projections. The distance between electrodes 1 and 8 of the octapolar electrode catheter was approximately 25 mm. LV, left ventricle; RVA, right ventricular apex; RVOT, right ventricular outflow tract. (*From Nogami A, Naito S, Tada H, et al. Demonstration of diastolic and presystolic Purkinje potential as critical potentials on a macroreentry circuit of verapamil-sensitive idiopathic left ventricular tachycardia.* J Am Coll Cardiol. *2000;36:811–823. With permission.*)

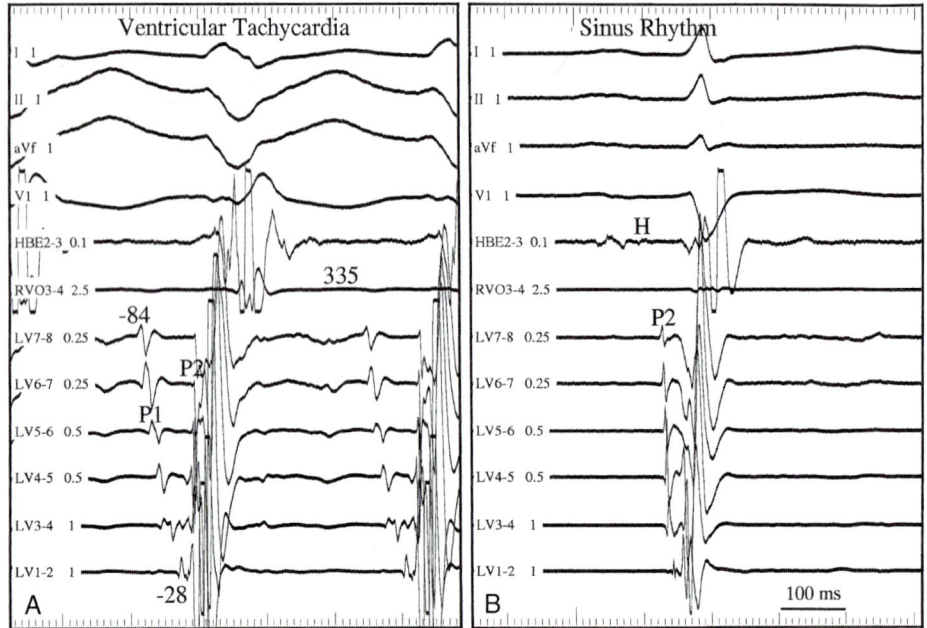

FIGURE 27-5. Intracardiac recordings from an octopolar electrode catheter. **A,** During left posterior fascicular ventricular tachycardia, a diastolic potential (P1) and a presystolic Purkinje potential (P2) were recorded. While P1 was recorded earlier from the proximal rather than the distal electrodes, P2 was recorded earlier from the distal rather than the proximal electrodes. **B,** During sinus rhythm, recording at the same site demonstrated the P2, is now recorded before the onset of the QRS complex and is earliest on the proximal electrodes. HBE, His bundle electrogram; RVO, right ventricular outflow; LV, left ventricle; 7-8, proximal bipole; 1-2, distal bipole; H, His. *(From Nogami A, Naito S, Tada H, et al. Demonstration of diastolic and presystolic Purkinje potential as critical potentials on a macroreentry circuit of verapamil-sensitive idiopathic left ventricular tachycardia.* J Am Coll Cardiol. *2000;36:811–823. With permission.)*

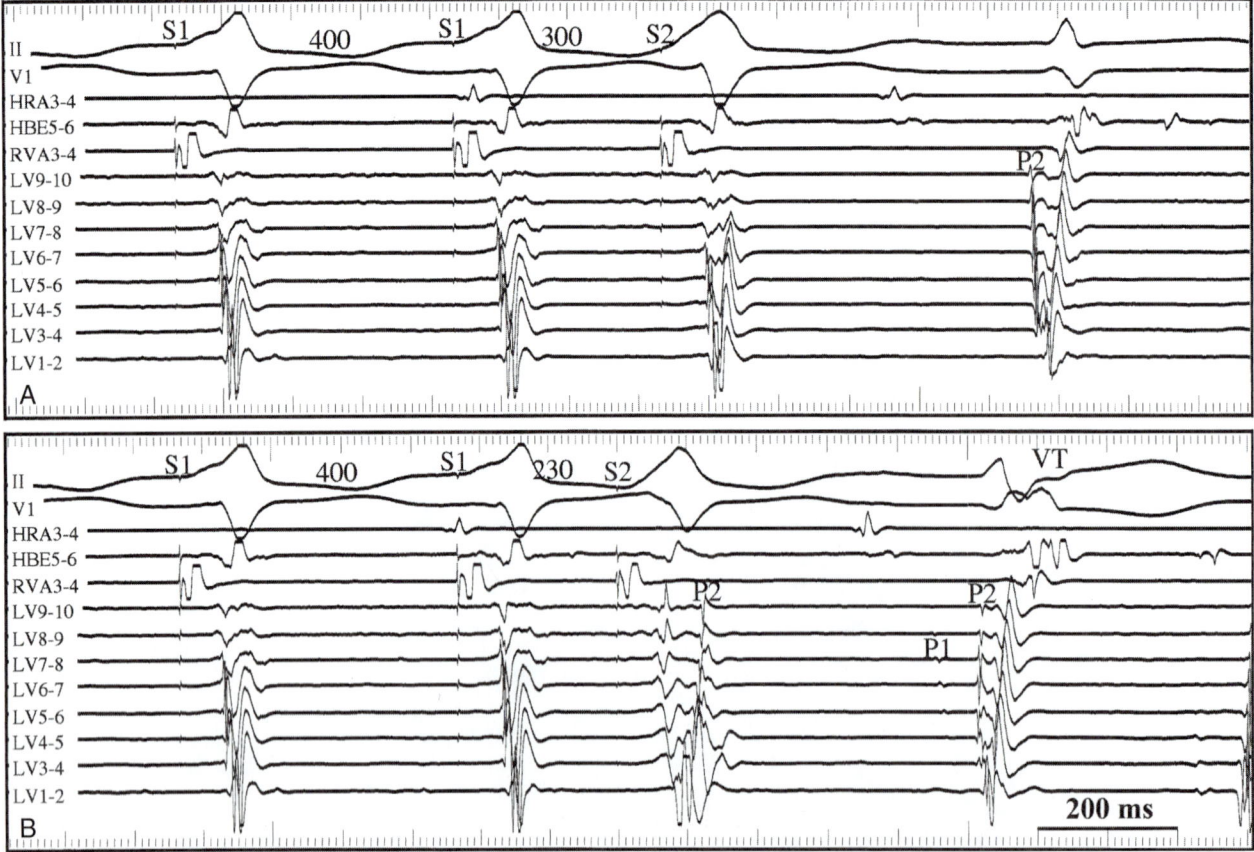

FIGURE 27-6. Induction of left posterior fascicular ventricular tachycardia (VT) by ventricular extrastimulation from the right ventricular apex. **A,** During the basic drive (S1) and at a coupling interval of 300 msec (S2), sharp electrical potentials (P2) were recorded just before the ventricular electrograms. These potentials were recorded earlier from the proximal than the distal electrodes. **B,** When the coupling interval was decreased to 230 msec, the activations of P2 were delayed and the sequence of P2 was reversed, resulting in initiating ventricular tachycardia. This sequence may be interpreted as development of antegrade unidirectional block in the fascicle generating P2, which is now activated by a distal connection with the fascicle generating P1. HBE, His bundle electrogram; HRA, high right atrium; LV, left ventricle; RVA, right ventricular apex.

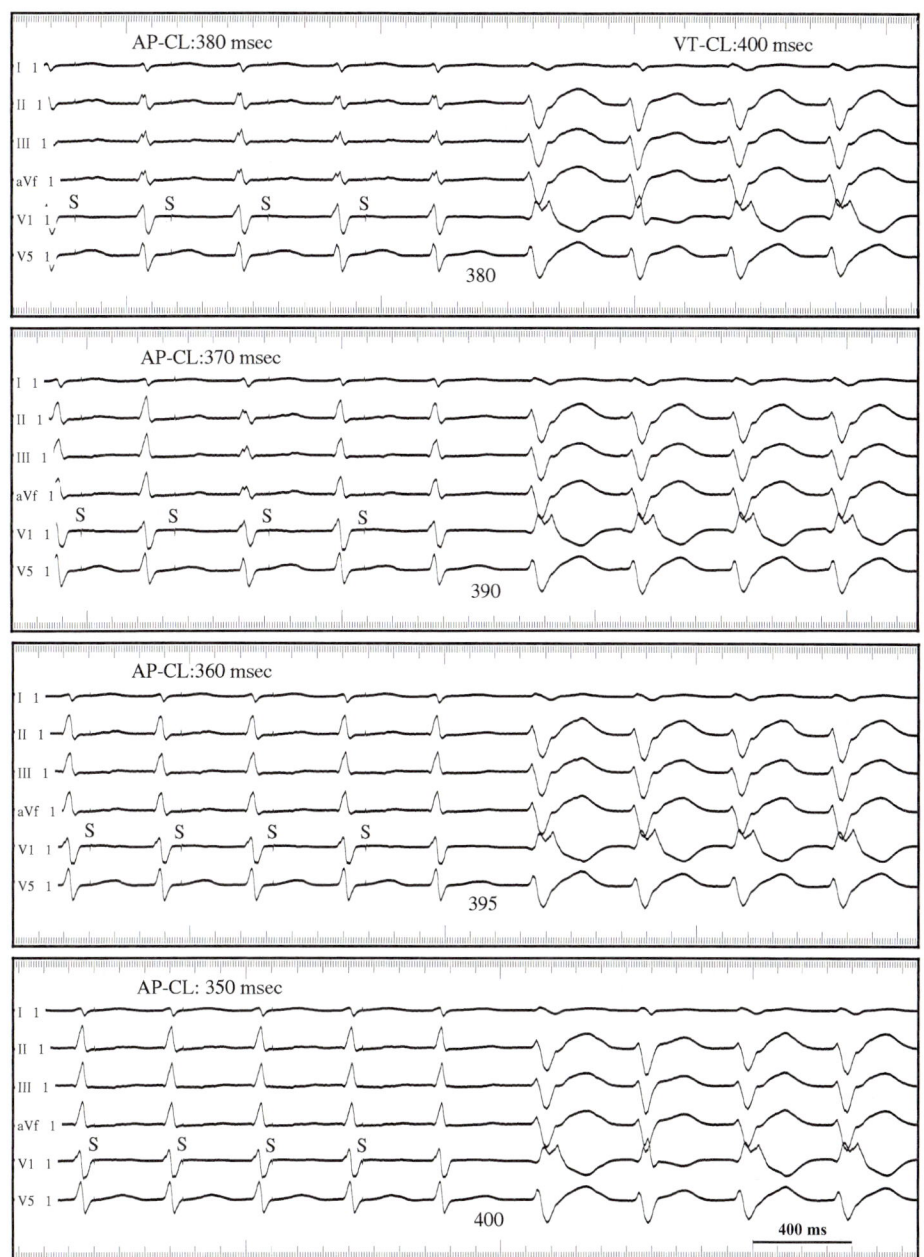

FIGURE 27-7. Surface electrocardiograms showing entrainment pacing from the high right atrium during left posterior fascicular ventricular tachycardia (VT). The QRS morphology exhibited constant fusion and progressive fusion. The subsequent VT had been reset because the interval between the last entrained QRS and VT was less than the VT cycle length. The interval between the last captured QRS and VT was prolonged with shortening of the pacing cycle length, presumably owing to decremental conduction within the reentry circuit. AP, atrial pacing; CL, cycle length; S, pacing stimulus.

tricle. Entrainment pacing from the atrium or ventricle captured P1 orthodromically and reset the VT (Figs. 27-8 and 27-9). The interval from the stimulus to P1 was prolonged as the pacing rate increased. The effect of verapamil on P1 and P2 is shown in Figure 27-10. The intravenous administration of 1.5 mg of verapamil significantly prolonged the cycle length of the VT, from 305 to 350 msec. Both the P1-P2 and P2-P1 intervals were proportionally prolonged after verapamil administration. However, the interval from P2 to the onset of the QRS complex remained unchanged. This study demonstrated that P1 is a critical potential in the circuit of the verapamil-sensitive left posterior fascicular VT and suggested the presence of a macroreentry circuit involving the normal Purkinje system and abnormal Purkinje tissue with decremental properties and verapamil sensitivity.

Although P1 has proved to be a critical potential in the VT circuit, whether the left posterior fascicle or Purkinje fiber (P2) is involved in the retrograde limb of the reentrant circuit remains unclear.[10,13,14] Morishima and associates[14] reported a case with negative participation of the proximal left posterior fascicle to the VT circuit. Although selective capture of left posterior fascicle by sinus beat did not affect the cycle length of VT, the postpacing interval after the entrainment from left ventricular septal myocardium was equal to the cycle length of VT (Fig. 27-11). Ouyang and coworkers[15] suggested that idiopathic left VT reentry might be a small macro-reentry circuit consisting of one anterograde Purkinje fiber with a Purkinje potential, one retrograde Purkinje fiber with retrograde Purkinje potential, and the ventricular myocardium as the bridge.

FIGURE 27-8. Intracardiac recordings during entrainment pacing from the high right atrium (HRA) during left posterior fascicular ventricular tachycardia (VT). Right atrial pacing (CL: 320 msec) during VT (CL: 345 msec) resulted in a narrowing of the QRS width without VT interruption. While the diastolic potential (P1) was orthodromically captured, the presystolic Purkinje potential (P2) was antidromically captured. The activation sequence of P2 was identical to that observed during sinus rhythm. CL, cycle length; H, His; HBE, His bundle electrogram; LV, left ventricle; S, pacing stimulus.

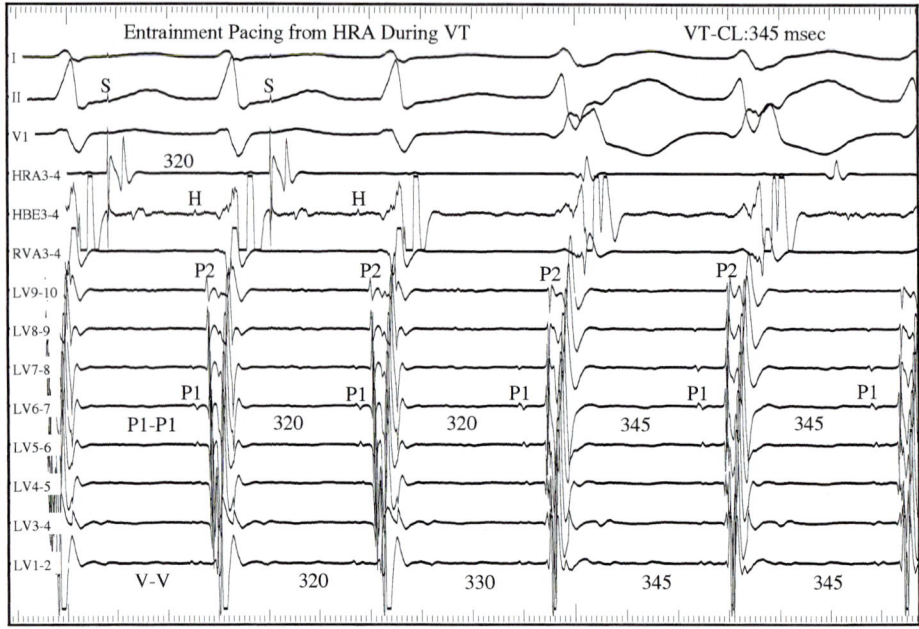

FIGURE 27-9. Concealed entrainment by pacing from the ventricular tachycardia (VT) exit site. During left posterior fascicular VT, the earliest ventricular electrogram with the fused Purkinje potential (P2) was recorded from the distal two electrodes. **A,** Pacing from the distal two electrodes at a cycle length and a starting coupling interval of 400 msec captured P1 orthodromically and produced QRS configurations similar to that of the VT. The postpacing interval (PPI) (S-P2) was equal to the VT cycle length. **B,** Pacing from the VT exit site at a cycle length of 380 msec also captured P1. A diastolic potential was simultaneously observed with a pacing artifact from left ventricle (LV) 7-8. The pacing stimulus P1 interval was prolonged. **C,** Pacing from the VT exit at a cycle length of 400 msec but with a starting coupling interval of 300 msec terminated the VT. A diastolic potential was not observed during pacing because it might have been captured antidromically and masked in the ventricular electrogram. HBE, His bundle electrogram; P1, diastolic potential; P2, presystolic Purkinje potential; RVO, right ventricular outflow tract; S, pacing stimulus. *(From Nogami A, Naito S, Tada H, et al. Demonstration of diastolic and presystolic Purkinje potential as critical potentials on a macroreentry circuit of verapamil-sensitive idiopathic left ventricular tachycardia.* J Am Coll Cardiol. *2000;36:811–823. With permission.)*

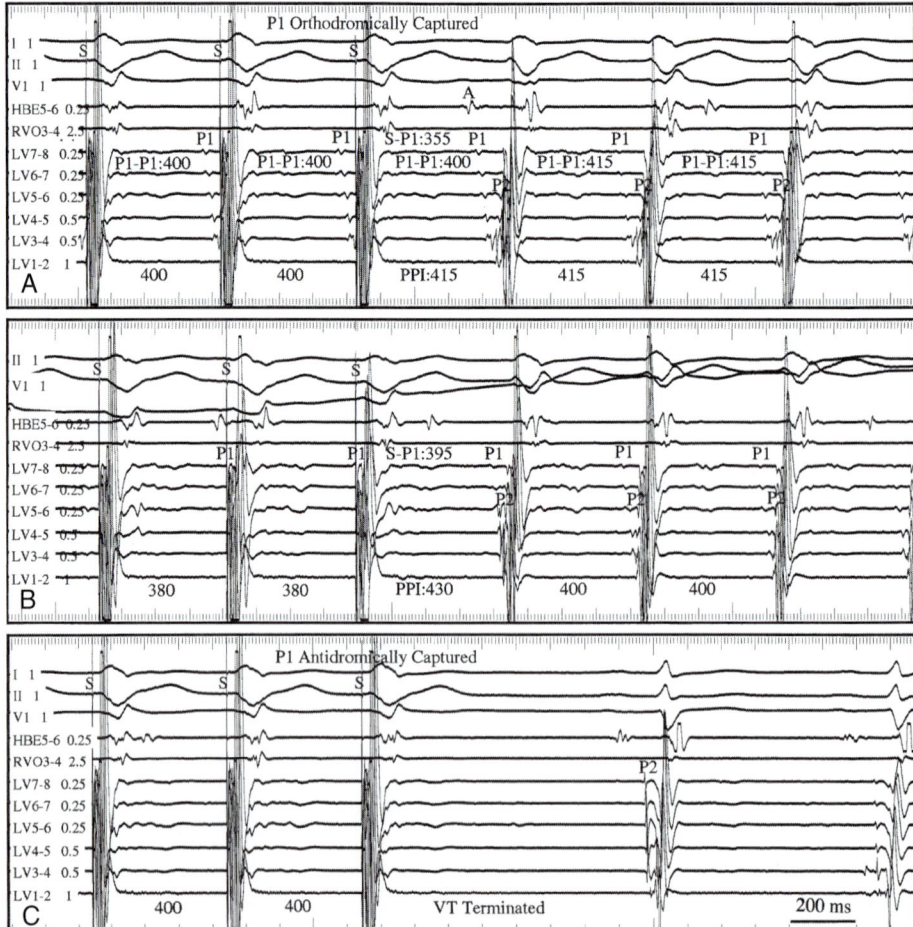

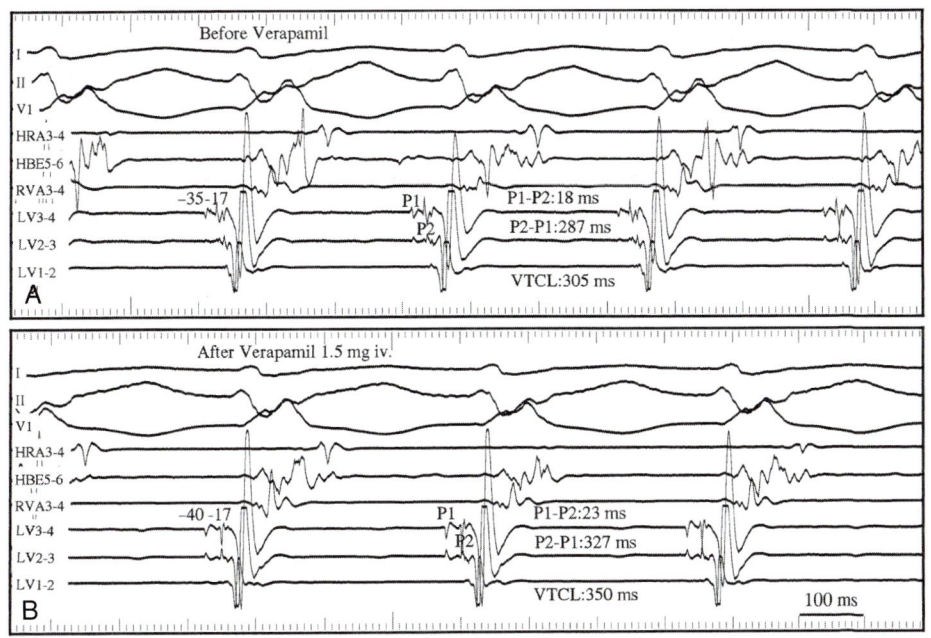

FIGURE 27-10. Effect of verapamil on the circuit of the left posterior fascicular ventricular tachycardia (VT). Intravenous administration of 1.5 mg of verapamil significantly prolonged the cycle length of the VT from 305 msec (**A**) to 350 msec (**B**). Both the P1-P2 and P2-P1 intervals were prolonged by similar proportions after verapamil, and the greatest absolute prolongation is from P2 to P1. However, the interval from P2 to the onset of the QRS complex remained unchanged. HBE, His bundle electrogram; HRA, high right atrium; LV, left ventricle; RVA, right ventricular apex; VTCL, cycle length of ventricular tachycardia. (*From Nogami A, Naito S, Tada H, et al. Demonstration of diastolic and presystolic Purkinje potential as critical potentials on a macroreentry circuit of verapamil-sensitive idiopathic left ventricular tachycardia. J Am Coll Cardiol. 2000;36:811-823. With permission.*)

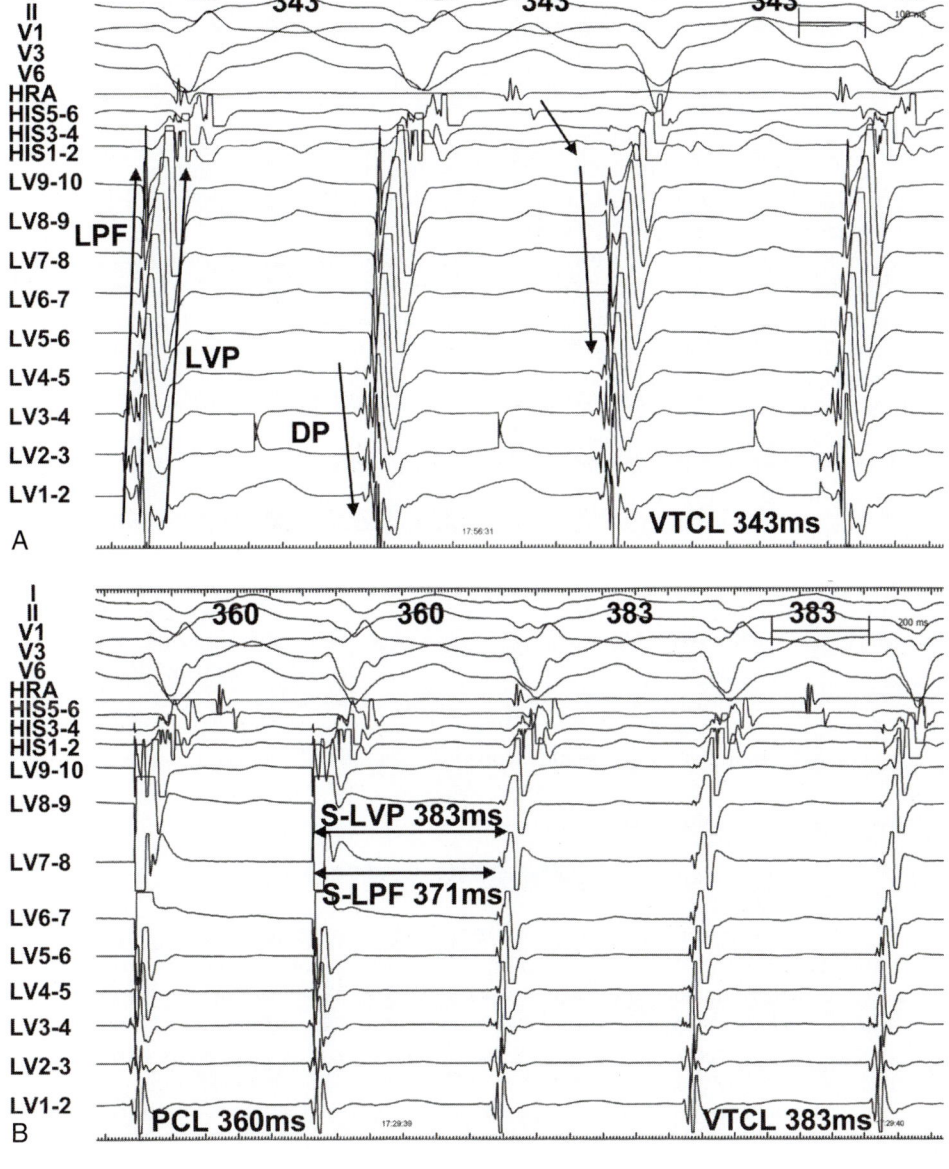

FIGURE 27-11. Negative participation of the proximal left posterior fascicle to the ventricular tachycardia (VT) circuit. **A,** Selective capture of left posterior fascicle by sinus beat did not affect the cycle length of VT. **B,** During entrainment pacing from left ventricle (LV) 7-8, both left posterior fascicle and left ventricular myocardium were simultaneously captured. While the postpacing interval at the left ventricular septal myocardium was equal to the VT cycle length (VTCL), the postpacing interval at the left posterior fascicle was shorter than the VT cycle length. CL, cycle length; LPF, left posterior fascicle; LVP, left ventricular myocardium potential; PCL, pacing cycle length; S, pacing stimulus. (*From Morishima I, Nogami A, Tsuboi H, et al. A case with negative participation of the left posterior fascicle to the reentry circuit of verapamil-sensitive idiopathic left ventricular tachycardia [abstract]. Heart Rhythm. 2009;6(Suppl):S387. With permission.*)

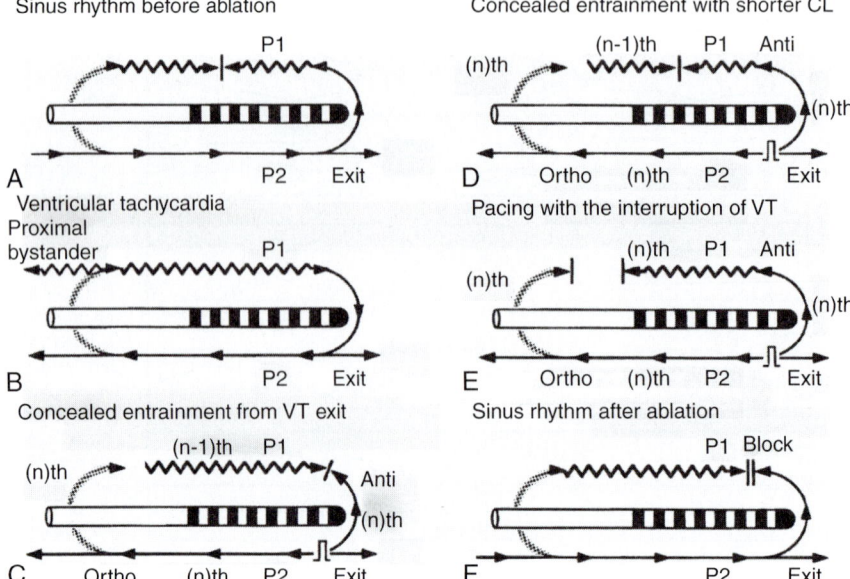

FIGURE 27-12. Schematic representation of the mechanism of left posterior fascicular ventricular tachycardia (VT). See the text for a discussion. Anti, antidromic wavefront; CL, cycle length; ortho, orthodromic wavefront; P1, diastolic potential; P2, presystolic Purkinje potential; VT, ventricular tachycardia. The dotted lines indicate the ventricular myocardium as the bridge between P1 and P2. The undulating line represents a zone of slow conduction. *(From Nogami A, Naito S, Tada H, et al. Demonstration of diastolic and presystolic Purkinje potential as critical potentials on a macroreentry circuit of verapamil-sensitive idiopathic left ventricular tachycardia.* J Am Coll Cardiol. 2000;36:811-823.)

Circuit Diagram

The hypothesized circuit of left posterior fascicular VT is depicted in Figure 27-12. In this circuit, P1 represents the activation potential in the distal portion of the specialized Purkinje tissue; it has decremental properties and verapamil sensitivity. P2 represents the activation of the left posterior fascicle or Purkinje fiber near the left posterior fascicle. P1 represents the antegrade limb of the circuit in VT and may represent longitudinal dissociation of the posterior fascicle, contiguous tissue coupled to the fascicle (false tendon), or ventricular myocardium interposed in the circuit. There is a distal link (network) between P1 and P2, and ventricular myocardium may act as a proximal bridge.

During sinus rhythm, the activation goes from P2 to P1 at the point of the fusion; therefore, P1 is buried in the local ventricular activation (Fig. 27-12A). During VT, P1 and P2 activate in the reverse direction (Fig. 27-12B). This explains why the activation sequences of P2 are reversed during sinus rhythm and VT. During concealed entrainment from the VT exit (e.g., at a cycle length of 400 msec as in Fig. 27-9A), P2 and P1 are activated orthodromically and the antidromic wavefront blocks, presumably in the connection between P1 and P2 (Fig. 27-12C). The orthodromic wavefront of the preceding (n - 1)th beat also blocks in the connection between P1 and P2 because it encounters the refractoriness created by the antidromic wavefront from the (n)th pacing impulse. The orthodromic wavefront from the last pacing impulse continues the tachycardia with resetting. During entrainment pacing with a shorter cycle length (e.g., at 380 msec as in Fig. 27-9B), the distal portion of P1 activates antidromically, and the antidromic wavefront blocks at the middle portion of P1 in the area of slow conduction (Fig. 27-12D). The orthodromic wave-

front from the last pacing impulse continues and resets the tachycardia. However, the interval from the last pacing stimulus to the orthodromically activated P1 is prolonged because of rate-dependent conduction delay in the area of slow conduction. During entrainment pacing with an even shorter cycle length or a shorter starting coupling interval (e.g., at a starting coupling interval of 300 msec as in Fig. 27-9C), P1 activates antidromically, and the antidromic wavefront blocks at the proximal portion of P1 in the area of slow conduction (Fig. 27-12E). However, the orthodromic wavefront from the previous paced beat also blocks. It blocks independent of either the collision with, or refractoriness secondary to, the previous antidromic wavefront. Because both the antidromic and the orthodromic wavefronts of the same beat are blocked, the VT is interrupted. Radiofrequency (RF) catheter ablation results in elimination of the conduction between P1 and P2. Figure 27-13 shows the position of the schematic fascicular VT circuits and the Purkinje potentials during sinus rhythm. The circuit of the left posterior fascicular VT was shown in Figure 27-13C. P1 and P2 can be recorded during the VT from the mid-septum. This type of VT can be named as *left posterior slow-fast type fascicular VT.*

Diagnostic Criteria

Surface Electrocardiogram

Based on the QRS morphology, verapamil-sensitive fascicular VT can be classified into three subgroups. The 12-lead electrocardiogram (ECG) of the left posterior fascicular VT exhibits an RBBB and a superior axis (left-axis deviation or northwest axis) (Fig. 27-1). This is the common type of verapamil-sensitive fascicular VT and may

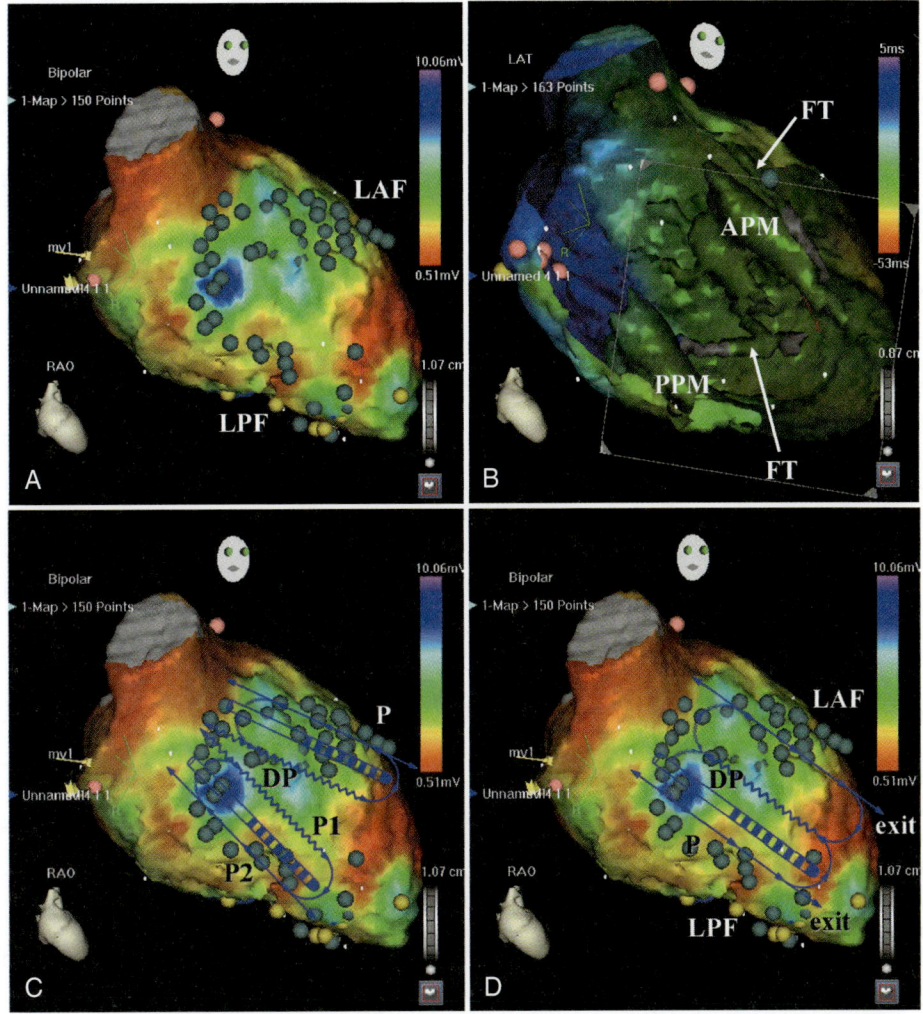

FIGURE 27-13. The position of fascicular ventricular tachycardia (VT) circuits and the Purkinje potentials during sinus rhythm. **A,** The tags in this CartoMerge image (Biosense Webster, Diamond Bar, CA) indicate the potentials of the left anterior fascicle (LAF), posterior fascicle (LPF), and distal Purkinje fiber during sinus rhythm. **B,** In the left ventricular cavity, anterior papillary muscle (APM), posterior papillary muscle (PPM), and false tendons (FT) were observed (endoscopic view). **C,** The circuits of the left posterior fascicular VT and left anterior fascicular VT (proximal type) were shown. Diastolic and presystolic Purkinje potentials can be recorded during the VT from the mid-septum. The *dotted lines* indicate the ventricular myocardium as the proximal bridge between diastolic and presystolic Purkinje potentials. The *undulating line* represents a zone of slow conduction. **D,** The circuit of the left upper septal fascicular VT was shown. See the text for a discussion.

account for up to 90% of cases. The uncommon type of this VT is a left anterior fascicular VT whose QRS morphology exhibits an RBBB configuration and right-axis deviation (Fig. 27-2).[5,16] The last type of VT is an upper septal fascicular VT, whose QRS morphology exhibits a relatively narrow QRS configuration and normal or right-axis deviation (Fig. 27-3).[6] This type of VT is very rare.

Intracardiac Electrograms

With left posterior fascicular VT, the earliest ventricular activation is recorded from the apical septum, and diastolic potentials are recorded from the mid-septum (Fig. 27-5). His activation follows QRS onset by 5 to 30 milliseconds.[17] During sinus rhythm, recording from the same site demonstrates the Purkinje potentials after the His bundle potential and before the onset of the QRS complex.

With left anterior fascicular VT, the earliest ventricular activation is recorded from the anterolateral left ventricle (Fig.

27-14), and diastolic potentials are recorded from the mid-septum (Fig. 27-15). There have been several reports that describe a left VT with an RBBB configuration, right-axis deviation, and a different mechanism. Yeh and colleagues[18] reported four cases with an RBBB configuration and right-axis deviation. This VT was adenosine sensitive and was successfully ablated from the anterobasal left ventricle. The chest leads exhibited an atypical RBBB configuration with wide "R" morphology. Crijns and colleagues[19] reported a rare case of interfascicular reentrant VT with an RBBB configuration and right-axis deviation. In their patient, the VT circuit used the anterior fascicle as the anterograde limb and the posterior fascicle as the retrograde limb. Interfascicular VT usually has a His bundle potential recorded in the diastolic phase during the VT as well as posterior fascicular potentials. However, it may be difficult to distinguish between interfascicular VT and intrafascicular VT (verapamil-sensitive left anterior fascicular VT).[16] The diagnostic criteria for left VTs are given in Table 27-1.

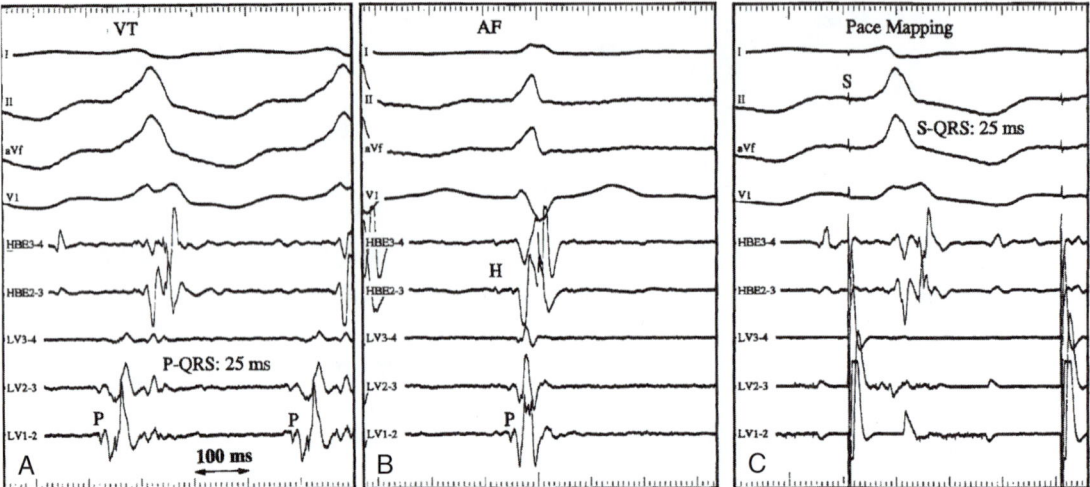

FIGURE 27-14. Intracardiac electrograms at the ventricular tachycardia (VT) exit site during left anterior fascicular VT. **A,** During the VT, the Purkinje potential preceded the QRS (P-QRS) by 25 msec. **B,** During the basal rhythm (atrial fibrillation [AF]), a Purkinje potential was recorded after the His-bundle potential (H) and before the QRS complex. **C,** Pace mapping at that site produced a similar QRS complex with an interval between the pacing stimulus and QRS (S-QRS) of 25 msec, equal to the P-QRS interval during the VT. The radiofrequency current delivered at that site terminated the VT; however, the VT was still induced. HBE, His bundle electrogram; LV, left ventricle. *(From Nogami A, Naito S, Tada H, et al. Verapamil-sensitive left anterior fascicular ventricular tachycardia: results of radiofrequency ablation in six patients. J Cardiovasc Electrophysiol. 1998;9:1269-1278. With Permission.)*

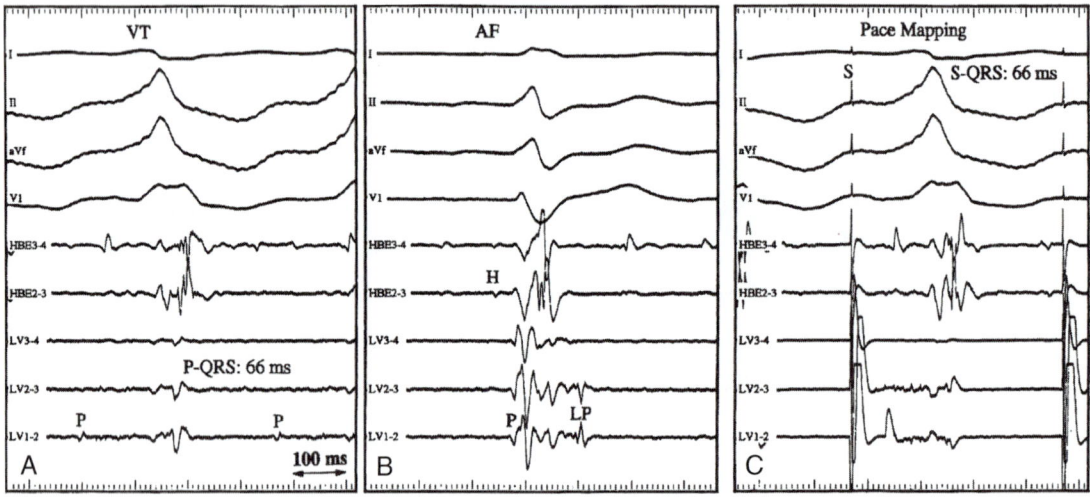

FIGURE 27-15. Intracardiac electrograms at the zone of slow conduction during left anterior fascicular ventricular tachycardia (VT). **A,** During the VT, the Purkinje potential (P) preceded the QRS (P-QRS) by 66 msec. **B,** During atrial fibrillation (AF), a Purkinje potential was recorded after the His bundle potential (H) and before the QRS complex, and a late potential (LP) was also recorded after the QRS complex. **C,** Pace mapping at that site produced a similar QRS complex with an interval between the pacing stimulus and QRS (S-QRS) of 66 msec, equal to the P-QRS interval during the VT. The radiofrequency current delivered at that site terminated the VT and suppressed the reinduction of the VT. *(From Nogami A, Naito S, Tada H, et al. Verapamil-sensitive left anterior fascicular ventricular tachycardia: results of radiofrequency ablation in six patients. J Cardiovasc Electrophysiol. 1998;9:1269-1278. With permission.)*

The differential diagnosis includes supraventricular tachycardias with bifascicular block aberrancy. With left upper septal fascicular VT, the retrograde activation of the His bundle is recorded before the onset of the QRS complex (Fig. 27-16). If there is retrograde ventriculoatrial conduction during the tachycardia, it mimics atrioventricular nodal reentry tachycardia or atrioventricular reciprocating tachycardia. The response of these tachycardias to verapamil and the ability to initiate and entrain them by atrial pacing may also lead to diagnostic confusion. To avoid a misdiagnosis, recognition of the retrograde sequence of the His bundle activation and measurement of a shorter His-to-ventricular (HV) interval during the tachycardia than

in sinus rhythm is important. An earlier potential than the His bundle potential is recorded from the left ventricular upper septum, where the left bundle potential is recorded during sinus rhythm. VT can be slowed or terminated by the intravenous administration of verapamil; however, it is unresponsive to β-blockers or Valsalva maneuvers. Class Ia and class Ic drugs are also effective. Rare cases of adenosine responsiveness occur, but only if the tachycardia shows catecholamine dependency.

In bundle branch reentry, the His activation precedes activation of the left bundle to produce a RBBB QRS morphology. In idiopathic left VT, the HV interval is shorter (negative) and follows left fascicular activation.

TABLE 27-1

DIAGNOSTIC CRITERIA FOR IDIOPATHIC LEFT VENTRICULAR TACHYCARDIAS

Verapamil-Sensitive Left Fascicular Tachycardia	Focal Purkinje Ventricular Tachycardia (Verapamil Insensitive)
• Characteristic surface ECG appearance • RBBB and superior axis configuration (common type) • RBBB and inferior axis configuration (uncommon type) • Narrow QRS and inferior axis configuration (rare type)	Characteristic surface ECG appearance • RBBB and either a left- or right-axis deviation • (Faster VT is prone to exhibit wider QRS)
Tachycardia dependence on left ventricular fascicular reentry • Purkinje potentials and diastolic potentials preceding ventricular activation • Changes in tachycardia rate preceded by similar changes in Purkinje and diastolic potentials • His activation follows QRS onset (short positive HV in rare type) • Induction and entrainment with ventricular and/or atrial pacing	Mechanism of tachycardia consistent with abnormal automaticity • Induction by exercise and that is catecholamines • Unable to induce or entrain by ventricular stimulation • Transient suppression by adenosine and with overdrive pacing or faster supraventricular rhythm
Verapamil-sensitive termination or slowing of tachycardia due to conduction slowing or block in fascicular system	Responsive to lidocaine, β-blockers, and class Ia drugs No response to verapamil
	Negative HV interval in tachycardia

ECG, electrocardiogram; HV, His-to-ventricular; RBBB, right bundle branch block; VT, ventricular tachycardia.

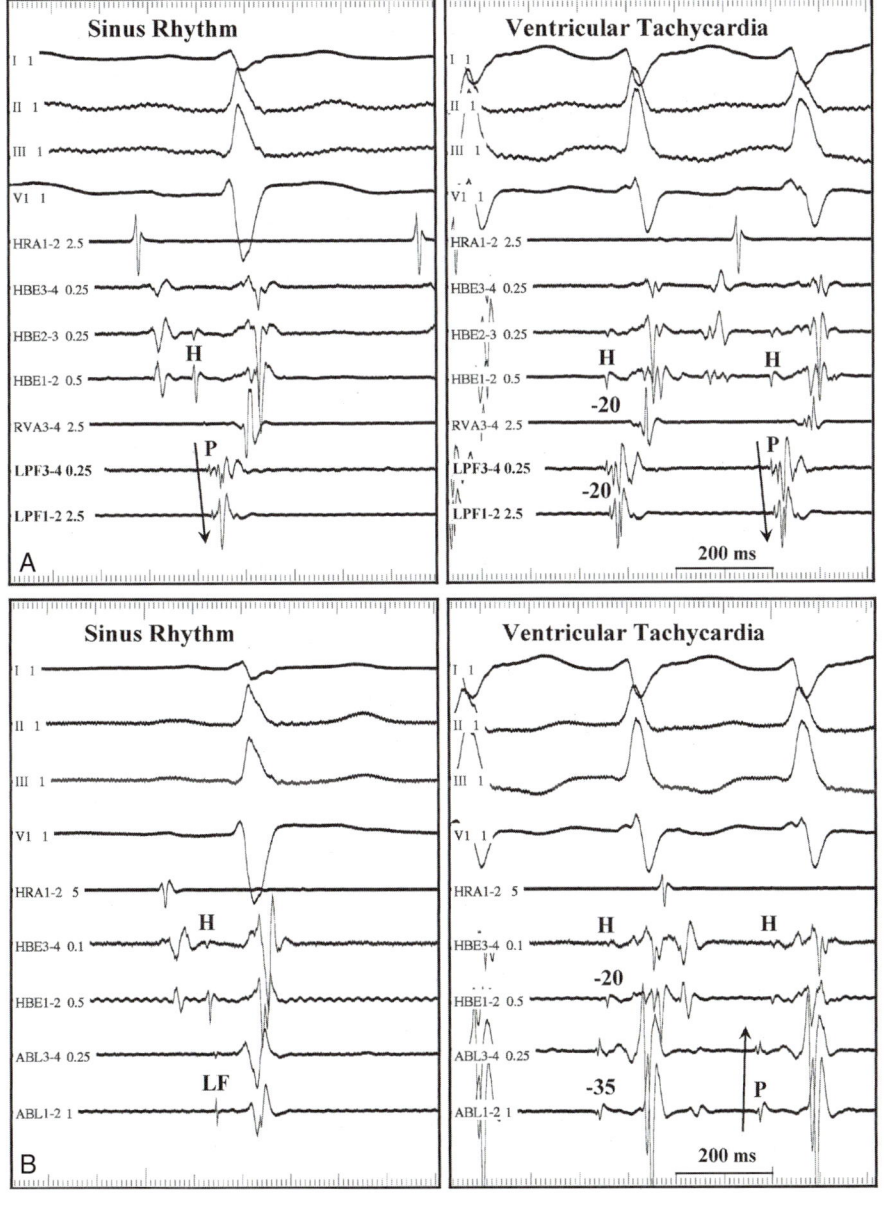

FIGURE 27-16. Intracardiac electrograms of a left upper septal fascicular ventricular tachycardia (VT). During the VT, there was a retrograde activation of the His bundle (H). The activation sequence of the His bundle potentials was reverse to that during sinus rhythm. The His-ventricular interval is short during the VT. **A,** During sinus rhythm, a fused Purkinje potential was recorded at left posterior fascicular (LPF) area. During the VT, recording at the same site also demonstrated a fused Purkinje potential, which preceded the onset of QRS by 20 msec. The activation sequences of Purkinje potentials are similar during sinus rhythm and VT. This site at the left posterior fascicular area is one of exit during VT because a fused presystolic ventricular potential was recorded. And the other exit during VT might be the left anterior fascicular area because the QRS morphology during VT is narrow and exhibited inferior axis. **B,** The VT was successfully ablated at the left ventricular upper septum. At that site, a left bundle branch (LF) potential was recorded during sinus rhythm, and the potential preceded the QRS by 35 msec during the VT. The radiofrequency application eliminated the VT without making left bundle branch block or atrioventricular block. ABL, ablation catheter; HBE, His bundle electrogram; HRA, high right atrium; RVA, right ventricular apex. *(From Nogami A. Idiopathic left ventricular tachycardia: assessment and treatment. Card Electrophysiol Rev. 2002;6:448-457. With permission.)*

Mapping and Ablation

RF catheter ablation may be considered a potential first-line therapy for patients with idiopathic VT because these VTs can be eliminated by ablation in a high percentage of patients.

Left Posterior Fascicular Ventricular Tachycardia

Conventional left ventricular septal mapping using a multipolar electrode catheter is useful in patients with left posterior fascicular VT.[12] Electroanatomic activation mapping is not typically required, but the ability to tag catheter positions of interest is often helpful. Two distinct potentials, P1 and P2, can be recorded during the VT from the mid-septum (Fig. 27-5). Because the diastolic potential (P1) has been proved a critical potential in the VT circuit, this potential can be targeted to cure the tachycardia. Nakagawa and coworkers[17] first reported the importance of Purkinje potentials in the ablation of this VT, and Tsuchiya and associates[20] reported the significance of a late diastolic potential and emphasized the role of late diastolic and presystolic potentials in the VT circuit. However, the successful ablation sites identified by these two research groups were different. Whereas Nakagawa's ablation sites were at the apical-inferior septum of the left ventricle, Tsuchiya's ablation sites were at the basal septal regions close to the main trunk of the left bundle branch. These findings suggest that any P1 during VT can be targeted for catheter ablation. We usually target the apical third of the septum, to avoid the creation of left bundle branch block (LBBB) or atrioventricular block (Fig. 27-17).

Using the retrograde aortic approach, the ablation catheter crosses the aortic valve with a tight curve oriented to the right side of the fluoroscopic view in RAO. Once in the left ventricular chamber, the catheter is rotated toward the septum, then the curvature is opened, allowing the tip of the catheter to fall toward the inferior septum toward the apex. In our study, P1 was recorded during the VT in 15 of 20 patients. RF ablation was successfully performed at this site in all 15 patients. During energy application, the P1-P2 interval was gradually prolonged, and the VT was terminated by block between P1 and P2 (Fig. 27-18). After termination of the tachycardia, the P1 was noted to occur after the QRS complex during sinus rhythm, whereas the P2 was still observed before the QRS complex. Figure 27-19 shows the potentials during sinus rhythm before and after the successful ablation. After successful ablation, the P1 occurred after the QRS complex, with an identical activation sequence to that observed during the VT. Figure 27-12F explains why P1 appears after ablation in the mid-diastolic period and with the same activation sequence as during the VT. When the distal segment of P1 is ablated, the P1 activation proceeds orthodromically around the circuit and subsequently blocks from a proximal to distal direction during sinus rhythm. The P1 that appears after ablation exhibits decremental properties during atrial pacing or ventricular pacing, or both (Fig. 27-20), and the intravenous administration of verapamil significantly prolongs the His-to-P1 interval during sinus rhythm (Fig. 27-21). Pace-mapping at the successful ablation site is usually not good because the selective pacing of P1 is difficult and there is an antidromic activation of the proximal P1 potential.

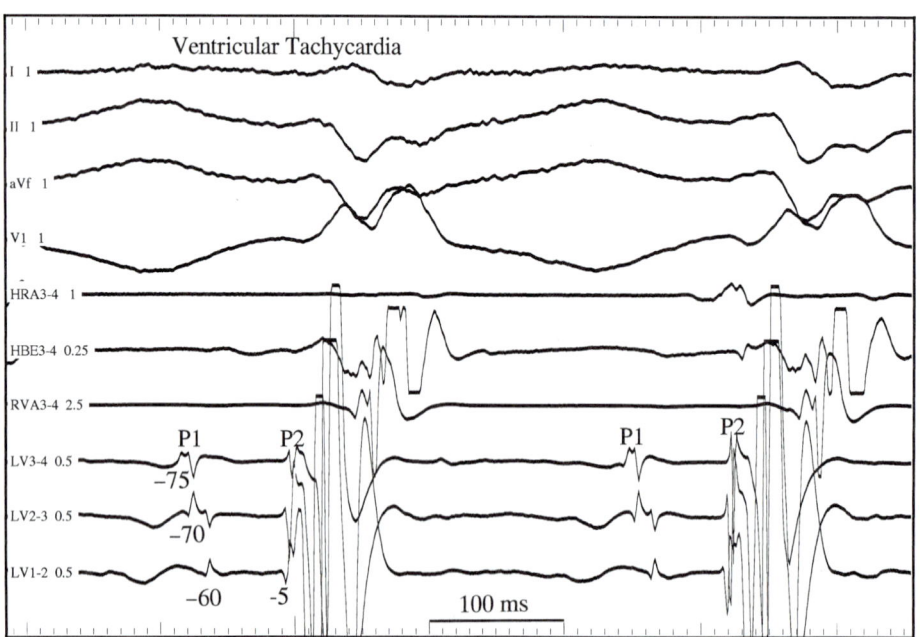

FIGURE 27-17. Recordings from the site of successful ablation during left posterior fascicular ventricular tachycardia (VT). A diastolic potential (P1) and presystolic Purkinje potential (P2) were recorded in the mid-septal area. The proximal two electrodes of the ablation catheter (LV) recorded the diastolic potential (P1) 15 msec earlier than the distal pair of electrodes. HBE, His bundle electrogram; HRA, high right atrium; RVA, right ventricular apex. (*From Nogami A, Naito S, Tada H, et al. Demonstration of diastolic and presystolic Purkinje potential as critical potentials on a macroreentry circuit of verapamil-sensitive idiopathic left ventricular tachycardia.* J Am Coll Cardiol. *2000;36:811-823. With permission.*)

Pace-mapping after successful ablation is sometimes better than before ablation because the antidromic activation of P1 is blocked.[21]

In the remaining 5 of our 20 patients, the diastolic potential (P1) could not be detected, and a single fused P2 was recorded only at the VT exit site. Successful ablation was performed at this site in all 5 patients. We can speculate that the circuit in these patients may have involved less of the Purkinje system or that the area of slow conduction may not have been close to the endocardial surface. The targets for catheter ablation are given in Table 27-2.

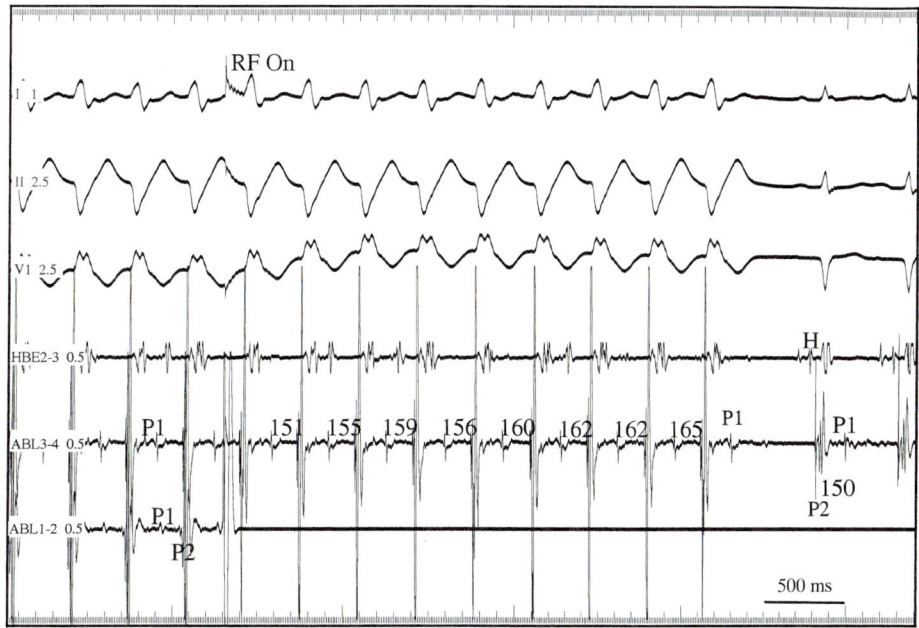

FIGURE 27-18. An application of radiofrequency current (RF) delivered during left posterior fascicular ventricular tachycardia (VT). During the energy application, the P1-P2 interval gradually prolonged, and the VT was terminated by block between P1 and P2. After the ablation, the P1 occurred after the QRS complex during sinus rhythm. ABL, ablation catheter; H, His recording; HBE, His bundle electrogram. *(From Nogami A, Naito S, Tada H, et al. Demonstration of diastolic and presystolic Purkinje potential as critical potentials on a macroreentry circuit of verapamil-sensitive idiopathic left ventricular tachycardia.* J Am Coll Cardiol. *2000;36:811-823. With permission.)*

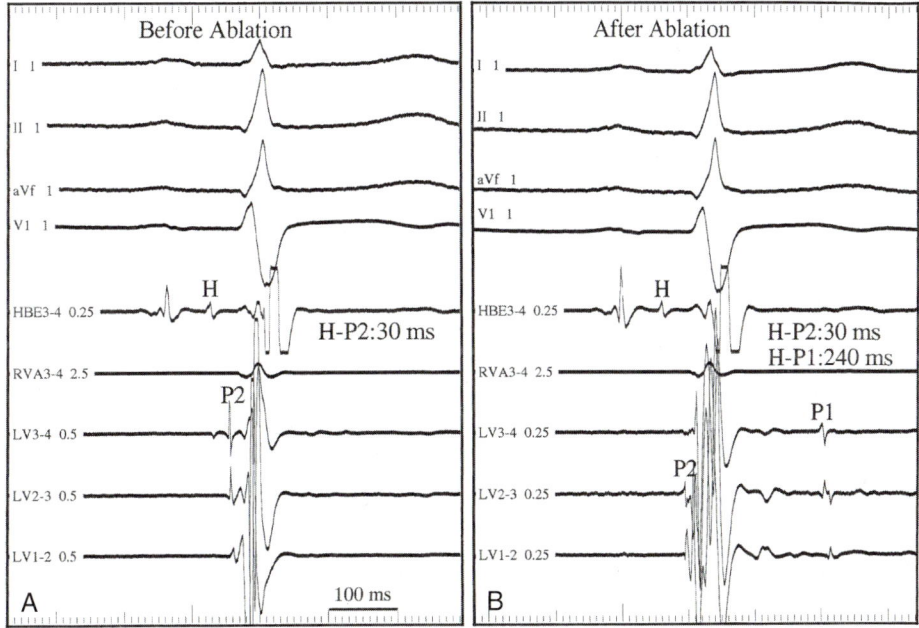

FIGURE 27-19. Intracardiac recordings during sinus rhythm before and after the successful ablation of left posterior fascicular ventricular tachycardia (VT). **A,** Before the ablation, no diastolic potential was observed during sinus rhythm. **B,** After the ablation, the P1 occurred after the QRS complex. The activation sequence of P1 was identical to that observed during the VT shown in Figure 27-17. HBE, His bundle electrogram; LV, left ventricle; RVA, right ventricular apex. *(From Nogami A, Naito S, Tada H, et al. Demonstration of diastolic and presystolic Purkinje potential as critical potentials on a macroreentry circuit of verapamil-sensitive idiopathic left ventricular tachycardia.* J Am Coll Cardiol. *2000;36:811-823. With permission.)*

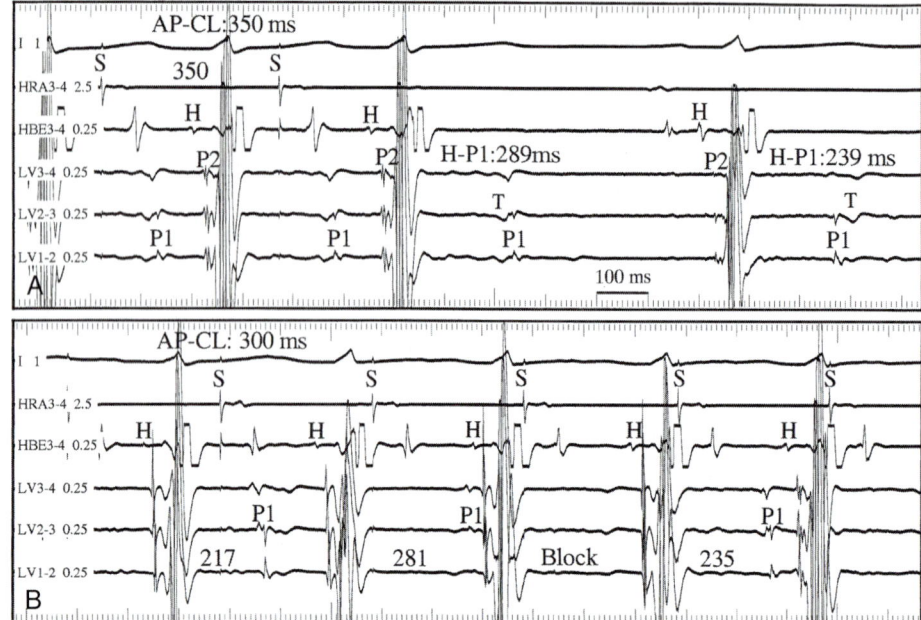

FIGURE 27-20. Decremental properties of P1, which occurred after the QRS complex. Intracardiac recordings during right atrial pacing after successful ablation of left posterior fascicular VT. **A,** The His-P1 (H-P1) interval increased during right atrial pacing at a cycle length of 350 msec. **B,** At a cycle length of 300 msec, the P1 demonstrated a Wenckebach-type block pattern. HBE, His bundle electrogram; HRA, high right atrium; LV, left ventricle; T, T-wave repolarization artifact. *(From Tada H, Nogami A, Naito S, et al. Retrograde Purkinje potential activation during sinus rhythm following catheter ablation of idiopathic left ventricular tachycardia.* J Cardiovasc Electrophysiol. *1998;9:1218-1224. With permission.)*

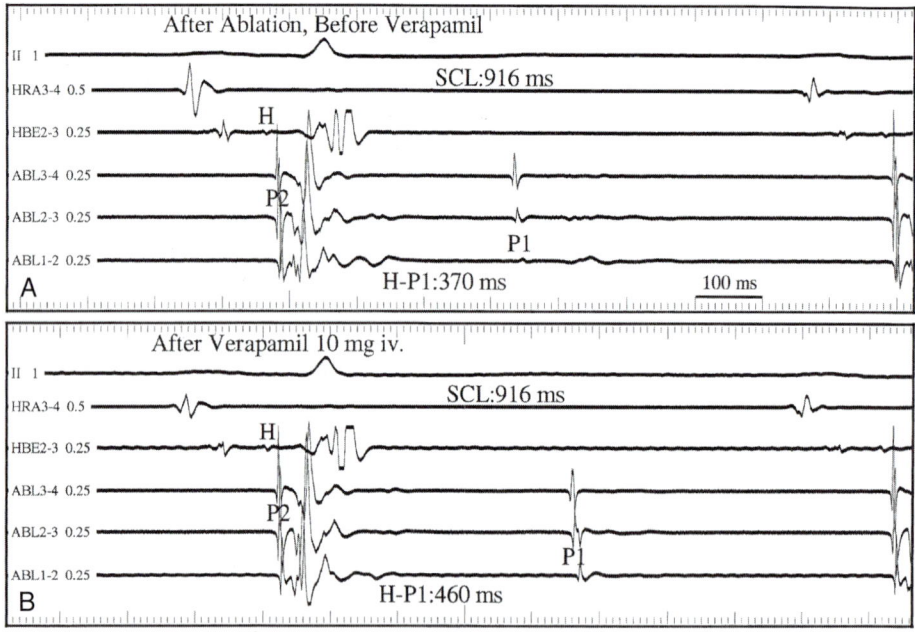

FIGURE 27-21. Verapamil sensitivity of P1, which occurred after the QRS complex. **A,** The His-P1 (H-P1) interval during sinus rhythm was 370 msec. **B,** The H-P1 interval significantly prolonged after the intravenous administration of 10 mg of verapamil. ABL, ablation catheter; HBE, His bundle electrogram; HRA, high right atrium; SCL, sinus cycle length. *(From Tada H, Nogami A, Naito S, et al. Retrograde Purkinje potential activation during sinus rhythm following catheter ablation of idiopathic left ventricular tachycardia.* J Cardiovasc Electrophysiol. *1998;9:1218-1224. With permission.)*

Left Anterior Fascicular Ventricular Tachycardia

Figure 27-2 shows the 12-lead ECGs of verapamil-sensitive left anterior fascicular VTs that we experienced.[16] The mean cycle length of the VT was 390 ± 62 milliseconds, and the mean electrical axis during the VT was 120 ± 16 degrees. Patient 3 also had a typical left posterior fascicular VT. Left ventricular endocardial mapping during left anterior fascicular VT identified the earliest ventricular activation in the anterolateral wall of the left ventricle. RF current delivered to this site suppressed the VT in three patients (patients 1, 2, and 3; the distal type). The

TABLE 27-2

TARGETS FOR ABLATION

Verapamil-Sensitive Left Fascicular Tachycardia

Diastolic potential (P1) in the antegrade limb of the VT circuit (middle septum). The earliest diastolic potential (P1) is not needed. The distal third of P1 potentials is usually targeted, to avoid the creation of LBBB or atrioventricular block (P1 - QRS = 28 to 130 msec).

Presystolic fused Purkinje potential (P2) at the VT exit (apical septum), if diastolic potential (P1) could not be recorded.

Pace mapping (a perfect QRS match during pace mapping is not needed)

Anatomic linear ablation to transect the involved middle to distal left fascicular tract.

Focal Purkinje Ventricular Tachycardia (Verapamil Insensitive)

The earliest Purkinje potential during VT

Site of perfect QRS match

LBBB, left bundle branch block; VT, ventricular tachycardia.

fused Purkinje potential was recorded at that site and preceded the QRS complex by 20 to 35 milliseconds, with pace-mapping exhibiting an optimal match between the paced rhythm and clinical VT. In the remaining three patients, RF catheter ablation at the site of the earliest ventricular activation was unsuccessful. In these patients, a Purkinje potential was recorded in the diastolic phase during the VT at the mid-anterior left ventricular septum. The Purkinje potential preceded the QRS during VT by 56 to 66 milliseconds, and catheter ablation at these sites was successful (patients 4, 5, and 6; the proximal type).

Figure 27-14 shows the intracardiac recording from the VT exit (anterolateral wall) in patient 4. The Purkinje potential preceded the QRS (P-QRS interval) by 25 milliseconds during the VT, and pace-mapping at that site produced a similar QRS complex with an interval between the pacing stimulus and QRS (S-QRS) of 25 milliseconds, equal to the P-QRS interval during VT. RF current delivered at this site terminated the VT; however, the VT was still induced. Figure 27-15 shows the intracardiac recordings from patient 4 at the zone of slow conduction during the VT. The ablation catheter was positioned in the mid-septal area, where the diastolic Purkinje potential was recorded. The Purkinje potential was recorded during the VT. Pace-mapping at that site produced a similar QRS complex, with an S-QRS interval of 66 milliseconds, equal to the P-QRS interval during the VT. RF current delivered at this site terminated the VT and suppressed the reinduction of the VT. There was a significant difference in the 12-lead ECGs between the distal type (patients 1 through 3) and the proximal type (patients 4 through 6) of this tachycardia. Although the distal type of left anterior fascicular VT exhibited a "QS" morphology in leads I, V_5, and V_6, the proximal type exhibited an "RS" morphology in those leads.

One of our patients with the proximal type of the left anterior fascicular VT also had a typical left posterior fascicular VT. Kottkamp and colleagues[22] also reported one patient who had two left VT configurations with right- and left-axis deviation. In this patient, RF catheter ablation delivered to the single site between the left anterior and posterior fascicles successfully eliminated both VTs. This suggests that the anterior limb is the common pathway.

The circuit of the proximal type of the left anterior fascicular VT was shown in Figure 27-13C. In this circuit, DP represents the activation potential in the proximal portion of the specialized Purkinje tissue with a decremental property. The P represents the activation in the Purkinje fibers near the left anterior fascicle. During VT, the antegrade limb is the DP, and the retrograde limb is the P. This type of VT can be named as *left anterior slow-fast type fascicular* VT. The circuit of distal type of this VT may be small or contains the small portion of normal and abnormal Purkinje fibers.

Left Upper Septal Fascicular Ventricular Tachycardia

Figure 27-16 shows the intracardiac electrograms of the upper septal fascicular VT. A fused Purkinje potential was recorded at left posterior fascicular (LPF) area during sinus rhythm (Fig. 27-16A). And during VT, recording at the same site also demonstrated a fused presystolic Purkinje potential, which preceded the onset of QRS by 20 milliseconds. The activation sequences of Purkinje potentials at LPF area are similar during sinus rhythm and VT. This site is one of exit during VT because a fused presystolic ventricular potential was recorded. And the other exit site during VT might be left anterior fascicular area because the QRS morphology during VT is quite narrow and exhibited an inferior axis. This VT was successfully ablated at the left ventricular upper septum (Fig. 27-16B). At this site, a left bundle branch (LF) potential was recorded during sinus rhythm and the Purkinje potential preceded the QRS by 35 milliseconds during the VT. The RF application eliminated the VT without creating an LBBB or atrioventricular block. The 12-lead ECG configuration in a case reported by Shimoike and associates[6] was different from ours. Their case showed LBBB configurations and a normal axis during the VT. However, the QRS width was narrow, and the successful ablation site was similar to ours.

The hypothesized VT circuit is depicted in Figure 27-13D. In this circuit, DP represents the activation potential of the specialized Purkinje tissue at left ventricular upper septum. P represents the activation of the left fascicles or Purkinje fiber near the left fascicles. Both left anterior and posterior fascicles are the antegrade limbs of the reentrant circuit in VT. This explains why this VT exhibits a narrow QRS configuration and inferior axis. DP represents the common retrograde limb of the circuit in VT and can be ablation target. This type of VT can be named as *fast-slow type fascicular VT*.

Radiofrequency Energy Delivery and the End Point of Ablation

With catheter ablation of verapamil-sensitive idiopathic left VT, no special mapping or ablation system is typically needed. We usually use a 7-French quadripolar steerable electrode catheter with a 4-mm tip and 2-mm interelectrode spacing between the distal two electrodes. RF energy is delivered using maximum power of 50 W and a maximum electrode-tissue interface temperature of 55° to 60°C. We deliver RF energy during the tachycardia of left posterior and anterior fascicular VTs. If the VT is terminated or slowed within 15 seconds, additional current is applied for another 60 to 120 seconds. If the initial RF current is ineffective, ablation is directed to a more proximal site with the earlier diastolic potential. If the mid-diastolic potential cannot be detected, RF current is applied at the VT exit site showing a single fused presystolic Purkinje potential. With upper septal fascicular VT, we deliver RF energy for 30 to 60 seconds during sinus rhythm to avoid atrioventricular block. We perform catheter ablation in this region using a low power output (i.e., 10 W), which can gradually be increased while carefully monitoring for development of a junctional rhythm or atrioventricular block.

After the ablation, programmed stimulation should be repeated. Other than the noninducibility of VT, there are several electrophysiologic findings that can serve as end points of RF applications for left posterior fascicular VT. After ablation of the distal attachment between P1 and P2, P1 appears after the QRS complex (Figs. 27-12F and 27-19). However, this phenomenon is not sufficient for an end point because this only indicates conduction block in the direction from P2 to P1 only. This unidirectional block can be seen during the baseline state[15] or after an insufficient RF application.[21] Figure 27-22 shows an example of residual conduction from P1 to P2. After the first RF application, the VT became noninducible, and P1 appeared after the QRS complex during sinus rhythm. However, 1 hour after the first RF application, a premature ventricular complex was observed, and its QRS morphology was similar to that observed during the

VT. The activation sequence of P2 before the premature ventricular complex was different from that during sinus rhythm but identical to that during the VT. This means that there was residual unidirectional conduction from P1 to P2. During isoproterenol infusion, an incessant form of nonsustained VT was initiated, and it was successfully ablated by additional RF applications at this site.[21] To confirm the creation of bidirectional block between P1 and P2, we do atrial pacing with various cycle lengths after the ablation (Fig. 27-23). If there is residual conduction from P1 to P2, a premature ventricular complex (i.e., ventricular echo beat) with a similar QRS morphology as that observed during the VT can be observed repeatedly.

Success and Recurrence Rates

Our experience at the time of this writing includes 75 patients with left posterior fascicular VT, 10 patients with left anterior fascicular VT, and 2 patients with left upper septal fascicular VT. The success and recurrence rates are 97% and 4%, respectively, for left posterior fascicular VT; 90% and 11% for left anterior fascicular VT; and 100% and 0% for left upper septal fascicular VT.

Complications

Aside from the complications that may result from any left ventricular electrophysiologic procedure (e.g., thrombophlebitis, damage to the femoral artery, ventricular perforation), the only complication that has been associated with catheter ablation of idiopathic left VT has been LBBB and atrioventricular block. Tsuchiya and associates[20] reported that 2 patients (12.5%) had transient LBBB after

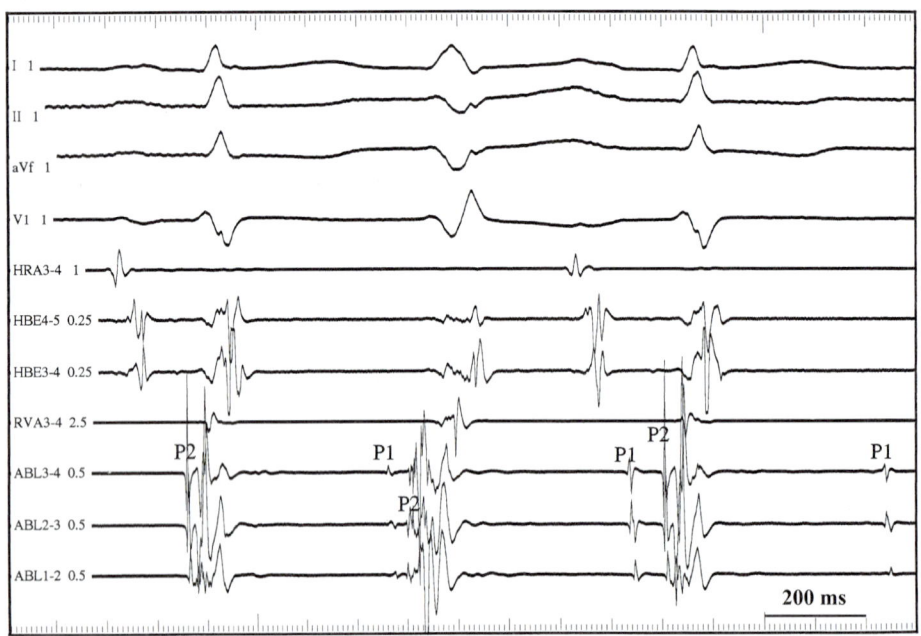

FIGURE 27-22. Intracardiac recordings from the site of catheter ablation obtained during sinus rhythm 1 hour after the first radiofrequency application. The premature ventricular complex was observed, and its QRS morphology was similar to that during the ventricular tachycardia (VT). The activation sequence of P2 before the premature ventricular complex was different from that during sinus rhythm, but identical to that during the VT. ABL, ablation catheter; HBE, His bundle electrogram; HRA, high right atrium. *(From Tada H, Nogami A, Naito S, et al. Retrograde Purkinje potential activation during sinus rhythm following catheter ablation of idiopathic left ventricular tachycardia. J Cardiovasc Electrophysiol. 1998;9:1218-1224. With permission.)*

ablation in their series of 16 patients. They targeted the left basal septum, and the LBBB disappeared within 10 minutes without VT recurrence. In our experience, 1 (1.1%) of 87 patients had a transient atrioventricular block. This patient had a left posterior fascicular VT, and the diastolic potential (P1) at the mid-septum was targeted for the ablation. Before the ablation, the patient had catheter-induced RBBB. About 15 seconds into the RF delivery, the VT terminated, and second-degree atrioventricular block was observed. The atrioventricular block disappeared immediately after discontinuation of the RF energy delivery.

Troubleshooting the Difficult Case

Common problems encountered with left VT ablation, and their solutions are given in Table 27-3. Inability to reliably induce VT is a formidable obstacle to successful ablation. Isoproterenol facilitates induction of sustained VT in 60% to 70% of those patients without inducible sustained VT at baseline. In some patients, the administration of small doses of class Ia drugs enhances the slow conduction at the specialized Purkinje tissue and facilitates induction of stable sustained VT. Catheter mapping sometimes mechanically suppresses the conduction in the VT circuit ("bump" phenomenon). In such cases, a ventricular echo beat during sinus rhythm or atrial pacing is useful (Figs. 27-22 and 27-23). If premature ventricular complexes with a similar QRS morphology to that observed during the VT are repeatedly seen, activation mapping can be performed. If no ventricular echo beats are inducible, the empirical anatomic approach can be an effective strategy for ablation of left posterior fascicular VT.[23] First, the VT exit site is sought by pace-mapping

TABLE 27-3

TROUBLESHOOTING THE DIFFICULT CASE (VERAPAMIL-SENSITIVE FASCICULAR TACHYCARDIA)

Problem	Causes	Solution
Unable to induce VT	Adrenergic dependency Insufficient slow conduction "Bump" phenomenon during mapping	Use isoproterenol Give small dose of class Ia drug Find ventricular echo beat with a similar QRS morphology as that observed during the VT Use pace mapping and the anatomic (linear) approach
Unable to find a good electrogram	Poor catheter contact	Improve the contact with a different catheter or approach, use multipolar mapping catheter
Unable to find a diastolic potential during VT	Unknown	Use pace mapping and the anatomic (linear) approach
Poor catheter stability	Excessive heart motion during the VT Frequent ventricular premature beats during the RF application	Ablate during sinus rhythm or overdrive pacing, change catheter reach and stiffness, use cryoablation Use verapamil IV (after which the noninducibility of VT becomes invalid as an end point), use cryoablation or overdrive pacing

RF, radiofrequency energy; VT, ventricular tachycardia.

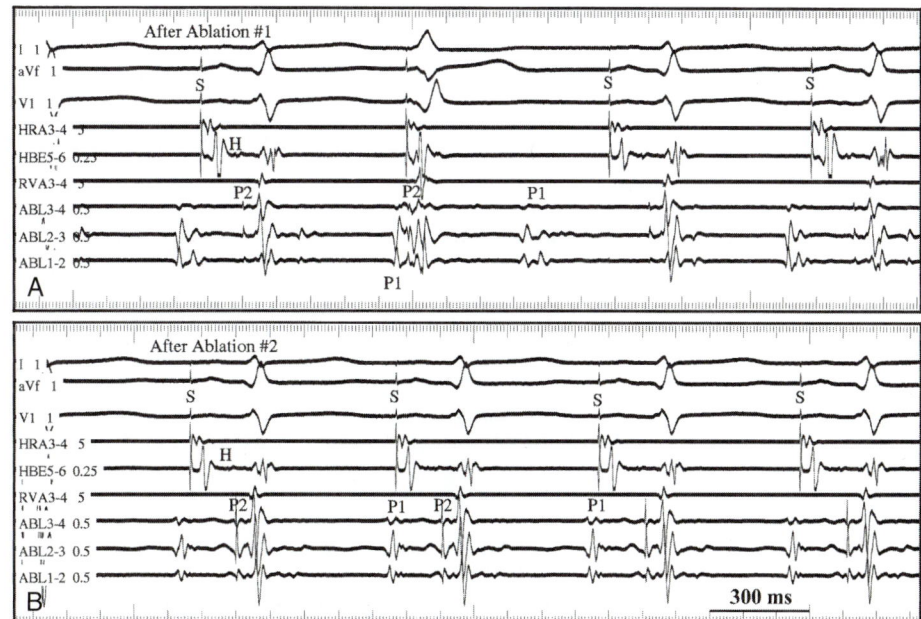

FIGURE 27-23. *Confirmation* of bidirectional block between P1 and P2 after the ablation. **A,** During atrial pacing (S), the premature ventricular complex with a similar QRS morphology as that during the ventricular tachycardia was repeatedly observed. The activation sequence of P2 before the premature ventricular complex was different from that during sinus rhythm. **B,** After the additional radiofrequency application, this ventricular echo beat was abolished. ABL, ablation catheter; HBE, His bundle electrogram; HRA, high right atrium; RVA, right ventricular apex.

during sinus rhythm, and RF energy is delivered to that site. Second, a linear lesion is placed at the mid-septum, perpendicular to the long axis of the left ventricle, about 10 to 15 mm proximal to the VT exit. During anatomic linear ablation, P1 suddenly appears after the QRS complex if the ablation site is on the descending limb of the VT circuit (Fig. 27-24). This anatomic approach is also useful in patients in whom diastolic Purkinje potential cannot be recorded during VT. Figure 27-25 shows activation mapping during VT. Although the earliest myocardial activation site was observed at the inferoapical septum, diastolic potential could not be recorded. RF energy application

to this exit site was ineffective. A linear RF lesion about 10 mm proximal to the VT exit was also ineffective. And finally, more proximal linear lesion successfully suppressed the VT.

If a good electrogram is not found at the septum, one possible reason is poor catheter contact with the septum. Figure 27-26 shows examples of poor and good catheter contact with the mid-septum. The left anterior oblique fluoroscopic view is used to guide the catheter toward the septum, and the right anterior oblique view to guide the catheter posteriorly and toward the apical third of the septum.

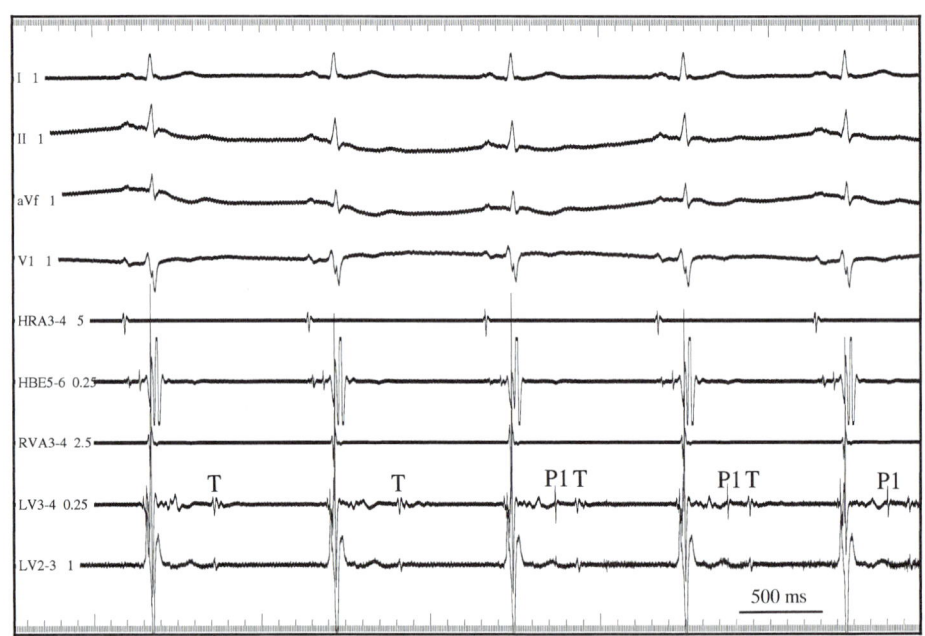

FIGURE 27-24. *Anatomical* linear approach during sinus rhythm in left posterior fascicular ventricular tachycardia (VT). A linear lesion is placed at the mid-septum perpendicular to the long axis of the left ventricle, about 10 to 15 mm proximal to the site of the best QRS match by pace mapping. During anatomic linear ablation, P1 suddenly appears after the QRS complex, if the ablation site is on the descending limb of the VT circuit. HBE, His bundle electrogram; HRA, high right atrium; LV, left ventricle; P1, diastolic potential; RVA, right ventricular apex; T, T-wave repolarization artifact.

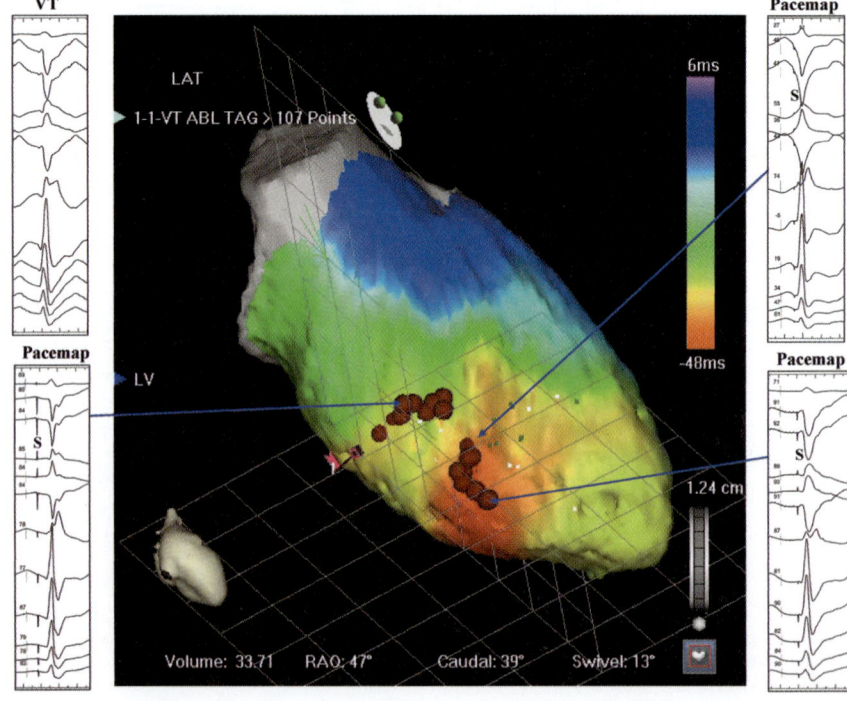

FIGURE 27-25. Anatomic approach when diastolic Purkinje potential cannot be recorded during ventricular tachycardia (VT). While the earliest myocardial activation site was observed at the inferoapical septum, diastolic potential could not be recorded. First, radiofrequency (RF) energy was delivered to the exit site, but that was ineffective. Second, a linear RF lesion about 10 mm proximal to the VT exit was created, but that was also ineffective. Finally, more proximal linear lesion successfully suppressed VT induction. LAT, lateral projection; LV, left ventricle; RAO, right anterior oblique projection.

If ablation catheter stability is poor during the VT because of excessive heart motion, RF energy can be delivered during sinus rhythm. However, even during sinus rhythm, frequent ventricular premature beats (with a similar QRS morphology to that observed during the VT) and VT are sometimes induced during the RF energy application. In such cases, overdrive pacing or intravenous administration of verapamil is effective for suppressing the ventricular premature beats and VT during the RF energy application. However, after such an infusion, the noninducibility of the VT becomes invalid as an end point for the ablation. Cryoablation of left VT has not been reported but may be effective given the superficial nature of the reentrant circuit. Cryoablation may offer the advantages of no induction of premature ventricular complexes and extreme catheter stability during ablation.

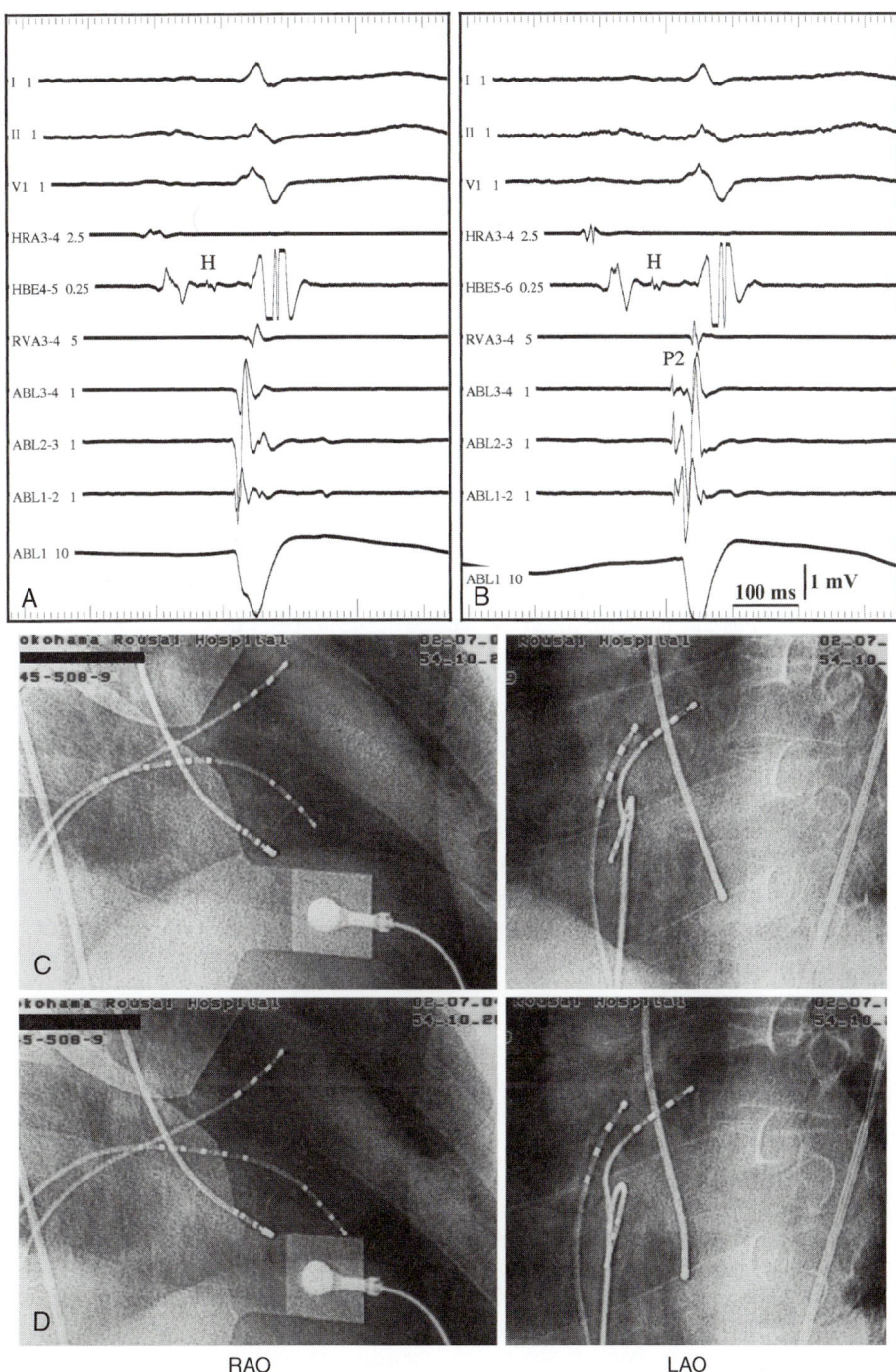

RAO   LAO

FIGURE 27-26. Representation of poor catheter contact (**A**) and good catheter contact (**B**) to the mid-septum. **C** and **D**, The left anterior oblique (LAO) fluoroscopic view is used to guide the catheter toward the septum. When the catheter has good contact with the septum, significant Purkinje potentials (P2) can be recorded after the His-bundle potential (H) and before the onset of the QRS complex. The right anterior oblique (RAO) view is used to guide the catheter posteriorly and toward the apical third of the septum.

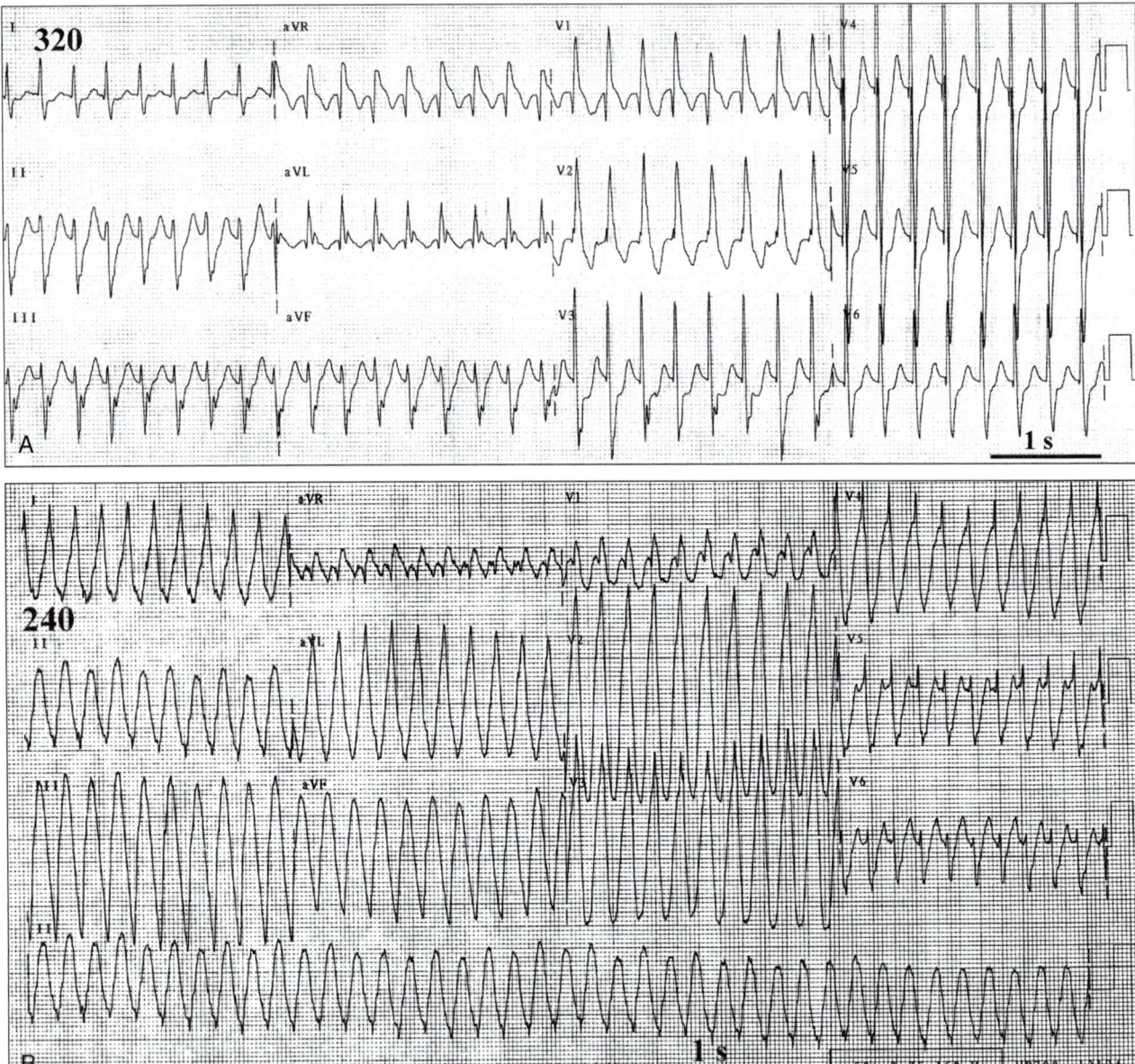

FIGURE 27-27. Twelve-lead electrocardiograms (ECGs) of focal Purkinje ventricular tachycardias (VTs) from the left posterior fascicle. **A,** This VT presents with right bundle branch block (RBBB) and left-axis deviation. It is difficult to distinguish the focal Purkinje VT from verapamil-sensitive left posterior fascicular VT by 12-lead ECG. **B,** This VT also presents with an RBBB and a left-axis deviation; however, the cycle length of VT is shorter and the QRS interval is wider than in **A.**

Focal Purkinje Ventricular Tachycardia

Clinical and Electrophysiologic Characteristics

Another type of Purkinje-related VT is the focal tachycardia from the Purkinje system (Table 27-1). This VT is classified as propranolol-sensitive automatic VT.[1] Although this VT is usually observed in patients with ischemic heart disease,[24] it is also observed in patients with structurally normal hearts.[25,26] Focal Purkinje VT from the left ventricle can present with an RBBB configuration and either a left- or right-axis deviation on the 12-lead ECG, depending on the origin (Fig. 27-27). It

is difficult to distinguish this VT from reentrant fascicular VT by 12-lead ECG. This VT can be induced by exercise and catecholamines (e.g., isoproterenol and phenylephrine); however, it cannot be induced or terminated by programmed ventricular stimulation. Although this VT is responsive to lidocaine and β-blockers, it is usually not responsive to verapamil. This can be used as a differentiation from verapamil-sensitive fascicular VT. This VT is transiently suppressed by adenosine and with overdrive pacing. Slow focal Purkinje VT can be also suppressed by faster supraventricular rhythm (Fig. 27-27C). The clinical and electrophysiologic characteristics of this VT have not been well defined.[25,26] Gonzalez and colleagues[25] reported the electrophysiologic spectrum of

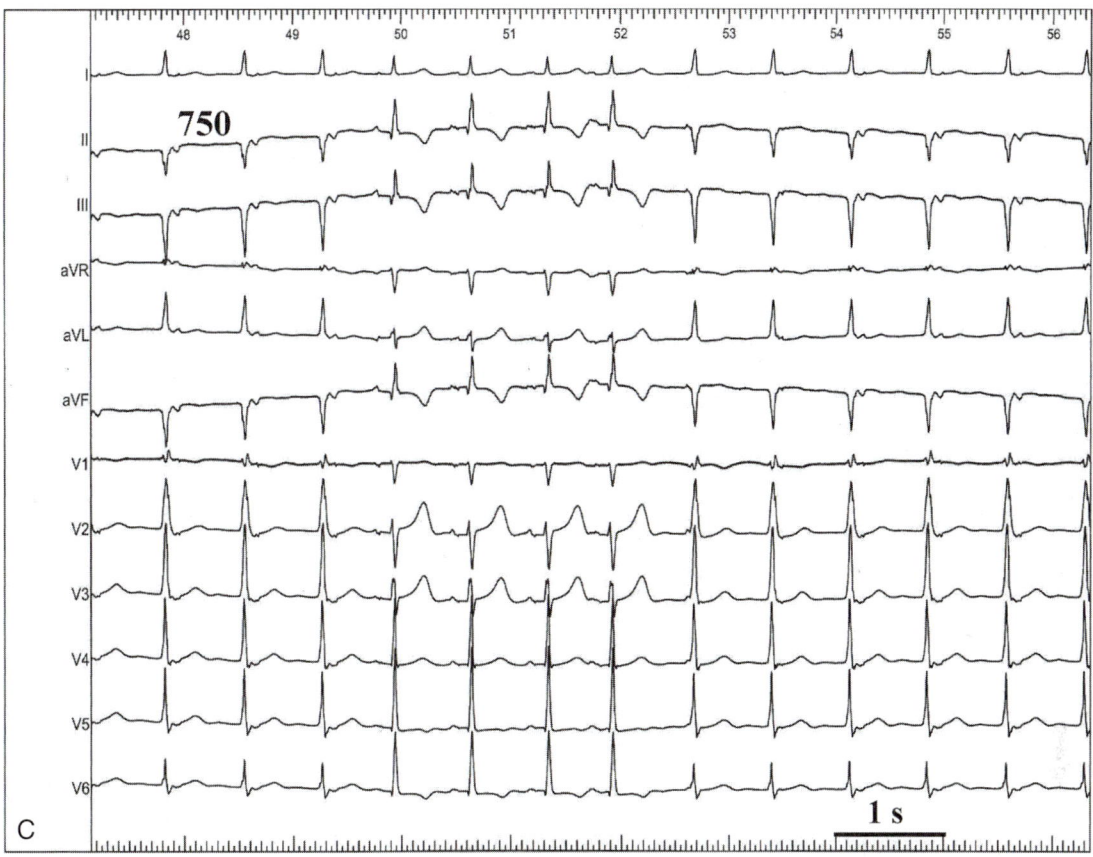

FIGURE 27-27, cont'd. C, The QRS interval during this slow VT with an RBBB configuration and left-axis deviation is very narrow and was transiently suppressed by faster sinus rhythm.

Purkinje-related VT in 8 patients and showed the mechanism to be consistent with abnormal automaticity or triggered activity in 5 patients. The 12-lead ECG during VT in these patients showed RBBB with left-axis deviation. A distinct His deflection was recorded with an HV interval during VT that was shorter than that during sinus rhythm. The authors speculated that this VT arises from a fascicular focus at some distance from the myocardial site of origin of the VT based on the varying ECG morphologies and a poor response to catheter ablation.

Recently, monomorphic premature ventricular complexes have been shown to initiate ventricular fibrillation (VF) in patients with no structural heart disease[27,28] and ischemic heart disease.[29] However, the difference in the clinical and electrophysiologic characteristic between VF triggered by premature ventricular complex from Purkinje system and monomorphic focal Purkinje VT has been undetermined. Tsuchiya and associates[30] reported a patient who exhibited the transition from Purkinje-related polymorphic VT to monomorphic VT. The intravenous administration of pilsicainide (class Ic) provoked incessant nonsustained polymorphic VT, and the polymorphic VT changed to monomorphic VT after the additional administration of pilsicainide. RF current application to the Purkinje system at the left ventricular septum suppressed both polymorphic and monomorphic VTs.

Mapping and Ablation

The ablation target of focal Purkinje VT is the earliest Purkinje activation during VT, whereas that of verapamil-sensitive fascicular VT is not necessarily the earliest Purkinje activation. Figure 27-28 shows the mapping and ablation of the focal VT from the distal Purkinje system of the left posterior fascicle. Presystolic Purkinje potentials were recorded from various sites in the left ventricle; however, the earliest Purkinje potential was recorded at the basal inferior wall (Fig. 27-28A). The Purkinje potential preceded the QRS during VT by 70 milliseconds, and the recording at the same site demonstrated a fused Purkinje potential during sinus rhythm (Fig. 27-28B and C). Pace-mapping at this site produced an identical QRS complex, with an S-QRS interval of 70 milliseconds, equal to the P-QRS interval during the VT (Fig. 27-28D). RF current delivered to this site suppressed the VT, whereas previous RF applications to other sites with a presystolic Purkinje potential were not effective.

Figure 27-29 shows the successful ablation site for focal Purkinje VT with an RBBB configuration and right-axis deviation. Because the VT could not be induced by ventricular stimulation and catecholamines, isolated premature ventricular complex with a similar QRS morphology to that observed during the VT was targeted. Left ventricular endocardial mapping during premature ventricular complex

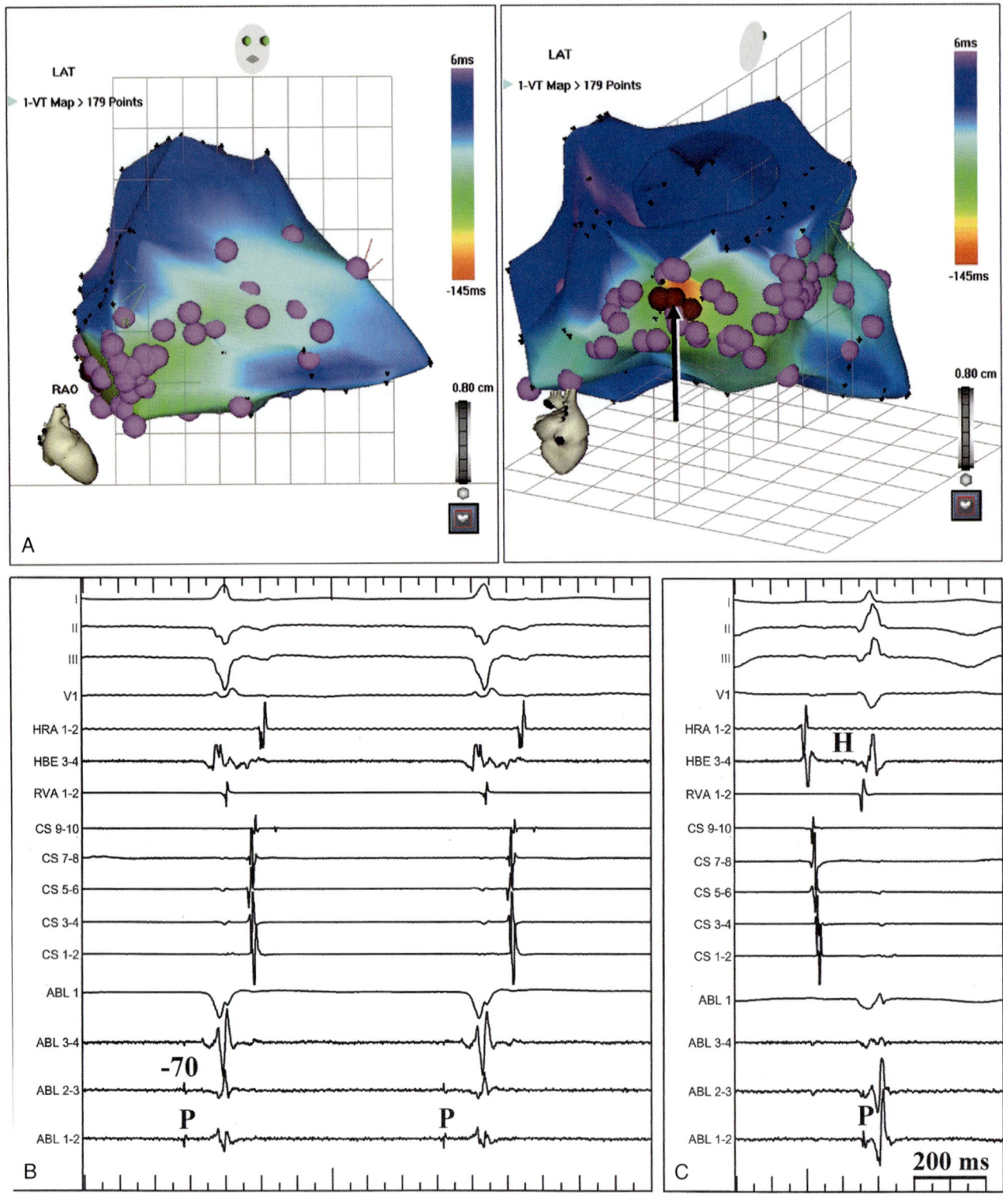

FIGURE 27-28. Ablation of the focal Purkinje ventricular tachycardia (VT) with right bundle branch block (RBBB) and left-axis deviation. **A,** Electroanatomic mapping during VT. Tags indicate the sites with the presystolic Purkinje potential during VT. The earliest Purkinje potential was recorded at the basal inferior wall, and radiofrequency (RF) current delivered to this site suppressed the VT (*arrow*). **B,** The Purkinje potential preceded the QRS during VT by 70 msec. **C,** The recording at the same site demonstrated a fused Purkinje potential during sinus rhythm.

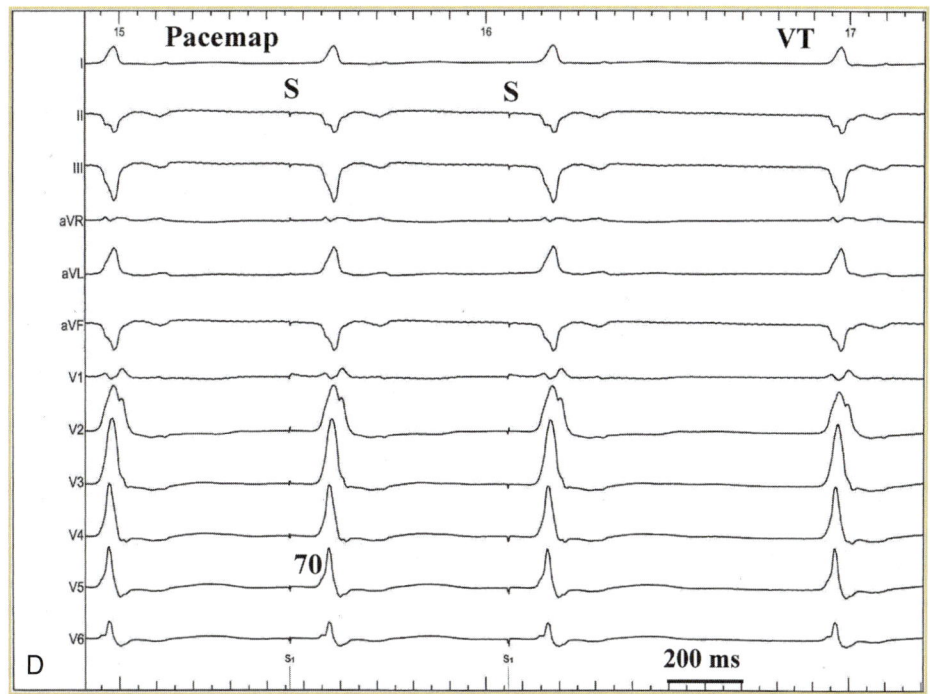

FIGURE 27-28, cont'd. D, Pace mapping at this site produced an identical QRS complex, with an S-QRS interval of 70 msec. ABL, ablation catheter; CS, coronary sinus; HBE, His bundle electrogram; HRA, high right atrium; LAT, local activation time; RAO, right anterior oblique projection; RVA, right ventricular apex.

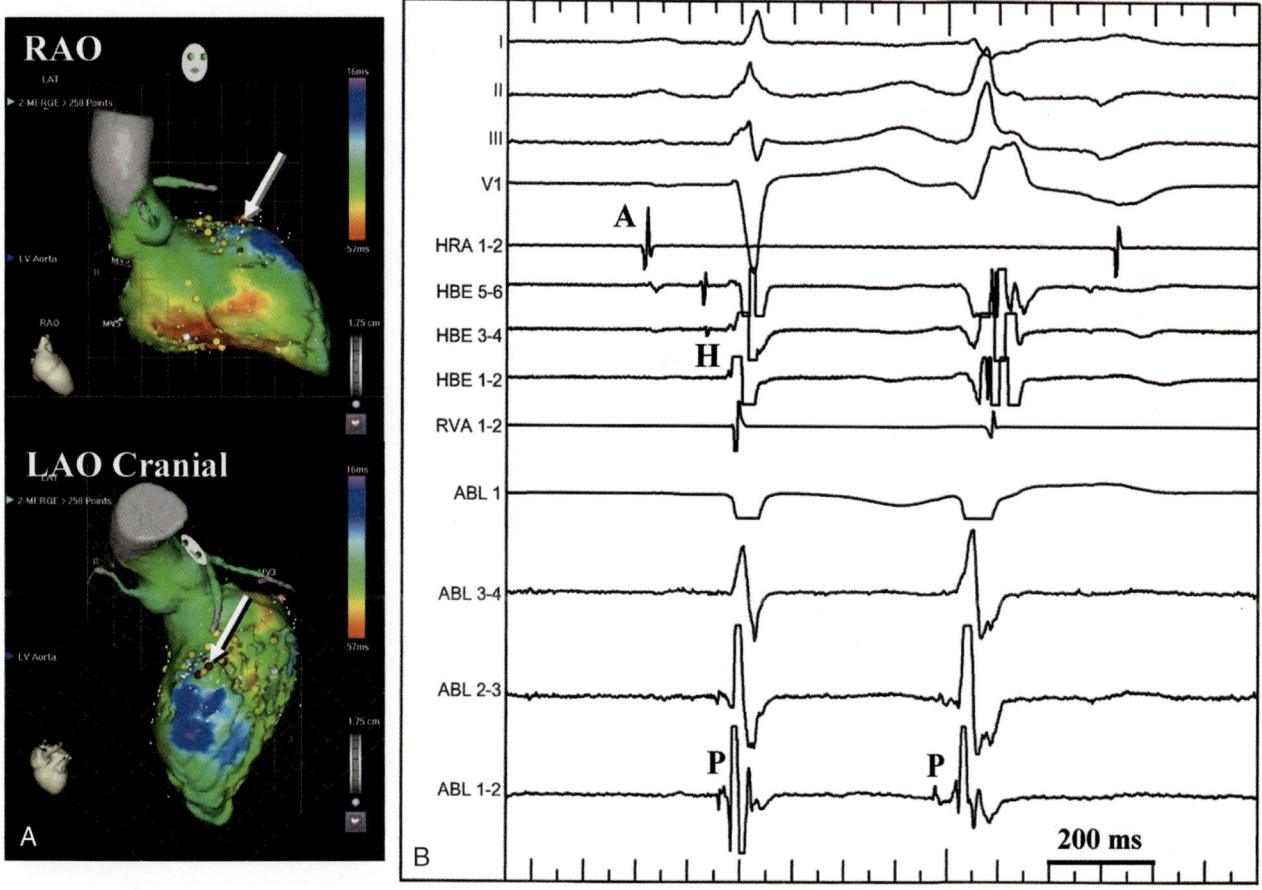

FIGURE 27-29. *Ablation* of the focal Purkinje ventricular tachycardia (VT) with right bundle branch block (RBBB) and right-axis deviation. **A,** Electroanatomic mapping during sinus rhythm. Tags in this CartoMerge image (Biosense Webster) indicate the sites with the fused Purkinje potential during sinus rhythm, and the arrow indicates the site of successful ablation. **B,** From the successful ablation site, presystolic Purkinje potentials were recorded both during sinus rhythm and during premature ventricular complex with a similar QRS morphology to that observed during the VT. ABL, ablation catheter; HBE, His bundle electrogram; HRA, high right atrium; LAO, left anterior oblique projection; RAO, right anterior oblique projection; RVA, right ventricular apex.

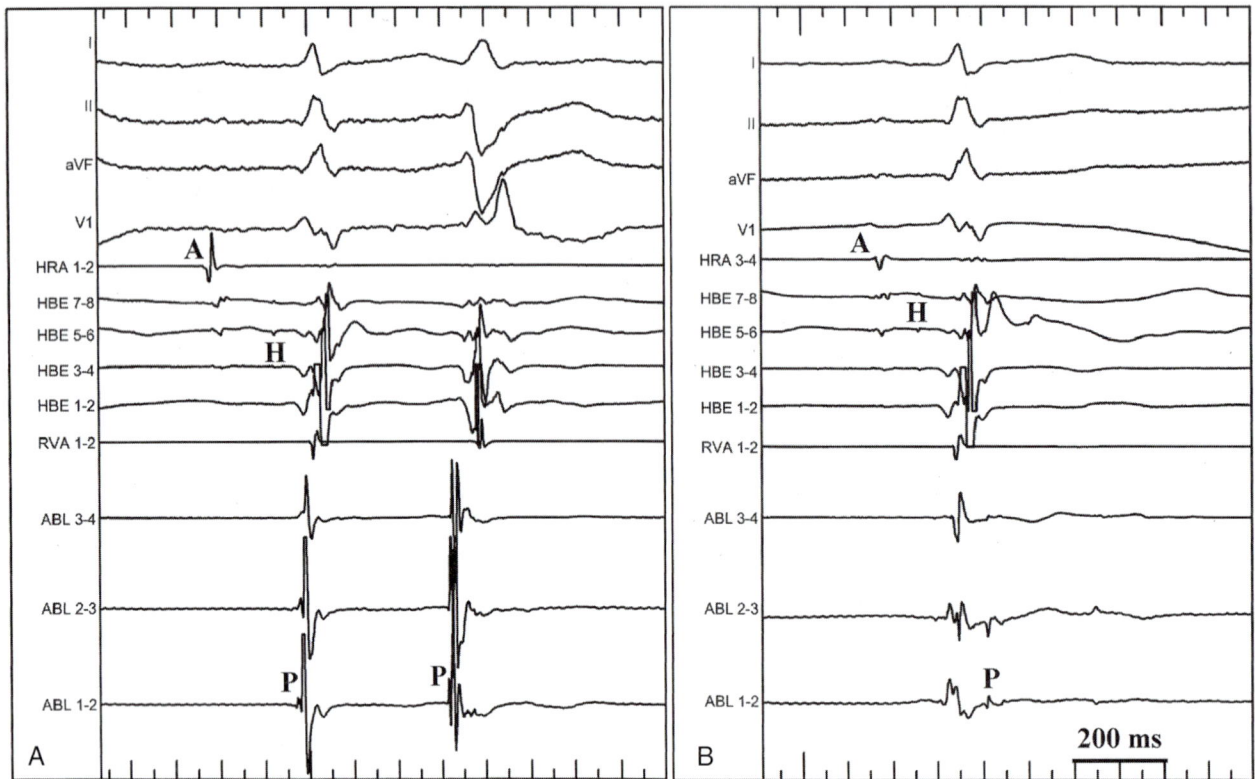

FIGURE 27-30. *Electrograms* before and after successful ablation for the focal Purkinje ventricular tachycardia (VT) at the distal portion of the left posterior fascicle. **A,** presystolic Purkinje potentials were recorded both during sinus rhythm and during premature ventricular complex with a similar QRS morphology to that observed during the VT. **B,** After successful ablation, Purkinje potential appeared after the diminished myocardial potential. There was no change in the surface QRS morphology or the His-ventricular (H-V) interval after ablation.

identified the earliest Purkinje activation in the anterolateral wall of the left ventricle. The fused Purkinje potential was also recorded at that site during sinus rhythm.

Complications

The complication that has been associated with catheter ablation of focal Purkinje VT has been LBBB and atrioventricular block. In verapamil-sensitive fascicular VTs, the creation of LBBB or atrioventricular block as the complication is quite rare because the ablation target is the diastolic "abnormal" Purkinje potential (P1) during VT, and the abolition of the normal Purkinje potential (P2) is not needed to suppress the VT. On the other hand, the abolition of the Purkinje system is usually necessary to suppress the focal Purkinje VT. Figure 27-30 shows the electrograms before and after successful ablation for the focal Purkinje VT with an RBBB configuration and a left-axis deviation. After successful ablation, the amplitude of the local myocardium has been diminished, and Purkinje potential appeared after the myocardial potential. Because this site was located at the distal portion of the left poste-

rior fascicle, there has been no change in the surface QRS morphology or HV interval after ablation. If the VT arises from a more proximal portion of the fascicle, there is a potential risk for creating LBBB or atrioventricular block by ablation. Rodriguez and colleagues[26] reported the focal Purkinje VT with an RBBB configuration and right-axis deviation in whom left anterior fascicular block occurred after the ablation. Lopera and associates[24] reported two focal Purkinje VT cases with ischemic heart disease in whom complete atrioventricular block occurred after the successful ablation of VT.

Success and Recurrence Rates

Our experience at the time of this writing includes 12 patients with idiopathic focal Purkinje VT. In all 12 patients, VT and ventricular premature complex were suppressed by catheter ablation; however, the true acute success rate is unclear because this VT is difficult to induce. Therefore, the recurrence rate is high (33%). Left posterior fascicular block occurred in 2 patients after ablation; however, no atrioventricular block occurred in our patients.

References

1. Lerman BB, Stein KM, Markowitz SM. Mechanism of idiopathic ventricular tachycardia. *J Cardiovasc Electrophysiol.* 1997;8:571–583.
2. Okumura K, Tsuchiya T. Idiopathic left ventricular tachycardia: clinical features, mechanism and management. *Card Electrophysiol Rev.* 2002;6:61–67.
3. Zipes DP, Foster PR, Troup PJ, Pedersen DH. Atrial induction of ventricular tachycardia: reentry versus triggered automaticity. *Am J Cardiol.* 1979;44:1–8.
4. Belhassen B, Rotmensch HH, Laniado S. Response of recurrent sustained ventricular tachycardia to verapamil. *Br Heart J.* 1981;46:679–682.
5. Ohe T, Shimomura K, Aihara N, et al. Idiopathic sustained left ventricular tachycardia: clinical and electrophysiological characteristics. *Circulation.* 1988;77:560–568.
6. Shimoike E, Ueda N, Maruyama T, Kaji Y. Radiofrequency catheter ablation of upper septal idiopathic left ventricular tachycardia exhibiting left bundle branch block morphology. *J Cardiovasc Electrophysiol.* 2000;11:203–207.
7. Gallagher JJ, Selle JG, Svenson RH, et al. Surgical treatment of arrhythmias. *Am J Cardiol.* 1988;61:27A–44A.
8. Suwa M, Yoneda Y, Nagao H, et al. Surgical correction of idiopathic paroxysmal ventricular tachycardia possibly related to left ventricular false tendon. *Am J Cardiol.* 1989;64:1217–1220.
9. Thakur RK, Klein GJ, Sivaram CA, et al. Anatomic substrate for idiopathic left ventricular tachycardia. *Circulation.* 1996;93:497–501.
10. Maruyama M, Terada T, Miyamoto S, Ino T. Demonstration of the reentrant circuit of verapamil-sensitive idiopathic left ventricular tachycardia: direct evidence for macroreentry as the underlying mechanism. *J Cardiovasc Electrophysiol.* 2001;12:968–972.
11. Lin FC, Wen MS, Wang CC, et al. Left ventricular fibromuscular band is not a specific substrate for idiopathic left ventricular tachycardia. *Circulation.* 1996;93:525–527.
12. Nogami A, Naito S, Tada H, et al. Demonstration of diastolic and presystolic Purkinje potential as critical potentials on a macroreentry circuit of verapamil-sensitive idiopathic left ventricular tachycardia. *J Am Coll Cardiol.* 2000;36:811–823.
13. Kuo JY, Tai CT, Chiang CE, et al. Is the fascicle of left bundle branch involved in the reentrant circuit of verapamil-sensitive idiopathic left ventricular tachycardia? *Pacing Clin Electrophysiol.* 2003;26:1986–1992.
14. Morishima I, Nogami A, Tsuboi H, et al. A case with negative participation of the left posterior fascicle to the reentry circuit of verapamil-sensitive idiopathic left ventricular tachycardia [abstract]. *Heart Rhythm.* 2009;6(suppl):S387.
15. Ouyang F, Cappato R, Ernst S, et al. Electroanatomic substrate of idiopathic left ventricular tachycardia: Unidirectional block and macroreentry within the Purkinje network. *Circulation.* 2002;105:462–469.
16. Nogami A, Naito S, Tada H, et al. Verapamil-sensitive left anterior fascicular ventricular tachycardia: Results of radiofrequency ablation in six patients. *J Cardiovasc Electrophysiol.* 1998;9:1269–1278.
17. Nakagawa H, Beckman KJ, McClelland JH, et al. Radiofrequency catheter ablation of idiopathic left ventricular tachycardia guided by a Purkinje potential. *Circulation.* 1993;88:2607–2617.
18. Yeh SJ, Wen MS, Wang CC, et al. Adenosine-sensitive ventricular tachycardia from the anterobasal left ventricle. *J Am Coll Cardiol.* 1997;30:339–345.
19. Crijns HJ, Smeets JL, Rodriguez LM, Meijer A. Cure of interfascicular reentrant ventricular tachycardia by ablation to anterior fascicle of the left bundle branch. *J Cardiovasc Electrophysiol.* 1995;6:486–492.
20. Tsuchiya T, Okumura K, Honda T, et al. Significance of late diastolic potential preceding Purkinje potential in verapamil-sensitive idiopathic left ventricular tachycardia. *Circulation.* 1999;99:2408–2413.
21. Tada H, Nogami A, Naito S, et al. Retrograde Purkinje potential activation during sinus rhythm following catheter ablation of idiopathic left ventricular tachycardia. *J Cardiovasc Electrophysiol.* 1998;9:1218–1224.
22. Kottkamp H, Hindricks G, Willems S, et al. Idiopathic left ventricular tachycardia: new insights into electrophysiological characteristics and radiofrequency catheter ablation. *Pacing Clin Electrophysiol.* 1995;18:1285–1297.
23. Lin D, Hsia HH, Gerstenfeld EP, et al. Idiopathic fascicular left ventricular tachycardia: Linear ablation lesion strategy for noninducible or nonsustained tachycardia. *Heart Rhythm.* 2005;2:934–939.
24. Lopera G, Stevenson WG, Soejima K, et al. Identification and ablation of three types of ventricular tachycardia involving the His-Purkinje system in patients with heart disease. *J Cardiovasc Electrophysiol.* 2004;15:52–58.
25. Gonzalez RP, Scheinman MM, Lesh MD, et al. Clinical and electrophysiologic spectrum of fascicular tachycardias. *Am Heart J.* 1994;128:147–156.
26. Rodriguez LM, Smeets JL, Timmermans C, et al. Radiofrequency catheter ablation of idiopathic ventricular tachycardia originating in the anterior fascicle of the left bundle branch. *J Cardiovasc Electrophysiol.* 1996;7:1211–1216.
27. Haïssaguerre M, Shah DC, Jaïs P, et al. Role of Purkinje conducting system in triggering of idiopathic ventricular fibrillation. *Lancet.* 2002;359:677–678.
28. Nogami A, Sugiyasu A, Kubota S, Kato K. Mapping and ablation of idiopathic ventricular fibrillation from the Purkinje system. *Heart Rhythm.* 2005;2:646–649.
29. Bänsch D, Ouyang F, Antz M, et al. Successful catheter ablation of electrical storm after myocardial infarction. *Circulation.* 2003;108:3011–3016.
30. Tsuchiya T, Nakagawa S, Yanagita Y, Fukunaga T. Transition from Purkinje fiber-related rapid polymorphic ventricular tachycardia to sustained monomorphic ventricular tachycardia in a patient with a structurally normal heart: a case report. *J Cardiovasc Electrophysiol.* 2007;18:102–105.

28
Ablation of Ventricular Tachycardia in Coronary Artery Disease

Haris M. Haqqani and David J. Callans

Key Points

The mechanism of ventricular tachycardia (VT) in coronary artery disease is reentry within the infarct scar and scar-border zone.

Diagnosis is made by tachycardia persistence independent of both supraventricular and His-Purkinje activation (except for bundle branch reentry).

Ablation targets include presystolic electrical activity within the infarct zone that demonstrates concealed entrainment and a reproducible relationship to the VT circuit. For substrate ablation, voltage mapping is used to define scar zone, scar-border zone, and higher voltage channels; pace mapping to determine putative VT exit sites and channels of slow conduction constrained by electrically unexcitable scar; and electrogram mapping to locate isolated potentials representing late-activated channels within scar. Linear lesions are created through these presumed channels and VT exit sites.

Three dimensional mapping systems are essential for linear ablation and often helpful for entrainment mapping. Irrigated ablation catheters create larger lesions.

The acute success rate for individual VT morphologies is more than 90%; however, new morphologies may develop in follow-up.

Ablation for ventricular tachycardia (VT) in patients after myocardial infarction is important, not for its relative frequency, but for the profound influence this procedure has on quality of life.[1,2] Most patients who undergo VT ablation have implantable cardioverter–defibrillators (ICDs) and have frequent episodes leading to ICD shocks. Patients who present with uniform tolerated VT typically receive ICDs after successful ablation because even after the most complete form of substrate modification, subendocardial resection, there is a significant residual risk for sudden death (2.1% per year).[3] This is consistent with the observation from the Electrophysiologic Study Versus Electromagnetic Monitoring (ESVEM) trial that presentation with uniform tolerated VT does not predict presentation with recurrent tolerated VT as opposed to cardiac arrest.[4] Antiarrhythmic therapy, although commonly used to complement ICD therapy in patients with recurrent VT, is incompletely successful in preventing VT episodes and may cause important cardiac and noncardiac side effects.[5] Although properly viewed as adjuvant therapy, most patients with frequent VT episodes have a single morphology (or a few dominant morphologies), and successful ablation significantly reduces the frequency of VT recurrence in follow-up.

Anatomy

The typical anatomic substrate for monomorphic VT is extensive healed infarction with resultant left ventricular (LV) dysfunction. The extent of myocardial necrosis, infarct involvement of the interventricular septum, and degree of LV dysfunction are the most important determinants of arrhythmia risk after infarction. Patients with tolerated sustained VT have more extensive infarction, more frequent aneurysm formation, and more pronounced LV dysfunction than patients with nonsustained VT or sudden cardiac death.[6] Increasing treatment with revascularization intervention whenever appropriate and medical therapy to prevent LV remodeling has decreased the incidence of VT after infarction to about 1%.[7] Nonetheless, this decreased incidence may be balanced by an increased prevalence as improved therapies prolong longevity in patients after infarction.

Pathophysiology

The electrophysiologic substrate for VT gradually develops in the first 2 weeks after myocardial infarction and, once established, appears to remain indefinitely. During the infarct healing process, necrotic myocardium is replaced with fibrous tissue. This results in a reduction in the number of gap junctions connecting surviving myocytes. In addition, there are molecular changes induced by the infarct changing the composition and the function of remaining gap junctions.[8] Because of abnormalities in cellular coupling, conduction is slow and discontinuous, despite the fact that normal sodium-dependent action potentials are recorded from living myocytes within the infarct zone. These conduction abnormalities provide the electrophysiologic substrate for VT.[9,10] Endocardial recordings from sites of VT origin during sinus rhythm consistently demonstrate low-amplitude, prolonged, multicomponent potentials (Fig. 28-1).[6] The individual components of fractionated electrograms are generated by individual "islets" of myocyte groups, isolated from neighboring cells by in-growth of fibrous tissue. The duration of the local electrogram represents the abnormally slow, fractionated conduction within the electrode field of view.

Although the relationship between inducible VT and spontaneous VT is poorly understood, inducible VT signifies the presence of an anatomic VT substrate and confirms increased susceptibility for arrhythmic events.[11] In addition to the presence of the anatomic substrate, spontaneous VT may occur only if a specific trigger is provided, such as ventricular ectopy, ischemia, heart failure, or changes in autonomic tone.[12–15]

The mechanism for most sustained monomorphic VTs in coronary artery disease is reentry in the setting of the conduction abnormalities provided by the anatomic substrate of the infarct (Fig. 28-2). The evidence leading to this conclusion is listed in Table 28-1. Reentrant circuits appear to have a fairly consistent relationship to the anatomic substrate (Fig. 28-3). A discrete, protected zone of slow conduction is contained within the dense infarct and proves important for many mapping techniques, as discussed later. The exit site of the circuit is consistently located at the border zone of the dense infarct, and activation at this site

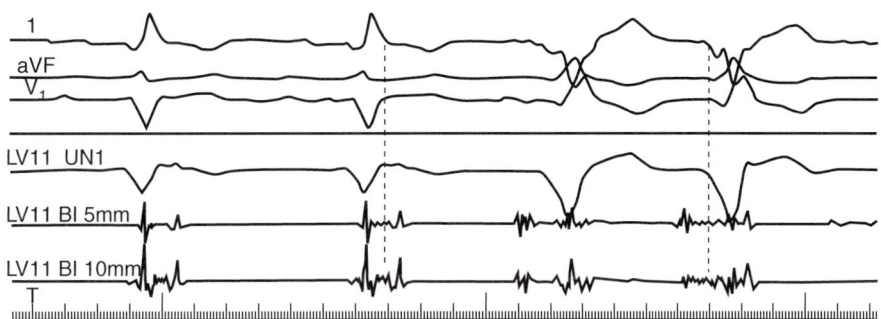

FIGURE 28-1. Electrogram recording from a ventricular tachycardia (VT) site of origin. Three surface electrocardiogram leads are shown with three intracardiac recordings from a catheter positioned within the infarct zone. During sinus rhythm, a fractionated, multicomponent signal is recorded; the final component of this electrogram is recorded after the end of the surface QRS. During VT (final two beats of the tracing), isolated diastolic potentials are observed, preceding the QRS by 90 msec. BI, bipolar; LV, left ventricle; UN, unipolar. *(From Josephson ME. Clinical Cardiac Electrophysiology: Techniques and Interpretations, 3rd ed. Philadelphia: Lippincott Williams & Wilkins; 2002. With permission.)*

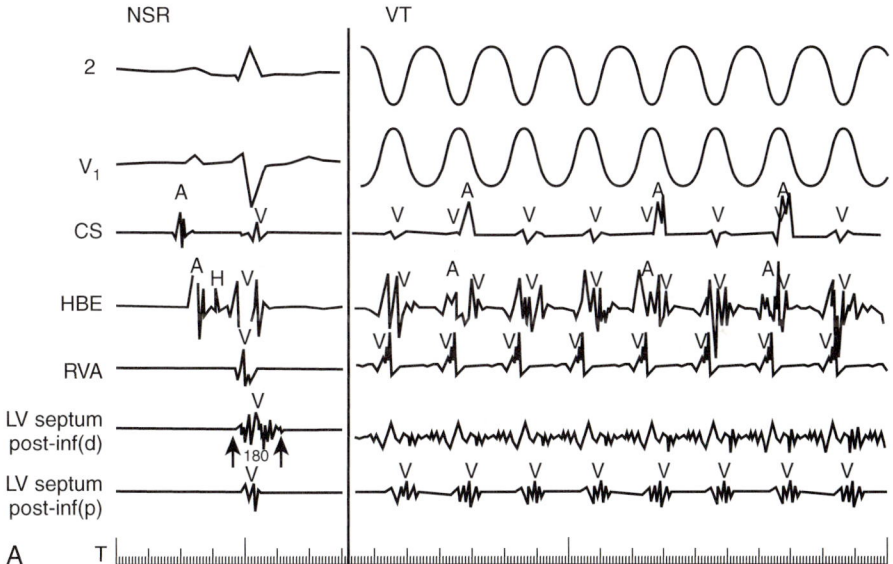

FIGURE 28-2. Observations supporting a reentrant mechanism for ventricular tachycardia (VT) in the setting of healed infarction. **A,** Continuous electrical activity. Electrogram recordings from the infarct (left ventricular [LV] septum after infarction [post-inf(d) and post-inf(p)]) and during sinus rhythm and VT. Continuous activity is demonstrated in the LV recording during VT. This is consistent with a reentrant mechanism, with activation of some portion of the circuit throughout the entire cycle length, all within the field of view of a single recording site. CS, coronary sinus; HBE, His bundle electrogram; NSR, normal sinus rhythm; RVA, right ventricular apex.

Continued

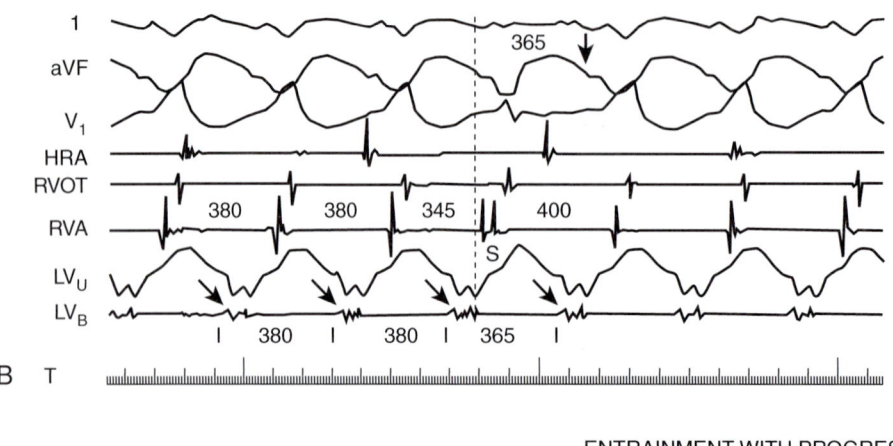

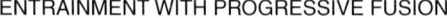

ENTRAINMENT WITH PROGRESSIVE FUSION

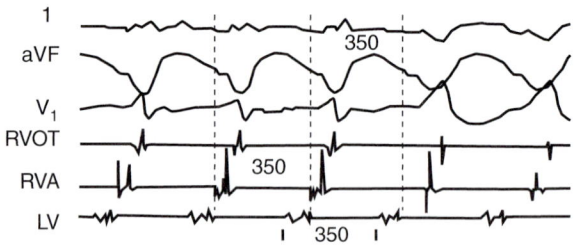

V. TACHYCARDIA

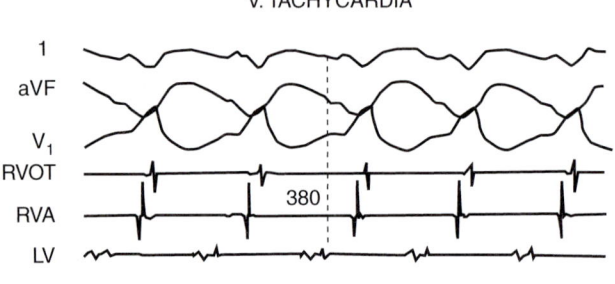

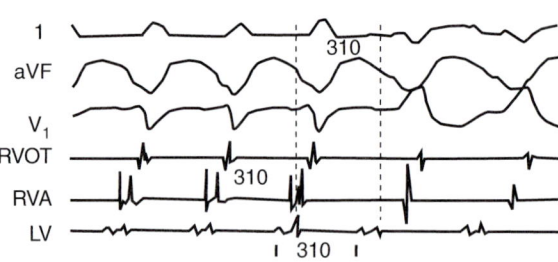

PACING

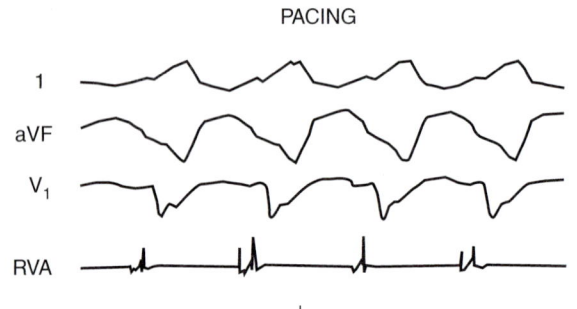

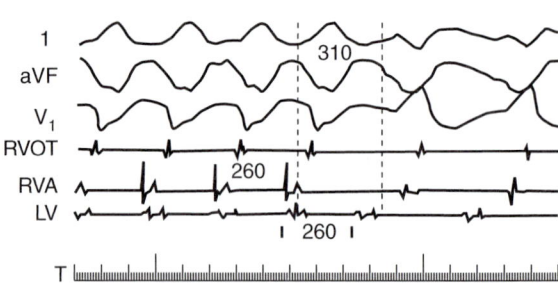

FIGURE 28-2, cont'd. B, Resetting with fusion. Surface electrocardiogram (ECG) and intracardiac recordings during VT. A single extrastimulus is delivered from the RVA after the inscription of the LV electrogram at the site of origin and the onset of the surface QRS. Nonetheless, surface fusion is observed, and the tachycardia is reset (i.e., the return cycle beat occurs earlier in time [345 + 400 msec < 380 + 380 msec] than it would have had the extrastimulus not been delivered). This is inconsistent with a focal mechanism and suggests reentry within a circuit with a distinct entrance and exit site. B, ; HRA, high right atrium; RVOT, right ventricular outflow tract; T, ; U, . **C,** Entrainment with progressive fusion. Surface ECG and intracardiac recordings during VT, RVA pacing, and entrainment at three different cycle lengths. Entrainment at faster cycle lengths changes the nature of the surface ECG fusion to more greatly resemble the paced QRS morphology. (**A,** *From Josephson ME, Horowitz LN, Farshidi A. Continuous local electrical activity: a mechanism of recurrent ventricular tachycardia. Circulation. 1978;57:659;* **B,** *from Almendral JM, Rosenthal ME, Stamato NJ, et al. Analysis of the resetting phenomenon in sustained uniform ventricular tachycardia: incidence and relation to termination.* J Am Coll Cardiol. *1986;8:294–300;* **C,** *from Almendral JM, Gottlieb CD, Rosenthal ME, et al. Entrainment of ventricular tachycardia: explanation for surface electrocardiographic phenomena by analysis of electrograms recorded within the tachycardia circuit. Circulation. 1988;77:569–580. With permission.*)

TABLE 28-1

OBSERVATIONS SUPPORTING REENTRY AS THE MECHANISM OF VENTRICULAR TACHYCARDIA IN HEALED INFARCTION

Induction and termination of ventricular tachycardia (VT) with programmed ventricular stimulation

Site-specificity of induction

Inverse relationship between the extrastimulus coupling interval and the onset of the first tachycardia beat

Continuous electrical activity demonstrated to be related to VT initiation and maintenance

Response to programmed stimulation during VT: resetting with fusion, entrainment

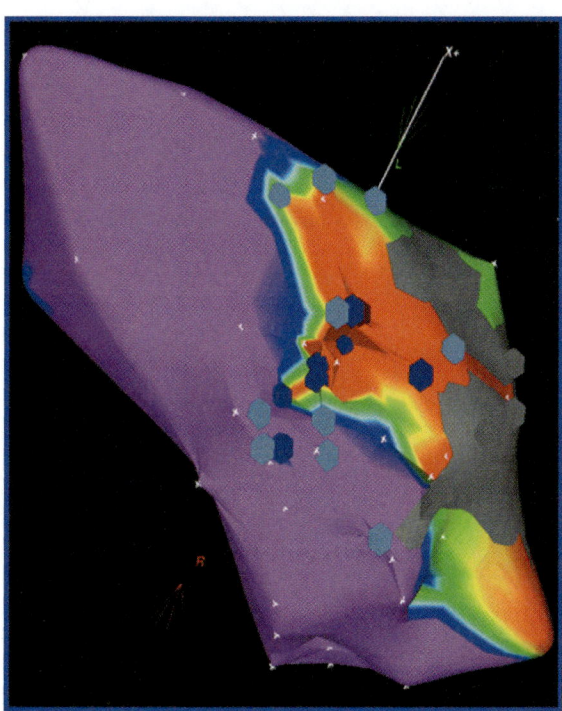

FIGURE 28-3. Relationship of the ventricular tachycardia (VT) circuit and the infarct anatomy. View of an electroanatomic voltage map in an inferior infarct (*red* signifies electrogram voltage <1 mV, identifying the dense infarct). On top of the voltage map, entrainment mapping was performed at multiple sites to demonstrate sites within (*dark blue dots*) and outside (*light blue dots*) the circuit. The onset of the QRS corresponded to the exit of the circuit from the infarct scar.

corresponds to the onset of the QRS complex in VT. In some cases, the protected zone is bounded by scar and an anatomic structure such as the mitral valve annulus. Nonreentrant mechanisms can also cause VT in patients with healed infarction. Repetitive monomorphic nonsustained VT may occur in this setting and may even arise from the infarct zone.

The relationship of the underlying infarct substrate is not as clearly defined for polymorphic ventricular tachycardias (PMVTs). Reports by Haïssaguerre and colleagues, however, have demonstrated that ablation can target the mechanism of initiation of PMVT in well-selected patients.[16] Reproducible arrhythmia triggers responsible for the initiation of PMVT

have been found in small patient groups with frequent arrhythmia episodes. Furthermore, typical electrocardiogram (ECG) signatures and anatomic locations for these triggers exist, facilitating pattern recognition and mapping. Often, triggers originate from the Purkinje system near the infarct border zone. The importance of these triggers for a more generalized group of patients after myocardial infarction remains to be determined.

Diagnosis

In patients with sustained VT, the diagnosis is often made by analysis of the ECG. VT is a wide QRS complex tachycardia, driven by the ventricles, and as such, atrioventricular (AV) dissociation may be evident. Several algorithms deal with the subject of differential diagnosis of wide complex tachycardias.[17-19] All are based on the concept that VT originates in diseased myocardium potentially away from the conduction system, whereas supraventricular arrhythmias with aberrancy arise from the His-Purkinje system. Because of this, SVT with aberrancy has to resemble either right or left bundle branch block (LBBB) and has rapid initial forces, but VT can arise from anywhere in the ventricle and thus can have any possible QRS morphology and slow initial forces. Nonetheless, the predictive value of these observations and the algorithms is negatively affected by the presence of antiarrhythmic drugs, electrolyte imbalances, or preexisting conduction system disease. More difficult differential diagnoses include atrial flutter with 1:1 aberrant conduction (Fig. 28-4) and preexcited tachycardias. Review of stored electrograms provides essential diagnostic information regarding the etiology of tachycardias that trigger ICD therapy (Fig. 28-5). The morphology of the ICD electrogram is rather specific.[20] Although supraventricular tachycardia with right bundle branch block (RBBB) (i.e., ipsilateral to the ICD lead, changing the vector with which it is activated) can change the electrogram morphology,[21] in most instances, this is diagnostic of VT. Furthermore, each different VT morphology produces different electrogram morphology; thus, careful review of stored electrograms before consideration of VT ablation can help to determine how many different VT morphologies are clinically relevant. Correlating ICD electrograms recorded during induced VT morphologies with those from spontaneous episodes can also help to determine clinical relevance.

The electrophysiologic criteria for diagnosing VT related to ischemic heart disease are given in Table 28-2. In general, the diagnosis is confirmed by demonstrating that the tachycardia is not dependent on atrial, AV nodal, or His-Purkinje activation. The occurrence of bundle branch reentry is an exception. Tachycardias related to prior myocardial infarction usually meet classic criteria for a reentrant mechanism.

Decision-Making Process for Ablation

The number of patients considered for ablation is relatively small compared with the denominator of patients with ventricular arrhythmias. Morady and coworkers estimated that

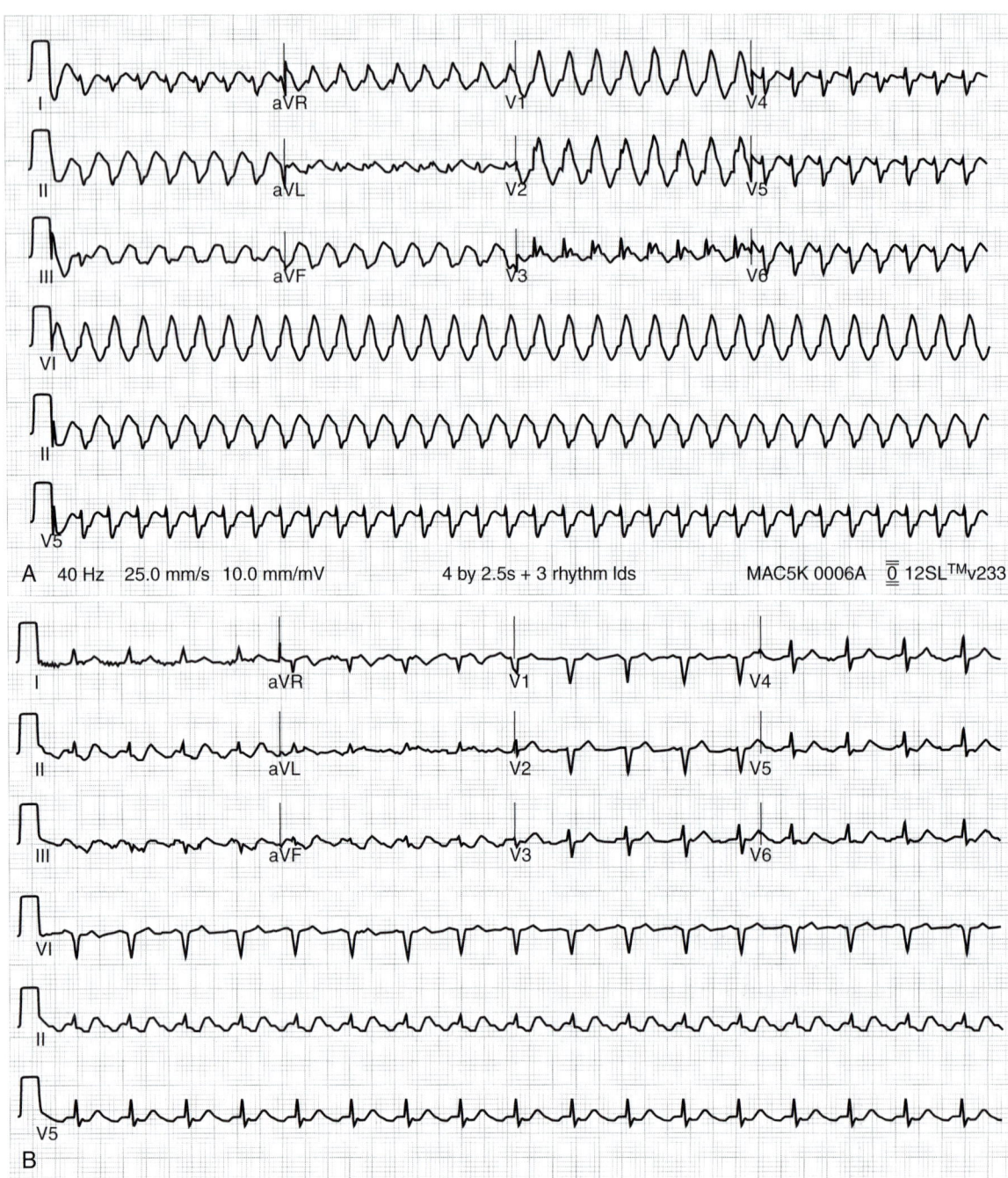

FIGURE 28-4. Atrial flutter with 1:1 conduction. **A,** The first electrocardiogram (ECG) was recorded when an elderly woman without structural heart disease presented to the emergency with chest pain. She had a history of atrial fibrillation and was treated with propafenone. A wide complex tachycardia with a QRS morphology and axis consistent with ventricular tachycardia is shown. **B,** The second ECG, however, shows atrial flutter with a narrow QRS; the atrial flutter cycle length is identical to the cycle length of the wide complex tachycardia. She was treated with catheter ablation of atrial flutter and continuation of propafenone.

10% of patients with VT are appropriate candidates for VT ablation.[22] This number may be significantly smaller with the current post-infarction therapy strategy. For the purposes of this discussion, the risk-benefit analysis of VT will be considered in ICD recipients with frequent symptomatic VT. Ablation alone (without ICD therapy) is considered by some investigators as the primary therapy for VT in patients who present with tolerated VT; however, because coronary heart disease is progressive and unpredictable, most agree that ablation therapy is palliative and adjunctive to ICD therapy.[23]

The typical patient considered for VT ablation has frequent VT episodes resulting in multiple ICD shocks due to rapid VT or ineffective antitachycardia pacing therapy or who has severe symptoms (palpitations, presyncope) despite effective antitachycardia pacing. Every attempt should be made to optimize pharmacologic and antitachycardia pacing therapy in such patients.[24–26]

The next important consideration in deciding about the relative merits of VT ablation is determining the number of clinically relevant VT morphologies. In patients with

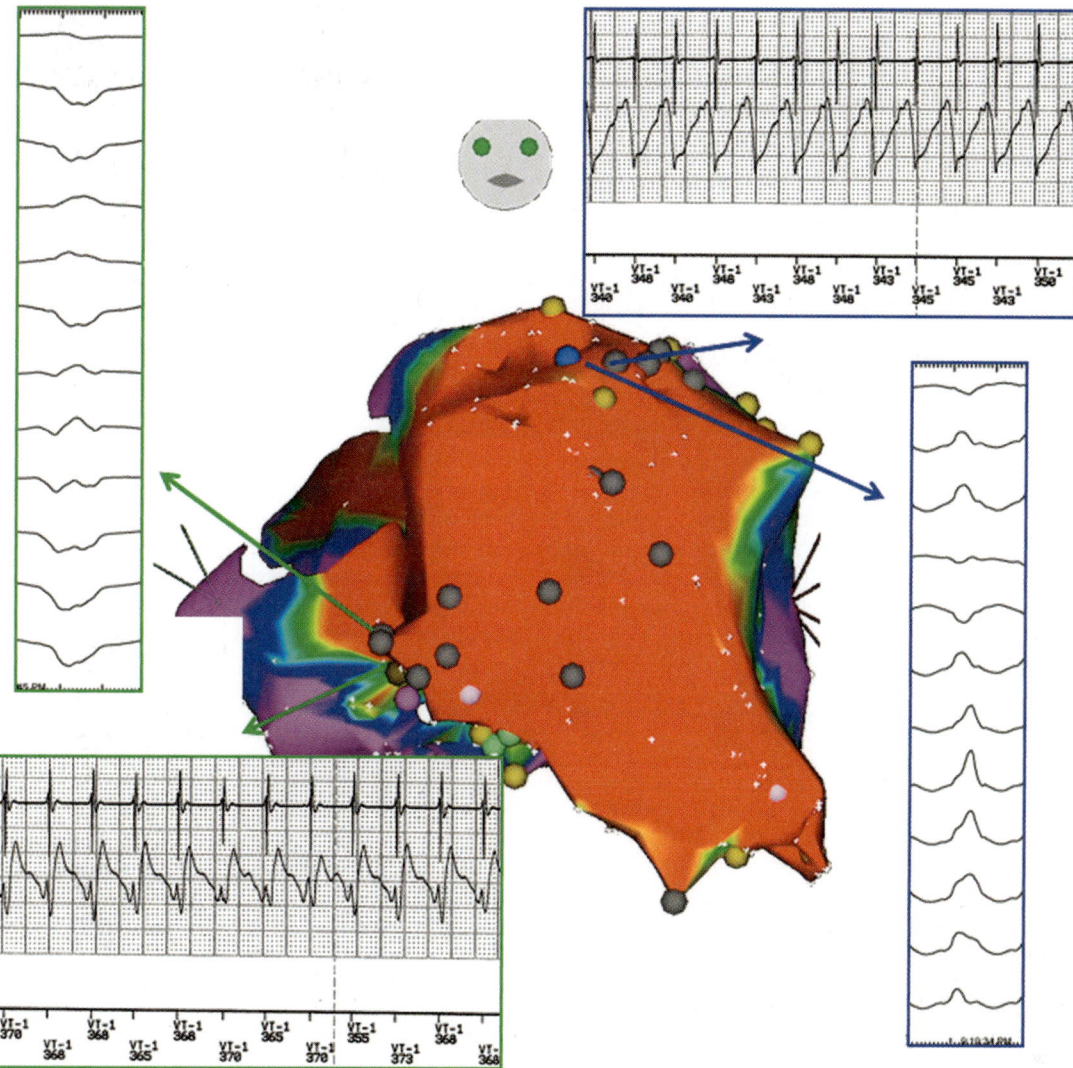

FIGURE 28-5. Electrograms recorded during implantable cardioverter-defibrillator (ICD) therapy correlate with different ventricular tachycardia (VT) morphologies. The color electroanatomic voltage map from a patient with a large anteroseptal infarction is shown in the anteroposterior projection and displays points of very low bipolar voltage (<0.5 mV) in *red*, corresponding to the dense scar zone, whereas *purple* corresponds to normal myocardium (bipolar voltage >1.5 mV). Depicted are two clinical VT morphologies with their recorded ICD electrograms. In the *top green panel* is the surface 12-lead electrocardiogram of an atypical left bundle branch block morphology VT, which exits the scar at its mid-inferoseptal aspect. Its accompanying ICD electrograms are displayed in the *lower green panel* with the local tip bipolar electrogram shown in the top channel, whereas the bottom channel shows the far-field right ventricular coil to ICD can electrogram. These electrograms are seen to have a completely different morphology to the ICD recordings from the right bundle branch block morphology VT (which exits at the opposite aspect of the scar) displayed in the *blue boxes.*

large infarctions, multiple VT morphologies are typically induced with programmed stimulation. Although programmed stimulation identifies "what is possible," many of these morphologies may not be clinically relevant (i.e., they may not ever occur spontaneously). Often the decision regarding which morphologies to ablate is made on the basis of VT cycle length and the reproducibility of induction (slower, reproducibly induced VT is thought more likely to be recurrent). Nonetheless, the gold standard for preprocedural planning is careful review of the ICD electrograms recorded during spontaneous VT episodes. As discussed previously, the electrograms inscribed during VT episodes are fairly specific: different electrogram morphologies signify different VT morphologies

TABLE 28-2
DIAGNOSTIC CRITERIA FOR ISCHEMIC SCAR-RELATED VENTRICULAR TACHYCARDIA
Tachycardia independent of atrial and atrioventricular nodal activation
Activation of His-Purkinje system follows ventricular myocardial activation (exception bundle branch reentry) • Dissociation of His-Purkinje system from tachycardia • His-ventricular interval shorter in tachycardia than sinus rhythm if 1:1 relationship
Meets criteria for reentrant tachycardia
Exclusion of preexcited tachycardias

(Fig. 28-5). Despite this, VT morphologies may be "paired" and represent different exit sites from the same circuit.[27] Still, ablation is more favorable if limited to a small number of spontaneous VT morphologies and is less attractive as this number increases.

Finally, the patient's medical condition must be taken into account. Patients with end-stage heart failure may be intolerant to protracted procedures. Peripheral vascular disease may limit vascular access and increase the risks for complications. The patient must also be willing to accept the risk for major complications such as stroke and cardiogenic shock.

Mapping

Independent of the strategy employed, the concept guiding VT ablation is similar to other arrhythmia substrates: detailed mapping should precede ablation to minimize the number of radiofrequency (RF) deliveries and the incidence of associated side effects (particularly stroke and heart failure). Several strategies are helpful in mapping VT in the setting of healed infarction, depending on the arrhythmia presentation, including (1) entrainment mapping for hemodynamically tolerated VT, (2) substrate mapping for unstable VT, and (3) mapping of triggers for polymorphic VT. Each of these strategies is described next.

Entrainment Mapping

Entrainment refers to pacing during a reentrant arrhythmia to transiently accelerate the arrhythmia to the pacing cycle length, restoring the unchanged tachycardia at the conclusion of pacing. Seminal work by Okumura and coworkers[28–30] as well as others[31–34] developed the concept of entrainment, applied it to the circumstances of VT after infarction, and used these techniques to demonstrate important properties of reentrant circuits. The concept of entrainment mapping for ablation of VT is targeting a single site that will interrupt the VT circuit. This site must therefore be located not only within the circuit but also in a protected and relatively narrow isthmus or channel. Although many of the mapping strategies to determine these characteristics had been developed by previous investigators, a computer model and ablation verification study by Stevenson and coworkers helped to crystallize our understanding of these relationships (Fig. 28-6).[35,36] Detailed mapping is performed during stable VT based on activation and response of pacing at multiple sites during VT (Table 28-3). The location of the protected isthmus is within the infarct zone and is typically predicted by bipolar electrogram voltages of 0.5 mV or less.[37,38] This anatomic construct provides for both the slow conduction necessary for the circuit and its narrow geometry (i.e., bounded by unexcitable areas) so that RF lesions can interrupt the circuit.

Before the planned VT ablation procedure, the patient's coronary anatomy and infarction pattern should be ascertained by coronary angiography, positron emission tomography (PET), or magnetic resonance imaging (MRI). This knowledge may help in selecting areas of interest for mapping and may influence the interpretation of ECGs. In addition, programmed ventricular stimulation is usually performed to initiate the clinical tachycardia and to determine the number of VT morphologies that are inducible. The process of entrainment mapping then proceeds in several steps. First, the general location of the VT circuit can be determined by analysis of the 12-lead ECG morphology during spontaneous and induced VT (Table 28-4).[39,40] Under the best circumstance, this exercise resolves the area of VT origin to about 4 cm². This technique has been recently reviewed.[40] Briefly, VT morphologies are examined for bundle branch pattern and axis, in the context of infarct location. LBBB morphologies typically originate from the interventricular septum (or rarely in patients with coronary disease, from the right ventricle); RBBB morphologies originate from the parietal left ventricle. Superior axis VT arises from the inferior LV (the inferior wall or inferior portion of the septum), and inferior axis VT from the superior LV (anterior basal wall or superior septum). The precordial R-wave transition helps to determine the site of origin in an apex-to-base dimension. VTs with positive R waves across the precordium arise from the mitral annulus, a posterior structure; VTs with negative QRS complexes across the precordium arise from the apex, which is an anterior site. VTs with rightward axis usually arise from the lateral wall, or from the apex. However, ECG localization is very difficult in patients with anterior infarction and right bundle VT morphologies because there are no consistent discriminating features between apical lateral and septal sites of origin. Recent work by Patel and coworkers[41] has demonstrated that relative timing of right ventricular apical activation may distinguish these sites.

Programmed stimulation is performed to induce all "clinically relevant" VT morphologies and assess for hemodynamic tolerance. Different investigators have defined clinical relevance in different ways; variables to be considered include matching induced to spontaneous morphologies (on the surface ECG or ICD electrograms) and cycle length. There is some precedent to using a cutoff of 270 milliseconds for VT cycle length, which was used in determining efficacy after surgical ablation and for some trials of catheter ablation as well.[42] In addition, slow VT tends to recur more frequently than rapid VT. Programmed stimulation typically yields more VT morphologies than have occurred spontaneously. Studies that have focused on induction of all possible morphologies of uniform VT yield an average of three or four per patient.[42,43] However, different morphologies are often related in pairs and can be ablated with the same lesion set.[27] An example of this is the combination of LBBB with a left superior axis and RBBB with a right superior axis VT pair commonly observed in the setting of inferior infarction, in which both use the "mitral isthmus."[44,45] In this case, the RBBB morphology tachycardia exits toward the lateral wall, and the LBBB morphology exits toward the septum.

Second, detailed activation mapping (and voltage mapping if applicable) is performed. If the patient is in hemodynamically stable VT, mapping is directed toward sites within the infarct zone that have high frequency, isolated components that occur in mid-diastole and drive, rather than follow, the VT QRS. This relationship can be determined by observing a constant electrogram-to-QRS relationship with spontaneous alterations in cycle length or during the return cycle following pacing from a distant source (Fig. 28-7).[33] If the patient is in sinus rhythm due to poorly tolerated VT, mapping can proceed by pace-mapping to generally reproduce the VT QRS morphology, starting at sites suggested by the ECG analysis that show fractionated potentials occurring after the end of the QRS. During pacing in sinus rhythm, sites of abnormal stimulus to QRS intervals (>40 milliseconds, and ideally >70 milliseconds) are targeted as well.[46]

Third, the relationship of the individual site to the circuit is assessed with pacing at that site during VT (Figs. 28-6 and 28-7). If the patient is in sinus rhythm, VT must be induced at this point. Important technical considerations include pacing just faster (usually 20 milliseconds less) than the VT cycle length at a current just sufficient to reliably capture; some investigators insist that unipolar pacing should be used, to prevent the confounding influence

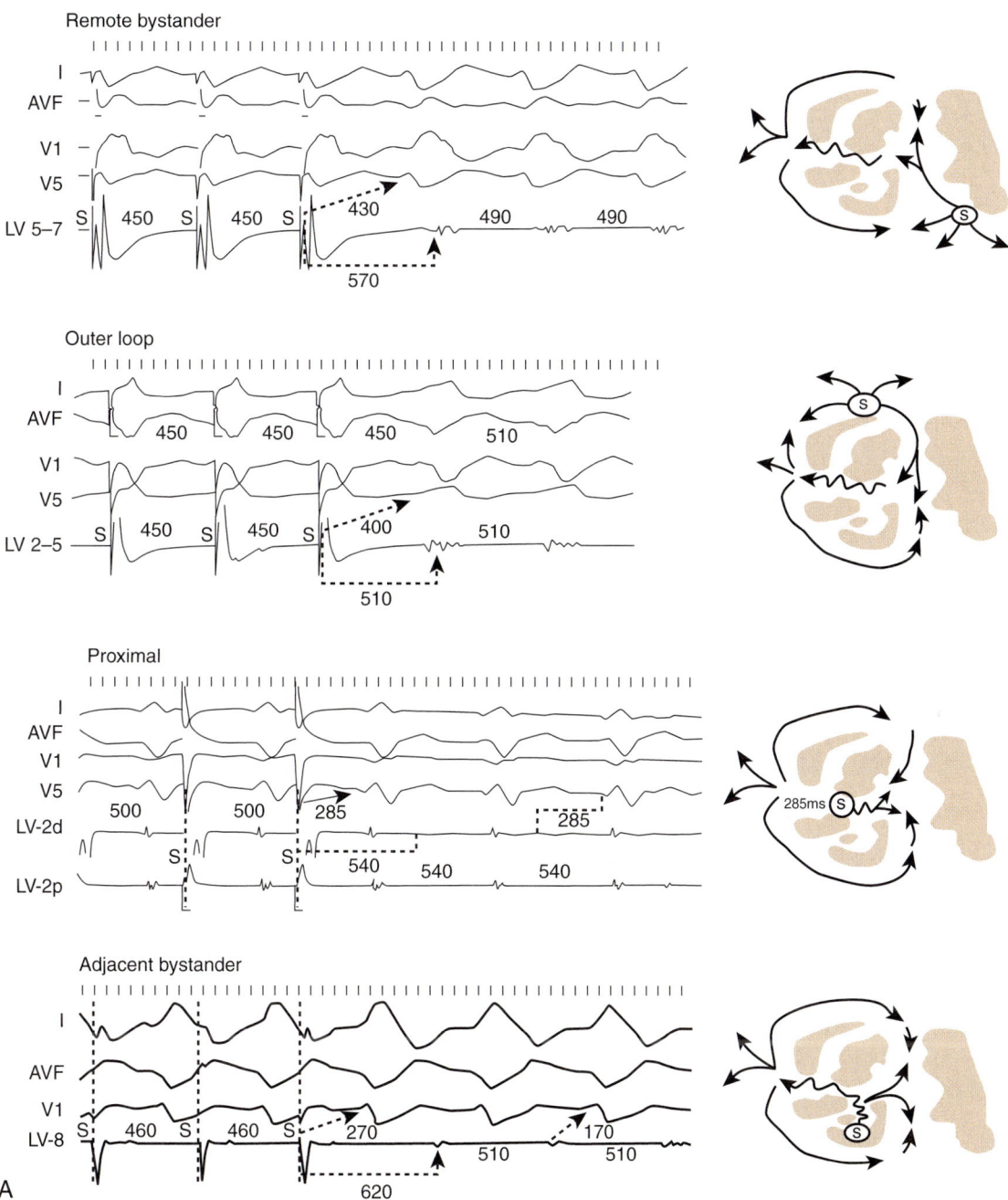

FIGURE 28-6. A, Computer model of ventricular tachycardia (VT) within unexcitable infarct scar (*tan areas, right panels*), demonstrating the response to entrainment with pacing at different sites within the circuit. The circuit is depicted as a figure-of-eight activation using a central common pathway with slow conduction. Pacing from remote bystander areas (*top*) shows some degree of fusion, and the return cycle is longer than the VT cycle length (by twice the conduction time from the site to the VT circuit). Pacing from outer loop sites (*second from top*) shows manifest entrainment because the pacing site has access to recruit areas away from the circuit and is not bounded by the infarct. Pacing from sites within the central pathway (*third from top*) demonstrates concealed entrainment with a stimulus-electrocardiogram interval equal to the electrogram-QRS interval during VT; the return cycle measured at this electrogram is equal to the VT cycle length. Pacing from adjacent bystander sites (*bottom*) results in concealed entrainment, but the return cycle is longer than the VT cycle length (by twice the conduction time from the site to the VT circuit).

Continued

ABLATION OF SCAR-RELATED VT

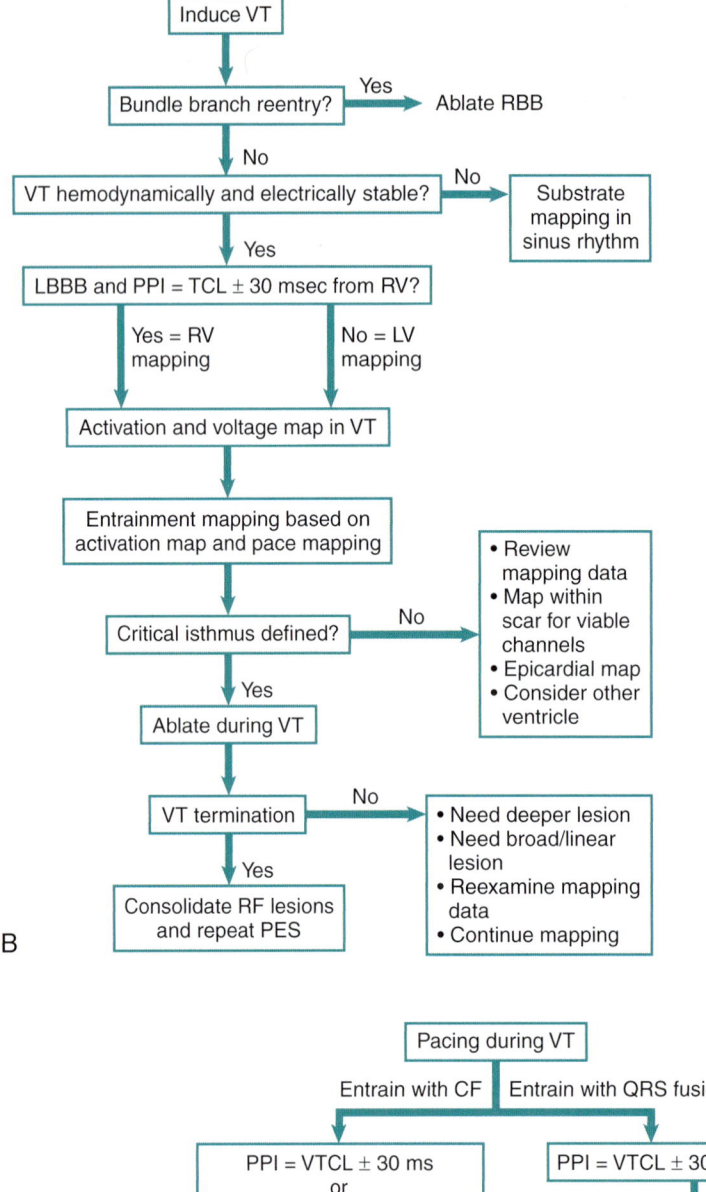

B

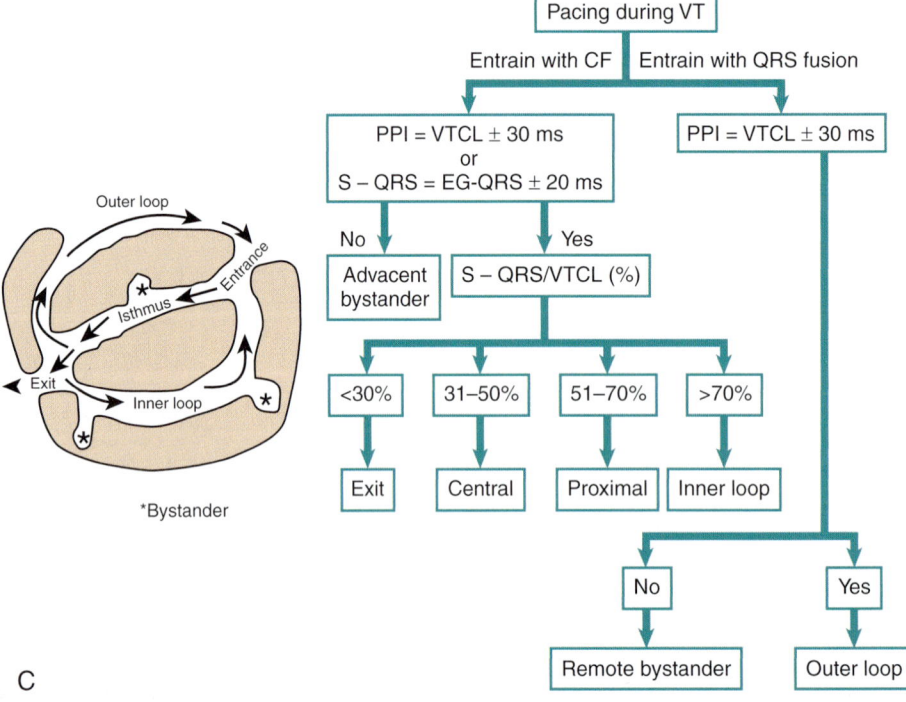

C

FIGURE 28-6, cont'd. **B,** Algorithm for ablation of scar-related VT. **C,** Algorithm to determine catheter position relative to a reentry circuit. CF, concealed fusion; EG, electrogram; LBBB, left bundle branch block; LV, left ventricle; PES, programmed electrical stimulation; PPI, post-pacing interval; RBB, right bundle branch; RV, right ventricle; S, stimulus; TCL, tachycardia cycle length; VTCL; ventricular tachycardia cycle length. (**A,** *From Stevenson WG. Catheter ablation of ventricular tachycardia. In Zipes DP, Jalife J [eds]: Cardiac Electrophysiology: From Cell to Bedside, 3rd ed. Philadelphia: Saunders; 2004:1091.*)

TARGETS FOR ABLATION

Entrainment mapping strategy: ideal target sites are within the infarct zone (bipolar voltage <0.5 mV) and during VT have components inscribed early in diastole (<70% of the VT cycle length before the onset of the QRS)

Entrainment pacing from these target sites results in the following:
- Concealed entrainment on pace mapping
- PPI = VT cycle length ± 30 msec
- Stimulus-QRS interval during pacing = electrogram – QRS during VT ± 20 msec

Substrate mapping strategy: "anchor points" for linear lesions are determined by pace mapping to match VT morphologies in the infarct border zone. Linear ablation is applied through these anchor points from the dense scar (<0.5 mV) to normal tissue (>1.5 mV) or anatomic barrier. Also target in sinus rhythm:
- Slow conduction areas
- Stimulus-QRS interval > 40-70 msec
- Sites showing QRS morphology 10/12 with pace map
- Isolated diastolic potentials
- Late potentials
- Channels between or within dense scar

Mapping triggers for PMVT: pace mapping at sites to match the surface ECG morphology of trigger beats. Sites typically display early Purkinje activation, both in sinus rhythm and during trigger PVCs.

ECG, electrocardiogram; PPI, postpacing interval; PMVT, polymorphic ventricular tachycardia; PVC, premature ventricular contraction; VT, ventricular tachycardia.

LOCALIZATION OF VENTRICULAR TACHYCARDIA BASED ON 12-LEAD ELECTROCARDIOGRAM

ECG Feature	Localization
Bundle Branch Morphology	
Right	Parietal LV
Left	Septum of right ventricle
Frontal Plane Axis	
Superior	LV inferior wall or inferior septum
Inferior	LV anterior wall or anterior septum
Right	LV lateral wall or apex
Precordial Transition (R > S)	
Early	Basal LV
Late	Apical LV
Concordant upright	Mitral valve annulus
QRS Upstroke	
Slurred	Epicardial

LV, left ventricle.

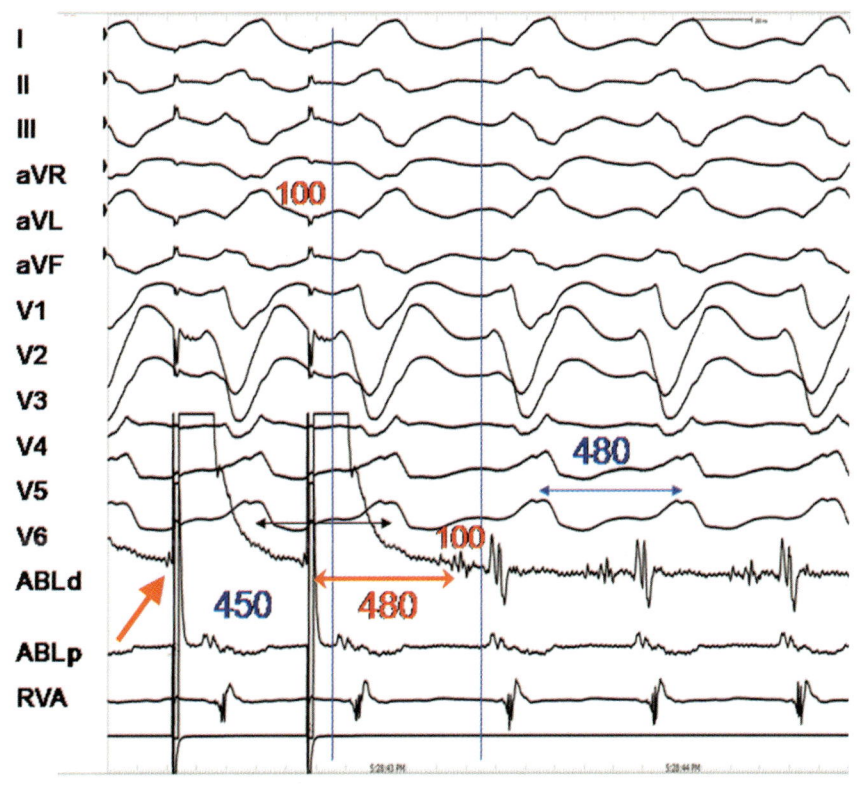

FIGURE 28-7. Characteristics of the "perfect map" for ablation of ventricular tachycardia (VT). The optimal single ablation site for VT has the following characteristics: (1) entrainment from the site will produce an exact match of the spontaneous VT QRS in all 12 leads; (2) the return cycle (the duration from the pacing stimulus to the first nonpaced beat, measured at the pacing site) will equal the VT cycle length, both 480 msec in this example; and (3) the stimulus to QRS will equal the electrogram to QRS both equal to 100 msec. With multicomponent fractionated signals, it can be difficult to know with certainty which component has been locally captured by pacing, and hence where to measure the return cycle length. In this case, the *arrowhead* shows the component of the fractionated electrogram, which is not captured orthodromically, and hence the *horizontal red calipers* measure the return cycle to the second component. ABLd, distal ablation catheter; ABLp, proximal ablation catheter; RVA, right ventricular apex.

of anodal capture at high output.[43] If the site is within the VT circuit and within a relatively protected zone of slow conduction, the following characteristics should be observed (Fig. 28-7). First, the surface 12-lead ECG during entrainment pacing from this site should be an exact match with that recorded during spontaneous VT. This is referred to as *entrainment with concealed fusion*, or *concealed entrainment*.[34] As discussed previously, entrainment pacing from outside the protected isthmus produces a fusion QRS. If the pacing site is within a protected zone within the circuit, both the pacing site and the activation of the circuit from the pacing site are equivalently activating the heart through the VT exit site, so that no ECG fusion is observed. After pacing is stopped, the electrogram at the pacing site should again be activated one VT cycle length after the last pacing stimulus. This follows from the idea that if this site is within the circuit, after the last pacing stimulus, the stimulated wavefront will traverse the VT circuit to again reach this site. A return cycle or postpacing interval (PPI) longer than the tachycardia cycle length indicates pacing from a bystander site. The formal way of expressing this concept is that the PPI at the pacing site should equal the VT cycle length ± 30 milliseconds, if the pacing site is within the circuit. The PPI may be difficult to measure because of artifact on the ablation channel from pacing. This problem may be overcome by pacing measuring the PPI from the proximal ablation electrodes after pacing from the distal electrode. This technique is well correlated with the true PPI but usually introduces some error. The PPI can also be estimated as well by comparing the interval of the two cycles after pacing to twice the tachycardia cycle length or by the "N + 1" method reported by Soejima and associates.[47] Finally, the relationships of orthodromically captured electrogram components should keep identical relationships during pacing and spontaneous VT. In other words, the S (stimulus)-QRS interval during pacing should equal the electrogram-QRS interval during VT ± 20 milliseconds. When expressed as a percentage of the VT cycle length, the S-QRS interval also localizes the pacing site within the reentrant circuit. Sites with an S-QRS interval of less than 30% of the tachycardia cycle length are considered near the circuit exit site, whereas those greater than 70% are within an inner loop.

Stevenson and coworkers provided the first "field testing" of these concepts in a unique study using VT termination during RF ablation to assess the importance of the characteristics described previously.[35] RF lesions were more likely to terminate VT at sites that demonstrated concealed entrainment, a PPI approximating the VT cycle length, and an S-QRS interval greater than 60 milliseconds but less than 70% of the VT cycle length. Concealed entrainment alone was not sufficient to guide ablation as 25% of sites where concealed entrainment was demonstrated were found to be bystander sites by analysis of the PPI and the S-QRS interval to the electrogram-QRS relationship. Sites with isolated diastolic potentials or continuous electrical activity were also demonstrated to be successful ablation targets; this observation has been expanded in subsequent work by other investigators.[48,49] Ablation at sites that demonstrated combinations of these favorable characteristics (entrainment with concealed fusion, PPI, S-QRS interval, and isolated diastolic potentials or concealed entrainment) resulted in VT termination in 35% of applications, compared with 4% when these characteristics were absent. VT termination did not consistently correlate with elimination of that morphology in this study; this potential dichotomy is discussed later. Subsequent work addressed the question of why these favorable characteristics were not absolutely predictive of successful VT ablation sites. Theoretically, three possibilities exist why ablation at these "ideal" sites would not result in VT termination: (1) the lesion is not effective (considered in detail later), (2) the protected isthmus is broader than the volume of a single lesion, or (3) mapping was insufficiently detailed. In a study by Bogun and coworkers,[38] the predictive value of a combination of these favorable characteristics for VT termination increased to 70% to 90%; the most favorable of these characteristics was an isolated mid-diastolic potential that could not be dissociated from the tachycardia with pacing techniques (Table 28-5). El-Shalakany and associates demonstrated uniform success of ablation at a single site if all of the following were fulfilled:

TABLE 28-5

SENSITIVITY AND SPECIFICITY OF INTRACARDIAC MAPPING CRITERIA FOR VENTRICULAR TACHYCARDIA ABLATION

Mapping Criterion	Sensitivity (%)	Specificity (%)	Positive-Predictive Value (%)	Negative-Predictive Value (%)
Concealed entrainment	—	—	54	—
IMDP				
• Overall	40	76	67	53
• Not dissociable from VT	32	95	89	54
PPI = VT CL	58	19	45	29
S-QRS/VT CL <0.7	96	52	71	92
S-QRS = EGM QRS				
Excluding IMDP	32	86	73	51
Including IMDP	56	86	82	62

CL, cycle length; EGM, electrogram; IMDP, isolated mid-diastolic potential; PPI, postpacing interval; VT, ventricular tachycardia.
From Bogun F, Bahu M, Knight BP, et al. Comparison of effective and ineffective target sites that demonstrate concealed entrainment in patients with coronary artery disease undergoing radiofrequency ablation of ventricular tachycardia. *Circulation.* 1997;95:183-190.

(1) an exact QRS match in all 12 leads during entrainment, (2) PPI less than 10 milliseconds different from the VT cycle length, and (3) S-QRS interval within 10 milliseconds different from the electrogram-QRS interval and less than 70% of the VT cycle length.[50] These studies strengthen the conceptual model and emphasize that successful VT ablation can be performed with ablation at a very limited number of sites using this strategy.

To apply entrainment mapping techniques, VT must be reproducibly inducible, hemodynamically well tolerated to allow prolonged mapping during VT, and stable (i.e., not accelerating or changing to different VT morphologies) during entrainment. This applies to a minority of patients with VT, estimated at about 10%[22]; however, this population is reasonably well represented in the population of patients with large infarcts and frequent VT recurrences. Strategies to improve hemodynamic tolerance during VT to facilitate mapping include use of antiarrhythmic drugs to slow the VT rate (intravenous procainamide during, or oral amiodarone before, the procedure), triggered atrial pacing during VT to provide AV synchrony, or circulatory support with inotropes or intra-aortic balloon counterpulsation, or both.

Substrate Mapping

The prerequisite conditions for entrainment mapping are often not met in contemporary patients referred for catheter ablation. In a consecutive series of patients referred for ablation for clinically tolerated VT, up to 25% of patients could not be treated successfully with entrainment mapping techniques,[51] and recent multicenter trials[52,53] have confirmed that only one third of patients have exclusively mappable VTs. The primary reason for procedural failure in these patients is the inability to induce sustained, tolerated VT to allow detailed entrainment mapping.

The development of a new procedural strategy for ablation of unmappable VT was based on experience from surgical ablation of VT. Surgical ablation established the obligate relationship of the VT circuit and the infarct anatomy. Subendocardial resection prevented recurrent VT in more than 90% of patients who survived surgery.[54] Importantly, extension of the surgical lesion outside of the visible infarct to anatomic barriers, such as the mitral annulus, further improved results.[44]

In attempting to recapitulate the surgical experience with catheter mapping, there were two immediate problems. First, although the surgeon could visualize the infarct anatomy by direct vision, imaging techniques to represent the infarct would be necessary during catheter mapping. Cassidy and coworkers[55] validated the concept of using bipolar electrogram characteristics (voltage, duration) to determine the underlying substrate at individual LV sites. We hypothesized that electroanatomic mapping could display the spatial orientation of the voltage information from many endocardial sites, allowing accurate representation of the infarct anatomy (Fig. 28-8). This concept has been validated by statistical analysis of normal bipolar electrograms (similar to the logic of the Cassidy analysis), by comparison with radiologic imaging and in a porcine model of anterior infarction.[56,57] In the animal model, infarct size and topography by voltage mapping correlated well with the area of regional wall motion abnormality (as assessed with intracardiac echocardiography) when using a bipolar peak-to-peak amplitude cutoff of 2 mV or less, and with pathologic measurements at a cutoff of 1 mV or less. In clinical cases, 95% of endocardial recordings from patients with normal, nonhypertrophied left ventricles had a bipolar voltage of more than 1.55 mV. Confluent sites with bipolar electrogram amplitude of 0.5 mV or less represent dense scar, and areas with voltages between 0.5 and 1.5 mV represent the infarct border zone. It is important to appreciate that the zone of dense scar frequently contains surviving myocyte bundles that can form critical isthmuses for VT circuits, and so is not entirely dead in any sense. In patients with prior myocardial infarction, the area of low bipolar voltage tends to be very discrete, with sharp demarcation from the normal, noninfarcted ventricle. Although systematic human pathologic studies are lacking, isolated autopsy studies[58,59] suggest that bipolar voltages of less than 1.5 mV do correspond to scarred myocardium. There is, however, an increasing body of radiologic data that also validates these voltage definitions in humans. Bello and coworkers[60] correlated scar imaging with both contrast-enhanced computed tomography (CT) and PET, with the zone of bipolar voltage 1 mV or less. Fahmy and associates[61] extended this approach by image-integration of fused PET and CT images with bipolar voltage maps. They were able to closely correlate this combined metabolic-anatomic scar definition with the bipolar isopotential area of 0.9 mV or less. However, the highest-resolution imaging of three-dimensional scar geometry is currently obtained by examining the zone of delayed gadolinium enhancement (DGE) on MRI. Recently, Codreanu and colleagues[62] have shown that the zone of bipolar voltage of less than 1.54 mV showed the optimal receiver operating characteristic curve

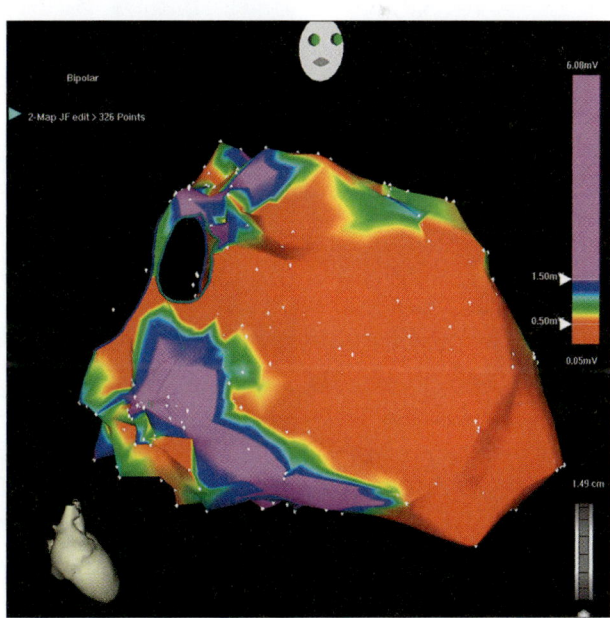

FIGURE 28-8. Electroanatomic voltage mapping. The left ventricular endocardium is mapped in sinus rhythm to define the anatomy of the infarct scar. The color scheme is arranged so that confluent areas of *red* correspond to the dense infarct (bipolar voltage <0.5 mV), *purple* corresponds to normal tissue (bipolar voltage >1.5 mV), and the border zone in the "rainbow" of colors is in between.

for DGE-defined infarction. The ability to integrate these images into a real-time electroanatomic map has the potential to streamline the substrate mapping and ablation process, but currently this approach is limited by the difficulties posed by the widespread prevalence of ICDs in this patient population.

The characteristics of the critical isthmus as defined by electroanatomic mapping during VT have been explored in detail by de Chillou and colleagues.[63] In patients with prior myocardial infarction and VT, the average isthmus length was 31 ± 7 mm, and width was 16 ± 8 mm. During VT, the isthmus encompasses only diastolic potentials, and conduction time through the isthmus accounts for 57% to 81% of the VT cycle length. Excluding perimitral circuits, the isthmus is usually oriented perpendicular to the mitral annulus in the septal, anteroapical, and inferolateral locations. In this study, double potentials indicating lines of block accounted for at least one boundary of the isthmus in 94% of VTs. Most VTs showed a double loop reentry pattern.

Second, subendocardial resection removed 5 to 8 cm² of infarct substrate; the amount of substrate modification with current catheter ablation technology is orders of magnitude or less. We hypothesized that linear lesions, delivered from the area of dense scar through the border zone and connecting out to anatomic barriers or normal myocardium, would represent the closest approximation that could be accomplished in the electrophysiologic laboratory. Linear lesions are constructed by individual RF point lesions and are directed to the area of the VT circuit by identifying the presumed exit site of the VT circuit by pace-mapping to match the 12-lead ECG morphology of the targeted VT. Single-point ablation guided by analysis of individual electrograms during sinus rhythm or pace-mapping has proved insufficient to guide VT ablation; ablation of regions of the border zone using multiple contiguous lesions mapped can successfully interrupt individual VT circuits. Again, unlike surgical ablation, which can remove the substrate for all possible VT circuits, the linear ablation technique is focused on individual VT morphologies. The steps used in a linear ablation procedure are detailed in Figure 28-9.

More recent developments in substrate mapping and ablation have focused on the precise targets within scar that

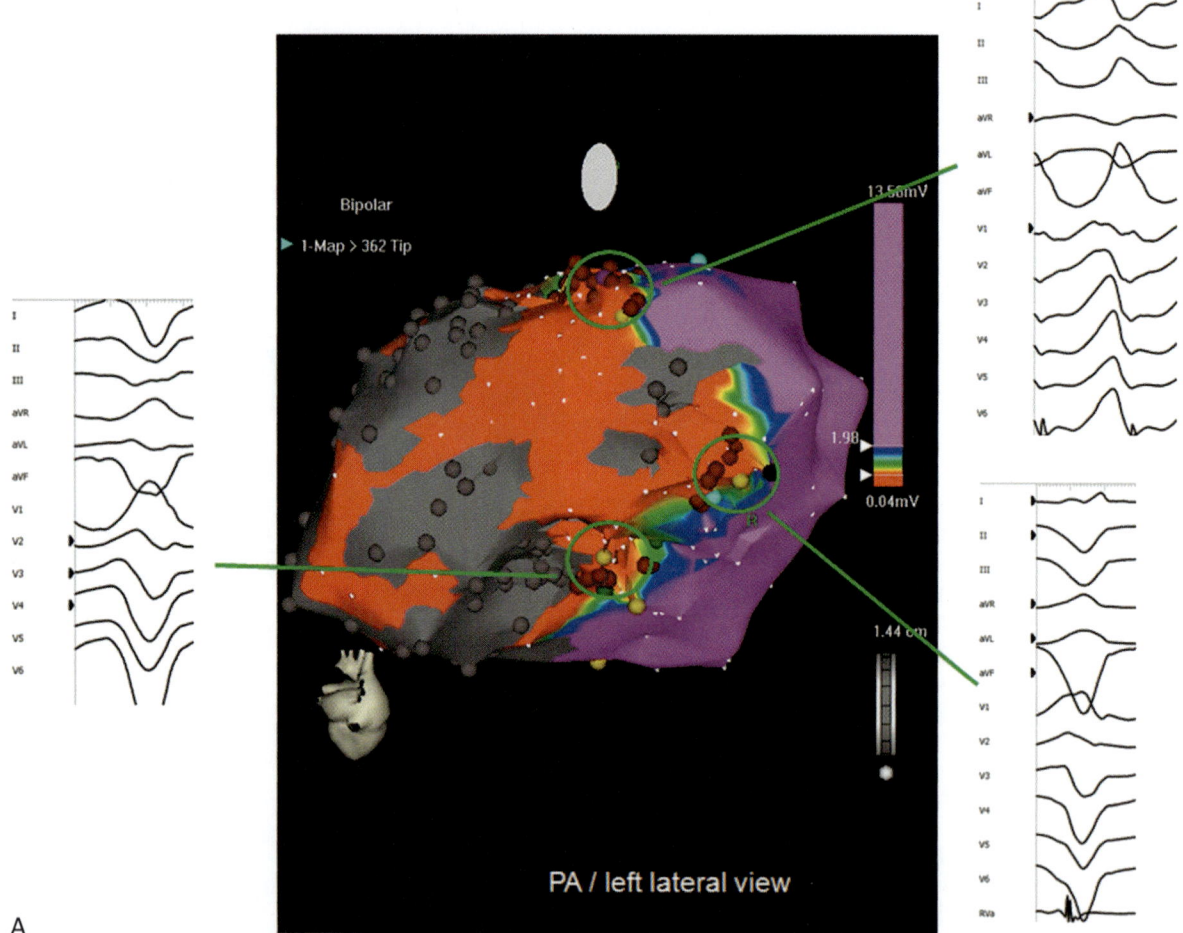

A

FIGURE 28-9. Linear lesions for ventricular tachycardia (VT) ablation. Two electroanatomic mapping projections (**A** and **B**) are shown to detail the sites of best pace-map match for four clinical VTs, right bundle branch block right superior axis (RBRS), and right bundle branch block left superior axis (RBLS) morphologies. The exit site of each VT morphology is approximated by pace mapping in the infarct border zone. Using the site of closest pace-map match as an "anchor," a linear lesion is fashioned as a radial line from the dense infarct out to normal tissue or an anatomic obstacle such as the mitral annulus.

Continued

can be used to guide linear lesion placement. Essentially, this means trying to define the critical components of the scar zone that can form conducting channels and support reentry. In this regard, pace-mapping has been especially useful for several reasons. First, as described previously, a good pace map from the scar border zone can give a reasonable approximation to the exit site of a particular VT. This, however, is not necessarily specific because good pace maps can be recorded from a more than 3.5-cm distance along the scar border,[64] and hence long linear lesions parallel to the scar border would seem necessary to ensure successful exit site ablation. Second, high-output pacing[65,66] can define areas of dense electrically unexcitable scar, and such regions act as conduction barriers to constrain diastolic isthmuses and channels within the infarct zone. Linear ablation to join these areas to each other or to other barriers is associated with good outcomes. Third, pace-mapping deep within scar can also identify slowly conducting channels by the long stimulus to QRS times (>40 milliseconds),[46] particularly when associated with a good pace map of a targeted VT .

Voltage mapping can also define channels by adjustment of the voltage representation on color isopotential maps.[67,68] Corridors of signals with more preserved voltages within the dense scar zone can be appreciated with this approach,

and these potential conducting channels may form diastolic isthmuses during VT and may appear evident during VT mapping using unipolar, noncontact mapping systems (Fig. 28-10).

Substrate mapping also relies heavily on other electrogram characteristics apart from voltage. Although fractionated electrograms are indicative of slow conduction and transverse cell-cell uncoupling resulting from interdigitation fibrosis, such signals are recorded throughout the scar and are not specific for VT circuit components. On the other hand, isolated and late potentials are likely to be more specific markers of small putative conducting channels that may form critical VT circuit components. Surviving fiber bundles at these sites are activated late in sinus rhythm by slowly percolating wavefronts propagating through dense scar. As such, the local isolated potential may be recorded well after the often higher-amplitude far-field potential, and usually well after the surface QRS or even the T wave (where they have been arbitrarily designated as very late potentials). Bogun and coworkers[69] showed that confirmed VT isthmuses almost always contained such potentials, whereas Miller and colleagues[70] demonstrated their disappearance after clinically successful surgical subendocardial resection. Recent data[71] have shown that the scars of myocardial infarction patients with no clinical arrhythmias are

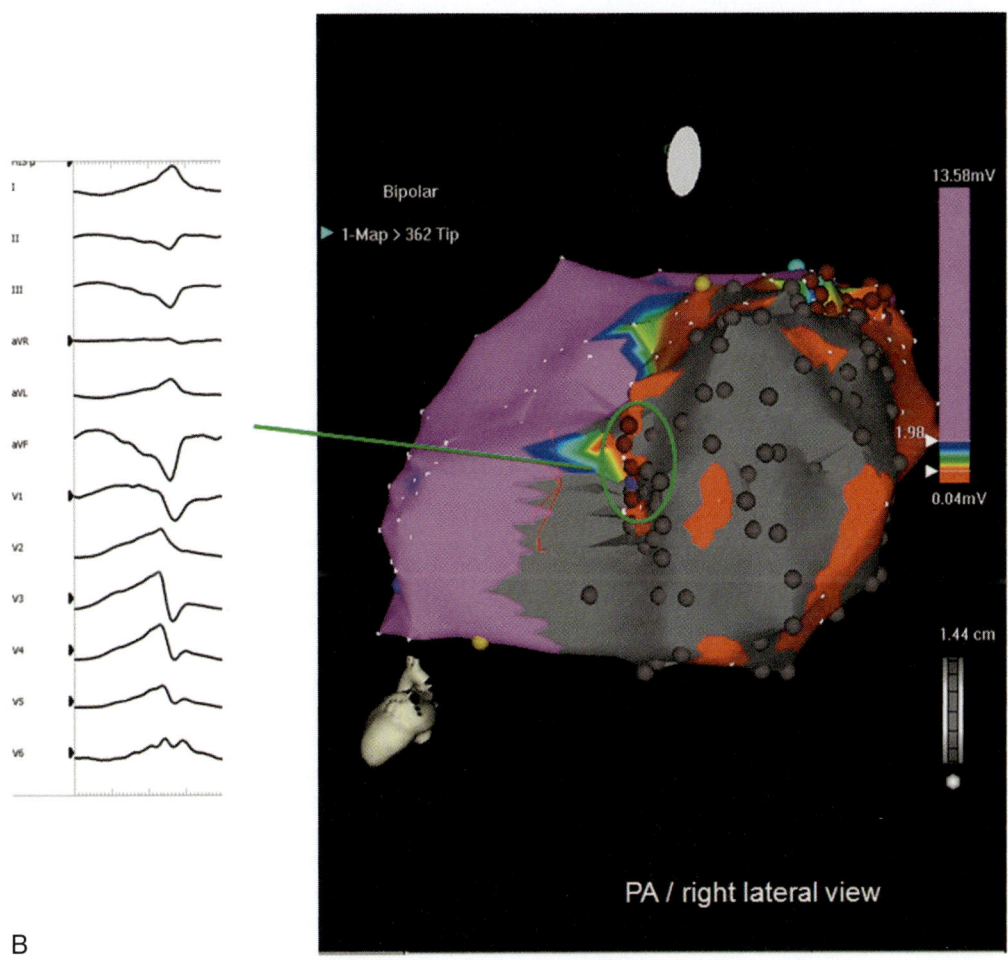

B

FIGURE 28-9, cont'd

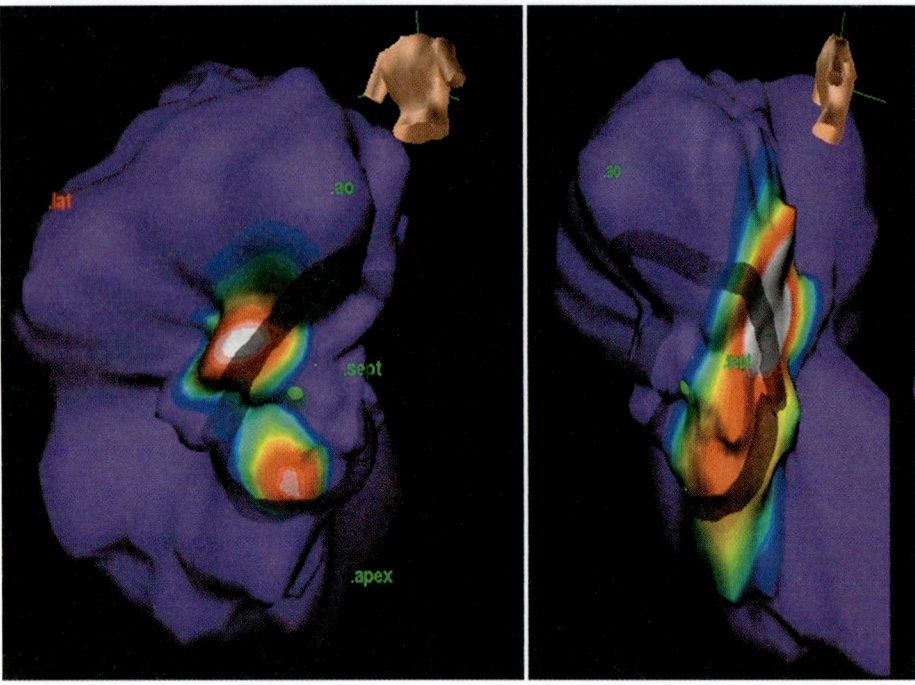

VT circuit entrance   VT circuit exit

FIGURE 28-10. Noncontact mapping to demonstrate "channels" in the ventricular tachycardia (VT) circuit. A cast of the left ventricle is shown with a color scheme denoting isopotential mapping. Resting tissue is shown in *purple*; as sites are activated and generate negative unipolar voltage, colors from *blue* to *white* (depending on voltage) are displayed. Two segments of an isopotential map recorded during VT in a patient with a small basal inferior infarction (outlined by the *thick black line*). Conduction seems to enter (*left panel*) and exit (*right panel*) the infarct zone in specific zones. The exit from the infarct always occurs at the onset of the surface QRS; often there is considerable delay, perhaps owing to impedance mismatch between the small mass of myocardium in the infarct and the healthy tissue outside.

not only smaller than matched patients with spontaneous VT but also have a much lower prevalence of isolated and very late potential per unit scar area. Because of the potentially critical role that such signals may play in multiple VT circuits, some centers[72] have commenced performing a substrate modification procedure that targets all isolated and late potentials. The limitations of this approach relate to the likely bystander cul-de-sac nature of a large proportion of these potentials and to the fact that the critical ones may be obscured by noise or adverse wavefront direction. The long-term outcome from such a strategy is presently unclear.

Mapping of Triggers for Polymorphic Ventricular Tachycardia

Electrophysiologic mapping techniques cannot be applied to nonuniform arrhythmias such as polymorphic VT. Although substrate mapping could potentially be applied, this technique is typically anchored by location of a specific uniform VT morphology. Haïssaguerre and associates[73] demonstrated that premature ventricular beats from relatively predictable anatomic locations may serve as the initiating events in patients with idiopathic ventricular fibrillation. This group extended these original observations in patients with healed infarction.[16] Five patients with myocardial infarction and depressed ejection fraction were observed to have multiple episodes of PMVT initiated by repetitive uniform premature beats (Fig. 28-11). Interestingly, three of the patients had very recently experienced myocardial

infarction, a stage at which automaticity in the surviving Purkinje network surrounding infarcted tissue is thought to play an important role in arrhythmogenesis. Activation and pace-mapping of these inciting beats demonstrated that they consistently arose from Purkinje fibers at the infarct border. Often, Purkinje spikes had varying intervals to the earliest ventricular activation, and the morphology of successive triggering beats changed in turn. Splitting of the Purkinje signal and Purkinje-ventricular block was also observed. Ablation targeting these sites resulted in freedom from recurrent arrhythmias in all patients over a follow-up period of 16 ± 5 months, documented by ICD monitoring in all patients. A similar strategy was employed by Marrouche and colleagues[74] and Bansch and associates,[75] who also targeted Purkinje-like potentials at the border of the scar in the patients with insufficient ectopy to allow activation mapping.

Ablation

Traditionally, VT mapping and ablation have been performed with 4-mm-tip catheters, using standard, temperature-controlled RF ablation. The precision of mapping, particularly as it applies to the electrode field of view during pacing, is better with smaller electrodes. The obvious tradeoff is the reduction in lesion size with smaller electrodes. Although only limited data are available on this issue, it is clear that this effect is even more important in infarcted tissue (Fig. 28-12).[76] As discussed later, this often limits procedural efficacy, and

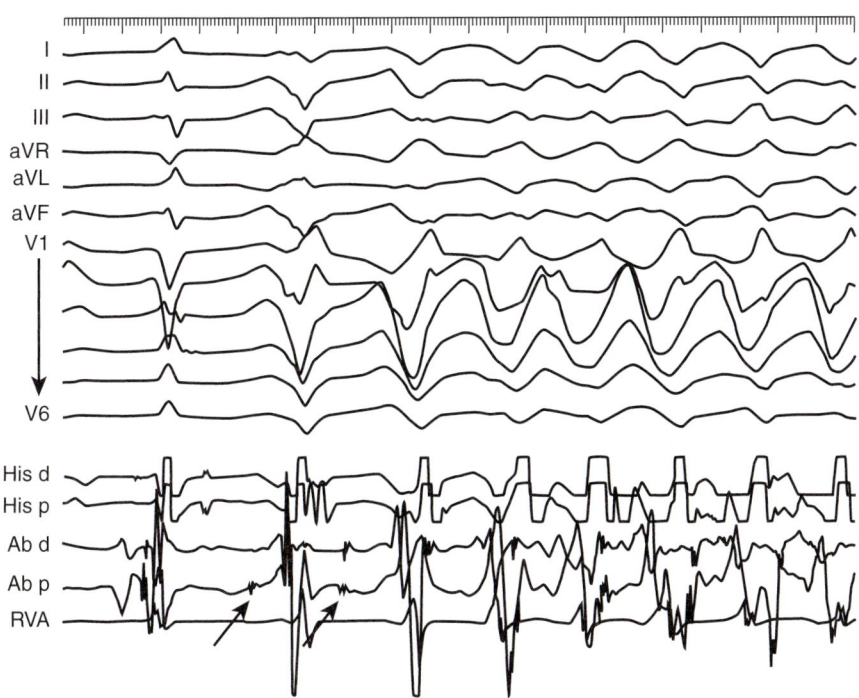

I
II
III
aVR
aVL
aVF
V1
↓
V6

His d
His p
Ab d
Ab p
RVA

FIGURE 28-11. Mapping and ablation of Purkinje triggers of polymorphic ventricular tachycardia (VT). This recording was made in a patient with frequent episodes of polymorphic VT, all preceded by right bundle branch block (RBBB) premature ventricular contractions (PVCs). In the electrophysiology laboratory, a run of RBBB PVCs was observed. Note the Purkinje potentials (*arrows*) recorded on the mapping catheter (labeled Ab d and Ab p), present on PVC beats and during sinus. Both the Purkinje-ventricular interval and the morphology of the PVCs change from beat to beat. Ablation of the Purkinje system trigger resulted in freedom from recurrent polymorphic VT. His, His bundle electrogram; RVA, right ventricular apex.

the use of irrigated ablation has been an important step forward. Typical power and temperature settings with standard 4-mm-tip catheters are similar to those used for other left-sided ablation procedures (50 W, 52°C, 60 seconds). In our laboratory, a temperature cutoff of 52° C is used because we observed an increased incidence of coagulum (without consistent evidence of impedance rise) when higher temperatures were reached. Impedance is also carefully monitored because excessive drop in impedance (>10 to 15 ohms) may also predict impending rise. Irrigated-tip RF ablation systems are typically used as the primary ablation modality as an alternative to standard-tip RF ablation. Compared with standard-tip RF, irrigated-tip or cooled-tip systems may show greater efficacy in VT termination, suggesting larger lesion sizes.[76–82] For irrigated catheters, the temperature limit is typically 40° to 45°C and power up to 50 W. Large-tip (8 mm) catheters are also able to achieve larger lesions but require high-output generators. In addition, the larger electrode reduces the resolution for mapping.

RF energy is usually applied during VT (if the tachycardia is tolerated) to determine whether ablation at an individual site leads to VT termination, verifying the site's importance in VT circuit maintenance. Although this information is critical, ablation during VT does present additional difficulties, including catheter stability at higher heart rates and on sudden VT termination. Termination during ablation is a good sign but is not equivalent to permanent destruction of the VT circuit. The adequacy of lesion formation can also be assessed by monitoring for impedance drop (target, 5 to 10 ohms) during RF delivery and electrogram amplitude reduction and by inability to pace the ablation site at 10 mA of output after ablation. Programmed electrical stimulation must be repeated after apparent acute success, both to determine whether the targeted VT has been eliminated and to assess the presence of additional VT morphologies. Some investigators argue for

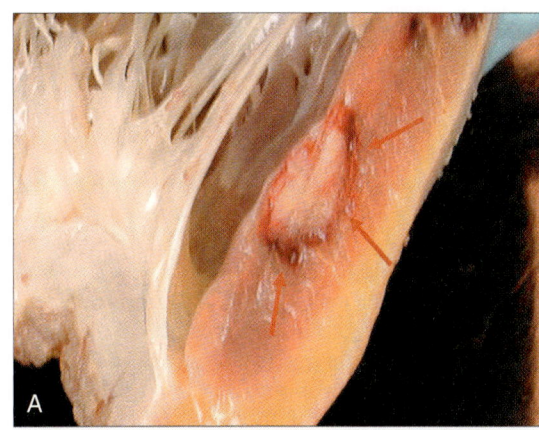

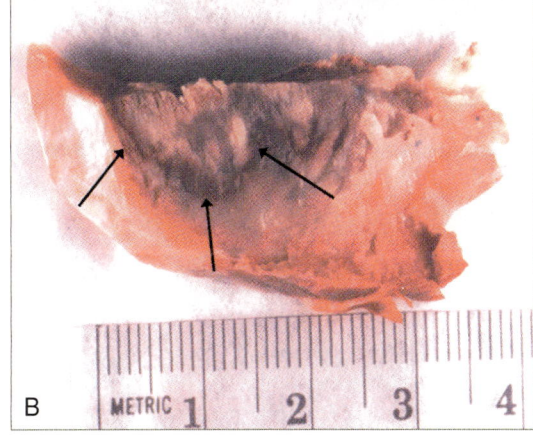

FIGURE 28-12. Effect of irrigated radiofrequency ablation in normal versus infarcted myocardium. **A,** Typical irrigated ablation lesion delivered to normal porcine ventricular myocardium. Lesion is typically 1 cm in diameter and about 7 mm in depth. **B,** Irrigated ablation in infarcted tissue results in smaller lesions. Here, a series of lesions was delivered to create a linear lesion. Individual lesions were 5 to 7 mm in diameter and 4 to 6 mm deep. (**B,** *From Callans DJ, Ren JF, Narula N, et al. Effects of linear, irrigated-tip radiofrequency ablation in porcine healed anterior infarction.* J Cardiovasc Electrophysiol. *2001;12:1037-1042. With permission.*)

late follow-up programmed stimulation to assess efficacy[42] because programmed stimulation during the index procedure may be less reliable because of the effects of lesion recovery and anesthesia. The end points for ablation in substrate mapping may be noninducibility of the relevant VTs or elimination of all suspected channels and abnormal electrograms within the infarct zone. During substrate ablation, lesions are given in a linear fashion perpendicularly across suspected channels. Lesions may also be given parallel to the area of dense scar within the border zone, incorporating sites defined by pace-mapping.

The success of VT ablation as a management strategy is less than completely clear. Most reports on ablation concentrate on technical details of mapping and ablation and are limited by short-term observation of highly selected patients. Nonetheless, the acute success of entrainment mapping and morphology specific ablation is reasonable, ranging from 67% to 96% of VTs in recent published trials.[22,35,38,42,43,50,77,83–85] These trials represent, for the most part, "on treatment" analysis, with "enrollment" only after tolerated VT is reproducibly induced in the laboratory. Limited data suggest that intention-to-treat analysis yields less favorable results.[51] Clinical follow-up in these trials is typically over a 2- to 3-year horizon. Most patients (about 90%) have freedom from targeted VT morphologies that were successfully ablated; however, the risk for developing new clinical VTs is fairly high. Some investigators advocate ablation of all mappable VTs (i.e., rather than just the "clinical" VT) to decrease the incidence of "new" VT morphologies in follow-up.[42,43,77] Even in these series, however, the risk for recurrence is 30% to 46%, despite multiple procedures and continued antiarrhythmic drug therapy in selected patients. The lingering effect of antiarrhythmic drugs, particularly amiodarone, during the ablation procedure is another confounding influence on intermediate-term results. In our experience, after apparently successful VT ablation, the freedom from any VT recurrence in follow-up (mean, 28 months) was higher in patients maintained on the same antiarrhythmic drug regimen compared with patients in whom drugs were discontinued after ablation (64% versus 32%).[86] Another important observation in series of VT ablation is the high all-cause mortality in patients who require VT ablation after myocardial infarction. Data from ablation series range from 12% to 30% mortality at 36 to 40 months, to 51% at 5 years.[43,84,85] Most of these deaths are due to progressive structural heart disease and refractory heart failure, although sudden, presumably arrhythmic death is also observed, arguing for adjunctive ICD therapy.[23]

The initial experience with substrate-based VT ablation was in 16 patients with drug-refractory, unmappable VT (9 patients had healed infarction). Before ablation, patients had experienced 6 to 55 episodes of VT/month, resulting in frequent ICD shocks. Ablation was performed with a 4-mm-tip catheter and standard RF energy (up to 50W; temperature, 52°C; duration, 60 seconds). Delivery of a median of 55 RF lesions to construct four linear lesions (each linear lesion through the exit site of a specific VT morphology) resulted in successful arrhythmia control in all but one patient over 8 months of mean follow-up.[56] Importantly, ventricular function did not change after the procedure, despite extensive ablation in patients with advanced structural heart disease. More extensive follow-up in a larger population including 36 patients with healed infarction demonstrated freedom from arrhythmia recurrence in 64% and infrequent VT recurrence in 25%.[87] Even in the 11% who had frequent VT episodes (defined as >1 VT episode in a 3-month period), there was a considerable reduction in episodes (mean, 30 per month before ablation) and ICD shocks after the procedure. These results were obtained largely with standard RF technology and 4-mm-tip catheters.

More recently, large multicenter series have reported postablation outcomes following combined entrainment and substrate mapping approaches. The Multicentre Thermocool Ventricular Tachycardia Ablation trial reported the outcomes in 231 patients who underwent VT ablation with an open irrigated catheter.[52] This was a representative population of postinfarction VT patients because they had a median ejection fraction of 25% and a median of three VTs induced, with only 31% having only mappable VTs. The targeted VT was ablated successfully in 81% of patients, and in 49%, VTs were rendered noninducible. Although at 6 months, 51% of patients had a recurrent episode, the frequency of episodes was markedly reduced in most. Similar acute procedural and short-term clinical outcomes were reported in the Euro-VT study in 63 postinfarction patients.[53] The randomized controlled Substrate Mapping and Ablation in Sinus Rhythm to Halt Ventricular Tachycardia (SMASH-VT) trial looked at the feasibility of using substrate-based ablation as a prophylactic strategy in 128 patients with ischemic cardiomyopathy who had received secondary prevention ICDs. At a mean follow-up of 23 months, appropriate ICD therapy was significantly lower in the ablation group compared with the control group (12% versus 33%) with a nonsignificant trend to lower all-cause mortality.

Complications

The procedural risk associated with VT ablation is higher than most other electrophysiology procedures. This is due to the inherent risk for extensive ablation in the left circulation, but more importantly to the presence of significant structural heart disease and comorbidities in a sick patient population. Before catheter mapping and ablation, an assessment to exclude active coronary ischemia or LV thrombus is essential. Recognized procedural risks for postinfarction VT ablation include stroke (either from mechanical dislodgment of atheromatous material or thrombus formation secondary to the ablation process), coronary artery embolism or injury, mechanical trauma to the aortic valve, cardiogenic shock, tamponade, heart block, and vascular complications and death. Cardiogenic shock may be a consequence of the requisite prolonged duration of VT episodes required for mapping, or because of "stunning" of healthy myocardium due to ablation of adjacent infarcted myocardium. Recent multicenter trials reported a more realistic incidence of 8% major complications (including death in 2.7%) and 6% minor complications.[77] The incidence of complications varies greatly with operator experience as well as patient comorbidities, particularly peripheral or cerebral vascular disease and active ischemia.

Troubleshooting the Difficult Case

There are several factors that can make a procedure more difficult than initially expected (Table 28-6). First, even in patients with VT that has been well tolerated clinically, there are instances in which only poorly tolerated VT is induced or the patient is noninducible. As discussed previously, substrate mapping during sinus rhythm can be performed if VT is unmappable, but most strategies require at least documentation of the 12-lead ECG morphology to provide some aspect of the VT circuit to target. Other strategies may be used, such as empirical ablation based on the infarct anatomy, the presence of relatively high-voltage conducting channels, or ablation of fractionated potentials within the infarct. Although these strategies may be effective, they cannot be verified in the case of inability to induce VT in the first place.

Second, repeated ablation lesions can fail to produce the desired effect of VT termination or elimination. There are two possibilities in this circumstance. The most likely is inadequate power delivery. This can be recognized in temperature-control mode by achieving target temperature at very low (often several watts) power settings. In this situation, there is also minimal change in the electrogram recorded by the distal ablation electrode after ablation. In my opinion, the temptation to increase the temperature limit should be avoided, owing to the increased risk for thromboemboli. Instead, more power can be safely delivered if irrigated ablation is used. Irrigated RF lesions are routinely larger than standard RF lesions, particularly in infarcted tissue, because more current can be delivered when the limitation of high temperature at the catheter-tissue interface is removed.[76–82] It should be remembered, however, that apparent ineffective ablation can be caused by inaccuracies of mapping and that relying solely on activation mapping data provided by sophisticated three-dimensional mapping systems may leave one particularly susceptible to this error. These systems can easily identify the earliest activation in the chamber mapped. Apparent early activation due to bystander sites needs to be discerned with entrainment

mapping techniques. In addition, VT that comes from a source outside the chamber being evaluated (RV, intramural, epicardial, papillary muscle) can often not be ablated at the site of earliest activation in that chamber. Careful attention to unipolar electrogram morphologies, the diffuse nature of early activation, and the proportion of the tachycardia cycle length mapped to one chamber may be helpful in this regard.

Techniques for percutaneous epicardial ablation, developed by Sosa and coworkers initially for treatment of VT in the setting of Chagas cardiomyopathy,[88] may be helpful in selected patients with healed infarction.[89,90] Initially, this seemed contrary to the conventional wisdom formed largely with the surgical ablation experience that VT circuits were primarily endocardial. Nonetheless, even if most of the circuit is endocardial, it is conceivable that individual vulnerable circuit sites may be epicardial or intramyocardial. Experience with this technique may be helpful in selected patients.

Some of the uncertainties of VT mapping and ablation may be resolved with improved imaging capabilities. Intracardiac echocardiography and magnetic resonance imaging may be helpful in providing more anatomically relevant imaging during VT ablation, allowing real-time visualization of catheter contact, relationship with the infarct scar, and validation of lesion creation. The impact of these adjunctive modalities is presently being assessed.

Conclusion

Ablation of VT in the setting of healed myocardial infarction may have a profound influence on clinical care in patients with frequent recurrence or incessant VT. Such patients typically receive multiple ICD shocks, and often multiple attempts at antiarrhythmic therapy have failed. VT ablation is more technically difficult and subject to a higher risk for complications than many other ablation procedures. Operators should have considerable experience with VT mapping techniques (both entrainment and substrate mapping) before embarking on these procedures, especially in patients with severe structural heart disease.

TABLE 28-6

TROUBLESHOOTING THE DIFFICULT CASE

Problem	Causes	Solution
Unmappable VT		
Poor hemodynamic stability during VT	Ventricular dysfunction	Slow VT rate with drugs, support BP with atrial pacing, pressors, balloon pump, noncontact mapping, substrate mapping, optimize filling pressures
Noninducible	Autonomically or ischemically mediated	Programmed stimulation on dopamine or isoproterenol, substrate mapping during sinus rhythm, linear ablation
Ineffective radiofrequency delivery	Small lesion size	Irrigated radiofrequency ablation or large-tip catheter and high-output generator
	Poor catheter contact	Change catheter reach, stiffness, change approach (transseptal from retrograde aortic)
	Low current delivery	Irrigated radiofrequency ablation
	Wide isthmus	Linear lesion or irrigated catheter
	Wrong site	Continue mapping
	Misdiagnosis	Consider bundle branch or fascicular reentry
Diffuse area of early activation	Intramural or epicardial site of origin	Transcutaneous pericardial approach for epicardial mapping, map right ventricular septum, papillary muscle

The results of VT ablation in terms of elimination of targeted VT morphologies are fairly favorable; however, the disease process following index infarction is progressive, and new VT circuits can develop over time. VT ablation is palliative at present because of this consideration; optimally, ICD therapy is concurrently employed to attempt to prevent the residual risk for sudden cardiac death. Ongoing research should address this limitation, specifically whether new technology and understanding will allow development of true substrate modification to prevent both present and future VT circuits.

References

1. Strickberger SA, Man KC, Daoud EG, et al. A prospective evaluation of catheter ablation of ventricular tachycardia as adjuvant therapy in patients with coronary artery disease and an implantable cardioverter-defibrillator. *Circulation.* 1997;96:1525–1531.
2. Calkins H, Bigger JTJ, Ackerman SJ, et al. Cost-effectiveness of catheter ablation in patients with ventricular tachycardia. *Circulation.* 2000;101: 280–288.
3. Sarter BH, Finkle JK, Gerszten RE, et al. What is the risk of sudden cardiac death in patients presenting with hemodynamically stable sustained ventricular tachycardia after myocardial infarction? *J Am Coll Cardiol.* 1996;28: 122–129.
4. Caruso AC, Marcus FI, Hahn EA, et al. Predictors of arrhythmic death and cardiac arrest in the ESVEM trial. Electrophysiologic Study Versus Electromagnetic Monitoring. *Circulation.* 1997;96:1888–1892.
5. Connolly SJ, Dorian P, Roberts RS, et al. Comparison of beta-blockers, amiodarone plus beta-blockers, or sotalol for prevention of shocks from implantable cardioverter defibrillators. The OPTIC Study: a randomized trial. *JAMA.* 2006;295:165–171.
6. Josephson ME. *Clinical Cardiac Electrophysiology: Techniques and Interpretations.* Philadelphia: Lippincott Williams & Wilkins; 2008.
7. de Bakker JMT, Janse MJ. Pathophysiological correlates of ventricular tachycardia in hearts with a healed infarct. In: Zipes DP, Jalife J, eds. *Cardiac Electrophysiology: From Cell to Bedside.* Philadelphia: Saunders; 2000: 415–421.
8. Peters NS, Coromilas J, Severs NJ, et al. Disturbed connexin43 gap junction distribution correlates with the location of reentrant circuits in the epicardial border zone of healing canine infarcts that cause ventricular tachycardia. *Circulation.* 1997;95:988–996.
9. de Bakker JM, van Capelle FJ, Janse MJ, et al. Reentry as a cause of ventricular tachycardia in patients with chronic ischemic heart disease: electrophysiologic and anatomic correlation. *Circulation.* 1988;77:589–606.
10. de Bakker JM, van Capelle FJ, Janse MJ, et al. Slow conduction in the infarcted human heart: "zigzag" course of activation. *Circulation.* 1993;88:915–926.
11. Buxton AE, Lee KL, DiCarlo L, et al. Electrophysiologic testing to identify patients with coronary artery disease who are at risk for sudden death. Multicenter Unsustained Tachycardia Trial Investigators. *N Engl J Med.* 2000;342: 1937–1945.
12. Echt DS, Liebson PR, Mitchell LB, et al. Mortality and morbidity in patients receiving encainide, flecainide, or placebo. The Cardiac Arrhythmia Suppression Trial. *N Engl J Med.* 1991;324:781–788.
13. Gomes JA, Mehta D, Ip J, et al. Predictors of long-term survival in patients with malignant ventricular arrhythmias. *Am J Cardiol.* 1997;79:1054–1060.
14. Exner DV, Pinski SL, Wyse DG, et al. Electrical storm presages nonsudden death: the antiarrhythmics versus implantable defibrillators (AVID) trial. *Circulation.* 2001;103:2066–2071.
15. Wyse DG, Friedman PL, Brodsky MA, et al. Life-threatening ventricular arrhythmias due to transient or correctable causes: high risk for death in follow-up. *J Am Coll Cardiol.* 2001;38:1718–1724.
16. Szumowski L, Sanders P, Walczak F, et al. Mapping and ablation of polymorphic ventricular tachycardia after myocardial infarction. *J Am Coll Cardiol.* 2004;44:1700–1706.
17. Wellens HJ, Bar FW, Lie KI. The value of the electrocardiogram in the differential diagnosis of a tachycardia with a widened QRS complex. *Am J Med.* 1978;64:27–33.
18. Kindwall KE, Brown J, Josephson ME. Electrocardiographic criteria for ventricular tachycardia in wide complex left bundle branch block morphology tachycardias. *Am J Cardiol.* 1988;61:1279–1283.
19. Antunes E, Brugada J, Steurer G, et al. The differential diagnosis of a regular tachycardia with a wide QRS complex on the 12-lead ECG: ventricular tachycardia, supraventricular tachycardia with aberrant intraventricular conduction, and supraventricular tachycardia with anterograde conduction over an accessory pathway. *Pacing Clin Electrophysiol.* 1994;17:1515–1524.
20. Callans DJ, Hook BG, Marchlinski FE. Use of bipolar recordings from patch-patch and rate sensing leads to distinguish ventricular tachycardia from supraventricular rhythms in patients with implantable cardioverter defibrillators. *Pacing Clin Electrophysiol.* 1991;14:1917–1922.
21. Sarter BH, Hook BG, Callans DJ, et al. Effect of bundle branch block on local electrogram morphologic features: implications for arrhythmia diagnosis by stored electrogram analysis. *Am Heart J.* 1996;131:947–952.
22. Morady F, Harvey M, Kalbfleisch SJ, et al. Radiofrequency catheter ablation of ventricular tachycardia in patients with coronary artery disease. *Circulation.* 1993;87:363–372.
23. Callans DJ. Patients with hemodynamically tolerated ventricular tachycardia require implantable cardioverter defibrillators. *Circulation.* 2007;116: 1196–1203.
24. Wathen MS, Sweeney MO, DeGroot PJ, et al. Shock reduction using antitachycardia pacing for spontaneous rapid ventricular tachycardia in patients with coronary artery disease. *Circulation.* 2001;104:796–801.
25. Pacifico A, Hohnloser SH, Williams JH, et al. Prevention of implantable-defibrillator shocks by treatment with sotalol. d,l-Sotalol Implantable Cardioverter-Defibrillator Study Group. *N Engl J Med.* 1999;340:1855–1862.
26. Dorian P, Borggrefe M, Al-Khalidi HR, et al. Placebo-controlled, randomized clinical trial of azimilide for prevention of ventricular tachyarrhythmias in patients with an implantable cardioverter defibrillator. *Circulation.* 2004;110:3646–3654.
27. Fitzgerald DM. Two for the price of one: identifying shared circuits in postinfarction reentrant ventricular tachycardia. *J Cardiovasc Electrophysiol.* 2002;13:242–243.
28. Okumura K, Henthorn RW, Epstein AE, et al. Further observations on transient entrainment: importance of pacing site and properties of the components of the reentry circuit. *Circulation.* 1985;72:1293–1307.
29. Okumura K, Olshansky B, Henthorn RW, et al. Demonstration of the presence of slow conduction during sustained ventricular tachycardia in man: use of transient entrainment of the tachycardia. *Circulation.* 1987;75:369–378.
30. Henthorn RW, Okumura K, Olshansky B, et al. A fourth criterion for transient entrainment: the electrogram equivalent of progressive fusion. *Circulation.* 1988;77:1003–1012.
31. Callans DJ, Hook BG, Josephson ME. Comparison of resetting and entrainment of uniform sustained ventricular tachycardia: further insights into the characteristics of the excitable gap. *Circulation.* 1993;87:1229–1238.
32. Almendral JM, Gottlieb CD, Rosenthal ME, et al. Entrainment of ventricular tachycardia: explanation for surface electrocardiographic phenomena by analysis of electrograms recorded within the tachycardia circuit. *Circulation.* 1988;77:569–580.
33. Fontaine G, Frank R, Tonet J, et al. Identification of a zone of slow conduction appropriate for VT ablation: theoretical and practical considerations. *Pacing Clin Electrophysiol.* 1989;12:262–267.
34. Morady F, Kadish A, Rosenheck S, et al. Concealed entrainment as a guide for catheter ablation of ventricular tachycardia in patients with prior myocardial infarction. *J Am Coll Cardiol.* 1991;17:678–689.
35. Stevenson WG, Khan H, Sager P, et al. Identification of reentry circuit sites during catheter mapping and radiofrequency ablation of ventricular tachycardia late after myocardial infarction. *Circulation.* 1993;88:1647–1670.
36. Stevenson WG, Friedman PL, Sager PT, et al. Exploring postinfarction reentrant ventricular tachycardia with entrainment mapping. *J Am Coll Cardiol.* 1997;29:1180–1189.
37. Stevenson WG, Weiss JN, Wiener I, et al. Fractionated endocardial electrograms are associated with slow conduction in humans: evidence from pace-mapping. *J Am Coll Cardiol.* 1989;13:369–376.
38. Bogun F, Bahu M, Knight BP, et al. Comparison of effective and ineffective target sites that demonstrate concealed entrainment in patients with coronary artery disease undergoing radiofrequency ablation of ventricular tachycardia. *Circulation.* 1997;95:183–190.
39. Miller JM, Marchlinski FE, Buxton AE, et al. Relationship between the 12-lead electrocardiogram during ventricular tachycardia and endocardial site of origin in patients with coronary artery disease. *Circulation.* 1988;77:759–766.
40. Josephson ME, Callans DJ. Using the twelve-lead electrocardiogram to localize the site of origin of ventricular tachycardia. *Heart Rhythm.* 2005;2:443–446.
41. Patel VV, Rho RW, Gerstenfeld EP, et al. Right bundle-branch block ventricular tachycardias: septal versus lateral ventricular origin based on activation time to the right ventricular apex. *Circulation.* 2004;110:2582–2587.
42. Rothman SA, Hsia HH, Cossu SF, et al. Radiofrequency catheter ablation of postinfarction ventricular tachycardia: long-term success and the significance of inducible nonclinical arrhythmias. *Circulation.* 1997;96:3499–3508.
43. Stevenson WG, Friedman PL, Kocovic D, et al. Radiofrequency catheter ablation of ventricular tachycardia after myocardial infarction. *Circulation.* 1998;98:308–314.
44. Hargrove WC, Miller JM, Vassallo JA, et al. Improved results in the operative management of ventricular tachycardia related to inferior wall infarction: importance of the annular isthmus. *J Thorac Cardiovasc Surg.* 1986;92:726–732.
45. Wilber DJ, Kopp DE, Glascock DN, et al. Catheter ablation of the mitral isthmus for ventricular tachycardia associated with inferior infarction. *Circulation.* 1995;92:3481–3489.
46. Brunckhorst CB, Stevenson WG, Soejima K, et al. Relationship of slow conduction detected by pace-mapping to ventricular tachycardia re-entry circuit sites after infarction. *J Am Coll Cardiol.* 2003;41:802–809.
47. Soejima K, Stevenson WG, Maisel WH, et al. The N + 1 difference: a new measure for entrainment mapping. *J Am Coll Cardiol.* 2001;37:1386–1394.
48. Bogun F, Bahu M, Knight BP, et al. Response to pacing at sites of isolated diastolic potentials during ventricular tachycardia in patients with previous myocardial infarction. *J Am Coll Cardiol.* 1997;30:505–513.

49. Bogun F, Hohnloser SH, Bender B, et al. Mechanism of ventricular tachycardia termination by pacing at left ventricular sites in patients with coronary artery disease. *J Interv Card Electrophysiol.* 2002;6:35–41.

50. El-Shalakany A, Hadjis T, Papageorgiou P, et al. Entrainment/mapping criteria for the prediction of termination of ventricular tachycardia by single radiofrequency lesion in patients with coronary artery disease. *Circulation.* 1999;99:2283–2289.

51. Callans DJ, Zado E, Sarter BH, et al. Efficacy of radiofrequency catheter ablation for ventricular tachycardia in healed myocardial infarction. *Am J Cardiol.* 1998;82:429–432.

52. Stevenson WG, Wilber DJ, Natale A, et al. Irrigated radiofrequency catheter ablation guided by electroanatomic mapping for recurrent ventricular tachycardia after myocardial infarction: the Multicenter Thermocool Ventricular Tachycardia Ablation trial. *Circulation.* 2008;118:2773–2782.

53. Aliot EM, Stevenson WG, Almendral-Garrote JM, et al. EHRA/HRS Expert Consensus on Catheter Ablation of Ventricular Arrhythmias: developed in a partnership with the European Heart Rhythm Association (EHRA), a Registered Branch of the European Society of Cardiology (ESC), and the Heart Rhythm Society (HRS); in collaboration with the American College of Cardiology (ACC) and the American Heart Association (AHA). *Heart Rhythm.* 2009;6:886–933.

54. Miller JM, Kienzle MG, Harken AH, et al. Subendocardial resection for ventricular tachycardia: predictors of surgical success. *Circulation.* 1984;70:624–631.

55. Cassidy DM, Vassallo JA, Miller JM, et al. Endocardial catheter mapping in patients in sinus rhythm: relationship to underlying heart disease and ventricular arrhythmias. *Circulation.* 1986;73:645–652.

56. Marchlinski FE, Callans DJ, Gottlieb CD, et al. Linear ablation lesions for control of unmappable ventricular tachycardia in patients with ischemic and nonischemic cardiomyopathy. *Circulation.* 2000;101:1288–1296.

57. Callans DJ, Ren JF, Michele J, et al. Electroanatomic left ventricular mapping in the porcine model of healed anterior myocardial infarction: correlation with intracardiac echocardiography and pathological analysis. *Circulation.* 1999;100:1744–1750.

58. Koa-Wing M, Ho SY, Kojodjojo P, et al. Radiofrequency ablation of infarct scar-related ventricular tachycardia: correlation of electroanatomical data with post-mortem histology. *J Cardiovasc Electrophysiol.* 2007;18:1330–1333.

59. Deneke T, Muller KM, Lemke B, et al. Human histopathology of electroanatomic mapping after cooled-tip radiofrequency ablation to treat ventricular tachycardia in remote myocardial infarction. *J Cardiovasc Electrophysiol.* 2005;16:1246–1251.

60. Bello D, Kipper S, Valderrabano M, et al. Catheter ablation of ventricular tachycardia guided by contrast-enhanced cardiac computed tomography. *Heart Rhythm.* 2004;1:490–492.

61. Fahmy TS, Wazni OM, Jaber WA, et al. Integration of positron emission tomography/computed tomography with electroanatomical mapping: a novel approach for ablation of scar-related ventricular tachycardia. *Heart Rhythm.* 2008;5:1538–1545.

62. Codreanu A, Odille F, Aliot E, et al. Electroanatomic characterization of postinfarct scars comparison with 3-dimensional myocardial scar reconstruction based on magnetic resonance imaging. *J Am Coll Cardiol.* 2008;52:839–842.

63. de Chillou C, Lacroix D, Klug D, et al. Isthmus characteristics of reentrant ventricular tachycardia after myocardial infarction. *Circulation.* 2002;105:726–731.

64. Alcalde O, Latif S, Scollan D, et al. Pacemapping around the edge of the scar substrate: 12 lead ECG spatial resolution (abstract). *Heart Rhythm.* 2009;6:S176.

65. Soejima K, Stevenson WG, Maisel WH, et al. Electrically unexcitable scar mapping based on pacing threshold for identification of the reentry circuit isthmus: feasibility for guiding ventricular tachycardia ablation. *Circulation.* 2002;106:1678–1683.

66. Sarrazin JF, Kuehne M, Wells D, et al. High-output pacing in mapping of postinfarction ventricular tachycardia. *Heart Rhythm.* 2008;5:1709–1714.

67. Arenal A, del Castillo S, Gonzalez-Torrecilla E, et al. Tachycardia-related channel in the scar tissue in patients with sustained monomorphic ventricular tachycardias: influence of the voltage scar definition. *Circulation.* 2004;110:2568–2574.

68. Hsia HH, Lin D, Sauer WH, et al. Anatomic characterization of endocardial substrate for hemodynamically stable reentrant ventricular tachycardia: identification of endocardial conducting channels. *Heart Rhythm.* 2006;3:503–512.

69. Bogun F, Good E, Reich S, et al. Isolated potentials during sinus rhythm and pace-mapping within scars as guides for ablation of post-infarction ventricular tachycardia. *J Am Coll Cardiol.* 2006;47:2013–2019.

70. Miller JM, Tyson GS, Hargrove WC, et al. Effect of subendocardial resection on sinus rhythm endocardial electrogram abnormalities. *Circulation.* 1995;91:2385–2391.

71. Haqqani HM, Kalman JM, Roberts-Thomson KC, et al. Fundamental differences in electrophysiologic and electroanatomic substrate between ischemic cardiomyopathy patients with and without clinical ventricular tachycardia. *J Am Coll Cardiol.* 2009;54:166–173.

72. Nault I, Maury P, Sacher F, et al. Characterization of later ventricular potentials as ventricular tachycardia substrate and impact of ablation. *Heart Rhythm.* 2009;6:S227.

73. Haïssaguerre M, Shoda M, Jais P, et al. Mapping and ablation of idiopathic ventricular fibrillation. *Circulation.* 2002;106:962–967.

74. Marrouche NF, Verma A, Wazni O, et al. Mode of initiation and ablation of ventricular fibrillation storms in patients with ischemic cardiomyopathy. *J Am Coll Cardiol.* 2004;43:1715–1720.

75. Bansch D, Oyang F, Antz M, et al. Successful catheter ablation of electrical storm after myocardial infarction. *Circulation.* 2003;108:3011–3016.

76. Callans DJ, Ren JF, Narula N, et al. Effects of linear, irrigated-tip radiofrequency ablation in porcine healed anterior infarction. *J Cardiovasc Electrophysiol.* 2001;12:1037–1042.

77. Calkins H, Epstein A, Packer D, et al. Catheter ablation of ventricular tachycardia in patients with structural heart disease using cooled radiofrequency energy: results of a prospective multicenter study. Cooled RF Multi Center Investigators Group. *J Am Coll Cardiol.* 2000;35:1905–1914.

78. Nakagawa H, Yamanashi WS, Pitha JV, et al. Comparison of in vivo tissue temperature profile and lesion geometry for radiofrequency ablation with a saline-irrigated electrode versus temperature control in a canine thigh muscle preparation. *Circulation.* 1995;91:2264–2273.

79. Delacretaz E, Stevenson WG, Winters GL, et al. Ablation of ventricular tachycardia with a saline-cooled radiofrequency catheter: anatomic and histologic characteristics of the lesions in humans. *J Cardiovasc Electrophysiol.* 1999;10:860–865.

80. Soejima K, Delacretaz E, Suzuki M, et al. Saline-cooled versus standard radiofrequency catheter ablation for infarct-related ventricular tachycardias. *Circulation.* 2001;103:1858–1862.

81. Ren JF, Callans DJ, Michele JJ, et al. Intracardiac echocardiographic evaluation of ventricular mural swelling from radiofrequency ablation in chronic myocardial infarction: irrigated-tip versus standard catheter. *J Interv Card Electrophysiol.* 2001;5:27–32.

82. Watanabe I, Masaki R, Min N, et al. Cooled-tip ablation results in increased radiofrequency power delivery and lesion size in the canine heart: importance of catheter-tip temperature monitoring for prevention of popping and impedance rise. *J Interv Card Electrophysiol.* 2002;6:9–16.

83. Kim YH, Sosa-Suarez G, Trouton TG, et al. Treatment of ventricular tachycardia by transcatheter radiofrequency ablation in patients with ischemic heart disease. *Circulation.* 1994;89:1094–1102.

84. O'Callaghan PA, Poloniecki J, Sosa-Suarez G, et al. Long-term clinical outcome of patients with prior myocardial infarction after palliative radiofrequency catheter ablation for frequent ventricular tachycardia. *Am J Cardiol.* 2001;87:975–979; A4.

85. Della Bella P, De Ponti R, Uriarte JA, et al. Catheter ablation and antiarrhythmic drugs for haemodynamically tolerated post-infarction ventricular tachycardia: long-term outcome in relation to acute electrophysiological findings. *Eur Heart J.* 2002;23:414–424.

86. Marchlinski FE, Zado E, Callans DJ, et al. Hybrid therapy for ventricular arrhythmia management. In: Miller JM, ed. *Cardiology Clinics: Ventricular Arrhythmias.* Philadelphia: Saunders; 1999:391–406.

87. Alonso C, Lin D, Poku J, et al. The role of transcatheter ablation in the prevention of sudden death. In: Santini M, ed. *Sudden Death: Nonpharmacological Treatment.* Rome: Adrianna Editirice; 2002.

88. Sosa E, Scanavacca M, d'Avila A, et al. A new technique to perform epicardial mapping in the electrophysiology laboratory. *J Cardiovasc Electrophysiol.* 1996;7:531–536.

89. Sosa E, Scanavacca M, d'Avila A, et al. Nonsurgical transthoracic epicardial catheter ablation to treat recurrent ventricular tachycardia occurring late after myocardial infarction. *J Am Coll Cardiol.* 2000;35:1442–1449.

90. Schweikert RA, Saliba WI, Tomassoni G, et al. Percutaneous pericardial instrumentation for endo-epicardial mapping of previously failed ablations. *Circulation.* 2003;108:1329–1335.

29
Ablation of Ventricular Tachycardia Associated with Nonischemic Cardiomyopathies

Mark A. Wood

Key Points

The mechanisms of bundle branch reentry is reentry. The mechanisms of ventricular tachycardia (VT) associated with right ventricular dysplasia, dilated cardiomyopathy, sarcoidosis, and Chagas disease are reentry and possibly automatic or triggered activity.

Ablation targets include the specialized conduction system for bundle branch reentry and sites defined by activation, entrainment, substrate, or pace-mapping for other VTs.

No special equipment is needed for ablation of bundle branch reentry. In other cases, computerized mapping systems are essential, and large-tip or irrigated-tip ablation systems may be needed.

Sources of difficulty include the following: for bundle branch reentry, ablation of broad left bundle; for right ventricular dysplasia, multiple inducible morphologies and high recurrence rates; for dilated cardiomyopathy, multiple morphologies with epicardial or intramyocardial circuits, noninducibility, and high recurrence rates; and for Chagas disease, epicardial foci.

Success rates are 100% for bundle branch reentry and variable (often 50% to 60%) for other etiologies.

Ventricular tachycardias (VTs) may occur in any condition that results in ventricular mechanical or electrical dysfunction. Ablation of VT has been most thoroughly investigated for patients with coronary artery disease, and the techniques developed from this experience are applicable to nonischemic cardiomyopathies as well. The clinical experience with ablation of VT related to nonischemic cardiomyopathies is more limited than with coronary artery disease. Like ablation of VT with coronary artery disease, VT ablation in nonischemic cardiomyopathies is almost entirely palliative and adjunctive because most cases are also managed with implantable defibrillators and drug therapy.

Bundle Branch Reentry

Bundle branch reentry (BBR) VT accounts for about 6% of sustained monomorphic VTs induced at electrophysiologic testing.[1-3] The incidence of the arrhythmia is much greater in certain patient populations.[4,5] In patients with nonischemic dilated cardiomyopathy (DCM), this mechanism may be responsible for up to 41% of inducible sustained monomorphic VTs.[1] This mechanism may be under-recognized clinically and at electrophysiologic testing. With the current trend toward early defibrillator implantation without electrophysiologic testing in patients with VTs, under-recognition is likely to continue. The diagnosis is important to make because BBR VT is highly amenable to catheter ablation.[2]

Anatomy

The atrioventricular (AV) node crosses the central fibrous body to become the penetrating portion of the AV bundle (Fig. 29-1). This penetrating portion of the bundle of His emerges from the central fibrous body to rest on the crest of the muscular ventricular septum.[6-8] This portion of the bundle enters the lower region of the pars membranacea, then courses for a variable distance to become the branching portion of the bundle.[6] The branching bundle lies at the lower part of the membranous ventricular septum, above the ventricular summit and below the noncoronary (posterior) aortic cusp. This portion of the bundle varies considerably in its dimensions, usually from 6.5 to 20 mm in length and 1 to 3 mm in width.[7] As it courses apically, it first gives rise to the fascicles of the left bundle branch (LBB). In general, the LBB fibers are subendocardial and very superficial. The main LBB is about 1 cm in width at

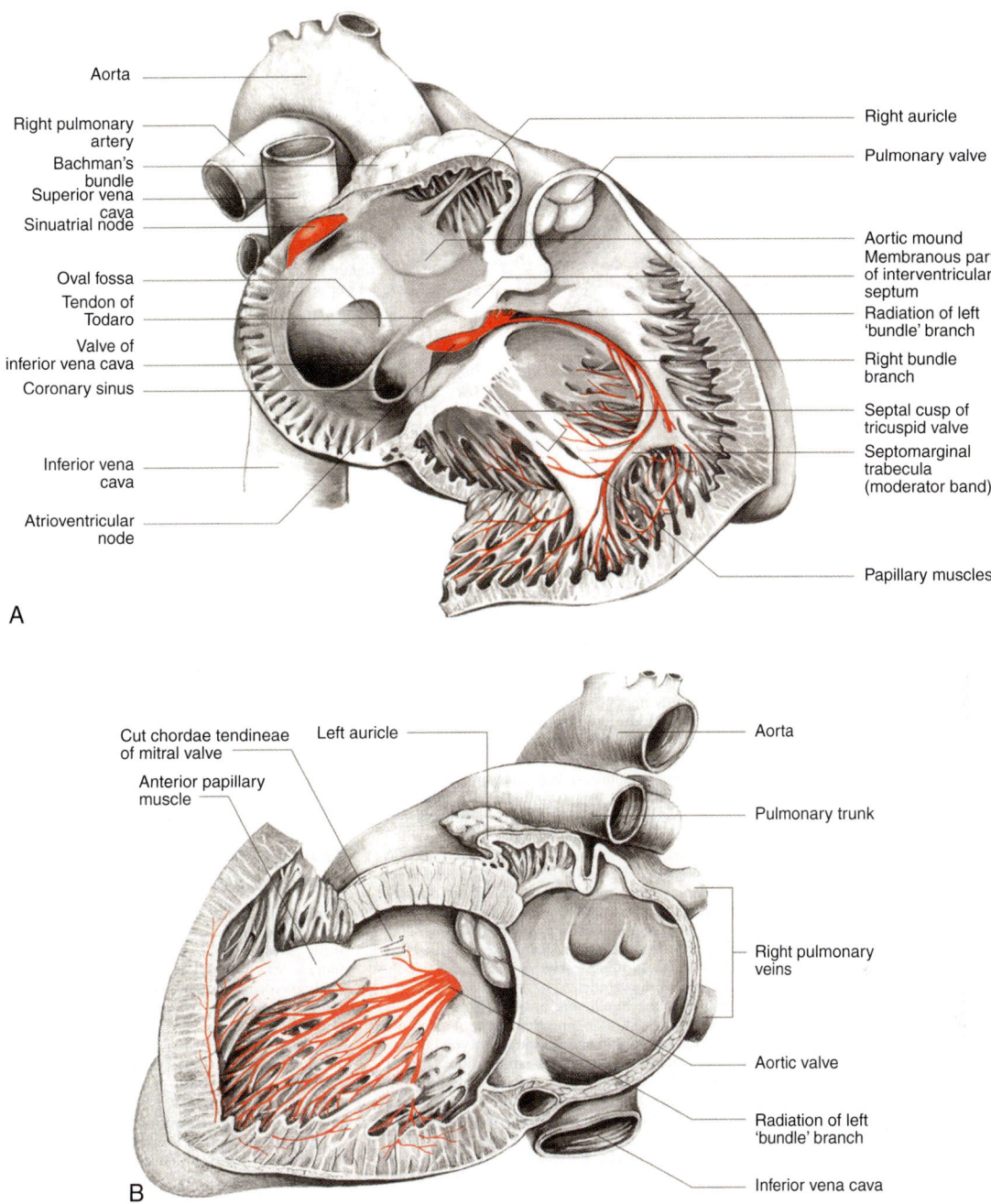

FIGURE 29-1. Anatomy of the specialized conduction system. **A,** The cordlike right bundle branch is a continuation of the bundle of His extending to the papillary muscle on the interventricular septum. **B,** The left bundle branch is short and broad before branching extensively to form the anterior and posterior fascicles. *(From Shah P. Heart and great vessels. In Standring S (ed):* Gray's Anatomy, *39th ed. Edinburgh: Elsevier; 2005:995-1029. With permission.)*

its origin and extends 1 to 3 cm in length before giving rise to the posterior and anterior fascicles.[7] The main LBB first gives rise to the larger posterior fascicle and then to the smaller anterior fascicle. Fibers from these two fascicles merge at the mid-septal level to form the septal branch of the left bundle.[6,7] The anterior fascicle courses along the anterior septal wall of the left ventricle to the base of the anterior papillary muscle. The posterior fascicle runs inferiorly from the His bundle to course along the posterior septum to the posterior papillary muscle. The left bundle is made up of one or more large bands of fibers, and the fascicles are networks of fine strands rather than single discrete structures. In some cases, the entire left-sided conduction system is an extensive network of fibers without discrete fascicles. In contrast, the right bundle branch (RBB) is a discrete entity formed by the continuation of the His bundle beyond the septal crest (Fig. 29-1). As the right bundle emerges from the membranous septum, it proceeds along the lower portion of the septal band to reach the moderator band. It then reaches the anterolateral papillary muscle, where it ramifies into branches. At least the midportion of the right bundle, and sometimes its entire extent, is intramyocardial. Mapping of the distal right bundle is often made difficult by its passage within the substance of the septomarginal trabeculation. The right bundle is usually about 50 mm long and 1 mm wide.[7]

Pathophysiology

As the name indicates, BBR VT involves sustained macro-reentry using the bundle branches as obligatory limbs of the circuit connected proximally by the bundle of His and distally by the ventricular myocardium (Fig. 29-2).[1-3,9] At electrophysiologic testing, right ventricular premature stimuli introduced after a drive train of long cycle length results in retrograde conduction to the His bundle by way of the RBB.[1] At shorter coupling intervals, retrograde block occurs in the right bundle because of its longer refractory period, and retrograde conduction occurs solely over the LBB. As the coupling interval shortens even further, progressive delay in transseptal myocardial conduction and the retrograde left bundle results in prolongation of the V_2H_2 interval. With a sufficiently long V_2H_2 interval, the right bundle may recover excitability, allowing antegrade conduction past the site of initial retrograde block and resulting in a reentrant beat of ventricular activation. These single BBR beats (V_3 phenomenon) are noted in 50% of patients with normal His-Purkinje conduction systems undergoing electrophysiologic testing.[9,10] With abrupt changes in cycle length, up to three consecutive BBR beats may be inducible in normal patients.[10] The rapid conduction and long refractory periods of the His-Purkinje system prevent sustained BBR in normal hearts, usually by retrograde block in the LBB.[11] In the setting of conduction delay in the His-Purkinje system, sustained BBR may occur. As described previously, the induced tachycardia would have a left bundle branch block (LBBB) morphology owing to antegrade conduction and ventricular activation over the RBB. The LBBB morphology is the most commonly induced and spontaneously occurring form of BBR VT.[1,12] This most likely results from the shorter LBB refractoriness, preferential retrograde LBB conduction in most patients,[1,12] and the common use of right ventricular pacing at electrophysiologic testing. BBR VT with right bundle branch block (RBBB) morphology is less common and results from reversal of the direction of activation in the reentrant circuit (Fig. 29-2). During right ventricular pacing, this may result from earlier retrograde block in the LBB or from recovery of retrograde RBB conduction after bilateral bundle branch block (BBB) due to the gap phenomenon.[1] Excellent detailed descriptions of the pathophysiology of BBR have been published by Blanck and colleagues.[1,13]

In addition, interfascicular reentry involving the anterior and posterior fascicles of the LBB system has been described (Fig. 29-2).[14-16] In this tachycardia, one of the fascicles serves as the antegrade limb and the other as the retrograde circuit. The distal link between the fascicles occurs through the ventricular myocardium. Interfascicular VT may be the clinical arrhythmia, or it may be inducible after ablation for BBR VT.[16] Finally, VT arising from automaticity in the right and left fascicular systems may occur.[16] Idiopathic left VT using portions of the left fascicular systems is described in Chapter 27.

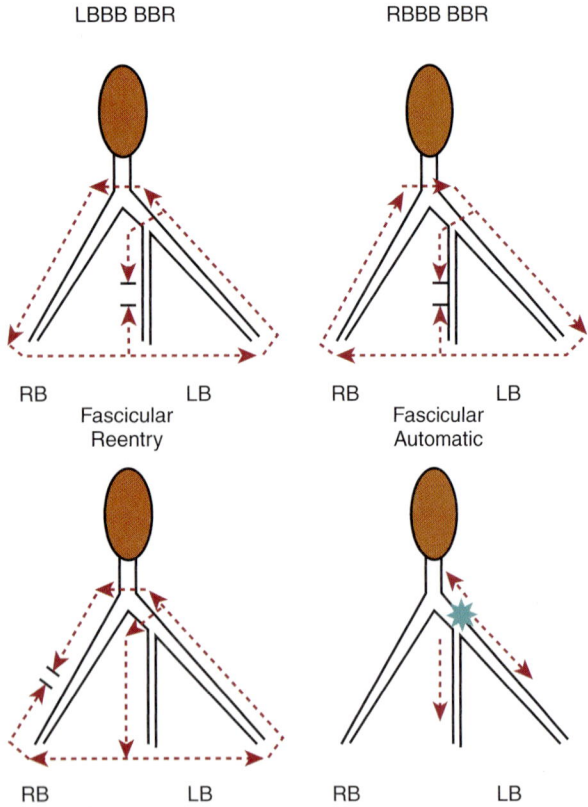

FIGURE 29-2. Schematics of reentrant circuits for bundle branch reentry (BBR), interfascicular reentry, and automatic fascicular tachycardia. LB, left bundle branch; LBBB, left bundle branch block; RB, right bundle branch; RBBB, right bundle branch block. *(Modified from Tchou P, Mehdirad AA. Bundle branch reentry ventricular tachycardia.* Pacing Clin Electrophysiol. *1995;18:1427-1437. With permission.)*

Diagnosis and Differential Diagnosis

Virtually all patients with BBR VT have underlying structural heart disease and evidence of His-Purkinje system disease. Dilated cardiomyopathy is present in 45% of these patients.[1] Coronary artery disease is also a frequent diagnosis. Other diagnoses associated with BBR are aortic valve replacement and muscular dystrophies.[4,5] BBR has also been described in association with mitral valve disease, Ebstein anomaly, and hypertrophic cardiomyopathy.[17-20] BBR may occur without structural heart disease in association with fixed or functional His-Purkinje conduction delays.[13,21]

Surface Electrocardiogram

Virtually all patients with BBR VT demonstrate intraventricular conduction delays in sinus rhythm. These abnormalities may be RBBB or LBBB, but nonspecific delays are common as well. The presence of RBBB or LBBB on the electrocardiogram (ECG) may indicate conduction delay rather than complete block in a bundle branch that would preclude BBR VT.[22-26] Complete antegrade bundle branch block may be present with intact retrograde conduction over the bundle to allow for BBR VT. Because ventricular activation occurs by antegrade conduction through the RBB or LBB, the ECG appearance is that of a typical LBBB or RBBB tachycardia and may be identical to the QRS morphology in sinus rhythm (Fig. 29-3). In BBR VT, an LBBB configuration is far more common and may be associated with a normal or leftward axis. Right-axis deviation is rare and is seen only with preexisting right-axis deviation in sinus rhythm. RBBB VT is usually associated with a left-axis deviation, but normal and right-axis deviation may occur as well. The cycle length of BBR VT is typically short (<300 milliseconds), and the tachycardia is usually poorly tolerated hemodynamically. Interfascicular reentry has an RBBB pattern owing to ventricular activation antegrade through one of the left fascicles. The direction of antegrade conduction in the left anterior or posterior fascicle determines the electrical axis.[1,16] VT from fascicular automaticity may have an LBBB or RBBB pattern, depending on the fascicle of origin.[16] In all three types of VT, the VT QRS often closely resembles the QRS in sinus rhythm, providing a clue to the diagnosis.[16]

Electrophysiologic Testing

At baseline, virtually all patients have prolongation of the His-ventricle (HV) interval, averaging 75 to 80 milliseconds (range, 60 to 110 milliseconds).[12,16] BBR VT has been reported in patients with a normal HV interval and ECG at baseline who demonstrated functional HV prolongation at higher rates.[21] The tachycardia is typically induced with ventricular extrastimulus testing, especially with the use of short-long-short protocols, but it may be induced with atrial pacing in some patients.[1,12] The abrupt cycle length prolongation by the long interval may result in more distal retrograde block

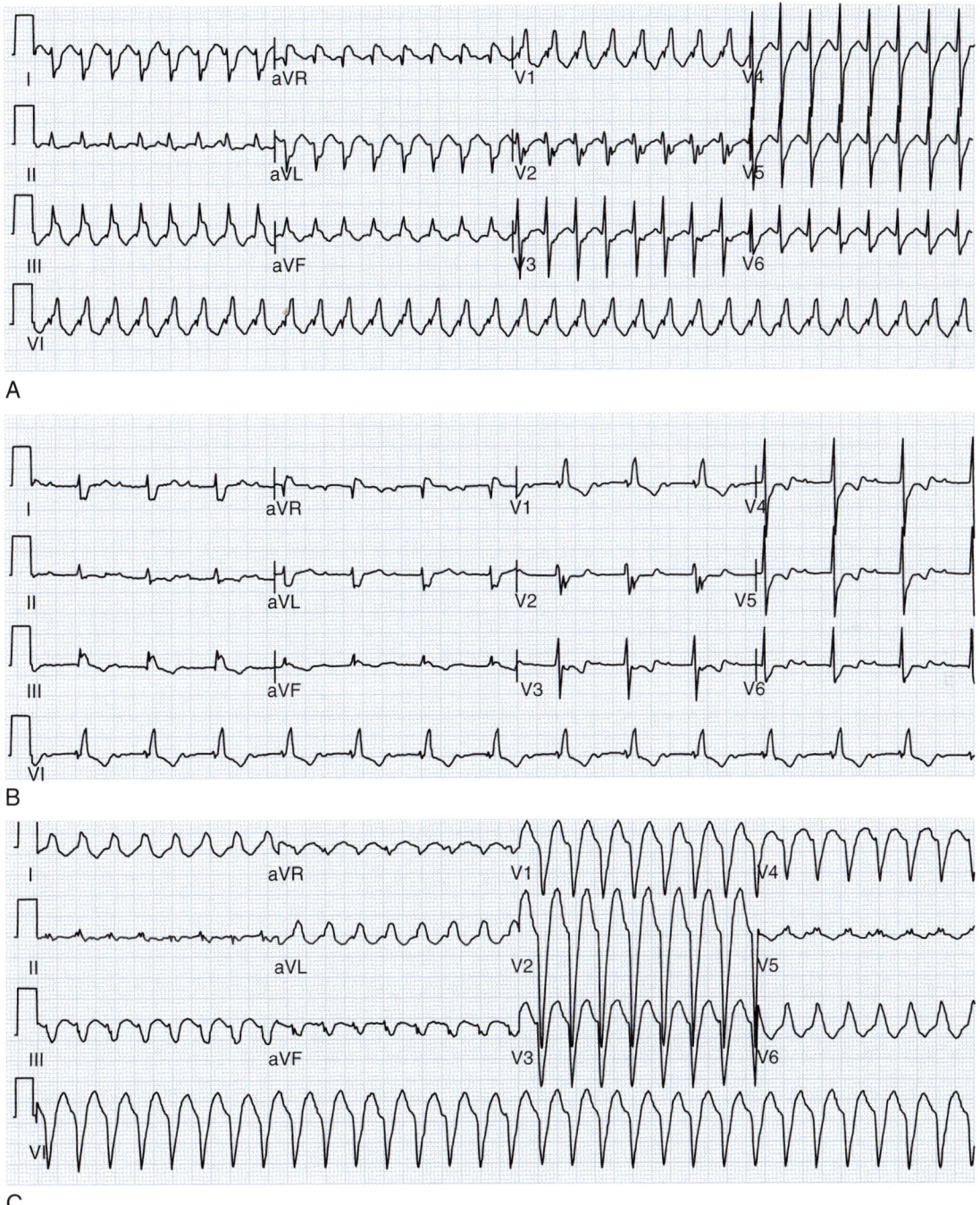

FIGURE 29-3. Electrocardiograms from the same patient during bundle branch reentry (BBR) with right bundle branch block morphology (**A**), sinus rhythm (**B**), and bundle branch reentry with left bundle branch morphology (**C**). The patient presented with sustained right bundle branch block BBR after aortic valve replacement. Note that the right bundle branch block QRS morphology in tachycardia is identical to that in sinus rhythm. The left bundle branch block BBR was induced at electrophysiologic testing.

in the His-Purkinje system, allowing more time to recover excitability in the antegrade direction. LBBB morphology VT is most commonly induced in the laboratory. Rarely, left ventricular pacing is required to induce this pattern.[1,12] RBBB morphology may be inducible in about 10% of patients but more commonly requires left ventricular pacing to initiate.[1,12] The induced BBR VT morphology may not match the clinical VT morphology (i.e., the contralateral bundle branch morphology is induced), especially if the clinical VT has an RBBB pattern (Fig. 29-3).[1,12] Isoproterenol or class IA drug infusion (to prolong His-Purkinje conduction delays) may be needed for induction.[1] The diagnostic criteria for BBR VT are given in Table 29-1.

The QRS morphology in VT must be consistent with ventricular activation through the RBB or LBB. Each ventricular depolarization should be preceded by depolarization of the His, RBB, and LBB. For LBBB VT, RBB activation immediately precedes ventricular activation. Ventricular activation is followed by LBB activation and then activation of the His bundle (Fig. 29-4). For RBBB pattern VT, LBB activation immediately precedes ventricular activation, which in turn is followed by activation of the RBB and then the His. The exact timing of His and antegrade conducting bundle branch activation depends on the relative conduction velocities of each of these structures.

The HV interval during VT is characteristically similar to or slightly longer (by 10 to 20 milliseconds) than the interval in sinus rhythm. This may result from rate-related changes in conduction velocity or from anisotropic conduction during retrograde activation of the His.[22] Occasionally, the HV is shorter because the retrograde activation to the His bundle is more rapid than antegrade conduction down the bundle branch. For RBBB pattern BBR VT, the changes in HV interval from sinus rhythm may be more marked.[1]

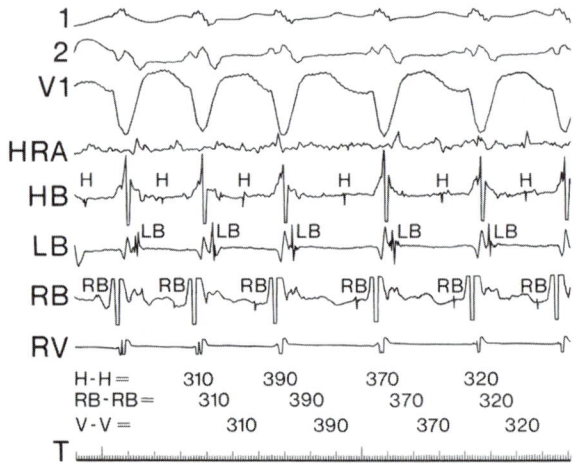

FIGURE 29-4. Intracardiac recordings demonstrating the sequence of activation of His-Purkinje system during bundle branch reentry. The tachycardia has a left bundle branch block morphology. The right ventricle is activated by conduction antegrade in the right bundle (RB). The RB potential precedes the ventricular activation. The right ventricular apex activation follows the retrograde activation of the left bundle (LB). The His bundle (H) is then activated to complete the circuit. Note that changes in the H-H interval are followed by similar changes in the V-V interval. The atria are in fibrillation. 1, 2, V$_1$, surface electrocardiogram leads; HB, His bundle; HRA, high right atrium; RV, right ventricle. *(From Blanck Z, Sra J, Dhala A, et al. Bundle branch reentry: mechanisms, diagnosis and treatment. In Zipes DP, Jalife J (eds): Cardiac Electrophysiology: From Cell to Bedside, 2nd ed. Philadelphia: Saunders; 1995:878-885. With permission.)*

TABLE 29-1

DIAGNOSTIC CRITERIA FOR BUNDLE BRANCH REENTRY AND FASCICULAR TACHYCARDIAS

Bundle Branch Reentry

QRS morphology in tachycardia demonstrates an LBBB or RBBB pattern consistent with ventricular activation through the appropriate bundle branch.

Each ventricular depolarization is preceded by His, left bundle, or right bundle activation with the appropriate sequence of activation for the tachycardia QRS morphology and with stable bundle electrogram-to-ventricle intervals.

Spontaneous variations in the V-V interval are preceded by similar changes in the H-H or bundle-to-bundle interval.

Tachycardia induction depends on achieving a critical conduction delay in the His-Purkinje system. The HV interval in tachycardias is typically longer than in sinus rhythm.

The tachycardia can be terminated by block in the His-Purkinje system and rendered noninducible by ablation of the RBB or LBB.

A short PPI (<30 msec) is obtained from the RVA.

Left Interfascicular Reentry

QRS morphology in tachycardia demonstrates an RBBB consistent with ventricular activation antegrade over the left anterior or posterior fascicle.

Each ventricular depolarization is preceded by a left fascicular potential, and activation of the His and right bundle follows left fascicular activation in tachycardia.

The HV interval is shorter than that recorded in sinus rhythm.

Tachycardia induction depends on critical delay within the left fascicular system.

The tachycardia can be terminated by block in the left fascicular system and rendered noninducible by ablation of the left anterior or posterior fascicle.

Automatic Fascicular Tachycardia

QRS morphology in tachycardia demonstrates a LBBB or RBBB pattern consistent with ventricular activation through the appropriate bundle branch.

Tachycardia is induced by catecholamine administration but not by programmed stimulation; classic entrainment criteria are not met.

Each ventricular depolarization in tachycardia is preceded by a Purkinje potential, and activation of the His and bundle branch occurs after Purkinje activation.

The HV interval during tachycardia as measured to the start of the QRS may be variable.

H-H, His bundle–His bundle; HV, His-ventricle; LBBB(B), left bundle branch (block); RBB(B), right bundle branch (block); V-V, ventricle-ventricle; PPI, postpacing interval; RVA, right ventricular apex.

Because of the obligatory involvement of the His-Purkinje system, changes in tachycardia cycle length should be preceded by changes in the His bundle–His bundle (HH) interval. Cycle length variation may be most common immediately after induction of the tachycardia. In addition, tachycardia induction depends on a critical degree of conduction delay in the conduction system and is terminated by block within the His-Purkinje system. The tachycardia may be advanced by premature activation of the His, RBB, or LBB. The tachycardia should be entrained from the right ventricular apex, which produces a short postpacing interval of less than 30 milliseconds.[23] BBR VT may show concealed entrainment from the atrium if AV nodal conduction is enhanced with atropine.[24]

Interfascicular reentry similarly demonstrates variations in the RR interval preceded by changes in the HH interval. In contrast to BBR, the HV interval in interfascicular reentry is shorter than that in sinus rhythm (Fig. 29-5).[14] Also in left interfascicular reentry, an RBBB QRS morphology should be recorded. In BBR, the His bundle activation should precede the left fascicular activation. In interfascicular reentry, however, activation of the His bundle follows that of the left fascicular potentials (Fig. 29-5).[14] Reentry can occur in opposite directions within the circuit in the same patient.[14]

Fascicular automaticity arising in the fascicular system appears to be a rare phenomenon.[16] The tachycardia may arise from either the RBB or the LBB. Clues to this diagnosis are failure to induce the tachycardia with programmed extrastimuli with, instead, dependence on catecholamines. Importantly, the HV interval as measured to the start of the QRS during tachycardia is variable. Purkinje potentials are recorded near the focus and demonstrate a short and consistent relationship to the QRS (Fig. 29-6).

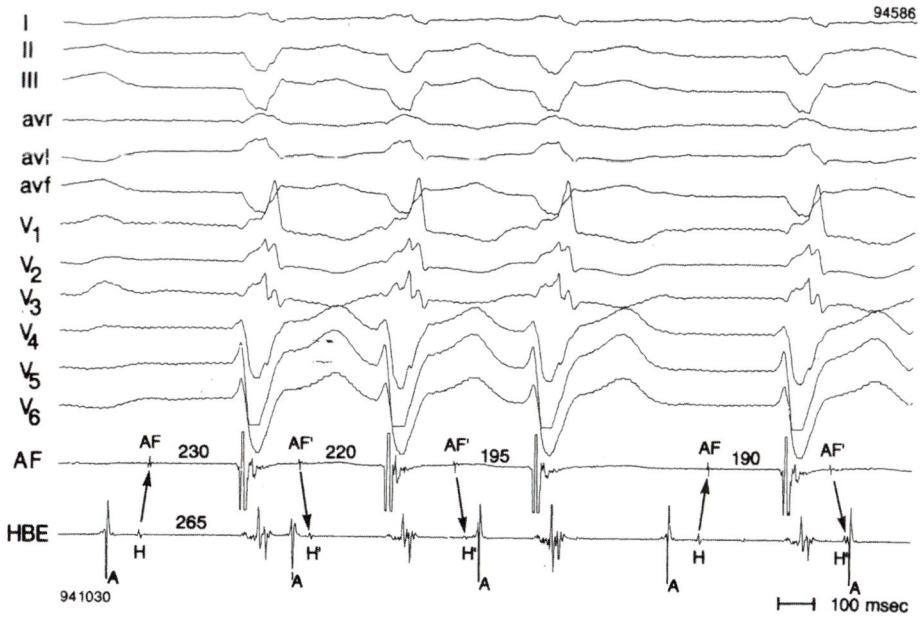

FIGURE 29-5. Electrocardiograms (ECGs) and electrograms demonstrating interfascicular reentry. From *top* to *bottom*: all 12 surface ECG leads. The first beat is sinus rhythm with block in the anterior fascicle distal to the recording site given the left axis deviation. Two beats of interfascicular reentry follow antegrade conduction in the posterior fascicle and retrograde activation of the anterior fascicle. After activation of the His, antegrade conduction over the left posterior fascicle activates the ventricle. Note the reversal of the sequence of activation of the His and anterior fascicle (AF) potentials during reentry. After the second reentry beat, retrograde conduction block occurs in the anterior fascicle. The QRS complex is identical in sinus and fascicular reentry.', indicates retrograde activation; A, atrial electrogram; AF, anterior fascicular recording; H, His electrogram; HBE, His bundle electrogram. *(From Crijns HJGM, Smeets JLRM, Rodriguez LM, et al. Cure of interfascicular reentrant ventricular tachycardia by ablation of the anterior fascicle of the left bundle branch. J Cardiovasc Electrophysiol. 1995;6:486–492. With permission.)*

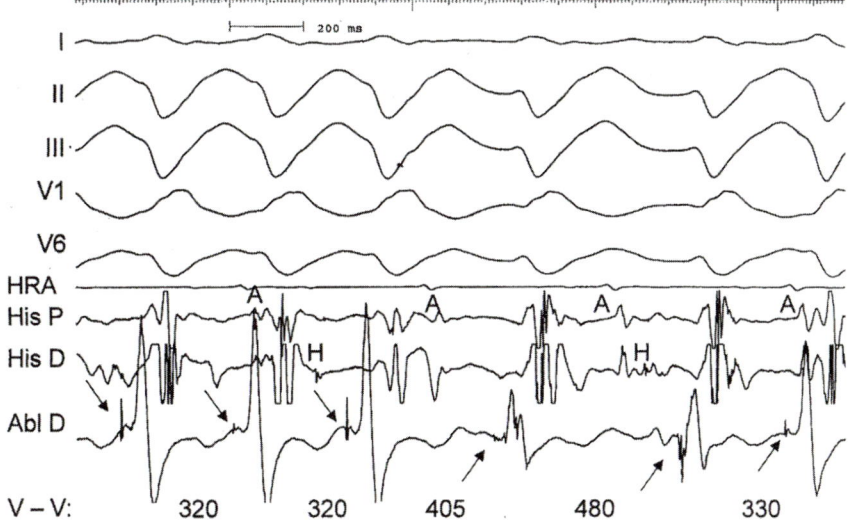

FIGURE 29-6. Electrograms of focal automatic fascicular tachycardia arising from the distal left bundle branch Purkinje system. The successful ablation site shows a sharp, discrete potential (*arrows*) preceding ventricular activation. Note the irregularity of the V-V intervals that are preceded by changes in the interval between these early potentials. I, II, III, V_1, V_6, surface electrocardiograms; A, atrium; Abl, ablation electrogram; D, distal; H, His bundle electrogram; HRA, high right atrium; P, proximal; V, ventricle. *(From Lopera G, Stevenson WG, Soejima K, et al. Identification and ablation of three types of ventricular tachycardia involving the His-Purkinje system in patients with heart disease. J Cardiovasc Electrophysiol. 2004;15:52-58. With permission.)*

Differential Diagnosis

The differential diagnosis of BBR VT includes interfascicular VT, automatic fascicular VT, idiopathic left ventricular VT, intramyocardial VT, supraventricular tachycardia with aberrancy, and atriofascicular reciprocating tachycardia. Interfascicular reentry is diagnosed by an RBBB VT pattern with an HV interval shorter than the HV interval in sinus rhythm and left fascicular activation before His activation.[14,16] Fascicular automaticity is catecholamine dependent, is not induced with programmed stimulation, and shows a variable HV interval in tachycardia.[16] Idiopathic left ventricular VT has a negative or short HV interval in tachycardia and a normal baseline QRS and HV interval.[25] As with interfascicular VT, the His activation follows activation of the left fascicles, which is inconsistent with RBBB pattern BBR VT. VT arising from myocardial foci rarely produces entirely typical RBBB or LBBB patterns on surface ECG, as is expected with BBR. In addition, the His activation is usually late in the QRS complex and may be dissociated from the tachycardia.

Supraventricular tachycardias with BBB aberrancy can be distinguished from BBR by the antegrade activation of both bundle branches. Reciprocating tachycardias show an obligatory 1:1 atrium-to-ventricle (A/V) relationship that is not present in BBR. AV nodal reentry may be terminated with adenosine. The ventricular postpacing interval after entrainment of the tachycardia from the right ventricular apex may differentiate BBR VT from myocardial VT and from AV nodal reentry.[23] The postpacing interval with BBR is short (<30 milliseconds) because the RBB inserts into the ventricular apex. For myocardial VT (unless originating in the apex) and AV nodal reentry with aberrancy, the postpacing intervals greatly exceed 30 milliseconds. For atrial tachycardias, dependency on atrial activation and AV nodal conduction is diagnostic. Features differentiating BBR from other wide-complex tachycardias are listed in Table 29-2.

Mapping

Bundle Branches

BBR VT may be prevented by ablation of either the right or left main bundle branch.[1,2] Even though most patients demonstrate more conduction system disease in the left bundle, the right bundle is typically the target for ablation.[26,27] This is because of the technical ease of ablation of the right bundle, in contrast to the difficulties involved in ablation of the left bundle. Left bundle ablation requires arterial access, increased risk for complications, and potentially more extensive ablation to transect this broad structure. In patients with complete antegrade block in the left bundle, RBB ablation necessitates permanent pacing. Complete antegrade LBBB is likely if left bundle potentials are recorded intermittently or after the ventricular electrogram in sinus rhythm or if catheter-induced trauma to the right bundle results in transient complete heart block.[27] In these cases, LBB ablation may be preferred if there is no other indication for pacemaker or implantable cardioverter-defibrillator (ICD) implantation. Induction of complete LBBB by ablation of both the anterior and posterior fascicles is curative for patients with both BBR and interfascicular VT.

The RBB is usually easily identified along the basilar right ventricular septum.[27] After a large His potential is recorded, the catheter is advanced apically in the right anterior oblique view to record the RBB (Fig. 29-7). The RBB must be differentiated from the His potential in this region. The RBB is identified by the absence or minimal amplitude of an atrial electrogram and by a His-RRB interval of greater than 15 milliseconds in sinus rhythm.[2,27] If RBB conduction delay is present, the RBB potential may be obscured by the local ventricular activation in sinus rhythm. In this case, the right bundle potential may not be identifiable in sinus rhythm and may be evident only during retrograde conduction during sustained BBR or BBR echo beats (Fig. 29-8).[28] If the RBB is not well recorded at the basilar septum, mapping the apical course of the RBB may be effective.

As described earlier, the LBB arises as a broad band of fibers directed inferiorly from the bundle of His. The left main bundle is typically about 1 to 3 cm in length and 1 cm wide but shows great individual variation. Methods for recording the LBB potential have been reported.[2,27] After crossing the aortic valve, the ablation catheter is directed toward the inferior apical septum, then withdrawn toward the His bundle until the LBB potential is recorded beneath the noncoronary aortic cusp (Figs. 29-9 and 29-10). This position is typically 1 to 1.5 cm inferior to the optimal His bundle recording site.[2,27] The LBB potential is identified by a potential-to-ventricular electrogram interval of less than or equal to 20 milliseconds, and an A/V electrogram ratio of 1:10 or less.[2,27] As mentioned, the LBB is typically a broad band that is not transected by a single RF lesion.

Left Fascicles

The left anterior fascicular network is located by extending the catheter further along the ventricular septum, toward the apex, from the area recording an LBB potential (Figs. 29-1, 29-9, and 29-10).[2,27] In patients with BBR VT, potentials from the left anterior fascicle may be absent, likely reflecting more extensive disease involvement than the posterior fascicle.[26] The left posterior fascicular network extends from the His bundle toward the inferior diaphragmatic wall (Figs. 29-1, 29-9, and 29-10). These structures are not discrete entities, and mapping is complex. Ablation of either the antegrade or the retrograde limb of the circuit should terminate the tachycardia. It may be possible to ablate "bystander" fibers within each respective fascicular system without termination of the tachycardia.[16] Although not described, determination of the postpacing intervals after entrainment at various sites may help to identify fascicular potentials that are critical to the reentry circuit. Ablation of the left main bundle would not be expected to terminate the tachycardia because the circuit is distal to this point. Similarly, ablation of one left-sided fascicle would not be expected to prevent BBR in a patient with both interfascicular and BBR VTs. In this situation, either both left-sided fascicles or the RBB and one of the left fascicles must be ablated.

Automatic Fascicular Tachycardia

This tachycardia may arise from either the right or left distal fascicular system, and mapping is directed at identifying

TABLE 29-2

DIFFERENTIAL DIAGNOSTIC FEATURES OF BUNDLE BRANCH REENTRY AND RELATED TACHYCARDIAS

Tachycardia Type	Baseline QRS	QRS in Tachycardia	HV in Tachycardia	His-Fascicular Activation	V-A Dissociation	Response to Adenosine	Response to Verapamil	V-V Changes Preceded by	Reset by	Onset Dependent on
BBR	Prolonged	Typical RBBB or LBBB	Prolonged or same as HV in sinus	LBBB VT: RB-V-LB-H RBBB VT: LB-V-RB-H	Common	No	No	Similar change in H-H interval	Advancing His or BB	Critical delay in His-Purkinje system
Interfascicular	Prolonged	Typical RBBB	Shorter than in sinus	LBB before His	Possible	Unknown	Unknown	Similar changes in fascicular activation	Advancing left fascicular system	Critical delay in left fascicular system
Fascicular automatic	Prolonged	RBBB or LBBB	Variable	RBBB VT: LBB before His LBBB VT: RBB before His	Possible	Unknown	Unknown	Changes in distal fascicular potentials	Advancing distal fascicular activation but not entrained	Catecholamine stimulation
Idiopathic LV VT	Normal	Typical RBBB	Negative (occurring after V)	Left fascicles or Purkinje fibers before His	Possible	Yes	Yes	Changes in presystolic P potential interval	Advancing left fascicular activation or P potential	Critical delay in left fascicular and/or involved myocardium
Intramyocardial VT	Normal or prolonged	Atypical BBB patterns	Negative or very short	Fascicles before His if measurable	Common	No	No	Unrelated to His-Purkinje system	Advancing ventricular myocardium	Critical V-V coupling intervals
Aberrant SVT	Normal or prolonged	Typical RBBB or LBBB	Same as in sinus or slightly prolonged	His before fascicles	AT: A > V possible AVNRT: unlikely AVRT: not possible	Common	Common	Changes in H-H	AT: advancing A AVNRT: possibly advancing septal AAVRT: advancing A or V activation	AT: critical A-A interval AVNRT: critical AH interval AVRT: critical AV interval
Atriofascicular AP	Normal or minimal preexcitation	LBBB	Shorter than in sinus or negative value	RBB before His	Not possible	Yes	Yes	Changes in AM or MM potential interval	Advancing atrial insertion site	Antegrade AV nodal block and critical delay in AV

A, atrium; AH, atrial-His interval; AP, accessory pathway; AM, atrium-to-Mahaim potential; AVNRT, atrioventricular nodal reentrant tachycardia; AVRT, atrioventricular reciprocating tachycardia; BB(B), bundle branch block; BBR, bundle branch reentry; H, His bundle; HV, His-ventricular interval; LB, left bundle; LBB(B), left bundle branch (block); LV, left ventricular; MM, Mahaim-to-Mahaim potential; P, Purkinje; RB, right bundle; RBB(B), right bundle branch (block); SVT, supraventricular tachycardia; V, ventricle; VT, ventricular tachycardia.

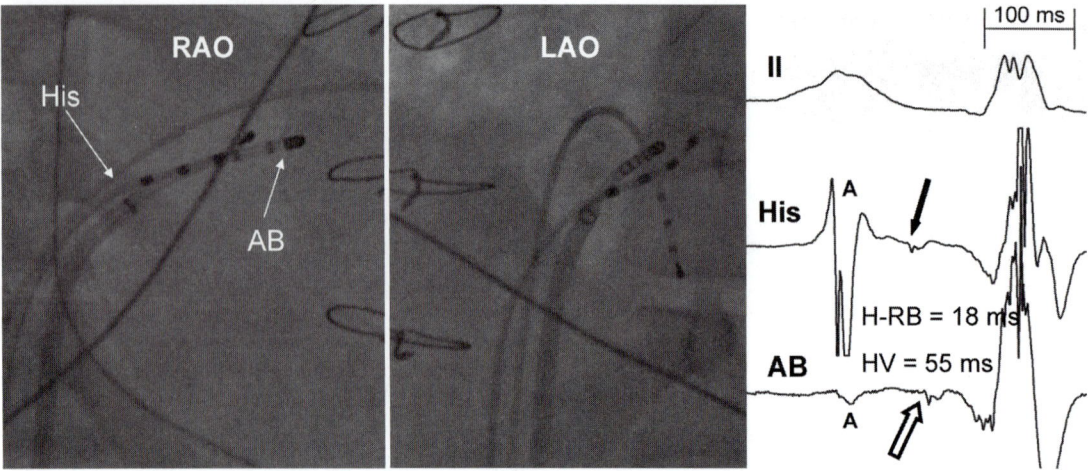

FIGURE 29-7. Right bundle branch recording. Right and left anterior oblique (RAO and LAO) views of the His and ablation (AB) catheters are shown. The *far right panel* shows electrograms recorded from these catheter positions. The right bundle (RB, *open arrow*) recording occurs >15 msec later than the His, (*solid arrow*) and a very small atrial electrogram is recorded. H, His.

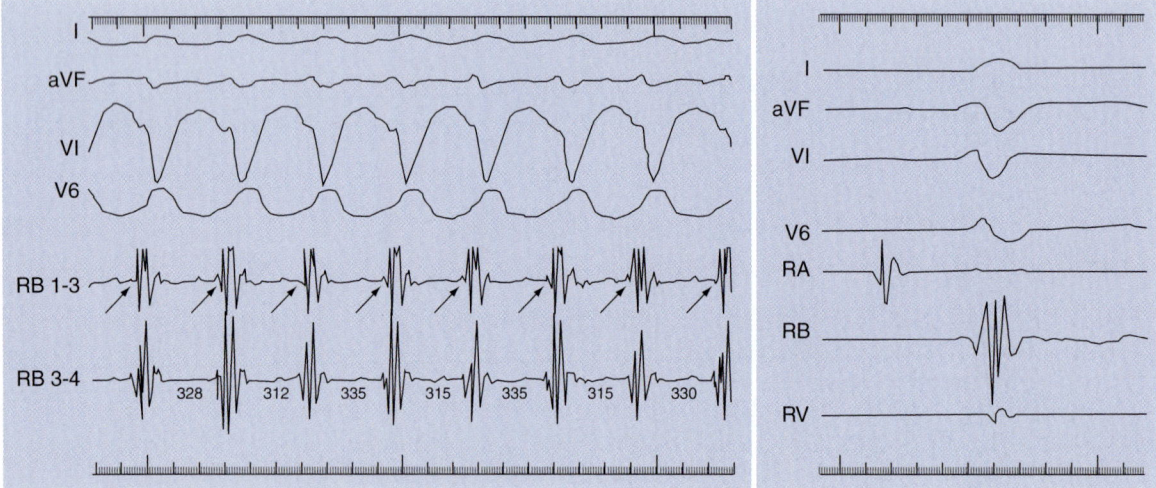

FIGURE 29-8. Inability to record antegrade right bundle potential in sinus rhythm. In sinus, the *right panel* shows the absence of a His or right bundle (RB) potential. In bundle branch reentry, however, the retrograde conduction is evident by the recording of the RB potential. RV, right ventricle. *(From Wang C-W, Sterba R, Tchou P. Bundle branch reentry ventricular tachycardia with 2 distinct left bundle branch block morphologies. J Cardiovasc Electrophysiol. 1997;8:688-693. With permission.)*

the earliest Purkinje potential preceding the QRS onset (Fig. 29-6).[16] The interval between the Purkinje potential and QRS onset is short.

The target sites for ablation of BBR and related arrhythmias are listed in Table 29-3.

Ablation

Because of the superficial nature of the His-Purkinje system in most patients, standard 4-mm-tip radiofrequency (RF) ablation catheters are sufficient.[12,16,27] The need for cooled ablation systems has not been described. Energy settings of 20 to 60 W with target temperatures of 60°C are reported.[12,16] For ablation of the cordlike RBB, a single RF lesion is usually effective. If the RBB cannot be identified, anatomically guided lesions or a linear ablation line placed perpendicularly to the axis of the RBB distal to the His recording may be effective.[28]

The LBB is infrequently ablated with a single RF lesion, owing to its width of about 1 cm.[7] Ablation of the LBB may require creation of a linear lesion distal to the His bundle that extends from the anterior superior septum, radiographically near the RBB in the right anterior oblique view, to the inferior basal septum. Care must be taken to avoid ablation of the His bundle itself because the LBB can have a very short course. This linear lesion across the left septum may be used to transect both the left anterior and posterior fascicles in patients with BBR and interfascicular reentry.[27] A less extensive line can be directed at the anterior or posterior fascicular regions if ablation of single fibers is ineffective. For ablation in tachycardia, termination and noninducibility should result. In sinus rhythm, complete RBB or LBB develops with successful ablation, although the QRS changes may be subtle in patients with preexisting conduction abnormalities.[27] Electrical axis changes may be the only manifestation of fascicular ablation. Elimination of retrograde V_2H_2 conduction may be used as a marker of successful ablation.[1]

For automatic fascicular tachycardias, successful ablation produces automaticity followed by quiescence.[16] Because automaticity is a feature of heating from any Purkinje tissue, the patient must be rechallenged for inducibility to ensure ablation at the proper site.

After ablation, all patients should be assessed for indications for permanent pacemaker or ICD implantation, based on the status of the residual conduction system and severity of underlying structural heart disease. In addition, VT of myocardial origin may be inducible in 36% to 60% of patients after successful ablation of BBR.[12,16]

100%.[12,16] Recurrence of these arrhythmias appears to be uncommon but has not been thoroughly documented with follow-up testing.[12,16] The long-term prognosis for these patients is more guarded, however, reflecting their underlying heart disease. Of 20 patients treated for BBR or fascicular automatic VT, Lopera and associates[16] reported need for pacing or ICD implantation in 19. Of the 14 patients who required an ICD, 7 (50%) had VT recurrences within 16 months. Five of these patients had VT of myocardial origin inducible at the time of ablation, and the recurrent VTs appeared to be different from the BBR VTs. In this series, cardiac transplantation or death from progressive heart failure occurred in 4 patients.

Clinical Outcomes
Acute and Long-Term Results

In the two largest series reported, the acute success rates for BBR (total, 44 patients), interfascicular reentry (4 patients), and automatic fascicular tachycardia (2 patients) were all

Complications

The most common complication of ablation for BBR is high-grade AV block, which is reported to occur in 10% to 30% of patients after successful ablation.[16,27] In a recent series of 20 patients with BBR VT, 15 patients had per-

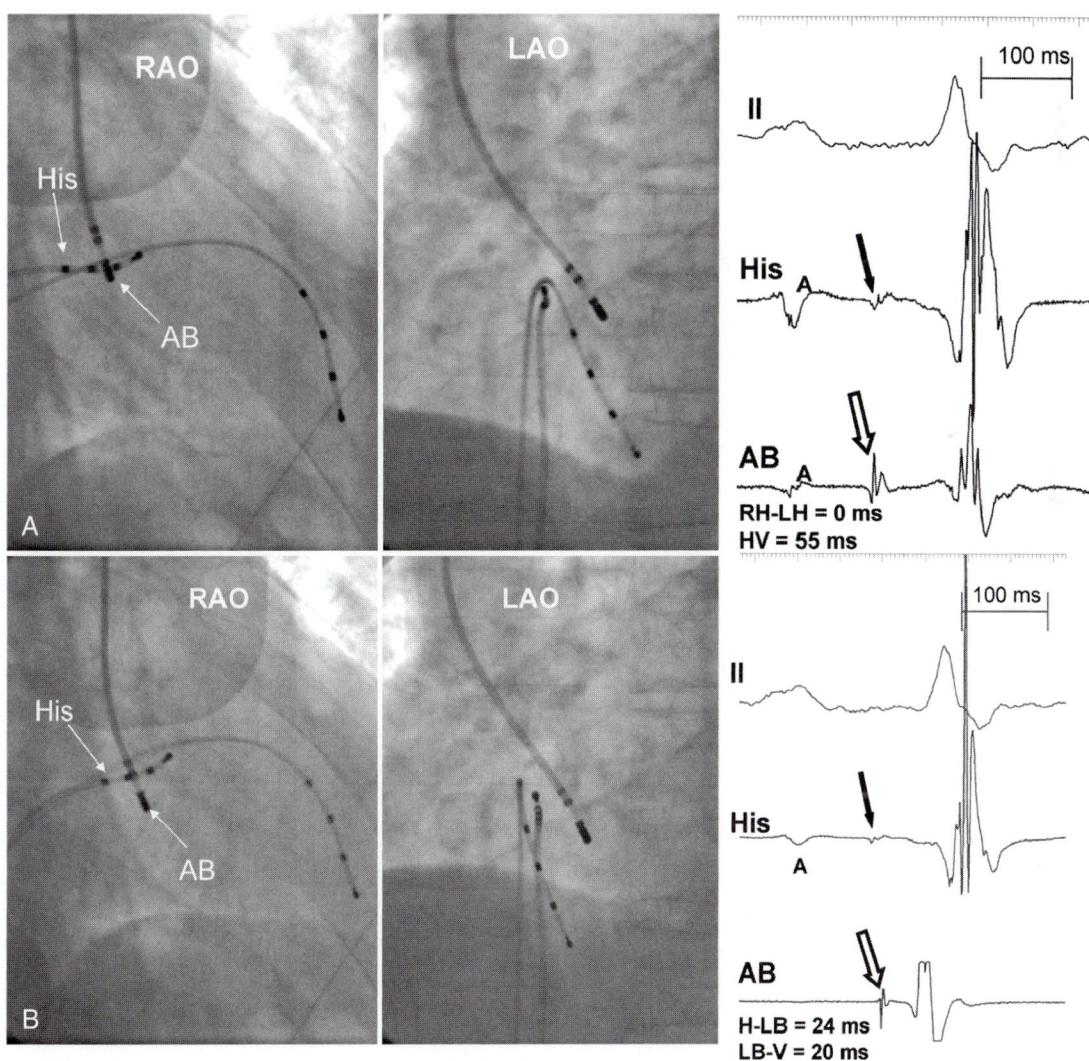

FIGURE 29-9. Recording potentials from the left-sided conduction system. **A,** His recording from the left ventricle. The *far right panel* shows the electrograms from the right-sided His catheter and the ablation catheter in the left ventricle. Note the proximity of the distal ablation electrodes to the His catheter, the equal timing of the left-sided (LH, *open arrow*) and right-sided (RH, *solid arrow*) His potentials, and the small atrial electrogram on the ablation recording. **B,** Left bundle branch recording. By advancing the ablation catheter slightly, toward the apex, the left bundle potential (*open arrow*) is identified by a timing interval 24 msec after the right-sided His recording (*solid arrow*). Note the absence of an atrial electrogram on the ablation recording.

Continued

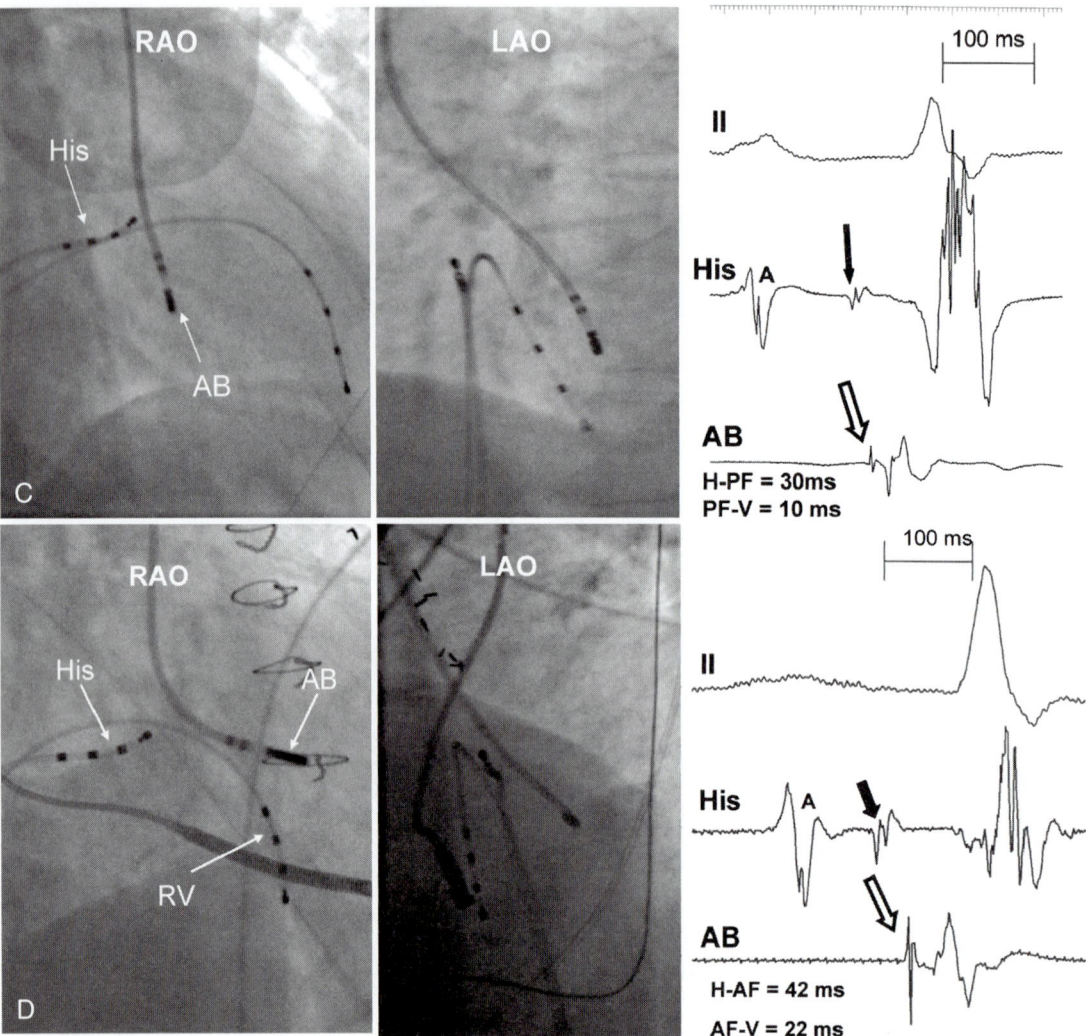

FIGURE 29-9, cont'd. C, Left posterior fascicle recording. Advancing the ablation catheter toward the inferior septum records a potential from the left posterior fascicular (PF, *open arrow*) system that precedes the local ventricular electrogram by only 10 msec. **D,** This anterior fascicular potential (*solid arrow*) is recorded directly apical from the His catheter in the mid-septum. This patient has an implantable cardioverter-defibrillator lead in the right ventricle. A, atrium; AB, ablation catheter; AF, anterior fascicular potential; H, His bundle electrogram; LAO, left anterior oblique; LB, left bundle; RAO, right anterior oblique; V, ventricle.

manent pacemakers or ICDs at the time of ablation, and 2 of the remaining 5 patients had indications for ICD implantation after ablation due to myocardial VTs.[16] Only 2 patients underwent pacemaker implantation alone for impaired AV conduction. Otherwise, complications have not been reported in the largest series of patients, but of course they may include the usual problems resulting from vascular access and left ventricular mapping.[12,16]

Troubleshooting the Difficult Case

Problems with ablation of BBR VT are relatively uncommon and are listed in Table 29-4. Noninducibility is rarely a problem and can be addressed by infusing catecholamines or procainamide, by using short-long-short pacing protocols, and by left ventricular pacing. Inability to record electrograms from the targeted bundle branch can be overcome by mapping in VT or echo beats or by anatomically guided ablation attempts. Linear lesions are

usually needed to ablate the left bundle and the left fascicles. The risk for high-grade AV block after ablation should be assessed by a thorough conduction study before ablation. Intramyocardial VTs induced during testing may require additional ablation or other forms of management. After ablation, the need for a pacemaker or ICD should be considered for all patients.

Right Ventricular Dysplasia (Cardiomyopathy)

Right ventricular dysplasia (RVD) is a sporadically occurring or hereditary condition involving primarily the right ventricle.[29,30] In this condition, portions of the right ventricle are replaced by fibrous or fatty tissue, or both. Focal inflammation and necrosis can be seen at histologic study. The interventricular septum and left ventricle may also show involvement. The involvement of the right ventricle

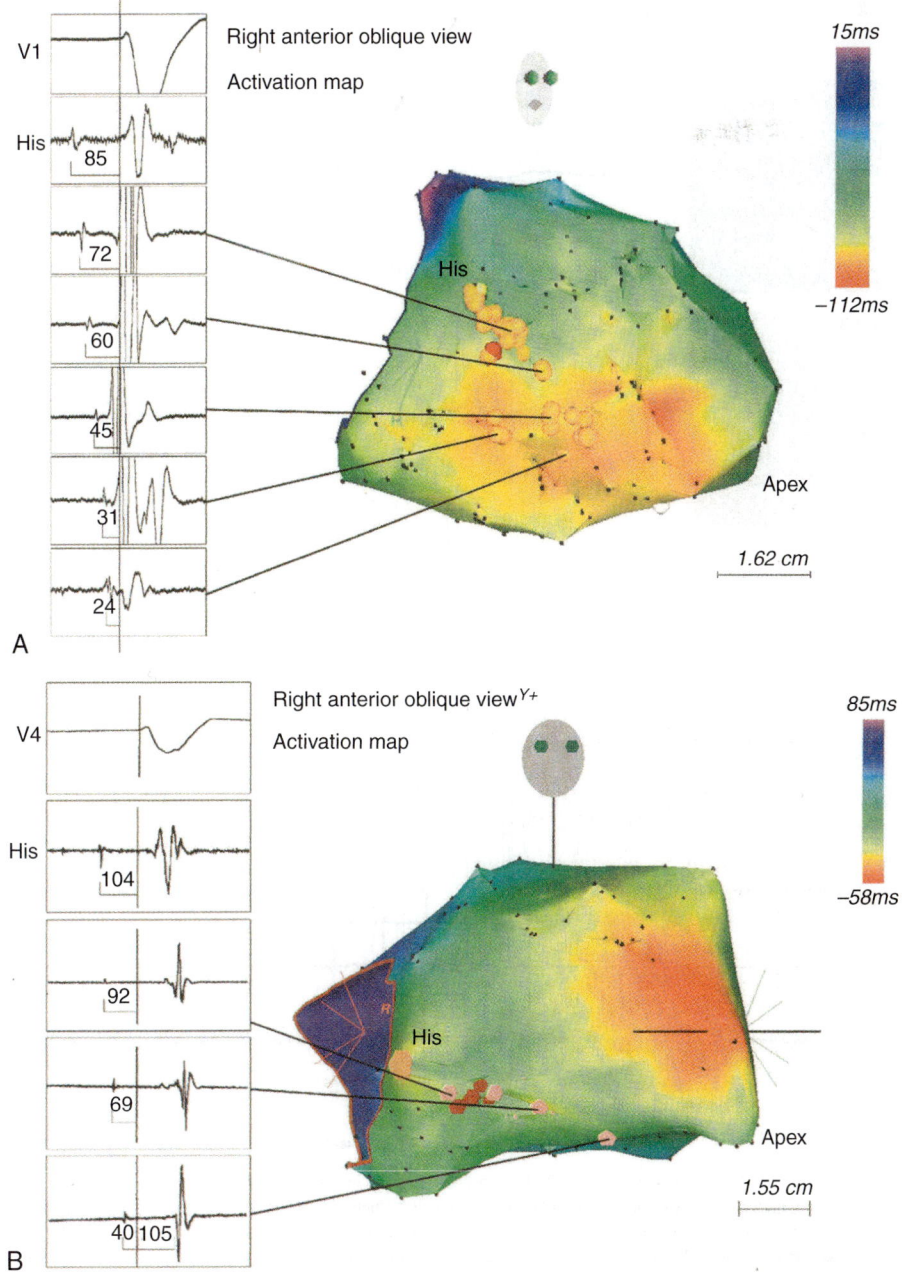

FIGURE 29-10. A, Electroanatomic map of the left ventricle during sinus rhythm in a patient with complete left bundle branch block (QRS duration, 135 msec). Color bar indicates onset of local ventricular activation relative to reference lead V₁ on the surface electrocardiogram (ECG), from –112 msec *(red)* to 15 msec *(purple).* Sites with *orange tags* indicate the left-sided conduction system presenting as a short, sharp, high-frequency, low-amplitude potential preceding ventricular activation *(left box).* The His bundle is depicted by *orange tags* recorded from the noncoronary aortic sinus. Note the absence of Purkinje activation in the area of the left anterior fascicular Purkinje fiber and slow conduction over the left bundle branch (His bundle activation to the latest Purkinje activation in the left posterior fiber is 61 msec). Earliest left ventricular activation is at the site of latest left posterior fascicle potentials, indicating intact antegrade left bundle conduction. *Dark red tag* indicates site of successful ablation of the left bundle branch. **B,** Electroanatomic map of the left ventricle during sinus rhythm in a patient with left bundle branch block (QRS duration, 225 msec). Color bar indicates onset of local ventricular activation relative to reference lead V₄ on the surface ECG, from –58 msec *(red)* to 85 msec *(purple).* The sites with *pink tags* indicate the left-sided conduction system. The His bundle is depicted by the two *orange tags* recorded from the noncoronary aortic sinus. Note again the absence Purkinje activation was recorded in the area of the left anterior fascicular Purkinje fiber and slow conduction (64 msec) over the left bundle. The earliest activation *(red)* of the left ventricle at the apical portion of the left septum is about 3 cm away from the sites with latest Purkinje potentials, which indicates left ventricular activation through a transseptal route and the absence of antegrade left bundle conduction. *Dark red tags* indicate site of successful ablation. *(From Schmidt B, Tang M, Chun KR, et al. Left bundle branch-Purkinje system in patients with bundle branch reentrant tachycardia: lessons from catheter ablation and electroanatomic mapping. Heart Rhythm. 2009;6:51-58. With permission.)*

TABLE 29-3

TARGETS FOR ABLATION OF BUNDLE BRANCH REENTRY AND RELATED TACHYCARDIAS

Bundle Branch Reentry

RBB usual primary target

LBB

Bundle Branch Reentry and Interfascicular VT

RBB and left anterior or posterior fascicle

Both left anterior and posterior fascicles

Interfascicular Reentry Tachycardia

Left anterior or posterior fascicle

Automatic Fascicular Tachycardia

Site of earliest Purkinje potential associated with tachycardia

LBB, left bundle branch; RBB, right bundle branch; VT, ventricular tachycardia.

is usually concentrated in the anterior infundibulum and basilar inferior walls.[31] The dysplastic areas of right ventricular involvement can best be imaged by magnetic resonance imaging (MRI) or right ventriculography.[29,32]

Anatomy and Pathophysiology

VTs are common in RVD because of the extensive myocardial fibrosis that provides the substrate for reentry.[29,30] Most patients demonstrate LBBB morphology VT, and most have multiple VT morphologies, either spontaneous or inducible.[31–42] RBBB VT may indicate left ventricular involvement or a left septal breakthrough site. At electrophysiology study, patients with RVD have very high rates of inducible VT, and the induction is highly reproducible as well. Both clinical and nonclinical VTs are usually initiated by programmed stimulation.[41] Up to 12 VT morphologies have been reported in a single patient.[35] In the electrophysiology laboratory, VTs in patients with RVD share many features with VTs in patients with coronary artery disease.

These features include response to entrainment reflecting a reentrant mechanism in most patients.[31] Right ventricular endocardial mapping typically demonstrates extensive areas of low-voltage electrograms around the tricuspid and pulmonary valve annuli, free wall, inferior wall, and inferior septum.[31–41] Late potentials are often seen in sinus rhythm.

Diagnosis and Differential Diagnosis

The diagnostic criteria for RVD are listed in Table 29-5.[29] VTs associated with RVD must be differentiated from other etiologies of LBBB tachycardias. VT related to RVD may be confused with right ventricular outflow tract tachycardia due to the LBBB morphology in the setting of normal left ventricular function. Features distinguishing between these two conditions are listed in Table 29-6.[32] The diagnosis of RVD is usually made by clinical findings outside the electrophysiology laboratory, but right ventriculography in the laboratory may be an important maneuver.[32] RVD must also be differentiated from cardiac sarcoidosis. Common to both conditions are multiple inducible VT morphologies, peritricuspid annular scar, and reentry around the tricuspid annulus.[42]

Mapping and Ablation

Mapping of VT related to RVD is largely analogous to mapping of VT in coronary artery disease (Table 29-7).[31–42] Because of the reliable and reproducible inducibility of VT, entrainment and activation mapping are commonly employed.[31–42] Electroanatomic mapping is useful to define areas of scar and low-voltage electrograms as well as to delineate reentry circuits and critical isthmuses of conduction. Focal activation patterns are found in up to one third of VTs; however, these arrhythmias still demonstrate reentry mechanisms.[42] Activation mapping demonstrates earliest ventricular electrograms averaging 38 to 112 milliseconds before QRS onset.[32] With entrainment mapping, the classic

TABLE 29-4

TROUBLESHOOTING THE DIFFICULT CASE OF BUNDLE BRANCH REENTRY ABLATION

Problem	Cause	Solution
Unable to record RBB	RBB intramyocardial or local scarring	Map/ablate LBB Anatomically guided ablation RBB
	Complete antegrade RBBB	Map/ablate in VT or during echo beats
Unable to ablate LBB	Broad band or multiple fibers	Linear ablation across LBB or both anterior and posterior fascicles
VT noninducible	Intermittent complete bidirectional BBB Insufficient conduction slowing	Facilitate conduction with isoproterenol Slow conduction with class IA agent (e.g., procainamide)
VT inducible after successful bundle branch ablation	Interfascicular reentry Automatic fascicular tachycardia Intramyocardial tachycardia Initial diagnosis incorrect	Ablate left anterior or posterior fascicle Ablate automatic focus Map/ablate VT or treat with ICD if appropriate Review differential diagnosis
Risk for AV block with ablation	Diffuse conduction system disease	Ablate bundle with worst conduction status Evaluate indication for pacemaker/ICD after ablation

AV, atrioventricular; BBB, bundle branch block; ICD, implantable cardioverter-defibrillator; LBB, left bundle branch; RBB(B), right bundle branch (block); VT, ventricular tachycardia.

TABLE 29-5

DIAGNOSTIC CRITERIA FOR RIGHT VENTRICULAR DYSPLASIA*

Cardiac Dysfunction and Structural Alterations

Major

Severe RV dilation or reduction RV ejection fraction with minimal or no LV impairment

Localized RV aneurysms

Severe segmental RV dilation

Minor

Mild global RV dilation or reduction in RV ejection fraction with normal LV function

Mild segmental RV dilation

Regional RV hypokinesis

Tissue Characterization of Wall

Major

Fibrofatty replacement of myocardium on endomyocardial biopsy

Repolarization Abnormalities

Minor

Inverted T waves in right precordial leads (V_2-V_3) with age >12 yr and in absence of right bundle branch block

Depolarization Abnormalities

Major

Epsilon waves or localized prolongation (>110 msec) of the QRS in right precordial leads (V_1-V_3)

Minor

Late potentials on signal-averaged ECG

Arrhythmias

Minor

Left bundle branch type ventricular tachycardia, sustained or nonsustained

Frequent ventricular extrasystoles (>1000/24 hr)

Family History

Major

Familial disease confirmed at necropsy or surgery

Minor

Family history of premature sudden death (<35 yr old) due to suspected RV dysplasia

Family history of clinical diagnosis

*Diagnosis requires the presence of two major, one major plus two minor, or four minor criteria.
ECG, electrocardiogram; LV, left ventricle; RV, right ventricle.
From Marcus F, Towbin JA, Zareba W, et al. Arrhythmogenic right ventricular dysplasia/cardiomyopathy (ARVD/C): a multidisciplinary study—design and protocol. *Circulation*. 2003;107:2975-2978.

TABLE 29-6

DIFFERENTIATING RIGHT VENTRICULAR DYSPLASIA FROM RIGHT VENTRICULAR OUTFLOW TRACT TACHYCARDIA*

Feature	RVD (N = 17)	RVOT Tachycardia (N = 33)
Epsilon wave or QRS >110 msec	30%	0%
Right precordial T-wave inversion	36%	0%
Family history of arrhythmias	53%	0%
VT mechanism in electrophysiology laboratory	Reentry	Automatic or triggered
Number of VT morphologies	Average, 1.8; range, 1-6	Single
Any major criteria for RVD	41%	0%
Any minor criteria for RVD	41%	3%
Major abnormalities on cardiac MRI	88%	6%
Minor abnormalities on MRI	12%	48%

*The values indicate the percentage of patients in each group demonstrating the study feature.
MRI, magnetic resonance imaging; RVD, right ventricular dysplasia; RVOT, right ventricular outflow tract; VT, ventricular tachycardia.
From O'Donnell D, Cox D, Bourke J, et al. Clinical and electrophysiologic differences between patients with arrhythmogenic right ventricular dysplasia and right ventricular outflow tract tachycardia. *Eur Heart J.* 2003;24:801-810, 2003.

TABLE 29-7

ABLATION TARGETS FOR VENTRICULAR TACHYCARDIA ASSOCIATED WITH NONISCHEMIC CARDIOMYOPATHIES (EXCLUDING BUNDLE BRANCH REENTRY)

Sites of earliest presystolic ventricular activation

Sites of concealed entrainment in tachycardia

- S-QRS–EGM-QRS < 20 msec
- PPI–TCL < 30 msec
- Concealed entrainment

Pace map sites with ≥10/12 lead match

Sites of continuous diastolic electrical activity

Sites of late potentials occurring after surface QRS

Electrical isthmuses defined by electroanatomic mapping for unstable VT

EGM-QRS, electrogram-QRS interval; PPI, postpacing interval; S-QRS, stimulus-QRS interval; TCL, tachycardia cycle length; VT, ventricular tachycardia.

entrance, exit, inner loop, outer loop, and bystander sites are identifiable.[31] The critical isthmus for identifiable reentry circuits invariably occurs between areas of scar or between scars and the tricuspid or pulmonic valves (Fig. 29-11).[36-42] Reentry circulating around the tricuspid valve as occurs with sarcoidosis has been described.[42] For unstable VTs, linear ablation between scars or from scar to other anatomic barriers (often tricuspid valve) at sites of satis-

factory pace-mapping is useful (Fig. 29-12).[36] Ablation is performed with standard 4-mm-tip ablation catheters or with irrigated catheters. Despite the frequency of epicardial involvement histologically, epicardial ablation is rarely reported.[36]

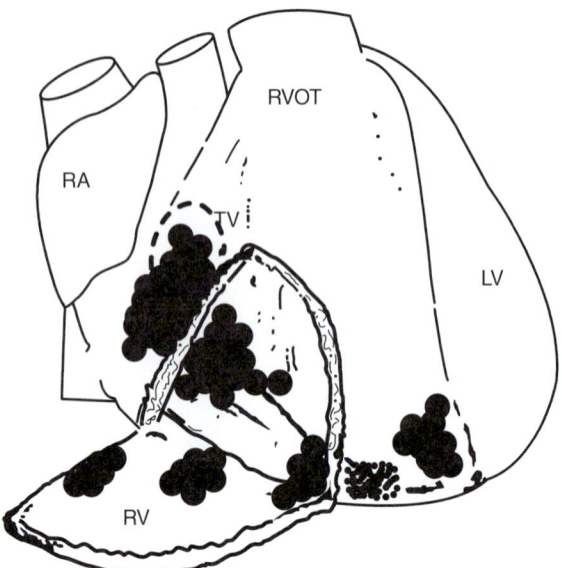

FIGURE 29-11. Location of 67 ventricular tachycardia (VT) ablations in 32 patients with right ventricular dysplasia. Most VTs arise near the tricuspid valve. LV, left ventricle; RA, right atrium; RV, right ventricle; RVOT, right ventricular outflow tract; TV, tricuspid valve. *(From Yao Y, Zhang S, Sheng D, et al. Radiofrequency ablation of the ventricular tachycardia with arrhythmogenic right ventricular cardiomyopathy using non-contact mapping.* Pacing Clin Electrophysiol. *2007;30:526-533. With permission.)*

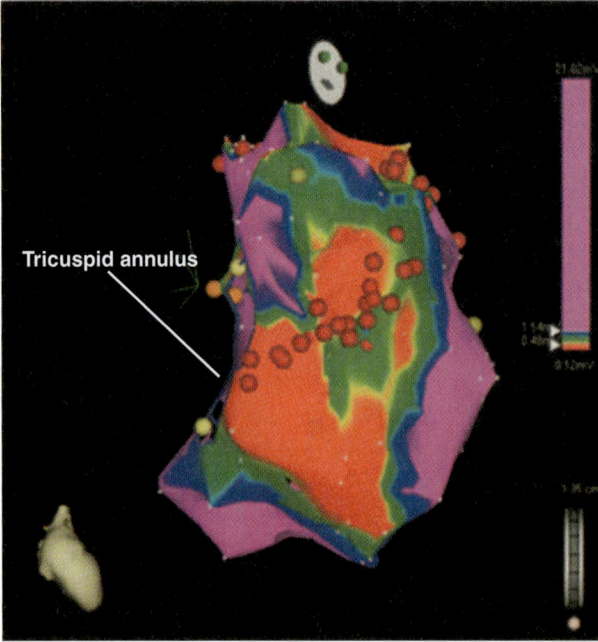

FIGURE 29-12. Right anterior oblique caudal electroanatomic map of right ventricle in a patient with ventricular tachycardia due to sarcoidosis. Areas of normal myocardial voltage are shown in *purple.* A linear lesion delivered (*red dots*) across islands of scar and to the tricuspid annulus rendered the patient's arrhythmia noninducible. *(From Verma A, Kilicaslan F, Schweikert R, et al. Short- and long -term success of substrate-based mapping and ablation of ventricular tachycardia in arrhythmogenic right ventricular dysplasia.* Circulation. *2005;111:3209-3216.)*

Clinical Outcomes

The clinical experience with catheter ablation of VT related to RVD is given in Table 29-8. Notable from this experience are the multiple VT morphologies inducible in

most patients and the high recurrence rates. Acute success, usually defined as absence of any inducible VT, is typically 70% to 80%. Recurrence of new or previously ablated VTs is usually more than 40% at 2 to 3 years despite continued antiarrhythmic drug therapy.[37–42] Death and cardiac tamponade have been reported with RVD ablation.[35,37,39]

In summary, catheter ablation is considered palliative or adjunctive therapy in patients with RVD. Most patients remain on drug therapy or have an ICD implanted after ablation because of incomplete elimination of VTs, recurrent VT, or concerns for the progressive nature of the disease process.

Dilated Cardiomyopathy

Anatomy and Pathophysiology

Sustained monomorphic VT is an uncommon clinical finding in patients with dilated cardiomyopathy (DCM) and is infrequently induced at electrophysiologic studies.[43] Primarily for these reasons, the clinical experience with catheter ablation of VT in patients with DCM is very limited. The electrophysiologic substrate for VT in DCM appears to be heterogeneous.[43] Scarring is common and occurs as endocardial plaques and patchy areas of interstitial fibrosis.[43] In addition, variable degrees of myofiber disarray, hypertrophy, and atrophy are common. The potential mechanisms for VT in this substrate include reentry and triggered VT.[43] At electrophysiologic study, patients with DCM demonstrate less frequent abnormal endocardial electrograms than do patients with ischemic cardiomyopathy (Fig. 29-13).[43] In addition, the abnormal electrograms in patients with DCM are less likely to show fragmentation and tend to be concentrated in the basal left ventricular endocardial region. DCM patients also show a higher frequency of abnormal epicardial electrograms than do patients with coronary artery disease.[43]

Mapping and Ablation

Given this wide distribution of abnormal myocardial substrate, VTs in patients with DCM may arise from the left ventricular endocardium, epicardium, middle myocardium, septum, or right ventricle.[44–47] The clinical experience with mapping of VTs in this patient group is very limited but has used activation mapping, pace-mapping, and entrainment mapping as the inducibility, duration, and tolerance of the VTs have allowed (Table 29-7). The reports on ablation of these arrhythmias contain small numbers of selected DCM patients.[44–46] Kottkamp and colleagues[44] attempted ablation for 9 VTs in 8 DCM patients with incessant or frequent monomorphic VTs that were reproducibly induced at testing. With the use of activation, pace, and entrainment mapping, the acute success rate was 66%, with a recurrence rate of 66%. Of 7 patients reported by Wilber and coworkers,[45] entrainment, pace, and activation mapping resulted in ablation of VT in 3 patients who had reproducible sustained arrhythmias but in none of the 4 patients with apparent non-reentrant mechanisms. The largest series was reported by Soejima and associates.[46] Of 28 DCM patients with a history of recurrent sustained monomorphic VT, most had endocardial or epicardial scar

TABLE 29-8

ABLATION OF RIGHT VENTRICULAR DYSPLASIA

Study	No. of Patients	No. of VTs	Mapping Techniques	Acute Success Rate	Complications	Recurrence Rate	Comments
Reithmann et al, 2003[34]	5	1 clinical each, 1–2 inducible	Electroanatomic and entrainment	80% for clinical VTs	None	40% at 7 ± 3 mo	Nonclinical VTs not targeted
Ellison et al, 1998[31]	5	3.8 average	Entrainment	42% of all morphologies	None	0% at 11–24 mo	All inducible VTs targeted
O'Donnell et al, 2003[32]	17	1.8 average; range, 1–6	Activation and entrainment	41% of patients noninducible	None	47% after 56 mo average (range, 13–92 mo)	Results compared with RVOT VT patients
Harada et al, 1998[33]	7	8 VTs in 7 patients	Entrainment	100%	None	0% after 19 ± 7 mo	1 patient with chemical ablation
Fontaine et al, 2000[35]	50	1–12 per patient	Not given	46% noninducible	2 deaths, 2 tamponade, 1 hemopericardium after DC ablation	54% after 5.4 yr average	DC ablation for patients failing RF
Marchlinski et al, 2004[36]	19	3.7 VT per patient	Electroanatomic and pace mapping	74% patients non-inducible with ≥ 1 procedure	None	16% after 27 ± 22 mo	Left ventricular mapping in 18 patients, 68% patients with repeat procedures
Verma et al, 2005[37]	22	3 ± 2	Electroanatomic and pace mapping	82% patients non-inducible	1 tamponade	47% at 3 years	Ablation to encircle scar 13 patients
Riethman et al, 2008[38]	11	23 VT in 11 patients	Entrainment and Stim-QRS >40 msec	9/11 patients	None	45% at 27 ± 17 mo	Target only stable MMVT
Dalal et al, 2007[39]	24	77% patients with ≥2 VTs	Pace, activation, entrainment, and electroanatomic	46% of all VTs, 31% clinical VT only	1 death	96% at 32 + 36 mo	4 mm tip only, recurrence rate same for repeat ablations
Satomi et al, 2006[40]	17	1.5 ± 0.8; range 1–4	Activation, electroanatomic, pace, entrainment	88% with no inducible MMVT	Not reported	4/17 patients at 26 ± 15 mo	Unstable VTs in 9 patients all ablated
Yao et al, 2007[41]	32	67 VT in 32 patients	Noncontact activation and entrainment	75%	None	10/32 at 3 mo	Noncontact mapping
Miljoen et al, 2005[42]	11	12	Electroanatomic and activation only	75% noninducible	None	50% successfully ablated VTs at 9–50 mo	Reentry around TV in 5 patients, only stable VTs targeted

DC, direct current; MMVT, monomorphic ventricular tachycardia; RF, radiofrequency energy; RVOT, right ventricular outflow tract; VT, ventricular tachycardia.

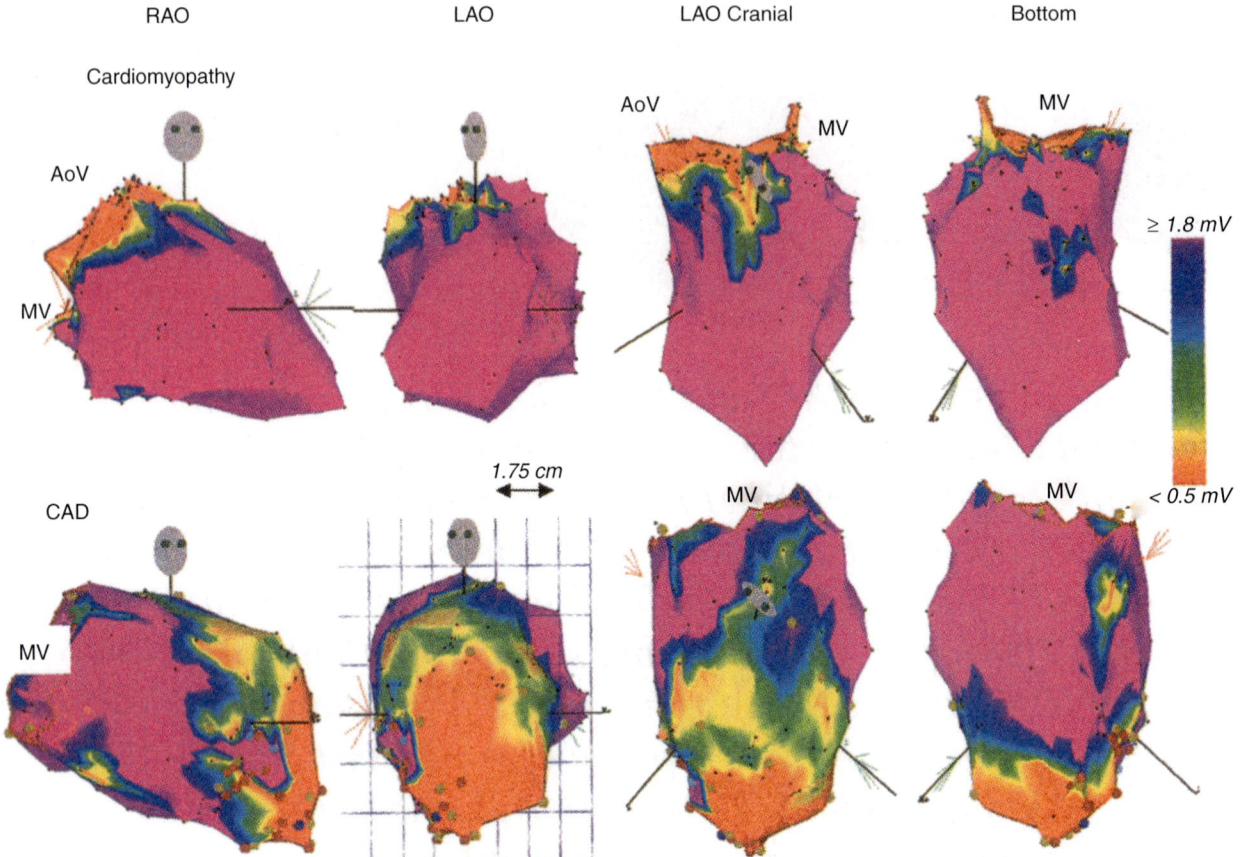

FIGURE 29-13. Distribution of abnormal left ventricular endocardial electrograms in patients with sustained tachycardia and idiopathic dilated cardiomyopathy (cardiomyopathy, *top*) and ischemic cardiomyopathy (coronary artery disease [CAD], *bottom*). Multiple views are shown. Normal voltages (>1.8 mV) are shown in *purple*, and scar (<0.5 mV) is shown in *red*. In the dilated cardiomyopathy patient, the small area of scar and abnormal electrogram voltages is confined to the base of the left ventricle near the mitral valves (MV) and aortic valves (AoV). In contrast, the patient with ischemic cardiomyopathy demonstrates an extensive apical scar over the anterior, septal, and posterior segments. LAO, left anterior oblique; RAO, right anterior oblique. *(From Hsia HH, Marchlinski FE. Characterization of the electroanatomic substrate for monomorphic ventricular tachycardia in patients with nonischemic cardiomyopathy. Pacing Clin Electrophysiol. 2002;25:1114-1127. With permission.)*

by electroanatomic mapping (20 and 7 patients, respectively). Virtually all patients had ICDs implanted before or after the ablation procedure. The endocardial scars were most frequently near a valve annulus. For stable sustained VT, entrainment and activation mapping were employed. For hemodynamically unstable VT, pace-mapping and substrate mapping were used to define potential exit sites. Electroanatomic mapping, entrainment mapping, and pace-mapping identified 19 VT circuit isthmuses in 22 patients with intramyocardial reentry. Five patients had automatic VTs, and 2 had BBR. An epicardial isthmus was found in 7 patients and an endocardial isthmus location in 12 patients with myocardial reentry (Fig. 29-14). Ablation was performed using an irrigated-tip or 8-mm-tip catheter if initial attempts with a 4-mm-tip electrode failed. Seventy-three VTs were induced in the 22 patients. An average of 18 ± 9 lesions were delivered to endocardial ablation sites and 11 ± 8 to endocardial sites. No serious complications occurred. All VTs were ablated in 12 (54%) of 22 patients, and VT induction was modified in 4 patients (18%). Only 54% of patients were free of VT recurrence after follow-up of 348 ± 345 days. The limited acute success rate was believed to be the result of a high incidence of intramyocardial reentry circuits.

Delayed-enhancement MRI demonstrates ventricular scar in about 50% of patients with nonischemic cardiomyopathy. The location of this scar may be a guide to mapping of ventricular arrhythmias.[48] In patients with predominantly intramyocardial scar, catheter ablation appears ineffective. In contrast, endocardial scar on MRI is associated with successful ablation from the endocardial approach, whereas epicardial scar is associated with successful epicardial ablation. Problems and potential solutions during ablation of VT in nonischemic cardiomyopathy are given in Table 29-9.

These studies suggest that scar-related reentry is the mechanism underlying sustained monomorphic VT in many patients with DCM. Automatic VT and BBR are not uncommon, however. Multiple VT morphologies are usually induced at electrophysiologic testing.[45] Preprocedural MRI may guide ablation to endocardial or epicardial sites.[48] Electroanatomic mapping is useful to define the regions of scar and to direct pace mapping and entrainment mapping.[46] Large-tip or irrigated-tip catheters are sometimes necessary for successful ablation.[46] Epicardial mapping and ablation is an important technique for many DCM patients.[46] Hemodynamically unstable VTs may be addressed by pace-mapping or noncontact mapping and can respond to substrate modification.[46] The limited acute

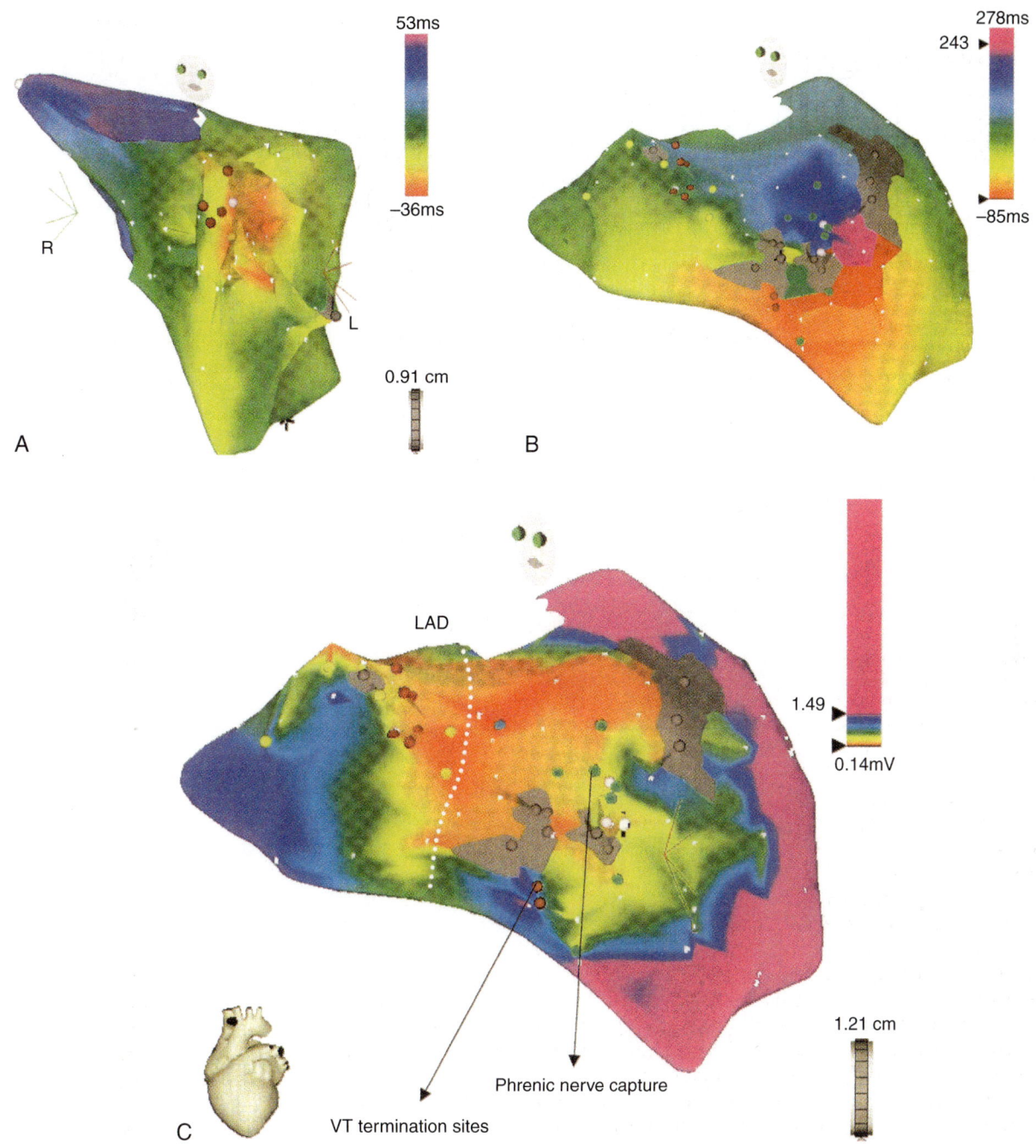

FIGURE 29-14. Endocardial (**A**) and epicardial (**B**) left ventricular activation maps from a patient with dilated cardiomyopathy and sustained ventricular tachycardia (VT). The earliest sites (*red*) in the endocardial map (**A**) are discrete, suggesting a focal origin. Ablation at these sites failed to terminate tachycardia. The epicardial map (**B**) was obtained for the same VT and demonstrated a large reentry circuit with a "head-meets-tail" sequence. The *green tags* represent areas of phrenic nerve stimulation with pacing. **C,** Epicardial voltage map from the same patient with normal voltages (>1.5 mV) shown in *purple* and scar (<0.14 mV) in *red*. The voltage map identified an isthmus between dense scars (*gray*). The VT was terminated by a line of radiofrequency lesions from the dense scar across the exit site and into the area of normal myocardial voltage. LAD, left anterior descending artery; R, right. *(From Soejima K, Stevenson WG, Sapp L, et al. Endocardial and epicardial radiofrequency ablation of ventricular tachycardia associated with dilated cardiomyopathy.* J Am Coll Cardiol. *2004;43:1834-1842. With permission.)*

success rate possibly reflects an epicardial or intramyocardial circuit in many patients.

Chagas Disease

Chagas disease is a major cause of cardiac disease in Latin America and is being recognized in North America as

well, owing to increasing emigration from endemic areas.[49] The causative organism is *Trypanosoma cruzi*, which is spread by an insect vector. Chronic heart disease develops in 10% to 40% of patients after acute infection and is manifested as DCM, heart failure, bradycardia, tachyarrhythmias, and sudden death. The diagnosis is made based on serologic testing and clinical findings.[49] Classically, patients with chronic chagasic heart disease may have

TABLE 29-9

TROUBLESHOOTING ABLATION FOR VENTRICULAR TACHYCARDIA WITH NONISCHEMIC CARDIOMYOPATHY

Problem	Cause	Solutions
Ventricular tachycardia noninducible	Non-reentrant mechanism	Test on catecholamine infusion, pace mapping, substrate mapping
Ventricular tachycardia hemodynamically unstable	Rapid rate Low ejection fraction, heart failure	Slow rate with procainamide or amiodarone Support with inotropes/pressors, intra-aortic balloon pump, volume repletion, pace mapping or substrate mapping, and ablation
No target sites	Origin in contralateral ventricle, outflow areas or above semilunar valves Epicardial origin Intramyocardial focus	Map contralateral ventricle, outflow areas, or above semilunar valves Map epicardium Consider ethanol ablation

RBBB, ST-segment elevation, and premature ventricular contractions on surface ECG. Left ventricular dilation, systolic dysfunction, and sometimes ventricular segmental aneurysms may be present. Sustained monomorphic VTs occurring in these patients are usually highly reproducible at electrophysiologic testing, suggesting a reentrant mechanism.[50–53] Multiple VT morphologies may be induced in individual patients.[50] Induction of sustained VT has been associated with the presence of conduction disturbances on ECG and left ventricular aneurysms (Fig. 29-15).[51,52] The arrhythmogenic potential of ventricular aneurysms is demonstrated by abolition of VT after surgical aneurysmectomy.[51]

There are limited data on catheter ablation of VTs associated with Chagas disease.[50,52] The largest series has been reported by Tavora and colleagues,[52] who studied 31 patients with a history of sustained VT and chronic Chagas disease. Activation and entrainment mapping were used to identify sites for ablation. Sites with electrograms preceding QRS onset by 30 milliseconds or longer were sought. The VT in all patients was believed to be reentrant in nature. An endocardial site of the reentrant circuit was identified in 70% of cases. Epicardial mapping was not performed. The utility of epicardial mapping in patients with Chagas disease was demonstrated by Sosa and associates.[50] In 10 patients, an epicardial circuit was identified in 14 of 18 inducible VTs (Fig. 29-16). Epicardial ablation was performed in 6 patients. The earliest epicardial sites were 107 ± 60 milliseconds before QRS onset. In 7 patients, epicardial mid-diastolic potentials or continuous activity was seen. Ablation was acutely successful in all patients receiving epicardial ablation, with no recurrences reported after 5 to 9 months of follow-up. In the 4 patients undergoing endocardial ablation, the VT remained inducible. Treatment of Chagas disease VT by chemical ablation has also been reported.[54]

These limited data suggest that ablation for VT associated with Chagas disease may have a limited success rate of about 50%. The ability to perform epicardial mapping and ablation appears important to procedural success. The long-term outcomes after ablation in this patient population are unknown.

Papillary Muscle Ventricular Tachycardia

Ventricular tachycardia originating from the left ventricular papillary muscles may account for 3% of idiopathic ventricular tachycardias[55] and may occur in patients with or without structural heart disease. In the absence of structural heart disease, the tachycardia shows automatic or triggered behavior, and frequent PVCs are more common than sustained ventricular tachycardia. When associated with previous myocardial infarction involving the papillary muscle regions, a reentrant mechanism may be found.[56] The infarct-unrelated arrhythmias originating from the papillary muscles are more commonly nonsustained ectopy (frequent PVCs) than sustained tachycardias. Tachycardias originating from the anterolateral papillary muscle demonstrate a right bundle branch block with inferior axis, whereas those from the posteromedial muscle show a right bundle branch block with superior axis. A precordial lead transition before lead V_4 is common.[56] In most series, the posteromedial muscle is more frequently arrhythmogenic.

Ventricular arrhythmias arising from the papillary muscles must be differentiated from left ventricular fascicular tachycardias.[57] Papillary muscle arrhythmias tend to have a wider QRS (150 ± 15 versus 127 ± 11 milliseconds) and monophasic R or qR patterns in V_1. Fascicular tachycardias have typical right bundle branch block; anterior or posterior fascicular block patterns with Q waves in the limb leads are rarely seen in papillary muscle tachycardias.

At electrophysiologic study, activation or pace-mapping determines the optimal sites for ablation. In the absence of myocardial infarction, the arrhythmias may present with catecholamine infusion but are not initiated with programmed stimulation. Activation mapping reveals local ventricular electrograms preceding QRS onset by up to 34 ± 15 milliseconds.[57] Pace maps can typically reproduce 12-lead morphology at successful ablation sites. The optimal sites for ablation are usually at the base or midportion of the papillary muscle. Intracardiac echocardiography is useful to localize the papillary muscle and to facilitate catheter stability during ablation, which is often difficult to achieve (Fig. 29-17). Alternatively, left ventricular angiography may allow visualization of the papillary muscles

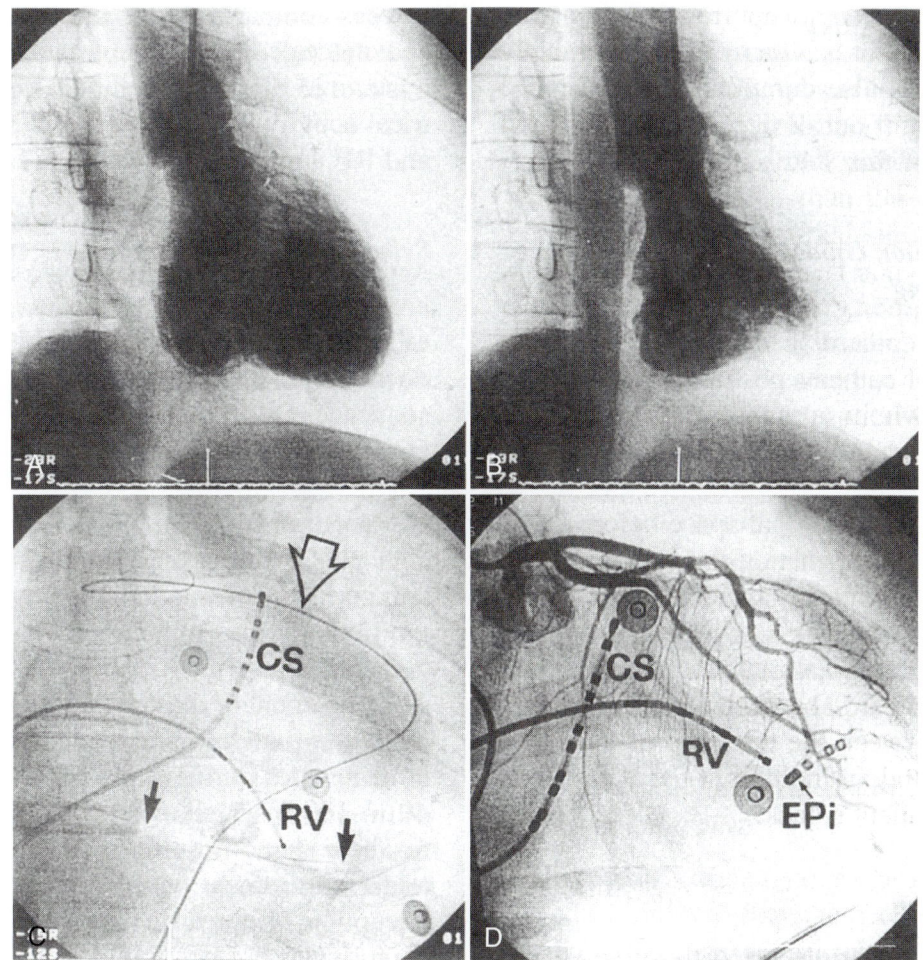

FIGURE 29-15. Right ventricular venography and catheter positions during mapping of ventricular tachycardia in a patient with Chagas disease. Right anterior oblique projection right ventriculogram in systole (**A**) and diastole (**B**) showing characteristic inferolateral ventricular aneurysm. **C,** Guidewire (*large open arrow*) introduced percutaneously into the pericardial space for epicardial mapping. The *small black arrows* show radiographic contrast injected percutaneously to visualize the pericardial space. **D,** With the epicardial mapping catheter (EPi) at a potential ablation site, coronary angiography is performed to evaluate the risk for coronary artery injury from the radiofrequency energy. CS, coronary sinus catheter; RV, right ventricular endocardial catheter. *(From Sosa E, Scanavacca M, D'Avila A, et al. Endocardial and epicardial ablation guided by nonsurgical transthoracic epicardial mapping to treat recurrent ventricular tachycardia.* J Cardiovasc Electrophysiol. *1998;9:229–239.)*

(Fig. 29-17). High-energy radiofrequency deliveries with irrigated ablation systems are required for consistent success.[55,58] Even so, the recurrence rates may be 60% in small series, and complete elimination of all ectopies may be uncommon. Up to three morphologies of ventricular ectopy may arise from a single papillary muscle.

Sarcoidosis

Sarcoidosis is a multisystem disease characterized by non-caseating granuloma formation in the involved tissues, including the heart in 20% to 30% of cases at autopsy. Cardiac sarcoidosis accounted for 8% of monomorphic ventricular tachycardias in patients with nonischemic cardiomyopathies at a large referral center.[59] At electrophysiologic study, these patients typically had multiple (4 ± 2) morphologies of inducible ventricular arrhythmias.[59] These arrhythmias show characteristics of reentry in most cases and are amenable to activation, pace, or entrainment mapping.[59–61]

Endocardial mapping in sinus rhythm typically demonstrates areas of slow conduction and low electrogram voltage amplitude in the right ventricular free wall and septum as well as along the annulus of the tricuspid valve (Fig. 29-18). Low-amplitude left ventricular endocardial electrograms were described in the inferior and basal areas.[59] Both left and right bundle branch block morphology tachycardias can be induced. Epicardial mapping may be necessary in some patients.[60] Jefic and associates[60] described that the single most common reentry location for VT was the tricuspid annulus, allowing for reentry around this structure. Peritricuspid VTs displayed a left bundle branch block morphology and either a superior or inferior axis. Ablation was successful for this arrhythmia by connecting ablation lines across areas of low voltage with good pace maps to the tricuspid annulus.[60] Both irrigated and nonirrigated catheters have been used.[59,60] Ablation eliminated about 70% of VTs with 50% rates of recurrence.[59,60] The intramyocardial location of granulomas may contribute to the inaccessibility to endocardial and epicardial ablation.

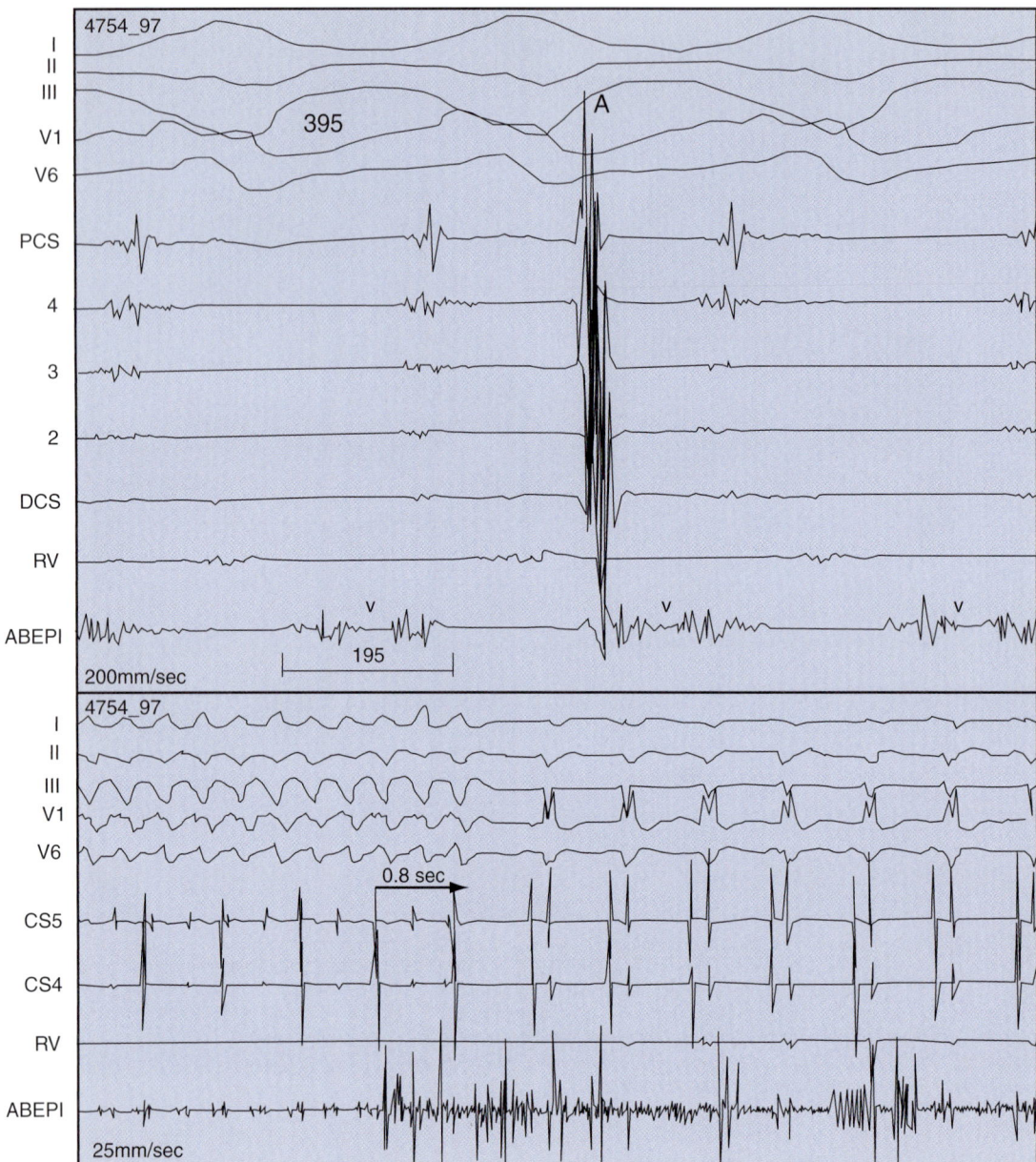

FIGURE 29-16. Epicardial activation mapping during sustained ventricular tachycardia from a patient with Chagas disease. The *top five tracings* on each panel are surface electrocardiogram leads. *Top panel,* The epicardial ablation electrogram precedes the QRS onset by 195 msec, and there is continuous electrical activity throughout diastole. The tachycardia cycle length is 395 msec. *Bottom panel,* Radiofrequency energy delivered to this site terminated the tachycardia in 0.8 second. 4-2, proximal to distal coronary sinus bipoles; A, atrial electrogram; ABEPI, epicardial ablation catheter; CS, coronary sinus; DCS, distal coronary sinus; PCS, proximal coronary sinus; RV, right ventricle; V, ventricular electrogram. *(From Sosa E, Scanavacca M, D'Avila A, et al. Endocardial and epicardial ablation guided by nonsurgical transthoracic epicardial mapping to treat recurrent ventricular tachycardia. J Cardiovasc Electrophysiol. 1998;9:229-239. With permission.)*

Valvular Heart Disease

Sustained monomorphic VT has been described in 4% of patients undergoing aortic or mitral valve surgery in the absence of myocardial infarction or congenital heart disease.[62] Monomorphic VT within 30 days of surgery is frequently noninducible or due to bundle branch reentry. In patients with VT late (1 to 16 years) after surgery, multiple VTs are often inducible and are due to scar-related reentry. The scar is typically periannular, with successful ablation sites concentrated in these areas. Electroanatomic, pace-mapping, and entrainment techniques result in ablation of 98% of VTs. Recurrent VT has been reported in 25% of patients.[62]

Miscellaneous

A series of case reports for the ablation of VT associated with miscellaneous etiologies of heart disease, including hypertrophic cardiomyopathy, are described in Table 29-10.[63–67]

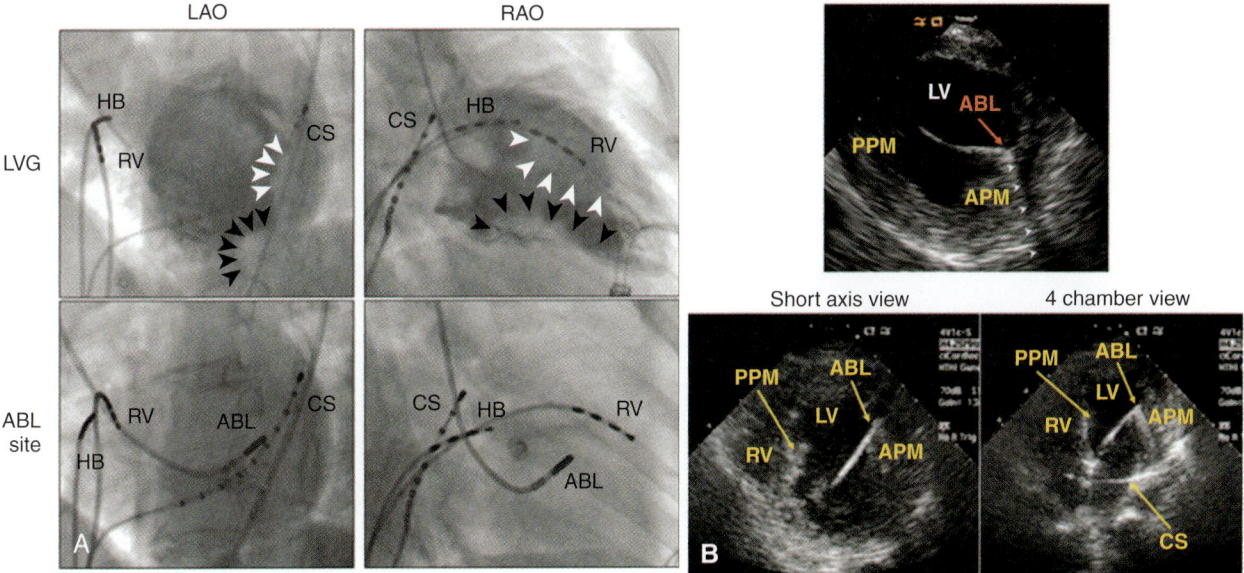

FIGURE 29-17. A, The *top figures* show fluoroscopic views of left ventriculograms (LVG), showing the anterior papillary muscle (*white arrowheads*) and posterior papillary muscle (*black arrowheads*). The *bottom panels* show ablation (ABL) catheter position for ablation of ventricular tachycardia arising from the midportion of the anterior papillary muscle. **B,** Intracardiac echocardiography images showing the ablation catheter (ABL) in contact with the anterior (APM) and posterior (PPM) papillary muscles. CS, coronary sinus; HB, His bundle catheter, LV, left ventricle, RV, right ventricle. *(From Yamada T, McElderry HT, Okado T, et al. Idiopathic focal ventricular arrhythmias originating from the anterior papillary muscle in the left ventricle.* J Cardiovasc Electrophysiol. *2009;20:866-872. With permission.)*

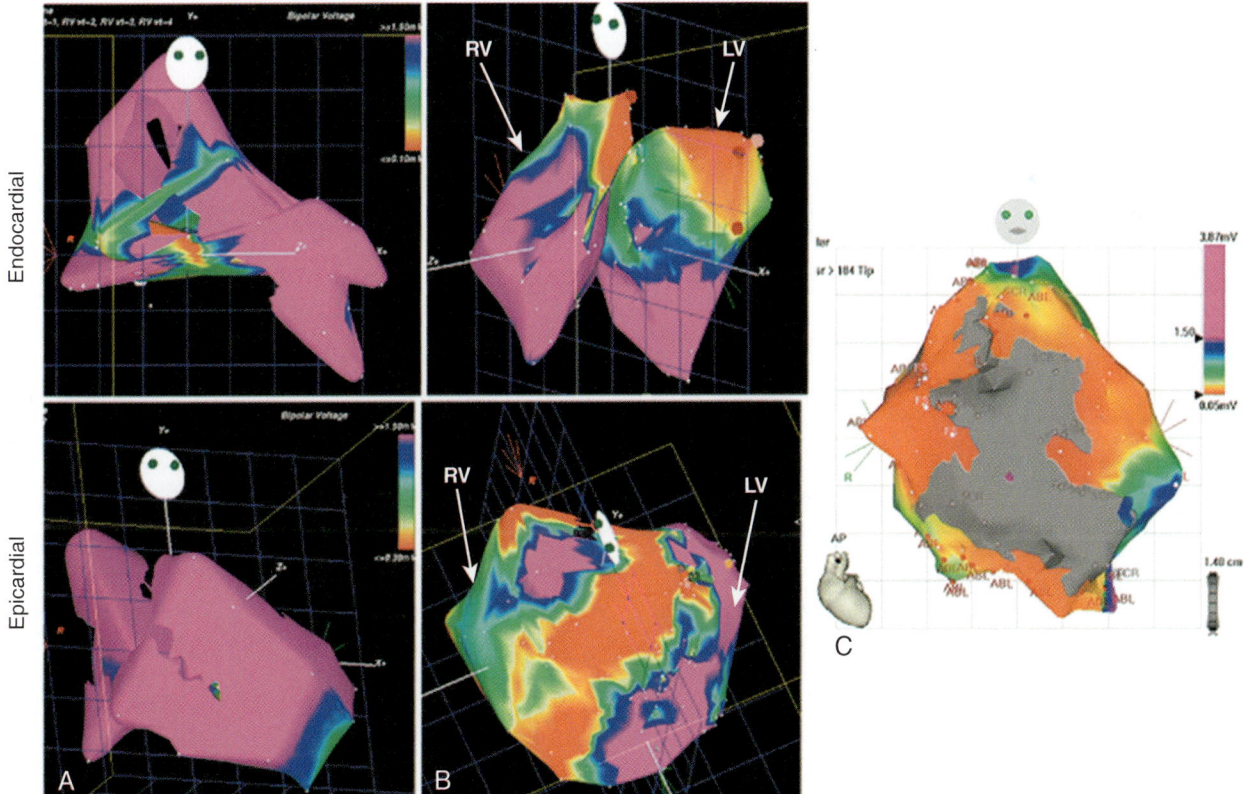

FIGURE 29-18. Electroanatomic voltage maps from three patients with sarcoidosis. Normal myocardium (bipolar voltage > 1.5 mV) is represented in *purple* and *gray* and indicates scar. Endocardial maps are shown in the *top panels* for patients A and B, and epicardial maps are shown in the *bottom panels*. **A,** Right ventricular inferior endocardial scar with minimal epicardial abnormalities. **B,** Basilar involvement of both the right and left ventricles (RV and LV). **C,** Extensive low-voltage electrograms over most of this left ventricular map. *(From Koplan BA, Soejima K, Baughman K, et al. Refractory ventricular tachycardia secondary to cardiac sarcoidosis: electrophysiologic characteristics, mapping and ablation.* Heart Rhythm. *2006;3:924-929. With permission.)*

TABLE 29-10

MISCELLANEOUS ETIOLOGIES OF NONISCHEMIC CARDIOMYOPATHY

Etiology	Reference(s)	VT Morphology	Comments
Hypertrophic cardiomyopathy	63-65	Variable	Epicardial ablation in 50% of patients, scar and entrainment mapping
Ventricular noncompaction	66	RBBB, right inferior axis (1 patient)	Reentrant mechanism, epicardial ablation from anterolateral LV
Giant cell myocarditis	67	RBBB, inferior axis (1 patient)	Reentrant mechanism, epicardial ablation at LV base

LV, left ventricle; RBBB, right bundle branch block.

References

1. Blanck Z, Sra J, Dhala A, et al. Bundle branch reentry: mechanisms, diagnosis and treatment. In: Zipes DP, Jalife J, eds. *Cardiac Electrophysiology: From Cell to Bedside.* 2nd ed. Philadelphia: Saunders; 1995:878–885.
2. Tchou P, Mehdirad AA. Bundle branch reentry ventricular tachycardia. *Pacing Clin Electrophysiol.* 1995;18:1427–1437.
3. Caceres J, Jazayeri M, McKinnie J, et al. Sustained bundle branch reentry as a mechanism of clinical tachycardia. *Circulation.* 1989;79:256–270.
4. Narasimhan C, Jazeyeri MR, Sra J, et al. Ventricular tachycardia in valvular heart disease: facilitation of sustained bundle branch reentry by valve surgery. *Circulation.* 1997;96:4307–4313.
5. Merino JL, Carmona JR, Fernandez-Lozano I, et al. Mechanisms of sustained ventricular tachycardia in myotonic dystrophy: implications for catheter ablation. *Circulation.* 1998;98:541–546.
6. Anderson RH, Ho SY. The morphology of the specialized atrioventricular junctional area: the evolution of understanding. *Pacing Clin Electrophysiol.* 2002;25:957–966.
7. Bharati S, Lev M. Anatomy of the normal conduction system, disease-related changes, and their relationship to arrhythmogenesis. In: Podrid PJ, Kowey PR, eds. *Cardiac Arrhythmia: Mechanisms, Diagnosis and Management.* Baltimore: Williams & Wilkins; 1995:1–15.
8. Shah P. Heart and great vessels. In: Standring S, ed. *Gray's Anatomy.* 39th ed. Edinburgh: Elsevier; 2005:995–1029.
9. Akhtar M, Damato AN, Batsford WP, et al. Demonstration of reentry within the His-Purkinje system in man. *Circulation.* 1974;50:1150–1162.
10. Denker S, Shenasa M, Gilbert C, et al. Effects of abrupt changes in cycle length on refractoriness of the His-Purkinje system in man. *Circulation.* 1983;67:60–68.
11. Josephson M. Electrophysiologic investigation: general concepts. In: Josephson M, ed. *Clinical Cardiac Electrophysiology: Techniques and Interpretations.* 3rd ed. Philadelphia: Lippincott Williams & Wilkins; 2002:19–67.
12. Blanck Z, Dhala A, Deshpande S, et al. Bundle branch reentrant ventricular tachycardia: cumulative experience in 48 patients. *J Cardiovasc Electrophysiol.* 1993;4:253–262.
13. Blanck Z, Jazayeri M, Dhala A, et al. Bundle branch reentry: a mechanism of tachycardia in the absence of valvular dysfunction. *J Am Coll Cardiol.* 1993;22:1718–1722.
14. Crijns HJGM, Smeets JLRM, Rodriguez LM, et al. Cure of interfascicular reentrant ventricular tachycardia by ablation of the anterior fascicle of the left bundle branch. *J Cardiovasc Electrophysiol.* 1995;6:486–492.
15. Berger RD, Orias D, Kasper EK, et al. Catheter ablation of coexistent bundle branch and interfascicular ventricular tachycardias. *J Cardiovasc Electrophysiol.* 1996;7:341–347.
16. Lopera G, Stevenson WG, Soejima K, et al. Identification and ablation of three types of ventricular tachycardia involving the His-Purkinje system in patients with heart disease. *J Cardiovasc Electrophysiol.* 2004;15:52–58.
17. Tchou P, Jazayeri M, Denker S, et al. Transcatheter electrical ablation of the right bundle branch: a method of treating macro-reentrant ventricular tachycardia due to bundle branch reentry. *Circulation.* 1988;78:246–257.
18. Youboul P, Kirkorian G, Atallah G, et al. Bundle branch reentrant tachycardia treated by electrical ablation of the right bundle branch. *J Am Coll Cardiol.* 1986;7:1404–1409.
19. Cohen T, Chien W, Lurie K, et al. Radiofrequency catheter ablation for treatment of bundle branch reentry: results and long term follow up. *J Am Coll Cardiol.* 1991;18:1767.
20. Andress JD, Vander Salm TJ, Huang SKS, et al. Bidirectional bundle branch reentry tachycardia associated with Ebstein's anomaly: cured by extensive cryoablation of the right bundle branch. *Pacing Clin Electrophysiol.* 1991;14:1639–1647.
21. Li Y-G, Gronefeld G, Isreal C, et al. Bundle branch reentrant tachycardia in patients with apparent normal His-Purkinje conduction: the role of functional conduction impairment. *J Cardiovasc Electrophysiol.* 2002;13:1233–1239.
22. Fisher JD. Bundle branch reentry tachycardia: why is the HV interval often longer than in sinus rhythm. The critical role of anisotropic conduction. *J Interv Card Electrophysiol.* 2001;5:173–176.
23. Merino JL, Peinado R, Fernandez-Lozano I, et al. Bundle-branch reentry and the postpacing interval after entrainment by right ventricular apex stimulation. *Circulation.* 2001;103:1102–1108.
24. Merino JL, Peinado R, Fernandez-Lozano I, et al. Transient entrainment of bundle-branch reentry by atrial and ventricular stimulation. *Circulation.* 1999;100:1784–1790.
25. Nakagawa H, Beckman KJ, McClelland JH, et al. Radiofrequency catheter ablation of idiopathic left ventricular tachycardia guided by a Purkinje potential. *Circulation.* 1993;88:2607–2617.
26. Schmidt B, Tang M, Chun KR, et al. Left bundle branch-Purkinje system in patients with bundle branch reentrant tachycardia: lessons from catheter ablation and electroanatomic mapping. *Heart Rhythm.* 2009;6:51–58.
27. Mehdirad AA, Tchou P. Catheter ablation of bundle branch reentrant ventricular tachycardia. In: Huang SKS, Wilber DJ, eds. *Radiofrequency Catheter Ablation of Cardiac Arrhythmias.* 2nd ed. Armonk, NY: Futura; 2000:653–667.
28. Wang C-W, Sterba R, Tchou P. Bundle branch reentry ventricular tachycardia with 2 distinct left bundle branch block morphologies. *J Cardiovasc Electrophysiol.* 1997;8:688–693.
29. Marcus F, Towbin JA, Zareba W, et al. Arrhythmogenic right ventricular dysplasia/cardiomyopathy (ARVD/C): a multidisciplinary study—design and protocol. *Circulation.* 2003;107:2975–2978.
30. Basso C, Thiene G, Corrado D, et al. Arrhythmogenic right ventricular cardiomyopathy: dysplasia, dystrophy or myocarditis? *Circulation.* 1996;94:983–991.
31. Ellison KE, Friedman PL, Ganz LI, et al. Entrainment mapping and radiofrequency catheter ablation of ventricular tachycardia in right ventricular dysplasia. *J Am Coll Cardiol.* 1998;32:724–728.
32. O'Donnell D, Cox D, Bourke J, et al. Clinical and electrophysiologic differences between patients with arrhythmogenic right ventricular dysplasia and right ventricular outflow tract tachycardia. *Eur Heart J.* 2003;24:801–810.
33. Harada T, Aonuma K, Yamauchi Y, et al. Catheter ablation of ventricular tachycardia in patients with right ventricular dysplasia: Identification of target sites by entrainment mapping techniques. *Pacing Clin Electrophysiol.* 1998;21:2547–2550.
34. Reithmann C, Hahnefeld A, Remp T, et al. Electroanatomic mapping of endocardial right ventricular activation as guide for catheter ablation in patients with arrhythmogenic right ventricular dysplasia. *Pacing Clin Electrophysiol.* 2003;26:1308–1316.
35. Fontaine G, Tonet J, Gallais Y, et al. Ventricular tachycardia catheter ablation in arrhythmogenic right ventricular dysplasia: a 16 year experience. *Curr Cardiol Rep.* 2000;2:498–506.
36. Marchlinski FE, Zado E, Dixit S, et al. Electroanoatomic substrate and outcome of catheter ablative therapy for ventricular tachycardia in setting of right ventricular cardiomyopathy. *Circulation.* 2004;110:2293–2298.
37. Verma A, Kilicaslan F, Schweikert R, et al. Short- and long -term success of substrate-based mapping and ablation of ventricular tachycardia in arrhythmogenic right ventricular dysplasia. *Circulation.* 2005;111:3209–3216.
38. Riethman C, Ulbrich M, Hahnefeld A, et al. Analysis during sinus rhythm and ventricular pacing of reentry circuit isthmus sites in right ventricular cardiomyopathy. *Pacing Clin Electrophysiol.* 2008;31:1535–1545.
39. Dalal D, Jain R, Tandri H, et al. Long-term efficacy of catheter ablation of ventricular tachycardia in patients with arrhythmogenic right ventricular dysplasia/cardiomyopathy. *J Am Coll Cardiol.* 2007;50:432–440.
40. Satomi K, Kurita T, Suyama K, et al. Catheter ablation of stable and unstable ventricular tachycardias in patients with arrhythmogenic right ventricular dysplasia. *J Cardiovasc Electrophysiol.* 2006;17:469–476.
41. Yao Y, Zhang S, Sheng D, et al. Radiofrequency ablation of the ventricular tachycardia with arrhythmogenic right ventricular cardiomyopathy using noncontact mapping. *Pacing Clin Electrophysiol.* 2007;30:526–533.
42. Miljoen H, State S, de Chillou C, et al. Electroanatomic mapping characteristics of ventricular tachycardia in patients with arrhythmogenic right ventricular cardiomyopathy/dysplasia. *Europace.* 2005;7:516–524.
43. Hsia HH, Marchlinski FE. Characterization of the electroanatomic substrate for monomorphic ventricular tachycardia in patients with nonischemic cardiomyopathy. *Pacing Clin Electrophysiol.* 2002;25:1114–1127.

44. Kottkamp H, Hindricks G, Chen X, et al. Radiofrequency catheter ablation of sustained ventricular tachycardia in idiopathic dilated cardiomyopathy. *Circulation*. 1995;92:1159–1168.
45. Wilber DJ, Glascock DN, Kall JG, et al. Radiofrequency catheter ablation of sustained ventricular tachycardia associated with idiopathic dilated cardiomyopathy [abstract]. *Circulation*. 1995;92(suppl):I165.
46. Soejima K, Stevenson WG, Sapp L, et al. Endocardial and epicardial radiofrequency ablation of ventricular tachycardia associated with dilated cardiomyopathy. *J Am Coll Cardiol*. 2004;43:1834–1842.
47. Marchlinski FE, Callans DJ, Gottlieb CD, et al. Linear lesions for control of unmappable ventricular tachycardia in patients with ischemic and nonischemic cardiomyopathy. *Circulation*. 2000;101:1288–1296.
48. Bogun FM, Desjardins B, Good E, et al. Delayed-enhanced magnetic resonance imaging in nonischemic cardiomyopathy: utility for identifying the ventricular arrhythmia substrate. *J Am Coll Cardiol*. 2009;53:1138–1145.
49. Acquatella H. Chagas' heart disease. In: Crawford MH, DiMarco JP, eds. *Cardiology*. London: Mosby; 2001:5.13.2–5.13.4.
50. Sosa E, Scanavacca M, D'Avila A, et al. Endocardial and epicardial ablation guided by nonsurgical transthoracic epicardial mapping to treat recurrent ventricular tachycardia. *J Cardiovasc Electrophysiol*. 1998;9:229–239.
51. Milei J, Pesce R, Valero E, et al. Electrophysiologic-structural correlations in chagasic aneurysm causing malignant arrhythmias. *Int J Cardiol*. 1991;32:65–73.
52. Tavora MZ, Mehta N, Silva RM, et al. Characteristics and identification of sites of chagasic ventricular tachycardia by endocardial mapping. *Arq Bras Cardiol*. 1999;72:451–474.
53. De Paola AA, Horowitz LN, Miyamoto MH, et al. Angiographic and electrophysiologic substrates of ventricular tachycardia in chronic chagasic myocarditis. *Am J Cardiol*. 1990;65:360–363.
54. De Paola AA, Gomes JA, Miyamoto MH, et al. Transcoronary chemical ablation of ventricular tachycardia in chronic chagasic myocarditis. *J Am Coll Cardiol*. 1992;20:480–482.
55. Doppalapundi H, Yamada T, McElderry HT, et al. Ventricular tachycardia originating from the posterior papillary muscle in the left ventricle: a distinct clinical syndrome. *Circ Arrhythmia Electrophysiol*. 2008;1:23–29.
56. Bogun F, Desjardins B, Crawford T, et al. Post-infarction ventricular arrhythmias originating in papillary muscles. *J Am Coll Cardiol*. 2008;51:1794–1802.
57. Good E, Desjardins B, Jongnarangsin K, et al. Ventricular arrhythmias originating from a papillary muscle in patients without prior infarction: a comparison with fascicular arrhythmias. *Heart Rhythm*. 2008;5:1530–1537.
58. Yamada T, McElderry HT, Okado T, et al. Idiopathic focal ventricular arrhythmias originating from the anterior papillary muscle in the left ventricle. *J Cardiovasc Electrophysiol*. 2009;20:866–872.
59. Koplan BA, Soejima K, Baughman K, et al. Refractory ventricular tachycardia secondary to cardiac sarcoidosis: electrophysiologic characteristics, mapping and ablation. *Heart Rhythm*. 2006;3:924–929.
60. Jefic D, Joel B, Good E, et al. Role of radiofrequency catheter ablation of ventricular tachycardia in cardiac sarcoidosis: report from a multicenter registry. *Heart Rhythm*. 2009;6:189–195.
61. Furushima H, Chinushi M, Sugiura H, et al. Ventricular tachyarrhythmia associated with cardiac sarcoidosis: Its mechanisms and outcome. *Clin Cardiol*. 2004;27:217–222.
62. Eckart RE, Hruczkowski TW, Tedrow U, et al. Sustained ventricular tachycardia associated with corrective valve surgery. *Circulation*. 2007;116:2005–2011.
63. Rodriguez L-M, Smeets JLRM, Timmermans C, et al. Radiofrequency catheter ablation of sustained monomorphic ventricular tachycardia in hypertrophic cardiomyopathy. *J Cardiovasc Electrophysiol*. 1997;8:803–806.
64. Lim K-K, Maron BJ, Knight BP. Successful catheter ablation of hemodynamically unstable monomorphic ventricular tachycardia in a patient with hypertrophic cardiomyopathy and apical aneurysm. *J Cardiovasc Electrophysiol*. 2009;20:445–447.
65. Santangeli P, Di Biase L, Lakkireddy D, et al. Radiofrequency catheter ablation of ventricular arrhythmias in patients with hypertrophic cardiomyopathy: safety and feasibility. *Heart Rhythm*. 2010;7:1036–1042.
66. Lim HE, Pak HN, Shim WJ, et al. Epicardial ablation of ventricular tachycardia associated with isolated ventricular noncompaction. *Pacing Clin Electrophysiol*. 2006;29:797–799.
67. Chauhan VS, Hameedullah I, Kumaraswamy N, Downar E. Epicardial ablation of incessant ventricular tachycardia in giant cell myocarditis. *J Cardiovasc Electrophysiol*. 2008;19:1219.

30

Ablation of Unstable Ventricular Tachycardia and Idiopathic Ventricular Fibrillation

Srinivas Dukkipati and Vivek Y. Reddy

Key Points

Substrate mapping is performed to delineate the infarcted myocardial tissue and ventricular tachycardia (VT) exit sites. For ventricular fibrillation, mapping the right and left ventricles is performed to identify the focal origin of the PVC triggers.

Targets for substrate ablation are sites of pace maps to identify the VT exit sites, sites of brief resetting and entrainment mapping, sites of late and fractionated potentials within the infarcted tissue, sites of latency mapping (long stimulus-to-QRS duration), and channels between dense ("electrically unexcitable") scar.

Targets for focal ventricular fibrillation (VF) triggers are premature ventricular contraction (PVC) triggers preceded by Purkinje potentials (about 80%) or located in ventricular outflow tract (about 20%) for structurally normal heart and, after myocardial infarction, PVC triggers preceded by Purkinje potentials.

Special equipment includes an electroanatomic mapping system, which is necessary to construct a three-dimensional rendering of the ventricular geometry and infarct location; an irrigated-tip radiofrequency ablation catheter, which is ideal to permit optimal mapping and ablation; intracardiac echocardiography, which may facilitate transseptal access to perform transmitral left ventricular mapping and monitoring for complications such as cardiac tamponade; and an intra-aortic balloon pump, which may be used to optimize the hemodynamic state.

Sources of difficulty include epicardial location of the VT circuit, deep septal location of the VT circuit and for VF ablation, and premature ventricular contraction (PVC) triggers that are difficult to induce.

During the past decade, our ability to successfully treat ventricular arrhythmias with catheter ablation has markedly improved. This is due in part to a better understanding of the pathophysiology of these arrhythmias and in part to improvements in technology related to the ablation procedure. From a procedural perspective, ventricular tachycardias (VTs) can be broadly divided into two groups: stable and unstable. In this context, a VT is considered stable if the ventricular chamber can be mapped during the arrhythmia of interest to permit identification of critical portions of the circuit. As described earlier in this book, a combination of activation and resetting and entrainment criteria can be employed to permit catheter mapping and ablation of these stable VTs with high success rates. However, in any given patient, a VT can be unstable because of hemodynamic intolerance during the arrhythmia of interest. In addition, the tachycardia can be unstable because of either nonsustained runs of the target arrhythmia or the presence of multiple morphologies of VT. Although these unstable VTs were typically not amenable to catheter ablation in the past, this chapter discusses the advances in technology and methodology that now allow for successful catheter ablation of most scar-related ventricular tachycardias regardless of their stability, hemodynamic or otherwise. In addition, this chapter discusses the recent demonstration that in some patients, ventricular fibrillation (VF) can also be targeted for catheter ablation.

Anatomy and Pathophysiology

Mechanism of Post–Myocardial Infarction Ventricular Tachycardia

In most patients with a prior myocardial infarction (MI), the pathogenesis of VT is reentry in the area of the scarred myocardium.[1,2] That is, after an MI, the tissue can be broadly divided into three zones: the dense scar, the surrounding live myocardial tissue, and the intervening "border zone." It is important to note that this border zone is not necessarily physically located only at the periphery of the scar, but is rather located at any of the interfaces between the normal tissue and dense scar. In the border zone, electrically active live myocardial fibrils are interspersed among the bed of infarcted, fibrotic tissue. These fibrils are characterized by abnormal electrophysiologic properties, including slower conduction velocity and decreased cell-to-cell electrical coupling (e.g., due to altered connexin activity at the gap junction). As with reentrant circuits located in other regions of the heart, the initiation of VT is dependent on the development of unidirectional block and conduction that is slow enough to allow the recovery of excitability of the initially blocked region to initiate a self-perpetuating reentrant circuit. The initiators of scar-related VT are not well understood. Presumably, a well-timed premature beat or series of premature beats arises as a result of triggered activity from discrete regions of the heart, and this allows for the unidirectional block and slow conduction required to initiate reentrant VT.

Once initiated, to maintain the reentrant circuit, the wavelength of the tachycardia circuit must be short enough, or the path of myocardial circuit long enough, such that the wavefront is constantly encountering excitable tissue. This can occur because of either an anatomically determined circuit of the appropriate length or a partial anatomic barrier combined with a functional barrier. For example, a functional barrier may result from ischemia, electrophysiologic changes resulting from treatment with antiarrhythmic drugs, or electrolyte and pH changes (Fig. 30-1). The anatomic compartmentalization, combined with altered cell-to-cell electrical coupling of the diseased tissue, sets the stage for local micro-reentrant or macro-reentrant circuits that result in VT and have the potential to culminate in VF.

Hemodynamically stable monomorphic VT circuits can be studied by careful transcatheter endocardial mapping of the electrical activity during the tachycardia. The "anatomy" of the path of surviving myocardial tissue within the scar that comprises the VT circuit can be characterized in detail using resetting and entrainment criteria. The "exit" point of the VT circuit from the scar (often located at the border of the scarred myocardium) can be identified, and radiofrequency (RF) catheter ablation can be performed at this region to eliminate the arrhythmia. At experienced centers, this can be accomplished with high (80% to 90%) success rates and few recurrences (0% to 30%) or complications.[3–7]

Only about 10% of patients, however, have a sustained VT that is hemodynamically tolerated to allow for adequate activation mapping.[8] Further, even in those patients with a stable VT that is mappable, it is almost invariably true that other unstable (i.e., "unmappable") VTs can also be induced. This is not surprising when one considers that the arrhythmogenic substrate is not a simple single circuit, but rather an extensive sheet of surviving myocardial fibers in a bed of scar tissue with multiple potential entry and exit points, allowing for different reentrant paths (i.e., different VTs) to be operative at any given time (Fig. 30-2).[9] From a procedural perspective, it may be most appropriate to regard this substrate as a mass of arrhythmogenic tissue with multiple tracts of surviving tissue traversing through scar— many, or perhaps even most, of which might be appropriate to target for ablation to completely eliminate VT.

Surgical Experience with Post–Myocardial Infarction Ventricular Tachycardia

The approach to ablation of unstable VTs developed directly from the extensive experience since the late 1970s with surgical modification of the arrhythmogenic substrate in post-MI patients. Because the location of the reentrant circuit is most often located in the subendocardium at the junction of normal and scarred myocardium, the initial surgical experience with simple aneurysmectomy was disappointing.[10,11] However, two effective general strategies were developed over time: (1) subendocardial resection involving surgical removal of the subendocardial layer containing the arrhythmogenic substrate in this border zone,[12–14] and (2) encircling endocardial ventriculotomy consisting of the placement of a circumferential surgical lesion through the border zone and, presumably, interrupting potential VT circuits.[15,16] Because of its distinct advantage in destroying myocardial cells without disrupting the fibrous stroma, cryoablation has also been used both as a stand-alone intervention during surgery and as an adjunct to subendocardial resection. Encircling cryoablation is an efficacious procedure incorporating cryoablation into the concept of an encircling endocardial ventriculotomy.[17,18] When performed at experienced centers, the long-term freedom from malignant VT and VF after surgery is greater than 90% (Fig. 30-3).

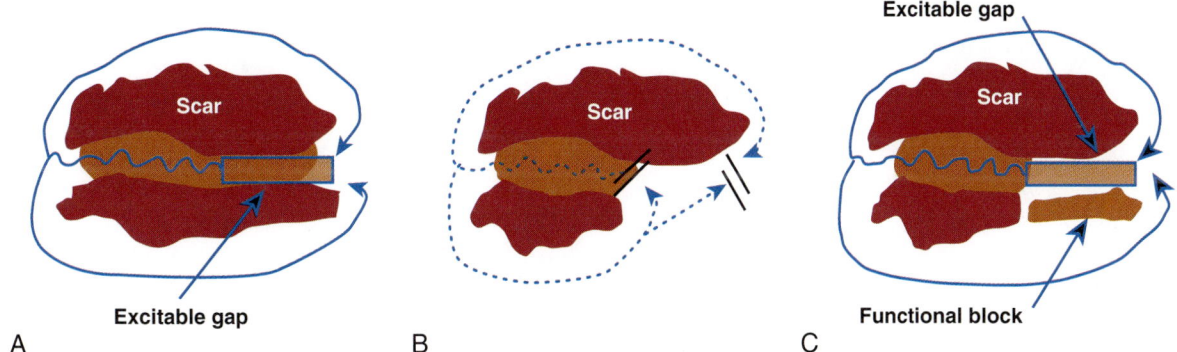

FIGURE 30-1. The importance of the excitable gap to maintain a reentrant tachycardia circuit. **A,** The wavefront traverses within the scarred tissue along a surviving tract of myocardial tissue. Conduction through this pathway is slow because of a number of potential factors, including the arrangement of the myocardial fibers (side to side instead of end to end), alterations in gap junctions between myocardial fibrils, a meandering path of the tract, and slow conduction velocity at certain regions (e.g., areas of extreme wavefront curvature). The wavelength of the circuit is short enough that the leading edge of the wavefront constantly encounters excitable myocardial tissue. This "excitable gap" allows the circuit to perpetuate and manifest as ventricular tachycardia (VT). **B,** The wavelength of the tachycardia circuit is longer than the tissue tract that it must follow. The leading edge of the wavefront encountered refractory tissue, so the circuit extinguished, and VT was not maintained. **C,** However, functional block can supervene in certain situations such as ischemia, increased heart rate, administration of drugs that alter conduction velocity or ventricular repolarization, electrolyte changes, and acid-base imbalances. In this situation, the combination of functional block to the preexisting anatomic block creates an excitable gap, allowing for sustained VT.

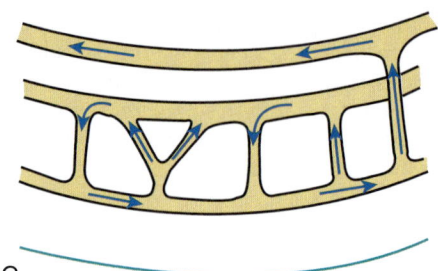

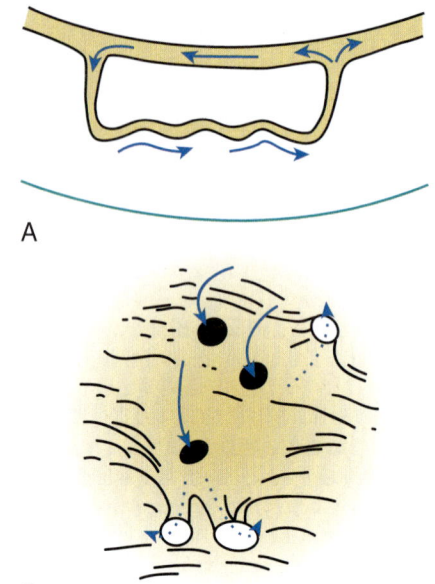

FIGURE 30-2. The substrate for ventricular tachycardia (VT) in post–myocardial infarction (MI) patients. Instead of a single bundle of myocardium forming the tachycardia circuit (**A**), surgical mapping studies of post-MI VT have revealed an extensive sheet of surviving myocardial fibers linked in the subendocardium through multiple "entrance" and "exit" points (**B** and **C**). This accounts for multiple potential reentrant paths (i.e., different VT morphologies) at different times, all originating from the same mass of infarcted tissue. *(From Downar E, Harris L, Michleborough LL, et al. Endocardial mapping of ventricular tachycardia in the intact human heart: evidence for reentrant mechanisms.* J Am Coll Cardiol. *1988;11:783-791. With permission.]*

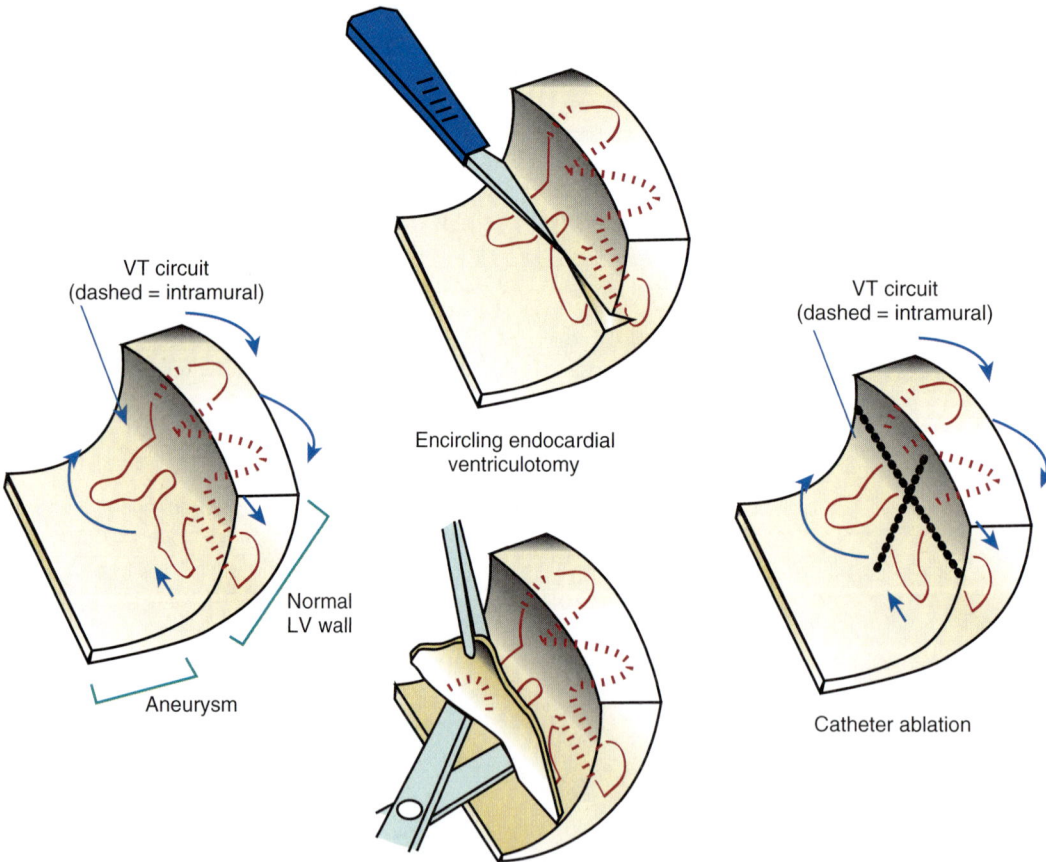

FIGURE 30-3. Surgical substrate modification to eliminate ventricular tachycardia (VT). The border between the normal and infarcted or aneurysmal wall contains a stylized VT circuit, predominantly endocardial and partially intramural. The surgical procedures, subendocardial resection and ventriculotomy, are thought to either remove or transect critical endocardial portions of the VT circuit, respectively. During catheter ablation, the border zone is mapped using the electroanatomic mapping system, the putative exit site of the VT is identified by pace mapping, and catheter-based linear lesions are placed in an attempt to interrupt the circuit. Because mapping is performed during sinus rhythm instead of during VT, greater patient safety and comfort are achieved. LV, left ventricle. *(From Miller J, Rothman SA, Addonizio VP. Surgical techniques for ventricular tachycardia ablation. In Singer I [ed]:* Interventional Electrophysiology. *Baltimore: Williams & Wilkins; 1997:641-684. With permission.)*

It is interesting to note that in the initial surgical experience, intraoperative mapping was performed to help guide the surgical resection. During open surgical bypass, multielectrode plaques were used to precisely identify the origin of the VT. This area of endocardium was either surgically removed or surgically transected using a scalpel blade. However, VT surgery then evolved such that in many cases, equivalent results were obtained by visualizing the scar and either simply resecting it or placing surgical cryoablation or laser ablation lesions along its border.[16-18] These empirical lesions are thought to eliminate critical portions of the circuit and thus render VT noninducible (Fig. 30-4).

The effect of arrhythmia surgery on the myocardial substrate was examined in a study of 18 patients undergoing successful subendocardial resection procedures.[19] These patients had all previously sustained anterior wall MIs and manifested multiple morphologies of drug-refractory monomorphic VT. During the operative procedure, a 20-electrode rectangular plaque array was used to obtain electrical data from the apical septum during VT as well as during normal sinus rhythm immediately before and immediately after resection of subendocardial tissue (Fig. 30-5).

Electrograms (EGMs) could be compared from 298 of 360 (83%) of the electrodes. Before resection, split EGMs were present in 130 (44%) and late potentials in 81 (27%) of the recordings. However, the post-resection recordings revealed a complete absence of the split EGMs as well as elimination of all the previously recorded late potentials. The mean EGM duration decreased from 112 ± 38 to 65 ± 27 milliseconds, primarily because of the loss of these split and late potentials. Histologic studies revealed that the subendocardial tissue removed in this procedure contained bundles of surviving muscle fibrils separated by dense connective tissue. These data suggest that the direct effect of the subendocardial resection procedure is to eliminate the tissue containing these abnormal EGM components.

The significant morbidity and mortality (3% to 14%) associated with arrhythmia surgery, as well as the safety and efficacy of implantable defibrillators to terminate life-threatening VT and VF, has severely curtailed its use in general practice. However, the surgical experience provided several important lessons that are relevant for modern catheter ablation of VT: (1) critical portions of the VT circuit reside on the endocardial surface of the

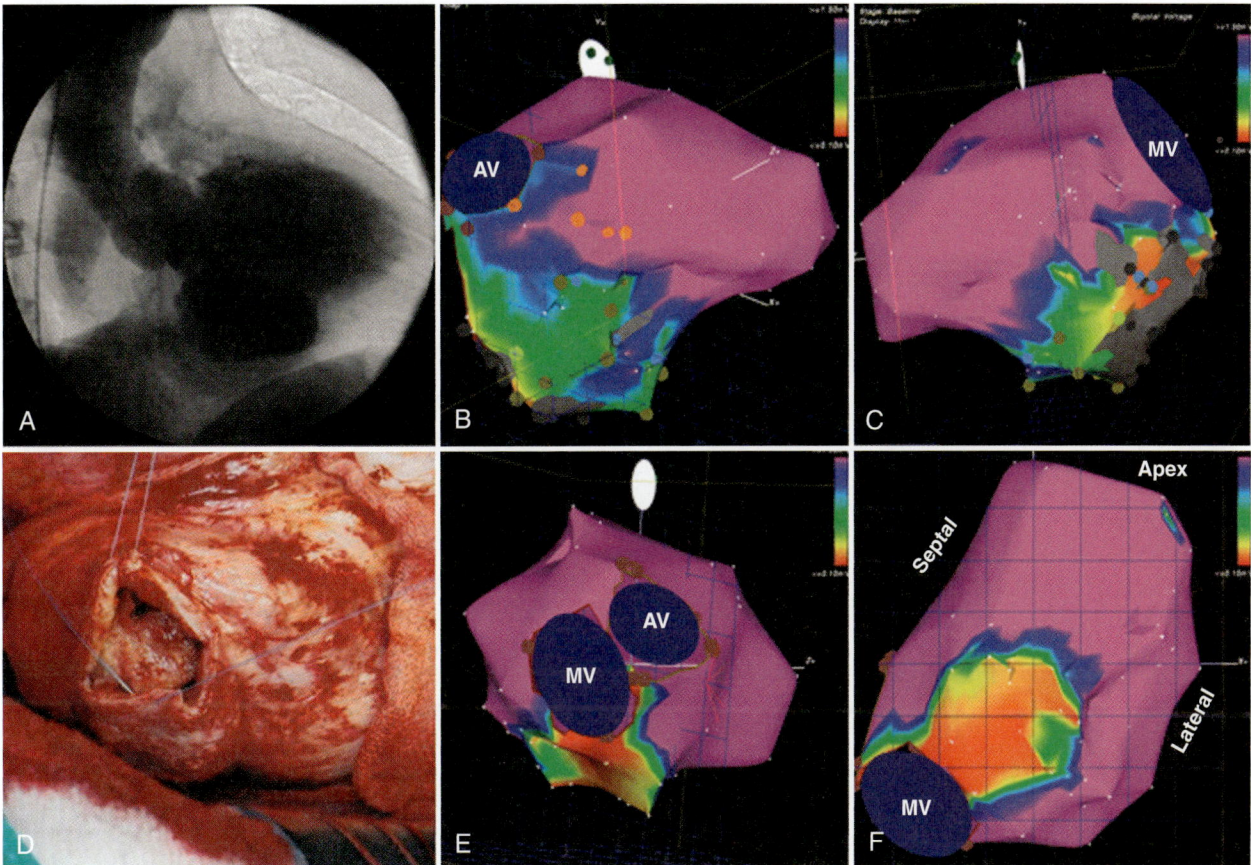

FIGURE 30-4. Electroanatomic mapping of the effect of arrhythmia surgery. **A,** Left ventriculography reveals a large inferobasal aneurysm in the setting of three-vessel coronary artery disease and clinical ventricular tachycardia (VT). During a presurgical electrophysiology study, programmed ventricular stimulation revealed easily inducible VT. Left ventricle (LV) electroanatomic mapping was performed during sinus rhythm (using the Carto system). The bipolar voltage amplitude maps shown in right anterior oblique caudal (**B**) and left lateral caudal (**C**) projections reveal a large inferobasal aneurysmal scar with electrograms containing abnormal fractionated and late potentials (not shown). **D,** During surgery, the LV was opened through the aneurysm, the aneurysm was resected, cryoablation was applied to the margins of the scar, and the ventricle was closed with the support of a patch. Months after the surgery, a repeat electrophysiology study revealed (1) a smaller homogeneous scar without evidence of fractionated and late potentials (right posterior oblique and inferior projections in **E** and **F**, respectively), (2) a more favorable ventricular geometry without an aneurysmal component, and (3) no inducible VT with programmed ventricular stimulation. The color range is set such that *purple* represents normal tissue (>1.5 mV), *red* the most severely disease tissue (<0.1 mV), and *gray* pure scar with no identifiable electrical activity. AV, aortic valve; MV, mitral valve.

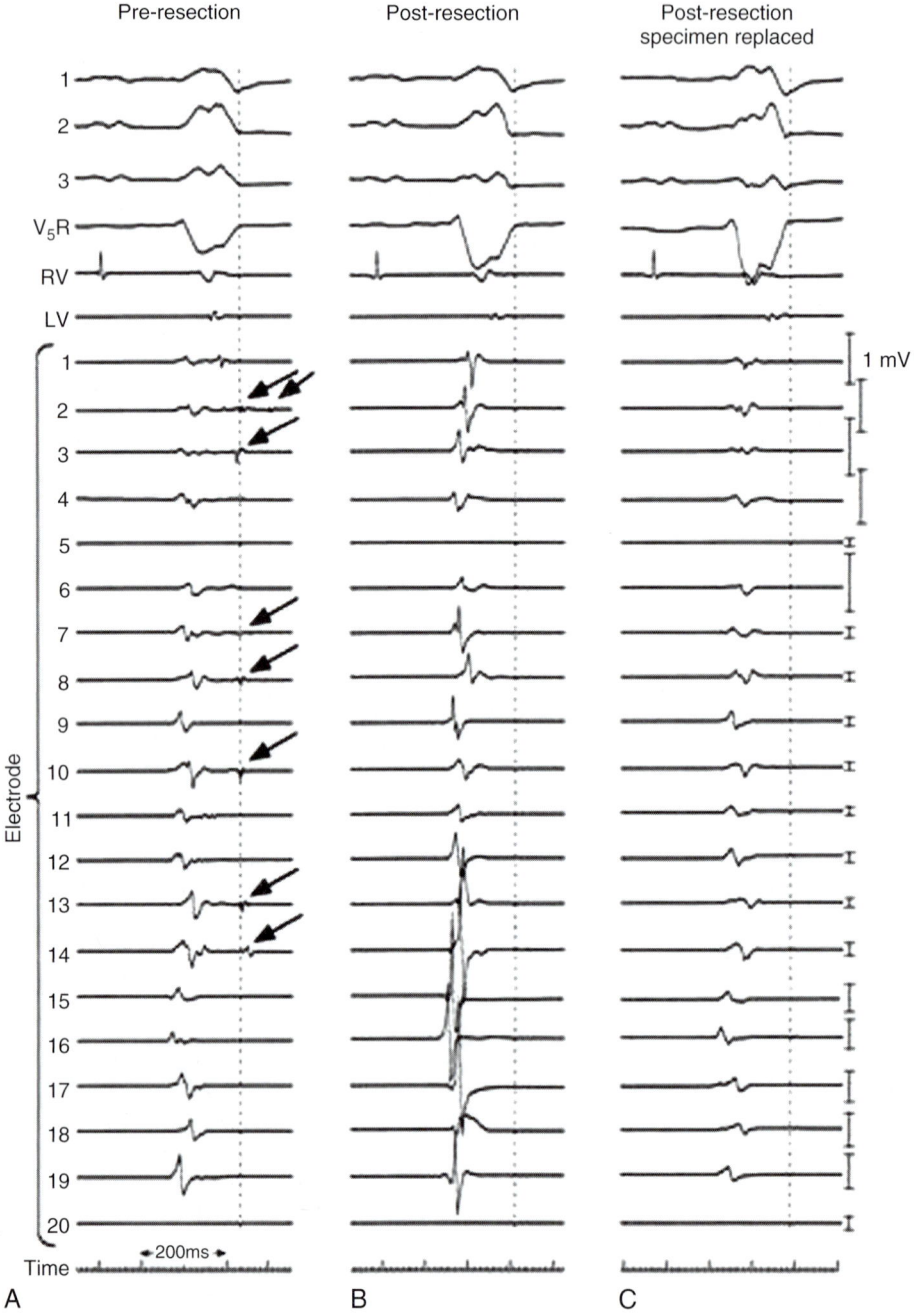

FIGURE 30-5. The electrophysiologic effect of subendocardial resection surgery. Recordings were made using a 20-bipole plaque array before (**A**) and after (**B**) resection as well as after replacement of (and recording through) the resected tissue specimen (**C**). The *dotted line* in **A** denotes the end of the QRS complex. The split and late electrogram (EGM) components (*arrows*) before resection are absent in the post-resection recordings. In addition, most channels show an increase in amplitude of the remaining early EGM component, which maintains the same general morphology as before resection. After replacement of the specimen, these early EGMs appear similar to those obtained before resection, but note the absence of split and late electrograms (channels 5 and 20 did not record properly). LV, left ventricle; RV, right ventricle. *(From Miller JM, Tyson GS, Hargrove WC, et al. Effect of subendocardial resection on sinus rhythm endocardial electrogram abnormalities. Circulation. 1995;91:2385-2391. With permission.)*

scar (allowing access through a percutaneous endoluminal approach); (2) most VTs exit from the border of the scarred myocardium; (3) during normal sinus rhythm, the "anatomy" of the scar can be delineated by certain distinguishing endocardial EGM criteria, including low-voltage amplitude, prolonged EGM duration, and the presence of late potentials[20]; and (4) empirical disruption of this arrhythmogenic substrate containing these abnormal fractionated, discrete, split, or late potentials in this border zone area can eliminate VT.

Mapping and Ablation

There are two broad groups of strategies that one can employ to eliminate unstable VTs. The first, substrate-based catheter ablation, attempts to replicate the success of the substrate modification strategy seen with arrhythmia surgery. The second relies on improvements in mapping technology that now allow one to perform rapid activation mapping during the VTs of interest to identify critical portions of the circuit to target for ablation.

Substrate-Based Ablation of Ventricular Tachycardia

This therapeutic strategy can be divided into three steps: (1) characterization of target VT morphologies, (2) delineation of the scarred myocardial substrate, and (3) identification and ablation of the arrhythmogenic myocardium, that is, those portions of the myocardial scar that are most likely to contribute to tachycardia formation (Table 30-1).

The first step is to define the many morphologies of VT that can potentially manifest from the infarct. The stimulation protocol typically includes programmed ventricular stimulation at two right ventricular (RV) and, if this does not induce VT, one left ventricular (LV) site at two cycle lengths (typically 600 and 400 milliseconds). In addition, burst pacing can also be performed until either 2:1 capture or a pacing cycle length of 250 milliseconds is reached. When a VT is induced, it is pace-terminated, and the stimulation protocol is continued to induce other VTs. Stimulation is continued until either the same VTs are repeatedly induced or electrical cardioversion needs to be performed to terminate VT (to minimize patient discomfort). It is useful to catalogue all induced VTs by bundle branch morphology, axis, precordial transition, cycle length, and induction and termination methods. From a safety perspective, it is important to remember that with depressed LV function, there is an increased risk for worsening congestive heart failure during the stimulation protocol. To mitigate against this, adequate time should be given between each stimulation train. In most patients undergoing VT ablation, particularly those with severely depressed ejection fraction or preexisting significant congestive heart failure, periprocedural intra-aortic balloon counterpulsation should be considered. In our experience, this minimizes the adverse hemodynamic effects of the stimulation protocol and mitigates periprocedural heart failure. Additionally, in some patients, hemodynamically unstable VT may convert to a more stable VT with additional intravenous pressors for hemodynamic support and allow mapping during arrhythmia. However, a second arterial puncture is required, and the risk for vascular and embolic complications may be increased in patients with severe arterial atherosclerotic disease.

The next step involves delineation of the myocardial scar. Catheter access for LV mapping can be achieved using either a retrograde aortic approach or a transseptal approach across the mitral valve. Typically, the mapping and ablation catheter is easily prolapsed across the aortic valve into the right ventricle after first deflecting the catheter into a U-shaped opening to the right of the fluoroscopy screen in the right anterior oblique projection. Several important aspects to transseptal LV mapping bear mentioning. First, because abnormal ventricular anatomy is frequently encountered in VT ablation patients, atrial dilation and cardiac rotation are not uncommon and should be anticipated. Second, because VT ablation patients often have implantable defibrillators, one must be careful not to dislodge the pacing and defibrillation leads. Third, there are no transseptal sheaths particularly suited for ventricular mapping; a simple Mullins-type curve often serves well to allow easy manipulation across the mitral valve into the left ventricle. Fourth, as during any prolonged transseptal access, it is prudent to maintain continuous flushing of the sheath with heparinized saline; a pump should be employed because the elevated ventricular pressures might otherwise preclude flow at times when the sheath is advanced over the catheter into the ventricular chamber proper. To save on mapping time, we typically use both the retrograde aortic and transseptal approaches. We find that when a particular region cannot be readily mapped using one approach, temporarily switching to the alternative approach often allows facile mapping of this region. Of course, in the presence of aortic stenosis, severe arterial tortuosity, extensive aortic atheroma, or a mechanical aortic valve, the transseptal approach alone would be preferred. Conversely, a mechanical mitral valve mandates retrograde mapping.

Based on surgical mapping studies in patients with post-MI VT, there are several EGM characteristics during sinus rhythm that help to differentiate normal from abnormal myocardial tissue—abnormal tissue is marked by EGMs of low-voltage amplitude, prolonged EGM duration, and fractionated EGMs with late and split potentials (Table 30-2 and Fig. 30-6).[19,20] In the past, the difficulties in appreciating three-dimensional (3D) anatomy using fluoroscopy alone precluded a systematic approach to targeting these abnormal EGMs.[21] However, this changed dramatically with the advent of a number of advanced 3D cardiac mapping systems: basket catheters,[22] electrode-mounted balloon catheters (EnSite, St. Jude Medical Center, St. Paul, MN),[23] and electroanatomic mapping systems that are based upon electrical impedance (NavX, St. Jude Medical),[24,25]

TABLE 30-1

SUBSTRATE-BASED VENTRICULAR TACHYCARDIA ABLATION

Programmed Stimulation: Characterize Target VTs

Obtain 12 leads spontaneous VTs
Two RV sites or RV and LV site; 2 cycle lengths; rapid pacing
Programmed stimulation from within scar
Catalogue BB morphology, axis, transition, CL, initiation, termination for each VT

Electroanatomic Mapping: Delineate Scar Substrate

Voltage range, 0.5-1.5 mV
Fill threshold at least 10 mm low-voltage tissue
Collect 150-400 points (concentrate mapping in areas of low voltage)
Tag sites of late potentials, fractionation, long stimulus-QRS interval

Targeting and Ablation

Defining Sites for Ablation

Pace mapping ≥10/12 match
Early VT activation during brief VT induction
Entrainment mapping during brief VT induction
Stimulus-QRS interval >40-70 msec (latency)
Late potentials

Ablation

Irrigated catheter: 5-10 ohm impedance drop, <40°C; up to 50 W at: VT exit sites
From dense scar to anatomic barrier
Parallel to scar border connecting sites of good pace maps
Crossing lesions parallel and perpendicular to scar at exit site
Channels within dense scar (defined by latency, entrainment, pace mapping, late potentials)

BB, bundle branch; CL, cycle length; LV, left ventricle; RV, right ventricle; VT, ventricular tachycardia.

low-level magnetic fields (Carto, Biosense Webster, Diamond Bar, CA).[26,27] These mapping systems serve critical purposes during substrate mapping, including (1) identification of the catheter tip during catheter mapping to minimize fluoroscopy exposure, (2) creation of 3D electroanatomic maps to electronically depict the ventricular normal and infarcted anatomy, and (3) cataloguing both important sites to target for ablation as well as the ablation sites themselves.

Most of the experimental and clinical experience with the use of electroanatomic mapping to identify the abnormal infarcted myocardium has been with magnetic

electroanatomic mapping (MEAM; using the Carto system).[26] The accuracy of the system has been estimated at 0.8 mm and 5 degrees. Using this system to guide catheter movement, an endocardial cast of the ventricle can be constructed, and the various EGM characteristics (bipolar and unipolar EGM voltage amplitude, activation sequence, and EGM duration) are annotated to each point displayed (Fig. 30-7).[28,29] The animals in the study underwent detailed ventricular electroanatomic mapping during normal sinus rhythm to reconstruct the chamber anatomy and display the EGM characteristics. Animal data demonstrated that the myocardial scar borders can be identified and targeted for ablation using electroanatomic mapping techniques.

Clinical work in patients revealed that a bipolar voltage EGM amplitude cutoff of 1.5 mV serves well to separate normal from infarcted tissue (Fig. 30-8).[30,31] Of note, some patients are not in sinus rhythm but are chronically ventricular paced (either RV or biventricular). The effect of this change in wavefront direction on bipolar EGM amplitude and subsequent identification of myocardial infarct architecture during electroanatomic mapping was assessed at 819 LV sites during atrial or ventricular pacing in 11 post-MI patients.[32] This study revealed that only 8% of sites had a bipolar EGM amplitude that was "reclassified" from abnormal (≤1.5 mV) to normal (>1.5 mV) or vice versa. Thus, substrate maps generated using bipolar EGM amplitude provide robust representations of the infarct morphology despite variations in the direction of wavefront propagation that would result from different rhythms. Bipolar voltage amplitude values lower than 0.5 mV are typically arbitrarily defined as dense scar, and values between 0.5 and 1.5 mV are defined as abnormal tissue, which represents the border zone. This tissue often contains surviving fibrils that can be identified as split or late potentials in sinus rhythm or mid-diastolic potentials during VT.

TABLE 30-2

SINUS RHYTHM ELECTROGRAM CHARACTERISTICS FOR SUBSTRATE ABLATION

Feature	Definition
Dense scar	Amplitude <0.5 mV
Low voltage	Amplitude ≥0.5 and ≤1.5 mV
Normal myocardium	Amplitude >1.5 mV
Fractionated electrogram	Amplitude <0.5 mV and duration >130 msec, multicomponent without isoelectric interval
Isolated diastolic potential	Electrogram component occurs after termination surface QRS and separated by isoelectric interval
Late potential	Any electrogram component occurring after termination surface QRS (includes isolated diastolic potentials)
Wide electrogram	Duration >100 msec with or without fractionation

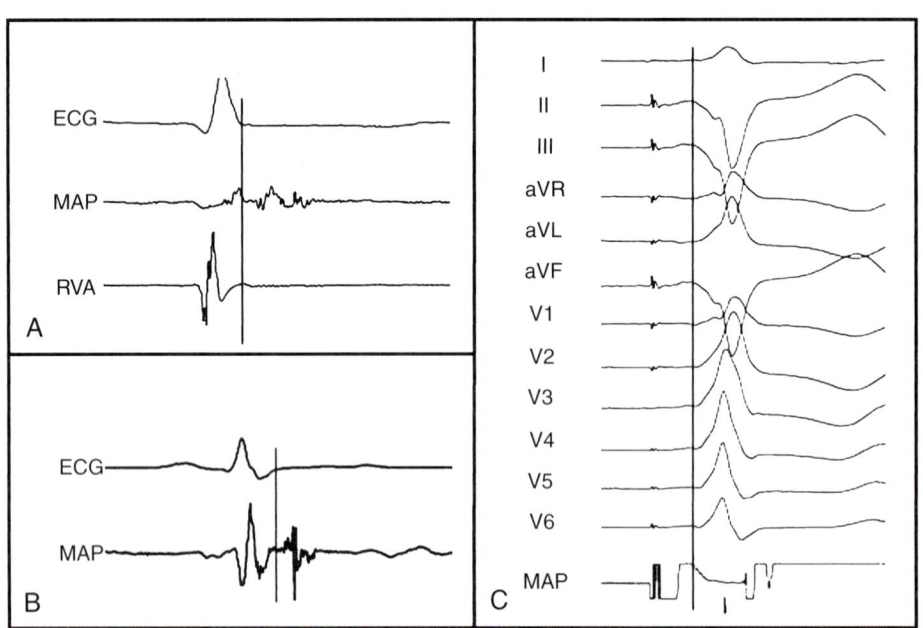

FIGURE 30-6. *Abnormal electrograms.* An example of a normal electrogram (EGM) is recorded from a catheter placed at the right ventricular apex (**A**); it is characterized by high-amplitude, short EGM duration, and no electrical activity noted after the end of the QRS complex (denoted by the *line*). Examples of fractionated and late potentials are shown on the mapping (MAP) catheter EGMs in **A** and **B**. **C,** When pacing from a location at which a late potential was recorded, there is a delay between the timing of the stimulus and the beginning of the QRS complex (again denoted by a *line*). This latency represents the time required for the wavefront to traverse from the surviving myocardial tissue within the infarct to the normal myocardium. ECG, electrocardiogram; RVA, right ventricular apex.

Recently, imaging studies using contrast enhanced computed tomography (CT) combined with positron emission tomography (PET) and magnetic resonance imaging (MRI) have evaluated, and largely validated, this classification based on bipolar voltage amplitude criteria.[33–38] Mapping based on bipolar EGM duration (using the MEAM system's double-annotation function) has also proved capable of delineating the scarred myocardium (>50 milliseconds and >100 milliseconds in porcine and human ventricles, respectively).[29] Because one must manually annotate the points to generate an EGM duration map, the practical utility of this approach may be limited. However, it is of interest that certain points that appear to be of artifactually low voltage amplitude because, for example, of poor catheter-tissue contact, are often shown to be of normal EGM duration.[29] We do not routinely perform EGM duration maps, but the information is often used to help determine the validity of low-amplitude signals during 3D bipolar voltage mapping. In clinical studies, the number of points sampled in the electroanatomic map averaged 285 ± 110 (range, 166 to 535).[31] The mapping should be most concentrated in areas of low EGM voltage. The fill threshold for electroanatomic mapping is set to at least 10 mm in low-voltage tissue and at least 20 mm in normal myocardium.

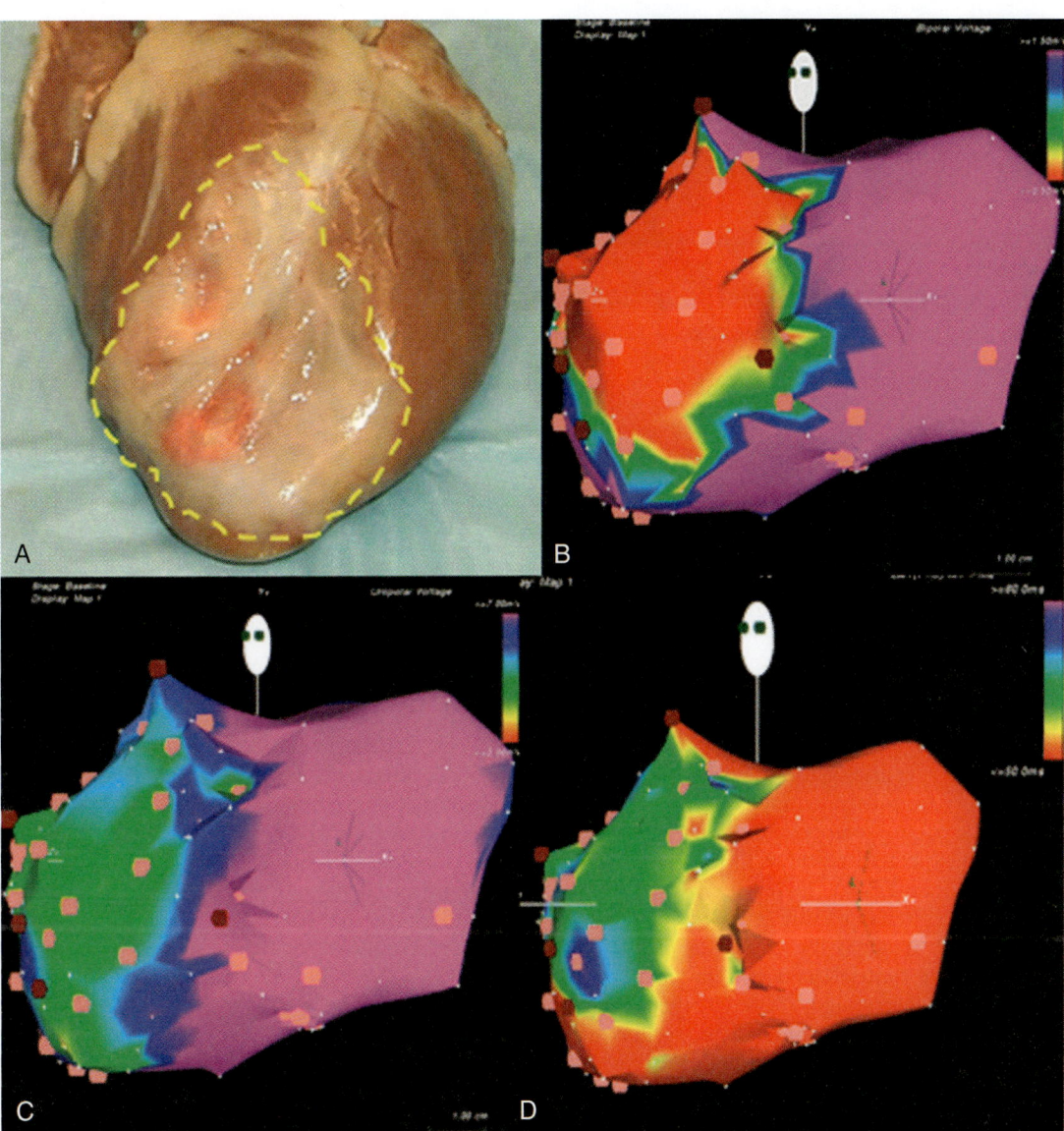

FIGURE 30-7. Electroanatomic mapping of a porcine model of chronic anterior wall myocardial infarction. This infarction model is created by injection of agarose microspheres into the mid-LAD. Eight weeks later, the electroanatomic mapping procedure is performed using the Carto system. The transmural anterior wall infarct is visible upon gross pathologic examination (**A**); the scar is outlined by the *dotted line*. In vivo electroanatomic mapping identified this anterior wall infarct by bipolar voltage amplitude criteria (**B**), unipolar voltage amplitude criteria (**C**), or bipolar electrogram (EGM) duration criteria (**D**). The projections are left anterior oblique in **B** to **D**; note the characteristic leftward rotation of the porcine heart. The color ranges in the bipolar voltage, unipolar voltage, and EGM duration maps are 0.5 to 1.5 mV, 2 to 7 mV, and 50 to 80 msec, respectively; *purple* and *red* represent normal and severely diseased tissue in the bipolar and unipolar voltage maps, respectively, whereas the opposite is true for the ECG duration map. The EGM duration maps were generated using the "double-annotation" caliper function.

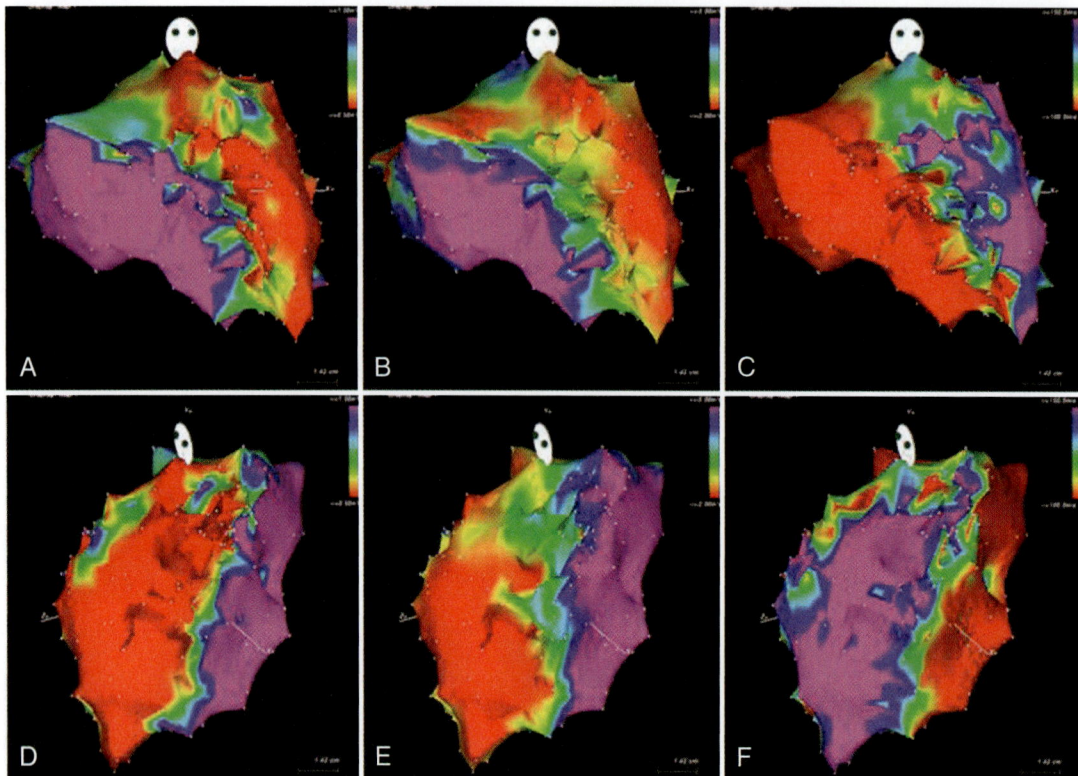

FIGURE 30-8. Substrate mapping of the left ventricular (LV) endocardium. Electroanatomic mapping (Carto) of the LV in this patient revealed a large anterior wall myocardial infarction based on bipolar voltage amplitude (**A, D**), unipolar voltage amplitude (**B, E**), and electrogram (EGM) duration (**C, F**) mapping (right anterior oblique projection in **A, B,** and **C** and left anterior oblique cranial projection in **D, E,** and **F**). The scale ranges from 0.5 to 1.5 mV, 2 to 5 mV, and 100 to 150 msec in the bipolar voltage, unipolar voltage, and EGM duration maps, respectively.

It is also important to note that any single mapped site with voltage amplitude greater than 1.5 mV (or EGM duration <100 milliseconds in human ventricles) is not necessarily normal. However, although such a site may be incorrectly identified as normal (or abnormal) based on EGM criteria, constructing a map using a large number of locations has the effect of minimizing the effects of these outliers and identifying the scar and border zone in a clinically useful manner. In fact, the use of these voltage amplitude cutoffs was described in patients without significant LV hypertrophy and may not be the most appropriate strategy for substrate mapping in all patients. For example, in a patient with ventricular hypertrophy, it is unrealistic to expect all tissue with a bipolar EGM amplitude higher than 1.5 mV to represent normal tissue. In this setting, a reference value of 1.6 to 2.0 mV may be more appropriate to use as the cutoff for normal tissue.[33] Similarly, in the ventricle of a patient with dilated cardiomyopathy demonstrating a "low-voltage" electrocardiogram (ECG) and superimposed scar, certain sites with a bipolar EGM amplitude lower than 1.5 mV are not likely to represent infarcted tissue. It is entirely possible that future studies may reveal alternate means to individualize EGM criteria in a patient-specific manner. In the interim, it is prudent to employ these arbitrary EGM criteria only as a guide to the location and morphology of the myocardial scar, and not as the final arbiter of normal versus abnormal tissue.

Marchlinski and colleagues examined the use of electroanatomic mapping in a seminal study involving patients with drug-refractory unstable VT.[30] This study demonstrated that after identifying the infarcted myocardium using bipolar voltage amplitude criteria, catheter-based RF ablation lesions directed in a linear fashion were able to control VT in nine post-MI patients. Using this high-density electroanatomic mapping system, we and others have since demonstrated that (1) a substrate-mapping strategy can be used to localize the arrhythmogenic substrate in most patients with a history of MI and sustained ventricular tachyarrhythmias, and (2) RF catheter ablation can be effectively and safely used to modify the arrhythmogenic substrate to render VT noninducible even in the presence of multiple hemodynamically unstable VT morphologies.[31,34–37] Common to all of these studies is the concept of substrate mapping, that is, delineation of the infarcted myocardium based on local EGM criteria.

Identification and Ablation of the Ventricular Tachycardia Exit Sites

There are a number of approaches to identifying and targeting the arrhythmogenic substrate, the third step of substrate-based VT ablation. These can be broadly divided into two categories: targeting the sites of VT exit from the scarred myocardium and targeting the myocardial channels of activation within the scarred myocardium. By definition, a reentrant rhythm is always depolarizing some quantity of myocardial tissue. Because the small mass of myocardial tissue in the protected myocardial channels within the scar contribute negligibly to the surface QRS, the QRS complex of a VT initiates when the wavefront of activation emanates from the border of the scar. Accordingly, once the myocardial scar is defined, a brief examination of the surface QRS morphology of the target VTs can generally regionalize the VT exit site to a scar border.[38,39] Most VTs in the setting of structural heart disease originate from the left ventricle. Accordingly, a left bundle branch block–like morphology in lead V_1 indicates that the VT is exiting from the LV septum or, rarely, from the right ventricle proper.[40] The remaining VTs exiting from other regions of the left ventricle typically have right bundle branch block morphology in lead V_1. However, a right bundle branch morphology VT can still have a septal exit site—a situation in which the frontal plane axis is typically leftward (positive in leads I and aVL). Determining septal versus lateral exit for an apical LV VT with right bundle branch block–type QRS morphology can also be assessed by examining the activation time to a fixed-reference endocardial recording at the RV apex.[41] For any right bundle branch block–type QRS morphology, created by pace mapping or VT in the setting of an apical infarct, the QRS–RV apex activation time is less than 100 milliseconds for an apical septal origin and more than 125 milliseconds for an apical lateral origin. Similar values are seen in the setting of nonapical infarcts, albeit with some degree of overlap.

The ECG frontal plane axis can help differentiate an anterior versus inferior exit; the former is characterized by an inferiorly directed QRS axis with positive complexes in leads II, III, and aVF, and the latter is characterized by a superiorly directed QRS axis (negative II, III, and aVF leads). An apical exit is characterized by predominantly negative QRS complexes in the precordial leads, whereas basal exit sites tend to be predominantly positive in these leads. Although these "rules" are helpful, a number of factors can influence the QRS complex in any given patient, including the size and location of the myocardial scar, the orientation of the heart in the thorax (horizontal versus vertical), and intrinsic conduction system disease that can modify the wavefront of activation.

Based on the ECG morphology of the VT, pace mapping is performed at the suspected borders of the scar during normal sinus rhythm to precisely localize the exit point. Unlike during VT, pacing during sinus rhythm results in omnidirectional spread of activation, which one may expect to result in a different paced-QRS morphology than the VT-QRS morphology even when pacing from the proper exit site. However, the optimal paced-QRS morphology is often only slightly different than the target VT-QRS morphology. This is likely because when pacing at a scar border, activation proceeding into the scar is slower and contributes little to overall ventricular activation when compared with the "orthodromic" wavefront that rapidly emanates in the opposite direction into normal tissue. Not surprisingly, less optimal matches of the pace-map exit sites are found when pacing along the borders of smaller scars as opposed to larger scars.

Pace mapping is also affected by the rate, stimulus strength, and electrode polarity during pacing. At faster pacing rates, the "antidromic" wavefront of activation into the scar may contribute less to the QRS morphology than during slow pacing. In addition, ventricular repolarization may fuse into and modify the QRS morphology during faster pacing rates. Because it is difficult to predict the effect of these variables, pacing is ideally performed at a rate similar to the target VT rate. By presumably capturing more distant (i.e., far-field) tissue, increasing the stimulus strength can also affect the QRS morphology. We typically start pacing at low output and increase the output until several QRS complexes are captured in succession. It is interesting to note that if multiple QRS morphologies are seen at varying outputs, this is indicative of a protected region (or channel) of tissue. That is, at the lower output, only this region is captured by pacing, whereas at higher output, the far-field tissue is also captured. In the ideal situation, pacing would be performed using unipolar pacing so that only the distal electrode could stimulate the myocardium and one could avoid inadvertent pacing capture by the proximal electrode. However, unipolar pacing typically results in a larger stimulus artifact that can preclude accurate QRS morphology interpretation. In addition, from a practical perspective, it is unusual for bipolar and unipolar pacing to be of markedly different morphologies, likely because the ablation catheter is typically not parallel to the tissue surface, resulting in the proximal electrode not being in contact with the tissue.

As with the difficulty in trying to predict the VT exit site from the QRS morphology, it is also difficult to predict the paced-QRS morphology from different LV sites. However, in any given patient, the previously mentioned ECG morphology rules work well to predict the paced-QRS morphology of a given site in relation to another site (Fig. 30-9). That is, if a particular pace site reveals a superior axis in the frontal QRS plane, it is fairly well predictable that pace sites progressively superior to this location would reveal an intermediate and then inferior axis in the frontal QRS plane.

After a VT exit site is identified, linear lesions are placed using one of a number of strategies: (1) extending from the dense scar (defined as <0.5 mV) to anatomic boundaries or normal myocardium, (2) extending along the borders of the scar traversing these optimal pace sites, or (3) a pair of crossing linear lesions extending from the exit site into the scar and the other along the border of the scar. Irrigated catheters are favored and the use of F-curve (Biosense Webster) or equivalent is usually best. Lesions are typically applied at one spot until one of the following criteria is realized: (1) a decrease of the contact impedance by 5 to 10 ohms, (2) a reduction in the EGM voltage amplitude by at least 75%, or (3) doubling of the pace-capture threshold after ablation. Linear lesions are generated by point-to-point spot applications with interpoint distances not exceeding 10 mm, and ideally 5 mm. The range of the number of lesions delivered per patient is about 8 to 86, with the average of about 20 to 30.[30,31] Because of the depth of ventricular tissue, we do not attempt to achieve, or check for, conduction block traversing these linear lesions. The strategy is not to contain or isolate the VT circuit because this is both unlikely given current ablation technology and possibly undesirable because of potential adverse effects. These lesions are instead delivered to transect critical portions of the circuit that are important for tachycardia maintenance.

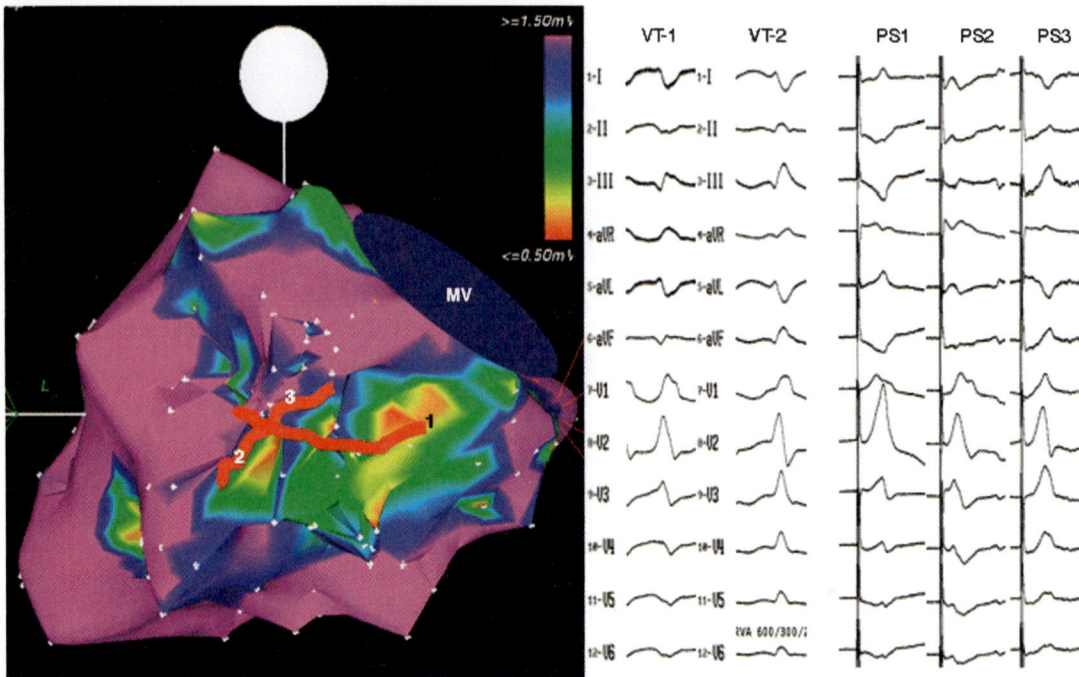

FIGURE 30-9. Substrate mapping and radiofrequency ablation. Sinus rhythm electroanatomic mapping in this post–myocardial infarction patient revealed a localized posterobasal infarct as shown in this bipolar voltage map (posteroanterior projection). Two ventricular tachycardias (VTs) were induced during programmed stimulation; note the differences in leads III and V$_3$ to V$_6$. Pacing during sinus rhythm from site 1 was too septal to the exit sites of these two VTs; leads I and aVL are positive in the pace map but negative during the VTs. Accordingly, pacing performed from the lateral aspect of the infarct from sites 2 and 3 revealed morphologies consistent with VT-1 and VT-2. The short stimulus-QRS duration indicates that these sites represent VT exit points. (The pacing artifact caused an initial distortion of the QRS complex during pace mapping.) Pacing between sites 2 and 3 generated a QRS morphology that alternated between VT-1 and VT-2, but with a longer stimulus-QRS time; this latency likely represents a common pathway for the two VT circuits. A series of radiofrequency ablation lesions was placed in a linear fashion along the scar border incorporating these two pacing sites (represented by the *short red line*). However, programmed stimulation induced a slower VT of similar morphology to VT-1 (not shown). After placing a second linear lesion extending into the scar (represented by the intersecting *darker red line*), no VT was inducible. MV, mitral valve.

The placement of catheter-based ablation lesions completely around the scar (mimicking the surgical partial encircling endocardial ventriculotomy procedure) may be predicted to be of equal if not superior efficacy, potentially obviating the pace-mapping step (Fig. 30-10). This procedure could certainly be performed in some patients, but there are two aspects to this strategy that must be considered. First, generating continuous linear lesions along the entire length of the tissue can be technically difficult with larger scars. Second, the placement of multiple ablation lesions at the scar border near normal tissue has the potential to adversely affect LV function (further discussed under "Minimizing Complications," below). Accordingly, a more limited "cross-hair" lesion set may be desirable for patients with more severe LV dysfunction.

Instead of large homogeneous infarcts, one may instead encounter patchy myocardial scars that preclude rapid identification of the VT exit zones (Fig. 30-11). These cases are particularly challenging but can still be approached using this strategy. Interestingly, these patchy scars are relatively uncommon (<10% in our experience), even in the presence of severe ventricular dysfunction.

Targeting the Myocardial Channels

Even in the setting of hemodynamically unstable VT, a number of strategies may be employed to identify and target putative myocardial channels within the scarred tissue, including (1) resetting and entrainment mapping (in those patients with stable as well as unstable VTs), (2) ablation of fractionated and late potentials within the scarred myocardium, (3) latency mapping, and (4) pace mapping to identify densely scarred tissue with intervening channels of activation.

The most direct and reliable means to identify a channel of activation is to employ entrainment and resetting criteria during VT. For hemodynamically unstable VT, this can be accomplished first by performing pace mapping at the scar border to identify the putative exit site, followed by a brief induction of the unstable VT. This is followed by quickly performing resetting and entrainment maneuvers to define the relevance of that location to the VT circuit, followed by pace termination of the VT (Fig. 30-12). As mentioned previously, this can be facilitated by use of intravenous pressors and an intra-aortic balloon pump to both support arterial perfusion during tachycardia and prevent worsening heart failure after termination of the rhythm. To perform resetting or entrainment of unstable VT, however, it is necessary to be able to reproducibly initiate the very same morphology of tachycardia. Additional sites of potentially arrhythmogenic myocardium related to the resetting and entrainment sites may be identified and incorporated into the ablation strategy. For example, in addition to a VT exit site, one may identify a site deeper within the scar demonstrating a similar QRS morphology when pace mapping during sinus rhythm, albeit with a longer stimulus-QRS

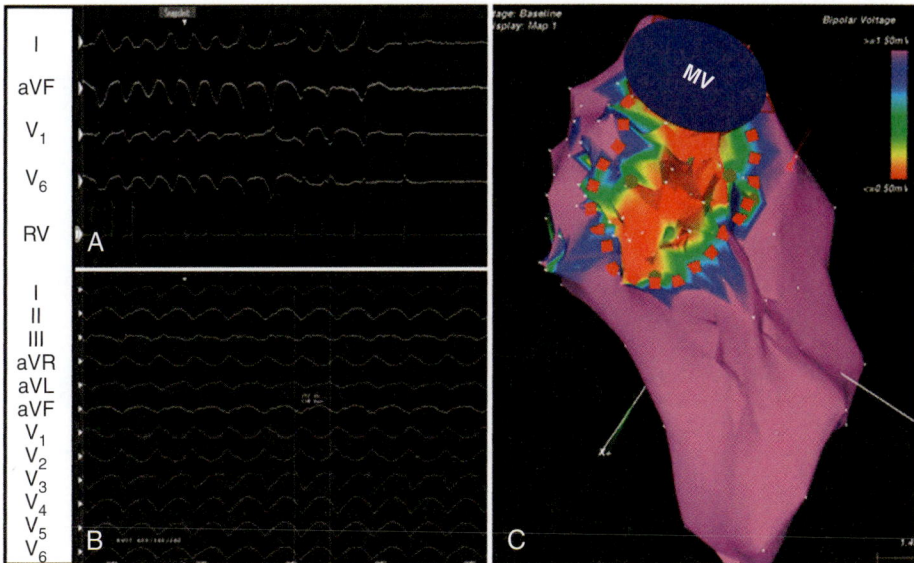

FIGURE 30-10. Catheter ablation to "encircle" the myocardial scar. In this patient with post–myocardial infarction (MI) ventricular tachycardia (VT), programmed ventricular stimulation induced only nonsustained polymorphic VT (**A**). Repeat stimulation after infusion of intravenous ajmaline (a class I antiarrhythmic agent) revealed an easily inducible monomorphic VT (**B**). The bipolar voltage map (**C**) identified an inferoposterior MI (right posterior oblique caudal projection; color range, 0.5 to 1.5 mV). Because pace mapping identified a suboptimal "best" exit site and the scar was relatively small, radiofrequency ablation lesions were placed along the full border of the scar (*dashed red line*). VT was no longer inducible at the end of the procedure. MV, mitral valve.

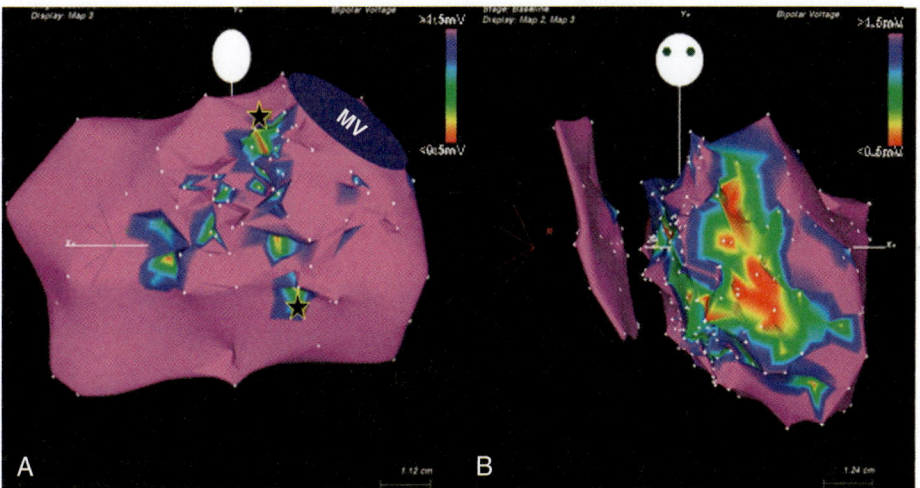

FIGURE 30-11. Post–myocardial infarction (MI) scar morphologies. A range of post-MI scar morphologies is seen, including small patchy scars (**A**) and large anterior wall scars with interventricular septal wall involvement (**B**). In the former situation, two VTs were induced, and pace-mapping revealed the exits to be located at the superior and inferior aspects of the scar (*black stars*); radiofrequency ablation lesions were placed, spanning between these two sites to render VT noninducible. In the latter situation, mapping the right ventricular (RV) aspect of the septum should be considered; in this patient, the RV septum displayed normal bipolar voltage amplitude. Shown are left posterior oblique and anterior projections in **A** and **B**, respectively (bipolar voltage map; color range, 0.5 to 1.5 mV). MV, mitral valve.

interval (latency). These regions of latency can be graphically represented to create a latency map (Fig. 30-13). These sites likely represent surviving myocardial fibrils within the body of scar that may be critical for the target or other VTs arising from the arrhythmogenic mass of tissue. Resetting and entrainment can also be used at these sites to determine their relevance to the particular VT circuit. Whether or not these sites are critical to the particular VT circuit, they should be targeted for ablation as well.

Although it is certainly true that the benefits of substrate-based VT ablation are greatest during ablation of hemodynamically *unstable* VT, this strategy can also be useful in ablation of stable VT.[31,42] Another strategy involves targeting of fractionated and late potentials during sinus or paced rhythm, based on the observation that the late and long-duration EGMs, despite a low sensitivity, were highly specific for identifying VT circuits.[20] This criterion required recording low-amplitude, high-frequency EGMs

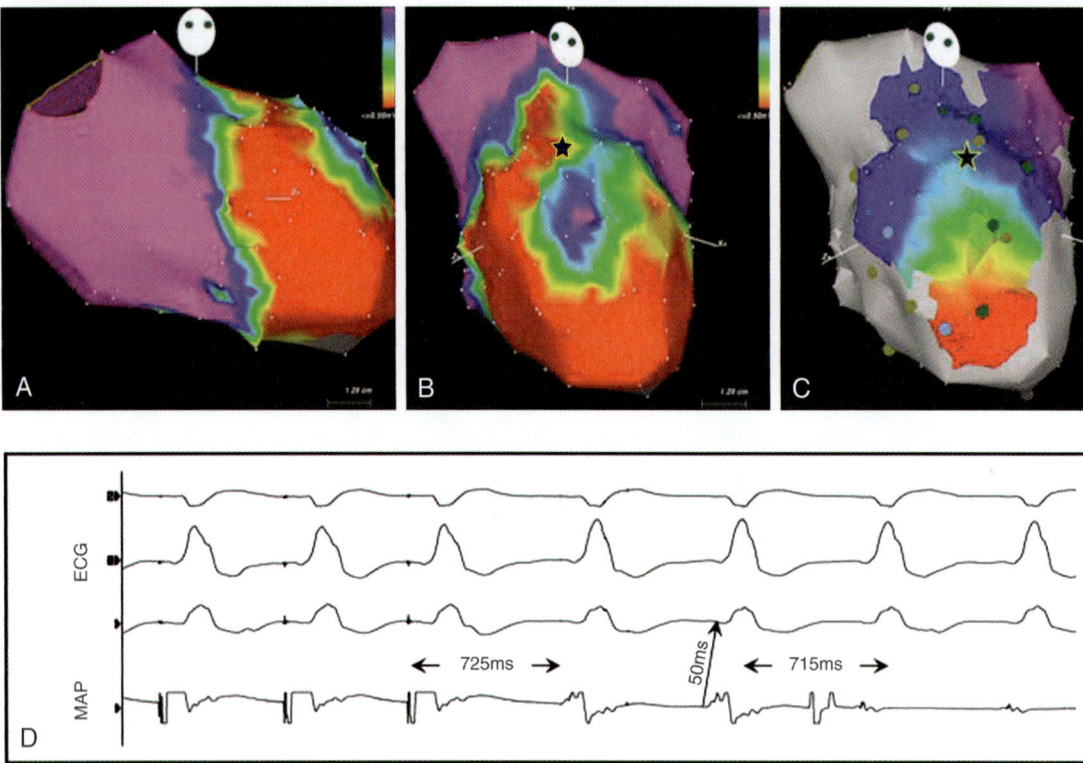

FIGURE 30-12. Role of substrate mapping in hemodynamically stable ventricular tachycardia (VT). This patient with a large anterior wall myocardial infarction (MI) presented with repetitive monomorphic slow VT resulting in congestive heart failure. Sinus rhythm bipolar voltage mapping revealed the large anterior infarct (right and left anterior oblique cranial projections in **A** and **B**, respectively; color range, 0.5 to 1.5 mV). Pace mapping identified a good putative exit site (*black star* in **B**). Then, the VT was induced and brief activation mapping (**C**) was performed. Entrainment performed at the optimal pace site (*black star* in **C**) revealed a postpacing interval only 10 msec longer than the tachycardia cycle length, and the stimulus-QRS and electrogram-QRS durations were short. Radiofrequency ablation at this site eliminated the arrhythmia; in addition, further lesions were placed extending into the scar to ablate other potential reentrant circuits. ECG, electrocardiogram; MAP, mapping catheter.

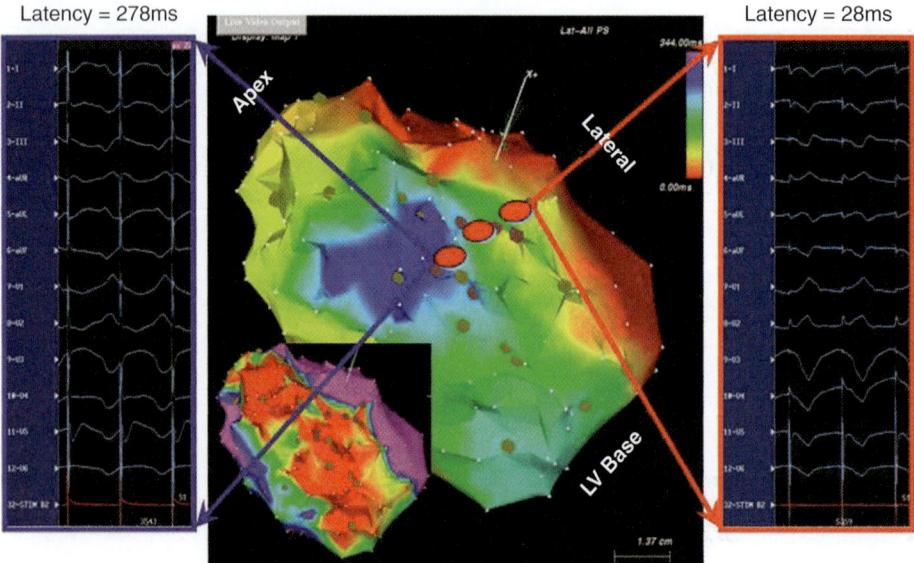

FIGURE 30-13. Latency mapping. Sinus rhythm substrate mapping in this patient with ventricular tachycardia (VT) revealed a large inferior wall myocardial infarction on bipolar voltage mapping (*inset;* color range, 0.5 to 1.5 mV). Pace mapping at various sites within and outside of the scar revealed varying degrees of delay between the pacing stimulus and the onset of the QRS complex. A latency map was generated by plotting these values onto the left ventricle (LV) anatomic construct (*main image;* range, 0 to 344 msec). Two examples of these pacing sites with varying degrees of latency and identical morphology to the target VT are shown. Radiofrequency catheter ablation extending between these sites eliminated the VT (*red dots*).

with multiple components of prolonged duration (fractionated potential) or a component recorded after the surface QRS that is separated by an isoelectric segment (late potential), similar to the EGMs recorded at the central common pathways, inner loops, or adjacent bystander locations (Fig. 30-14). Some investigators have labeled late potentials as isolated potentials and further defined the length of the isoelectric segment (≥20 or ≥50 milliseconds).[42,43] These late or isolated potentials are particularly interesting in that they are thought more likely to represent critical portions of the VT circuit (isthmus) and are excellent targets for ablation.[42,44] It is certainly true that targeting these EGMs would invariably result in ablation of bystander sites that may not be operative in any VTs (e.g., a "dead-end" pathway), but this approach has the advantage of placing ablation lesions at regions far from the normal tissue. Thus, ablation at these sites would not result in any adverse effect on ventricular function. However, fractionated and late EGMs are underappreciated during sinus rhythm. One potential reason is that overlapping of EGMs or a particular orientation of a line of block with respect to the activation wavefront may preclude the identification of multiple components during sinus rhythm. The sensitivity of identifying these components during catheter mapping can be increased by changing the propagation wavefront during catheter mapping by RV pacing or LV pacing (e.g., from within a ventricular branch of the coronary sinus).[42,45] From a practical perspective, this can be accomplished by pacing whenever the EGM at the site being mapped is suggestive of, but does not conclusively identify, a late potential site. As a corollary to this approach, by performing high-density mapping of the scar, channels of activation percolating into the scar may be mapped in great detail. Then, these channels of activation can be targeted for ablation at the borders of the scar such that fractionated or late potentials at the center of the scar are eliminated without being directly ablated.

The approach is limited by the facts that this does increase procedural time and technical difficulty, that the complexity of the arrays of myofibrillar bundles surviving within the infracted tissue may preclude one's ability to precisely map these multiple and potentially overlapping activation pathways, and that this approach is unlikely to be efficacious in patients with smaller infarcts and faster VTs resulting from smaller circuits.

The alternative, or "inverse," strategy to identify these protected isthmus sites is to stimulate directly within the infarcted tissue at target sites of questionable significance (i.e., sites at which it is difficult to determine whether a late potential is present). Because of the limited myocardial tissue depolarized, activation of the isthmus contributes negligibly to the surface ECG until the wavefront of activation exits to the normal myocardium, thereby producing the observed QRS complex. Therefore, pace mapping from a site more proximally located within the isthmus should produce a QRS complex similar to the VT QRS morphology, albeit with a longer stimulus-QRS interval. Accordingly, the duration of the stimulus-QRS interval can serve as a surrogate to late potentials and can be targeted for catheter ablation to eliminate VT circuits.[46] Another approach is pace mapping to identify regions of dense scar based on the inability of pacing stimuli to capture any myocardium at a particular site (using pulses of 2 milliseconds' duration, 10 mA of amplitude, unipolar stimuli).[47] These areas of electrically unexcitable scar can delineate isthmuses for VT circuits that can be transected with ablation lesions connecting these various dense scar regions to each other and to fixed anatomic barriers (e.g., mitral valve). Recently, it has been suggested that potential VT isthmus sites are located in areas of electrically unexcitable tissue, as defined previously, and that even higher outputs are required to delineate these potential channels (2 to 10 milliseconds' duration, 20 mA of amplitude, bipolar stimuli).[48]

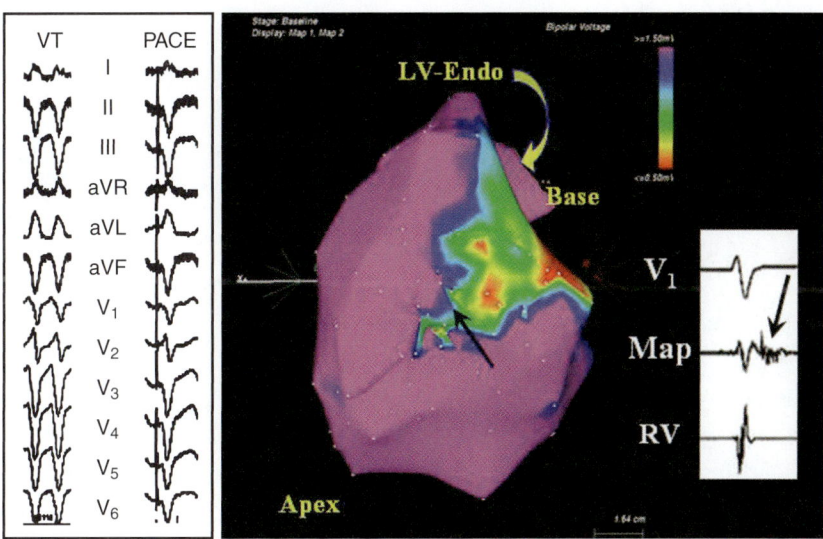

FIGURE 30-14. Substrate mapping followed by targeting of late potentials. In this patient with a post–myocardial infarction ventricular tachycardia (VT), endocardial substrate mapping revealed a small myocardial scar without fractionated or late components and a suboptimal "best" pacing site (not shown). However, epicardial substrate mapping using the subxyphoid puncture approach (see below) revealed an inferobasal scar (color range, 0.5 to 1.5 mV). The optimal pace site at the apex of this epicardial scar matched the VT QRS morphology well (electrocardiograms shown at left; pacing site indicated by *black arrow* in center). Also, this site demonstrated a late potential with fractionated components during sinus rhythm (*inset at right*). Catheter ablation at this site eliminated the VT. Endo, endocardium; LV, left ventricle; Map, mapping catheter.

Which Ablation Targets or Strategy Should Be Used?

The relative efficacy of these various criteria to guide identification and targeting of the arrhythmogenic portion of the scar is unknown and will be fully appreciated only with future comparative studies. However, certain general principles can be stated. Trying to minimize the number of ablation lesions placed at the border zone would be advantageous to minimize adverse effect on LV function. Indeed, a strategy targeting fractionated and late potentials is particularly attractive in patients with depressed ventricular function or congestive heart failure. Conversely, in patients with preserved ventricular function and small or patchy scars, it is not necessarily possible to identify channels of activity, and ablation lesions based in large part on pace mapping would be appropriate.

Ideally, the ablation procedure is considered complete when all VTs inducible at the beginning of the procedure are eliminated and no additional VTs are inducible. Because the substrate modification procedure in theory could inadvertently create new arrhythmogenic channels of activity, one is obligated to rule out this possibility. Inducibility at the end of the procedure should minimally include one RV and one LV site. In addition, if nonsustained monomorphic VT is induced, one should strongly consider infusion of a sympathetic agent such as isoproterenol to determine whether the VT then becomes sustained (Fig. 30-15). However, complete noninducibility is not necessarily achievable in every patient, particularly those with severe ventricular dysfunction in whom a sine wave–like VT (i.e., a morphologically indeterminate VT with no isoelectric segment) is often inducible with aggressive ventricular stimulation (Fig. 30-16).[31] In this situation, after all the late potentials are eliminated, the procedure is terminated.

Radiofrequency Ablation Catheter Technology

An important variable to address is the type of RF catheter ablation catheter used. In Marchlinski's seminal study, one of the patients experienced a cerebrovascular accident associated with an impedance rise during RF energy delivery.[30] The ablation catheter used in that study was a 4-mm-tip non–temperature-controlled catheter, which has limited ability to monitor for signs of excessive heating

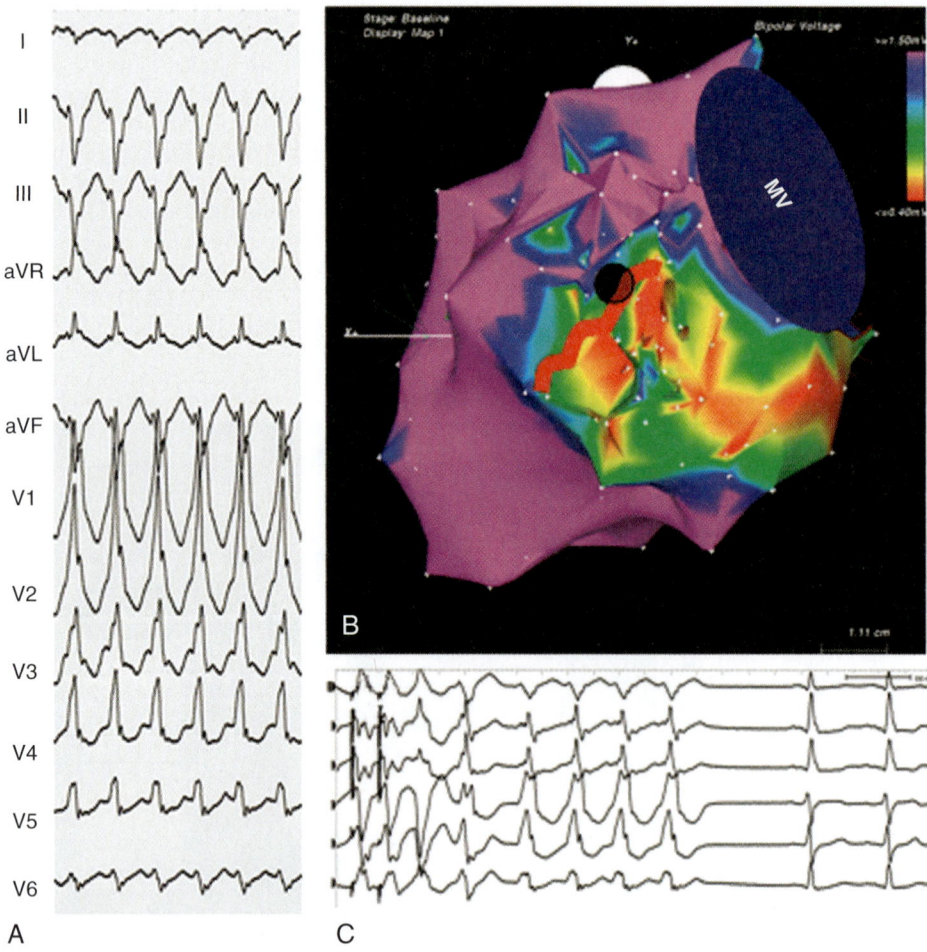

FIGURE 30-15. Postablation inducibility of nonsustained ventricular tachycardia (VT). Monomorphic VT was inducible in this patient with a prior inferior wall myocardial infarction (**A**). Sinus rhythm substrate mapping revealed an inferoposterior basal scar (bipolar voltage map in **B**; color range, 0.4 to 1.5 mV), and a pace site identical to the VT (*black circle*). Radiofrequency ablation lesions were placed in a linear fashion incorporating this pacing site (*red line* in **B**). Repeat programmed stimulation induced only nonsustained VT, but of identical morphology to the sustained VT induced at baseline (**C**). However, repeat stimulation after infusion of intravenous isoproterenol caused this VT to sustain. Accordingly, additional RF lesions were placed to extend the ablation line to the mitral valve annulus; then, VT was no longer inducible at baseline or after intravenous isoproterenol infusion.

of the electrode tip that can lead to coagulum formation. Unlike that early-generation catheter, ablation catheters are now able to not only monitor the temperature at the electrode tip but also cool the ablation electrode in either a passive or active fashion. Passive cooling is achieved by use of an 8-mm-tip temperature-controlled catheter; that is, if the distal end of the catheter is in contact with the tissue, the proximal end is cooled by the ambient blood flow to allow greater delivery of ablative energy into the tissue without excessive temperature rises.[49] However, this catheter is limited both because of its only modest cooling efficiency and because the electrode size limits one's ability to perform detailed ventricular mapping. An alternative family of RF ablation catheters is the temperature-sensing saline-irrigated catheters—both externally irrigated catheters and internally cooled catheters.[50] Active cooling of the ablation electrode by saline irrigation of the catheter tip has been shown to allow greater

RF energy delivery into the target tissue.[51,52] With the externally irrigated catheter, saline is constantly infused through a central lumen through openings in the electrode tip at 15 to 30 mL/minute during RF energy delivery or at 2 mL/minute during catheter manipulation to maintain lumen patency. In contrast, with the internally cooled catheter, the saline is circulated within the electrode tip. An ex vivo comparison of the two types of saline-irrigated catheters demonstrated a lower risk for thrombus formation and incidence of steam pops with the externally irrigated catheter.[53] Additionally, in patients undergoing VT ablation, there was a 2.7% incidence of procedure-related stroke or transient ischemic attack with the internally cooled catheter and a 0% incidence with the externally irrigated catheter.[54,55] Because of its better safety profile, the externally irrigated catheter is widely favored. With this catheter, it is our practice to deliver RF lesions in 60-second intervals under power control of 25

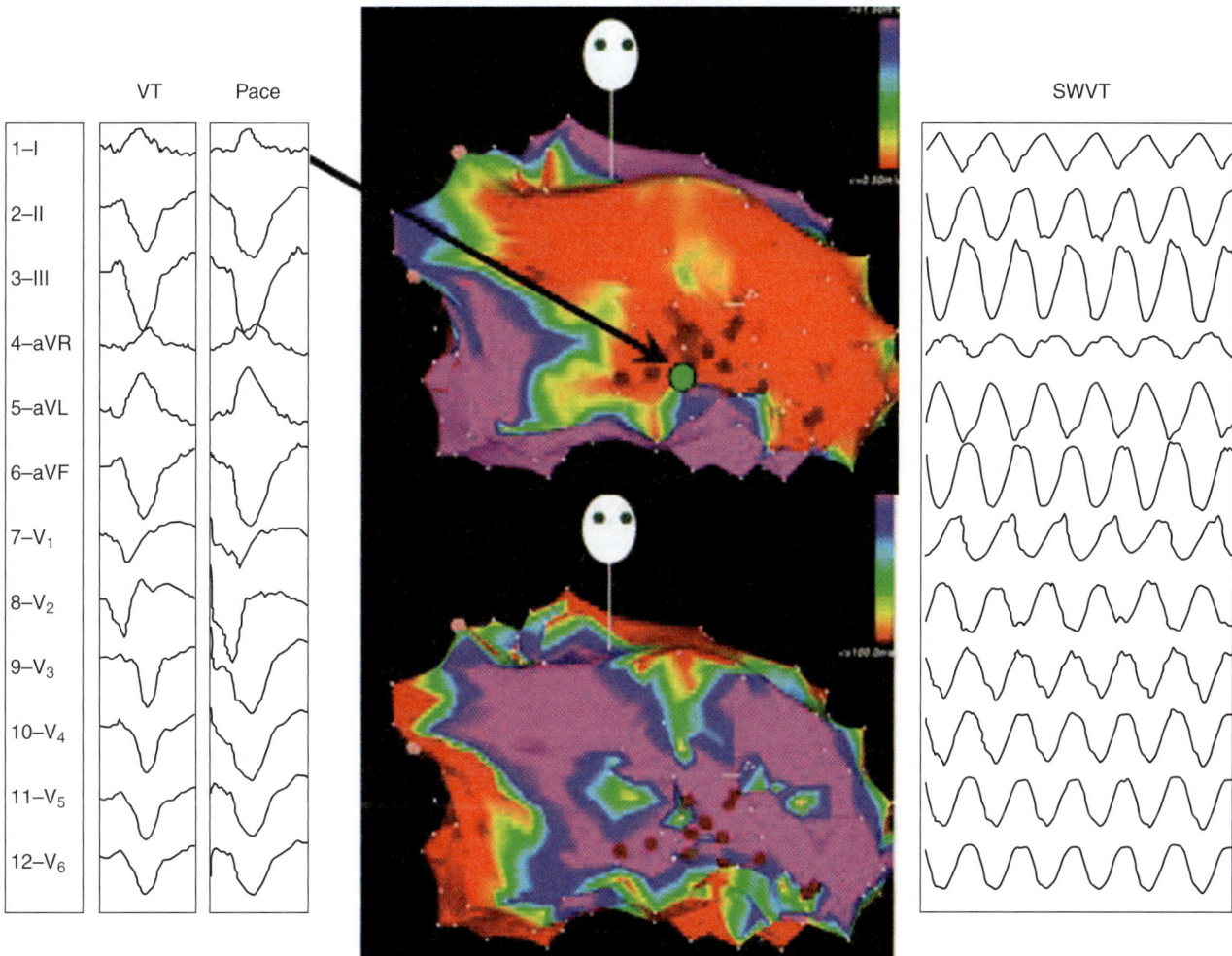

FIGURE 30-16. Induction of sine-wave ventricular tachycardia (SWVT). A large anteroseptal and apical aneurysm is seen in the right anterior oblique view on both the bipolar voltage (*top*; color range, 0.5 to 1.5 mV) and electrogram duration (*bottom*; 100 to 150 msec) maps obtained during sinus rhythm. Programmed stimulation induced a hemodynamically tolerated ventricular tachycardia (VT) (shown at *left*) as well as several untolerated VTs. Pace mapping (at the site noted by the *arrow*) produced a QRS morphology similar to the tolerated VT. Concealed entrainment was noted at this point, with a postpacing interval 25 msec greater than the VT cycle length. VT could not be induced when mechanical pressure was applied just inferior to this site (*green dot*). Ablation at this site eliminated the VT; additional lesions were placed in a linear fashion to incorporate pace-map latency sites and fractionated potentials. Further programmed stimulation from the right and left ventricles induced only a sine-wave–like VT (cycle length, 311 msec; electrocardiogram at *right*) that rapidly degenerated into ventricular fibrillation (VF); note the indeterminate nature of this arrhythmia's electrocardiogram morphology. Despite the relatively slow rate, this arrhythmia could not be targeted for ablation. The clinical significance of postablation inducible SWVT (as well as inducible VF) is unclear and can be assessed only by prospective clinical trials.

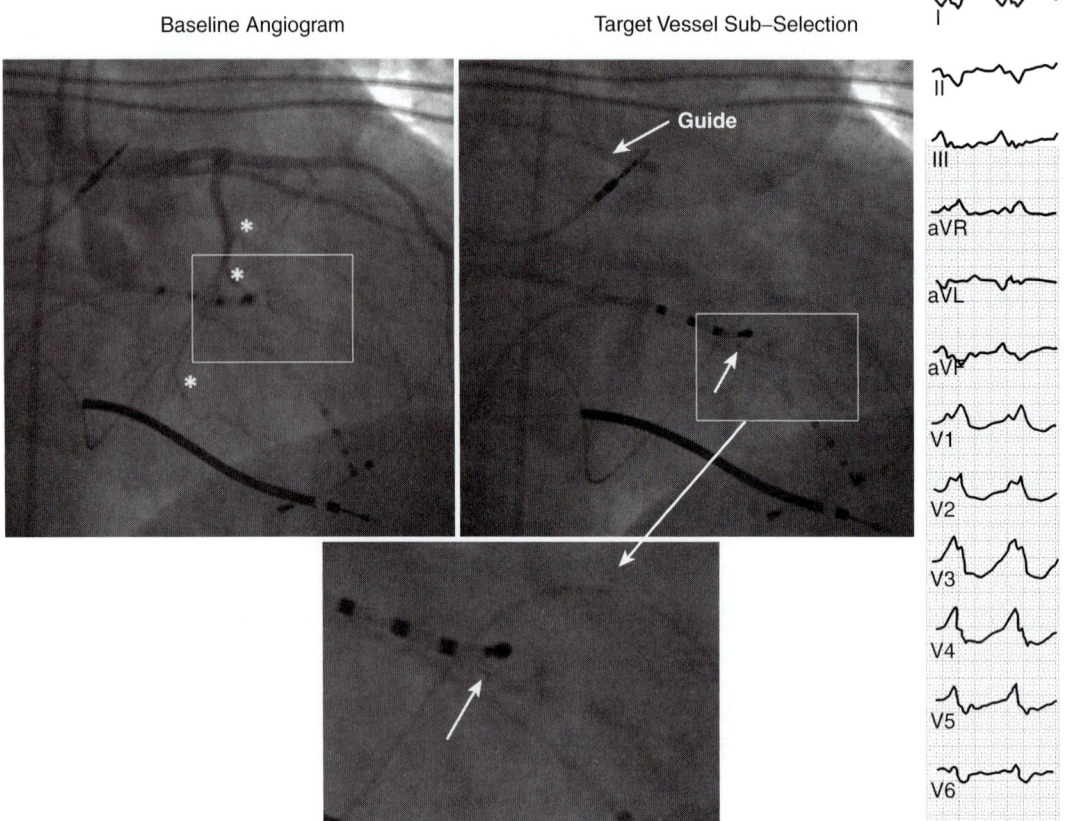

Baseline Angiogram   Target Vessel Sub–Selection

FIGURE 30-17. Alcohol ablation for ventricular tachycardia (VT) refractory to three attempts at endocardial and epicardial ablation. The VT is shown at the *far right* and was pace-mapped to the posterior basal left ventricle. Baseline angiography showed three marginal branches (*) from the circumflex artery feeding the area of interest. Each vessel was cannulated with a 1.5-mm balloon catheter and iced saline injection of the middle vessel (highlighted in *box* and shown with subselective contrast injection) resulted in tachycardia termination. Injection of 2-mm sterile absolute ethanol into this vessel rendered the VT noninducible. The *short arrows* indicate the end of the balloon catheter.

to 50 W with careful impedance and temperature monitoring to achieve an impedance fall of 10 to 15 ohms and limit catheter-tip temperature to 40°C. Excessively rapid impedance decreases often portends a steam pop.

Ablation sites not responding to endocardial and epicardial ablation may represent intramyocardial or broad circuits.[56] The use of ethanol ablation to treat these resistant circuits has been described primarily for stable VTs. After a tachycardia is localized to a region of myocardium, coronary angiography is used to identify the vasculature feeding that area. The feeding vessel is subselected as distally as possible (Fig. 30-17). The VT is induced, and 2 to 3 mL of iced saline is injected through a occlusive balloon catheter as distal in the artery as possible. If the VT reliably terminates with iced saline, 1 mL of sterile absolute alcohol is injected, and complete vessel occlusion is maintained for 10 minutes to prevent leaking of alcohol into nontarget vessels. Up to 5 mL of alcohol can be injected into any single vessel to prevent VT reinduction.

Substrate-based VT ablation is a viable strategy only if placement of the requisite multiple lesions does not adversely affect ventricular pump function. This is particular true when contemplating use of more powerful ablation technologies such as the saline-irrigated ablation catheter. Accordingly, it is imperative that ablation lesions be largely, if not exclusively, confined to the infarcted myocardium. In clinical studies of substrate-based catheter ablation, no

change in ventricular function has been noted (see later under "Minimizing Complications").

Clinical Results of Substrate-Based Ventricular Tachycardia Ablation

Regarding the efficacy of this approach, most of the published studies using a substrate-based approach have been nonrandomized studies with historical controls (Table 30-3).[57,58] One single-center study in patients with coronary artery disease and VT showed that the success rates of substrate-based ablation (54%) were similar to those of mapping during VT (60%) with a mean follow-up of 24 ± 12 months.[59] Although these data are encouraging, there is a high degree of variability in the methods used for substrate-based ablation, and the actual efficacy is largely unknown. Prospective randomized clinical trials are needed to delineate the optimal method for substrate-based ablation and to properly assess clinical efficacy.

Rapid Single-Beat Activation Mapping

Instead of the substrate-based approach, there is one mapping technology that can perform noncontact mapping of far-field EGM activity such that global chamber activation can be visualized during a single cardiac cycle (EnSite)[23] (Fig. 30-18). Because the system theoreti-

TABLE 30-3

CATHETER ABLATION OF UNSTABLE VENTRICULAR TACHYCARDIA

Study	Myocardial Pathology	No. of Patients	VT Ablation Approach	Follow-Up (mo)	Clinical Success (%)
Marchlinski et al, 2000[30]	CAD, ARVC	21	Substrate based	8 ± 7	75
Merino et al, 1996[40]	CAD	40	Substrate based	10 ± 8	63
Patel et al, 2004[41]	CAD	19	Substrate based	7 ± 2	66
Reddy et al, 2003[31]	CAD	11	Substrate based	13 ± 2	82
De Chillou et al, 2002[42]	CAD	24	Substrate based	9 ± 4	79
Bogun et al, 2006[43]	CAD	28	Substrate based	15 ± 8	64
Kriebel et al, 2007[65]	CAD	25	Substrate based	26 ± 14	54
Schilling et al, 1999[23]	CAD, DCM	24	Single-beat mapping	18	64
Roberts et al, 1987[69]	CAD, DCM	15	Single-beat mapping	1	71
Hsia et al, 2003[70]	CAD, DCM, ARVC	17	Single-beat mapping	20 ± 5	59
McKenna et al, 1994[76]	DCM	19	Substrate based	22 ± 12	68
Marchlinski et al, 2004[77]	DCM	28	Substrate based	11 ± 9	54
Bogun et al, 2009[74]	ARVC	21	Substrate based	27 ± 22	89
Maguire et al, 1987[79]	ARVC	21	Substrate based	36	53
Soejima et al, 2004[71]	TOF repair	10	Single-beat mapping	35	75
Della Bella et al, 2002[64]	Chagas CM	17	Substrate based	11 ± 3	79

ARVC, arrhythmogenic right ventricular cardiomyopathy/dysplasia; CAD, coronary artery disease; CM, cardiomyopathy; DCM, dilated cardiomyopathy; TOF, tetralogy of Fallot.

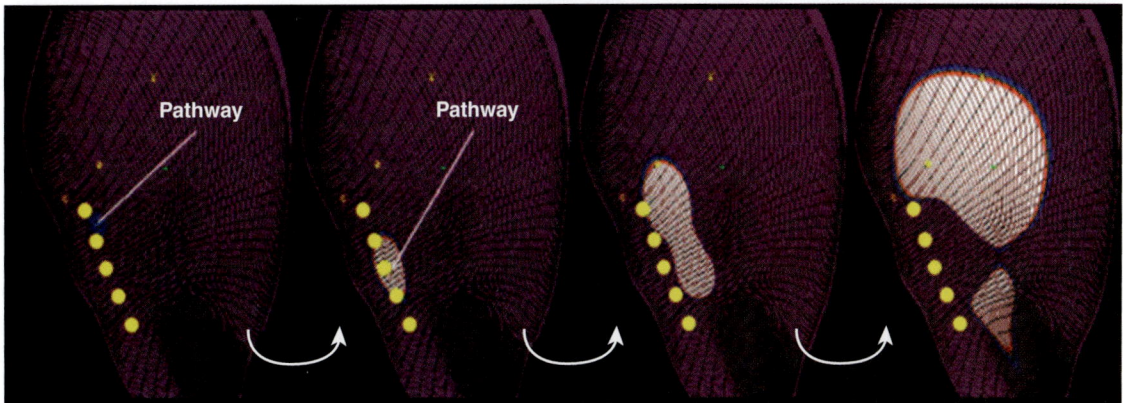

FIGURE 30-18. Single-beat noncontact mapping of ventricular tachycardia (VT). Noncontact mapping of hemodynamically unstable VT is possible by analysis of a few beats, or as little as a single beat of tachycardia (EnSite). The wavefront of activation is represented by *white*.

cally requires only a single beat of VT to create an isopotential map, even hemodynamically unstable VTs are mappable. A number of investigators have assessed the use of this technology to identify and ablate hemodynamically tolerated and untolerated VTs in patients with scar-related arrhythmias (post-MI, arrhythmogenic right ventricular cardiomyopathy-dysplasia [ARVC], dilated cardiomyopathy, and after surgical repair of teratology of Fallot).[23,60-65] After deploying this balloon catheter into the left ventricle to record several beats of the target VT, diastolic pathways of activation are identified and targeted for ablation. However, this noncontact mapping system has several limitations: (1) the presence of the mapping balloon catheter within the ventricle can complicate one's ability to maneuver the ablation catheter to the region of interest; (2)

the location accuracy of this system is inferior to the electroanatomical mapping system; (3) voltage amplitude maps cannot be accurately constructed from recording the far-field potentials,[66] which limits substrate mapping with this system; and therefore (4) only VTs that are induced can be targeted for catheter ablation—that is, one may potentially be limited to identifying only those arrhythmogenic zones that are operative during the VTs induced during that particular procedure. However, recent work by Ciaccio and associates[67] demonstrated that it is possible to use sinus rhythm activation times to determine the isthmus of VT circuits that overlapped with the diastolic pathways of the VTs, with 84% sensitivity and 89% specificity. The relative merits of VT ablation based on single-beat activation mapping versus substrate-based mapping have been studied in only one prospective, randomized study.[66] Substrate-based mapping and single-beat mapping were found to be equally efficacious; however, for unstable VTs, the acute success rate was higher for the latter (30% versus 83%; P < .05). Klemm and colleagues[61] demonstrated a benefit to using a combination of substrate-based and single-beat mapping. Using this approach, 77% of induced VTs were rendered noninducible, and after a follow-up period of 15 months, 67% of patients remained free of recurrence.

Other Scar-Related Ventricular Tachycardias

Because of its frequency, most of the literature regarding scar-related reentrant VT has been devoted to the study of post-MI VT. However, reentrant VT also occurs from myocardial scar in the setting of other forms of cardiac pathology, such as dilated cardiomyopathy (DCM). Histologic studies of myocardial tissue from patients with DCM have revealed multiple patchy areas of interstitial and replacement fibrosis and myofibrillar disarray with variable degrees of myocyte hypertrophy and atrophy.[68] A necropsy study in patients with idiopathic DCM revealed that despite a relative paucity of visible scar (14%), a high

incidence of mural endocardial plaque (69% to 85%) and myocardial fibrosis (57%) was found.[69] As with post-MI VT, the mechanism of VT related to DCM is most commonly reentrant and is related to this scarred substrate. Accordingly, scar-related VT in the setting of DCM may be expected on the endocardial surface, on the epicardial surface, or in a deep intramural region of the heart. Clinical studies of VT mapping and ablation in the setting of DCM have revealed that a substrate-based approach is also useful to eliminate these arrhythmias.[39,70,71] Interestingly, the location of the myocardial scar by delayed contrast-enhanced MRI is not necessarily restricted to the endocardium; it is commonly found in the mid-myocardium and epicardium.[72–74] In our experience, and in the experience of other investigators, the scar tends to be predominantly localized by electroanatomic mapping to the basal regions of the left ventricle and the ventricular septum.[39,75–77] Of importance, when a myocardial scar is identified, this abnormal area can be targeted for ablation based on mapping strategies similar to those for post-MI VT, including pace mapping and targeting of late potentials (Fig. 30-19).

Another pathologic state associated with scar-related VT that lends itself to a substrate mapping approach is ARVC. The precise pathophysiology of ARVC is not fully

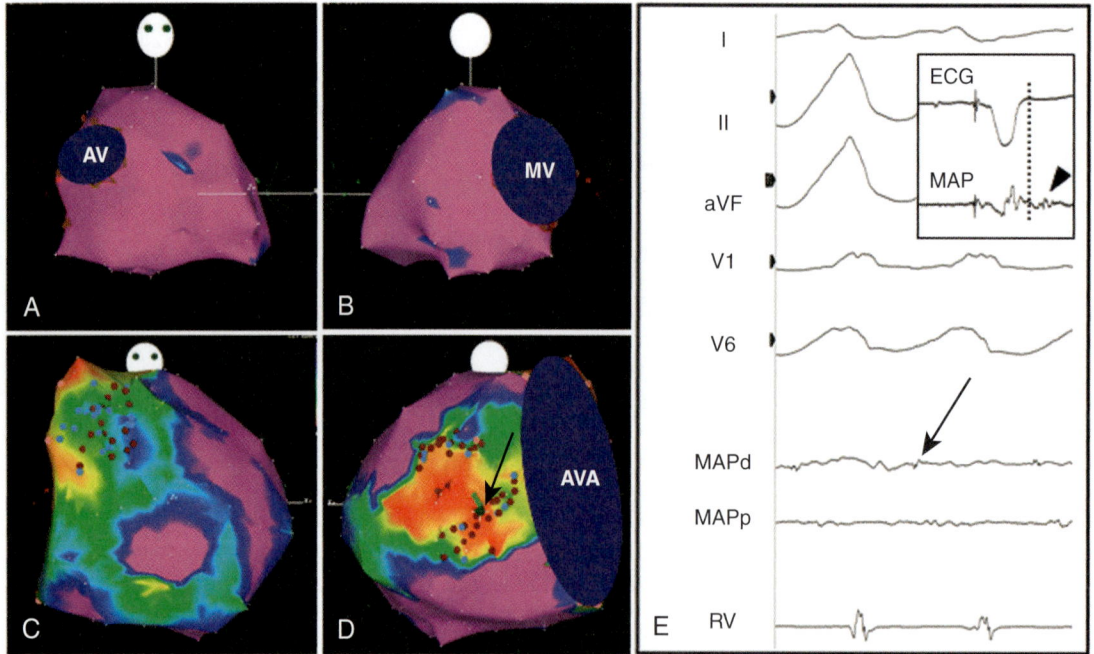

FIGURE 30-19. Substrate mapping and ablation of hemodynamically unstable ventricular tachycardia (VT) in a patient with dilated cardiomyopathy. This patient with dilated cardiomyopathy presented with defibrillator shocks due to fast VTs. Programmed ventricular stimulation revealed five hemodynamically unstable VTs. Left ventricle (LV) endocardial substrate mapping during atrioventricular sequential pacing (right anterior oblique [**A**] and posteroanterior [**B**] projections) revealed no significant patches of diseased myocardium based on bipolar voltage criteria or electrogram characteristics (fractionated or late potentials). After pericardial access using a subxyphoid puncture approach, the ventricular epicardial surface was mapped during atrioventricular pacing (anteroposterior [**C**] and posteroanterior [**D**] projections). Two large patches of abnormal myocardium were identified by substrate mapping based on both low bipolar voltage amplitude and abnormal electrogram components (*blue dots* indicate late potentials): one right anterior overlying the right ventricle (RV), and the other left lateral overlying the LV near the atrioventricular groove. The low-voltage area overlying the RV acute margin likely represents an area of normal myocardium with overlying epicardial fat; notice the lack of late potentials at this region. At one of the late potential sites (*black arrow* in **D**; and *black arrowhead* in **E**, *inset*), an optimal pace map was obtained for one of the VTs. With the catheter placed at this position, VT was briefly induced (**E**); an intra-aortic balloon pump was placed for hemodynamic support. A diastolic component was noted at this site (*black arrow* in **E**), and entrainment maneuvers identified this as the exit site of the circuit. RF ablation at this site eliminated the VT. Additional radiofrequency ablation lesions were applied along areas of late potentials along the inferior and superior borders of the LV epicardial scar (**D**) and the RV epicardial scar (**C**); no further VT was inducible at the end of the procedure (color range, 0.1 to 1.5 mV). AV, aortic valve; AVA, atrioventricular annulus; d, distal; ECG, electrocardiogram; MAP, mapping catheter; MV, mitral valve; p, proximal.

understood, but its hallmark is the presence of fibrosis and fatty infiltrate of the RV myocardium.[76] VT that occurs in the setting of ARVC usually originates from within the scarred myocardium of the right ventricle and is of a reentrant mechanism. Substrate mapping of the right ventricle in these individuals typically reveals abnormal myocardial tissue that involves the perivalvular tricuspid valve, pulmonic valve, or both valves.[77] The abnormal myocardium virtually always involves the RV free wall (epicardium more than endocardium), frequently involves the septum, and rarely involves the apex.[78-83] A substrate-based approach is also successful in eliminating VT in these patients.[30,63,83,84]

Chronic Chagas-related cardiomyopathy is another important myocardial disease process with a high incidence of scar-related reentrant VT.[39,79] Histologic studies have again revealed myofibrillar disarray and diffuse fibrosis resulting in scar formation in two characteristic distributions: the inferolateral LV wall and the apical septal and apical inferior walls. The pathophysiologic mechanism of scar formation in this disease state is not fully understood but is thought to be a cell-mediated autoimmune reaction with autonomic denervation. As with other scar-related VTs, the mechanism of Chagas-related VT is reentry.[39,80] Unlike other substrates, however, the VT circuits in the setting of Chagas disease have an extremely high incidence of epicardial origin.[39,81]

Are All Scar-Related Ventricular Tachycardias Located at the Subendocardium?

Because only the endocardial surface of the scarred myocardium traditionally underwent catheter mapping, it was typical for little to be known regarding the electrophysiologic characteristics of the epicardial extent of the scar in any particular patient. By necessity, the infarcted substrate was typically viewed by the electrophysiologist as a two-dimensional surface, with little consideration given to its character throughout the thickness of the wall. Fortunately, in most patients with post-MI VT, the arrhythmogenic substrate is located on the endocardial surface of the heart. However, surgical mapping studies have revealed all VT circuits could be eliminated by endocardial ablative strategies alone. In one study, 15% of the patients undergoing arrhythmia surgery for VT required epicardial laser ablation to eliminate the target VT.[82] For reasons still not fully understood, most of these patients requiring epicardial ablative lesions (90%) had inferior wall MIs with no identifiable aneurysm. Thus, only a minority of post-MI patients would require an epicardial ablation approach to eliminate it.

In those post-MI patients with VT in whom an endocardial approach is unsuccessful, it has been demonstrated that one can perform pericardial mapping of the epicardial surface of the heart using a percutaneous subxiphoid puncture approach.[83-87] This approach has been employed to eliminate hemodynamically stable VT in a variety of clinical settings.[39,77,81,84,87] In a porcine model of healed myocardial infarction, the feasibility of substrate mapping of the ventricular epicardial surface has been demonstrated (Fig. 30-20).[85] Accordingly, just as with endocardial substrate mapping and ablation, epicardial substrate mapping and ablation can be employed to eliminate VT.

It is prudent to consider an epicardial approach in patients in whom an endocardial attempt at VT ablation has failed. However, the decision about whether to consider a primary epicardial-endocardial approach has not been studied in any prospective fashion. Epicardial mapping should certainly be considered in the setting of cardiac pathologies that appear to have a high incidence of epicardial scar, including Chagas-related, DCM-related, and ARVC-related VT. The morphology of a target

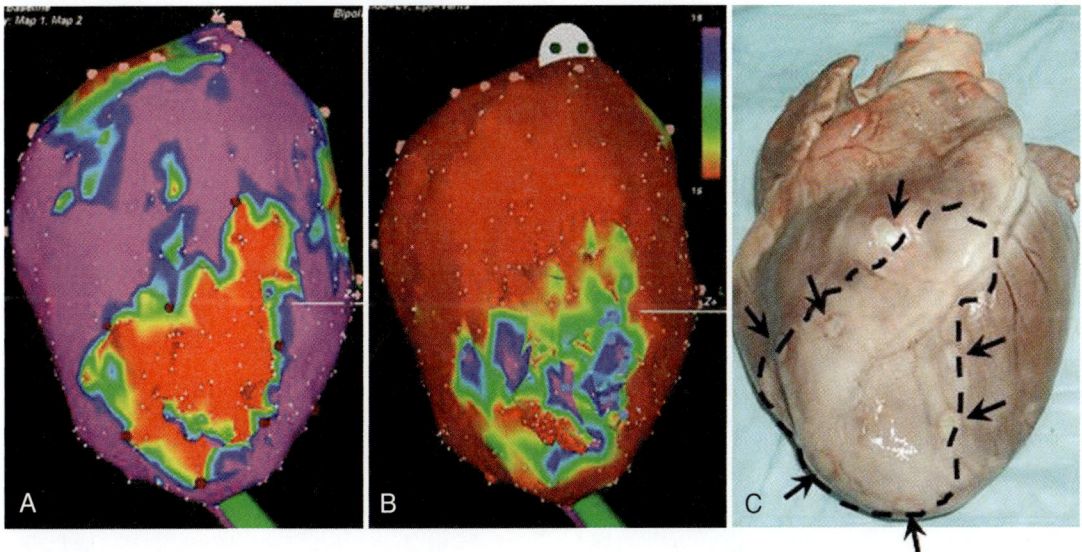

FIGURE 30-20. Epicardial substrate mapping of porcine infarcts. A porcine chronic myocardial infarction (MI) model underwent epicardial electroanatomic mapping using a percutaneous subxyphoid puncture approach. Using either bipolar voltage (**A**; range, 0.5 to 1.5 mV) or electrogram duration (**B**; 50 to 80 msec) criteria, the epicardial extent of the myocardial scar could be mapped. Of note, sites over normal tissue with corresponding falsely low bipolar voltage values were frequently correctly defined as normal based on electrogram duration criteria. Based solely on the bipolar voltage electroanatomic map, radiofrequency ablation lesions were placed to "tag" the scar border (*red dots* in **A**). Gross pathologic examination revealed that the ablation lesions (*black arrows* in **C**) were indeed situated at the scar periphery. The *purple-green* tube represents the pericardial access sheath.

VT might provide additional clues to its exit from the infarcted tissue. In a systematic study of the ECG pattern of VTs eliminated from the endocardial versus epicardial surface of the heart, an epicardial origin was predicted by the following characteristics of the VT: (1) a longer pseudo-delta wave as measured from the earliest ventricular activation to the earliest fast deflection in any precordial lead; (2) a longer intrinsicoid deflection time in lead V_2; (3) a longer "shortest RS complex," defined as the interval from the earliest ventricular activation to the nadir of the first S wave in any precordial lead; and (4) a wider QRS complex.[86] This study concluded that an epicardial VT origin can be identified by a pseudo-delta wave of 34 milliseconds or longer (sensitivity 83%, specificity 95%), intrinsicoid deflection time of 85 milliseconds or longer (sensitivity 87%, specificity 90%), and shortest RS complex of 121 milliseconds or longer (sensitivity 76%, specificity 85%). As relates to substrate-based VT ablation, an important caveat that must be considered is that the ECG morphology only addresses the exit point of VT from the scar; little can be derived regarding the location of the critical protected portion of the circuit. For example, despite an epicardial exit, endocardial ablation may eliminate a critical portion of the circuit (and vice versa, a "narrow" QRS VT may be eliminated by epicardial ablation). Thus, for any patient with a prior inferior wall MI VT without a history of cardiac surgery, it is our practice to consider a primary combined epicardial-endocardial approach (Fig. 30-21). In patients with prior cardiac surgery, epicardial mapping can nonetheless be performed using a percutaneous[87] or surgical[88] subxyphoid approach, but this is reserved for patients who have failed an endocardial approach.

Future of Unstable Ventricular Tachycardia Ablation

During the next several years, technologic advances will likely allow us to improve the clinical efficacy of unstable VT ablation. Improved hemodynamic support during unstable VT would allow us to directly map VT using activation mapping and resetting and entrainment criteria. Although intra-aortic balloon pumps are useful to prevent acute congestive heart failure as a result of the procedure, they rarely provide enough hemodynamic support to allow mapping of otherwise unstable VTs. Currently, there are two percutaneous LV assist devices that are available. The TandemHeart system (CardiacAssist, Pittsburgh, PA) provides hemodynamic support by delivering oxygenated blood from the left atrium directly to the ascending aorta. A 21-French (21F) cannula is placed in the left atrium with a transseptal approach, and a 17F arterial cannula is placed in the aorta with a retrograde aortic approach.[89] During unstable VT, the device is capable of providing up to 5 L/minute of cardiac output to allow mapping and ablation of the VT (Fig. 30-22). The Impella device (ABIOMED, Danvers, MA) is placed in the left ventricle through a retrograde aortic approach. The 12F device is advanced over a guidewire into the ascending aorta and across the aortic valve into the left ventricle. The tip of the catheter contains a pigtail to minimize trauma. The device is capable of unloading the left ventricle by transporting up to 2.5 L/minute of blood from the LV cavity into the ascending aorta. Mapping may be done during unstable VT with this additional hemodynamic support. The main limitation is maneuvering the mapping catheter around the device. These devices require large-caliber arterial

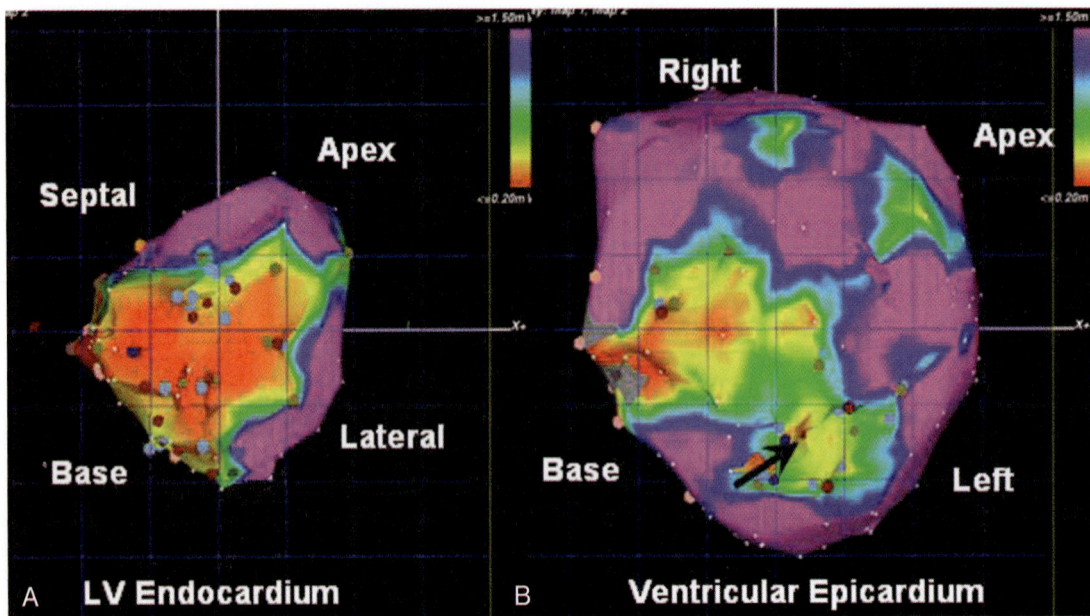

FIGURE 30-21. Combined endocardial-epicardial substrate mapping of post–myocardial infarction (MI) ventricular tachycardia (VT). In this patient with a prior inferior wall MI, endocardial (**A**) and epicardial (**B**) substrate mapping in sinus rhythm revealed a large area of infarcted tissue (color range, 0.2 to 1.5 mV). Extensive endocardial mapping failed to identify an isthmus site for the clinical VT, but epicardial mapping identified a site (*arrow* in **B**) with a late potential during sinus rhythm and a diastolic component during tachycardia. Catheter ablation at this point eliminated this VT; additional radiofrequency ablation lesions at endocardial and epicardial sites of fractionated and late potentials eliminated inducible VT. LV, left ventricle.

and venous access and should be reserved for patients who have previously failed multiple ablations with unstable VTs or for patients with VT storm.

During substrate-based VT ablation, 3D electroanatomic mapping is used to identify scar based on voltage criteria. A more ideal paradigm would be to directly visualize scar with delayed contrast-enhanced MRI and PET-CT imaging, and to incorporate that information into the electroanatomic maps. Delayed contrast-enhanced MRI can distinguish normal from chronically infarcted cardiac tissue with millimeter spatial resolution (Fig. 30-23).[90] By defining the scar morphology in post-MI patients, a preprocedural cardiac MRI could serve as a useful "road map" to guide substrate-based catheter ablation. Of course, MRI is currently not routinely performed in patients with preexisting implantable defibrillators or pacemakers. However, PET can also detect myocardial scar and can be combined with CT imaging to allow both anatomic and metabolic visualization of myocardium and scar.[33] This imaging modality can be safely used in patients with implantable defibrillators and pacemakers. Recently, investigators have shown that it is possible to successfully incorporate these MRI and PET-CT studies into the electroanatomic voltage maps to better define

scar and to guide ablation.[33–38] In the future, with even more advances in imaging, we may be able to visualize the arrhythmogenic channels within the scar, which would be expected to improve clinical efficacy.

Minimizing Complications

By the very nature of the cardiac function in patients in whom substrate-based VT ablation is performed, an important potential complication of the procedure is worsening or new congestive heart failure. This can occur as a result of programmed stimulation or catheter ablation. To mitigate against worsening heart failure, programmed stimulation should be performed with an adequate pause between stimulus trains, and in patients with severe LV dysfunction an intra-aortic balloon pump should be strongly considered. Given that these patients often enter the electrophysiology laboratory in a worsened heart failure state, and this is further exacerbated by the stimulation and inductions of VT, our threshold for using the balloon pump is quite low. We typically place the balloon pump at the beginning of the procedure and remove it at the end before the patient

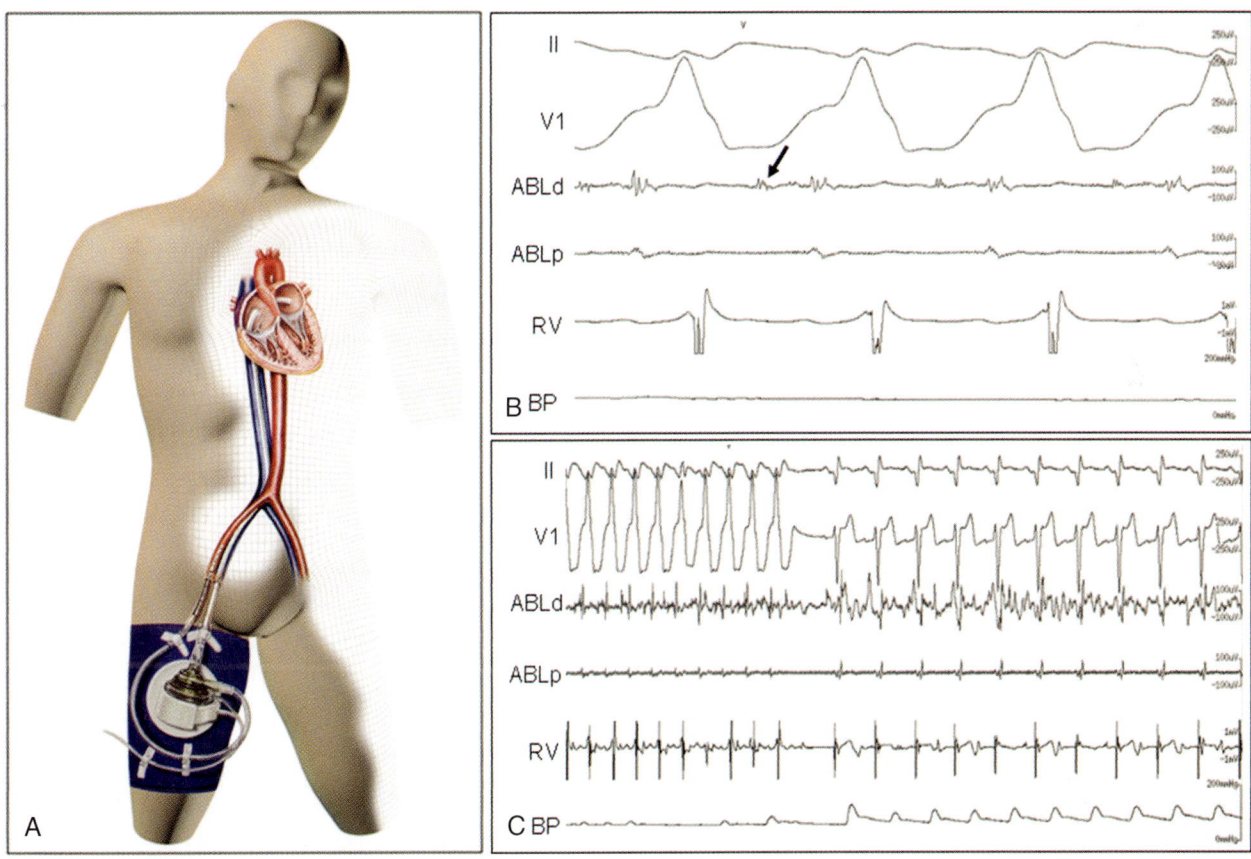

FIGURE 30-22. Using hemodynamic support to map unstable ventricular tachycardias. **A,** Schematic representation of the TandemHeart percutaneous left ventricular device. The pump is positioned at the patient's leg and attached to a control console (not shown). The pump is connected to a venous cannula that is positioned in the left atrium by transseptal puncture and also to an arterial cannula positioned in the aorta. The pump circulates oxygenated blood from the left atrium and delivers it to the aorta, bypassing the left ventricle. The device is capable of circulating blood up to 5 L/min. **B,** The patient is left in otherwise unstable VT, which can then be mapped. Blood pressure (BP) during hemodynamic support and VT is displayed. There is minimal pulsation in the arterial waveform, but the mean BP was about 70 mm Hg. During this time, the patient was receiving hemodynamic support through the TandemHeart device. The VT was mapped, and mid-diastolic potentials (*arrow*) were identified. **C,** Ablation at this site slowed and then terminated the VT. Shown on the *left side* of the tracing is BP during VT. The minimally pulsatile arterial waveform is better appreciated (mean pressure was about 70 mm Hg). With ablation (ABL), the VT terminated, and the arterial waveform returned to normal morphology and pressure. RV, right ventricle.

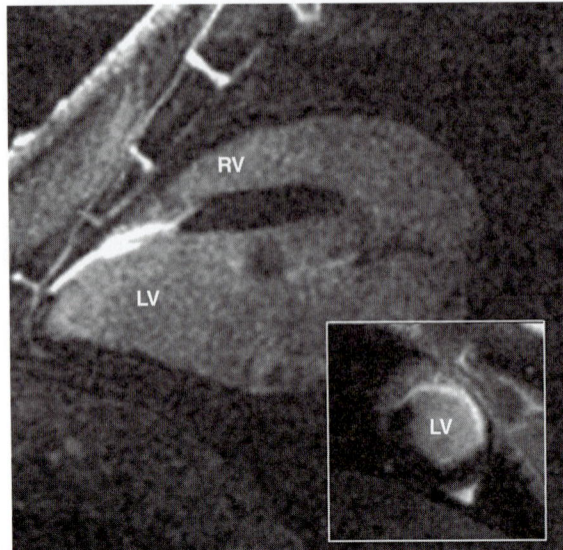

FIGURE 30-23. Contrast-enhanced magnetic resonance imaging (MRI) of infarcted tissue. Contrast enhancement observed relatively quickly (within tens of seconds) after injection of the MRI contrast agent, gadolinium, is related to vascular perfusion. Delayed enhancement (defined as appearing >5 minutes after bolus injection) is selectively observed in infarcted tissue because of the relatively larger extracellular space and therefore larger volume of distribution of gadolinium within this tissue. Long- and short-axis views (*main view* and *inset*, respectively) of the infarcted left ventricle (LV) are shown after gadolinium delayed enhancement MRI: the infarcted interventricular septum and anterior wall are enhanced. RV, right ventricle.

leaves the electrophysiology laboratory. Also, it is important to note that during substrate-based VT ablation, the patient is typically in sinus rhythm and not in VT throughout most of the procedure. Accordingly, this procedure is well tolerated even by patients with severe ventricular dysfunction. With externally irrigated catheter ablation, it is crucial to note the patient's fluid balance during the procedure. Because it is our practice to routinely map the left ventricle with a transseptal approach (in addition to a retrograde aortic approach), we often measure left atrial pressure before and after the procedure to assess for fluid overload and administer diuretic therapy as necessary.

There is also the potential for transient worsening of ventricular function due to catheter ablation. An experimental porcine study was performed in which linear RF ablation lesions were placed along the borders of a healed myocardial infarct.[91] In this study, intracardiac ECG revealed that linear lesions caused significant systolic dysfunction (38.5% decrease in fractional shortening) in the normal myocardium adjacent to the infarct border (1 cm from the ablation site). The mechanism of this phenomenon is unknown but is probably related to myocardial stunning resulting from microvascular dysfunction. Consistent with this hypothesis, systolic function recovered to baseline function in this porcine model within 30 minutes. Furthermore, in a separate clinical study, the impact of catheter ablation on LV function was examined in a series of 62 post-MI patients who underwent VT ablation.[92] Digitized echocardiography performed within 1 week before and less than 72 hours after the procedure revealed no significant changes in LV function in the entire group, the patients who received more than 25 lesions, or the patients who received more than 40 lesions. However, the LV ejection fraction increased more

than 5% in 12 of 62 (19.4%) patients and decreased 5% or more in 14 of 62 (22.5%) patients; there was no relation to the number of RF lesions. Thus, when the ablation lesions are confined to the area of abnormal EGMs, most patients do not experience any appreciable change in LV function. Accordingly, we rarely place ablation lesions in tissue with bipolar EGM amplitude higher than 1.0 mV.

As with all left-sided ablation procedures, it is important to minimize the risk for embolic complications by using adequate anticoagulation during and after the procedure. During the procedure, intravenous heparin is infused to achieve an activated clotting time of more than 250 seconds. When using the transseptal approach, an intravenous heparin bolus (5000 to 8000 units) is infused at least 5 minutes before the transseptal puncture procedure; both the transseptal needle and the traumatized, denuded tissue at the puncture site are extremely thrombogenic. In addition, continuous flushing of the transseptal sheath helps prevent air or thrombotic emboli from being expelled. Because of the number of ablation lesions typically delivered during substrate-based VT ablation, we always use an irrigated catheter because of the favorable safety profile with respect to thrombus formation and impedance pops.

Pericardial effusion resulting in cardiac tamponade physiology is another potential complication of substrate ablation. This can occur during the transseptal puncture procedure, a risk that is minimized by the use of intracardiac ultrasound imaging at least during the "difficult" punctures. Perforation of the LV by the ablation catheter is rare because of the thickness of this chamber; when the wall is thin due to a chronic MI, the fibrous tissue is difficult to perforate. However, the thinner-walled right ventricle may be perforated by either the ablation catheter during mapping or the RV quadripolar pacing catheter. This is particularly prone to happen when the patient is receiving intravenous inotropic agents such as isoproterenol. Perforation of the right ventricle related to catheter ablation has also been reported in a patient with ARVC.[56]

Damage to the aortic or mitral valves can also occur, particularly if the ablation catheters are forcibly manipulated across these structures. Damage to the coronary arteries can occur as a result of embolization from an RF ablation lesion–related thrombus. The coronary artery can also be damaged by inadvertent introduction of the ablation catheter into a coronary vessel, which could traumatize an atherosclerotic coronary plaque. This is of particular concern in patients with coronary artery bypass grafts because of the difficulty in knowing the locations of the origins of these vessels. One means to avoid entering these vessels is to deflect the catheter into a U shape when advancing into the ascending aorta and crossing the aortic valve so that the catheter tip does not enter a coronary vessel. Inadvertent delivery of RF energy within the coronary would be disastrous.

Complications of epicardial mapping and ablation (covered in detail elsewhere in this book) can be divided into those related to pericardial access and ablation. Certainly, the location of the coronary arteries relative to the ablation catheter must be assessed before pericardial energy delivery. Although it is rare to find a surviving coronary vessel traversing an epicardial scar in post-MI patients, this is of particular concern in patients with nonischemic cardiomyopathy. Specifically relating to substrate-based VT ablation, it should be recognized that if multiple lesions are

TABLE 30-4

TROUBLESHOOTING THE DIFFICULT CASE

Problem	Solution
Preprocedural echo reveals left ventricular thrombus	Postpone procedure if possible. After anticoagulation for 4-6 weeks to allow organization of the thrombus, perform procedure. Consider an epicardial-alone approach.
During ventricular mapping, frequent premature ventricular contractions complicate substrate mapping	Consider intravenous infusion of antiarrhythmic drugs to suppress ectopy (e.g., lidocaine)
During programmed stimulation, only polymorphic ventricular tachycardia is inducible	Consider repeat stimulation after infusion of a class I antiarrhythmic drug such as intravenous procainamide (but not if significantly depressed left ventricular ejection fraction) Obtain 12 leads of spontaneous ventricular tachycardias to generalize regions of interest
Left ventricular mapping reveals a large septal scar	Consider right ventricular septal mapping to assess for arrhythmogenic tissue on the right side of the septum
Unable to find suitable endocardial pace-map site or abnormal electrograms (e.g., late potentials)	Perform epicardial mapping using a subxyphoid approach If previous cardiac surgery, can use either subxyphoid puncture approach or direct surgical subxyphoid exposure
Difficult to cross aortic valve with ablation catheter, poor catheter motion	Use a transseptal approach to left ventricle mapping
Severely depressed ventricular function (especially in association with preexisting congestive heart failure)	Aggressive patient monitoring, including Foley catheter to monitor urine output, and left atrial pressure monitoring, either direct transseptal sheath or Swan-Ganz catheter (wedge) Judicious use of intravenous diuretic agents Judicious use of intravenous pressor agents Consider intra-aortic balloon pump support for the duration of the procedure Minimize the number of ablation lesions placed near normal ventricular myocardium

delivered, there is an increased risk for pericardial inflammation and pericarditis. To mitigate against this complication, one can lavage the pericardial space at the end of the procedure with fresh sterile saline to minimize the presence of blood (which is proinflammatory), and then administer a one-time dose of pericardial steroids (methylprednisolone or triamcinolone, 2 to 5 mg/kg) and intravenous antibiotics. In an animal model, we have shown that intrapericardial injection of 2 mg/kg of triamcinolone is effective at preventing postprocedure inflammatory adhesions.[93] There is no consensus on the optimal pericardial steroid dose that one should use, but our clinical experience indicates that higher doses of intrapericardial methylprednisolone or triamcinolone (5 mg/kg) are optimal to minimize significant pericarditis. Patients are also typically given oral nonsteroidal anti-inflammatory drugs as needed.

Troubleshooting the Difficult Case

Most of the problems associated with unstable VT ablation have been described previously and are summarized in Table 30-4. Multiple VT morphologies are usually inducible, and it is often difficult to identify the most clinically significant arrhythmia. Surface ECG recordings or implantable cardioverter-defibrillator EGM tracings of spontaneous arrhythmias may be helpful. Hemodynamic stability may be tenuous in these patients, even in sinus rhythm. The use of pressors, mechanical support, and attention to fluid balance can be critical. If no favorable ablation sites are identified in the LV endocardium, it is important to change strategies to include epicardial or RV mapping before the patient decompensates from lengthy unproductive mapping. Meticulous and efficient mapping is critical. Each EGM site should be scrutinized for proper annotation and features of late potentials. Even at favorable ablation sites,

energy delivery may be ineffective because of poor tissue contact, heavily scarred tissue, or intramyocardial circuits. Changing ablation approach (e.g., from retrograde aortic to transseptal or vice versa) or use of a different catheter curve can improve catheter contact. Irrigated ablation is generally necessary to create the large lesions required to interrupt VT circuits. Alcohol ablation is a rarely used approach to target otherwise refractory foci.

Ventricular Fibrillation

Just as atrial fibrillation can occur as the result of a focal mechanism with fibrillatory conduction, Haïssaguerre and colleagues were the first to demonstrate that there are certain patients with a focal mechanism of VF that can be treated by catheter ablation.[94] After being resuscitated from recurrent (10 ±12) episodes of primary VF, 27 patients without known structural heart disease underwent an electrophysiology procedure.[95] These patients were studied because of the presence of isolated premature ventricular beats of identical morphology and coupling interval (297 ± 41 milliseconds) to the first initiating beat of VF (Fig. 30-24). Endocardial mapping revealed that these triggers initiated from the RV or LV Purkinje system in 23 of 27 patients (85%) and from the myocardium of the RV outflow tract in 4 of 27 patients (15%). The interval from the Purkinje potential to ventricular activation varied from 10 to 150 milliseconds during the premature beat. A Purkinje potential was also seen at these same sites during sinus rhythm but preceded the QRS by only 11 ± 5 milliseconds. RF catheter ablation at these sites eliminated the triggering PVCs and subsequent VF in most of these patients. The mean number of RF ablation lesions required to eliminate these triggers was nine.

Focal PVC triggers of VF have also been described in two other groups of patients: those with channelopathies and otherwise structurally normal hearts, and those with

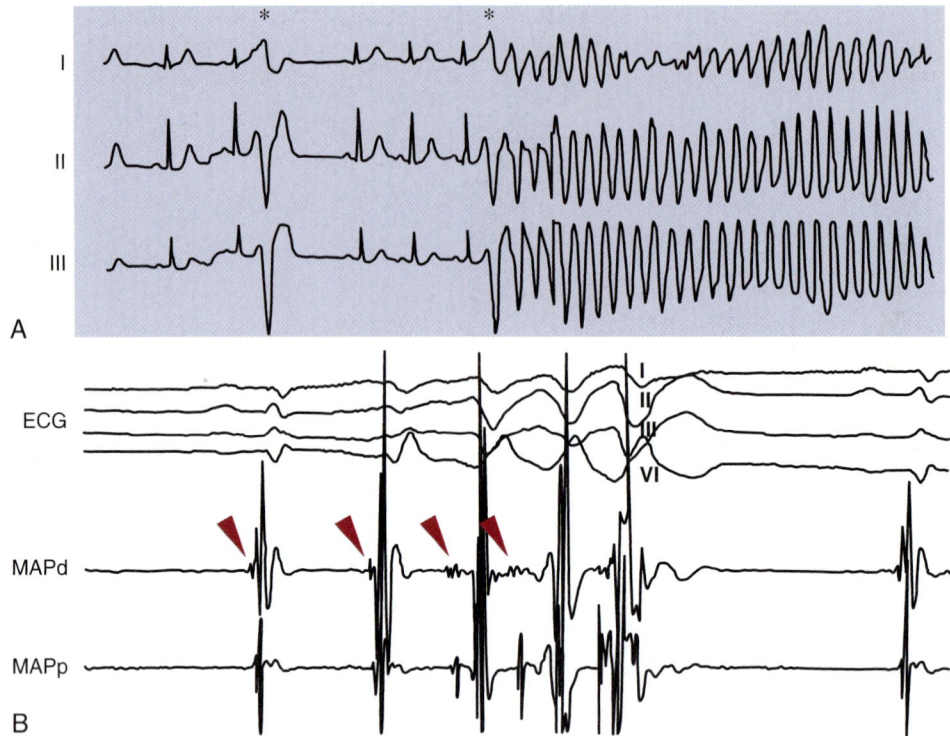

FIGURE 30-24. Catheter ablation of focal ventricular fibrillation. **A,** In this patient with a structurally normal heart and recurrent ventricular fibrillation (VF), an example of monomorphic premature ventricular contractions (PVCs) initiating VF is shown. **B,** In another patient with a structurally normal heart and VF, catheter mapping revealed a focal site with Purkinje potentials (*arrows*) preceding the initiating PVCs of the nonsustained polymorphic VT episode. Note that at this site, Purkinje potentials are also noted during sinus rhythm—albeit with a significantly shorter interval to the local ventricular electrogram. ECG, electrocardiogram; d, distal; MAP, mapping catheter; p, proximal. *(Courtesy of M. Haïssaguerre.)*

ischemic heart disease. Regarding the former, PVC triggers amenable to catheter ablation have been found in patients with either long QT syndrome or Brugada syndrome.[96] As with the other idiopathic VF patients, two types of PVC triggers have been found in both these clinical disease states: those with preceding Purkinje potentials, and those originating from the RV outflow tract.

Unlike the scar-related reentrant VT that is seen after an MI, it has recently been demonstrated that certain post-MI patients with drug-refractory primary VF (i.e., VF not preceded by monomorphic VT) have PVC triggers of the arrhythmia.[97-99] These post-MI patients can be divided into those with a recent MI (<1 week) and those with remote MI (>1 month). The PVC triggers were exclusively associated with Purkinje-like potentials and also successfully targeted for catheter ablation. In addition to VF, Bogun and colleagues showed that the Purkinje system may play a role in post-MI reentrant VT that was relatively narrow (QRS complex ± 145 milliseconds) and resembled fascicular VT.[100] Mapping during VT demonstrated a reentrant mechanism with Purkinje potentials noted at the exit site. Even in patients with VF or VT storm related to acute coronary syndromes, PVCs originating from the Purkinje network have been implicated as triggers and successfully ablated.[101]

Common to all these patients with VF amenable to catheter ablation is the clinical demonstration of frequent PVCs initiating the arrhythmia (Table 30-5). Recently, a multicenter study reported the long-term follow-up of 38 patients who underwent catheter ablation of PVC triggers for idiopathic VF.[102] During a median follow-up of 63 months, 7 patients (18%) had recurrent VF. Five of the 7 patients underwent a repeat procedure with successful ablation of PVC triggers. Different PVCs were demonstrated in 4 of 5 patients, and an identical PVC was demonstrated in the remaining. Despite the impressive clinical success rate of this therapeutic paradigm, an important practical limitation is the unknown frequency at which these patients can be identified. These patients appear to represent a highly selected cohort, thereby rendering VF ablation a rarity. Another limitation is the fact that frequent PVCs are necessary to map and target the Purkinje potentials. If frequent PVCs are absent, one is limited to pace-mapping techniques to identify the target site (assuming that a 12-lead ECG of the pathologic PVCs is available), a technique inferior to activation mapping of the pathologic PVCs.

Conclusion

Hemodynamically unstable ventricular arrhythmias are now amenable to catheter ablative approaches. Currently, both scar-related VTs and certain patients with primary VF can be treated well with catheter ablation. The demonstration that VF can be eliminated by catheter ablation in certain patients is an exciting option in the treatment of this sometimes intractable clinical situation. Our understanding of the role of catheter ablation in primary VF and the role of the Purkinje network is being refined with increased clinical experience. Regarding scar-related VT, a paradigm shift has occurred. Instead of only trying to

TABLE 30-5

CATHETER ABLATION OF FOCALLY TRIGGERED VENTRICULAR FIBRILLATION

Study	Cardiac Pathology	No. of Patients	Distribution of Foci	Follow-Up (mo)	Clinical Success (%)
Haïssaguerre et al[95]	Normal	27	Purkinje = 23 RVOT = 4	24 ± 28	89
Haïssaguerre et al[96]	LQTS, Brugada	7	Purkinje = 4 RVOT = 3	17 ± 17	100
Bransch et al[97]	CAD, MI	4	Purkinje = 4	15 ± 13	100
Marrouche et al[98]	CAD, MI	8	Purkinje = 8	10 ± 6	88
Szumowski et al[99]	CAD, MI	5	Purkinje = 5	16 ± 5	100
Knecht et al[102]	Normal	38	Purkinje = 33 RVOT = 4 Myocardium = 1	63	82

CAD, coronary artery disease; LQTS, long QT syndrome; MI, myocardial infarction; RVOT, right ventricular outflow tract.

identify the pathway of activation during the tachycardia of interest, the scarred myocardium is identified, and ablation lesions are strategically placed to eliminate potentially arrhythmogenic tissue. Because this substrate-based ablation strategy is performed in sinus rhythm, virtually any VT can be targeted for catheter ablation regardless of its hemodynamic effect. Indeed, regardless of the cardiac pathology underlying the formation of the myocardial scar, a substrate-based approach to VT ablation can still be employed. However, substrate-based catheter ablation of VT is a strategy in evolution, and the future will likely witness technologic advances in cardiac imaging to better visualize the arrhythmogenic substrate and perhaps increase clinical efficacy.

References

1. Josephson ME, Horowitz LN, Farshidi A, Kastor JA. Recurrent sustained ventricular tachycardia. 1. Mechanisms. *Circulation.* 1978;57:431–440.
2. Downar E, Harris L, Michleborough LL, et al. Endocardial mapping of ventricular tachycardia in the intact human heart: evidence for reentrant mechanisms. *J Am Coll Cardiol.* 1988;11:783–791.
3. El-Shalakany A, Hadjis T, Papageorgiou P, et al. Entrainment mapping criteria for the prediction of termination of ventricular tachycardia by single radiofrequency lesion in patients with coronary artery disease. *Circulation.* 1999;99:2283–2289.
4. Stevenson WG, Friedman PL, Kocovic D, et al. Radiofrequency catheter ablation of ventricular tachycardia after myocardial infarction. *Circulation.* 1998;98:308–314.
5. Strickberger SA, Man KC, Daoud EG, et al. A prospective evaluation of catheter ablation of ventricular tachycardia as adjuvant therapy in patients with coronary artery disease and an implantable cardioverter/defibrillator. *Circulation.* 1997;96:1525–1531.
6. Kim YH, Sosa-Suarez G, Trouton TG, et al. Treatment of ventricular tachycardia by transcatheter radiofrequency ablation in patients with ischemic heart disease. *Circulation.* 1994;89:1094–1102.
7. Rothman SA, Hsia HH, Cossu SF, et al. Radiofrequency catheter ablation of postinfarction ventricular tachycardia: long-term success and the significance of inducible non-clinical tachycardias. *Circulation.* 1997;96:3499–3508.
8. Morady F, Harvey M, Kalbfleisch SJ, et al. Radiofrequency ablation of ventricular tachycardia in patients with coronary artery disease. *Circulation.* 1993;87:363–372.
9. Downar E, Kimber S, Harris L, et al. Endocardial mapping of ventricular tachycardia in the intact human heart. II. Evidence for multiuse reentry in a functional sheet of surviving myocardium. *J Am Coll Cardiol.* 1992;20:869–878.
10. Harken AH, Horowitz LN, Josephson ME. Comparison of standard aneurysmectomy and aneurysmectomy with directed endocardial resection for the treatment of recurrent sustained ventricular tachycardia. *J Thorac Cardiovasc Surg.* 1980;80:527–534.
11. Mason JW, Stinson EB, Winkle RA, et al. Relative efficacy of blind left ventricular aneurysm resection for the treatment of recurrent sustained ventricular tachycardia. *Am J Cardiol.* 1982;49:241–248.
12. Miller JM, Kienzle MG, Harken AH, Josephson ME. Subendocardial resection for ventricular tachycardia: predictors for surgical success. *Circulation.* 1984;70:624–631.
13. Garan H, Nguyen K, McGovern B, et al. Perioperative and long-term results after electrophysiologically directed ventricular surgery for recurrent ventricular tachycardia. *J Am Coll Cardiol.* 1986;8:201–209.
14. Haines DE, Lerman BB, Kron IL, DiMarco JP. Surgical ablation of ventricular tachycardia with sequential map-guided subendocardial resection: electrophysiologic assessment and long-term follow-up. *Circulation.* 1988;77:131–141.
15. Ostermeyer J, Breithardt G, Borggrefe M, et al. Surgical treatment of ventricular tachycardias: Complete versus partial encircling endocardial ventriculotomy. *J Thorac Cardiovasc Surg.* 1984;87:517–525.
16. Miller J, Rothman SA, Addonizio VP. Surgical techniques for ventricular tachycardia ablation. In: Singer I, ed. Interventional Electrophysiology. Baltimore: Williams & Wilkins; 1997:641–684.
17. Guiraudon GM, Thakur RK, Klein GJ, et al. Encircling endocardial cryoablation for ventricular tachycardia after myocardial infarction: experience with 33 patients. *Am Heart J.* 1994;128:982–989.
18. Frapier JM, Hubaut JJ, Pasquie JL, Chaptal PA. Large encircling cryoablation without mapping for ventricular tachycardia after anterior myocardial infarction: long-term outcome. *J Thorac Cardiovasc Surg.* 1998;116:578–583.
19. Miller JM, Tyson GS, Hargrove WC, et al. Effect of subendocardial resection on sinus rhythm endocardial electrogram abnormalities. *Circulation.* 1995;91:2385–2391.
20. Cassidy DM, Vassallo JA, Buxton AE, et al. The value of catheter mapping during sinus rhythm to localize site of origin of ventricular tachycardia. *Circulation.* 1984;69:1103–1110.
21. Furniss S, Anil-Kumar R, Bourke JP, et al. Radiofrequency ablation of haemodynamically unstable ventricular tachycardia after myocardial infarction. *Heart.* 2000;84:648–652.
22. Eldar M, Fitzpatrick AP, Ohad D, et al. Percutaneous multielectrode endocardial mapping during ventricular tachycardia in the swine model. *Circulation.* 1996;94:1125–1130.
23. Schilling RJ, Peters NS, Davies DW. Feasibility of a noncontact catheter for endocardial mapping of human ventricular tachycardia. *Circulation.* 1999;99:2543–2552.
24. Wittkampf FHM, Wever EFD, Derksen R, et al. LocaLisa: new technique for real-time 3-dimensional localization of regular intracardiac electrodes. *Circulation.* 1999;99:1312–1317.
25. Ventura R, Rostock T, Klemm HU, et al. Catheter ablation of common-type atrial flutter guided by three-dimensional right atrial geometry reconstruction and catheter tracking using cutaneous patches: a randomized prospective study. *J Cardiovasc Electrophysiol.* 2004;15:1157–1161.
26. Gepstein L, Hayam G, Ben-Haim SA. A novel method for nonfluoroscopic catheter-based electroanatomical mapping of the heart in vitro and in vivo accuracy results. *Circulation.* 1997;95:1611–1622.
27. De Groot NMS, Bootsma M, van der Velde ET, et al. Three-dimensional catheter positioning during radiofrequency ablation in patients: first application of a real-time position management system. *J Cardiovasc Electrophysiol.* 2000;11:1183–1192.
28. Callans DJ, Ran J-F, Michele J, et al. Electroanatomic left ventricular mapping in the porcine model of healed anterior myocardial infarction: correlation with intracardiac echocardiography and pathological analysis. *Circulation.* 1999;100:1744–1750.
29. Wrobleski D, Houghtaling C, Josephson ME, et al. Use of electrogram characteristics during sinus rhythm to delineate the endocardial scar in a porcine model of healed myocardial infarction. *J Cardiovasc Electrophysiol.* 2003;14:524–529.

30. Marchlinski FE, Callans DJ, Gottlieb CD, Zado E. Linear ablation lesions for control of unmappable ventricular tachycardia in patients with ischemic and nonischemic cardiomyopathy. *Circulation.* 2000;101:1288–1296.

31. Reddy VY, Neuzil P, Taborsky M, Ruskin JN. Short-term results of substrate-mapping and radiofrequency ablation of ischemic ventricular tachycardia using a saline-irrigated catheter. *J Am Coll Cardiol.* 2003;41:2228–2236.

32. Brunckhorst CB, Delacretaz E, Soejima K, et al. Impact of changing activation sequence on bipolar electrogram amplitude for voltage mapping of left ventricular infarcts causing ventricular tachycardia. *J Interv Card Electrophysiol.* 2005;12:137–141.

33. Hsia HH, Marchlinski FE. Characterization of the electroanatomic substrate for monomorphic ventricular tachycardia in patients with nonischemic cardiomyopathy. *Pacing Clin Electrophysiol.* 2002;25:1114–1127.

34. Soejima K, Suzuki M, Maisel WH, et al. Catheter ablation in patients with multiple and unstable ventricular tachycardias after myocardial infarction: short ablation lines guided by reentry circuit isthmuses and sinus rhythm mapping. *Circulation.* 2001;104:664–669.

35. Sra J, Bhatia A, Dhala A, et al. Electroanatomically guided catheter ablation of ventricular tachycardias causing multiple defibrillator shocks. *Pacing Clin Electrophysiol.* 2001;24:1645–1652.

36. Arenal A, Glez-Torrecilla E, Ortiz M, et al. Ablation of electrograms with an isolated, delayed component as treatment of unmappable monomorphic ventricular tachycardias in patients with structural heart disease. *J Am Coll Cardiol.* 2003;41:81–92.

37. Kottkamp H, Wetzel U, Schirdewahn P, et al. Catheter ablation of ventricular tachycardia in remote myocardial infarction: substrate description guiding placement of individual linear lesions targeting noninducibility. *J Cardiovasc Electrophysiol.* 2003;14:675–681.

38. Miller JM, Marchlinski FE, Buxton AE, Josephson ME. Relationship between the 12-lead electrogram during ventricular tachycardia and endocardial site of origin in patients with coronary artery disease. *Circulation.* 1988;77:759–766.

39. Kuchar DL, Ruskin JN, Garan H. Electrocardiographic localization of the site of origin of ventricular tachycardia in patients with prior myocardial infarction. *J Am Coll Cardiol.* 1989;13:893–900.

40. Merino JL, Almendral J, Villacastin JP, et al. Radiofrequency catheter ablation of ventricular tachycardia from the right ventricle late after myocardial infarction. *Am J Cardiol.* 1996;77:1261–1263.

41. Patel VV, Rho RW, Gerstenfeld EP, et al. Right bundle branch block ventricular tachycardias: septal versus lateral ventricular origin based on activation time to the right ventricular apex. *Circulation.* 2004;110:2582–2587.

42. de Chillou C, Lacroix D, Klug D, et al. Isthmus characteristics of reentrant ventricular tachycardia after myocardial infarction. *Circulation.* 2002;12: 726–731.

43. Bogun F, Good E, Reich S, et al. Isolated potentials during sinus rhythm and pace-mapping within scars as guides for ablation of post-infarction ventricular tachycardia. *J Am Coll Cardiol.* 2006;47:2013–2019.

44. Hsia HH, Lin D, Sauer WH, et al. Relationship of late potentials to the ventricular tachycardia circuit defined by entrainment. *J Interv Card Electrophysiol.* 2009;26:21–29.

45. Brunckhorst CB, Stevenson WG, Jackman WM, et al. Ventricular mapping during atrial and ventricular pacing: relationship of multipotential electrograms to ventricular tachycardia reentry circuits after myocardial infarction. *Eur Heart J.* 2002;23:1131–1138.

46. Brunckhorst CB, Delacretaz E, Soejima K, et al. Identification of the ventricular tachycardia isthmus after infarction by pace mapping. *Circulation.* 2004;110:652–659.

47. Soejima K, Stevenson WG, Maisel WH, et al. Electrically unexcitable scar mapping based on pacing threshold for identification of the reentry circuit isthmus: feasibility for guiding ventricular tachycardia ablation. *Circulation.* 2002;106:1678–1683.

48. Sarrazin JF, Kuehne M, Wells D, et al. High-output pacing in mapping of postinfarction ventricular tachycardia. *Heart Rhythm.* 2008;5:1709–1714.

49. Langberg JJ, Gallagher M, Strickberger A, et al. Temperature-guided radiofrequency catheter ablation with very large electrodes. *Circulation.* 1993; 88:245–249.

50. Calkins H, Epstein A, Packer D, et al. Catheter ablation of ventricular tachycardia in patients with structural heart disease using cooled radiofrequency energy. *J Am Coll Cardiol.* 2000;35:1905–1914.

51. Nakagawa H, Yamanashi WS, Pitha JV, et al. Comparison of in vivo tissue temperature profile and lesion geometry for radiofrequency ablation with a saline-irrigated electrode versus temperature control in a canine thigh muscle preparation. *Circulation.* 1995;91:2264–2273.

52. Nakagawa H, Wittkampf FHM, Yamanashi WS, et al. Inverse relationship between electrode size and lesion size during radiofrequency ablation with active electrode cooling. *Circulation.* 1998;98:458–465.

53. Yokoyama K, Nakagawa H, Wittkampf FH, et al. Comparison of electrode cooling between internal and open irrigation in radiofrequency ablation lesion depth and incidence of thrombus and steam pop. *Circulation.* 2006; 113:11–19.

54. Stevenson WG, Wilber DJ, Natale A, et al. Irrigated radiofrequency catheter ablation guided by electroanatomic mapping for recurrent ventricular tachycardia after myocardial infarction: the Multicenter ThermoCool Tachycardia Ablation trial. *Circulation.* 2008;118:2773–2782.

55. Tanner H, Hindricks G, Volkmer M, et al. Catheter ablation of recurrent scar-related ventricular tachycardia using electroanatomical mapping and irrigated ablation technology: results of the prospective multicenter Euro-VT-study. *J Cardiovasc Electrophysiol.* 2009;21:54–55.

56. Sacher F, Sobieszczyk P, Tedrow U, et al. Transcoronary ethanol ventricular tachycardia ablation in the modern electrophysiology era. *Heart Rhythm.* 2008;5:52–68.

57. Verma A, Kilicaslan F, Schweikert RA, et al. Short- and long-term success of substrate-based mapping and ablation of ventricular tachycardia in arrhythmogenic right ventricular dysplasia. *O Circulation.* 2005;111:3209–3216.

58. Henz BD, do Nascimento TA, Dietrich CO, et al. Simultaneous epicardial and endocardial substrate mapping and radiofrequency catheter ablation as first-line treatment for ventricular tachycardia and frequent ICD shocks in chronic chagasic cardiomyopathy. *J Interv Card Electrophysiol.* 2009;26:195–205.

59. Volkmer M, Ouyang F, Deger F, et al. Substrate mapping vs. tachycardia mapping using CARTO in patients with coronary artery disease and ventricular tachycardia: impact on outcome of catheter ablation. *Europace.* 2006;8:968–976.

60. Pratola C, Baldo E, Toselli T, et al. Contact versus noncontact mapping for ablation of ventricular tachycardia in patients with previous myocardial infarction. *Pacing Clin Electrophysiol.* 2009;32:842–850.

61. Klemm HU, Ventura R, Steven D, et al. Catheter ablation of multiple ventricular tachycardias after myocardial infarction guided by combined contact and noncontact mapping. *Circulation.* 2007;115:2697–2704.

62. Carbucicchio C, Santamaria M, Trevisi N, et al. Catheter ablation for the treatment of electrical storm in patients with implantable cardioverter-defibrillators: short- and long-term outcomes in a prospective single-center study. *Circulation.* 2008;117:462–469.

63. Strickberger SA, Knight BP, Michaud GF, et al. Mapping and ablation of ventricular tachycardia guided by virtual electrograms using a noncontact, computerized mapping system. *J Am Coll Cardiol.* 2000;35:414–421.

64. Della Bella P, Pappalardo A, Riva S, et al. Non-contact mapping to guide catheter ablation of untolerated ventricular tachycardia. *Eur Heart J.* 2002;23:742–752.

65. Kriebel T, Saul JP, Schneider H, et al. Noncontact mapping and radiofrequency catheter ablation of fast and hemodynamically unstable ventricular tachycardia after surgical repair of tetralogy of Fallot. *J Am Coll Cardiol.* 2007; 50:2162–2168.

66. Thiagalingam A, Wallace EM, Campbell CR, et al. Value of noncontact mapping for identifying left ventricular scar in an ovine model. *Circulation.* 2004;110:3175–3180.

67. Ciaccio EJ, Chow AW, Kaba RA, et al. Detection of the diastolic pathway, circuit morphology, and inducibility of human postinfarction ventricular tachycardia from mapping in sinus rhythm. *Heart Rhythm.* 2008;5:981–991.

68. Nakayama Y, Shimizu G, Hirota Y, et al. Extent of myocardial fibrosis and cellular hypertrophy in dilated cardiomyopathy. *Am J Cardiol.* 1988;10:186–192.

69. Roberts WC, Siegel RJ, McManus BM. Idiopathic dilated cardiomyopathy: analysis of 152 necropsy patients. *Am J Cardiol.* 1987;60:1340–1355.

70. Hsia HH, Callans DJ, Marchlinski FE. Characterization of endocardial electrophysiological substrate in patients with nonischemic cardiomyopathy and monomorphic ventricular tachycardia. *Circulation.* 2003;108:704–710.

71. Soejima K, Stevenson WG, Sapp JL, et al. Endocardial and epicardial radiofrequency ablation of ventricular tachycardia associated with dilated cardiomyopathy. *J Am Coll Cardiol.* 2004;43:1834–1842.

72. McCrohon JA, Moon JC, Prasad SK, et al. Differentiation of heart failure related to dilated cardiomyopathy and coronary artery disease using gadolinium-enhanced cardiovascular magnetic resonance. *Circulation.* 2003;108:54–59.

73. Soriano CJ, Ridocci F, Estornell J, et al. Noninvasive diagnosis of coronary artery disease in patients with heart failure and systolic dysfunction of uncertain etiology, using late gadolinium-enhanced cardiovascular magnetic resonance. *J Am Coll Cardiol.* 2005;45:743–748.

74. Bogun FM, Desjardins B, Good E, et al. Delayed-enhanced magnetic resonance imaging in nonischemic cardiomyopathy: utility for identifying the ventricular arrhythmia substrate. *J Am Coll Cardiol.* 2009;53:1138–1145.

75. Cano O, Hutchinson M, Lin D, et al. Electroanatomic substrate and ablation outcome for suspected epicardial ventricular tachycardia in left ventricular nonischemic cardiomyopathy. *J Am Coll Cardiol.* 2009;54:799–808.

76. McKenna WJ, Thiene G, Nava A, et al. Diagnosis of arrhythmogenic right ventricular dysplasia/cardiomyopathy. Task force of the working group for myocardial and pericardial disease of the European Society of Cardiology and of the Scientific Council on Cardiomyopathies of the International Society and Federation of Cardiology. *Br Heart J.* 1994;71:215–218.

77. Marchlinski FE, Zado E, Dixit S, et al. Electroanatomic substrate and outcome of catheter ablative therapy for ventricular tachycardia in setting of right ventricular cardiomyopathy. *Circulation.* 2004;100:2293–2298.

78. Garcia FC, Bazan V, Zado ES, Ren JF, Marchlinski FE. Epicardial substrate and outcome with epicardial ablation of ventricular tachycardia in arrhythmogenic right ventricular cardiomyopathy/dysplasia. *Circulation.* 2009;120:366–375.

79. Maguire JH, Hoff R, Sherlock I, et al. Cardiac morbidity and mortality due to Chagas' disease: Prospective electrocardiographic study of a Brazilian community. *Circulation.* 1987;75:1140–1145.

80. Scanavacca M, Sosa E. Electrophysiologic study in chronic Chagas' heart disease. *Rev Paul Med.* 1995;113:841–850.

81. Sosa E, Scanavacca M, d'Avila A, et al. Endocardial and epicardial ablation guided by nonsurgical transthoracic epicardial mapping to treat recurrent ventricular tachycardia. *J Cardiovasc Electrophysiol.* 1998;9:229–239.

82. Svenson RH, Littmann L, Gallagher JJ, et al. Termination of ventricular tachycardia with epicardial laser photocoagulation: a clinical comparison with patients undergoing successful endocardial photocoagulation alone. *J Am Coll Cardiol.* 1990;15:163–170.

83. D'Avila A, Scanavacca M, Sosa E, et al. Pericardial anatomy for the interventional electrophysiologist. *J Cardiovasc Electrophysiol.* 2003;14:422–430.

84. Schweikert RA, Saliba WI, Tomassoni G, et al. Percutaneous pericardial instrumentation for endo-epicardial mapping of previously failed ablations. *Circulation.* 2003;108:1329–1335.

85. Reddy VY, Wrobleski D, Houghtaling C, et al. Combined epicardial and endocardial electroanatomic-mapping in a porcine model of healed myocardial infarction. *Circulation.* 2003;107:3236–3242.

86. Berruezo A, Mont L, Nava S, et al. Electrocardiographic recognition of the epicardial origin of ventricular tachycardias. *Circulation.* 2004;109:1842–1847.

87. Sosa E, Scanavacca M, D'Avila A, et al. Nonsurgical transthoracic epicardial approach in patients with ventricular tachycardia and previous cardiac surgery. *J Interv Card Electrophysiol.* 2004;10:281–288.

88. Soejima K, Couper G, Cooper JM, et al. Subxiphoid surgical approach for epicardial catheter-based mapping and ablation in patients with prior cardiac surgery or difficult pericardial access. *Circulation.* 2004;110:1197–1201.

89. Friedman PA, Munger TM, Torres N, et al. Percutaneous endocardial and epicardial ablation of hypotensive ventricular tachycardia with percutaneous left ventricular assist in the electrophysiology laboratory. *J Cardiovasc Electrophysiol.* 2007;18:106–109.

90. Kim RJ, Wu E, Rafael A, et al. The use of contrast-enhanced magnetic resonance imaging to identify reversible myocardial dysfunction. *N Engl J Med.* 2000;343:1445–1453.

91. Callans DJ, Ren J-F, Narula N, et al. Effects of linear, irrigated-tip radiofrequency ablation in porcine healed anterior infarction. *J Cardiovasc Electrophysiol.* 2001;12:1037–1042.

92. Khan HH, Maisel WH, Ho C, et al. Effect of radiofrequency catheter ablation of ventricular tachycardia on left ventricular function in patients with prior myocardial infarction. *J Interv Card Electrophysiol.* 2002;2:243–247.

93. d'Avila A, Neuzil P, Thiagalingam A, et al. Experimental efficacy of pericardial instillation of anti-inflammatory agents during percutaneous epicardial catheter ablation to prevent postprocedure pericarditis. *J Cardiovasc Electrophysiol.* 2007;18:1178–1183.

94. Haïssaguerre M, Shah DC, Jais P, et al. Role of Purkinje conducting system in triggering of idiopathic ventricular fibrillation. *Lancet.* 2002;359:677–678.

95. Haïssaguerre M, Shoda M, Jais P, et al. Mapping and ablation of idiopathic ventricular fibrillation. *Circulation.* 2002;106:962–967.

96. Haïssaguerre M, Extramiana F, Hocini M, et al. Mapping and ablation of ventricular fibrillation associated with long-QT and Brugada syndromes. *Circulation.* 2003;108:925–928.

97. Bansch D, Oyang F, Antz M, et al. Successful catheter ablation of electrical storm after myocardial infarction. *Circulation.* 2003;108:3011–3016.

98. Marrouche N, Verma A, Wazni O, et al. Mode of initiation and ablation of ventricular fibrillation storms in patients with ischemic cardiomyopathy. *J Am Coll Cardiol.* 2004;43:1715–1720.

99. Szumowski L, Sander P, Walczak F, et al. Mapping and ablation of polymorphic ventricular tachycardia after myocardial infarction. *J Am Coll Cardiol.* 2004;44:1700–1706.

100. Bogun F, Good E, Reich S, et al. Role of Purkinje fibers in post-infarction ventricular tachycardia. *J Am Coll Cardiol.* 2006;48:2500–2507.

101. Enjoji Y, Mizobuchi M, Muranishi H, et al. Catheter ablation of fatal ventricular tachyarrhythmias storm in acute coronary syndrome: role of Purkinje fiber network. *J Interv Card Electrophysiol.* 2009;26:207–215.

102. Knecht S, Sacher F, Wright M, et al. Long-term follow-up of idiopathic ventricular fibrillation ablation—a multicenter study. *J Am Coll Cardiol.* 2009;54:522–528.

31

Epicardial Approach to Catheter Ablation of Ventricular Tachycardia

Eduardo Sosa and Mauricio Scanavacca

Key Points

Epicardial ventricular tachycardia (VT) may occur in ischemic, nonischemic, and idiopathic VT.

Epicardial VTs are suggested by pseudo-delta waves and delayed ventricular activation times on the surface electrocardiogram (ECG) and by failure of endocardial mapping and ablation.

Percutaneous pericardial access is feasible in the electrophysiology laboratory.

Coronary angiography is routinely performed with epicardial ablation.

Irrigated-tip ablation and electroanatomic three-dimensional mapping systems may be required.

Catheter ablation of ventricular tachycardias (VTs) is still a great challenge. Ablation of supraventricular tachycardias and some types of idiopathic VTs is the first-line treatment of because of its high success rate and low complication rate.[1,2] However, catheter ablation of atrial fibrillation[3–5] and VTs associated with structural heart disease is a complex and laborious procedure.[2] Most VTs occur because of scar-related reentry. The scar-related VT is characterized by the presence of several bundles of surviving myocardial tissue surrounded by dense scar tissue. These surviving bundles of tissue may interconnect in a way that allows slow conduction and a reentry circuit to exist to an extent that VT can occur.[2] The ability to localize and destroy the bundles of surviving tissue inside the scar constitutes the basis for catheter-based ablation of scar-related VT. Its success in the treatment of rare VTs, such as focal[6] and bundle branch reentry VTs,[7] depends on the ability to identify the site of origin of the VT or bundle branch involved in the reentry circuit.

These different targets have usually been reached from the endocardium, but the success rate from this approach has not been homogeneous.[2] The presence of epicardial circuits has been considered one of the reasons for the failure of endocardial ablation, and epicardial circuits have been described in several types of cardiac disease in which surgical and nonsurgical techniques have been used.[8–19]

The recognition of epicardial VT is not new. Littmann and colleagues,[8] using epicardial laser photocoagulation during surgical ablation of 25 VTs in 10 patients, observed that post–myocardial infarction (MI) VT may result from epicardial macro-reentry. Slow conduction within the reentry circuit can be localized by epicardial mapping, and epicardial ablation can interrupt certain epicardial post-MI VTs. In studies of patients with nonischemic VT, Cassidy and coworkers[9] and Perlman and associates[10] found that abnormal fractionated or late endocardial electrograms, or both, are less frequently seen in patients with dilated cardiomyopathy than in those with post-MI VT. Svenson and colleagues[11] described the existence of epicardial circuits in post-MI VTs and suggested that they are particularly common in patients after inferior wall infarction.

Several techniques to map the epicardial surface of the heart in the electrophysiology laboratory have been described. The transseptal[12] and aortic coronary cusp approaches[13] are useful to map specific forms of idiopathic VT that originate in the left ventricular outflow tract. Coronary veins can be used to perform epicardial mapping, but the manipulation of the catheter is limited by the anatomic distribution of these vessels.[14] To the best of our knowledge, the subxiphoid percutaneous approach to the epicardial space is the only technique currently available that allows extensive and unrestricted mapping of the epicardial surface of both ventricles.[15,16]

At least two major reasons explain why epicardial VT ablation has become a matter of interest: one is that epicardial VT could be the source of failure for endocardial ablation even with the use of sophisticated mapping systems[17] and irrigated catheters; the other is that we are now able not only to reach the pericardial space easily but also to map and ablate epicardial VT in the electrophysiology laboratory.[16–25]

Subxiphoid Percutaneous Approach

The subxiphoid percutaneous approach has been previously described in detail.[16] The pericardial space is easily reached, and this is usually performed after positioning multipolar catheters in the coronary sinus and right ventricular apex through the femoral venous approach, before starting anticoagulation. The pericardial space is reached by using a commercially available needle, originally developed to perform a spinal tap (Fig. 31-1). The tip of this type of needle is shaped to reach a virtual space without damaging the spinal cord (epidural needle: 17 gauge × 3⁷⁄₈" inches [9.84 cm] × 5 inches [12.5 cm] Thin Wall (TW) with centimeter markings; Arrow International, Reading, PA). Because of its shape, this type of needle is considered safer for the transthoracic epicardial approach. Other types of needles can be used; however, the operator must be aware of the higher risk for perforation of the heart.

The puncture must be performed at the angle between the left border of the subxiphoid process and the lower left rib. The spatial orientation of the needle is an important step that will determine what portion of the ventricles will be reached. The needle usually has to point to the left shoulder, and it must be introduced more horizontally if the target is the anterior portion of the ventricles and more vertically if the diaphragmatic portion of the heart is the area of interest. After crossing the subcutaneous tissue, the needle movement should be monitored by fluoroscopy in the left anterior oblique view, 35 to 40 degrees (Fig. 31-2). The needle must be carefully moved toward the heart silhouette until the operator can detect the heart movement.

The injection of a small amount of contrast (about 1 mL) may demonstrate whether the needle tip is pushing or passing through the tissue. If the diaphragm has not been reached, the contrast will be seen in the subdiaphragmatic area. When the needle reaches the pericardial sac, the contrast will spread around the heart, restricted to its silhouette. The appearance of a "sluggish" layering of the contrast medium indicates that the needle is correctly positioned in

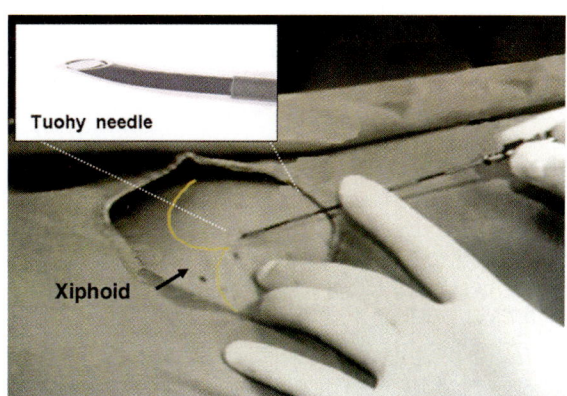

FIGURE 31-1. Technique used to perform subxiphoid approach. A regular Tuohy needle (*upper left corner*) is used to reach pericardial space.

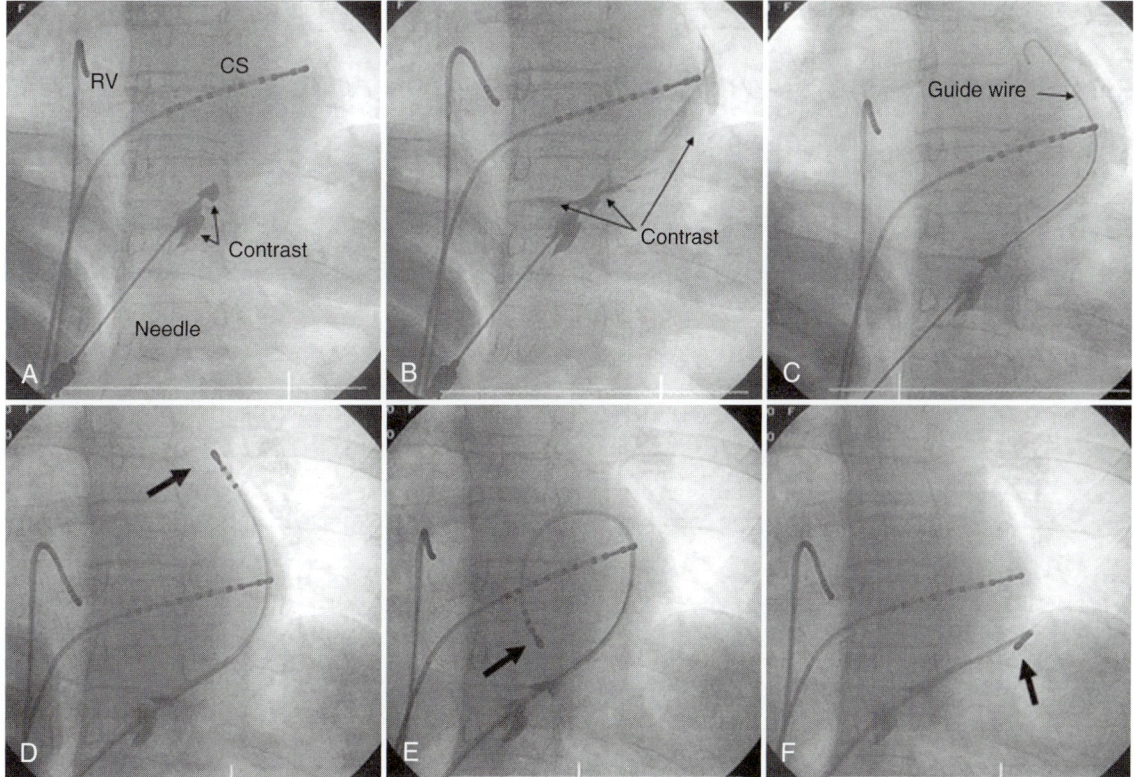

FIGURE 31-2. Left anterior oblique projection shown. **A,** Injection of contrast medium to check whether the needle tip is pushing or passing through the tissue. **B,** The moment at which the contrast medium is layering the heart silhouette. **C,** Guidewire around the heart silhouette correctly positioned inside the pericardial space. **D** to **F,** Images of catheter into the pericardial space. *Arrows* indicate the epicardial catheter. CS, coronary sinus catheter; RV, right ventricular catheter.

the pericardial space, and a soft floppy-tipped guidewire is then passed through the needle and an 8-French introducer is advanced. Then an ablation catheter is introduced into the pericardial space.

Using contrast media to demonstrate the precise site of the needle tip could be a problem. Sometimes, too much contrast is infused outside the pericardial space that infiltrates the mediastinum, creating an obscured image of the target area (Fig. 31-3). These fluoroscopic "dirty" images compromise the localization of the needle tip and its relationship with cardiac silhouette.

To avoid this problem, we use a soft guidewire rather than the contrast media. Hence, the needle is advanced very slowly toward the cardiac border, guided by the radioscopy image, until we feel the heart movement. Then, the needle tip is positioned tangential to the cardiac border and carefully advanced. Usually, it is possible to perceive when the needle tip crosses the parietal pericardium by an instantaneous resistance decrease when pushing the needle (like a transseptal puncture) or by feeling a "pop" when crossing it. At this moment, the guidewire is introduced to confirm the position. If the needle tip is in the pericardial space, the guidewire surrounds the heart silhouette, best observed in 30 to 45 degrees of left anterior oblique projection.

If the guidewire is outside the pericardial space, it twists around itself in the subdiaphragmatic region. Then, the

guidewire must be gently withdrawn to the interior of the needle that is slowly readvanced again to reach the pericardial space. This maneuver is carefully repeated until the guidewire is clearly inside the pericardial space.

Once the catheter is inside the pericardial space, epicardial ventricular electrograms can be nicely recorded during sinus rhythm and during VT (Fig. 31-4). The entire surface of the ventricles can be mapped and eventually ablated.

From the initial report in 1996[15] to December 2003, this approach has been performed in 215 consecutive patients with VT. VT was associated with Chagas disease in 138 patients. Fifty VTs were post-MI inferior wall VT, and 15 VTs were associated with idiopathic dilated cardiomyopathy (IDCM). Twelve idiopathic VTs are included in this series. The average numbers of inducible VTs ranged from 1.8 to 2.2. Unmappable VTs were observed in 40% to 44% of patients. Only one endocardial VT was induced in an average of 5% of patients, and only one epicardial VT was induced in an average of 3.5% of patients. In a group of mappable VTs, epicardial VT was present in 25% of IDCM VTs, 32% of post-MI VTs, and 36% of Chagas-related VTs. Successful radiofrequency (RF) ablation (termination and noninducibility) was obtained from the epicardium in 50% of post-MI VTs, 60% of Chagas-related VTs, and in 55% of IDCM VTs.

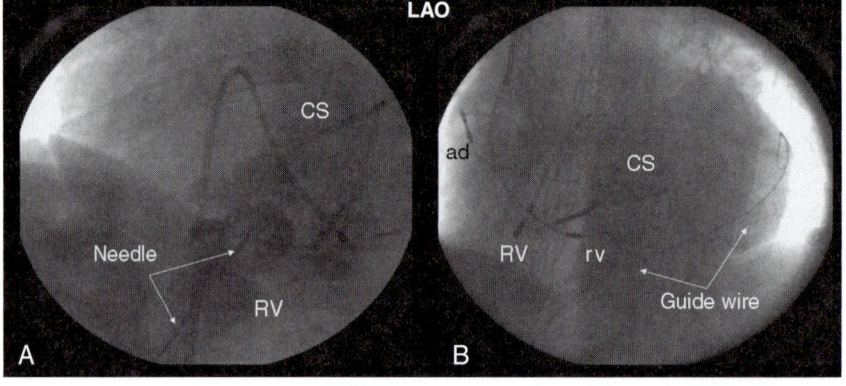

FIGURE 31-3. Radiographic image in left anterior oblique (LAO) projection. **A,** Contrast media infiltrated the tissue around the heart silhouette. Needle tip is difficult to localize. RV, right ventricle; CS, coronary sinus. **B,** The access to pericardial space without contrast media (see text). ad, ; CS, coronary sinus; rv, right ventricular catheter; RV, right ventricle.

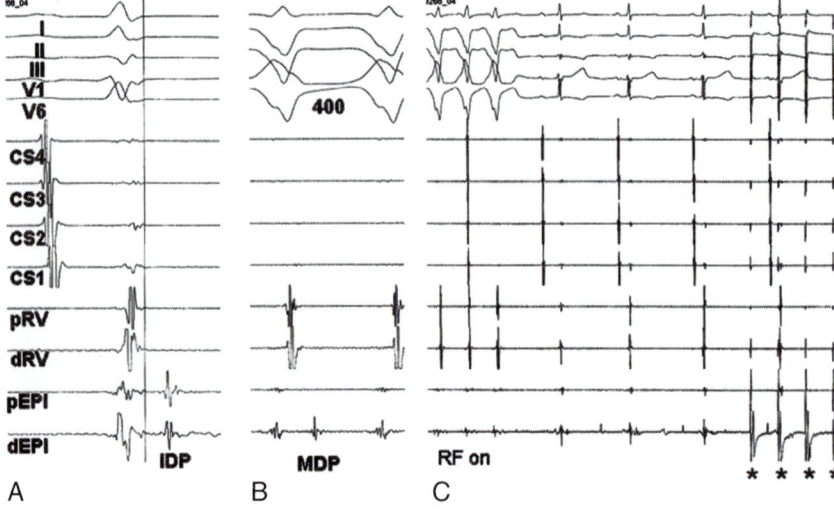

FIGURE 31-4. Electrocardiogram leads I, II, III, V$_1$, and V$_6$ are displayed with proximal-to-distal coronary sinus electrograms (CS4, CS3, CS2, CS1); proximal and distal right ventricular electrograms (pRV, dRV), and proximal and distal epicardial electrograms (pEPI, dEPI). **A,** Mapping during sinus rhythms: note the presence of isolated diastolic potential (IDP). **B,** Mapping during ventricular tachycardia: note the transformation of IDP in mid-diastolic potential (MDP). **C,** Radiofrequency (RF) interruption of ventricular tachycardia. Asterisks indicate artifact of epicardial stimulation in order to avoid phrenic nerve injury.

Epicardial VTs were defined as those with critical sites of the reentrant circuit (or with "origin" site) located exclusively in the subepicardial tissue as suggested by entrainment maneuvers or those that were terminated within 10 seconds with standard RF pulses (Fig. 31-5). We are aware that critical epicardial sites theoretically could be entrained or interrupted within 10 seconds from both the endocardial and epicardial surfaces, making it difficult to demonstrate the presence of a truly epicardial circuit in a given case. Epicardial VT may occur in patients with idiopathic VT[17,18,25] and in those with ischemic[23,26] or nonischemic VT.[17,18,22]

Problems Related to the Subxiphoid Epicardial Approach

Several concerns are raised regarding the use of this approach. The most common is related to the puncture accidents. Predictable and avoidable accidents were related to a "dry" right ventricular puncture in 4.5% of 215 consecutive patients who underwent epicardial ablation. Drainable hemopericardium of 200 ± 98 mL of blood was observed in 7% of patients. These predictable accidents are mostly related to the learning curve. One patient in this series had bleeding in the abdominal cavity from an injured diaphragmatic vessel, which required blood transfusion and laparotomy to achieve control.

Avoiding Coronary Artery Damage

The other main concern during epicardial mapping and ablation is coronary artery damage. In this regard, d'Avila and associates[27] reported experimental data from nine mongrel dogs in which linear and single RF lesions were applied on or near the coronary artery. The authors conclude that in an acute model, RF application delivery near the artery may result in intimal hyperplasia and thrombosis. The susceptibility to damage, however, was inversely proportional to the vessel size. No endothelial lesions were present in vessels with an internal perimeter larger than 2 mm.

The chronic effects of RF lesions on the epicardial coronary artery were also analyzed by Miranda[28] in seven young pigs observed for at least 70 days after RF ablation, and the results suggest that RF pulses delivered near the epicardial vessels do not provoke either myocardial infarction or vascular thrombosis. The endothelium was preserved in most of the animals, but intense intimal thickening was seen in only a few animals. The presence of fat and veins interposed between the epicardial coronary arteries and the ablation catheter tip may be protective and cause less intimal damaging and thickening; however, the precise reason is still unknown.

Our current approach to minimize the risk for damaging the coronary vessels is to obtain an angiogram before ablation in all patients. Based on the analysis of the anatomy of coronary arteries, safer or riskier areas can be found for epicardial ablation (Fig. 31-6). Depending on the area where the ablation site is located, another angiogram can

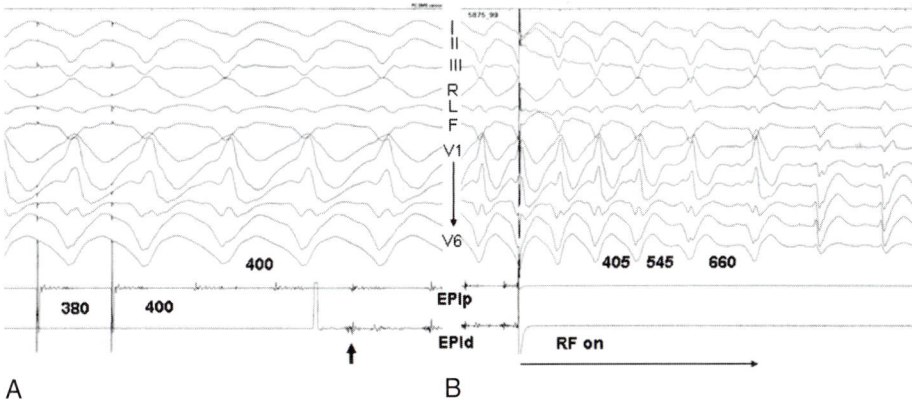

FIGURE 31-5. A, Activation mapping during ventricular tachycardia (VT). Note a mid-diastolic potential (*arrows*). Pacing at this site reproduced the VT QRS morphology. The postpacing interval is identical to VT cycle length, suggesting that this epicardial site is part of the VT circuit. **B,** One radiofrequency (RF) pulse applied at this site interrupted and rendered VT noninducible. EPIp and EPId, proximal and distal epicardial electrograms .

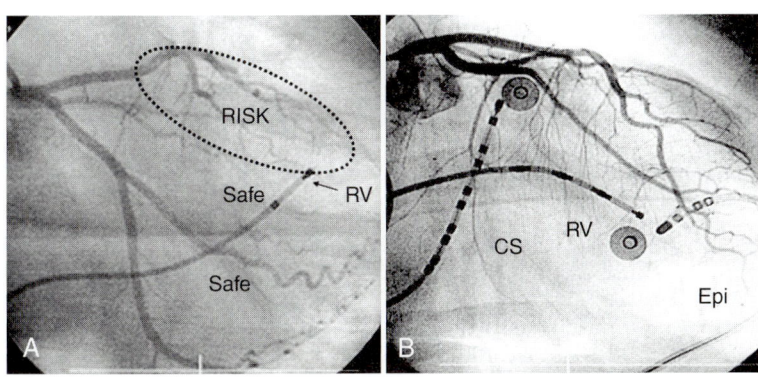

FIGURE 31-6. Avoiding coronary artery damage. **A,** Previous coronary angiography indicating areas of risk and safer areas for radiofrequency (RF) application. **B,** Coronary angiography just before RF application (see text). CS, coronary sinus catheter; Epi, epicardial catheter; RV, right ventricular catheter.

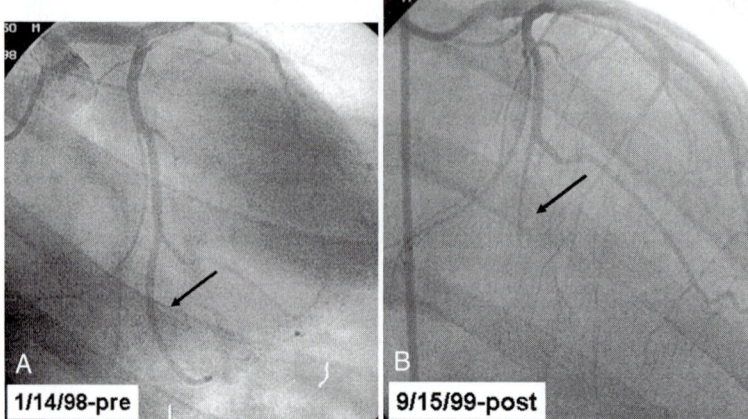

FIGURE 31-7. Coronary angiography before (**A**) and 1 year after (**B**) epicardial ablation to control Chagas cardiomyopathy with incessant ventricular tachycardia. The *arrows* indicate the coronary branch occluded.

be obtained during the procedure, right before ablation is begun (Fig. 31-6), but we do not routinely do this. As a general rule, we assume that a safe application could be delivered when the distance between the catheter tip and a visible coronary vessel is greater than 1 cm. However, if a critical site of the tachycardia circuit is identified close to a coronary artery despite extensive mapping, then, as in all clinical scenarios, a risk-benefit analysis should be undertaken.

In only 1 of 215 consecutive patients, RF application caused coronary artery occlusion of a marginal branch (see Fig. 31-7), resulting in non–Q-wave MI with a myocardial creatine kinase peak level of 35 U/L.

Effects of Epicardial Fat on Epicardial Mapping and Ablation

The presence of epicardial fat interposed between the catheter tip and an epicardial target also deserves special attention. Depending on its location and amount, the fat tissue may either minimize vascular damage during RF application or diminish the efficacy of epicardial catheter ablation (insulating effect). D'Avila and colleagues[29] compared the bipolar epicardial electrograms and ventricular epicardial stimulation threshold obtained with a 4-mm ablation catheter from 44 areas without and 45 areas with epicardial fat in 10 patients during open chest surgery. The authors observed that epicardial fat thickness of up to 5 mm interposed between the ablation catheter and the epicardium does not alter either the amplitude or duration of the bipolar epicardial electrogram or the epicardial ventricular stimulation threshold. In areas with a layer of epicardial fat thickness greater than 5 mm, ventricular stimulus capture was not possible even at maximum of 10 mA pulses.

The effect of epicardial fat on RF lesion formation was analyzed in animal models using standard and cooled-tip RF catheters.[30] This study suggested that fat attenuates epicardial lesion formation. The absence of blood flow in the epicardial space makes the catheter tip heat up excessively at a low-power delivery. The use of a cooled-tip ablation catheter allows for more energy to be delivered and a larger lesion to be created despite the presence of fat interposed between the catheter tip and the epicardium.

The same results[31] could be extrapolated to epicardial cryoablation. Epicardial cryoablation can create a very deep lesion, but the presence of a fat layer thicker than 5 mm strongly attenuates epicardial cryolesions. These data are important and may help to explain failures during epicardial RF ablation.

Pericarditis

Another potential complication seen after epicardial catheter ablation is postprocedure pericarditis. In the experimental study, animals mapped and ablated intrapericardially may develop an intense postpericarditis,[32] which can be eliminated by the pericardial infusion of 2 mg/kg of triamcinolone at the end of the procedure. Such an intense pericarditis has not been seen in patients in our series. Precordial distress and pain were observed in about 30% of our patients. However, pericardial effusion is minimal, and the symptoms are easily controlled with regular anti-inflammatory drugs in these patients. All 29 patients in our series who had more than one epicardial procedure, ranging from 1 week to 10 months after the first procedure, were free of pericardial effusion and pericardial adhesions.

Pericardial Adhesions

Postoperative pericardial adhesions may represent a limitation to the percutaneous transthoracic epicardial approach. In our series, five patients had monomorphic ventricular tachycardia 7 to 10 years after open chest surgery.[33] The ejection fraction was about 40%. Despite the presence of postoperative adhesions, all patients underwent endocardial and epicardial approaches of VT ablation simultaneously. In these patients, the pericardial puncture was directed to the inferior wall of the heart, where pericardial adhesions are thought to be less common than those in the anterior wall. The pericardial space was entered in all patients. Fourteen VTs were induced, and 8 VTs were unmappable. Three of six mappable VTs were successfully ablated from the endocardium, and two were successfully ablated from the epicardium (Figs. 31-8 and 31-9).

In one of our patients with Chagas-related VT who had a previous endocardial ablation failure, the presence of a

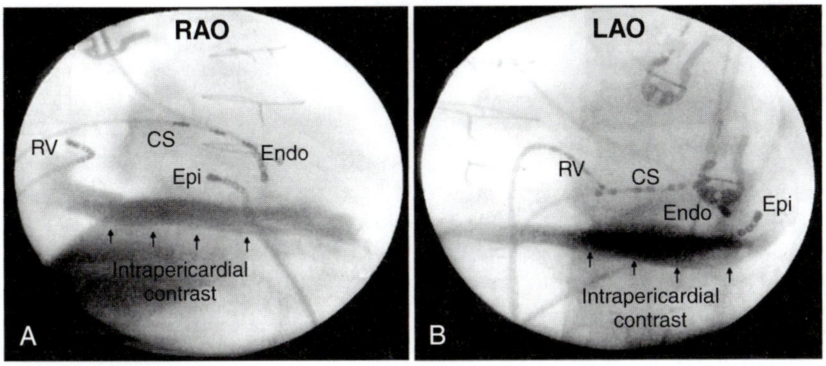

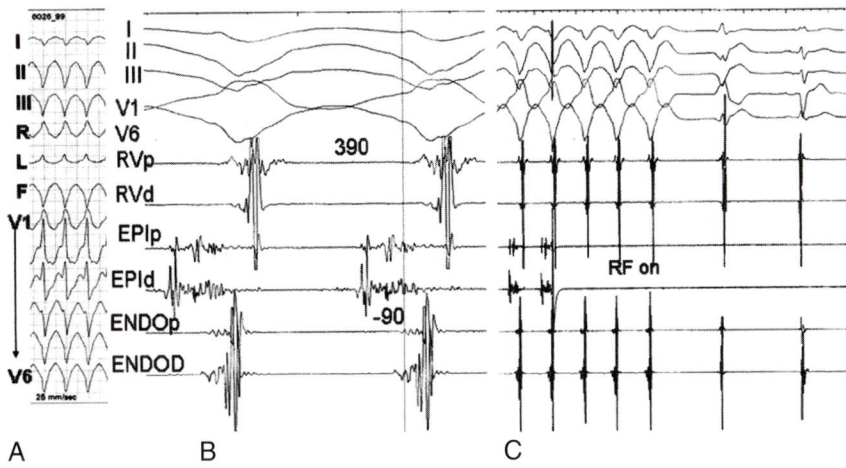

FIGURE 31-8. Right anterior oblique (RAO) (**A**) and left anterior oblique (LAO) (**B**) views of the heart showing the catheter position during simultaneous endocardial and epicardial mapping for ventricular ablation. Note that the contrast media accumulated at the inferior wall as a result of dense postoperative adhesions located at the high lateral and anterior walls of both ventricles.). CS, coronary sinus catheter; Endo, left ventricular catheter; Epi, epicardial catheter; RV, right ventricular catheter.

FIGURE 31-9. Shown are the electrocardiographic (ECG) patterns of inducible ventricular tachycardia (VT) (**A**), electrogram characteristics at the ablation site (**B**), and interruption of VT (**C**) in a patient with postoperative epicardial VT. The *dotted line* indicates the onset of the QRS complex (**B**). ECG leads I, II, III, V₁, and V₆ are displayed with proximal-to-distal right ventricle electrograms (RVp, RVd), proximal and distal epicardial electrograms (EPIp, EPId), and proximal (ENDOp) and distal (ENDOd) endocardial left ventricle electrograms. RF, radiofrequency.

large megacolon was thought to increase the risk for epicardial puncture (Fig. 31-10). Thus, a surgical window was created in the electrophysiology laboratory using the technique previously described.[38] This approach was essential for VT ablation, as depicted in Figure 31-10. An interesting mid-diastolic potential was used to guide RF ablation; VT was interrupted and rendered noninducible. This is the only patient in our experience in whom a surgical approach was needed to gain access to the epicardial space. The surgical approach can be used to gain access to the pericardial space for those less familiar with the percutaneous method.

Phrenic Nerve Injury

Injury of the phrenic nerve is a rare complication of endocardial atrial RF ablation. The phrenic nerves course through the upper chest, medial to the mediastinal pleura and the apex of the right or left lung. The right phrenic nerve lies laterally to the right brachiocephalic vein and the superior vena cava. The left phrenic nerve courses along the lateral aspect of the transverse arch of the aorta. The two nerves subsequently pass anteriorly to their respective pulmonary hila and then inferiorly in a broad vertical plane along the margin of the heart between the fibrous pericardium and the mediastinal pleura. The application of RF pulses in the lateral aspect of the heart silhouette can theoretically induce phrenic nerve injury.[34–36]

In our first 215 patients, we never observed this complication. We are aware, however, that the incidence of this complication could be underestimated because unilateral diaphragmatic paralysis usually does not cause significant shortness of breath unless underlying pulmonary disease is coexisting.

For prevention of phrenic nerve injury, high-output pacing (15 mA, 5 milliseconds pulse duration) at the ablation site (theoretically near the phrenic course) before the RF delivery and even between RF applications might be helpful (Fig. 31-11). This is not difficult because we usually do not apply many pulses to ablate epicardial VT. If necessary, the phrenic nerve can be displaced away from the ablation site with a second intrapericardial catheter or balloon.

Electroanatomic Mapping

The use of traditional electrophysiologic mapping systems to map and eventually to ablate several different types of VT has been demonstrated to control stable and scar-related monomorphic VT. This type of VT is found in no more than 20% of the VTs induced in the electrophysiology laboratory. In this subset of patients, the control of the recurrence at 2-year follow-up is about 50% with the combined endocardial and epicardial procedure (unpublished data). These results could be a consequence of disease progression or incomplete or reversible target elimination.

To provide more information about the localization and extension of the substrate of VT associated with Chagas

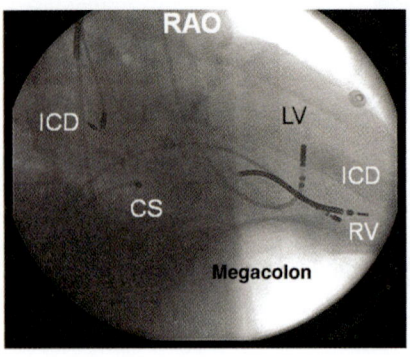

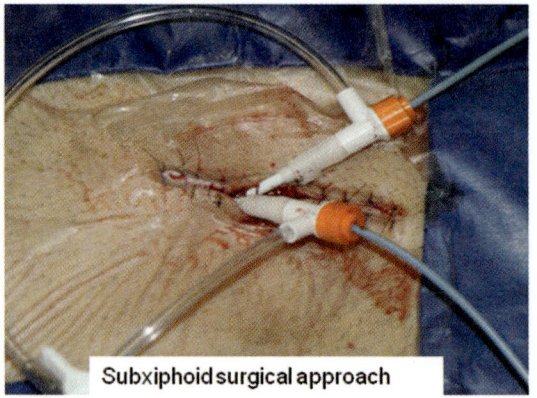

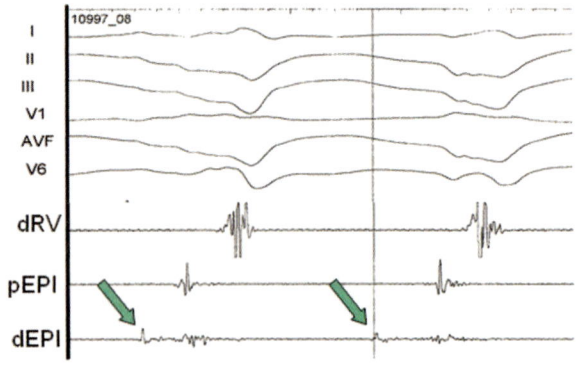

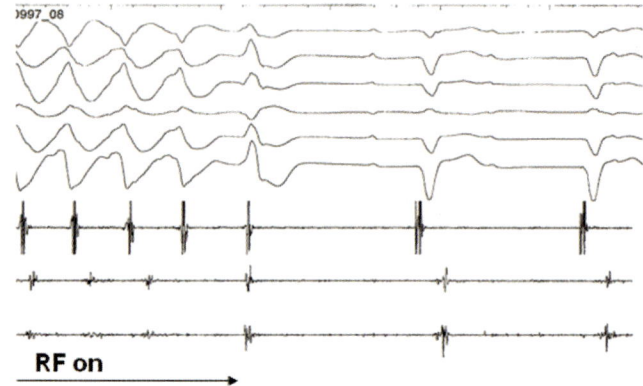

FIGURE 31-10. *Top left,* Radiographic image in right anterior oblique (RAO) projection showing the relationship between the heart silhouette and the megacolon. *Top right,* Two sheaths introduced through a minimal subxiphoid surgical incision. *Bottom left,* Electrocardiogram leads I to V$_6$. Note the middiastolic electrogram obtained during ventricular tachycardia (VT) and marked with *green arrows. Lower right,* The interruption on ventricular tachycardia with radiofrequency (RF) pulse. CS, coronary sinus; dRV, distal right ventricle; ICD, implantable cardioverter-defibrillator leads; LV, left ventricle; pEPI and dEPI, proximal and distal epicardial electrogram; RV, right ventricle.

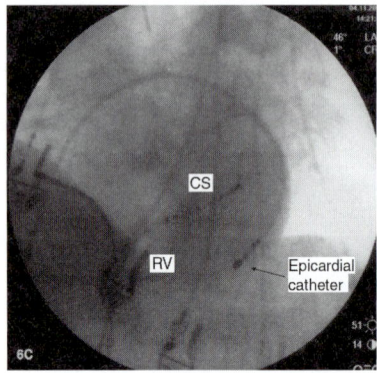

FIGURE 31-11. Left-anterior oblique view of the heart from the patient described in Fig. 31-4 showing the catheter positions during ventricular tachycardia ablation in site with phrenic nerve stimulation. CS, coronary sinus catheter; RV, right ventricular catheter.

disease, the more prevalent etiology at our institution, we started to use a Carto system (Biosense Webster, Diamond Bar, CA) associated with the traditional and combined electrophysiologic approaches.

Figures 31-12, 31-13, and 31-14 show a 55-year-old man taking amiodarone to control recurrent VT associated with Chagas disease with functional New York Heart Association class I and an echo ejection fraction of 31%. The ECG during sinus rhythm shows right bundle branch block with left axis deviation. During electrophysiologic study, only one monomorphic VT was induced. A coronary angiogram showed normal coronary arteries, diffuse left ventricular hypokinesia, and a lateral basal inferior left ventricular aneurysm. This is the usual substrate of Chagas-related VT. Electroanatomic mapping (Carto) of the left ventricle revealed a larger scar in the epicardial surface than in the endocardial surface. Despite a larger epicardial scar, the best electrogram was found in the endocardial portion of the scar, where a continuous electrical activity was seen. It is interesting to notice that the endocardial electrogram was nearly normal during sinus rhythm after application of one RF pulse. In other words, a very fractionated electrogram was seen during VT. However, an almost normal endocardial electrogram was seen in the same area during sinus rhythm.

Figure 31-15, 31-16, and 31-17 illustrate a 38-year-old woman taking amiodarone to control recurrent VT associated with Chagas disease with functional New York Heart Association class I and an echo ejection fraction of 55%. The electrophysiologic study induced only one monomorphic VT. In this patient, voltage mapping showed a much smaller endocardial left ventricular scar compared with its epicardial extension. An interesting site for ablation, represented by a continuous diastolic ventricular activity during VT, was found in the epicardial surface of the heart. Again, a nearly normal electrogram

11018

(Endocardial) ablation of Chagas VT

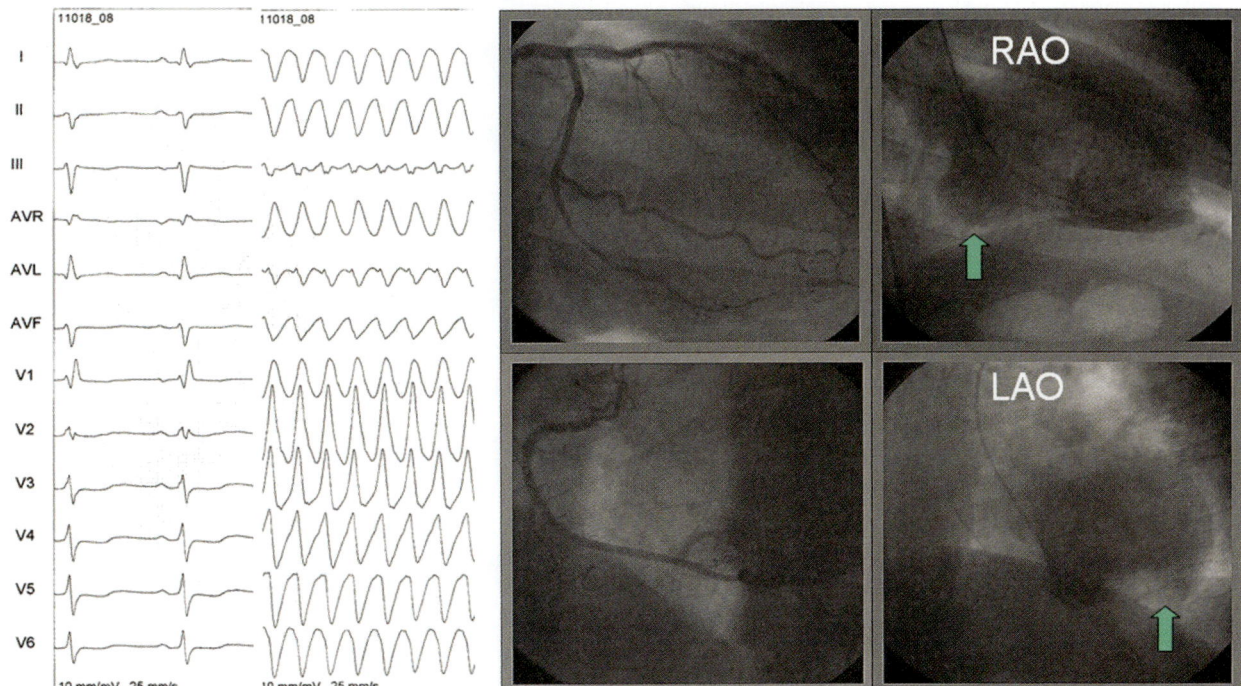

FIGURE 31-12. Endocardial ablation of Chagas ventricular tachycardia (VT). *Left*, 12-lead electrocardiogram (ECG) during sinus rhythm. *Middle*, 12-lead ECG during VT. *Right*, Radiographic image of left and right coronary angiography (*left*) and left ventricular angiography in right (RAO) and left anterior oblique (LAO) projections. *Arrow* points to the inferior aneurysm. bpm, beats per minute.

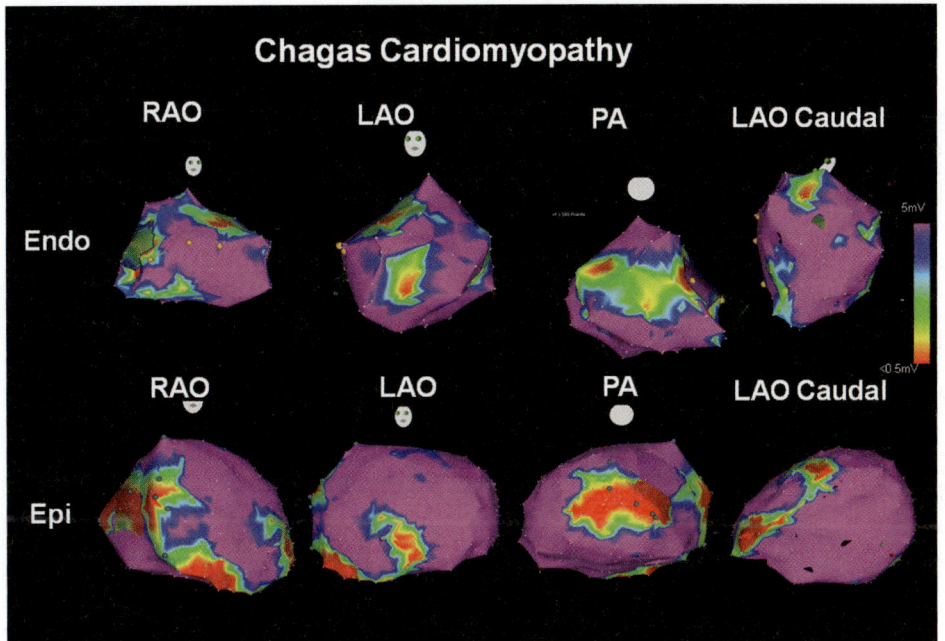

FIGURE 31-13. Endocardial and epicardial electroanatomic maps in the same patient with Chagas disease as in Fig. 31-12. Note the greater area of epicardial scarring. LAO, left anterior oblique; PA, posteroanterior; RAO, right anterior oblique.

was seen during sinus rhythm immediately after interruption of VT. These two cases suggest that substrate mapping and ablation in sinus rhythm may be difficult and inappropriate in some patients.

Another interesting finding in this case is the discrepancy between the big extensions of the left ventricular scar suggested by the contrasted angiography compared with the smaller scar suggested by the voltage mapping obtained with the Carto system. This curious finding suggested that fibrosis could predominate in the intramyocardial tissue rather than in the endocardial or epicardial surface.

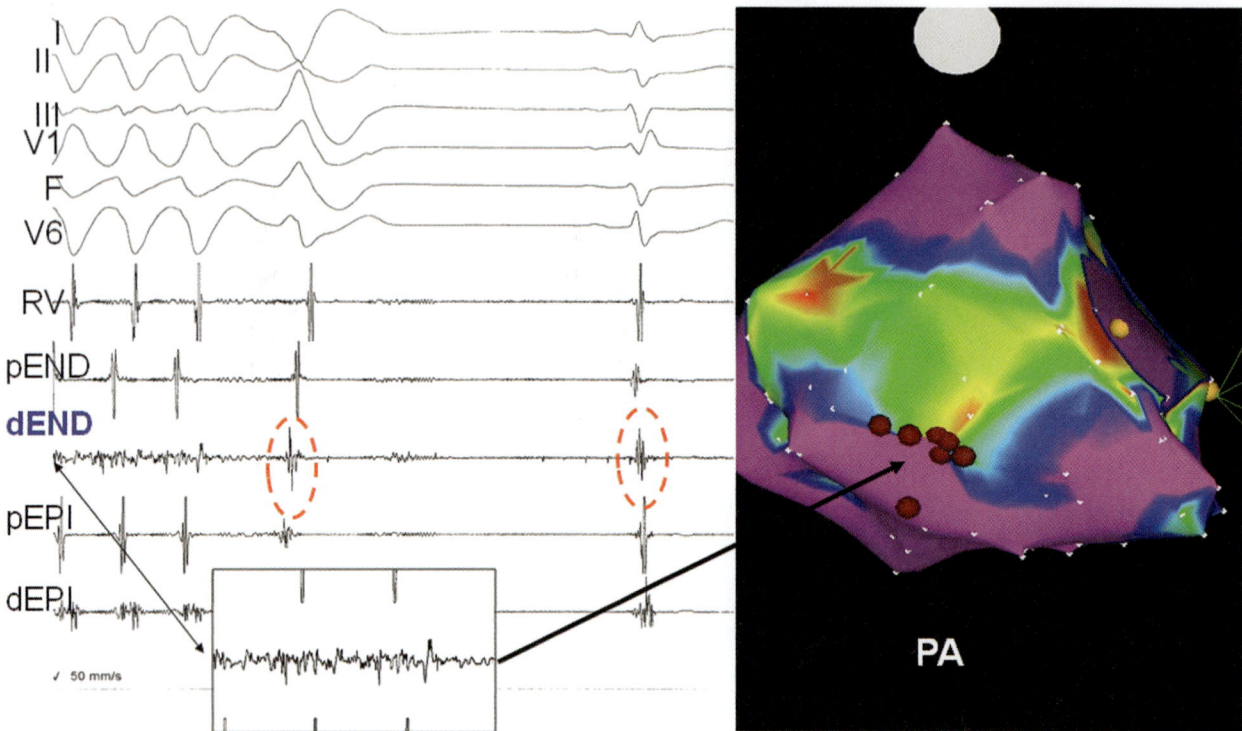

FIGURE 31-14. Electrophysiologic (*left*) and electroanatomic (*right*) voltage mapping from the same patient in Fig. 31-12. The best location for radiofrequency (RF) application is represented by continuous electrogram obtained in the endocardium of the left ventricle. At this location, one RF pulse terminated ventricular tachycardia (VT) and rendered VT noninducible. Note the near-normal ventricular electrogram during sinus rhythm at the location with continuous electrogram during VT (see text). dEND and pEND, distal and proximal endocardial electrograms; dEPI and pEPI, distal and proximal epicardial electrograms; PA, posteroanterior; RV, right ventricle.

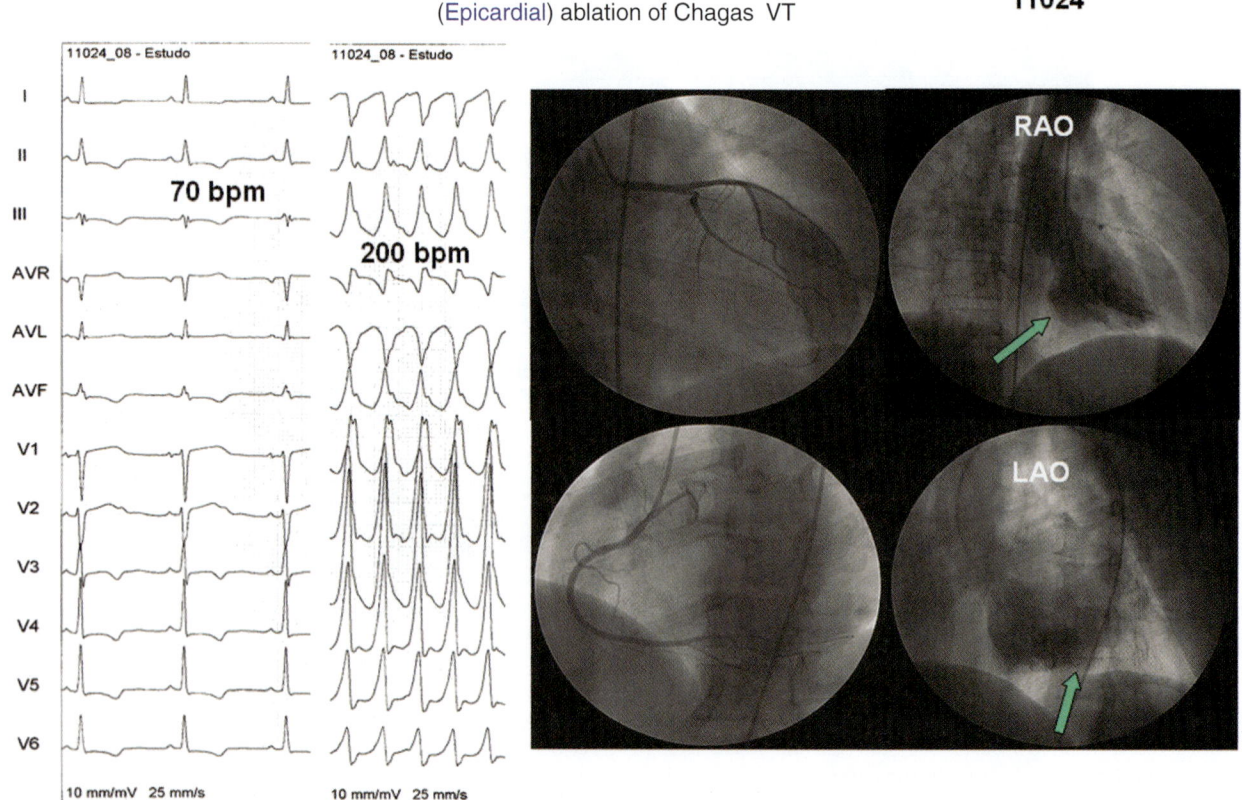

FIGURE 31-15. Epicardial ablation of Chagas ventricular tachycardia (VT). *Left,* 12-lead electrocardiogram (ECG) during sinus rhythm. *Middle,* 12-lead ECG during VT. *Right,* Radiographic image of left and right coronaries angiography (*left*) and left ventricular angiography in right (RAO) and left anterior oblique (LAO) projections. *Green arrows* points to the inferior aneurysm.

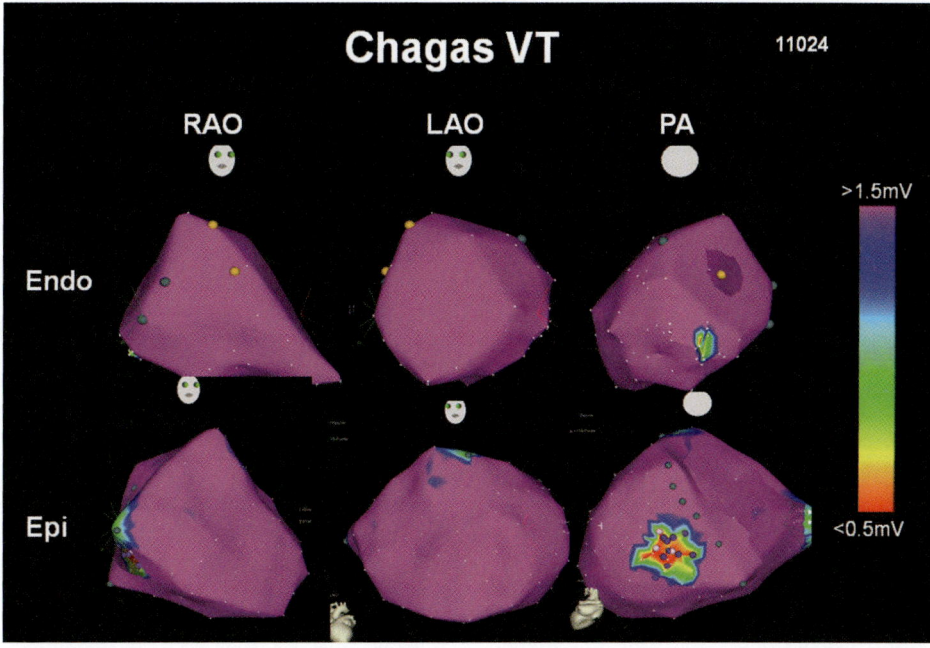

FIGURE 31-16. Electroanatomic voltage mapping from the patient in Fig. 31-15. The image depicts that the epicardial (Epi) scar is larger than endocardial (Endo) scar (see text). LAO, left anterior oblique; PA, posteroanterior; RAO, right anterior oblique.

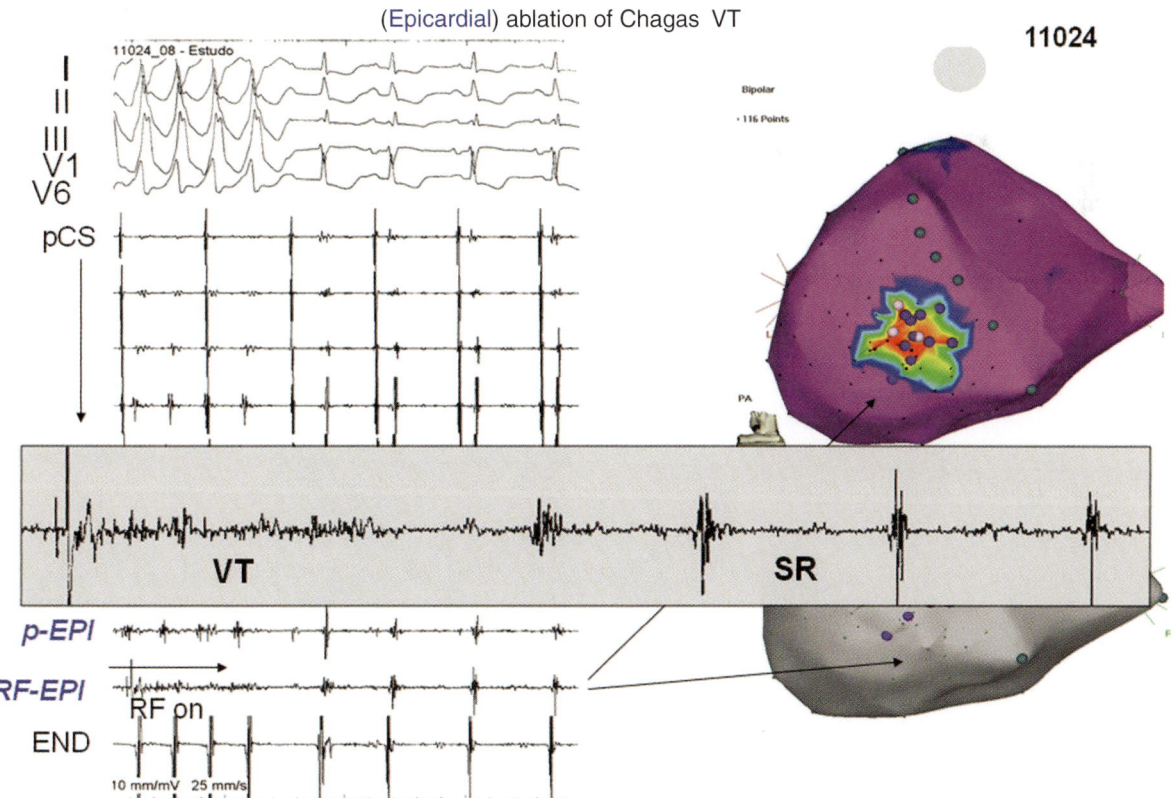

FIGURE 31-17. Epicardial recordings from the same patient as in Figs. 31-15 and 31-16. Note the continuous electrical activity recorded from the distal epicardial ablation (RF-EPI) electrodes shown in the inset. Radiofrequency (RF) energy application immediately terminates the tachycardia. The site of ablation is designated on the epicardial electroanatomic map. END, endocardial electrogram; pCS, proximal coronary sinus electrogram; p-EPI, proximal epicardial electrogram; SR, sinus rhythm; VT, ventricular tachycardia.

When Should the Epicardial Approach Be Used?

There remains the question of when the epicardial approach should be used, and the answer depends on the preference of the electrophysiologist. It is not clear whether one should use this approach only after endocardial failure or only when the ECG of clinical VT suggests an epicardial origin of VT. As a matter of fact, the simultaneous approach may have several advantages, including reduced cost, a better chance to map and ablate all inducible VT, and an opportunity to acquire more experience with the technique.

We analyzed the ECG pattern obtained during endocardial and epicardial ventricular stimulation in 40 stimulated sites (Fig. 31-18). The differences between the endocardial and epicardial QRS complex duration and the shortest RS complex were not statistically significant. However, the intrinsicoid deflection time and the presence of a pseudo-delta wave were statistically different.

Comparing the same parameter for the QRS complexes of endocardial and epicardial VTs (Fig. 31-19), we observed that the intrinsicoid deflection time was longer in the epicardial VT compared with the endocardial VT. The specificity and sensitivity for an epicardial VT were 80% and 50%, respectively, when the intrinsicoid deflection was longer than 97 milliseconds. A similar situation occurs with QRS duration (Fig. 31-20); QRS duration is longer in epicardial VT than in endocardial VT. A QRS complex longer than 198 milliseconds had a specificity of 86% and a sensitivity of 59% for epicardial circuits. The shortest RS time is also longer in epicardial VT, with a sensitivity of 82% and a specificity of 57% when longer than 122 milliseconds (Fig. 31-19).

The presence of a pseudo-delta wave is also suggestive of an epicardial VT. This parameter had a sensitivity and specificity of 80% for epicardial circuits (Fig. 31-20). Although these ECG characteristics are subtle, the epicardial origin of a given VT should be suspected when the QRS duration is longer than 200 milliseconds and a delta wave–like pattern is present. Berruezo and associates[37] recently reported similar findings. At electrophysiologic testing, an epicardial VT may be suggested by a broad area of "early" endocardial ventricular activation (representing endocardial breakthrough), the absence of early endocardial ventricular activation or satisfactory pace maps, or the failure of ablation at the most favorable endocardial sites (Table 31-1). In addition, in nonischemic cardiomyopathy patients, the presence of a Q wave in lead I and the absence of Q waves in the inferior leads suggest a basal lateral origin of VT (Fig. 31-21).[39]

Conclusion

Subepicardial VT may occur in ischemic, nonischemic, and idiopathic VT. Truly subepicardial VT can preferentially be ablated from the epicardial surface. A percutaneous subxiphoid approach to the pericardial space is easily and safely performed in the electrophysiology laboratory. Certain characteristics of QRS morphology and ventricular activation times on the surface ECG during VT (Table 31-1) may suggest the epicardial origin of VT. Simultaneous endocardial and epicardial approaches to VT mapping and ablation may improve the results of catheter ablation of difficult VTs.

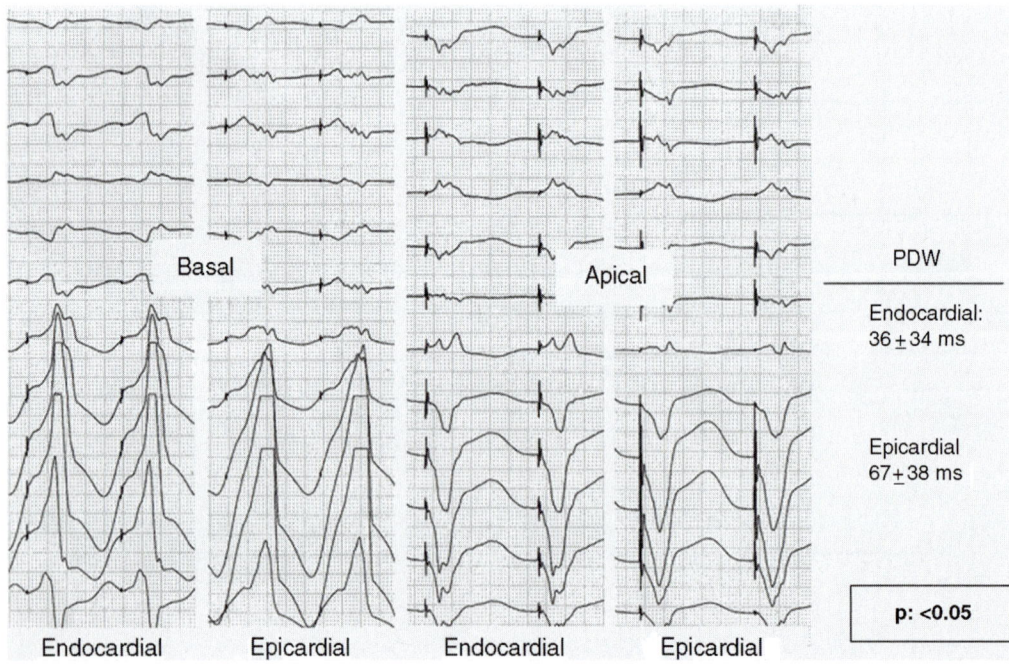

FIGURE 31-18. Endocardial versus epicardial stimulated QRS complex obtained in 40 sites at the basal and apical zone of the left ventricle (see text). PDW, pseudo-delta wave.

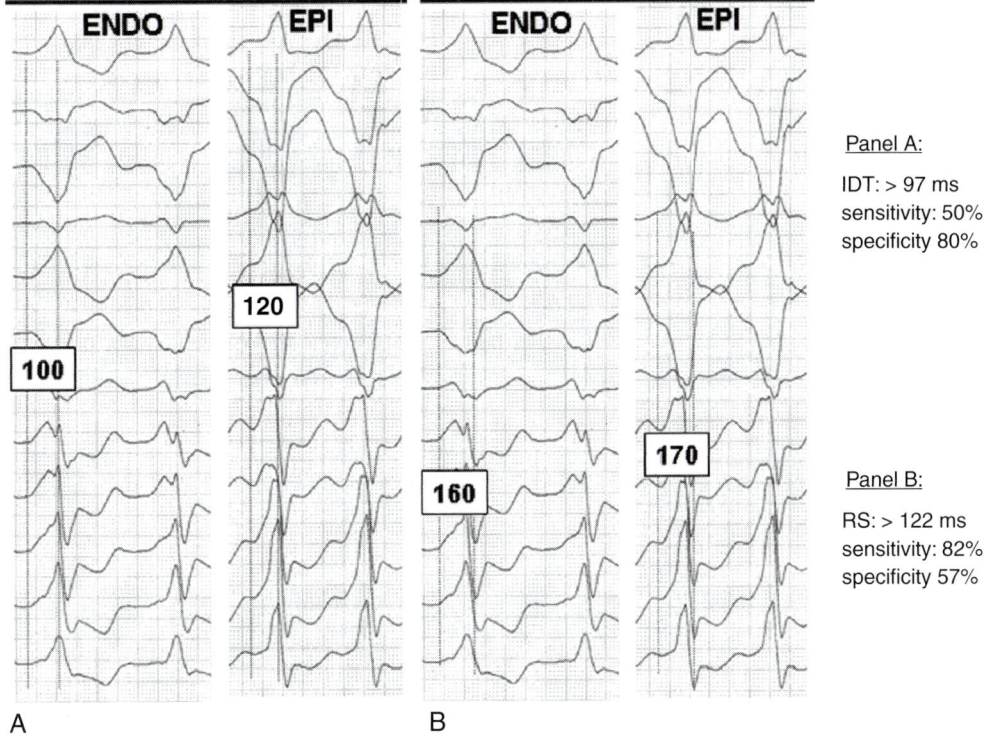

FIGURE 31-19. Twelve-lead electrocardiogram obtained during spontaneous endocardial and epicardial ventricular tachycardias (VTs). *Dotted lines* indicate the parameter measured. The numbers between the dotted lines show the interval measured in milliseconds in a specific case. **A,** Comparison of the intrinsicoid deflection time (IDT) in endocardial and epicardial VTs. **B,** Comparison of shorted RS duration (RS).

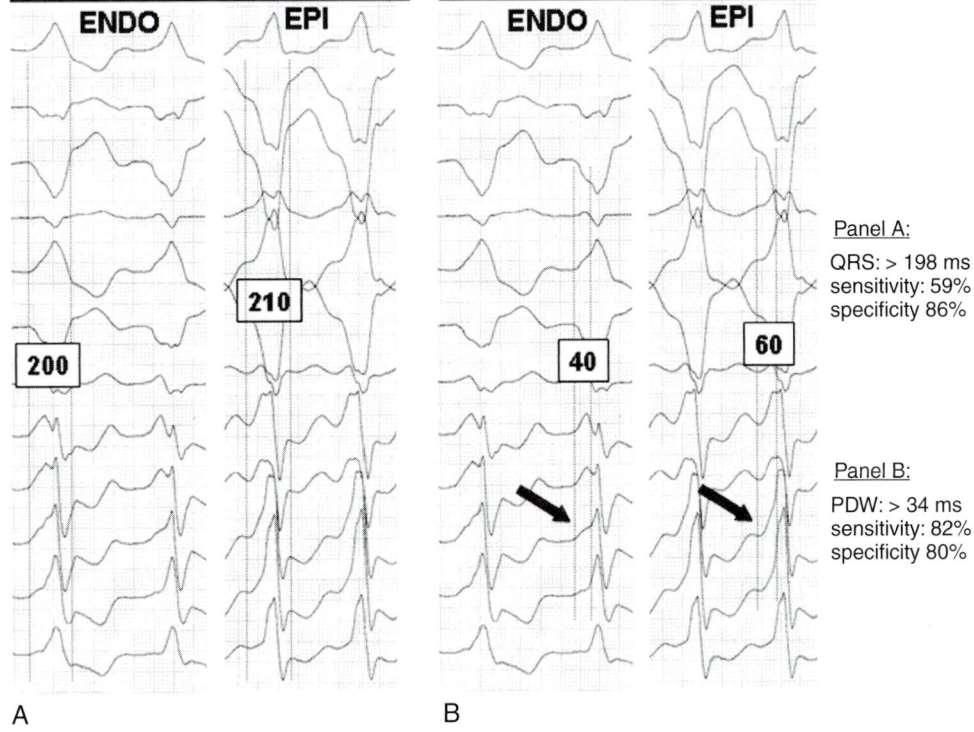

FIGURE 31-20. Identical case to Fig. 31-19. Electrocardiogram obtained during endocardial and epicardial spontaneous ventricular tachycardia. **A,** Total QRS duration. **B,** Pseudo-delta wave (PDW). *Arrows* indicate pseudo-delta wave.

TABLE 31-1

FINDINGS SUGGESTIVE OF EPICARDIAL VENTRICULAR TACHYCARDIA

Finding	Definition	Sensitivity (%)/ Specificity (%) of Ischemic Cardiomyopathy*	Sensitivity (%)/ Specificity (%) of Nonischemic Cardiomyopathy†
Surface Electrocardiogram			
QRS duration ≥198 msec	Total QRS duration		
Pseudo-delta wave >34 msec‡	Earliest ventricular activation to earliest fast deflection in any precordial lead	83/95	62/50
Intrinsicoid deflection time ≥85 msec‡	Interval from earliest ventricular activation to peak of R wave in V₂	87/90	69/50
RS complex duration ≥121 msec‡	Interval from earliest ventricular activation to nadir of the first S wave in any precordial lead	76/85	93/50
Delayed maximal peak deflection index ≥0.54§	Interval from earliest ventricular activation to peak of R or S wave divided by total QRS duration		33/75
Presence of Q wave in lead I	Initial negative deflection possibly preceded by short isoelectric segment of the QRS		88/88
Absence of Q waves in inferior leads	Initial positive deflection of QRS in inferior leads		94/63
Intracardiac Recordings			
Absence of early endocardial activation sites			
Diffuse area of earliest endocardial activation			
Poor endocardial pace maps			
Failed ablation at best endocardial sites			

* Values derived from patients with nonischemic cardiomyopathy by Valles E, Bazan V, Marchlinski F. ECG criteria to identify epicardial ventricular tachycardia in nonischemic cardiomyopathy. *Circ Arrhythmia Electrophysiol.* 2010;3:63-71.
† Values are to predict failure of endocardial ablation for VT in primarily ischemic heart disease patients from Berruezo A, Mont L, Nava S, et al. Electrocardiographic recognition of the epicardial origin of ventricular tachycardias. Circulation. 2004;109:1842-1847.
‡ Data from Berruezo A, Mont L, Nava S, et al. Electrocardiographic recognition of the epicardial origin of ventricular tachycardias. *Circulation.* 2004;109:1842-1847.
§ Diagnosis based on smallest ratio in any precordial lead.

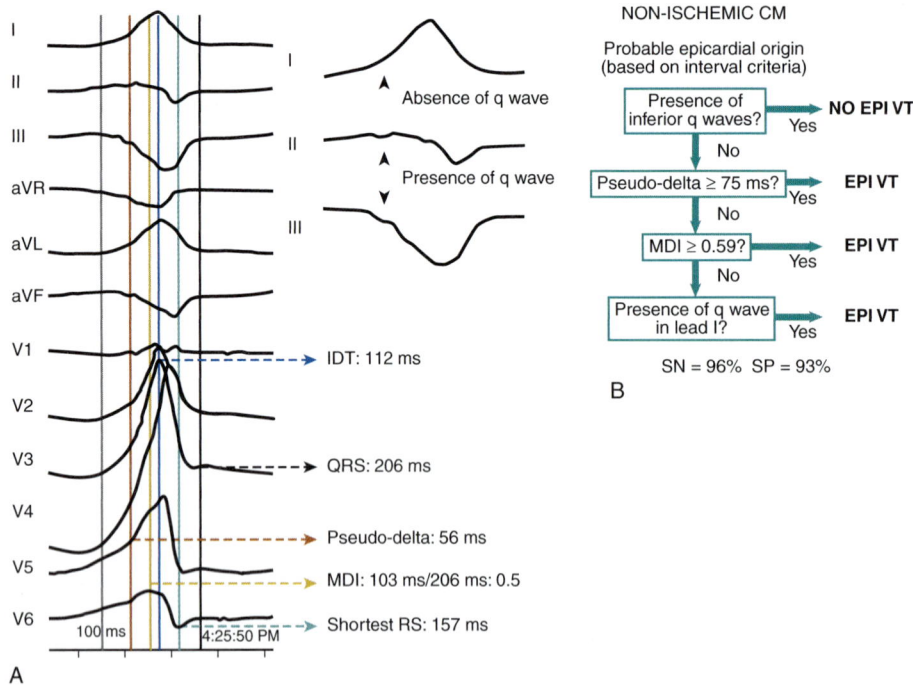

FIGURE 31-21. A, QRS from endocardial ventricular tachycardia (VT) showing discrepancy between interval and morphology criteria. This example demonstrates all interval and morphology criteria routinely assessed. The QRS from VT with endocardial site of origin in the example shown demonstrates interval criteria suggesting epicardial VT but morphology criteria (absence of a q wave in lead I and presence of small q waves in inferior leads) supporting an endocardial origin. **B,** Four-step algorithm for identifying epicardial origin from basal superior and lateral left ventricle in the setting of nonischemic cardiomyopathy. The three top steps have a high specificity, and the last step is the most accurate. The total sensitivity (SN) and specificity (SP) of the algorithm in the study population for pace-map localization reach 96% and 93%, respectively. IDT, intrinsicoid deflection time; MDI, maximum deflection index. *(Reproduced with permission from: Valles E et al. Circulation Arrhythmia and Electrophysiol 2010 ;3:63-71. With permission.)*

References

1. Morady F. Catheter ablation of supraventricular arrhythmias: state of the art. *Heart Rhythms*. 2004;1:67C–84C.
2. Stevenson WG. Catheter ablation of monomorphic ventricular tachycardia. *Curr Opin Cardiol*. 2005;20:42–47.
3. Jais P, Sanders P, Hsu LF, et al. Catheter ablation for atrial fibrillation. *Heart*. 2005;91:7–9.
4. Pappone C, Santinelli V. The who, what, why, and how-to guide for circumferential pulmonary vein ablation. *J Cardiovasc Electrophysiol*. 2004;15:1226–1230.
5. Hsu LF, Jais P, Sanders P, et al. Catheter ablation for atrial fibrillation in congestive heart failure. *N Engl J Med*. 2004;351:2373–2383.
6. Klein LS, Shih HT, Hackett FK, et al. Radiofrequency catheter ablation of ventricular tachycardia in patients without structural heart disease. *Circulation*. 1992;85:1666–1674.
7. Tchou P, Jazayeri M, Denker S, et al. Transcatheter electrical ablation of the right bundle branch: A method of treating macroreentrant ventricular tachycardia due to bundle branch reentry. *Circulation*. 1988;78:246–257.
8. Littmann L, Svenson RH, Gallagher JJ, et al. Functional role of the epicardium in postinfarction ventricular tachycardia: observations derived from computerized epicardial activation mapping, entrainment, and epicardial laser photoablation. *Circulation*. 1991;83:1577–1591.
9. Cassidy DM, Vassallo JA, Miller JM, et al. Endocardial catheter mapping in patients in sinus rhythm: relationship to underlying heart disease and ventricular arrhythmias. *Circulation*. 1986;73:645–652.
10. Perlman RL, Miller J, Kindwall KE, et al. Abnormal epicardial and endocardial electrograms in patients with idiopathic dilated cardiomyopathy: relationship to arrhythmias [abstract]. *Circulation*. 1990;82(suppl III):708.
11. Svenson RH, Littmann L, Gallagher JJ, et al. Termination of ventricular tachycardia with epicardial laser photocoagulation: a clinical comparison with patients undergoing successful endocardial photocoagulation alone. *J Am Coll Cardiol*. 1990;15:163–170.
12. Sosa E, Scanavacca M, d'Avila A. Catheter ablation of the left ventricular outflow tract tachycardia from the left atrium. *J Interv Card Electrophysiol*. 2002;7:61–63.
13. Hachiya H, Aonuma K, Yamauchi Y, et al. Successful radiofrequency catheter ablation from the supravalvular region of the aortic valve in a patient with outflow tract ventricular tachycardia. *Jpn Circ J*. 2000;64:459–463.
14. de Paola AA, Melo WD, Tavora MZ, Martinez EE. Angiographic and electrophysiological substrates for ventricular tachycardia mapping through the coronary veins. *Heart*. 1998;79:59–63.
15. Sosa E, Scanavacca M, d'Avila A, Pilleggi F. A new technique to perform epicardial mapping in the electrophysiology laboratory. *J Cardiovasc Electrophysiol*. 1996;7:531–536.
16. Sosa E, Scanavacca M. Epicardial mapping and ablation technique to control ventricular tachycardia. *J Cardiovasc Electrophysiol*. 2005;16:449–452.
17. Swarup V, Morton JB, Arruda M, Wilber DJ. Ablation of epicardial macroreentrant ventricular tachycardia associated with idiopathic nonischemic dilated cardiomyopathy by a percutaneous transthoracic approach. *J Cardiovasc Electrophysiol*. 2002;13:1164–1168.
18. Ouyang F, Bansch D, Schaumann A, et al. Catheter ablation of subepicardial ventricular tachycardia using electroanatomic mapping. *Herz*. 2003;28:591–597.
19. Soejima K, Stevenson WG, Sapp JL, et al. Endocardial and epicardial radiofrequency ablation of ventricular tachycardia associated with dilated cardiomyopathy: the importance of low-voltage scars. *J Am Coll Cardiol*. 2004;43:1834–1842.
20. Soejima K, Stevenson WG. Catheter ablation of ventricular tachycardia in patients with ischemic heart disease. *Curr Cardiol Rep*. 2003;5:364–368.
21. Schweikert RA, Saliba WI, Tomassoni G, et al. Percutaneous pericardial instrumentation for endo-epicardial mapping of previously failed ablations. *Circulation*. 2003;108:1329–1335.
22. Sosa E, Scanavacca M, D'Avila A, et al. Radiofrequency catheter ablation of ventricular tachycardia guided by nonsurgical epicardial mapping in chronic chagasic heart disease. *Pacing Clin Electrophysiol*. 1999;22:128–130.
23. Sosa E, Scanavacca M, d'Avila A, et al. Nonsurgical transthoracic epicardial catheter ablation to treat recurrent ventricular tachycardia occurring late after myocardial infarction. *J Am Coll Cardiol*. 2000;35:1442–1449.
24. Sosa E, Scanavacca M, d'Avila A. Transthoracic epicardial catheter ablation to treat recurrent ventricular tachycardia. *Curr Cardiol Rep*. 2001;3:451–458.
25. Sosa E, Scanavacca M, d'Avila A, et al. Nonsurgical transthoracic mapping and ablation in a child with incessant ventricular tachycardia. *J Cardiovasc Electrophysiol*. 2000;11:208–210.
26. Brugada J, Berruezo A, Cuesta A, et al. Nonsurgical transthoracic epicardial radiofrequency ablation: an alternative in incessant ventricular tachycardia. *J Am Coll Cardiol*. 2003;41:2036–2043.
27. d'Avila A, Gutierrez P, Scanavacca M, et al. Effects of radiofrequency pulses delivered in the vicinity of the coronary arteries: implications for nonsurgical transthoracic epicardial catheter ablation to treat ventricular tachycardia. *Pacing Clin Electrophysiol*. 2002;25:1488–1495.
28. Miranda RC. *Estudo dos efeitos das aplicações de radiofrequencia sobre as artérias coronárias, grandes artérias da base, esôfago e brônquio de suínos*. São Paulo, Brazil: Tese (Doutorado); 1999.
29. d'Avila A, Dias R, Scanavacca M, Sosa E. Epicardial fat tissue does not modify amplitude and duration of the epicardial electrograms and/or ventricular stimulation threshold [abstract]. *Eur J Cardiol*. 2002;109.
30. d'Avila A, Houghtaling C, Gutierrez P, et al. Catheter ablation of ventricular epicardial tissue: a comparison of standard and cooled-tip radiofrequency energy. *Circulation*. 2004;109(19):2363–2369.
31. d'Avila A, Holmvang G, Houghtaling C, et al. Focal and linear endocardial and epicardial catheter-based cryoablation of normal and infarcted ventricular tissue. *Heart Rhythms*. 2004;1:1S.
32. d'Avila A, Scanavacca M, Sosa E, et al. Pericardial anatomy for the interventional electrophysiologist. *J Cardiovasc Electrophysiol*. 2003;14:422–430.
33. Sosa E, Scanavacca M, D'Avila A, et al. Nonsurgical transthoracic epicardial approach in patients with ventricular tachycardia and previous cardiac surgery. *J Interv Card Electrophysiol*. 2004;10:281–288.
34. Rumbak M, Chokshi SK, Abel N, et al. Left phrenic nerve paresis complicating catheter radiofrequency ablation for Wolf-Parkinson-White syndrome. *Am Heart J*. 1996;132:1281–1285.
35. Durnate -ME, Vecchio D, Ruggiero G. Right diaphragm paralysis following cardiac ablation for inappropriate sinus tachycardia. *Pacing Clin Electrophysiol*. 2003;26:783–784.
36. Lee B-K, Choi K-J, Rhee K-S, et al. Right phrenic nerve injury following electrical disconnection of the right superior pulmonary vein. *Pacing Clin Electrophysiol*. 2004;27:1444–1446.
37. Berruezo A, Mont L, Nava S, et al. Electrocardiographic recognition of the epicardial origin of ventricular tachycardias. *Circulation*. 2004;109:1842–1847.
38. Soejima K, Couper G, Cooper JM, et al. Subxiphoid surgical approach for epicardial catheter-based mapping and ablation in patients with prior cardiac surgery or difficult pericardial access. *Circulation*. 2004;110:1197–1201.
39. Valles E, Bazan V, Marchlinski F. ECG criteria to identify epicardial ventricular tachycardia in nonischemic cardiomyopathy. *Circ Arrhythmia Electrophysiol*. 2010;3:63–71.

32
Ablation of Ventricular Tachycardia with Congenital Heart Disease

George F. Van Hare

Key Points

The mechanism of ventricular tachycardia with congenital heart disease is macro-reentry related to surgical scars.

Diagnosis is based on inducibility, demonstration of entrainment, and mapping.

Ablation targets include specific isthmuses of ventricular myocardium related to surgical and anatomic lines of block.

Substrate mapping using electroanatomic mapping is helpful, and cooled radiofrequency ablation may be essential to create deep lesions.

Ventricular tachycardia (VT) and its relationship to sudden death remain difficult management issues in patients who have previously undergone surgical repair of significant congenital heart defects. For the most part, the initial life-threatening hemodynamic problem in these patients has been successfully palliated or repaired by surgery, often years or decades previously. Although atrioventricular block has been implicated in the etiology of sudden death in a few patients, and atrial flutter with rapid conduction is certainly involved in the sudden death of those patients with extensive atrial surgery,[1,2] VT is an important contributor. Clinicians have observed the frequent occurrence of premature ventricular contractions and nonsustained and sustained ventricular arrhythmias in patients who have undergone complete repair of tetralogy of Fallot and related defects such as double-outlet right ventricle, and VT has been implicated in the etiology of sudden death in this patient group. Indeed, it has been reported that postoperative tetralogy of Fallot is the single most common condition in sudden death among children between the ages of 1 and 16 years,[3] although the risk for sudden death is also elevated in aortic stenosis, coarctation, and postoperative transposition of the great arteries.[4]

Pathophysiology

Substrate

By far the most information regarding patients with VT and congenital heart disease pertains to tetralogy of Fallot. Ventricular arrhythmias occur much more rarely in patients with other lesions.[5] However, for the purposes of management, tetralogy of Fallot can be viewed as a reasonable model for other lesions, when patients with other lesions present with ventricular arrhythmias in the setting of ventriculotomy or ventricular dysfunction. Surgery and chronic pressure-volume overload in these patients lead to myocardial scarring and fibrosis that are common substrates for VT in congenital heart disease.

Controversy still exists regarding the role of various risk factors for the occurrence of ventricular arrhythmias and sudden death, the exact relationship between ventricular arrhythmias and sudden death, the role of electrophysiologic study and other procedures for risk stratification, and, ultimately, the appropriate management of postoperative VT. Although major advances in understanding of the roles of antiarrhythmic agents and implantable cardioverter-defibrillators in patients with coronary disease have been made through the performance of large multicenter trials,[6] one faces a much greater challenge of answering similar questions in this much smaller patient population. Indeed, as Bricker[7] pointed out, sufficient numbers of operated patients may not be available to perform an adequately powered cohort study to sort out the various likely predictors of sudden death.

Pertinent Anatomy

An extensive review of congenital heart disease anatomy and surgical techniques is beyond the scope of this chapter. However, one must consider the changes in surgical technique that have taken place over the years to understand how patient age, age at repair, and method of repair may interact to increase the risk for arrhythmias. The first complete repair of tetralogy of Fallot was performed in 1954 by Dr. C. W. Lillehei, and starting in the 1960s, complete repair became quite common. Although infants were operated on from the beginning, the mortality rate was high, and it was more common for patients to undergo repair later, often as late as the second or even third decade of life. Starting in the 1970s, owing to improvements in both surgical technique and postoperative care, several centers chose to perform primary repair in infancy, with good results, and this is now the current practice at almost all centers.

Unoperated patients with tetralogy of Fallot have a ventricular septal defect with some degree, usually severe, of right ventricular outflow tract (RVOT) obstruction, leading to chronic cyanosis. The placement of a systemic-to-pulmonary artery shunt as a palliative procedure adds the element of potential left ventricular volume overload. Correction of the defect involves patch closure of the ventricular septal defect with relief of right ventricular obstruction. In almost all patients, this requires resection of a large amount of right ventricular muscle, and early in the experience, this was not done through the tricuspid valve but rather required a ventriculotomy. Finally, the pulmonary annulus is usually small, and repair with a transannular patch leads to chronic pulmonic insufficiency, which may be very severe if associated with downstream obstruction because of significant pulmonary arterial stenosis.

It has been hypothesized that ventricular arrhythmias are caused by the effect of years of chronic cyanosis, followed by the placement of a ventriculotomy, with right ventricular dysfunction. Dysfunction is a result of elevation of right ventricular pressures as a result of inadequate relief of obstruction and severe pulmonic regurgitation.[8–10] Such factors as wall stress and chronic cyanosis, coupled with the passage of time, may lead to myocardial fibrosis and result in the substrate for reentrant ventricular arrhythmias. This hypothesis is supported by histologic studies of the hearts of patients with tetralogy of Fallot who died suddenly, which have shown extensive fibrosis.[11] It is also supported by the observation that fractionated electrograms, late potentials, and areas of low voltage may be recorded from the right ventricle at electrophysiologic study, suggesting the presence of slow conduction.[12,13] Whereas there

is a 5% incidence of coronary artery abnormalities in tetralogy of Fallot, putting the left anterior descending coronary artery or other large branches at risk at the time of complete repair, such potential damage is manifest immediately after surgery and has never been seriously implicated in the etiology of ventricular arrhythmias or of sudden death in most patients.

Mechanism

Careful electrophysiologic studies in patients with clinical VT after tetralogy surgery have supported the concept that the mechanism of tachycardia is macro-reentry involving the RVOT, either at the site of anterior right ventriculotomy or at the site of a ventricular septal defect patch. Transient entrainment can often be documented, with constant fusion at the paced cycle length and progressive fusion at decreasing cycle lengths, and the evaluation of postpacing intervals strongly suggests that sites in the RVOT are part of a macro-reentrant circuit (Fig. 32-1).

Anatomically, one may imagine several long circuits that might support macro-reentry based on congenital and surgical anatomy, and there have been several circuits described in patients with tetralogy of Fallot after surgery. Whereas the simplest notion is a circuit that rotates around an RVOT patch, this is possible only if the patch does not extend all the way to the pulmonic annulus, as a transannular patch would. One well-delineated potential circuit was described by Horton and colleagues,[14] who used pacing techniques to document the importance of the right ventricular isthmus between the tricuspid annulus and the RVOT patch. Notably, these investigators did not map the entire circuit in their two patients, and thus the rest of the circuit was unknown. Their patients both had transannular patches, so there was no possible isthmus between the RVOT patch and the pulmonic annulus. Presumably, the circuit also involved the interventricular septum. Others, notably Downar coworkers,[15] have mapped VT intraoperatively and have found reentry involving the RVOT in all patients, but they only

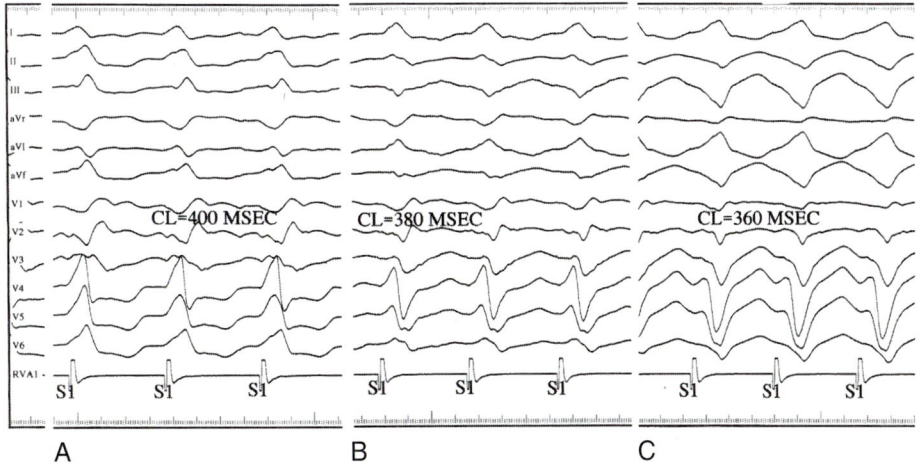

FIGURE 32-1. Tracings at electrophysiologic study of a 35-year-old man who was status postrepair of tetralogy of Fallot at 11 years of age. Ventricular tachycardia was induced by ventricular extrastimulation, with a tachycardia cycle length of 435 msec. Entrainment pacing is performed at 400 msec (**A**), 380 msec (**B**), and 360 msec (**C**). Note that there is progressive fusion at faster paced cycle lengths. CL, cycle length; MSEC, milliseconds.

identified sites of earliest ventricular activation, rather than the entire circuit. They noted early sites located in the septum, free wall, and parietal band.

Diagnostic Criteria

Surface Electrocardiogram

The criteria for the diagnosis of VT are the same as for other forms of macro-reentrant tachycardia (Table 32-1). There is a wide-complex tachycardia, often with atrioventricular dissociation. Despite the fact that most patients with tetralogy of Fallot have macro-reentry arising from the RVOT, the QRS morphology is often not indicative of this location. As described by Horton and colleagues,[14] QRS morphology of VT arising from the RVOT mainly depends on the direction of rotation (clockwise versus counterclockwise) around the circuit, which in their study involved the isthmus of tissue in the right ventricle between the tricuspid annulus and the RVOT patch (Fig. 32-2). They described a clockwise rotation giving rise to a negative QRS in lead I and biphasic QRS in V_1,

TABLE 32-1
KEYS TO DIAGNOSIS
Differentiate ventricular macro-reentry and focal tachycardia through entrainment (see Chapter 28).
Identify surgical and anatomic lines of block through substrate mapping and/or entrainment mapping.

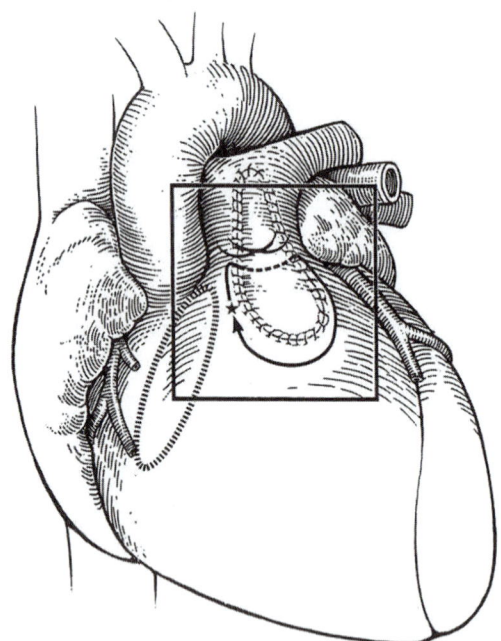

FIGURE 32-2. Right ventricle and right ventricular outflow tract with transannular patch across outflow tract and pulmonic valve. The location of the tricuspid valve annulus is shown with *hatched markings*. The proposed macro-reentrant circuit (*inset*) for ventricular tachycardia involves clockwise or counterclockwise activation between the patch and tricuspid annulus. The *arrow* demonstrates a hypothetical pathway for the remainder of the circuit. *(From Horton RP, Canby RC, Kessler DJ, et al. Ablation of ventricular tachycardia associated with tetralogy of Fallot: demonstration of bidirectional block. J Cardiovasc Electrophysiol. 1997;8:432-435.)*

whereas a counterclockwise rotation produces upright R waves in lead I and an entirely negative QRS (left bundle branch block morphology) in V_1.

Intracardiac Electrograms

As far as is known, there are no specific intracardiac electrogram features in patients with congenital heart disease. Low-amplitude and fractionated late potentials have been described, but it is uncertain whether these electrograms are involved in the substrate for VT. Still, Biblo and Carlson[16] used such mid-diastolic potentials to successfully ablate VT in a patient with tetralogy of Fallot in 1993. In addition, Stevenson and associates,[17] as well as Rostock and coworkers,[18] emphasized the usefulness of voltage maps for delineating the tachycardia circuit in such patients (see later discussion), and such maps depend on the presence of low-amplitude signals in association with myocardial scarring or patch material as barriers that support macro-reentry.

Diagnostic Maneuvers

The principal diagnostic maneuver that is useful in such cases is entrainment mapping, to prove the macro-reentrant nature of the tachycardia. Entrainment, of course, depends on the presence of an excitable gap, which might not exist in tachycardias that are very rapid. Such rapid tachycardias may not be tolerated hemodynamically. Furthermore, in one form of concealed entrainment, pacing close to the exit site from a zone of slow conduction does not allow one to satisfy any of the criteria for entrainment. This problem occurs, despite the existence of a macro-reentrant tachycardia, because of the lack of surface electrocardiogram fusion, as was pointed out by Waldo and Henthorn.[19] An inability to demonstrate manifest entrainment does not rule out a macro-reentrant mechanism.

Mapping and Ablation

Strategies for Basic Mapping

Because most evidence supports the concept of macro-reentry as the mechanism of such VT, it is desirable to use entrainment pacing and mapping techniques (Table 32-2). Several investigators have reported successful procedures using radiofrequency energy.[14,20–22] Stevenson and associates,[17] in particular, reported the utility of voltage maps to identify areas of scar in the right ventricle.

Although well-tolerated VT can be mapped in the electrophysiology laboratory, many patients have ventricular dysfunction or rapid VT, or both, and will not tolerate

TABLE 32-2
TARGETS FOR ABLATION
Sites of early ventricular activation
Sites of concealed entrainment
Anatomic isthmuses between surgical and structural lines of block

this. Several investigators have reported intraoperative mapping and ablation.[15,23-25] In particular, Downar and coworkers[15] used intraoperative mapping of the RVOT in the beating heart, employing an endocardial electrode balloon and a simultaneous epicardial electrode shock array. Ablation was carried out by cryotherapy lesions during normothermic cardiopulmonary bypass with the heart beating, or during anoxic arrest, with good success in three patients.

Use of Specialized Mapping Systems

Electroanatomic mapping of the arrhythmia circuit may be feasible if the tachycardia is inducible and is slow enough to be mapped completely. The Carto system (Biosense Webster, Diamond Bar, CA) allows the construction of isochronal and propagation maps. As with other arrhythmias, the process of construction of an electroanatomic map may be time-consuming and difficult. An additional available modality provided by the Carto system is the ability to construct three-dimensional voltage maps to better identify the anatomic barriers. Rostock and colleagues[18] reported a procedure in a 36-year-old patient after surgical repair of tetralogy by use of a homograft conduit, using electroanatomic voltage mapping methods. They used a combination of entrainment mapping and voltage maps

constructed in sinus rhythm, using the Carto system. They defined an area of scar by the recording of electrogram amplitudes of less than 0.5 mV, and created a Y-shaped incision blocking conduction of impulses between the RVOT and the homograft. Subsequently, Zeppenfeld and associates[22] demonstrated the use of these modalities in the successful mapping and ablation of right ventricular reentrant tachycardia in 16 adult patients after repair of congenital heart disease, of whom 14 were tetralogy of Fallot patients. They also included the failure to capture with high-output unipolar pacing as a criterion for the identification of scar or patch material, and employed both the identification of scar and low voltage myocardium in the identification of potential isthmuses supporting ventricular tachycardia. They then targeted these isthmuses using radiofrequency ablation, with either cooled-tip or irrigated-tip ablation in most cases. They demonstrated the usefulness of tagged ablation sites in constructing a broad line of block between the ventriculotomy scar and the tricuspid annulus (Fig. 32-3).

Targets for Ablation

Appropriate targets for ablation may be determined by relatively simple means, such as sites of early ventricular activation that precede surface QRS during tachycardia. Given

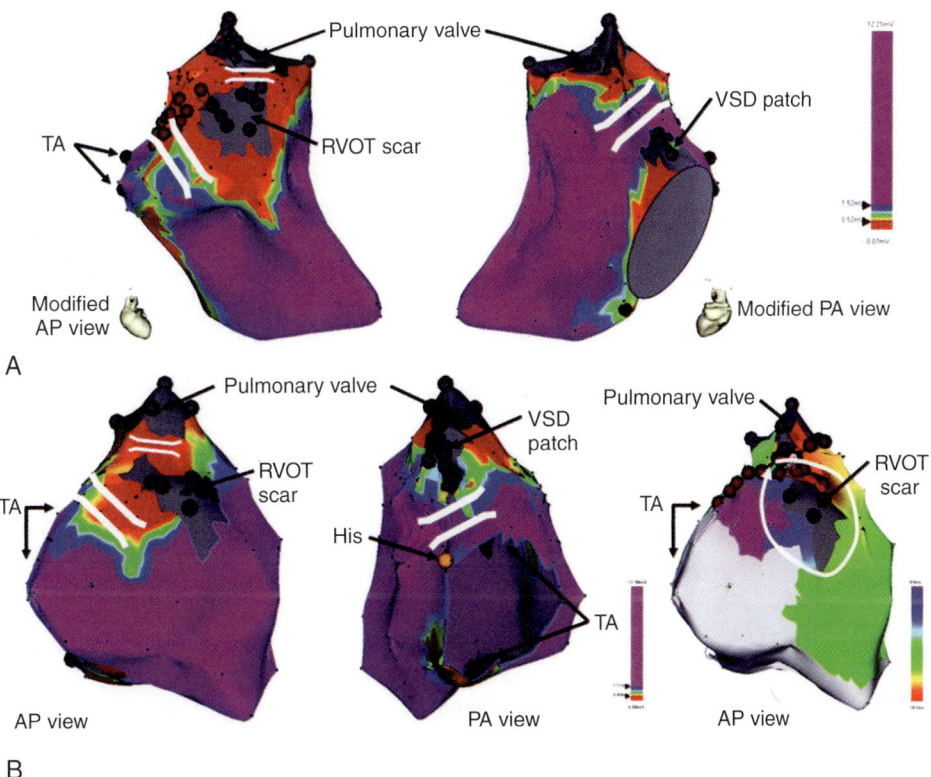

FIGURE 32-3. A, Voltage maps of the right ventricle (RV) in a modified anterior (AP) view and modified posterior (PA) view in a patient with tetralogy of Fallot. Three anatomic isthmuses were delineated (*white lines*). In this patient, the first isthmus is bordered by the pulmonary valve and right ventricular outflow tract (RVOT) scar. No muscular rim is present between the ventricular septal defect (VSD) patch and the tricuspid annulus (TA). Linear ablation lesions (*red tags*) the transect anatomic isthmus. **B,** Voltage maps of RV in an AP view (*left*) and PA view (*center*) in another tetralogy patient. In contrast to **A,** a muscular rim is present between the VSD patch and the tricuspid annulus. Activation map of ventricular tachycardia (*right,* AP view). Activation time is color coded; the activation time (270 msec) equals the VT cycle length. The macro-reentrant circuit propagates clockwise around the RVOT scar through the second isthmus and inferior to superior through the first isthmus. The catheter tip indicates the termination site. *(From Zeppenfeld K, Schalij MJ, Bartelings MM, et al. Catheter ablation of ventricular tachycardia after repair of congenital heart disease: electroanatomic identification of the critical right ventricular isthmus. Circulation. 2007;116:2241-2252. With permission.)*

the macro-reentrant nature of these rhythms, however, it makes sense to consider the entire circuit and to focus on sites that are found to be in the circuit by entrainment mapping techniques, and where barriers can be connected by a series of lesions with the effect of bridging the isthmus and creating bidirectional block. These techniques, of course, are well developed in the ablation of typical atrial flutter, as well as in the ablation of postsurgical intra-atrial reentrant tachycardia. An early demonstration of this concept was the report by Horton and colleagues,[14] in which two patients were found to have VT involving the isthmus between the RVOT patch and the tricuspid annulus. The important contribution made by this case report was the demonstration of a clear method for documenting isthmus block in both clockwise and counterclockwise directions. This capability provides a better criterion for ablation success than simple noninducibility. Horton and colleagues demonstrated that the creation of a line of block between the tricuspid annulus and RVOT patch is associated with a characteristic alteration in the paced QRS morphology, as well as a clear change in the order of ventricular activation with pacing from specific sites. Subsequently, Zeppenfeld and associates were able to define a total of only four anatomic isthmuses supporting right ventricular tachycardia in their series of 16 patients[22] (Fig. 32-4). This is an important observation because the limited number of potential isthmuses supporting VT holds the promise of allowing ablation procedures to be performed without needing to map or ablate during VT.

Alternate Ablation Sources

The potential for irrigated-tip or cooled-tip radiofrequency ablation to penetrate the myocardium more deeply is clearly an advantage when working in the right ventricle, which may well be thick because of the chronic pressure overload and pulmonic insufficiency that often exist in such patients. It was successfully employed in the study by Zeppenfeld and colleagues.[22] Second, as Morwood and coworkers[26] noted, occasionally the tachycardia circuit involves regions that are close to the

site where the His bundle potential is recorded. In such a situation, one might imagine the utility of cryoablation, in which "ice mapping" of lesions is possible, to avoid inadvertent complete atrioventricular block.

Success and Recurrence Rates

With a few notable exceptions, reports of ablation of VT in patients with congenital heart disease are single-center reports that involve one or two procedures. A listing of reported ablations in patients with tetralogy of Fallot or other congenital heart disease is found in Table 32-3. This includes one case, in 1986, in which DC ablation was attempted, as well as a number of other cases in which radiofrequency energy was used. Most procedures are reported as successful. The total success rate derived from these reports, 96%, should be treated with a great deal of caution, however. Centers that succeed in ablating this substrate are clearly more likely to report their results than are centers that have failed, and such "reporting bias" has the potential to skew the impression of expected results.

Somewhat more useful are reports of multiple cases from a single center, in which a large time frame is used and patients are included consecutively. Morwood and coworkers[26] reported the experience at the Children's Hospital in Boston with ablation for VT in young patients. They reported that, of 97 consecutive ablation procedures for VT over 13 years, 20 were in patients with congenital heart disease. In 8 of these patients, mapping or ablation, or both, was not considered to be feasible because of tachycardia noninducibility, tachycardia rate, hemodynamic instability, or location close to the His bundle. Ablation was attempted in the other 12 patients, with acute success in 10 (80%). Four of these 10 patients (40%) had experienced recurrence at last follow-up.

Another source for data concerning ablations in the pediatric population is the Pediatric Radiofrequency Ablation Registry. From 1991 to 2005, pediatric electrophysiologists at almost 50 centers periodically reported their acute results to the registry.[27-29] An analysis of data from both the early and the late registry experience found a total of 74 proce-

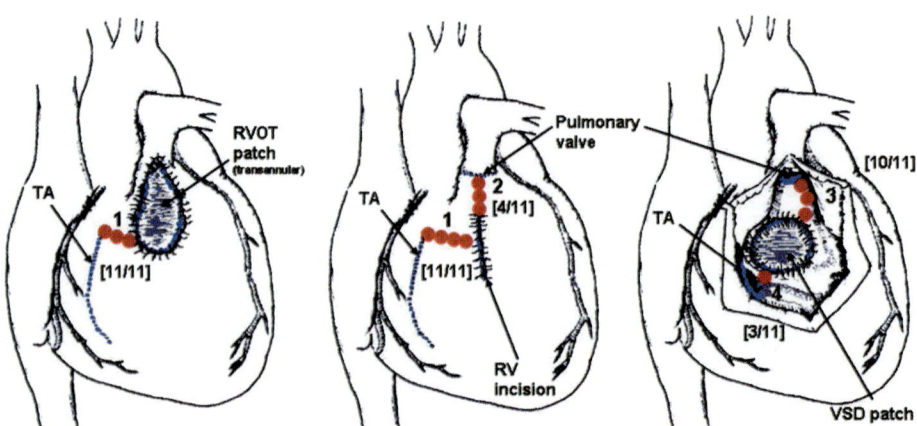

FIGURE 32-4. Schematic of the localization of anatomic boundaries for ventricular tachycardia after repair of congenital heart disease and the resulting anatomic isthmuses. Frequency of the distinct isthmuses in 11 patients are shown in brackets. RV, right ventricular; RVOT, right ventricular outflow tract; TA, tricuspid annulus; VSD, ventricular septal defect. (*From Zeppenfeld K, Schalij MJ, Bartelings MM, et al. Catheter ablation of ventricular tachycardia after repair of congenital heart disease: electroanatomic identification of the critical right ventricular isthmus. Circulation. 2007;116:2241-2252. With permission.*)

TABLE 32-3

ABLATION IN PATIENTS WITH TETRALOGY OF FALLOT OR OTHER CONGENITAL HEART DISEASE

Study	Method	No. of Procedures	No. Successful
Oda et al, 1986[30]	DC	1	1
Burton & Leon, 1993[31]	RF	2	2
Goldner et al, 1994[32]	RF	1	1
Biblo & Carlson, 1994[16]	RF	1	1
Chinushi et al, 1995[33]	RF	1	1
Gonska et al, 1996[20]	RF	16	15
Horton et al, 1997[14]	RF	2	2
Papagiannis et al, 1998[21]	RF	1	1
Stevenson et al, 1998[17]	RF/Carto	1	1
Saul & Alexander, 1999[34]	RF	2	2
Fukuhara et al, 2000[35]	RF	1	1
Arenal et al, 2003[36]	RF/Carto	1	1
Rojel et al, 2003[37]	RF	2	2
Morwood et al, 2004[26]	RF	12	10
Rostock et al, 2004[18]	RF/Carto	1	1
Furushima et al, 2006[38]	RF	8	8
Zeppenfeld et al, 2007[22]	Substrate mapping	11	11
Kriebel et al, 2007[39]	EnSite	8	8
Chinushi et al, 2009[13]	RF/Carto	1	1
Total reported procedures		73	70 (96%)

DC, direct current; RF, radiofrequency.

dures in patients with congenital heart disease for whom ablation of VT was attempted (D. L. Fairbrother and colleagues, unpublished data). Of the VTs in these patients, 50 or 74 (68%) were mapped to a morphologically right ventricle, and 24 or 74 (32%) were mapped to a left ventricle. The initial success rate for these ablation attempts was only 47 of 74, or 64%. These multicenter data highlight the difficulties in arriving at benchmarks for ablation success when one relies on single-center reports involving very few patients.

Complications

In general, complications of radiofrequency ablation for VT are rarely reported. Overall complication rates in this population have been estimated to be about 3%.[26,27,29] Specific reported complications are similar to those reported for other types of ablation, including hematomas and second-degree atrioventricular block.

Troubleshooting the Difficult Case

Because ablation of VT is only rarely attempted and so little is known about the substrate and the best methods for ablation, in truth all such cases can be thought of as difficult cases. That is, there is not really any case that would qualify as a "routine" case. Therefore, it is difficult to provide any additional advice concerning the approach to a "difficult"

TABLE 32-4

TROUBLESHOOTING THE DIFFICULT CASE

Problem	Causes	Solutions
Complex cardiovascular anatomy	Congenital heart disease and previous surgery	Thorough review of records and imaging studies Slow with antiarrhythmic drugs
Hemodynamically unstable ventricular tachycardia	Rapid rate, ventricular dysfunction	Substrate mapping
Unable to terminate with ablation	Dense scar	Cooled radiofrequency ablation
	Thick myocardial wall Broad channel	Create linear lesions

case than what has already been provided (Table 32-4). Perhaps the only thing to say is that each case of VT in a patient with congenital heart disease should be approached in a comprehensive fashion. One must start with a detailed knowledge of the congenital heart anatomy and perform a careful review of the details of the surgical repair that was performed, using the dictated operative report if possible. All imaging studies available should be reviewed, such as echocardiogram and angiogram, because they may provide more information concerning the underlying anatomy. In the laboratory, if sustained VT is inducible and is sufficiently well tolerated, entrainment should be performed in an attempt to make a diagnosis of a macro-reentrant tachycardia. Should the tachycardia be stable, entrainment mapping can be performed, searching for sites at which the postpacing interval is equivalent to the tachycardia cycle length, indicating that the site is in the macro-reentrant circuit. Electroanatomic mapping is an important adjunct, particularly with the use of voltage mapping and unipolar pacing to identify the scars and other important anatomic details. Lesions may be planned to connect surgical scars or anatomic barriers. It seems important that a complete line of block should be created, and the method of Horton and colleagues[14] is attractive. Alternatively, one might consider documentation of the line of block by the use of repeat electroanatomic mapping.

In the final analysis, as discussed earlier, it is by no means certain that successful ablation of a VT circuit in a patient with congenital heart disease will in any way decrease or eliminate the risk for sudden death, so many patients will be appropriate candidates for implantation of implantable cardioverter-defibrillators, most prominently in those with strong risk factors for sudden death such as severe right ventricular dilation and dysfunction, or pulmonic insufficiency.

References

1. Harrison DA, Siu SC, Hussain F, et al. Sustained atrial arrhythmias in adults late after repair of tetralogy of Fallot. *Am J Cardiol.* 2001;87:584–588.
2. Li W, Somerville J. Atrial flutter in grown-up congenital heart (GUCH) patients: clinical characteristics of affected population. *Int J Cardiol.* 2000;75:129–137; discussion 138-139.
3. Garson A, McNamara DG. Sudden death in a pediatric cardiology population, 1958 to 1983: relation to prior arrhythmias. *J Am Coll Cardiol.* 1985;5:134B–137B.
4. Silka MJ, Hardy BG, Menashe VD, Morris CD. A population-based prospective evaluation of risk of sudden cardiac death after operation for common congenital heart defects. *J Am Coll Cardiol.* 1998;32:245–251.
5. Vetter VL, Horowitz LN. Electrophysiologic residua and sequelae of surgery for congenital heart defects. *Am J Cardiol.* 1982;50:588–604.
6. The Antiarrhythmics versus Implantable Defibrillators (AVID) Investigators. A comparison of antiarrhythmic-drug therapy with implantable defibrillators in patients resuscitated from near-fatal ventricular arrhythmias. *N Engl J Med.* 1997;337:1576–1583.
7. Bricker JT. Sudden death and tetralogy of Fallot: risks, markers, and causes. *Circulation.* 1995;92:158–159.
8. Zahka KG, Horneffer PJ, Rowe SA, et al. Long-term valvular function after total repair of tetralogy of Fallot: relation to ventricular arrhythmias. *Circulation.* 1988;78:III14–III19.
9. Gatzoulis MA, Till JA, Somerville J, Redington AN. Mechanoelectrical interaction in tetralogy of Fallot: QRS prolongation relates to right ventricular size and predicts malignant ventricular arrhythmias and sudden death. *Circulation.* 1995;92:231–237.
10. Gatzoulis MA, Till JA, Redington AN. Depolarization-repolarization inhomogeneity after repair of tetralogy of Fallot: the substrate for malignant ventricular tachycardia? *Circulation.* 1997;95:401–404.
11. Deanfield JE, Ho SY, Anderson RH, et al. Late sudden death after repair of tetralogy of Fallot: a clinicopathologic study. *Circulation.* 1983;67:626–631.
12. Zimmermann M, Friedli B, Adamec R, Oberhansli I. Ventricular late potentials and induced ventricular arrhythmias after surgical repair of tetralogy of Fallot. *Am J Cardiol.* 1991;67:873–878.
13. Chinushi M, Komura S, Furushima H, Aizawa Y. Segmental conduction block in low-voltage area suppressed macro-reentrant ventricular tachycardia after surgical repair of tetralogy of Fallot. *Intern Med.* 2009;48:1021–1023.
14. Horton RP, Canby RC, Kessler DJ, et al. Ablation of ventricular tachycardia associated with tetralogy of Fallot: Demonstration of bidirectional block. *J Cardiovasc Electrophysiol.* 1997;8:432–435.
15. Downar E, Harris L, Kimber S, et al. Ventricular tachycardia after surgical repair of tetralogy of Fallot: results of intraoperative mapping studies. *J Am Coll Cardiol.* 1992;20:648–655.
16. Biblo LA, Carlson MD. Transcatheter radiofrequency ablation of ventricular tachycardia following surgical correction of tetralogy of Fallot. *Pacing Clin Electrophysiol.* 1994;17:1556–1560.
17. Stevenson WG, Delacretaz E, Friedman PL, Ellison KE. Identification and ablation of macroreentrant ventricular tachycardia with the CARTO electroanatomical mapping system. *Pacing Clin Electrophysiol.* 1998;21:1448–1456.
18. Rostock T, Willems S, Ventura R, et al. Radiofrequency catheter ablation of a macroreentrant ventricular tachycardia late after surgical repair of tetralogy of Fallot using the electroanatomic mapping (CARTO). *Pacing Clin Electrophysiol.* 2004;27:801–804.
19. Waldo AL, Henthorn RW. Use of transient entrainment during ventricular tachycardia to localize a critical area in the reentry circuit for ablation. *Pacing Clin Electrophysiol.* 1989;12:231–244.
20. Gonska BD, Cao K, Raab J, et al. Radiofrequency catheter ablation of right ventricular tachycardia late after repair of congenital heart defects. *Circulation.* 1996;94:1902–1908.
21. Papagiannis J, Kanter RJ, Wharton JM. Radiofrequency catheter ablation of multiple haemodynamically unstable ventricular tachycardias in a patient with surgically repaired tetralogy of Fallot. *Cardiol Young.* 1998;8:379–382.
22. Zeppenfeld K, Schalij MJ, Bartelings MM, et al. Catheter ablation of ventricular tachycardia after repair of congenital heart disease: electroanatomic identification of the critical right ventricular isthmus. *Circulation.* 2007;116:2241–2252.
23. Ressia L, Graffigna A, Salerno-Uriarte JA, Vigano M. The complex origin of ventricular tachycardia after the total correction of tetralogy of Fallot. *G Ital Cardiol.* 1993;23:905–910.
24. Frank G, Schmid C, Baumgart D, et al. Surgical therapy of life-threatening tachycardic cardiac arrhythmias in children. *Monatsschrift Kinderheilkunde.* 1989;137:269–274.
25. Lawrie GM, Pacifico A, Kaushik R. Results of direct surgical ablation of ventricular tachycardia not due to ischemic heart disease. *Ann Surg.* 1989;209:716–727.
26. Morwood JG, Triedman JK, Berul CI, et al. Radiofrequency catheter ablation of ventricular tachycardia in children and young adults with congenital heart disease. *Heart Rhythm.* 2004;1:301–308.
27. Kugler JD, Danford DA, Deal BJ, et al. Radiofrequency catheter ablation for tachyarrhythmias in children and adolescents. The Pediatric Electrophysiology Society. *N Engl J Med.* 1994;330:1481–1487.
28. Van Hare GF, Carmelli D, Smith WM, et al. Prospective assessment after pediatric cardiac ablation: design and implementation of the multicenter study. *Pacing Clin Electrophysiol.* 2002;25:332–341.
29. Van Hare GF, Javitz H, Carmelli D, et al. Prospective assessment after pediatric cardiac ablation: Demographics, medical profiles, and initial outcomes. *J Cardiovasc Electrophysiol.* 2004;15:759–770.
30. Oda H, Aizawa Y, Murata M, et al. A successful electrical ablation of recurrent sustained ventricular tachycardia in a postoperative case of tetralogy of Fallot. *Jpn Heart J.* 1986;27:421–428.
31. Burton ME, Leon AR. Radiofrequency catheter ablation of right ventricular outflow tract tachycardia late after complete repair of tetralogy of Fallot using the pace mapping technique. *Pacing Clin Electrophysiol.* 1993;16:2319–2325.
32. Goldner BG, Cooper R, Blau W, Cohen TJ. Radiofrequency catheter ablation as a primary therapy for treatment of ventricular tachycardia in a patient after repair of tetralogy of Fallot. *Pacing Clin Electrophysiol.* 1994;17:1441–1446.
33. Chinushi M, Aizawa Y, Kitazawa H, et al. Successful radiofrequency catheter ablation for macroreentrant ventricular tachycardias in a patient with tetralogy of Fallot after corrective surgery. *Pacing Clin Electrophysiol.* 1995;18:1713–1716.
34. Saul JP, Alexander ME. Preventing sudden death after repair of tetralogy of Fallot: complex therapy for complex patients. *J Cardiovasc Electrophysiol.* 1999;10:1271–1287.
35. Fukuhara H, Nakamura Y, Tasato H, et al. Successful radiofrequency catheter ablation of left ventricular tachycardia following surgical correction of tetralogy of Fallot. *Pacing Clin Electrophysiol.* 2000;23:1442–1445.
36. Arenal A, Glez-Torrecilla E, Ortiz M, et al. Ablation of electrograms with an isolated, delayed component as treatment of unmappable monomorphic ventricular tachycardias in patients with structural heart disease. *J Am Coll Cardiol.* 2003;41:81–92.
37. Rojel U, Cuesta A, Mont L, Brugada J. Radiofrequency ablation of late ventricular tachycardia in patients with corrected tetralogy of Fallot. *Arch Cardiol Mex.* 2003;73:275–279.
38. Furushima H, Chinushi M, Sugiura H, et al. Ventricular tachycardia late after repair of congenital heart disease: efficacy of combination therapy with radiofrequency catheter ablation and class III antiarrhythmic agents and long-term outcome. *J Electrocardiol.* 2006;39:219–224.
39. Kriebel T, Saul JP, Schneider H, et al. Noncontact mapping and radiofrequency catheter ablation of fast and hemodynamically unstable ventricular tachycardia after surgical repair of tetralogy of Fallot. *J Am Coll Cardiol.* 2007;50:2162–2168.

Miscellaneous Topics

PART VIII

33

Complications Associated with Radiofrequency Catheter Ablation of Cardiac Arrhythmias

Hugh Calkins

Key Points

Complications may result from any aspect of the diagnostic electrophysiologic study and ablation procedure.

The risk for stroke is highest during catheter ablation of atrial fibrillation.

The risks for radiation exposure are cumulative and usually occur days to weeks after an ablation procedure. Children are at greatest risk for radiation injury.

The precise types of risk and the incidence of risk vary greatly depending on the ablation target. Catheter ablation of atrial fibrillation and nonidiopathic ventricular tachycardia are associated with the greatest risk.

Because catheter ablation procedures are generally employed on patients without life-threatening conditions, it is particularly important to make every effort to minimize risk.

For most cardiac arrhythmias, medical therapy with antiarrhythmic drugs is not completely effective. In addition to poor or sporadic efficacy, such drugs can be associated with a number of bothersome side effects, proarrhythmia, high cost, and inconvenience. It is for these reasons that nonpharmacologic interventions, initially using a surgical approach and more recently with catheter ablation, have played an increasingly important role in the management of cardiac arrhythmias.

During the past two and one half decades, radiofrequency (RF) catheter ablation has evolved from a highly experimental technique to first-line therapy for many cardiac arrhythmias. During the 4-year period from 1989 to 1992, the number of patients undergoing catheter ablation procedures in the United States increased more than 30-fold from an estimated 450 procedures in 1989 to 15,000 procedures in 1993.[1] A great deal of information has been published that has focused on the acute and long-term efficacy of RF catheter ablation procedures. Perhaps of equal importance in determining the ultimate clinical role of a particular procedure are the type and incidence of complications. The purpose of this chapter, therefore, is to provide an update regarding the current understanding of the risks and complications that can occur during catheter ablation procedures. Particular attention will be focused on defining the risks associated with catheter ablation of atrial fibrillation (AF) and identifying those techniques that may reduce the incidence of complications.

Prior Studies of Complications during Catheter Ablation Procedures

Information concerning the type and incidence of complications during catheter ablation procedures can be derived from single-center experiences, registry data, and prospective multicenter clinical studies (Tables 33-1 to 33-4). Among these various sources, data obtained as part of a prospective multicenter clinical trial are generally the most relevant to clinical practice. Registry data are also a useful source of complication data. In contrast, information derived from a single center may be unique to that center and its staff and operators and is therefore less likely to reflect the types and incidence of anticipated complications when RF catheter ablation is applied on a widespread basis. For this reason, the data presented in the review have been obtained primarily from multicenter experiences and from registry information. We also review the results of meta-analyses when available. The results of four multicenter surveys of patients who underwent catheter ablation have been published.[1-4] The 1995 North American Society for Pacing and Electrophysiology (NASPE)

TABLE 33-1

COMPLICATIONS ASSOCIATED WITH CATHETER ABLATION OF ACCESSORY PATHWAYS (AP)

Complications	MERFS[2] (N = 2222)	NASPE 1995[1] (N = 5427)	NASPE 1998[3] (N = 654)	Calkins et al[4] (N = 500)	Spector et al[14] (N = 2267)*
Complete AV block	14 (0.63%)	9 (0.17%)	2 (0.3%)	5 (1%)	16 (0.8%)
Valve damage	1 (0.05%)	6† (0.11%)	0 (0%)	+	0 (0%)
Coronary artery injury, occlusion	0 (0%)	3 (0.06%)	1 (0.16%)	1 (0.2%)	0 (0%)
Tamponade	16 (0.72%)	7 (0.13%)	7 (1.1%)	+	8 (0.4%)
Venous thrombosis	4 (0.18%)	‡	0 (0%)	+	0 (0%)
Pulmonary embolism	2 (0.09%)	‡	1 (0.16%)	+	0 (0%)
Arterial thrombosis	4 (0.18%)	0 (0%)	0 (0%)	+	0 (0%)
CVA/TIA	11 (0.49%)	8 (0.15%)	0 (0%)	1 (0.2%)§	5 (0.3%)
Bleeding at puncture site, vascular injury	7 (0.32%)	3 (0.06%)	13 (1.99%)¶	+	8 (0.6%)
Death	3 (0.13%)	4 (0.08%)	0 (0.00%)	1 (0.2%)	2 (0.1%)

* Number of patients reported varies per complication.
† Aortic valve perforations in four and mitral valve damages in two.
‡ Reported but no number specified.
§ Left-sided anteroposterior with transseptal approach.
¶ Twelve left free wall anteroposterior and one septal anteroposterior.
+, Complications were presented for all arrhythmias and were not all categorized based on the target arrhythmia; AV, atrioventricular; CVA/TIA cerebrovascular accident/transient ischemic event.

TABLE 33-2

COMPLICATIONS ASSOCIATED WITH CATHETER ABLATION OF ATRIOVENTRICULAR NODAL REENTRY TACHYCARDIA

Complications	MERFS[2] (N = 815)	NASPE 1995[1] (N = 5423)	NASPE 1998[3] (N = 1197)	Calkins et al[4] (N = 373)	Spector et al[14] (N = 4748)*
Complete AV block	41 (5.07%)	6 (0.11%)	9 (0.74%)	5 (1.3%)	78 (1.7%)
Pneumothorax	0 (0%)	5 (0.09%)	1 (0.08%)	+	2 (0.1%)
Tamponade/ Pericarditis	2 (0.24%)	18 (0.33%)	0 (0%)	+	2 (0.1%)
Venous thrombosis	9 (1.11%)	5 (0.09%)	1 (0.08%)		2 (0.1%)
Pulmonary emboli	2 (0.24%)	0 (0%)	1 (0.08%))	+	5 (0.2%
CVA/TIA	1 (0.12%)	0 (0%)	0 (0%)	+	0 (0%)
Bleeding at puncture site, vascular injury	2 (0.24%)	3 (0.06%)	6 (0.49%)	+	12 (0.4%)
Death	0 (0%)	0 (0%)	0 (0%)	0 (0%)	0 (0%)

* Number of patients reported varies per complication.
+, Complications were presented for all arrhythmias and were not all categorized based on the target arrhythmia; AV, atrioventricular; CVA/TIA cerebrovascular accident/transient ischemic event.

survey retrospectively reviewed the results of about 37,000 catheter ablation procedures performed in 157 United States centers between 1989 and 1993.[1] The Multicenter European Radiofrequency Survey (MERFS) focused on the complications related to catheter ablation, surveying the ablation results at 68 European institutions between 1987 and 1992.[2] The 1998 NASPE registry prospectively enrolled 3357 patients who underwent catheter ablation procedures at 68 institutions in the United States.[3] The 2001 Spanish Registry on Catheter Ablation reviewed the results of 4374 catheter ablation procedures in 41 centers.[4] The 2002 Spanish Registry on Catheter Ablation reviewed the results of 4970 catheter ablation procedures in 4755 patients in 42 centers.[5] In addition, three prospective multicenter clinical trials focusing on the efficacy and safety of RF catheter ablation of accessory pathways, atrioventricular nodal reentrant tachycardia (AVNRT), and the atrioventricular (AV) junction, as well as ventricular tachycardia (VT), have been published.[6–8] Finally, there have also been several multicenter studies published on catheter ablation of atrial flutter.[9,10] This review will pay particular attention to these studies. We have also included extensive data derived from a variety of sources on the risks associated with catheter ablation of AF.

TABLE 33-3

COMPLICATIONS ASSOCIATED WITH CATHETER ABLATION OF THE ATRIOVENTRICULAR JUNCTION

Complications	MERFS[2] (N = 900)	NASPE 1995[1] (N = 2084)	NASPE 1998[3] (N = 646)	Calkins et al[4] (N = 121)
Tamponade	1 (0.11%)	2 (0.1%)	0 (0%)	+
Venous thrombosis	9 (1.00%)	0 (0%)	0 (0%)	+
Pulmonary emboli	2 (0.22%)	0 (0%)	0 (0%)	1 (0.82%)
Significant TR	1 (0.11%)	0 (0%)	1 (0.15%)	+
Bleeding at puncture site, vascular injury	0 (0%)	0 (0%)	2 (0.30%)	+
CVA/TIA	0 (0%)	2* (0.1%)	0 (0%)	1 (0.82%)*
Myocardial infarction	0 (0%)	1 (0.05%)	0 (0%)	0 (0%)
Sudden death, polymorphic VT	1 (0.11%)	3 (0.15%)	1† (0.15%)	2 (1.65%)
Death (total)	1 (0.11%)	4 (0.2%)	1 (0.15%)	2 (1.65%)

* All associated with left-sided approach.
† Death due to pacemaker malfunction.
+, Complications were presented for all arrhythmias and were not all categorized based on the target arrhythmia; AV, atrioventricular; CVA/TIA cerebrovascular accident/transient ischemic event; TR tricuspid regurgitation, VT ventricular tachycardia.

TABLE 33-4

COMPLICATIONS ASSOCIATED WITH RADIOFREQUENCY ABLATION OF VENTRICULAR TACHYCARDIA

Complications	MERFS[2] (N = 320)	NASPE 1995[1] (N = 844)	NASPE 1998[3] (N = 201)	Calkins et al[5] (N = 146)	Stevenson et al[8] (N = 231)
Complete AV block	1 (0.31%)	1 (0.12%)	+	2 (1.4%)	
Valve damage	+	+	+	1 (0.7%)	1 (0.4%)
Peripheral embolism	2 (0.63%)	3 (0.36%)	+	+	
Tamponade	1 (0.31%)	6 (0.71%)	2 (1.0%)	4 (2.7%)	1 (0.4%)
Arterial thrombosis	1 (0.31%)	1 (0.12%)	+	+	0
CVA/TIA	4 (1.26%)	+	+	4 (2.7%)	0
Pulmonary embolism	2 (0.63%)	+	+	+	
Bleeding at puncture site, vascular injury	2 (0.63%)	+	+	1 (0.7%)	11 (5%)
Death	1 (0.31%)	0 (0%)	3† (1.5%)	4 (2.7%)*	7 (3%)

* One from left main occlusion, one from tamponade, one from CVA and cerebral herniation, one from aortic valve perforation.
† During the follow-up.
+, Data not provided, AV, atrioventricular; CVA/TIA cerebrovascular accident/transient ischemic event.

Types and Classification of Complications

There are a large number of potential complications, which may occur during or after a catheter ablation procedure. Major complications are generally defined as those that result in permanent injury or death, require an intervention for treatment, or prolong the duration of hospitalization. All other complications are generally referred to as minor complications.

The complications that occur during RF catheter ablation procedures can result from any aspect of the procedure, including (1) placement of a peripheral intravenous catheter, (2) conscious sedation or anesthesia, (3) radiation exposure resulting from fluoroscopy, (4) obtaining vascular access, (5) intravascular and intracardiac catheter manipulation, (6) cardioversion, and (7) delivery of RF energy. Intravascular and intracardiac catheter manipulation can lead to several possible complications, including cardiac tamponade, vessel perforation, aortic dissection, traumatic valve damage, coronary artery dissection, and thromboembolism. It is also possible to inadvertently enter into a hepatic vein and cause traumatic damage to the liver. Complications that may be directly associated with delivery of RF energy include inadvertent AV block, coronary artery spasm or occlusion, thromboembolism, development of an atrial esophageal fistula, pulmonary vein stenosis, phrenic nerve paralysis, and myocardial perforation. It is notable that many of the complications that occur during catheter ablation procedures are not directly attributable to the delivery of RF energy.

Thromboembolism and Catheter Ablation

Other than death, perhaps one of the most feared complications that may result from catheter ablation procedures is stroke. Recent studies that have evaluated thrombin-antithrombin III and D-dimer levels before and during electrophysiology testing and catheter ablation have provided evidence that sheath placement and placement of catheters results in a prothrombotic state.[11] Despite this, the risk for stroke associated with catheter ablation procedures for most arrhythmias has been small. Perhaps the most notable exception is catheter ablation of AF, which is associated with a 0.5% to 1% risk for a stroke or transient ischemic attack (TIA). We discuss the stroke risks associated with catheter ablation of AF later.

The 1995 NASPE survey reported 8 cerebrovascular accidents among the 5427 patients (0.15%) who underwent catheter ablation of accessory pathways, 2 cerebrovascular accidents among the 2084 patients (0.10%) who underwent catheter ablation of the AV junction (both used a left-sided approach), no cerebrovascular accidents among the 5423 patients who underwent ablation of AVNRT, and 3 systemic emboli among the 844 patients (0.36%) who underwent catheter ablation of nonidiopathic VT.[1] In MERFS, Hindricks reported thromboembolic complications in 33 of 4398 patients (0.8%), including cerebral embolism (0.4%), pulmonary embolism (0.2%), arterial thrombosis (0.5%), and peripheral arterial embolism (0.06%).[2,11] A more recent registry has reported a lower incidence of thromboembolic complications, with only 1 cerebrovascular accident among the 3357 ablation procedures, which were reported in the 1998 NASPE survey.[3] In the 2002 Spanish Registry on Catheter Ablation, Álvarez Lopez and associates reported one case of pulmonary embolism (0.07%) resulting in one death out of 4755 patients.[5] This lower incidence of thromboembolic complications may represent, at least in part, the greater use of closed loop temperature control, which has been shown to decrease the incidence of coagulum formation from 2.2% with power control alone to 0.8% of RF applications with temperature control ($P < .01$).[12] However, systemic embolism can occur without temperature rise or coagulum formation.[13] A recently published meta-analysis reported no strokes or TIAs among 673 patients who underwent catheter ablation of atrial flutter, no strokes or TIAs among 992 patients who underwent catheter ablation of AVNRT, and two strokes and three TIAs among 2267 patients who underwent catheter ablation of an accessory pathway (0.3%).[14]

Catheter ablation of AF is associated with a significantly higher risk for a thromboembolic complication compared with catheter ablation of most other types of cardiac arrhythmias. An international survey of AF ablation procedures reported a 0.94% incidence of stroke or TIA.[15] A more recent single-center experience from our institution reported a similar risk for stroke or TIA of 1.1%.[16] A recent large meta-analysis of AF ablation studies reported an incidence of stroke of 0.3% and an incidence of a TIA of 0.2%.[14] Based on the results of these studies and on our clinical experience with AF ablation, we estimate that the current incidence of a stroke and/or TIA is about 0.5% to 1%. This incidence of stroke occurs despite adherence to the strict guidelines for anticoagulation of patients before, during, and after catheter ablation of AF.

Radiation Exposure

Although electrophysiologists are aware of the acute risks associated with catheter ablation procedures, the long-term risks that result from radiation exposure received by patients and electrophysiologists are less well recognized. There have been several case reports of serious radiation-induced skin injuries during fluoroscopy-guided interventional procedures (Fig. 33-1).[17] Because radiation can be neither felt nor seen and its detrimental effects may not appear until

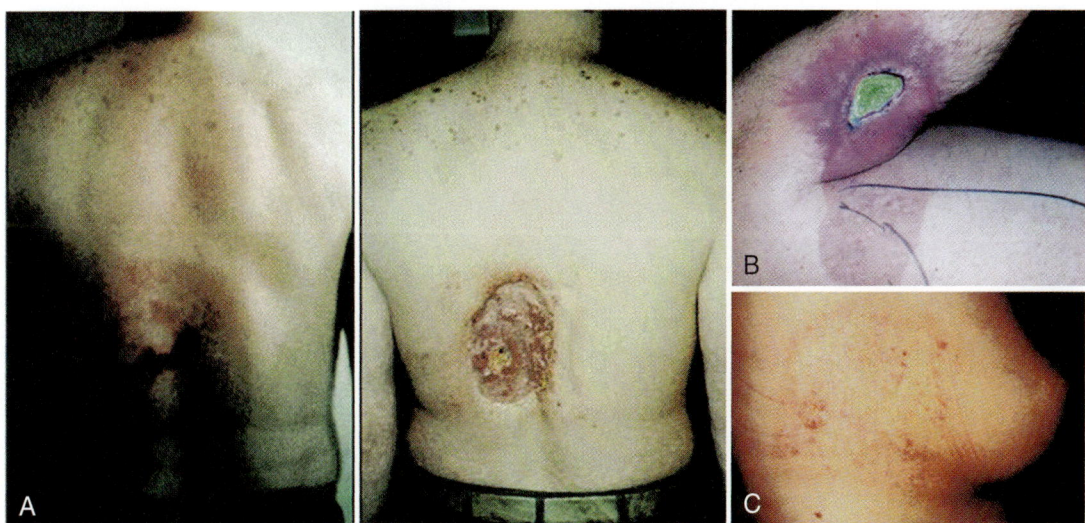

FIGURE 33-1. Radiation injuries following multiple coronary angioplasties (**A**) and radiofrequency ablation for supraventricular arrhythmia in two patients (**B** and **C**). The patient in **C** was a 17-year-old girl with total fluoroscopy time of 100 minutes. She had pain and atrophic skin changes even 2 years after the procedure. (*From Hirshfeld JW, Balter S, Lindsay BD, et al. ACCF/AHA/HRS/SCAI clinical competence statement on physician knowledge to optimize patient safety and image quality in fluoroscopically guided invasive cardiovascular procedures.* J Am Coll Cardiol. *2004;11:2259-2282. With permission.*)

decades later, these hidden risks of catheter ablation are easily ignored. As the number, complexity, and duration of catheter ablation procedures increase, the radiation-related risks of these procedures increase in importance.

Several studies have evaluated fluoroscopy time during catheter ablation procedures. Calkins and associates reported a fluoroscopy time of 44 ± 40 minutes during catheter ablation of accessory pathways; Lindsay and colleagues reported a fluoroscopy time of 50 ± 31 minutes during catheter ablation of AVNRT or accessory pathways; Park and coworkers reported a fluoroscopy time of 47 ± 31 minutes during catheter ablation of a wide variety of ablation targets; Macle and colleagues reported a fluoroscopy time of 57 ± 30 minutes for paroxysmal AF, 20 ± 10 minutes for common atrial flutter, and 22 ± 21 minutes for accessory pathways.[18–21]

Fluoroscopy uses x-radiation generated with kilovoltages typically between 65 and 100 kVp to image the heart and guide catheter placement (Table 33-5). These x-rays have low penetrating power, resulting in delivery of the maximal dose of radiation at the skin surface. To date, a number of studies have evaluated the radiation exposure received by patients during catheter ablation procedures. Despite differences in the techniques used to estimate patient radiation exposure, the radiation exposure estimates in these studies are remarkably consistent.[18–22] In the study by Calkins and colleagues, the site receiving the largest amount of radiation was the ninth thoracic vertebral body posteriorly, with a median exposure of 7.26 rem.[18] The mean entrance radiation dose received by the skin on the back in another trial was 1.3 ± 1.3 Sv. The threshold dose of radiation needed to cause the earliest sign of radiation injury (2 Sv) was exceeded in 19% of patients.[22] The absence of any clinical reports of skin erythema by patients in these studies may reflect a lack of awareness of this complication and the absence of formal follow-up to ascertain the effects of radiation, which may not appear for 2 to 3 weeks,[23] or the fact that the estimates of radiation exposure in these studies represent an upper limit of radiation dose. Children receive less radiation exposure than adults, women receive less radiation exposure than men, patients undergoing successful ablation procedures receive less radiation exposure than

TABLE 33-5

ESTIMATED RADIATION EXPOSURES BY DIFFERENT MEASUREMENTS

Quantity	Units of Measurement	What It Is	What It Measures	Why It's Useful	Conversion between Old and New Units
Absorbed dose	Gray (Gy) or milligray (mGy) [rad or millirad (mrad)]	The amount of energy locally deposited in tissue per unit mass of tissue	Measures concentration of energy deposition in tissue	Assesses the potential biologic risk to that specific tissue	1 rad = 10 mGy
Effective dose	Sievert (Sv) or millisievert (mSv) [rem or millirem (mrem)]	An attributed whole-body dose that produces the same whole-person stochastic risk as an absorbed dose to a limited portion of the body	Converts any localized absorbed or equivalent dose to a whole-body risk factor	Permits comparison of risks among several exposed individuals, even though the doses might be delivered to different sets of organs in these individuals	1 rem = 10 mSv
Air kerma*	Gray (Gy) or milligray (mGy) [rad or millirad (mrad)]	The sum of initial kinetic energies of all charged particles liberated by the radiographs per mass of air	Measures amount of radiation at a point in space	Assesses the level of hazard at the specific location†	1 rad = 10 mGy
Exposure	Millicoulomb·kg⁻¹ [roentgen (R) or milliroentgen (mR)]	The total charge of ions of one sign produced by the radiation per unit mass of air	Measures amount of radiation at a point in space	Assesses the level of hazard at the specified location†	1 millicoulomb·kg⁻¹ 4 Roentgen (R)
Equivalent dose‡	Sievert (Sv) or millisievert (mSv) [rem or millirem (mrem)]	A dose quantity that factors in the relative biologic damage caused by different types of radiation	Provides a relative dose that accounts for increased biologic damage from some types of radiation	This is the most common unit used to measure radiation risk to specific tissues for radiation protection of personnel‡	1 rem = 10 mSv

* Air kerma can be presented in two separate ways. Incident air kerma is the kerma to air from an incident x-ray beam measured on the central beam axis at the position of the patient and excludes backscattered radiation. Entrance surface air kerma is the kerma to air from an incident x-ray beam measured on the central beam axis at the position of the patient with backscattered radiation included. The two may differ from each other by up to about 40%.
† Exposure and air kerma are both used for the same purpose. Exposure used to be the most common measure, but with the switch to international units, air kerma is the preferred unit.
‡ For x-rays, gamma rays, and electrons, there is no difference between absorbed dose and equivalent dose, i.e., 1 mGy = 1 mSv. This is not the case for neutrons and α-particles, but these radiation types are not relevant to x-ray exposure. The important issue is that cardiologists recognize that for their interests there is no practical difference between a measurement of mGy and that of mSv.
From Hirshfeld JW, Balter S, Lindsay BD, et al. ACCF/AHA/HRS/SCAI clinical competence statement on physician knowledge to optimize patient safety and image quality in fluoroscopically guided invasive cardiovascular procedures. *J Am Coll Cardiol*. 2004;11:2259-2282.

those in whom catheter ablation failed, and patients undergoing ablation of accessory pathways receive more radiation than those undergoing ablation of AVNRT or the AV junction.[22] The mean peak skin dose received by patients undergoing AF ablation was more than threefold greater than that received by patients undergoing catheter ablation of atrial flutter and AVNRT.[24] The amount of radiation received by patients during RF catheter ablation is greater than has been previously reported during diagnostic catheterization procedures but similar to prior reports of radiation exposure during percutaneous transluminal coronary angioplasty procedures.

The risk for a fatal malignancy resulting from the radiation received during catheter ablation procedures has been estimated to be about 1 per 1000 patients per hour of fluoroscopy.[18,22] The significance of this risk must be considered in terms of the baseline 20% lifetime risk for a fatal malignancy in the general population. Because the risk for a fatal malignancy resulting from radiation exposure is age dependent, being greater in children than adults, the risk for a fatal malignancy in a child younger than 14 years of age would be about twice than of a 35-year-old patient. The risk for a genetic disorder resulting from 1 hour of fluoroscopy was estimated to be 5 per 1 million births for men and 20 per 1 million live births for women.[18] The risk for cancer development must be considered whenever radiation is applied. This is of particular concern following procedures, such as catheter ablation of AF, that require prolonged fluoroscopy times. Organs contributing most to the total risk were the lungs, stomach, and active bone marrow, as well as breast tissue in females. Despite the prolonged fluoroscopy durations, the risk for fatal malignancy resulting from catheter ablation of AF and by extrapolation of all other catheter ablation is low.

Another risk of catheter ablation procedures is the risk for radiation exposure to the operator. The amount of radiation received by the catheter operators during RF catheter ablation procedures is small and well below the occupational radiation exposure limits, which have been established by the National Council of Radiation Protection (NCRP).[18,25] The dose limit for whole-body irradiation is based on the tolerable risk to an individual of suffering stochastic effects. Dose limits for extremities and for the lens of the eye are based on the dose thresholds at which deterministic effects occur after prolonged exposure. Of particular concern is radiation exposure to the lens of the eye. Several cases of ophthalmologically confirmed lens injuries caused by occupational exposure to radiation during interventional radiologic procedures have been reported. The doses to the eye range from 450 to 900 mSv per year, which exceeds the threshold for lens opacities.[26] The mean equivalent doses to the cardiologists' left hand and forehead were 0.24 mSv and 0.05 mSv, respectively, per RF ablation procedure. The effective dose to the cardiologists was less than 0.15 mSv per month.[27]

Because of long fluoroscopy times, radiation exposure is a major concern during catheter ablation of AF. Lickfett and colleagues recently compared fluoroscopy times and radiation exposure during catheter ablation of AF, atrial flutter, and AVNRT.[24] The study included 15 patients with AF and 5 patients each with atrial flutter and AVNRT who underwent fluoroscopy-guided procedures on a biplane

x-ray system operated at a low frame pulsed fluoroscopy (7.5 fps). Radiation exposure was measured directly with 50 to 60 thermoluminescent dosimeters (TLDs). The position of TLDs within the radiation field was verified by the exposure of direct film. Peak skin doses, effective radiation doses, and risk for fatal malignancies were all computed. Mean fluoroscopy durations for AF procedures were 67.8 ± 21 minutes in the right anterior oblique (RAO) projection and 61.9 ± 16.6 minutes in the left anterior oblique (LAO) projection, significantly different from those required for atrial flutter and AVNRT. The mean peak skin doses measured with the TLDs were 1.0 ± 0.5 Gy in RAO and 1.5 ± 0.4 Gy in LAO projection. The lifetime risk for excess fatal malignancies normalized to 60 minutes of fluoroscopy was 0.07% for female patients and 0.1% for male patients. The relatively small amounts of patients' radiation exposure in this study, despite the prolonged fluoroscopy durations, can be attributed in large measure to the use of very low frame pulsed fluoroscopy, the avoidance of magnification, and optimal adjustments of the fluoroscopy exposure rates. The resulting lifetime risk for fatal malignancy is within the range previously reported for standard supraventricular arrhythmia types.

Complications Associated with Catheter Ablation of Supraventricular Arrhythmias

Accessory Pathways

The efficacy of catheter ablation of accessory pathways (APs) is between 91% and 95%.[1-3,6,14] Complications associated with catheter ablation of accessory pathways include complete AV block, coronary artery injury, valvular perforation or damage, pericardial effusion, cardiac tamponade, hematoma formation, cerebrovascular accident (CVA) or TIA, venous thrombosis, and death.

Table 33-1 summarizes the type and incidence of major complications during catheter ablation of accessory pathways. The procedure-related mortality rate has ranged from 0% to 0.2%. The MERFS reported data from 2222 patients who underwent catheter ablation of an accessory pathway.[2] The overall complication rate was 4.4%, including three deaths (0.13%). In the 1995 NASPE survey, out of the 5427 patients who underwent catheter ablations of an accessory pathway, a total of 99 (1.82%) had significant complications, including four procedure-related deaths (0.08%).[1] The 1998 NASPE registry included 654 patients with accessory pathways.[3] There were no procedure-related deaths. Calkins and coworkers reported the only data available from a multicenter clinical trial.[6] In this study, the results of catheter ablation in 1050 patients who underwent catheter ablation of an accessory pathway, AVNRT, and the AV junction were reported. Among the 500 patients undergoing ablation of an accessory pathway in this series, there was one death (0.2%). This patient died of a dissected left main coronary artery during an attempt at catheter ablation of a left free wall accessory pathway. In the 2001 Spanish Registry, 1084 patients underwent catheter ablation of accessory pathways. The procedure had a success rate of 93%. Major complications occurred in 17 patients (1.6%), the most frequent being vascular arterial complications (*n* = 9). There were no deaths.[4] In the 2002 Spanish Registry, 1416 procedures of catheter ablation were performed in 1350 patients. Major complications occurred in 12 patients (0.9%).[5] A recently published meta-analysis reported that among 2267 patients who underwent ablation of an accessory pathway, there were two deaths (0.1%), two strokes, and three TIAs; 8 patients with cardiac tamponade ((0.4%); and 16 patients with heart block (0.8%), among whom 3 required a pacemaker.[14]

The two most common types of major complications, which have been reported during catheter ablation of accessory pathways, are inadvertent complete AV block and cardiac tamponade. The incidence of inadvertent complete AV block ranges from 0.17% to 1.0 %.[1-3,6] Most instances of complete AV block occur in the setting of the ablation of septal and posteroseptal accessory pathways. Cryoablation may be associated with a lower risk for inadvertent AV block. The frequency of cardiac tamponade as a result of the ablation of accessory pathways varies between 0.13% and 1.1%.[1-3,6,14]

Atrioventricular Nodal Reentrant Tachycardia

Catheter ablation of AVNRT is performed by targeting the slow pathway.[28-30] Catheter ablation of AVNRT is effective in about 95% of patients.[1-3,6,14,28,30] The incidence of AV block is 1% or less.

Complications associated with catheter ablation of AVNRT include complete AV block, pneumothorax, tamponade, pulmonary emboli, CVA/TIA, and significant bleeding and vessel injury. There were no reported deaths from the ablation of AVNRT in MERFS, the 1995 NASPE survey, the 1998 NASPE registry, the study by Calkins, or the recent meta-analysis by Spector.[1-3,6,14]

Table 33-2 details the complications associated with catheter ablation of AVNRT. The most common type of major complication is inadvertent complete AV block. In the 1995 NASPE survey,[1] 6 of 5423 patients (0.11%) who underwent catheter ablation for AVNRT developed complete AV block. On the other hand, 41 of 815 patients (5.07%) in MERFS[2] developed complete heart block. The difference in the results between the two retrospective surveys was attributed to a higher incidence of complete AV block with the anterior approach (6.2%) than with the posterior approach (2.0%). In the 1998 NASPE registry,[3] 9 of 1197 patients (0.74%) who underwent ablation for AVNRT developed complete heart block. In the study by Calkins and coworkers,[6] complete AV block occurred in 5 of 373 patients (1.3%) who had the catheter ablation procedure for AVNRT. Delise and colleagues have compiled the results of a 10-year multicenter study on the risks of intraprocedural atrioventricular block. From February 1990 to December 2000, 510 patients were enrolled for AVNRT.[31] Intraprocedural second- and third-degree AV block occurred in 20 patients. The block was transient in 14 patients. Four patients had second-degree AV block, and 10 patients had third-degree AV block. Persistent second- and third-degree AV block occurred in 6 patients. Two patients had second-degree AV block, and 4 had

third-degree AV block. Transient late AV block occurred in 1 patient. One patient with transient intraprocedural third-degree AV block developed a persistent late third-degree AV block 2 days after the procedure. Another patient who had transient acute third-degree AV block developed a persistent late second-degree AV block. Chronic second- or third-degree AV block occurred in 7 of the patients. A pacemaker was implanted for permanent third-degree AV block in 5 patients. Two of the patients with second-degree AV block did not require a pacemaker because they had a good heart rate at rest and during effort. A recently published meta-analysis reported that among 4748 patients who underwent ablation of AVNRT, there were no deaths, no strokes or TIAs, two patients with cardiac tamponade, and 78 patients with heart block (1.7%) among whom 34 (0.7%) required a pacemaker.[14]

A number of techniques have been described to reduce the likelihood of developing inadvertent AV block. Several authors have reported the likelihood of developing AV block increases as the ablation catheter nears the His bundle. However, AV block has been reported even when RF energy is delivered at the level of the coronary sinus ostium. It is critical that AV conduction be continuously monitored during an application of RF energy. If AV block occurs, the application should be terminated immediately. If a junctional rhythm develops during an application of RF energy, as is often the case, ventriculoatrial (VA) conduction can be monitored. The development of VA block in association with a junctional rhythm is an indication of damage to the fast pathway and should prompt immediate termination of the application. We have employed an even more conservative approach, discontinuing RF energy delivery when a junctional rhythm is observed. Once AV conduction is confirmed, RF energy is reapplied to the same site. Using this method, longer and longer applications of RF energy are delivered until eventually no junctional rhythm is observed. With this technique, no patients have developed AV block during catheter ablation of AVNRT.

Cryoablation been reported to reduce the risk for AV block during catheter ablation of AVNRT. This potential for greater safety has to be balanced against longer procedure times, a somewhat lower acute success rate, and a higher recurrence rate. Most experienced electrophysiology laboratories continue to use RF energy as the preferred energy source for catheter ablation of AVNRT.[32-34]

Atrioventricular Junction

Catheter ablation of the AV junction is generally reserved for atrial arrhythmias that cannot be controlled with pharmacologic therapy and that result in a rapid ventricular response. The procedure is performed by positioning a steerable ablation catheter across the tricuspid annulus to record the largest His bundle electrogram associated with the largest atrial electrogram. A second electrode catheter is placed at the apex of the right ventricle for temporary pacing. Once an appropriate target site is identified, RF energy is delivered for 30 to 60 seconds. If unsuccessful, a left-sided approach can be used.[35] The efficacy of catheter ablation of the AV junction approaches 100%.[6,35-37] After catheter ablation of the AV junction, a permanent rate responsive pacemaker is inserted.

Complications associated with catheter ablation of the AV junction include pneumothorax, tamponade, arterial or venous thrombosis (or both), and sudden death. Sudden cardiac death, occurring early or late after catheter ablation of the AV junction, is by far the most feared complication of this procedure. The MERFS reported data from 900 patients who underwent catheter ablation of the AV junction.[2] The overall complication rate was 3.2%, including one sudden death 7 days after catheter ablation (0.11%). In the 1995 NASPE survey, out of the 2084 patients who had catheter ablations for AV junction, 3 patients (0.15%) developed polymorphic ventricular tachycardia or a cardiac arrest following the catheter ablation procedure.[1] The 1998 NASPE registry included 646 patients with AV junction ablation. There was one sudden death (0.15%) that resulted from pacemaker malfunction 3 hours after the procedure.[3] In a prospective multicenter trial by Calkins and colleagues, 2 of the 121 patients (1.65%) undergoing AV junction ablation and pacemaker implantation died suddenly within 30 days of the ablation procedure.[4] Table 33-3 summarized and categorized the rates of complications associated with catheter ablation of the AV junction. Recent studies have demonstrated that the risk for sudden death following catheter ablation of the AV junction can be reduced by an increased rate of ventricular pacing. Geelen and colleagues reported a 6% incidence of ventricular fibrillation or sudden death within 1 month after RF ablation of the AV junction when pacing rates were set to 60 beats/minute for the first 1 to 3 months after the procedure, compared with no incidence of sudden cardiac death, when pacing rates were programmed to 90 beats/minute for the first 1 to 3 months after the procedure, with subsequent reductions of the pacing rate to 70 beats/minute.[38] Based on the results of these and other studies, a general consensus exists that patients who undergo ablation of the AV junction should be paced at 90 beats/minute for at least 1 month after the catheter ablation procedure.

Inappropriate Sinus Tachycardia

The clinical presentation for patients with inappropriate sinus tachycardia is an elevated resting heart rate (>100 beats/minute) or an exaggerated increase in heart rate in response to exercise in the absence of identifiable causes for sinus tachycardia, or both. Man and associates studied 29 consecutive drug-refractory patients who underwent catheter ablation of inappropriate sinus tachycardia and reported an acute success rate of 76%.[39] There were two complications (7%) noted. One patient had a near syncope with sinus pauses up to 4 seconds in duration, and another patient developed right hemidiaphragm paralysis after catheter ablation. In the 1998 NASPE registry, there were a total of 40 patients who underwent catheter ablation of inappropriate sinus tachycardia. The acute success rate was 71.4%. There were two complications (5%).[3] The first was inadvertent complete heart block, and the second was damage to a previously implanted pacemaker. More recently, Marrouche and colleagues studied the usefulness of three-dimensional nonfluoroscopic mapping of inappropriate sinus tachycardia in 39 patients with debilitating inappropriate sinus tachycardia.[40] The sinus node was successfully modified in all patients (100%). The heart rate dropped from a mean of 99 ± 14 beats/minute to 72 ± 8 beats/minute. Twenty-one percent of the patients experienced recurrence of inappropriate sinus tachycardia and were successfully reablated. No complications occurred. Anecdotally, superior vena cava stenosis has been observed after sinus node modification (editor's note).

Atrial Flutter

Atrial flutter can be categorized as (1) isthmus dependent, (2) non–isthmus dependent, or (3) atypical.[41-43] Isthmus-dependent and non–isthmus-dependent atrial flutter can be cured with catheter ablation. In isthmus-dependent flutter, the lesions are placed in one or more lines across the isthmus from tricuspid annulus to the inferior vena cava.[47] In non–isthmus-dependent flutter, the slow conduction zone is identified with entrainment mapping and subsequently ablated.

Catheter ablation of typical atrial flutter is performed using a deflectable ablation catheter positioned in the inferior right atrium, usually through the right femoral vein. The end point for this procedure is demonstration of bidirectional conduction block through the isthmus after the procedure.[44,45] Use of this strategy has led to an acute success rate of 100% and a recurrence rate of about 7% in three published series.[44-46] At the present time, almost all flutter ablation procedures are performed either with ablation catheters with irrigated-tip technology or with high-power RF generators coupled with 8- to 10-mm-tip ablation electrodes.[47,48]

The complications associated with catheter ablation of atrial flutter, including complete AV block, tamponade, bleeding or hematoma, and hemopneumothorax, are similar to those associated with other catheter ablation procedures. Catheter ablation of atrial flutter is notable, however, because of infrequency with which complications occur. There have been no deaths reported during catheter ablation of atrial flutter.[1,3,9,10,14] The 1995 NASPE survey reported that among 570 patients undergoing atrial flutter ablation, the overall complication rate was 0.4%. Complete heart block occurred in 1 patient. The 1998 NASPE registry included 477 patients who underwent atrial flutter ablation. One patient developed tamponade (0.21%), 1 patient developed a hemopneumothorax (0.21%), 2 patients developed complete AV block (0.42%), and 3 patients developed bleeding or a hematoma, or both, at the site of vascular access (0.63%). There were no deaths. MERFS did not specifically examine the frequency with which complications developed during catheter ablation of atrial flutter.[2]

A meta-analysis including 10,719 patients in 158 studies of outcomes after atrial flutter ablation reported a 2.6% incidence of complications.[47] One third of all complications were vascular, 16% of complications were AV block, and 10% of complications involved pericardial effusion.

There are also two multicenter studies discussing the safety and efficacy of catheter ablation of atrial flutter. Feld and colleagues noted a complication rate of 3.6% in 169 patients.[9] They noted six major adverse events, including pulmonary embolism (*n* = 1), bilateral lower extremity ischemia due to systemic thromboembolism (*n* = 1), deep venous thrombosis (*n* = 1), right groin hematoma (*n* = 1), cerebral embolus with resolution of neurologic findings (*n* = 1), cerebral infarct (thrombotic) 5 days after the procedure with persistent mild aphasia ($n = 1$), and a fractured femur ($n = 1$). The fractured femur was accidental and unrelated to the procedure itself. The cerebral embolus and cerebral infarct were associated with a left atrial ablation procedure and intracranial occlusion of right and left middle cerebral arteries, respectively. Calkins and coworkers had a complication rate of 2.7%.[10] They noted four significant device or procedure related complications within 1 week of the procedure in 4 of 150 ablated patients. They were a small pericardial effusion ($n = 1$), ongoing right-sided pleural effusion that was present at baseline ($n = 1$), ventricular fibrillation during RF energy delivery ($n = 1$), and a large groin hematoma. In addition to these four significant complications, three patients developed second-degree skin burns occurring at the edge of the dispersive pad. This was subsequently remedied in the next 105 patients through the use of a dual dispersive pad system. In addition to this registry and multicenter information, there is a recent meta-analysis of previously published studies of catheter ablation of atrial flutter.[14] Among 671 patients, there were no deaths, strokes, TIAs, or cases of cardiac tamponade. AV block occurred in three patients (0.4%).

Atrial Tachycardia

In the 1998 NASPE registry, catheter ablation of ectopic atrial tachycardia was performed in 216 patients. An overall success rate of 73.0% was achieved.[3] Complications included cardiac tamponade in 2 patients, damage to the pacemaker lead in 1 patient, transient AV block in 1 patient, aspiration pneumonia in 1 patient, and right atrial to aortic fistula in 1 patient. In the 2001 Spanish Registry, 137 procedures of catheter ablation for focal atrial tachycardia were performed in 124 patients. An overall success rate of 82% was achieved. Successful results were obtained in 83% of the tachycardias located in the right atrium, compared with 71% of the tachycardias located in the left atrium. No complications were listed.[4]

Atrial Fibrillation

Catheter ablation of AF is a demanding and complex interventional electrophysiologic procedure associated with an important risk for major complications. An international survey of AF ablation procedures reported a 6% incidence of major complication.[15] In this study, the incidence of cardiac tamponade was 1.2 %, stroke or TIA was 0.94%, pulmonary vein stenosis was 1.3%, and death was 0.05%. A more recent single-center experience from our institution reported a major complication rate of 5%, including stroke or TIA (1.1%), cardiac tamponade (1.2%), pulmonary vein stenosis (0.2%), and vascular injury (1.7%).[16] A recent large meta-analysis of AF ablation studies and antiarrhythmic drug studies reported a major complication rate of catheter ablation of 4.9%.[49] Of particular note is a very recent report from the international survey of AF ablation of 162 centers, which reported details on 32 deaths that occurred during or after AF ablation procedures in 32,569 patients (0.1%).[50] Causes of death included tamponade in 8 patients (25% of deaths), stroke in 5 (16%), atrioesophageal fistula in 5 (16%), and

pneumonia in 2 (6%). A variety of miscellaneous causes accounted for each of the remaining deaths. Based on our review and knowledge of the literature, as well as our clinical experience with AF ablation, I would estimate that the current incidence of major complications lies between 2% and 6%. The incidence of cardiac tamponade is 0.5% to 2%, stroke or TIA is 0.5% to 1%, and vascular injury is 0.5% to 2%, and the risk for development of an atrial esophageal fistula or death is less than 0.1%. Another less common complication is phrenic nerve injury resulting in diaphragmatic paralysis. This is a rare complication with conventional RF and irrigated RF ablation catheters when used for wide area circumferential ablation. However, phrenic nerve paralysis may occur with isolation of the superior vena cava, even when high-output pacing is performed from the ablation catheter to locate the phrenic nerve. The problem of phrenic nerve paralysis appears to be greatest during ablation of the right superior pulmonary vein with a cryoballoon catheter. Great caution must be used in this situation. The section that follows provides more detail about phrenic nerve injury and some of the other rare but serious complications associated with AF ablation.

The development of an atrial esophageal fistula is one of the most serious complications of AF ablation. Although its precise incidence is unknown, it has been estimated to occur after less than 0.1% of AF ablation procedures. Early diagnosis of an atrial esophageal fistula is difficult because it typically presents 2 to 4 weeks after the ablation procedure. The most common symptoms are fever, chills, chest pain, and recurrent neurologic events. More dramatic presentations are septic shock and death. If suspected, the best diagnostic modalities are computed tomography and magnetic resonance imaging of the esophagus. Although a barium swallow may detect a fistula, its sensitivity is low. Endoscopy is a diagnostic modality that should be avoided because insufflation of the esophagus with air has resulted in a devastating massive CVA and death resulting from a large air embolus. It must be recognized that most patients who have developed an atrial esophageal fistula have died, and the survivors are often left with disability from cerebrovascular events. Nevertheless, early diagnosis is important because there have been a number of patients with esophageal perforation who have achieved full recovery by urgent surgical intervention. There has been one case report of a favorable outcome after placement of an esophageal stent. Because of the severe consequences of an atrial esophageal fistula, it is vital to avoid this complication. Currently, a number of different approaches are being employed to avoid the development of an atrial esophageal fistula. The most common practice decreases power delivery, limiting energy to 25 to 35 W; decreases tissue contact pressure; and moves the ablation catheter every 10 to 20 seconds when close to the esophagus. It is also now common to place a temperature probe in the esophagus to monitor for esophageal heating. If esophageal heating is seen, RF energy is immediately discontinued. Because of the rarity of this complication, it remains unproved whether these practices lower or eliminate the risk for esophageal perforation. Cryoablation for pulmonary vein isolation may produce esophageal irritation, but ulceration appears to be uncommon.

As noted previously, phrenic nerve injury is a rare but important complication of AF ablation. It results from direct thermal injury, usually to the right phrenic nerve, which is located near the right superior pulmonary vein and the superior vena cava. Less frequently, ablation within the left atrial appendage can result in left phrenic nerve damage. The development of phrenic nerve injury has resulted from AF ablation using RF, cryoablation, ultrasound, and laser ablation. The reported incidence of phrenic nerve injury varies from 0% to 0.48% with RF energy, especially when delivered in the superior vena cava or deep within the right superior pulmonary vein. Despite the rarity of this complication, it is important for those performing AF ablation to be aware of it and know how to avoid it. Right phrenic nerve injury has been seen more frequently with the use of balloon ablation catheters in the right superior pulmonary vein, irrespective of the energy source. Phrenic nerve damage can be asymptomatic or can cause dyspnea, hiccup, atelectasis, pleural effusion, cough, and thoracic pain. When suspected, the diagnosis can be confirmed by fluoroscopy showing unilateral diaphragmatic paralysis. Strategies to prevent phrenic nerve damage include high-output pacing to establish whether the phrenic nerve can be captured from the proposed ablation site before ablation; phrenic nerve mapping by pacing along the superior vena cava to identify the location of the phrenic nerve; ensuring proximal and antral ablation when ablating around the right upper pulmonary vein; and fluoroscopic monitoring of diaphragmatic excursion during ablation, with or without phrenic nerve pacing during energy delivery. Energy delivery should be interrupted immediately when diaphragmatic movement stops. In most reports, phrenic nerve function was recovered between 1 day and more than 12 months. However, there have been some cases of permanent phrenic nerve injury. There is no active treatment known to aid phrenic nerve healing.

Complications Associated with Catheter Ablation of Ventricular Tachycardia

Idiopathic Ventricular Tachycardia

Idiopathic ventricular tachycardia is defined as VT that occurs in patients without structural heart disease, metabolic abnormalities, or the long QT syndrome. In the United States, idiopathic VT typically arises in the right ventricular outflow tract (RVOT). A review of the results of catheter ablation of idiopathic VT arising in the RVOT reported an acute success rate of 93% (range, 85% to 100%) with the mean recurrence rate of 7%.[51,52] Complications included death from a perforated outflow tract in 1 patient (1%) and persistent right bundle branch block in 2 patients (2%). In the 1998 NASPE registry, 82 of 98 patients (85.7%) had successful catheter ablation for RVOT VT. In the 2001 Spanish Registry, 90 of 125 patients (78%) had successful catheter ablation in 30 centers. The RVOT was the most frequent location (76%), followed by fascicular (14%), left ventricular outflow tract (4%), and other locations (6%). Pericardial effusion in

one patient was the only major complication (0.8%).[4] The complications associated with catheter ablation of ventricular tachycardia were not categorized based on the specific type of VT.[3] Table 33-4 summarizes the overall complications that can occur during catheter ablation of all types of VT.

Nonidiopathic Ventricular Tachycardia

To date, there have been two published prospective multicenter clinical trials that have evaluated the safety and efficacy of catheter ablation of nonidiopathic VT.[7,8] Catheter ablation was acutely successful, as defined by elimination of all mappable VTs in 106 of 146 patients (75%) who participated in the first clinical trial. Sixteen patients (10.8%) had a major complication, including death (2.7%), myocardial infarction (0.7%), tamponade (2.7%), complete AV block (1.4%), CVA/TIA (2.7%), and valve injury (0.7%). The more recent clinical trial of RF ablation of VT with an irrigated ablation catheter in 231 patients reported elimination of all inducible VTs in 49% of patients. Fifty-three patients were free of recurrent VT at 6 months' follow-up. The procedure-related mortality rate was 3%, and the 1-year mortality rate was 18%. The major complication rate was 7.3%, including heart failure in 5 patients and 1 patient with mitral valve damage resulting in severe mitral regurgitation. Complications resulting from vascular access occurred in 4.7% of patients. There were no thromboembolic complications of strokes. In addition to these two prospective multicenter clinical trials, data regarding the safety of catheter ablation of VT was also examined in the MERFS and the two NASPE registries. The MERFS and the two NASPE registries did not subdivide patients based on whether they were undergoing catheter ablation of idiopathic versus nonidiopathic VT. In the 1995 NASPE survey, 170 of 257 patients (66%) who underwent catheter ablation for VT associated with coronary artery disease had successful ablation.[1] In the 1998 NASPE registry, acute success of catheter ablation for VT associated with coronary artery disease was achieved in 31 of 53 patients (58.5%).[3] Table 33-4 summarizes the complications associated with catheter ablation of VT. The 2001 Spanish Registry subdivided patients based on whether they had VT associated with postinfarction scar or macro-reentrant VT not associated with postinfarction scar. In VT associated with postinfarction scar, the substrate was treated in 24 centers, in which 125 procedures were performed in 99 patients. The procedure was successful in 70 patients (71%), and complications appeared in 4 patients (4%): two arterial vascular complications, one heart failure, and one death after a procedure.[55] In macro-reentrant VT not associated with postinfarction scar, the substrate was treated only in 16 centers, with 48 procedures performed in 43 patients. Fifteen ventricular tachycardias due to a bundle branch reentry mechanism were treated, 17 patients had dilated idiopathic cardiomyopathy, and 12 patients had an arrhythmogenic right ventricular dysplasia. The procedure was successful in 29 patients (67%). Complications occurred in 2 patients (5%): one arterial vascular complication and one AV block.[4]

Catheter Ablation in Pediatric Patients

The Pediatric Radiofrequency Ablation Registry reported the outcome of catheter ablation in 652 patients.[53] The median age was 13.5 years, with 41% of patients younger than 13 years and 8% of patients younger than 4 years. Major complications occurred in 35 patients (4.8%). Independent risk factors for complications, which were identified by multivariate analysis, included a body weight of less than 15 kg and the number of ablation procedures performed at a medical center. The complication rate among children weighing less than 15 kg was 10%. The results of this study suggest that catheter ablation procedures should be avoided in very small children unless other therapeutic options do not exist. Torres and associates looked at the treatment of supraventricular arrhythmias in 203 patients younger than 18 years.[54] The presence of an accessory pathway caused the tachyarrhythmia in 181 patients (89.1%) with a total of 187 accessory pathways; AV nodal reentry caused the arrhythmia in 18 patients (8.8%) and atrial flutter in only 4 patients (1.9%). They were able to eliminate the accessory pathway in 171 patients (91.4%). A total of 23 patients showed a recurrence of the tachycardia, and there were complications in 4 patients (2.1%). The procedure was successful in the treatment of the AV nodal reentry in the 18 cases, with ablation of the slow pathway in 17 cases and of the fast pathway in only 1 patient; also, 1 patient showed total AV block, and recurrence of the arrhythmia occurred in 3 patients (16.6%). The procedure was successful in the 4 patients with atrial flutter, with one recurrence (25%). All in all, the RF catheter ablation was successful in 193 patients (95%), with recurrence of the arrhythmia in 27 cases (13.3%) and with complications in only 5 patients (2.6%).[54] The results of this study suggest that catheter ablation is a safe and effective procedure for the treatment of supraventricular tachyarrhythmia in children. Celiker and coworkers, in a Turkish study, reported the outcome of catheter ablation in 73 pediatric patients with tachyarrhythmia ranging from 2 to 21 years of age.[55] The median age was 11 years. Procedure-related complications occurred in 8 patients (11%), and the overall final success rate for all the diagnoses was 82% ($n = 60$). These results suggest that radiofrequency catheter ablation has a good success rate and low risk for complication in children.

Conclusion

In conclusion, RF catheter ablation is a highly effective approach to the treatment of cardiac arrhythmias. Success rates of greater than 90% with complication rates of less than 3% should be anticipated for catheter ablation of AVNRT, accessory pathways, atrial flutter, idiopathic ventricular tachycardia, and the atrioventricular junction. For these arrhythmias, the safety and efficacy profile of catheter ablation would suggest that it should be considered first-line therapy and an alternative to pharmacologic therapy. In contrast, the safety and efficacy of RF catheter ablation is considerably lower than 90%, and the incidence of complications is generally greater than

3% during catheter ablation of AF and nonidiopathic VT. This safety and efficacy profile would suggest that the appropriate role of catheter ablation for these arrhythmias is as second-line therapy after attempts at pharmacologic therapy have failed.

References

1. Scheinman MM. NASPE survey on catheter ablation. *Pacing Clin Electrophysiol.* 1995;18:1474–1478.
2. Hindricks G. The Multicentre European Radiofrequency Survey (MERFS): complications of radiofrequency catheter ablation of arrhythmias. The Multicentre European Radiofrequency Survey (MERFS) investigators of the Working Group on Arrhythmias of the European Society of Cardiology [see comments]. *Eur Heart J.* 1993;14:1644–1653.
3. Scheinman MM, Huang S. The 1998 NASPE prospective catheter ablation registry. *Pacing Clin Electrophysiol.* 2000;23:1020–1028.
4. Álvarez Lopez M, Merino JL. Spanish Registry on Catheter Ablation. First official report of the Working Group on Electrophysiology and Arrhythmias of the Spanish Society of Cardiology (2001). *Rev Esp Cardiol.* 2002;55:1273–1285.
5. Álvarez Lopez M, Merino JL. Spanish Registry on Catheter Ablation. Second Official Report of the Working Group on Electrophysiology and Arrhythmias of the Spanish Society of Cardiology (2002). *Rev Esp Cardiol.* 2003;56:1093–1104.
6. Calkins H, Yong P, Miller JM, et al. Catheter ablation of accessory pathways, atrioventricular nodal reentrant tachycardia, and the atrioventricular junction: final results of a prospective, multicenter clinical trial. The Atakr Multicenter Investigators Group. *Circulation.* 1999;99:262–270.
7. Calkins H, Epstein A, Packer D, et al. Catheter ablation of ventricular tachycardia in patients with structural heart disease using cooled radiofrequency energy: results of a prospective multicenter study. Cooled RF Multi Center Investigators Group. *J Am Coll Cardiol.* 2000;35:1905–1914.
8. Stevenson WG, Wilber DJ, Natale A, et al, the Multicenter ThermoCool VT Ablation Trial Investigators. Irrigated radiofrequency catheter ablation guided by electroanatomic mapping for recurrent ventricular tachycardia after myocardial infarction: the multicenter ThermoCool ventricular tachycardia ablation trial. *Circulation.* 2008;118:2773–2782.
9. Feld G, Wharton M, Plumb V, et al, for the EPT-1000 XP Cardiac Ablation System Investigators. Radiofrequency catheter ablation of type 1 atrial flutter using large-tip 8- or 10-mm electrode catheters and a high-output radiofrequency energy generator: results of a multicenter safety and efficacy study. *J Am Coll Cardiol.* 2004;43:1466–1472.
10. Calkins H, Canby R, Weiss R, et al, for the 100W Atakr II Investigator Group. Results of catheter ablation of typical atrial flutter. *Am J Cardiol.* 2004;95:437–442.
11. Lee DS, Dorian P, Downar E, et al. Thrombogenicity of radiofrequency ablation procedures: what factors influence thrombin generation? *Europace.* 2001;3:195–200.
12. Calkins H, Prystowsky E, Carlson M, et al. Temperature monitoring during radiofrequency catheter ablation procedures using closed loop control. Atakr Multicenter Investigators Group. *Circulation.* 1994;90:1279–1286.
13. Epstein MR, Knapp LD, Martindill M, et al. Embolic complications associated with radiofrequency catheter ablation. Atakr Investigator Group. *Am J Cardiol.* 1996;77:655–658.
14. Spector P, Reynolds MR, Calkins H, et al. Meta-analysis of ablation of atrial flutter and supraventricular tachycardia [review]. *Am J Cardiol.* 2009;104:671–677.
15. Cappato R, Calkins H, Chen SA, et al. Worldwide survey on the methods, efficacy, and safety of catheter ablation for human atrial fibrillation. *Circulation.* 2005;111:1100–1105.
16. Spragg D, Dalal D, Cheema A, et al. Complications of catheter ablation for atrial fibrillation: incidence and predictors. *J Cardiovasc Electrophysiol.* 2008;19:627–631.
17. Hirshfeld JW, Balter S, Lindsay BD, et al. ACCF/AHA/HRS/SCAI clinical competence statement on physician knowledge to optimize patient safety and image quality in fluoroscopically guided invasive cardiovascular procedures. *J Am Coll Cardiol.* 2004;11:2259–2282.
18. Calkins H, Niklason L, Sousa J, et al. Radiation exposure during radiofrequency catheter ablation of accessory atrioventricular connections [see comments]. *Circulation.* 1991;84:2376–2382.
19. Lindsay BD, Eichling JO, Ambos HD, Cain ME. Radiation exposure to patients and medical personnel during radiofrequency catheter ablation for supraventricular tachycardia. *Am J Cardiol.* 1992;70:218–223.
20. Park TH, Eichling JO, Schechtman KB, et al. Risk of radiation induced skin injuries from arrhythmia ablation procedures. *Pacing Clin Electrophysiol.* 1996;19:1363–1369.
21. Macle L, Weerasooriya R, Jais P, et al. Radiation exposure during radiofrequency catheter ablation for atrial fibrillation. *Pacing Clin Electrophysiol.* 2003;26:288–291.
22. Rosenthal LS, Mahesh M, Beck TJ, et al. Predictors of fluoroscopy time and estimated radiation exposure during radiofrequency catheter ablation procedures. *Am J Cardiol.* 1998;82:451–458.
23. Wagner LK, Eifel PJ, Geise RA. Potential biological effects following high X-ray dose interventional procedures. *J Vasc Interv Radiol.* 1994;5:71–84.

24. Lickfett L, Mahesh M, Vasamreddy C, et al. Radiation exposure during catheter ablation of atrial fibrillation. *Circulation*. 2004;110:3003–3010.
25. National Council on Radiation Protection and Measurements. *Limitation on exposure to ionizing radiation*. NRCP Report No.116 Bethesda, MD: NCRP; 1993.
26. Vano E, Gonzalez L, Beneytez F, Moreno F. Lens injuries induced by occupational exposure in non-optimized interventional radiology laboratories. *Br J Radiol*. 1998;71:728–733.
27. McFadden SL, Mooney RB, Shepherd PH. X-ray dose and associated risks from radiofrequency catheter ablation procedures. *Br J Radiol*. 2002;75:253–265.
28. Langberg JJ, Leon A, Borganelli M, et al. A randomized, prospective comparison of anterior and posterior approaches to radiofrequency catheter ablation of atrioventricular nodal reentry tachycardia. *Circulation*. 1993;87:1551–1556.
29. Lee MA, Morady F, Kadish A, et al. Catheter modification of the atrioventricular junction with radiofrequency energy for control of atrioventricular nodal reentry tachycardia. *Circulation*. 1991;83:827–835.
30. Kottkamp H, Hindricks G, Willems S, et al. An anatomically and electrogram-guided stepwise approach for effective and safe catheter ablation of the fast pathway for elimination of atrioventricular node reentrant tachycardia [see comments]. *J Am Coll Cardiol*. 1995;25:974–981.
31. Delise P, Sitta N, Zoppo F, et al. Radiofrequency ablation of atrioventricular nodal reentrant tachycardia: the risk of intraprocedural, late and long-term atrioventricular block. The Veneto Region multicenter experience. *Ital Heart J*. 2002;3:715–720.
32. Chan NY, Mok NS, Lau CL, et al. Treatment of atrioventricular nodal reentrant tachycardia by cryoablation with a 6 mm-tip catheter vs. radiofrequency ablation. *Europace*. 2009;11:1065–1070.
33. Rivard L, Dubuc M, Guerra PG, et al. Cryoablation outcomes for AV nodal reentrant tachycardia comparing 4-mm versus 6-mm electrode-tip catheters. *J. Heart Rhythm*. 2008;5:230–234.
34. Sandilands A, Boreham P, Pitts-Cricks J, Cripps T. Impact of cryoablation catheter on success rates in the treatment of atrioventricular nodal re-entry tachycardia in 160 patients with long-term follow-up. *Europace*. 2008;10:683–686.
35. Sousa J, el-Atassi R, Rosenheck S, et al. Radiofrequency catheter ablation of the atrioventricular junction from the left ventricle. *Circulation*. 1991;84:567–571.
36. Morady F, Calkins H, Langberg JJ, et al. A prospective randomized comparison of direct current and radiofrequency ablation of the atrioventricular junction. *J Am Coll Cardiol*. 1993;21:102–109.
37. Trohman RG, Simmons TW, Moore SL, et al. Catheter ablation of the atrioventricular junction using radiofrequency energy and a bilateral cardiac approach. *Am J Cardiol*. 1992;70:1438–1443.
38. Geelen P, Brugada J, Andries E, Brugada P. Ventricular fibrillation and sudden death after radiofrequency catheter ablation of the atrioventricular junction. *Pacing Clin Electrophysiol*. 1997;20:343–348.
39. Man KC, Knight B, Tse HF, et al. Radiofrequency catheter ablation of inappropriate sinus tachycardia guided by activation mapping. *J Am Coll Cardiol*. 2000;35:451–457.
40. Marrouche NF, Beheiry S, Tomassoni G, et al. Three-dimensional nonfluoroscopic mapping and ablation of inappropriate sinus tachycardia. Procedural strategies and long-term outcome. *J Am Coll Cardiol*. 2002;39:1046–1054.
41. Kalman JM, Olgin JE, Saxon LA, et al. Activation and entrainment mapping defines the tricuspid annulus as the anterior barrier in typical atrial flutter [see comments]. *Circulation*. 1996;94:398–406.
42. Nakagawa H, Lazzara R, Khastgir T, et al. Role of the tricuspid annulus and the eustachian valve/ridge on atrial flutter: relevance to catheter ablation of the septal isthmus and a new technique for rapid identification of ablation success [see comments]. *Circulation*. 1996;94:407–424.
43. Poty H, Saoudi N, Abdel Aziz A, et al. Radiofrequency catheter ablation of type 1 atrial flutter: prediction of late success by electrophysiological criteria. *Circulation*. 1995;92:1389–1392.
44. Poty H, Saoudi N, Nair M, et al. Radiofrequency catheter ablation of atrial flutter: further insights into the various types of isthmus block. Application to ablation during sinus rhythm. *Circulation*. 1996;94:3204–3213.
45. Tai CT, Chen SA, Chiang CE, et al. Long-term outcome of radiofrequency catheter ablation for typical atrial flutter: risk prediction of recurrent arrhythmias. *J Cardiovasc Electrophysiol*. 1998;9:115–121.
46. Tai CT, Chen SA, Chiang CE, et al. Electrophysiologic characteristics and radiofrequency catheter ablation in patients with clockwise atrial flutter. *J Cardiovasc Electrophysiol*. 1997;8:24–34.
47. Perez FJ, Schubert CM, Parvez B, et al. Long-term outcomes after catheter ablation of cavo-tricuspid isthmus dependent atrial flutter: a meta-analysis. *Circ Arrhythmia Electrophysiol*. 2009;2:393–401.
48. Wu RC, Berger R, Calkins H. Catheter ablation of atrial flutter and macroreentrant atrial tachycardia. *Curr Opin Cardiol*. 2002;17:58–64.
49. Calkins H, Reynolds MR, Spector P, et al. Treatment of atrial fibrillation with antiarrhythmic drugs or radiofrequency ablation: two systematic literature reviews and metaanalyses. *Circ Arrhythmia Electrophysiol*. 2009;2:349–361.
50. Cappato R, Calkins H, Chen SA, et al. Prevalence and causes of fatal outcome in catheter ablation of atrial fibrillation. *J Am Coll Cardiol*. 2009;53: 1798–1803.
51. Calkins H. Role of invasive EP testing in the evaluation and management of right ventricular outflow tract tachycardias. *Card Electrophysiol Rev*. 2000;4:71–75.
52. Wen MS, Yeh SJ, Wang CC, et al. Radiofrequency ablation therapy in idiopathic left ventricular tachycardia with no obvious structural heart disease. *Circulation*. 1994;89:1690–1696.
53. Kugler JD, Danford DA, Deal BJ, et al. Radiofrequency catheter ablation for tachyarrhythmias in children and adolescents. The Pediatric Electrophysiology Society. *N Engl J Med*. 1994;330:1481–1487.
54. Torres Iturralde P, Garrido Garcia LM, Cordero A, et al. Radiofrequency ablation in the treatment of supraventricular arrhythmias in pediatrics: experience with 203 consecutive patients. *Arch Inst Cardiol Mex*. 1998;68:27–36.
55. Celiker A, Kafali G, Karagoz T, et al. The results of electrophysiological study and radio-frequency catheter ablation in pediatric patients with tachyarrhythmia. *Turk J Pediatr*. 2003;45:209–216.

34
Transseptal Catheterization

Westby G. Fisher and Alexander S. Ro

Key Points

Safe transseptal catheterization requires thorough familiarity with cardiac anatomy and the transseptal apparatus.

Contraindications to transseptal catheterization include left atrial thrombus, severe bleeding diathesis, atrial septal closure devices, significant anatomic abnormalities, and uncooperative patient.

Intracardiac echocardiography minimizes complications and greatly facilitates difficult cases.

The risks for complications are inversely related to operator expertise.

Transseptal catheterization has gained widespread acceptance in the electrophysiology community as a viable approach for ablation of left-sided arrhythmias. With intense interest in pulmonary vein isolation for atrial fibrillation, as well as the ability to map and ablate left focal atrial tachycardias and flutter, this technique is becoming an indispensable skill for the interventional electrophysiologist. First introduced in 1958 by Ross and colleagues[1] and Cope,[2] transseptal catheterization was seen as an alternative method to retrograde transaortic measurement of left-sided pressures. Despite subsequent modifications in the technique by Braunwald,[3] Brockenbrough and associates,[4] and Mullins,[5] its popularity quickly declined because of fear of cardiac perforation and the use of pulmonary artery flotation catheters as a surrogate for left atrial pressures. The advent of percutaneous mitral valve commissurotomy renewed interest in the procedure in the 1980s. However, its use remained restricted to a limited number of interventional cardiologists in high-volume cardiac catheterization laboratories.

With the development of radiofrequency catheter ablation, resurgence of transseptal catheterization developed as an alternative approach to left-sided accessory pathway ablation. Studies comparing transseptal to retrograde approaches for left-sided accessory pathway ablation have suggested at least comparable success and fewer complications with the transseptal approach.[6,7] The transseptal approach to accessory pathway ablation provides a nonobstructive path from the right atrium to the mitral valve annulus and avoids arterial system complications such as femoral arteriovenous fistula, femoral artery pseudoaneurysm, iliac-femoral thrombotic occlusion, papillary muscle disruption, aortic dissection, and aortic valvular perforation.[8]

Transseptal catheterization will continue to play a significant role in the field of electrophysiology. Lack of familiarity with the technique, however, makes performing the procedure a formidable task for many. Ultimately, the most important predictor for the likelihood of a successful procedure is operator experience. This chapter reviews the anatomy of the interatrial septum and vital surrounding structures; the technique of transseptal catheterization, including setup and adjunctive tools that we commonly use in our laboratory; and potential complications and pitfalls that should be avoided.

Anatomy

A thorough understanding of anatomy for both right and left atria and the interatrial septum is vital for a successful and safe transseptal catheterization.[9] The right atrium lies rightward, superior, and anterior to the left atrium. Its free wall has a smooth posterior portion and a muscular anterolateral portion, and its floor is the orifice of the tricuspid valve. In contrast, the left atrium lies leftward, posterior, and inferior to the right atrium at the base of the heart. The interatrial septum lies between the two and is bounded anteriorly by the sinus of Valsalva and posteriorly by pericardium. Access to the left atrium from the right side is obtained through the fossa ovalis by either a needle puncture or a patent foramen ovale (Fig. 34-1). The fossa ovalis lies in the posterior aspect of the intra-atrial septum and is bounded superiorly by the limbus, an arch-shaped outer muscular rim.

The fossa ovalis makes up roughly 25% to 30% of the total septal area and is usually the thinnest portion of the septum. The diameter of the fossa can vary dramatically

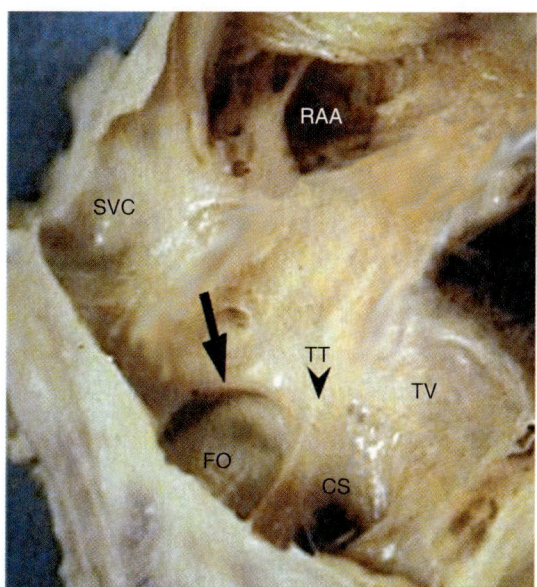

FIGURE 34-1. Right atrial septal anatomy. A postmortem right atrium is opened to expose the septal wall of the right atrium. Note that the right atrial free wall was incised and the superior portion of the atrium lifted superiorly to expose the endocardium of the right atrial appendage (RAA). The posterior aspect of the atrium lies to the left and the anterior aspect of the atrium to the right. Note that the fossa ovalis (FO) occupies a significant portion of the right atrial septum. The superior limbus of the fossa ovalis (*larger arrow*) is clearly demonstrated. CS, coronary sinus os; SVC, superior vena cava; TT, tendon of Todaro; TV, tricuspid valve.

a patent foramen ovale to ensure evacuation of air from the left atrium before terminating cardiopulmonary bypass. Because fluoroscopy allows only indirect assessment of the location of the fossa ovalis without good visual representation of these critical anatomic landmarks, advancement of the transseptal needle using only fluoroscopically guided techniques was associated with unpredictable outcomes. More recently, the introduction of intracardiac echocardiography (ICE) has added greatly to the appreciation of the anatomic variability and location of the fossa ovalis.[11-13] ICE has permitted many more electrophysiologists to gain confidence to perform the procedure, and its use adds valuable early insight to the development of complications such as pericardial tamponade.

Procedural Preparation

Laboratory Facilities and Staff

Although complications are rare, transseptal catheterization must be performed by doctors and laboratory personnel familiar with the administration of conscious sedation and the associated monitoring required, including electrocardiographic, hemodynamic, and pulse oximetry or end-tidal carbon dioxide measurements. Equipment for treatment of cardiovascular emergencies such as pericardial tamponade should also be readily available. With the close attention to administrative cost-saving measures at interventional laboratories, pressure to limit personnel performing this procedure exists. A minimum of three personnel should be present when transseptal catheterization is performed: (1) the physician performing the procedure, (2) the nurse or anesthesiologist, to monitor vital signs and monitor conscious sedation, and (3) a circulator, to bring equipment. Any fewer personnel might delay the rapid response required to manage acute tamponade occurring in the anticoagulated patient after transseptal catheterization. Apparatus for emergent pericardiocentesis should be immediately available.

Protamine Sulfate

Although it happens rarely, the operator must be prepared to deal with acute pericardial tamponade should cardiac perforation occur during the transseptal process. In the setting of significant systemic anticoagulation with heparin, tamponade can develop rapidly, and anticoagulation must be reversed expeditiously. Familiarity with protamine sulfate, an antidote to heparin, must be gained before proceeding with transseptal catheterization.

Protamine sulfate is itself a mild anticoagulant, but when it is given with heparin (which is strongly acidic), a stable, noncoagulating salt is created that inactivates the anticoagulant effect of heparin. On average, 1 mg of protamine will reverse about 90 USP units of heparin derived from beef lung or 115 USP units of heparin derived from porcine intestinal mucosa. Usually, it is advised that no more than 50 mg of protamine be given over 10 minutes. Rapid administration of protamine can result in severe hypotension, anaphylactoid reactions, and respiratory compromise. Medications should be available to deal with this emergency.

from patient to patient. In one series, the fossa diameters ranged from about 10 to 25 mm (average, about 16 mm).[10] The membrane consistency varies as well, usually becoming thicker and more fibrotic with age. From an embryologic standpoint, the interatrial septum arises from the development of two membranes in succession that separate the primitive left and right atria. The septum primum grows ventrally from the dorsal cranial wall, followed by the septum secundum, which grows from the ventral cranial wall. The fossa ovalis is the remnant of the foramen ovale, which acts as the communication between the two atria that allows well-oxygenated blood to move from the inferior vena cava to the left side of the heart during fetal life. In 20% of patients, this opening remains patent, allowing for access to the left heart without the use of a needle puncture.

Most complications that arise from transseptal catheterization occur as a result of inadvertent puncture of adjacent structures to the interatrial septum and fossa ovalis. As stated earlier, the interatrial septum is bounded posteriorly by the pericardium. The aortic root lies superior and anterior to the fossa ovalis, whereas the ostium of the coronary sinus (CS) lies inferior to the fossa ovalis and posterior to the tricuspid valve orifice. In pathologic hearts, there frequently is distortion of the atrial and interatrial septum anatomy, which can significantly alter the proximity of these structures. The septum tends to lie more horizontally in patients with left atrial enlargement, and it can be more vertical in patients with aortic valve disease or a dilated aortic root. Varying degrees of kyphoscoliosis can also alter intrathoracic cardiac rotation. In addition, prior open heart surgery can result in a thickened fossa ovalis because surgeons occasionally must oversew the fossa in patients with

Imaging Equipment

The importance of adequate (and preferably biplane) fluoroscopic equipment cannot be overstated. One must be able to visualize relatively small structures, such as the tip of the transseptal needle within the dilator of a long vascular transseptal sheath in obese patients. The ability to alter the angulation of the acquired fluoroscopic images to the right anterior oblique (RAO) or left anterior oblique (LAO) view should be present because imaging in multiple planes provides added assurance of needle location before the transseptal puncture.

Some centers routinely perform transesophageal echocardiography (TEE) to facilitate transseptal catheterization with real-time echocardiography. TEE has limited utility in facilitating transseptal catheterization because of the difficulty in reliably imaging the fossa ovalis and the transseptal needle.[14] TEE can readily image the fossa ovalis and needle assembly, but it requires a second operator and greater degrees of sedation and is not practical for long procedures. More recently, ICE has been employed to facilitate transseptal catheterization.[11-13] With this technology, a single operator can perform the procedure painlessly and continuously without sedation during invasive left atrial procedures, adding greatly to the safety of transseptal procedures.

A totally venous access approach to transseptal procedures is now commonly used in experienced electrophysiology laboratories.[15] Because electrophysiologic catheters are placed in strategic anatomic locations defined by their recorded electrograms, electrophysiologic recording equipment is required. Alternatively, if the laboratory is more comfortable with an arteriovenous approach—that is, an approach requiring arterial placement of a pigtail catheter—hemodynamic pressure recording equipment (e.g., pressure transducers, pressurized heparinized saline infusions, tubing) is required.

Finally, machines that can perform activated clotting time (ACT) measurements after the transseptal catheterization and heparinization should be readily available and calibrated before the procedure.

Patient Preparation

Patients undergoing transseptal catheterization must tolerate lying flat for the procedure and be psychologically capable of following directions if minimal sedation is used. Blood dyscrasias such as coagulopathies or thrombocytopenia should be evaluated before enlisting the patient for this procedure. Other contraindications to the procedure must also be considered (Table 34-1). Echocardiographic evaluation of the left atrium to exclude pathologic masses or anatomic variants should also be obtained. Preprocedure TEE should be considered in patients who are at high risk for atrial or left ventricular thrombus.

Transseptal Sheaths and Dilators

When assembling the sheaths and needles to perform transseptal catheterization, it is important for the electrophysiologist or interventionalist to be familiar with the relative lengths and diameters of the equipment. Most adult transseptal sheaths are 59 to 63 cm in length with dilators

TABLE 34-1
CONTRAINDICATIONS TO TRANSSEPTAL CATHETERIZATION
Absolute Contraindications
Presence of left atrial thrombus
Severe bleeding diathesis
Presence of significant anatomic anomalies (e.g., severe kyphoscoliosis, pneumonectomy)
Hemodynamically unstable patient
Patient unable to remain still during the procedure or intolerant to sedation
Relative Contraindications
Preexisting percutaneous septal closure devices implanted
Prior interatrial septal surgery

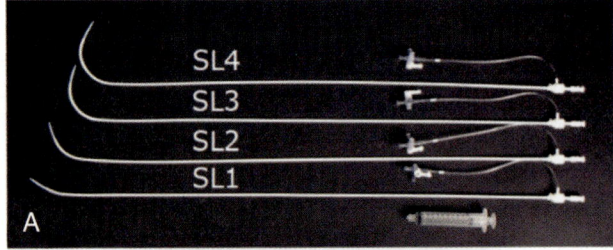
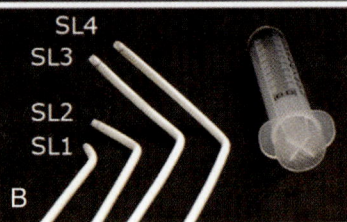

FIGURE 34-2. Transseptal sheath designs—compound curvatures. Multiple transseptal sheaths have been developed to provide improved catheter delivery in various portions of the left atrium. Longer distal curvatures are typically best for more inferoposterior aspects of the left atrium, whereas shorter curvatures reach the upper left atrium more efficiently. St. Jude Medical's Daig SL sheaths (Minnetonka, MN) not only have varying lengths of curvature in one plane (**A**) but also provide a second plane of curvature (SL1 through SL4) designed to orient the ablation catheter slightly anteriorly in close proximity to the mitral annulus (**B**).

67 cm in length (Fig. 34-2). These dilators accommodate a Brockenbrough needle 71 cm in length. Left-sided sheath dilators typically can only accommodate a guidewire of 0.032 inch or smaller.

Special transseptal sheaths exist for procedures in extremely tall patients. These sheaths are longer (73 cm) and are equipped with one or more hemostatic valves and longer dilators; they therefore require an 89-cm Brockenbrough needle if placed primarily during the transseptal procedure. The operator should ensure that the length of the Brockenbrough needle corresponds to the length of the sheath and its dilator before proceeding with the transseptal procedure. Specialized telescoping sheaths for compound ablation catheter angulations, deflectable sheaths, and sheaths for placement of multiple catheters through one transseptal puncture are also available (Figs. 34-3 and 34-4).

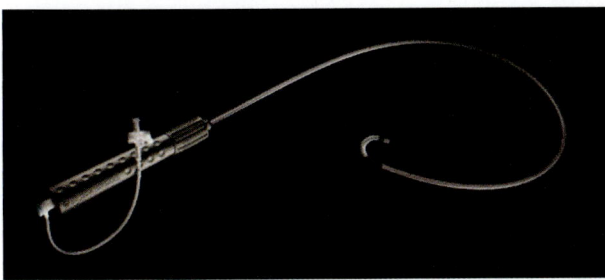

FIGURE 34-3. Deflectable sheath suitable for transseptal catheterization.(Courtesy of Daig, Minnetonka, MN.)

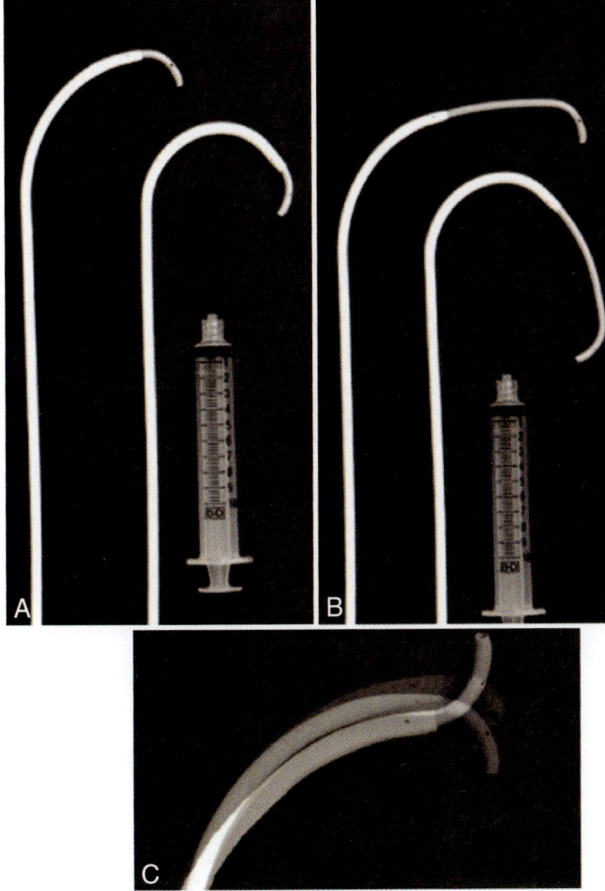

FIGURE 34-4. Telescoping sheath design. Another variation of transseptal sheath demonstrates an 11-French outer sheath through which a more conventional 8-French sheath passes. The outer sheath serves as a platform from which to guide the inner sheath to different portions of the left atrium. **A,** The outer sheath is demonstrated to have different degrees of curvature. Note that the inner sheath is retracted within the outer sheath. **B,** The inner sheath is shown extended and permits stable ablation catheter delivery to the far atrial walls in patients with left atrial enlargement. **C,** The multidirectional capabilities of the sheath-within-a-sheath design. One must use care when this system is deployed within the left atrium, however, because the double-sheath design is inherently stiff and unforgiving when manipulating an ablation catheter. Placement of this system within the left atrium requires conventional transseptal catheterization followed by a wire exchange (usually using a stiff 0.032-inch Amplatz guidewire) to place the sheath assembly within the left atrium.

Brockenbrough Needle

Varying curvatures of the Brockenbrough needle have been developed to accommodate variations in right atrial anatomy. Although most transseptal procedures are accomplished with a BRK-shaped (St. Jude Medical/Daig, St. Paul, MN) Brockenbrough needle, adult patients with marked right atrial enlargement may require the enhanced curvature of the BRK-1 Brockenbrough needle to reach the interatrial septum (Fig. 34-5). For children, a smaller BRK-2 curvature is available. The needles are malleable, allowing for manual modification of the curvature if desired to provide more or less reach. The proximal end of the Brockenbrough needle contains a flange with a flat and a pointed end, replicating an arrow. The pointed tip of the arrow points in the plane of the curvature of the needle. Additionally, all Brockenbrough needles are initially packaged with a thin stainless-steel wire stylet (Fig. 34-5B) that facilitates the passage of the needle into the dilator of the transseptal sheath. Although this stylet can be discarded, we have found that leaving it in place until the needle is just proximal to the distal end of the dilator prevents shearing of small filaments of plastic from the inner lumen of the transseptal sheath with complex curvatures. The stylet should be removed and the lumen of the needle flushed with heparinized saline before transseptal crossing.

Transseptal Catheterization

When performing transseptal catheterization in the electrophysiology laboratory, it is our practice to always begin by placing a His bundle catheter and a CS catheter to provide these critical anatomic landmarks fluoroscopically. A His bundle catheter *that is recording a His bundle electrogram* identifies the location of the central fibrous body at the most inferior aspect of the noncoronary aortic cusp. This obviates the need for an arterial puncture to place a pigtail catheter in the ascending aorta. One must remember that an electrophysiologic catheter that is *not* recording a His bundle electrogram cannot reliably determine the location of the aorta. Additionally, a CS catheter properly placed along the atrioventricular groove defines the intrathoracic cardiac rotation and demarcates the widest portion of the left atrium parallel and just posterior to the mitral annulus. One must ensure that the CS catheter courses near the mitral annulus, by ensuring that equal-amplitude atrial and ventricular electrograms exist throughout the course of the catheter. If not, the catheter may have inadvertently been placed in a posterolateral branch of the CS and should be repositioned before the transseptal catheterization is performed.

After selection of the appropriate sheath and dilator assembly and Brockenbrough needle, both the sheath and dilator should be flushed with heparinized saline. Using a modified Seldinger technique, an 8-French (8F), 15-cm side-port sheath is initially placed in the right femoral vein.[16] Under fluoroscopic guidance, a 0.032-inch J wire is positioned from the right femoral venous approach retrogradely to the superior vena cava (SVC). The 8F short sheath is then removed, and the transseptal sheath is placed over the 0.032-inch J wire into the SVC or left innominate vein. Once the sheath and dilator assembly are placed at this location, the guidewire is removed, and the dilator is flushed carefully with heparinized saline to remove all evidence of bubbles. The 71-cm Brockenbrough needle and its stylet are then placed through the sheath and dilator assembly until the stylet of the needle lies just proximal to the distal end of the sheath dilator (Fig. 34-6A). Because the Brockenbrough needle tapers slightly at its distal tip, care must be taken not to protrude the distal tip or needle stylet past the end of the sheath dilator to avoid inadvertent perforation of vascular structures.

Once the needle is located just proximal to the distal end of the sheath dilator, the needle is also flushed with heparinized saline, using care to first aspirate from the needle until a small amount of blood is visualized in the syringe chamber. On occasion, the sheath dilator presses against the wall of the SVC or innominate vein, and aspiration from the needle is met with difficulty. In this case, small rotation of the needle is required to free the distal tip

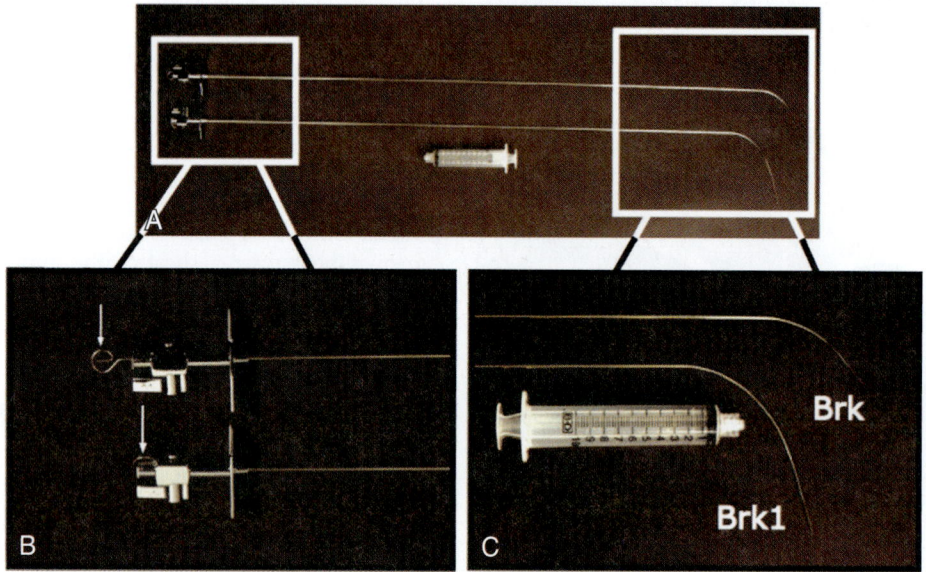

FIGURE 34-5. The Brockenbrough needle assembly. **A,** The Brockenbrough needle is typically 71 cm in length, although other long needles 89 cm in length (not shown) can be purchased for use with sheaths 73 cm in length or longer. A 10-mL syringe is shown for size comparison purposes. Note that the proximal end of the Brockenbrough needle has a hemostatic valve that contains a central thin stainless steel stylet (**B,** *arrow*), which should be removed before transseptal crossing. **C,** Two curvatures of the Brockenbrough needle are demonstrated: Brk is used for most patients with relatively normal right atria. In the patients with marked dilation of the right atria, a Brk1 needle, with its accentuated curvature, will provide improved contact with the fossa ovalis.

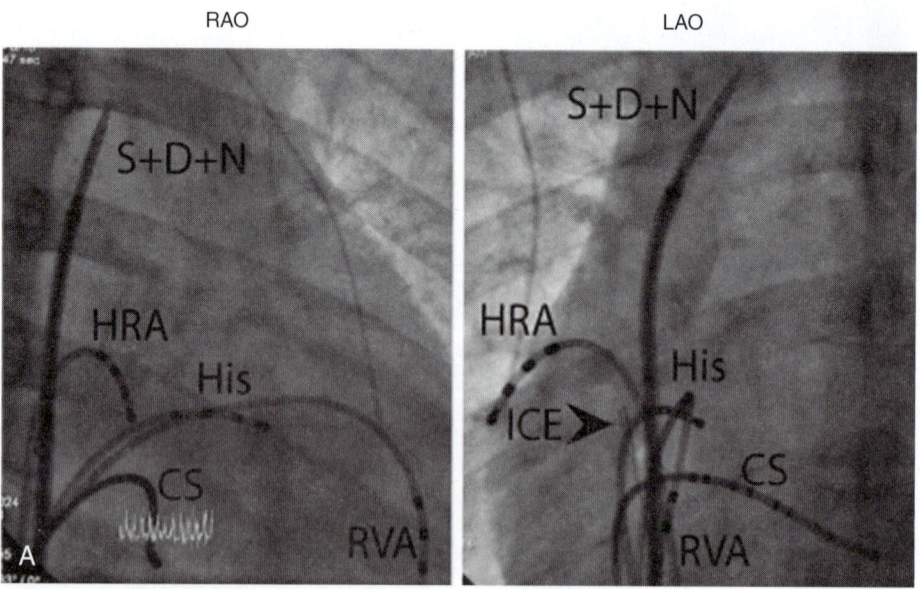

FIGURE 34-6. **A,** The transseptal catheterization procedure—fluoroscopy of initial catheter placement. Forty-degree right anterior oblique (RAO) and 40-degree left anterior oblique (LAO) views are demonstrated. The sheath (S), its dilator (D), and needle (N) (S + D + N) have been placed in the left innominate vein retrograde from the right femoral venous approach. The needle is kept just proximal to the end of the sheath's dilator. Note that the angulations of fluoroscopy are set so that the LAO view demonstrates the His bundle catheter (His) and right ventricular apical (RVA) catheter, which identify the interventricular septum and are pointed toward the viewer. The RAO fluoroscopic angulation is determined by the plane where the coronary sinus (CS) catheter fluoroscopically crosses the proximal electrode of the His catheter and is oriented away from the viewer. The sheath, dilator, and needle are then withdrawn as a single unit from this position into the right atrium, maintaining the orientation of the Brockenbrough needle at about 4 o'clock (posterior and leftward). HRA, high right atrium; ICE, intracardiac echocardiography catheter.

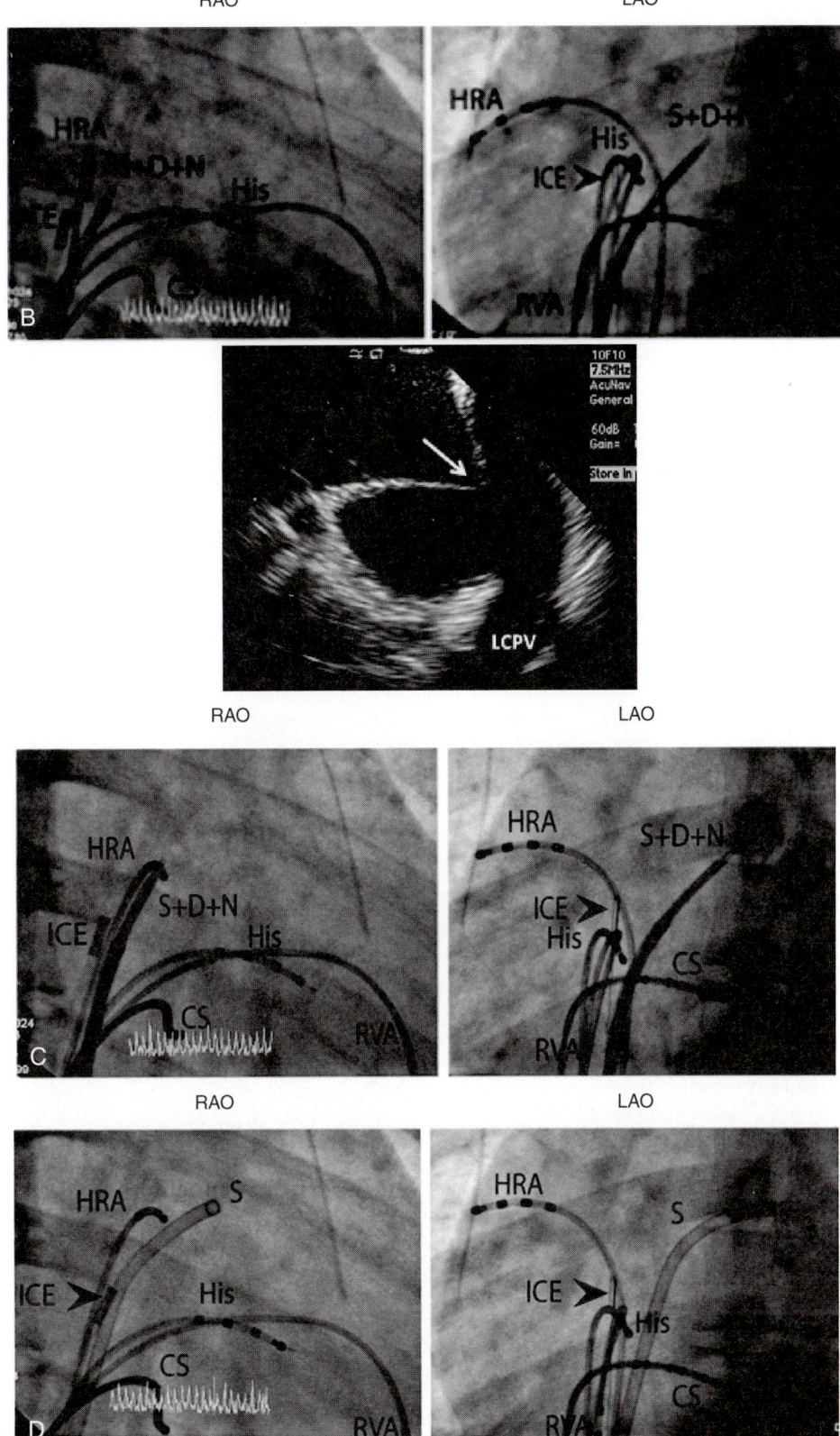

FIGURE 34-6, cont'd. B, Transseptal catheterization—sheath, dilator, and Brockenbrough needle at the fossa ovalis. Identical RAO and LAO fluoroscopic angulations to **A** demonstrate the sheath, dilator, and needle assembly at the level of the fossa ovalis. The intracardiac echocardiogram (ICE) (*black arrow*) sits just posterior to the His catheter in the LAO image. After withdrawing the sheath, dilator, and needle to the level of the fossa ovalis, the tip of the dilator moved distinctly leftward once the assembly reached the level of the His bundle catheter. The phased-array ICE at this location is also seen. Note that tenting of the fossa ovalis by the dilator and needle is clearly demonstrated (*arrow* in ultrasound image), and the angulation of the assembly appears to be pointing toward the mid-cavity of the left atrium. **C,** Transseptal catheterization— the sheath, dilator, and Brockenbrough needle in the left atrium. Again the fluoroscopic angulations are the same as in **A.** The needle was advanced slightly beyond the end of the sheath's dilator, and a palpable "pop" was noted, followed by an abrupt movement of the dilator into the left atrium. The needle has been withdrawn back into the sheath but maintained across the septum to provide support for delivery of the sheath over the dilator and needle into the left atrium. (Catheter labels as in **A.**) **D,** Transseptal catheterization—the sheath in the left atrium. RAO and LAO fluoroscopic images of the sheath after it has been delivered into the left atrium and the dilator and needle withdrawn. Fluoroscopic angulations and catheter labels as in **A.**

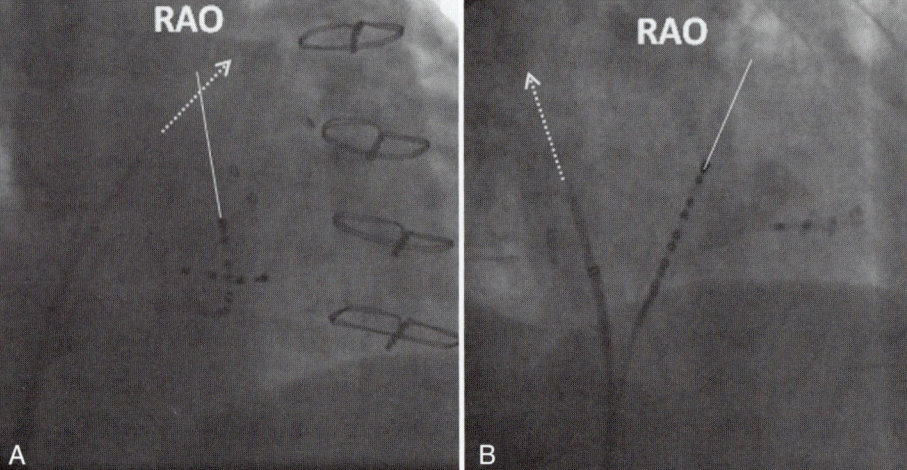

FIGURE 34-7. Directing the transseptal sheath parallel to the coronary sinus catheter. **A,** The trajectory of the sheath (*broken arrow*) is too anterior and crosses the extended line of the coronary sinus catheter (*solid line*). **B,** The trajectory of the sheath is too posterior, directed away from the coronary sinus catheter.

of the sheath dilator from the wall of the vessel, permitting flow of blood retrograde into the aspirating syringe. Once the blood is visualized and all bubbles have been removed from the chamber of the Brockenbrough needle, heparinized saline is flushed to clear the needle of any potential source of air embolus or thrombus. The Brockenbrough needle should be connected to hemodynamic measurement before transseptal crossing with the sheath.

The LAO fluoroscopic view is adjusted so that the His bundle catheter is pointing directly at the image intensifier. The RAO angulation is adjusted so that the projection of the CS catheter intersects the His bundle catheter at its midpoint and is directed perpendicular to the plane of the fluoroscopic image. Careful evaluation of the His bundle recording should be maintained to ensure an accurate anatomic reference relative to the inferior aspect of the aorta. The Brockenbrough needle and sheath assembly is withdrawn as a *single unit,* maintaining the relative positions of the needle and the sheath dilator from the SVC to the right atrium with the needle oriented in the 4-o'clock position (leftward and posterior). If the CS catheter has been placed from a superior approach, care must be used to ensure during torquing of the sheath that the CS catheter is not twisted around the sheath and needle assembly. If it is, the needle and sheath assembly should be rotated to free the CS catheter before being withdrawn into the right atrium, and the needle should be reoriented to a 4-o'clock position. Withdrawal of the assembly from the SVC should occur in the LAO projection with occasional verification of alignment in the RAO view.

As the needle and sheath assembly is withdrawn, an initial slight leftward movement of the assembly is noted as it enters the right atrium. As it is withdrawn further, a second, more significant leftward "jump" occurs when the tip of the assembly approaches the level of the His bundle catheter, signifying that the assembly has fallen below the superior limbus and into the fossa ovalis (Fig. 34-6, **Videos 34-1 and 34-2**). Once this level is located, the RAO fluoroscopic view should confirm that the assembly tip is well posterior to the site of the His bundle recording and that it is angled posterior and *parallel* to the projection of the CS

TABLE 34-2
CONFIRMING SHEATH LOCATION IN FOSSA OVALIS
Fluoroscopic motion and landmarks
Contrast staining
Intracardiac echocardiography
Right atrial angiography

catheter. This angle ensures that the assembly is not pointing posteriorly, which could perforate the posterior wall of the left atrium, and that it is not pointing too anteriorly, in which case the needle might enter the ascending aorta (Fig. 34-7). Adjustments of angulation between 3 and 5 o'clock may be necessary, with enlarged left atria often requiring a more posterior (or 5-o'clock) angulation and vertically oriented hearts requiring a more anterior (3-o'clock) angulation of the needle.

Once the angulation of the needle and sheath assembly is confirmed, the LAO projection is visualized to perform the transseptal crossing. The assembly is first withdrawn an additional 0.25 to 0.5 cm and then advanced to engage the limbus of the fossa ovalis (Fig. 34-6). Pressure measurements taken from any transseptal needle, if used, are usually damped or well off of a 40-mm Hg scale while the needle and dilator are juxtaposed to the intra-atrial septum. ICE or contrast injection through the needle to stain the septum can be performed to confirm the needle location (Table 34-2). Provided that the needle position is confirmed, the transseptal needle can be advanced 1 to 2 mm from within the sheath dilator to enter the left atrium, and often a tactile "pop" is felt **(Video 34-3)**. Once the needle enters the left atrium, this position can be confirmed by a pressure recording from the distal tip of the needle, by passing a 0.014-inch guidewire into a left pulmonary vein, by ICE findings (see later), or by a hand contrast injection (Fig. 34-8: Table 34-3). The sheath dilator assembly is then advanced over the needle to enter the left atrium (Fig. 34-6D).

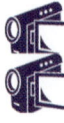

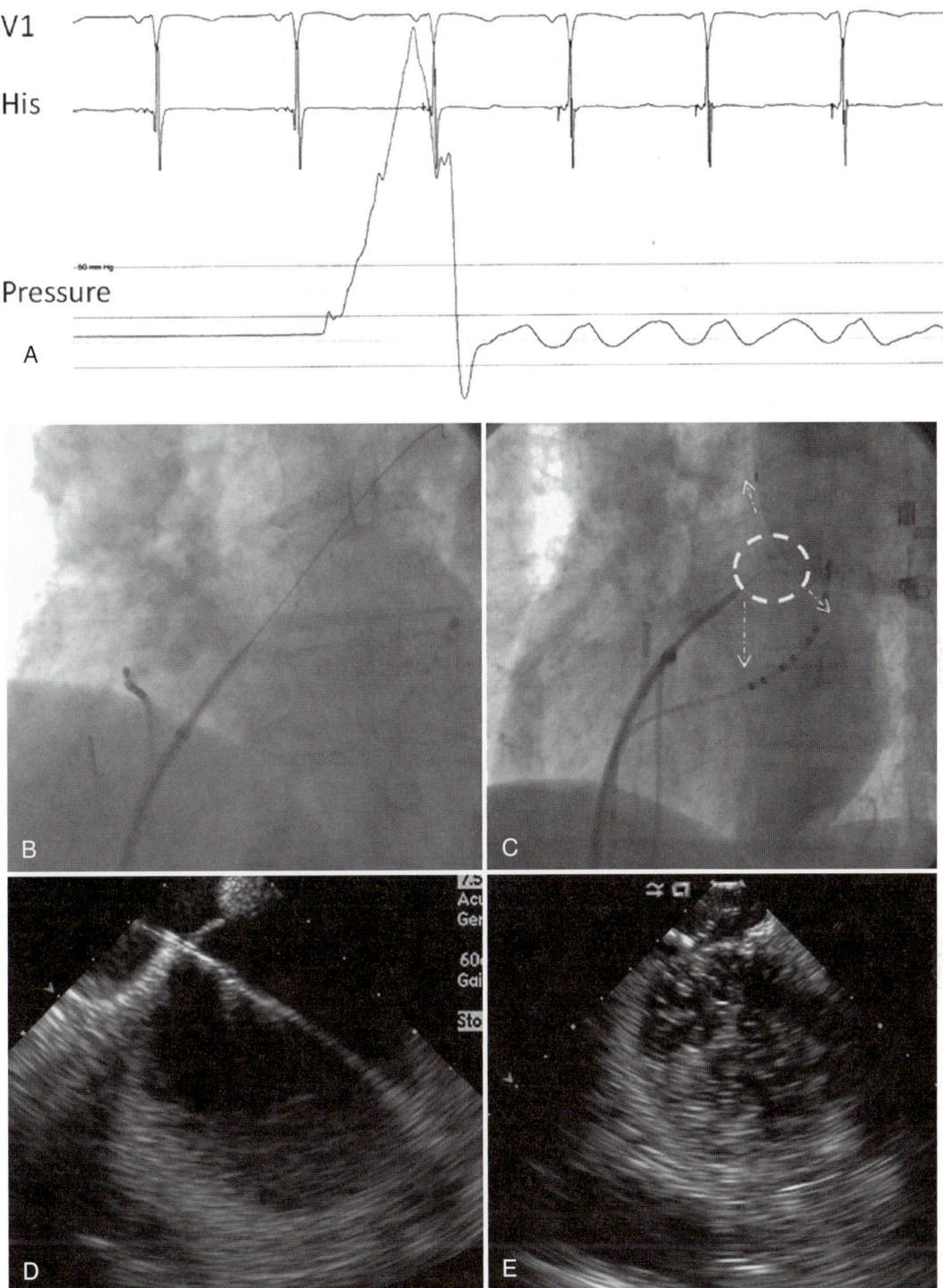

FIGURE 34-8. Confirming needle puncture into the left atrium. **A,** Left atrial pressure recording. Before transseptal puncture, the pressure recording from the transseptal needle is dampened. The recording pressure increases abruptly with advancement of the needle into the tissue of the foramen before giving way to a left atrial pressure waveform. **B,** A 0.014-mm guidewire passed from the transseptal needle into the left superior pulmonary vein. Note that the wire is well outside of the cardiac border. **C,** Contrast injection from the needle into the left atrium. There is dispersal of the contrast characteristic of blood flow patterns in the left atrium. **D,** Intracardiac echocardiographic visualization of the guidewire passage into the left superior pulmonary vein analogous to panel **B. E,** Intracardiac echocardiographic visualization of saline contrast injection from the needle into the body of the left atrium.

TABLE 34-3

CONFIRMING NEEDLE PUNCTURE TO LEFT ATRIUM

Left atrial pressure waveform

Contrast injection

0.014 guidewire passage into pulmonary vein

Intracardiac echocardiogram visualization

Intracardiac echocardiogram contrast injection

Blood O_2 saturation*

*Not specific for left atrium.

Once the dilator has been placed within the left atrium, the needle is left just proximal to the end of the dilator to provide support for the more proximal aspects of the sheath to be placed over the dilator and into the left atrium. If there is any question about the location of the needle after its advancement outside the sheath dilator, the dilator should never be advanced, to avoid catastrophic cardiac complications. A small contrast injection through the needle should be used if there is any question about its location. Puncture of the left atrium posteriorly or anteriorly *with the needle alone* has rarely resulted in significant cardiac complications. It is typically the dilation with the sheath dilator or sheath itself that can cause significant cardiac compromise. If there is aortic or pericardial staining after what is presumed to be transseptal puncture, the needle must be removed and the dilator withdrawn; then the 0.032-inch J wire is repositioned to the SVC, and the process is repeated until such time as proper transseptal crossing is performed.

Once the dilator and sheath have been safely placed in the left atrium, the needle and dilator are removed carefully and the sheath is aspirated to remove any evidence of thrombus or bubbles. The sheath is then carefully flushed with heparinized saline (Fig. 34-6). Systemic heparinization is then administered. At this point, in patients requiring single transseptal catheterization, it is our practice to place an ablation catheter into the left atrium, through the sheath, so that it lies within the pulmonary vein architecture outside the cardiac silhouette. Full curvature of the catheter is then employed, and the catheter is withdrawn from the pulmonary vein area until it falls into the body of the left atrium in a curled fashion. The ablation catheter can then be advanced carefully, with the catheter coiled so that it resembles a pigtail catheter and has a low potential to perforate cardiac structures. Confirmation of free movement of the ablation catheter to ensure that it is positioned within the chamber of the left atrium is obtained by torquing the sheath clockwise and counterclockwise to document free mobility. Once this is confirmed, the patient should be immediately administered heparin and followed to maintain an ACT of about 300 to 350 seconds. After the catheter ablation procedures, the ablation catheter and sheath are removed together without withdrawing the catheter into the sheath (to prevent shearing of thrombus and coagulum into the left atrium) by withdrawing the system back to the right atrium, and then the heparin is discontinued.

Intracardiac Echocardiography during Transseptal Catheterization

We have found cardiac ultrasound imaging to be invaluable during ablation procedures because it minimizes the risks for transseptal catheterization while affording the advantage of continuous monitoring of the patient's pericardial space for fluid. Early identification of pericardial effusion can be made with ICE, and prompt measures can be undertaken before hemodynamic compromise occurs. Perhaps the greatest assistance for the operator is in localization of the proper site of puncture during transseptal catheterization.

Two types of ultrasound catheters are available. One system uses a single rotating crystal ultrasound transducer based on either a 9F, 9-MHz rotating crystal or a 8F, 12.5-MHz ultrasound crystal (Boston Scientific CVIS, Sunnyvale, CA). Rotating crystal transducers (Fig. 34-9) image circumferentially for 360 degrees in the horizontal plane and view the intra-atrial septum well, but they do not have the capability to perform Doppler flow analysis and are not deflectable. However, the 360-degree images make it relatively easy to interpret catheter orientation relative to anatomic structures. The ideal imaging frequency of the rotating crystal ultrasound catheter for transseptal catheterization is 9 MHz.

The alternative is a 64-element, phased-array ultrasound system using an 8F or 10F transducer that images in a sector field oriented in the plane of the catheter rather than in a circumferential field of view (Fig. 34-10; see also Fig. 34-6). Although this catheter requires a steeper learning curve, the advantages of higher-resolution images, superior depth of imaging, and Doppler flow imaging capability make this a technology better suited for imaging left-sided anatomies. Once the catheter enters the right atrium, it should be rotated to visualize the tricuspid valve. Clockwise torque of the catheter from this image rotates the crystal array posteriorly, so that the ascending aorta comes into view, followed by the more posterior fossa ovalis (Fig 34-10). It is helpful to deflect the catheter slightly away from the intra-atrial septum, so that it does not lie immediately adjacent to the interatrial septum; this provides better imaging and less interference with the transseptal equipment. The greatest utility of the ultrasound approach can be seen in tenting and puncturing the desired portion of the foramen ovale **(Video 34-4)**. Care should be taken, however, to identify the tip of the *needle* because septal tenting can be seen when the needle is against the thicker portions of the intra-atrial septum. A pitfall is to see the body of the transseptal catheter transected by the echocardiographic beam and mistake this for the catheter tip.

Double Transseptal Technique

In some procedures, there is an advantage to having two transseptal sheaths placed through the interatrial septum simultaneously. There are generally two approaches to this procedure: (1) perform two separate punctures of the fossa ovalis as outlined previously, or (2) place two sheaths by separate skin punctures through the same single site of

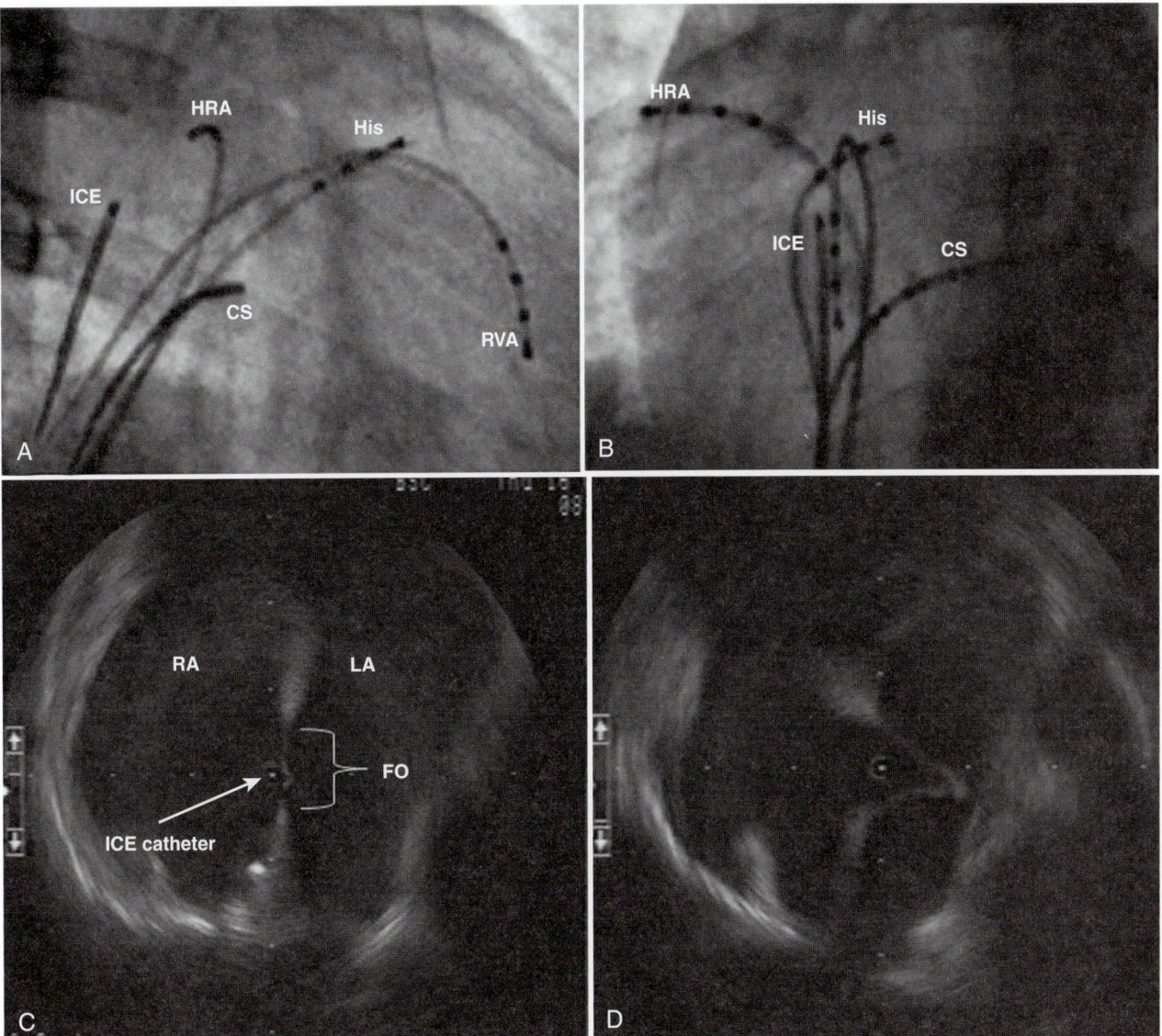

FIGURE 34-9. Example of rotating crystal intracardiac echocardiographic (ICE) images. **A** and **B** show the 40-degree right and left anterior oblique images of the ICE catheter at the level of the fossa ovalis. **C,** The fossa is well visualized before sheath placement. **D,** The transseptal sheath deeply indents the before extension of the needle. CS, coronary sinus catheter; FO, fossa ovalis; His, His bundle catheter; HRA, high right atrium; LA, left atrium; RA, right atrium; RVA, right ventricular apical catheter.

the initial transseptal puncture. Our laboratory typically performs the latter approach because of the ease of the exchange guidewire technique.

To place two sheaths through one transseptal puncture site, after the first sheath is safely placed into the left atrium, it is flushed with heparinized saline. Then the dilator of the first transseptal sheath is removed and flushed with heparinized saline. Next, an alternate 8F, 15-cm sheath, previously placed in the right femoral vein, is removed and replaced with the second transseptal sheath, which is again placed retrograde to the SVC or left innominate vein. The dilator of this second sheath is also flushed with heparinized saline to remove all evidence of bubbles. A Brockenbrough needle is placed into the second sheath and flushed carefully with heparinized saline.

Next, a 0.032-inch guidewire is passed through the dilator of the *first* transseptal sheath, and the guidewire and dilator are placed back into the first transseptal sheath, using care to pass the guidewire well into the left superior or left inferior pulmonary vein. Once the guidewire is placed well into the pulmonary vein, the first sheath and dilator are withdrawn back into the right atrium, leaving the 0.032-inch guidewire in the left atrium. The *second* sheath and dilator assembly is then withdrawn from the SVC in the same angle as the first transseptal crossing, using the Brockenbrough needle to torque the second sheath. Once the dilator falls to the level of the existing transseptal guidewire, the biplane orientation of the second sheath's dilator to the transseptal guidewire is adjusted until the dilator passes immediately adjacent to the guidewire into the left atrium. Needle puncture of the interatrial septum typically is not required. Alternatively, after withdrawal of the first transseptal sheath into the right atrium, an ablation catheter through the second sheath is used to steer across the hole in the foramen ovalis.

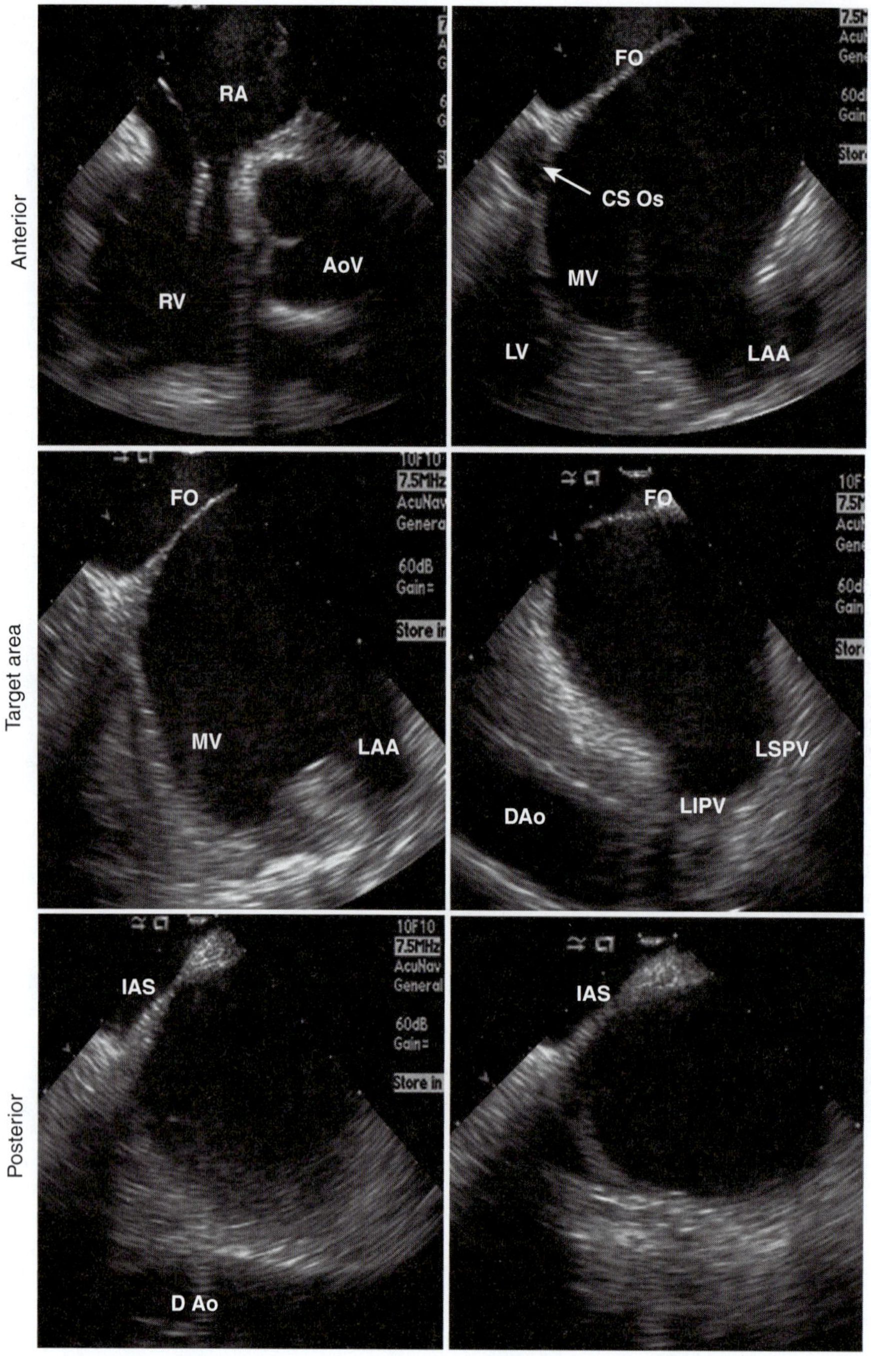

FIGURE 34-10. Intracardiac echocardiographic visualization of the atrial septum. The areas of the septum seen in the *upper two panels* are anterior to the center of the fossa ovalis (FO) as indicated by the visualization of the aortic valve (AoV), coronary sinus os (CS Os), and mitral valve (MV). The *upper right panel* may be suitable for approaches to the mitral annulus, however. The *middle panels* show the midportion of the foramen. Note the well-defined limbus and visualization of the left inferior (LIPV) and left superior (LSPV) pulmonary veins and appendage (LAA) without seeing the aortic valves. The *lower panels* show the inter-atrial septum (IAS) posterior to the fossa. There is no distinct fossa visualized, the body of the left atrium is small, and the descending aorta (DAo) is now seen. RA, right atrium; RV, right ventricle.

Troubleshooting the Difficult Case

Difficulty with the transseptal puncture typically arises from variations in the position of the fossa ovalis and from physical characteristics of the fossa itself. Anatomic variations in the location of the fossa include displacement inferiorly or posteriorly, or both, especially with dilated atria.

The fossa may appear anterior to the expected location in the vertically oriented heart. These situations are best resolved by imaging the interatrial septum with ICE or by formal angiographic visualization of the right atrium.[17]

The fossa may be very small in diameter and difficult to engage with the sheath (Fig. 34-11). Alternatively, the fossa can be very large and aneurysmal, making engagement easy but perforation difficult because of the highly compliant nature of the fossa tissue (Fig. 34-11). In some

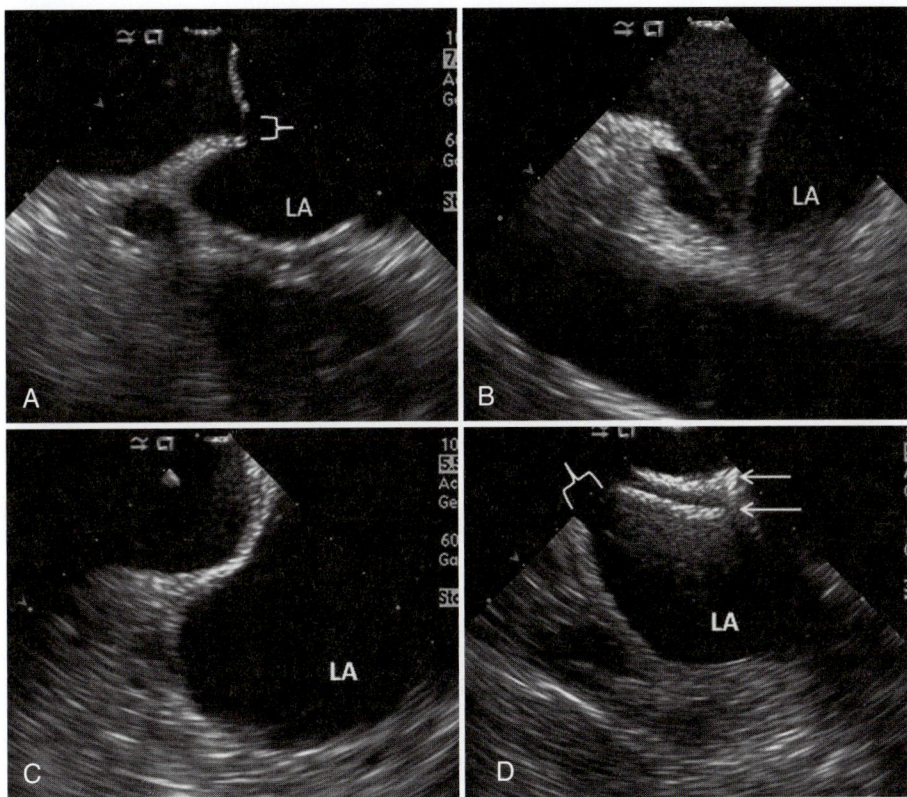

FIGURE 34-11. Intracardiac echocardiographic visualization of troublesome atrial septal anatomy for transseptal access. **A,** Small foramen ovale measuring only 4 mm in diameter in this view. **B,** Redundant, aneurysmal foramen ovale. The "floppy" foramen stretches under pressure from the transseptal sheath until there is contact with the posterior atrial wall. **C,** Scarred, thickened, poorly defined foramen ovale. **D,** Presence of a mechanical closure device for a patent foramen ovale (*arrows*). The only area of the atrial septum not covered is at the inferior aspect of the closure device (*marked*). LA, left atrium.

cases, the transseptal needle comes into close proximity to the atrial wall before the foramen is crossed (Fig. 34-11). Solutions to crossing the aneurysmal foramen include aggressive patient hydration to expand the left atrium and orientation of the transseptal needle toward the most lateral aspect of the left atrium to allow the greatest excursion of the apparatus before contacting the atrial wall. This situation may be most readily overcome, however, by the use of a radiofrequency-powered transseptal needle.[18] A commercially available system with dedicated needles and generator applies 10 W of radiofrequency energy to the tip of the needle (extended beyond the sheath) for 2 seconds.[18] The effects of this system have been replicated by application of the radiofrequency energy to the proximal end of standard transseptal needles from an ablation catheter or a handheld electrosurgical cautery.[19] Using the cautery probe, 10 to 20 W of power is delivered for 1 to 2 seconds in the cutting mode to the needle as it is extended from the sheath. A potential problem with the radiofrequency-powered transseptal technique is that a misdirected hole created by radiofrequency may not be self-sealing as with mechanical punctures. Alternatively, "extra-sharp" transseptal needles are available to facilitate passage through compliant tissue.

The foramen is often scarred and more difficult to cross after previous transseptal puncture.[20] In these cases, use of extra-sharp or radiofrequency-powered needles may be helpful. Patients with atrial septal defect or patent foramen ovale repair can present particular challenges. In these patients, the characteristic catheter "jump" into the fossa ovalis is absent. The use of intracardiac echocardiography is essential in these cases. Pericardial and Dacron patches may be crossed by directly, but Gore-Tex patches may be impassable.[21] Mechanical closure devices require septal puncture at the periphery of the device (Fig. 34-11).[21] The inferoposterior border of the device may be most amenable to puncture, but the device may encompass the entire septum without a suitable margin for access.

With large sheaths or with redundant foramen, there may be difficulty advancing the sheath through the septum despite successful puncture of the foramen. In this situation, rotating the sheath and dilator posteriorly (clockwise and ideally over a guidewire in the right superior pulmonary vein) while advancing will allow passage of the sheath.

For patients without inferior venous access to the heart, transseptal catheterization from the right internal jugular vein has been reported.[22] A guide to troubleshooting difficult transseptal procedures is given in Table 34-4.

Acknowledgments

The authors would like to thank Mr. Jonathan F. Hillebrand of Multimedia Services at Evanston Hospital, Evanston, Illinois, for his tireless efforts to secure the figures that accompany this chapter. In addition, we thank the staff of the Electrophysiology Division of Evanston Northwestern Healthcare for their exceptional professionalism and care rendered to our patients during the preparation of this manuscript.

TABLE 34-4

TROUBLESHOOTING THE DIFFICULT CASE

Problem	Cause	Possible Solutions
Fossa ovalis anatomically displaced	Anatomic variation, atrial dilation, cardiac rotation, congenital heart disease	Direct visualization of atrial septum with ICE or right atrial angiography
Aneurysmal fossa ovalis	Congenital	Hydrate patient to expand atrial volume ICE "Extra sharp" transseptal needle Direct needle toward far lateral atrial wall Radiofrequency-powered transseptal needle
Thick, scarred fossa ovalis	Congenital or previous transseptal puncture(s)	ICE "Extra sharp" transseptal needle Radiofrequency-powered transseptal needle
Repaired ASD/PFO	Congenital	ICE Cross pericardial or Dacron patches directly or at periphery Cross septum at periphery mechanical closure devices
Absence of inferior venous access	Anatomic variation, IVC filter/obstruction, tortuous vasculature, thrombosis	Right internal jugular approach

ASD, atrial-septal defect; ICE, intracardiac echocardiography; PFO, patent foramen ovale.

References

1. Ross J, Braunwald E, Morrow AG. Transseptal left atrial puncture: new technique for the measurement of left atrial pressures. *Am J Cardiol.* 1959;3:653–655.
2. Cope C. Technique for the transseptal catheterization of the left atrium: preliminary report. *J Thorac Surg.* 1959;37:482–486.
3. Braunwald E. Transseptal left heart catheterization. *Circulation.* 1968;37 (suppl 3):74–79.
4. Brockenbrough EC, Braunwald E, Ross J Jr. Transseptal left heart catheterization: a review of 450 studies and description of an improved technique. *Circulation.* 1962;25:15–21.
5. Mullins CE. Transseptal left heart catheterization: experience with a new technique in 520 pediatric and adult patients. *Pediatr Cardiol.* 1983;4:239–245.
6. Lesh MD, Van Hare GF, Scheinman MM, et al. Comparison of the retrograde and transseptal methods for left free wall accessory pathways. *J Am Coll Cardiol.* 1993;22:542–549.
7. Packer DL, Hammill SC, Holmes DR. Comparison of transaortic and transseptal approaches for the ablation of left-sided accessory pathways [abstract]. *Circulation.* 1992;86(suppl 1):I–783.
8. Seifort MJ, Morady F, Calkins HG, Langberg JJ. Aortic leaflet perforation during radiofrequency ablation. *Pacing Clin Electrophysiol.* 1991;14:1582–1585.
9. Anderson RH, Becker AE. *Cardiac Anatomy: An Integrated Text and Color Atlas.* London: Gower Medical Publishing; 1980.
10. Sweeney LJ, Rosenquist GC. The normal anatomy of the atrial septum in the human heart. *Am Heart J.* 1979;98:194–199.
11. Hung JS, Fu M, Yeh KH, et al. Usefulness of intracardiac echocardiography in complex transseptal catheterization during percutaneous transvenous mitral commissurotomy. *Mayo Clin Proc.* 1996;71:134–140.
12. Daoud EG, Kalbfleisch SJ, Hummel JD. Intracardiac echocardiography to guide transseptal catheterization for radiofrequency catheter ablation. *J Cardiovasc Electrophysiol.* 1999;10:358–363.
13. Epstein LM, Smith T, TenHoff H. Nonfluoroscopic transseptal catheterization: safety and efficacy of intracardiac echocardiographic guidance. *J Cardiovasc Electrophysiol.* 1998;9:625–630.
14. Sethi KK, Mohan JC. Transseptal catheterization for the electrophysiologist: modification with a "view." *J Interv Card Electrophysiol.* 2001;5:97–99.
15. Gonzalez MD, Otomo K, Shah N, et al. Transseptal left heart catheterization for cardiac ablation procedures. *J Interv Cardiac Electrophysiol.* 2001;5:89–95.
16. Swartz JF, Fisher WG, Tracy CM. Ablation of left-sided atrioventricular accessory pathways via the transeptal atrial approach. In: Huang SKS, ed. *Radiofrequency Catheter Ablation of Cardiac Arrhythmias: Basic Concepts and Clinical Applications.* Armonk, NY: Futura; 1995:255.
17. Rogers DPS, Lambiase PD, Dhinoja M, et al. Right atrial angiography facilitates transseptal puncture for complex ablation in patients with unusual anatomy. *J Interv Card Electrophysiol.* 2006;17:29–34.
18. Sakata Y, Feldman T. Transcatheter creation of atrial septal perforation using a radiofrequency transseptal system: novel approach as an alternative to transseptal needle puncture. *Cath Cardiovasc Interv.* 2005;64:327–332.
19. McWilliams MJ, Tchou P. The use of standard radiofrequency energy delivery system to facilitate transseptal puncture. *J Cardiovasc Electrophysiol.* 2009;20:238–240.
20. Marcus GM, Ren X, Tseng ZH, et al. Repeat transseptal catheterization after ablation for atrial fibrillation. *J Cardiovasc Electrophysiol.* 2007;18:55–59.
21. Lakkireddy D, Rangisetty U, Prasad S, et al. Intracardiac echo-guided radiofrequency catheter ablation of atrial fibrillation in patients with atrial septal defect or patent foramen ovale repair: a feasibility, safety and efficacy study. *J Cardiovasc Electrophysiol.* 2008;19:1137–1142.
22. Lim HE, Pak HN, Tse HF, et al. Catheter ablation of atrial fibrillation via superior approach in patients with interruption of the inferior vena cava. *Heart Rhythm.* 2009;6:174–179.

Videos

Video 34-1. Transeptal sheath engaging the foramen ovale. The LAO view is shown. A coronary sinus catheter, intracardiac echocardiography catheter, and His bundle catheter are in position. The needle is within the sheath apparatus. The sheath is directed toward the atrial septum and withdrawn from a cranial-to-caudal direction. The abrupt rightward motion of the sheath in this view represents the apparatus falling into the foramen.

Video 34-2. The same sequence as Video 34-1, except seen in the RAO view. Note that the falling motion of the sheath is much less apparent in this view compared with the LAO view. Also, observe that the trajectory of the sheath is parallel to the coronary sinus catheter.

Video 34-3. Extension of the transseptal needle to penetrate the foramen ovale. With the sheath apparatus firmly engaging the foramen, the needle is briskly advanced beyond the sheath. At this point, left atrial pressure should be recorded from the needle.

Video 34-4. Needle penetration of the foramen ovale as seen by intracardiac echocardiography. The sheath apparatus deeply indents the foramen. With extension of the needle in this patient, the dilator and sheath both enter the left atrium. Note that the foramen recoils to a neutral position after penetration.

35

Special Considerations for Ablation in Pediatric Patients

J. Philip Saul

Key Points

Children have the same variety of arrhythmia mechanisms as adults, but with a different distribution and often in different clinical settings.

Although older children are physically similar to adults, children are not just little adults when it comes to the choice to proceed with and techniques for performing ablation.

Ablation in infants and very small children carries a variety of special risks and should be undertaken only after failure of medical therapy and in the most experienced hands.

The presence of structural congenital heart disease significantly complicates any ablation procedure, demanding that the operator be familiar with both the structural and electrophysiologic issues at hand, particularly if atrioventricular discordance is present.

Atrial flutter and fibrillation are rare arrhythmias in the pediatric population in the absence of congenital heart disease.

Atrial ectopic tachycardia, junctional ectopic tachycardia, and the permanent form of junctional reciprocating tachycardia can all manifest as incessant tachyarrhythmias with a dilated cardiomyopathy in children. Ablation therapy may be particularly helpful in such cases, if it can be performed safely.

Coronary injury from RF ablation can occur when the ablation site is in close proximity to a small coronary artery, and is probably unrecognized in most cases in which it occurs. Consequently, coronary angiography should be considered before the use of RF ablation of all posteroseptal substrates, particularly in smaller children.

For ablation in children, safety should always take precedence over efficacy. Consequently, when cryotherapy can be effective, it is often the technology of first choice.

The explosion in understanding and management of most arrhythmias in adults during the past 20 years is both reflected and amplified in the field of pediatrics. The application of procedures or devices commonly used in the management of arrhythmias in adults remains somewhat delayed in children because of technical issues related to size or lack of regulatory approval. Other issues, such as smaller numbers of patients and a higher diversity of clinical characteristics and age, have limited the ability to perform controlled therapeutic trials, even multicenter ones. Despite these limitations, a combination of continued technical developments in the miniaturization of devices, multicenter retrospective reviews[1,2] and registries,[3-7] occasional controlled clinical trials, and the use of pharmacologic agents approved by the U.S. Food and Drug Administration for adults[8-9] has resulted in an equivalence in the armamentarium of adult and pediatric electrophysiologists. However, as is reviewed in this chapter, the parity of tools does not necessarily imply parity of disease and its management.

This chapter concentrates primarily on two categories of rhythm disorders: arrhythmias that are mechanistically similar or identical to those in adults, but whose presentation and management is complicated by the presence of young age or congenital heart disease, and arrhythmias that are either unique to pediatric patients or are observed only rarely in adults (Table 35-1). Some arrhythmias and their presentations are covered in other chapters and are mentioned here only briefly in the context of differences from the typical adult patient. Although many patients with congenital heart disease and arrhythmias are in fact adults, for the purposes of this chapter, the term *adult* will be used to refer to patients without congenital heart disease who are not usually cared for by a pediatric cardiologist.

TABLE 35-1

COMPARISON OF ARRHYTHMIAS IN CHILDREN AND ADULTS

Arrhythmias Not Typically Observed in Adults

Ectopic atrial tachycardia
Junctional ectopic tachycardia
Permanent junctional reciprocating tachycardia (PJRT)
Double atrioventricular nodes

Alternative Presentations of Arrhythmias Commonly Observed in Adults

Atrioventricular nodal reentrant tachycardia (AVNRT)
Preexcitation syndromes in infants
Preexcitation syndromes with congenital heart disease
Ventricular tachycardia with tetralogy of Fallot
Atrial reentry with congenital heart disease

Arrhythmias with Similar Management in Adults and Children

Preexcitation syndromes after infancy
Congenital long QT syndrome
Right ventricular outflow tract (RVOT) ventricular tachycardia
Arrhythmogenic right ventricular dysplasia
Benign accelerated idioventricular rhythm

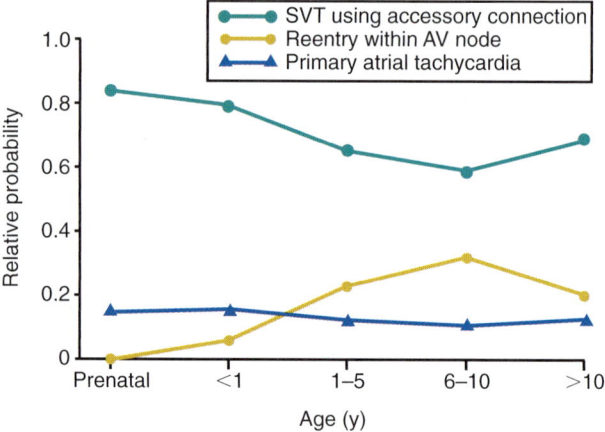

FIGURE 35-1. Distribution of supraventricular tachycardia (SVT) mechanisms as a function of age in pediatric patients. The percentage of patients with primary atrial tachycardias remains relatively constant, whereas there is a shift from accessory pathway mediated tachycardias to atrioventricular (AV) nodal reentry from infancy to adolescence. *(From Ko JK, Deal BJ, Strasburger JF, Benson DW Jr. Supraventricular tachycardia mechanisms and their age distribution in pediatric patients. Am J Cardiol. 1992;69:1028-1032. With permission.)*

Are Children Just Little Adults?

The notion that children are simply small adults is not entirely inaccurate, particularly when it comes to catheter ablation for some arrhythmias in relatively older and larger children, perhaps after 10 to 12 years of age. However, for many procedures, what seems like only a difference of scale can have dramatic implications, which begin with the diagnosis,[10] extend from the initial recommendation for an ablation to the technical performance of the procedure,[11] and end with the long-term risks of producing radiofrequency (RF) lesions in developing myocardium[12] and near coronary arteries.[13-17]

On average, children are obviously smaller than adults, which results in smaller cardiac chambers, thinner and perhaps more fragile tissues, smaller coronary arteries, and smaller distances between structures, such as the posterior septum and the atrioventricular (AV) node, or the AV ring and the coronary arteries. Not so obviously, children may be dissimilar from adults in ways other than size. Arrhythmia mechanisms overlap but are proportionately very different.[10,18-20] Incessant arrhythmias are much more common,[21-23] probably based on lack of symptom recognition in infants and small children, better early tolerance, and late morbidity and mortality if left untreated, which ensures that most patients will not reach adulthood with their arrhythmias. Accessory pathway (AP) locations are skewed toward the right side,[23-24] at least partially related to the simultaneous presence of structural congenital heart disease.[25-28] In addition, developing myocardium appears to have the potential for spontaneous cure of an arrhythmia[2] but also the potential for dramatic RF lesion growth with time.[12] Finally, children are generally less cooperative and tolerant than adults, a feature that necessitates special attention in all aspects of the ablation procedure. These issues are discussed in detail in this chapter, along with a review of possible solutions and the implications

for management of arrhythmias treatable by RF catheter ablation in both children and adults.

Arrhythmia Mechanisms

The arrhythmias seen in pediatric patients are typically the more treatable varieties. Ventricular tachycardia is relatively rare in children, accounting for fewer than 5% of all tachycardias and only 20% of wide-complex tachycardias.[29] In addition, when ventricular tachycardia does occur in a child without structural heart disease, it is more likely than in an adult to have one of the ablatable mechanisms.[30-32] Supraventricular tachycardia (SVT), which accounts for most arrhythmias in children, is most likely to result from a concealed or manifest accessory AV pathway (Fig. 35-1),[10] again portending well for possible catheter ablation therapy. In the absence of a history of surgery for structural congenital heart disease, APs probably underlie about 75% of all SVTs in children[10] and account for about 95% of SVTs in neonates,[33,34] compared with 30% to 40% of SVTs in adults.[19-20] Atrioventricular nodal reentrant tachycardia (AVNRT) and primary atrial tachycardias (both reentrant and automatic) each appear to account for about half of the remaining SVTs (Fig. 35-1).[10]

The Decision to Ablate: Safety Versus Efficacy

One overriding theme in the management of arrhythmias in children compared with adults is an emphasis on safety over efficacy. Although there are few cases at any age in which safety is not an important concern, the relatively benign course of many arrhythmic conditions in childhood, the potential disruption that therapies such as permanent pacing cause for a child, and the fact that parents are usually the decision-making surrogate for the child often lead to a different decision tree for children than for adults. Further, for some situations and technologies (e.g., the potential for coronary damage with RF energy application at the AV groove), the size of the patient and of the heart may really matter.

Ablation in patients with Wolff-Parkinson-White (WPW) syndrome is an excellent example of how decision making may be highly age dependent.[35] In this chapter, the term *WPW* will be used to describe the condition of preexcitation on the surface electrocardiogram (ECG), with or without coexisting tachycardia. As a result of a variety of concerns, even the most symptomatic infant with WPW and paroxysmal SVT is only rarely a candidate for ablation.[36-38] Myocardial injury[12] and potentially severe coronary injury[13-15,39] are more likely with RF ablation in this age group. Although the introduction of cryoablation has changed this situation somewhat, there remain a number of reasons to be cautious in managing infants with ablation procedures.[37,38] Perhaps most important is that about 40% of APs in infants spontaneously stop functioning during the first year of life,[2,40] and an additional one third of patients are unlikely to have symptoms between infancy and early childhood.[41] In children older than 4 years who have symptomatic arrhythmias, the balance between risks and benefits clearly shifts toward ablation therapy, but usually only if the ablation can be performed safely.[35] In contrast to the situation in infants, even asymptomatic WPW patients between the ages of 10 and 18 years may be managed more aggressively than adults. Unlike asymptomatic adults older than age 28 years, who are unlikely to ever have symptoms,[42,43] the older child with a high-risk pathway is exactly the type of patient who may present with sudden arrhythmic death as their initial symptom, leading to the recommendation that such patients undergo risk stratification, with those who are high risk being offered catheter ablation as a therapeutic option.[44] Further, the guidelines for sports participation in patients with WPW recommend considering risk stratification before approval for this age group.[45,46] Other age-dependent differences in management decisions are addressed in the discussions of individual arrhythmias.

Use of Cryoablation in Children

Catheter-based cryotherapy was approved for use in the United States in 2003 for ablation of a variety of cardiac arrhythmias.[47,53] Since then, there have been a variety of reports in children, primarily focused on its use in AVNRT and other septal substrates.[47,48,54-56] Cryoablation has several potential advantages over RF ablation, including (1) reversible cryomapping before the production of a permanent lesion,[50,57-59] (2) adherence of the catheter tip to the endocardium on freezing, (3) a well-defined edge of the cryolesion, (4) minimal effects on adjacent coronary arteries,[60] and (5) a lower incidence of thrombus.[61] The first four of these issues are particularly relevant to small children because of the close proximity of a variety of critical cardiac structures to the ablation target and the reported potential for RF lesion growth in immature myocardium.[12] In fact, the most common major complication during RF ablation in pediatric patients is AV block,[3,38,62] and there appears to be a higher potential for coronary artery injury in this patient group,[13-15,17,63] even during slow pathway modification[13] (see full discussion later under "Atrioventricular Nodal Reentrant Tachycardia in Children").

Typical cryotherapy systems allow for both *ice mapping* at a tip temperature of −30° to −40°C, whereby the catheter adheres and nearby tissue loses electrical activity but few cell are killed, and *ablation* at a tip temperature of less than −65°C, whereby a lesion will be formed. Once cells freeze, they expand and burst. After 4 minutes at the ablation temperature with a small-tip catheter, a typical lesion size is 3 to 6 mm in diameter, smaller than that seen with RF. One of the contrasting features of cryoablation compared with RF is that there is a much larger zone of reversibility as the lesion expands because tissue cooling above the freezing point will lead to loss of electrical activation well before the loss of viability. This feature has dramatically enhanced the safety profile in clinical trials to date. In fact, despite frequent use of the technology for septal tachycardia substrates, there are no reports of AV block with cryoablation,[47-50,64] even in children as small as 20 kg, in the presence of a His potential.[56]

The primary disadvantage of cryoablation is that inherent in its high level of safety is a smaller lesion size than for RF ablation. For ablation of septal tachycardia substrates (AV node modification, anterior and posterior septal pathways), cryoablation success rates have been statistically similar to those for RF techniques.[47-50,64] However, most operators are less aggressive with RF in septal areas and have had to be highly aggressive with cryotherapy to achieve success. Further, with one exception,[65] even aggressive application of cryoenergy has not yielded similar success rates to RF for ablation of nonseptal accessory pathways. Although the data are limited in very small children and infants, anecdotal evidence suggests that cryoablation may be effective for all accessory pathway locations in these unique patient groups. Given these considerations, as discussed later for individual arrhythmia substrates, the use of cryoablation is most important for septal substrates, small children, and patients with abnormal anatomy when the precise location of the AV conduction system is not known.

Alternative Presentations or Management of Arrhythmias Commonly Observed in Adults

The complexity of an arrhythmia and its management may result from either the nature of the abnormal rhythm or the setting in which it occurs. The latter aspect is addressed in this section of the chapter, including AVNRT in the child, preexcitation syndromes in the infant and small child, preexcitation syndromes in the patient with congenital heart disease, and atrial reentry (flutter or fibrillation) in the pediatric patient without congenital heart disease. Atrial and ventricular tachyarrhythmias in the patient with congenital heart disease are addressed in Chapters 14 and 32, respectively.

Atrioventricular Nodal Reentrant Tachycardia in Children

The issue, addressed earlier, of rebalancing safety and efficacy in the decision-making process for a child is particularly important in the management of AVNRT. A number of factors that are distinctly different in children compared with adults must be taken into account. These factors are related to particular risk in children that may affect the decision to ablate, the diagnosis of dual AV nodal physiology and AVNRT, and the technical aspects of the ablation procedure.

Medical Management

No natural history data exist for the medical management of AVNRT presenting in childhood. However, at presentation, AV node reentry appears easier to manage medically in children than in adults, and particularly in infants.[66]

Atrioventricular Node Physiology in Children

Based on the classic definition for dual AV node physiology (a 50-millisecond increase in the atrium–His bundle [AH] interval for a 10-millisecond decrement in the atrium-atrium (A-A) interval), many fewer pediatric[67-69] than adult[70] patients with inducible AVNRT have demonstrable dual AV nodal physiology (about 60% versus 90% to 100%, respectively). Because the mechanism of AVNRT induction is similar in children with or without demonstrable dual AV nodal physiology, the presence of two pathways must be assumed. The notion is that the difference in the baseline conduction properties of the two pathways does not reach the threshold for dual physiology in about 40% of children, suggesting that less stringent or more specific criteria may be necessary to define dual AV nodal physiology in children. For instance, the transition from fast to slow pathway conduction may occur with a change in the slope of the AH response to a change in A-A interval,[71] but without a change in AH interval that meets the 50-millisecond criterion.[72] In fact, a change in conduction pathway could theoretically take place without any change in the AH interval. One might speculate that the magnitude of the AH change at the transition from the fast to the slow pathway would indeed be related to heart size and therefore to age because normal AV nodal conduction times, expressed as either the AH or the PR interval, increase with age. Younger children have also been shown to have faster conduction in the slow pathway than older children and adults.[69] Consequently, in children, the slope change of AH versus AA is probably a more reliable and specific measure of the transition between the fast and slow pathways than the AH jump criterion alone.

Decision to Ablate and Safety Issues

Once a decision has been made to perform slow pathway modification in a child, identification of appropriate locations for modification is not particularly different from that in adults. Further, the ablation technique and end points for either RF ablation or cryoablation do not vary significantly in children and adults, with the exception that a smaller catheter should generally be used in smaller children (<20 kg or so), to minimize the lesion size. With the use of such techniques, it appears that more than 95% of AVNRT can be eliminated in adults or children.[23,24,68] However, two safety issues and their implications should make a significant difference between adults and children in the decision to use RF ablation: the risk for AV block and the risk for coronary damage.

Atrioventricular Block. The possibility of ablation-induced complete heart block deserves special attention in the pediatric patient for two reasons. First, the risk for heart block is theoretically higher in smaller patients. Because

the size of an average RF lesion does not depend on patient size,[12,73,74] the typical lesion is relatively large compared with the size of the heart in a smaller patient. The smaller the patient, the closer the AV node is to the area of the slow pathway and to the posterior and anterior septum. Further, the AV node itself is smaller in small hearts and therefore can be included in a typically sized lesion more easily than in an adult heart. Despite these potential problems, the reported incidence of ablation-induced complete heart block does not appear to be significantly higher in infants and children than in adults.[11,24,62,68,75-78] However, a second consideration is the technical details of pacing if heart block occurs. Superior vena caval thrombosis complicating transvenous pacing can occur with both single- and dual-chamber systems, leading most clinicians to place epicardial pacing systems in children who weigh less than 10 to 20 kg, and only single-chamber transvenous systems in patients weighing under 20 to 25 kg. For this reason, pacing may require chest surgery and may leave the patient physiologically compromised by asynchronous pacing. In addition, the pacing system in a child may need to be maintained for as many as 70 to 80 years, and its presence will almost certainly restrict the child from many competitive sports, thereby setting lifestyle limits that are of less concern for most adult patients. These issues should affect both the decision to ablate and the energy choice for the procedure itself when ablating near the normal AV conduction system, if either the AV node or an AP is targeted. In particular, there are still no reported cases in the literature of permanent AV block with the use of cryoablation; however, a theoretical risk does exist.

Coronary Artery Damage. Acute and late coronary artery injury has been reported after RF ablation for AP-mediated tachycardias in children, adults, and animals.[14,15,39,79-82] These cases have involved both left- and right-sided coronary arteries,[15,79,82] as well as a posterior descending branches of the right coronary artery during ablation of a right posteroseptal AP.[81]

In 2004, we reported a case of coronary damage during slow pathway modification in a 30-month-old, 15.5-kg child with recurrent AVNRT resistant to drug therapy.[13] About 100 seconds after a fourth application of RF energy, ST elevation was noted (Fig. 35-2); it lasted about 15 minutes and was not accompanied by hemodynamic compromise or echocardiographic abnormalities. Selective coronary angiography revealed a dominant right coronary artery giving off

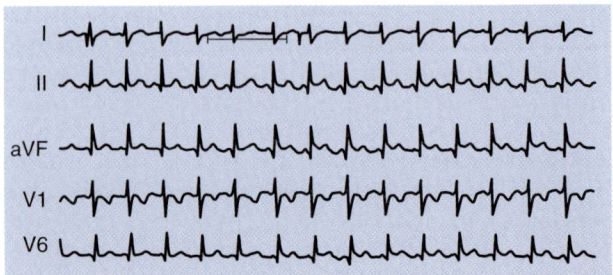

FIGURE 35-2. ST-segment elevation occurring about 100 seconds after the last radiofrequency application for slow pathway modification in a 2.5-year-old with atrioventricular nodal reentrant tachycardia. *(From Blaufox AD, Saul JP. Acute coronary artery stenosis during slow pathway ablation for atrioventricular nodal reentrant tachycardia in a child.* J Cardiovasc Electrophysiol. *2004;15:97–100. With permission.)*

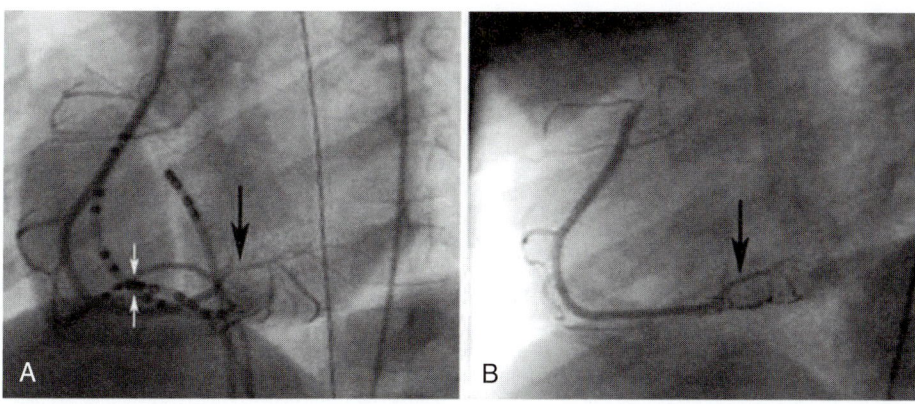

FIGURE 35-3. **A,** Left anterior oblique (LAO) projection of right coronary angiogram a few minutes after the ST-segment changes in Fig. 35-2 had spontaneously normalized. About 80% stenosis (*arrows*) is seen in a posterior left ventricular branch off a dominant right coronary. Ablation catheter was moved away from the septum at the time of angiogram, but had been immediately adjacent to the stenosis during the radiofrequency application. **B,** Similar LAO projection of right coronary angiogram 2 months after ablation. *Arrow* marks are of prior stenosis, which is now resolved. *(From Blaufox AD, Saul JP. Acute coronary artery stenosis during slow pathway ablation for atrioventricular nodal reentrant tachycardia in a child.* J Cardiovasc Electrophysiol. *2004;15:97-100. With permission.)*

a posterior left ventricular branch artery that had an 80% stenosis (Fig. 35-3). The vessel course was within 2 to 3 mm of where the catheter tip had been placed during the last RF application ablation. Acute management was conservative, and after 2 days, repeat angiography revealed some improvement, with an about 50% stenosis. Repeat selective right coronary angiography 2 months later revealed complete resolution of narrowing (Fig. 35-3) and repeat electrophysiologic studies with and without isoproterenol failed to induce any AVNRT. ST segments remained normal with the isoproterenol infusion. Follow-up off medical therapy has been unremarkable.

Although this case is anecdotal, it reveals several important issues regarding the potential for coronary artery injury during RF ablation in children. First, coronary artery injury may occur with slow pathway ablation for AVNRT. Second, acute coronary artery injury has the potential to be missed and is probably an underreported phenomenon. Third, infants and young children may be at particular risk. The inflammatory component of tissue injury caused by RF energy has been shown to invade layers of the right coronary artery, leading to acute narrowing, when RF energy is applied to the atrial side of the lateral tricuspid annulus in pigs.[39] Further maturation of this injury can result in significant late coronary stenosis.[63] Therefore, with RF energy application, coronary stenosis may occur acutely or be delayed. Our patient's injury was almost missed because ST-segment changes did not occur until 100 seconds after the last RF application and resolved spontaneously within minutes, despite a significant persistent stenosis of the involved artery. Other instances of coronary artery injury after RF ablation were also nearly missed because of this delay.[15,82] In large retrospective and prospective studies in which there were no coordinated attempts to investigate coronary injury after RF ablation, the reported incidences of injury were 0.03% in children[24] and 0.06% to 0.1% in adults.[77] However, in a study in which coronary angiography was performed before and after RF ablation for AP-mediated tachycardias, Solomon and associates[80] reported a 1.3% incidence of coronary artery injury in 70 patients. In fact, we have an unreported case of 95% occlusion of the posterior descending artery in a 41-kg, 10-year-old patient undergoing ablation of a left posteroseptal AP in the proximal coronary sinus. The stenosis was completely asymptomatic without ECG changes and was discovered only because we perform routine coronary angiography before and after ablation for posteroseptal AP locations. Therefore, unless evidence for coronary artery injury is actively sought, it will go undiagnosed and underreported.

Smaller children may be at particular risk for coronary injury because the distance between the ablation catheter and the coronary arteries is significantly less than in adults. Although coronary blood flow probably helps reduce this risk, the flow in small coronaries in any patient may be inadequate to prevent damage. Understanding these factors is critical to preventing injury.

Ablation with Cryoenergy versus Radiofrequency Energy. Although RF energy is the time-honored ablation technology for slow pathway modification to treat AVNRT, during the past several years the use of cryoenergy has gained gradual acceptance, particularly in the pediatric population for AVNRT. This growth in acceptance has come from a combination of the safety features of cryoablation discussed in the introductory sections previously and increasing evidence of equivalent acute success and recurrence rates to RF. Earlier reports did find lower acute success rates and higher recurrence rates for AVNRT therapy in both children and adults.[56,83,84] However, as experience has accumulated and technology has progressed,[85] both acute and long-term results have improved to the point that a recent report in 80 children demonstrated a 97% acute success rate and 2% recurrence with cryoablation, equivalent to their prior success with RF.[54] Further, as noted early, there are no reports of permanent AV block with cryoablation, despite its most common use being for ablation of septal arrhythmia substrates.

Summary and Recommendations. To absolutely minimize the chance of coronary injury and AV block in children undergoing slow pathway modification for AVNRT, we make the following recommendations. For all children, cryoablation is the preferred ablation methodology. In addition, for children who weigh less than 20 kg (Table 35-2), (1) selective coronary angiography

TABLE 35-2

PRECAUTIONS FOR ABLATION OF ATRIOVENTRICULAR NODAL REENTRANT TACHYCARDIA IN CHILDREN

Cryoablation is the preferred energy modality.

For children weighing less than 20 kg:

- Before ablation, coronary angiography of the artery supplying the posterior septum should be performed.

- If a small coronary artery is <2-3 mm from an RF ablation site, RF energy should NOT be delivered.

- After RF delivery, immediate repeat coronary angiography should be performed.

RF, radiofrequency energy.

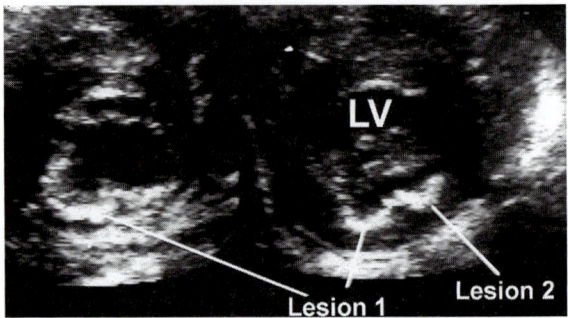

FIGURE 35-4. Short-axis echocardiogram of an infant who died suddenly 2 weeks after an ablation procedure for two left-sided accessory pathways. Immediately after resuscitation, two large echo-dense regions were seen in the left ventricle (LV) despite radiofrequency applications being placed from an atrial approach. These echo-dense lesions correlated with the findings on postmortem examinations. *(From Erickson CC, Walsh EP, Triedman JK, Saul JP. Efficacy and safety of radiofrequency ablation in infants and young children <18 months of age. Am J Cardiol. 1994;74:944-947. With permission.)*

of the artery supplying the posterior septum should be performed before ablation; (2) if a small coronary artery is within 2 to 3 mm of the expected ablation location, RF energy should not be delivered; (3) if any RF energy is delivered, acute follow-up angiography should be performed after ablation; and (4) postablation angiography should be performed whenever RF has been used.

Preexcitation Syndromes in Infants

There are three special considerations in infants that make management of symptoms secondary to an AP different from those in an older child or adult. First, the risk for a sustained reentrant primary atrial tachycardia, such as atrial fibrillation, is very close to zero in the small, structurally normal heart, making the risk for sudden death in infants with WPW very low.[2,86] Second, as noted earlier, AP function may spontaneously disappear by 1 year of age.[2,40] Finally, the known risks of any catheterization, combined with the specific risks of catheter ablation in this age group,[38,87-90] suggest that pharmacologic control should be aggressively pursued before ablation is attempted. This last issue deserves further discussion.

In humans, myocardial cell division probably occurs through about 6 months of age.[91] Although this finding could potentially protect the myocardium from long-term complications secondary to early injury, ventriculotomy scars produced in newborn puppies[92] and RF ablation lesions in immature lambs[12] appear to increase in size during subsequent development. In addition, in contrast to mature ablation scars from adult animals, late lesions from the neonatal lambs were often histologically invasive and poorly demarcated from the surrounding tissue.[12] The potential clinical importance of these results is underscored by a reported sudden death 2 weeks after an AP ablation in a 5-week-old, 3.2-kg infant.[11,87] An echocardiogram from the infant at the time of a brief resuscitation, as well as autopsy findings, revealed relatively large lesions extending into the left ventricle from the intended mitral groove ablation site (Fig. 35-4). Another heightened risk in infants is coronary artery damage due to the potentially close proximity of the coronaries to the ablation catheter and the reduced capacity for protective cooling during RF application in any small coronary artery. Although most reports of coronary damage in the literature have been limited to the posterior septum or a nondominant right coronary

TABLE 35-3

PRECAUTIONS FOR ABLATION OF ACCESSORY ATRIOVENTRICULAR CONNECTIONS IN INFANTS

Cryoablation is the preferred technique.

When RF ablation is necessary:

- Deliver energy as far on the atrial side as possible.

- Use a 5-French RF ablation catheter.

- Perform a test application with low-temperature RF delivery (50° to 55°C) before high-temperature delivery.

- Limit maximal target temperature to 60°C.

- Use short-duration RF delivery 7 to 10 times the time to effect, with 30 to 40 seconds of maximal delivery.

RF, radiofrequency energy.

artery,[13,15,39] complete occlusion of the left circumflex artery was reported in a 5-week-old, 5.0-kg infant undergoing RF ablation of a left lateral AP.[14]

Despite these disturbing cases, nonpharmacologic therapy will be necessary in a small subset of infants with AP-mediated tachycardia.[89,93] Until accurate methods are available to assess lesion size in real time, alternative methodologies should be used in all infants. As discussed earlier, data on the effects of cryotherapy suggest that this form of energy is much less harmful to coronary arteries, even when they are in very close contact,[94] owing to the differing effects of cold and heat on connective tissue and the vascular inflammatory response. Coronary artery flow also protects the vessel through local warming during cryotherapy, similar to the way in which blood flow protects through local cooling during RF energy application. If technical or other considerations require the use of RF energy, considerable caution should be used. RF lesion size is related to catheter-tip size, RF power, tip temperature, and lesion duration.[73,95] Therefore, the following technical modifications should be adopted (Table 35-3): (1) deliver energy in as atrial a location as possible; (2) use a 5-French (5F) catheter tip; (3) use *low temperature mapping* (50° to 55°C) to identify the correct location before higher-temperature RF application[96]; (4) use a lower temperature set point of

60°C for the ablation lesion; and (5) use lesions of shorter duration (7 to 10 times the time to effect, with a maximum of 30 to 40 seconds). The future development of real-time ultrasonographic or other modality monitoring of lesion size may also help reduce the procedural risks.[97]

Preexcitation Syndromes in Patients with Structural Congenital Heart Disease

Although it is not strictly a pediatric issue, the combination of structural heart disease and arrhythmia is clearly encountered more often by pediatric electrophysiologists than by others. In agreement with previous studies,[27,98] a review of this issue in unselected patients with congenital heart disease at the Children's Hospital in Boston found that preexcitation syndromes are statistically increased in patients with Ebstein malformation, L-transposition of the great arteries, or hypertrophic myopathy (Table 35-4).[26] Of course, preexcitation also occurs in other patients with congenital heart disease, but with an incidence not statistically higher than in the general population.

Anatomy

The association of WPW with Ebstein anomaly and with the left-sided tricuspid valve in L-transposition probably has its basis in the embryology of tricuspid valve formation.[99-101] The leaflets of the AV valves normally develop through a process of undermining or delamination of the interior surface of the embryonic ventricular myocardium. Separation of the atrium from the ventricle occurs through completion of this process and encroachment of fibrous tissue from the AV sulcus. The mitral valve and the anterior leaflet of the tricuspid valve are fully delaminated early in development; however, the posterior and septal leaflets of the tricuspid valve are not even fully formed by 3 months' gestation.[101] Ebstein anomaly appears to occur when there is arrested development of tricuspid valve formation sometime between delamination of the anterior and of the posterior leaflets. The high prevalence of preexcitation combined with anatomic findings of accessory connections in a number of selected cases of Ebstein anomaly[100,102] suggests that the arrested valve development results in remnants of muscular or specialized tissue connections that cross the AV groove. In fact, multiple pathways are common in these patients, often with a combination of a posteroseptal pathway and one or more additional free wall pathways.

Pathophysiology

The electrophysiology of the APs in patients with congenital heart disease is not particularly unique. Bidirectional, antegrade-only, and retrograde-only APs have been reported. Further, these patients have the same range of tachyarrhythmias found in patients with structurally normal hearts: orthodromic and antidromic AV reciprocating tachycardias

TABLE 35-4			
ASSOCIATIONS OF WOLFF-PARKINSON-WHITE SYNDROME AND CONGENITAL HEART LESIONS			
Lesion	**No. of Patients**	**No. of Patients with WPW Syndrome**	**Prevalence (%)**
Ebstein	234	21	8.97*
L-TGA	588	8	1.36*
HCM	300	3	1.00*
Pulmonary valve disease	424	2	0.47
Tricuspid atresia	458	2	0.44
VSD-membranous	2659	10	0.38
DORV	955	3	0.31
HLHS	666	2	0.30
MVP	1096	3	0.27
Dextrocardia	427	1	0.23
Trisomy 21	916	2	0.22
TOF-pulmonary atresia	556	1	0.18
TOF	2520	3	0.12
AV canal defect	2058	2	0.09
D-TGA (all)	2156	2	0.09
Coarctation	2862	1	0.04*
d-TGA/IVS	704	0	0.00
Mitral atresia	417	0	0.00
Total	20303	66	0.33

*$P < .01$ compared with general population estimate of 0.30%.
AV, atrioventricular; DORV, double-outlet right ventricle; HCM, hypertrophic cardiomyopathy; HLHS, hypoplastic left heart syndrome; IVS, intact ventricular septum; MVP, mitral valve prolapse; D-TGA, transposition of the great arteries with D-looped ventricles; L-TGA, "corrected" transposition of the great arteries; TOF, tetralogy of Fallot; VSD, ventricular septal defect.
Data from Children's Hospital, Boston, and New England Infant Regional Cardiac Program Computer Records.

and other SVTs (e.g., AVNRT, atrial flutter or fibrillation), with bystander participation of an antegrade conducting AP. However, the physiologic and clinical implications of the tachycardia may be markedly different in patients with congenital heart disease.

Abnormal hemodynamics, increased incidence of isolated atrial and ventricular ectopy, sometimes poor tolerance of antiarrhythmic therapy, and the need for surgical repair that accompanies congenital heart disease all contribute to an increased need for aggressive arrhythmia management in this patient population. However, abnormal anatomy and atypical conduction systems may also enhance the difficulty and risks of either surgical or catheter ablation (Fig. 35-5). Although RF catheter ablation is difficult in these patients, results have been good enough to recommend the procedure in all patients who require subsequent surgical repair to avoid postoperative arrhythmias as a complication and in most symptomatic patients older than 1 year of age who have significant structural lesions.

A review of the reported cases of RF ablation in patients with congenital heart disease revealed that most of the patients had Ebstein malformation of a right-sided tricuspid valve.[25,77,78,103,104] However, a significant proportion had more complex anatomy, with AV valve discordance (right atrium to left ventricle, left atrium to right ventricle—S, L, L or I, D, D) and often heterotaxy. Multiple pathways are extremely common in this group, occurring in 30% to 80% of patients,[25,78,102,103,105] compared with 5% to 10% of patients without congenital heart disease.[76-78,106,107] Like the patients with Ebstein malformation, those with AV discordance had all of their APs associated with the tricuspid valve regardless of atrial situs, AV relationship, or valve function. This finding is in contrast to the more random location of APs reported for patients without congenital heart disease.[76-78,106-110] Hypertrophic cardiomyopathy is the exception: APs are more likely to be on the normal left-sided mitral valve.

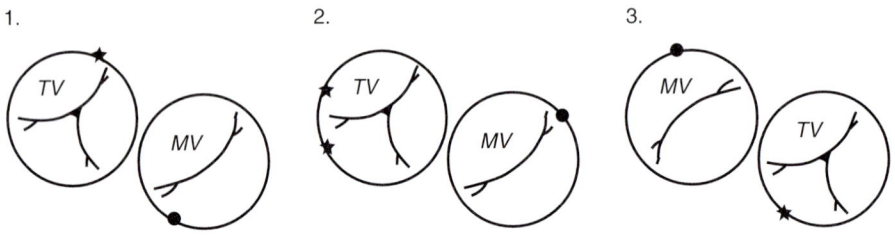

1. DORV {I, D, A}, situs inversus, pulmonary stenosis, PAPVC, dextrocardia

2. TGA {I, D, D}, situs inversus, subpulmonary stenosis

3. DORV {S, L, L}, situs inversus, pulmonary stenosis, straddling mitral valve

● HIS bundle
★ Accessory pathway

A

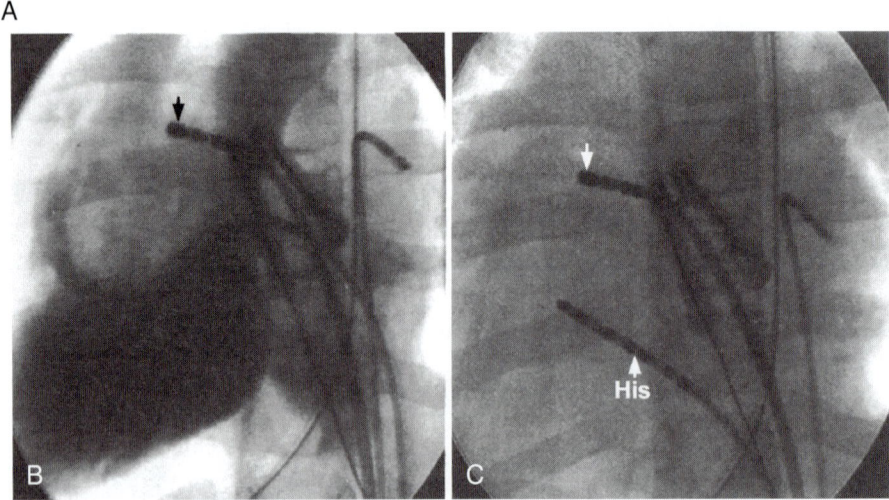

FIGURE 35-5. A, A cartoon demonstrating the locations of the mitral valve (MV), tricuspid valve (TV), His bundle, and accessory pathways in three patients with preexcitation syndromes and atrioventricular discordance. Patient 1 corresponds with **B** and **C**. The angiogram in the anteroposterior projection (**C**) illustrates the importance of defining the anatomy of the atrioventricular valves. The decapolar catheter (*bottom white arrow* in **C**) was advanced from the left-sided inferior vena cava across the mitral valve and positioned with the second pair of electrodes at the His bundle. The mapping catheter (*black arrow* in **B**, *upper white arrow* in **C**) was advanced from the inferior vena cava across the atrial septum to the right-sided (anatomic) left atrium and positioned at the location of the accessory pathway, which in this case was at the superior and anterior portion of the left-sided tricuspid valve. The unmarked catheter is an atrial pacing catheter in the left-sided right atrium. DORV, double outlet right ventricle; PAPVC, partial anomalous pulmonary venous connection; TGA, transposition of the great arteries. *(From Saul JP, Walsh EP, Triedman JK. Mechanisms and therapy of complex arrhythmias in pediatric patients.* J Cardiovasc Electrophysiol. *1995;6:1129-1148. With permission.)*

Mapping and Ablation in Patients with Ebstein Anomaly

Some aspects of the procedure in patients with Ebstein malformation are of special note. First, differentiation of atrial and ventricular signals and precise localization of the AV groove can be difficult, leading to a lack of specificity for what appear to be excellent signals in predicting a successful ablation site. In fact, very early ventricular activations, which might be termed *pseudo* AP potentials, can often be seen near the AV groove (Fig. 35-6). This issue is particularly important for older patients who have large hearts with poorly defined AV grooves. The true AV groove is best identified by the right coronary artery. Use of a right coronary electrode wire can be considered[76,111] but may be difficult because of a diminutive right coronary artery, and the

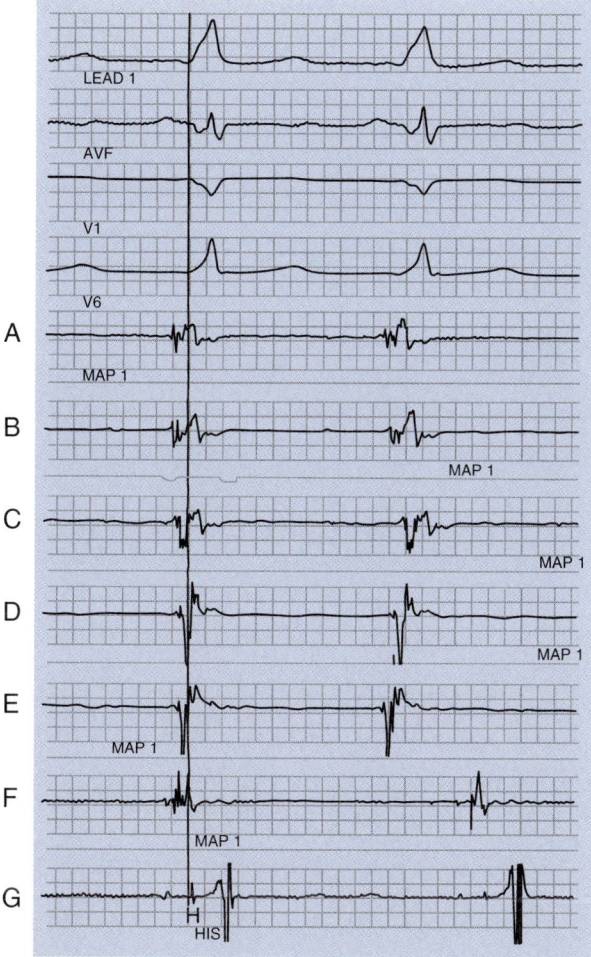

FIGURE 35-6. Electrograms near the accessory pathway in a patient with Ebstein malformation. Electrograms *A* through *F* were recorded with the distal pair of an ablating catheter very near the point of successful ablation shown in *F*. Note early ventricular activation in *A* through *D*, despite lack of success. Electrograms in *D* and *E* were not significantly different, but *E* had transient success. *F*, the point of permanent success, probably has the earliest activation; however, the differences are much more clear in retrospect. The *dark vertical line* marks the point of earliest surface QRS activation for all electrograms. *G* shows the position of the atrial and His electrograms. Pathway location was posterior septal. MAP, mapping catheter. *(From Saul JP. Ablation of atrioventricular accessory pathways in children with and without congenital heart disease. In Huang SK [ed]: Radiofrequency Catheter Ablation of Cardiac Arrhythmias: Basic Concepts and Clinical Applications. Mt. Kisko, NY: Futura; 1994:365-396. With permission.)*

wire may need to be in place for long periods if multiple pathways are present. A safer and recommended alternative is continual display of the relevant coronary angiogram using a real-time biplane image storage and display system. As with any AP, searching for balanced atrial and ventricular electrograms during mapping is important. Despite these maneuvers, it may still be very difficult to define the AV groove in these patients, necessitating more test applications of the ablation modality to identify the correct location. Catheter stabilization for free wall pathways in the largest hearts is difficult and is not sufficiently improved through the use of a long sheath or a variety of approaches.[11] The overall issue of patient size is addressed later.

As expected, it appears to be impossible to approach the ventricular side of the tricuspid valve in patients with Ebstein malformation. No specific reports have noted the use of nonstandard ablation technologies for these patients, but a few observations can be made. Coronary damage has been reported on multiple occasions in patients with Ebstein anomaly, probably because of the thin RV wall and often diminutive right coronary artery. Consequently, despite the tendency to use higher-power ablation systems with active or passive cooling for difficult cases, such technologies should be employed only if an adequate distance between the catheter tip and the artery has been documented. The definition of *adequate* here depends on the size of the nearby coronary artery: the larger the size, the safer the ablation. Further, strong consideration should be given to the use of cryotherapy, at least as a mapping tool. Safety is enhanced, and the adhesion of the catheter may be particularly useful in larger patients.

If multiple pathways are present, persistence may be the electrophysiologist's best weapon for successful ablation. In general, 80% to 90% of patients can be rendered arrhythmia free by the procedure, with relatively infrequent major complications such as permanent AV block.[23,25,78,103] However, recurrence rates have been reported to be as high as 40%, particularly if multiple pathways are present.[23,25,78,103]

Atrioventricular Discordance

Ablation procedures in patients with heterotaxy or AV discordance require special considerations. First, detailed echocardiography and angiography are instrumental in defining the complex anatomy of the atria, the AV ring, and the coronary sinus, so that the cameras and catheters can be positioned appropriately (Fig. 35-5). Second, careful attention must be given to locating the normal conduction system. In virtually all patients with AV discordance, the AP has been associated with the tricuspid valve, whereas the His bundle has been associated more closely with the mitral valve. As predicted by Ho and Andersen,[112] the normal conduction axis is often located at an anterior position along the AV groove. Once the "normal" and abnormal conduction fibers are located, electrophysiologic study and RF ablation of the APs can proceed with less risk for damage to the normal conduction system.

Mapping and ablation require detailed knowledge of the anatomy and often innovative approaches. For instance, in cases of atrial inversion (right atrium on the left, or vice versa) with AV discordance (I, D, D), an atrial approach to the right-sided tricuspid valve may require a *reverse* transseptal procedure from the left-sided inferior vena cava and right atrium to the right-sided left atrium. If present, the coronary sinus in such cases will also be reversed. AVNRT may also be present in these patients, requiring identification of the slow pathway of an AV node that is typically along the anterior mitral annulus. Clearly, the need for a detailed understanding of the anatomy in these cases cannot be overemphasized. Ablation technologies similar to those recommended for patients with Ebstein anomaly are applicable to patients with AV discordance as well.

Double Atrioventricular Nodes

In hearts with normal or inverted atrial situs, but discordant AV connections (S, L, L or I, D, D), the anterosuperior ventricle is a morphologic left ventricle that carries with it the mitral valve.[113] When all four valves are well formed in such hearts, the condition is often referred to as *corrected transposition* because the physiologic connections are all correct (i.e., systemic venous return flows to the lungs, and pulmonary venous return flows to the aorta). As Anderson and others[99,112] have described, the AV node in corrected transposition is typically situated superior and anterior in the atrial wall, near the anterolateral quadrant of the mitral valve (Fig. 35-7A). The penetrating bundle then runs in the fibrous continuity between the right-sided mitral valve and the anterior cusp of the posterior great artery, eventually linking to the left bundle branch on the right side of the ventricular septum. The right bundle branch then penetrates the ventricular septum to emerge in the inferior left-sided right ventricle. A second AV node that is often present more inferiorly, in the normal area of the triangle of Koch, can also link to the ventricular conduction fibers posteriorly, usually inferior to a ventricular septal defect. If the posterior and anterior ventricular bundle branches link together, a conduction sling (Fig. 35-7B), sometimes referred to as a *Mönckeberg sling*, is formed.[100-102] These anatomic findings provide the substrate for a host of different modes of ventricular excitation or preexcitation and AV reciprocating tachycardias. However, before 1999,[114] there had been no electrophysiologic documentation of this phenomenon.

In 2001, we reported on seven of these patients, all of whom had AV discordance (two S, L, L and one I, D, D) and characteristics consistent with the diagnosis of two separate AV nodes (twin or double).[115] Five of the seven patients also had a malaligned AV canal defect. The electrophysiologic findings included (1) the existence of two discrete, nonpreexcited QRS morphologies, each with an associated His bundle electrogram and a normal His bundle–ventricle (HV) interval; (2) decremental as well as adenosine-sensitive anterograde and retrograde conduction; and (3) inducible AV reciprocating tachycardia with anterograde conduction over one AV node and retrograde conduction over the other. Ventricular premature beats placed into tachycardia while the His was refractory could preexcite the atrium, indicating that the tachycardia involved two AV connections. In all cases, applications of RF energy at the site of the bidirectional pathway resulted in transient *junctional* acceleration with an identical QRS morphology to that generated by anterograde conduction over the targeted AV node, and modified or eliminated both antegrade and retrograde conduction at that site. Although there is a possibility that one or the other of these pathways

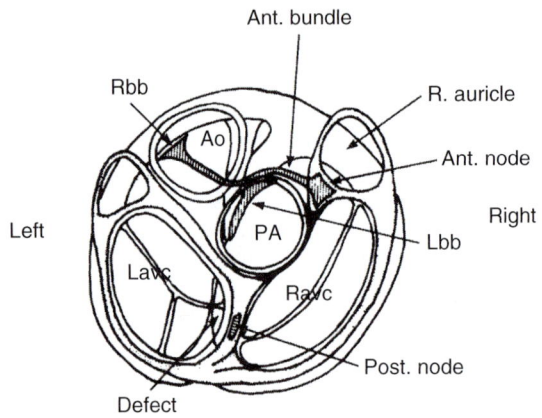

A

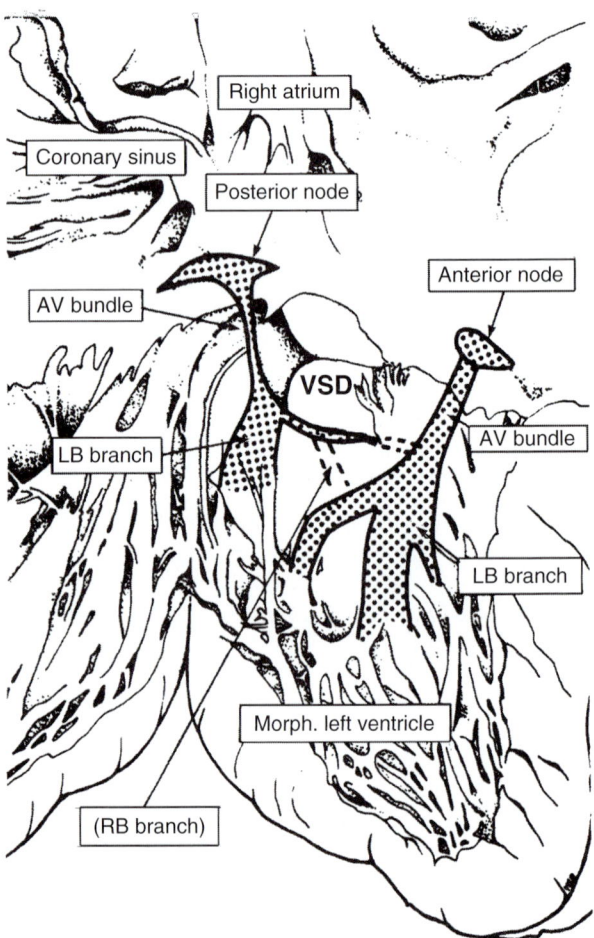

B

FIGURE 35-7. A, Diagram of the base of the heart and the atrioventricular (AV) conduction system in L-transposition of the great arteries (corrected) as seen from above. Note the bicommissural mitral valve on the *right* and the tricommissural tricuspid valve on the *left*. The AV node may either lie posteriorly (Post. node) in the septum in a somewhat normal location, anteriorly on the right-sided mitral valve (Ant. bundle), or in both places. Lbb, left bundle branch; Rbb, right bundle branch. **B,** Diagram of the conduction system from a patient with corrected transposition in a crisscross heart, with AV valve anatomy similar to that shown in **A**. Note the dual conduction system with both the posterior and anterior AV nodes penetrating into the ventricles, and near connection of the conduction systems within the ventricle. LB, left bundle; RB, right bundle; VSD, ventricular septal defect. *(A, From Anderson RH, Arnold R, Wilkinson JL. The conducting system in congenitally corrected transposition. Lancet. 1973;1:1286-1288; B, from Symons JC, Shinebourne EA, Joseph MC, et al. Criss-cross heart with congenitally corrected transposition: Report of a case with d-transposed aorta and ventricular preexcitation. Eur J Cardiol. 1977;5:493. With permission.)*

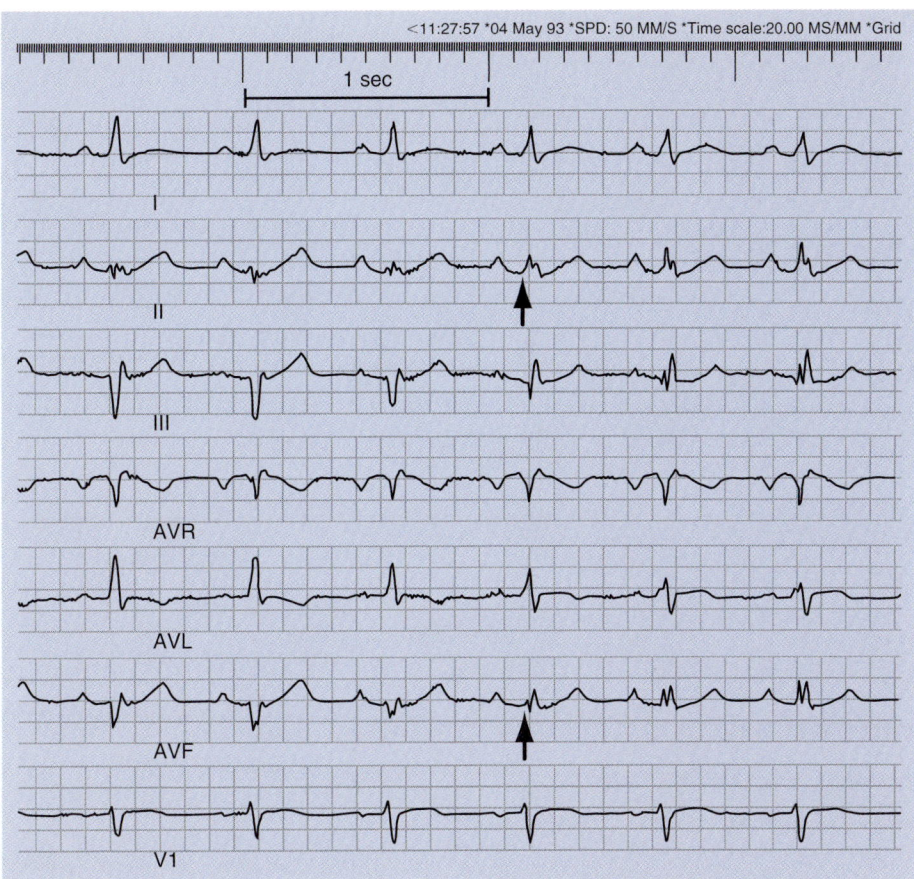

FIGURE 35-8. Six-lead electrocardiogram in a patient with L-looped ventricles and common atrioventricular (AV) canal. Note spontaneously changing QRS morphology without obvious changes in the PR interval (*arrows*). The first morphology has a superior axis consistent with non-preexcited rhythm from a posterior location as in common AV canal. The other morphology was presumed to be from a second anterior AV node as per the electrophysiologic study findings (see Fig. 35-9 and text). *(From Saul JP. Ablation of atrioventricular accessory pathways in children with and without congenital heart disease. In Huang SK [ed]:* Radiofrequency Catheter Ablation of Cardiac Arrhythmias: Basic Concepts and Clinical Applications. *Mt. Kisko, NY: Futura; 1994:365-396. With permission.)*

was a *Mahaim-type* AV fiber, their locations and the presence of near-normal HV intervals, retrograde conduction, *orthodromic* tachycardia, and *junctional*-type acceleration during RF ablation all favor a second AV node. The precise etiology may make little difference for the medical management of such patients, but is important if damage to the best of the two conduction systems is to be avoided during ablation procedures performed before surgery in these patients with complex anatomy.

One patient with AV discordance and complete common AV canal was particularly illustrative of the features described. Two QRS morphologies were seen during *normal* rhythm, each with a normal PR interval (Fig. 35-8). One of the QRS morphologies (#1) was more typical of an endocardial cushion defect with a superior axis. At electrophysiology study, QRS morphology #1 could be produced by posterior atrial pacing and had an HV interval of about 50 milliseconds, with the His potential found posteriorly in the ventricle (Fig. 35-9). The other QRS morphology (#2) could be produced by anterior atrial pacing and had an associated HV interval (from the posterior His) of only 20 milliseconds, but the QRS appearance did not strongly suggest preexcitation (Fig. 35-9). The antegrade effective refractory period (ERP) of this anterior pathway was about 200 milliseconds. Earliest ventricular activation was near the septal

remnant regardless of QRS morphology. A regular tachycardia involving (1) QRS morphology #1 (Fig. 35-9), (2) a 1:1 A/V relation, (3) a minimal ventriculoatrial (VA) interval of 70 milliseconds, and (4) earliest retrograde atrial activation at the left anterior AV groove near the midline (tricuspid side of common valve) could be reproducibly induced with ventricular pacing. Ventricular premature beats placed into tachycardia while the His was refractory could preexcite the atrium, indicating that the tachycardia involved two AV connections. Retrograde VA conduction was all through the anterior pathway, was decremental, and had an ERP of 230 milliseconds. Application of RF energy near the point of earliest retrograde conduction (anterior and to the left) resulted in transient junctional acceleration of QRS rhythm #2, followed by a sudden change to a regular slower rhythm of QRS #1 (Fig. 35-10; and see Fig. 35-18, later). After RF application, VA conduction was eliminated, and tachycardia was noninducible. These findings illustrate the following important features: (1) there were two antegrade conduction pathways, one posteroseptal and one anteroseptal; (2) both pathways were on the left (tricuspid) side of the common AV ring; (3) both pathways had slow conduction properties; (4) retrograde conduction occurred over only the anterior pathway; and (5) tachycardia was *orthodromic*, antegrade posterior, and retrograde anterior.

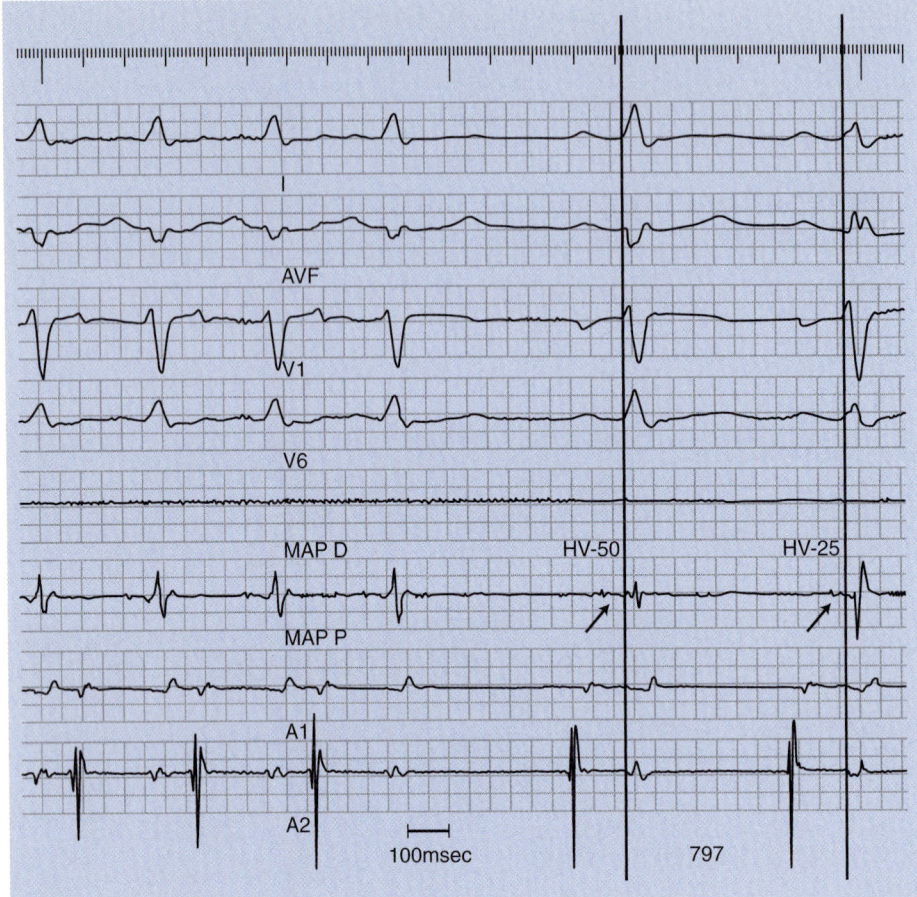

FIGURE 35-9. Intracardiac recordings in same patient as Fig. 35-8 with L-loop ventricles and common atrioventricular (AV) canal. Note HV interval of 50 msec during the tachycardia and the first sinus beat after spontaneous termination. QRS morphologies for the tachycardia and this beat were identical. Also note shorter HV interval of 25 msec during the last beat, which is the anterior AV node QRS morphology. *MAP, mapping catheter. (From Saul JP. Ablation of atrioventricular accessory pathways in children with and without congenital heart disease. In Huang SK [ed]:* Radiofrequency Catheter Ablation of Cardiac Arrhythmias: Basic Concepts and Clinical Applications. *Mt. Kisko, NY: Futura; 1994:365-396. With permission)*

Clearly, an extensive understanding of the anatomy and electrophysiology should be obtained in such patients before proceeding to mapping and ablation. Further, lack of clarity in defining the anatomy of AV conduction in these patients suggests that ablation should first be undertaken using cryotherapy, proceeding to RF energy only if cryotherapy is unsuccessful or after a recurrence. The one caveat to this recommendation is that low-power RF application may be helpful in identifying the location of the anterior and posterior AV nodes through their acceleration response when heated.

Patient Size and Structural Disease

One observation that is difficult to prove statistically but seems clear from our own experience is that the smaller chamber size in smaller patients with structural heart disease is a technical asset in catheter ablation. In our initial series,[25] a total of seven procedures lasting an average of 4.1 hours were required to ablate seven of nine accessory connections in six patients weighing less than 40 kg, whereas seven procedures lasting an average of 6.5 hours were used to ablate only three of seven connections in four patients who weighed more than 40 kg. Although larger patient size may be useful when the retrograde approach to left-sided accessory connections is used, smaller patient size appears

to be helpful for catheter stabilization during an atrial approach, particularly in patients with structural heart disease and potentially very large hearts. Consequently, earlier intervention during childhood is preferable to waiting for near-adult size.

Recurrence Risk

The incidence of recurrence of tachycardia or preexcitation in patients who were initially successfully ablated has been reported to be as high as 40%.[24,77,78,106,116] Although this recurrence risk is higher than the range of 8% to 12% reported in other large series, the authors did note an increased risk for recurrence with right-sided pathways and with multiple pathways.[24,106,116] Both these conditions occur with increased frequency in this patient population, and, in combination with the complex anatomy, this probably accounts for the high recurrence rate.

Summary

Based on our own observations and those in the literature, a few recommendations concerning catheter ablation in patients with congenital defects can be made: (1) an attempt should be made to carefully identify the location of the normal AV conducting system, particularly in patients with AV discordance; (2) the anatomic tricuspid valve is the

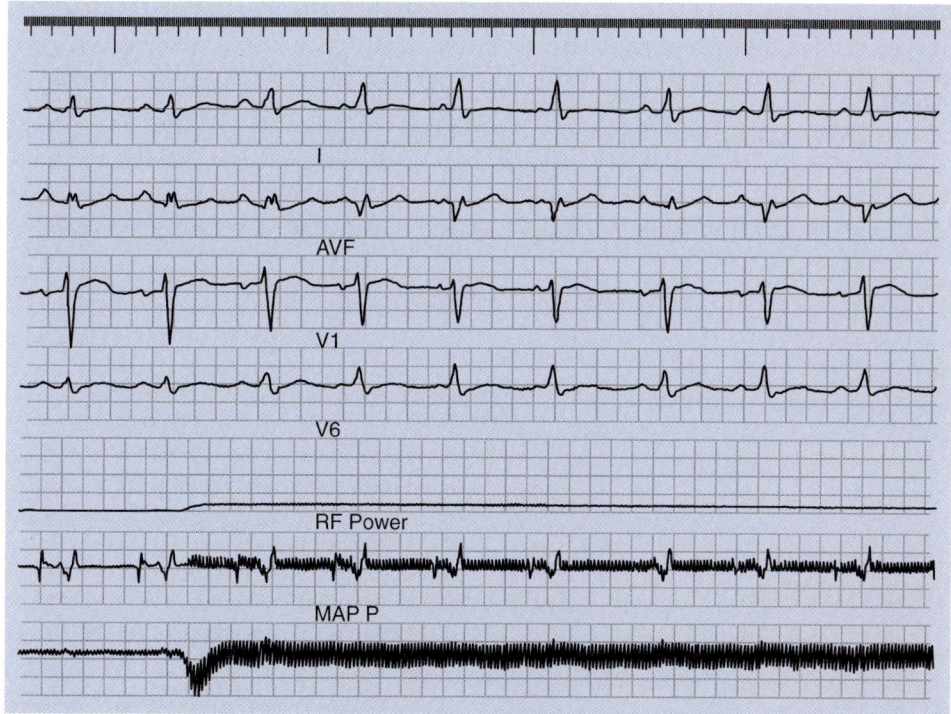

FIGURE 35-10. Response to radiofrequency (RF) ablation at the location of the anterior atrioventricular (AV) node in the same patient as in Figs. 35-8 and 35-9. Within 1 second after application of RF energy, the PR interval shortened, presumably owing to junctional acceleration. About 1 second later, the junctional acceleration stopped, and the PR interval lengthened with a change in QRS morphology consistent with loss of the morphology associated with the anterior AV node that had a shorter HV interval. MAP, mapping catheter. *(From Saul JP. Ablation of atrioventricular accessory pathways in children with and without congenital heart disease. In Huang SK [ed]: Radiofrequency Catheter Ablation of Cardiac Arrhythmias: Basic Concepts and Clinical Applications. Mt. Kisko, NY: Futura; 1994:365-396. With permission)*

most likely location for accessory connections; (3) smaller patient size may be an asset; (4) an atrial approach should probably be attempted first for connections around the tricuspid annulus (right- or left-sided); (5) the true AV groove should be well identified, using either atrial and ventricular electrogram balance, a coronary angiogram, or, if available, a coronary mapping wire in larger patients; and (6) consider double AV nodes as the substrate for reentrant tachycardia in patients with AV discordance and malaligned AV canal defects who have two distinct QRS morphologies that both have normal PR intervals. With these caveats in mind, it appears that, despite the difficulties of unusual anatomic landmarks and abnormally positioned conduction systems, most APs in patients with structural congenital heart disease can be safely and effectively ablated.

Atrial Flutter or Fibrillation in the Absence of Other Heart Disease

In children, atrial reentrant tachycardias are relatively rare in the absence of either structural or functional heart disease. The term *lone atrial flutter* or *fibrillation* has been applied here, referring to the isolated nature of the arrhythmia findings. However, both of these tachyarrhythmias are occasionally observed in pediatric patients. There are two age ranges for presentation. Perhaps the most common is during the third trimester of fetal life, when atrial flutter accounts for up to one third of fetal tachycardias,[10] often lasting through delivery and leading to ventricular dysfunction. Neonatal atrial flutter almost universally resolves without recurrence if it can be managed successfully

during fetal and early neonatal life.[117] Consequently, ablation therapy for such infants should not be necessary and has never been reported.

A second presentation peak occurs during adolescence, when both atrial flutter and fibrillation may occur in the absence of any identifiable structural, hormonal, or chemical cause. Although initial management should be conservative, in contrast to the cases in infants, the arrhythmia typically recurs multiple times in this age group despite medical therapy, creating a need for ablation therapy similar to the scenario in adults. The use of catheter ablation has been reported for both flutter and fibrillation in young patients. Success rates were greater than 90% for the flutter subgroup in a relatively large series of patients in the Pediatric Ablation Registry.[3] Acute success was also recently reported in seven of eight pediatric patients with paroxysmal fibrillation who underwent either ablation of a single ectopic atrial focus or pulmonary vein electrical isolation.[118] Further, one of the cases that we included in a series of ablations for patients with ectopic atrial tachycardia (EAT) in 1992[119] was a 12-year-old boy who presented with recurrent atrial fibrillation that was permanently eliminated after ablation of a single left pulmonary vein ectopic focus.

Specific technical details for ablation of either atrial flutter or fibrillation in the larger child are not particularly different from those in adults and are not repeated here; however, the decision of when to ablate can be quite different, particularly for fibrillation. After conversion from a first episode of one of these arrhythmias, either no therapy or a drug to block the AV node response is adequate. After recurrences, the threshold for ablation of atrial flutter can be similar to that in adults. The use of ablation therapy for the rare cases of atrial fibrillation in pediatric patients is also appealing, but the high emphasis on safety over efficacy for all children mandates that a decision to use RF ablation in this age group be considered only after failure of multiple antiarrhythmic agents. Further, the technique chosen should be the most conservative in terms of safety because complications such as pulmonary vein stenosis and stroke can be devastating to a child.

Atrial and Ventricular Tachycardias in Patients with Congenital Heart Disease

Atrial and ventricular tachycardias in patients with congenital heart disease are covered in Chapters 14 and 32.

Arrhythmias Unique to the Pediatric Patient

A variety of issues may account for differences between adults and children in the incidence or prevalence of an arrhythmia (Table 35-1).[10] For the arrhythmia labeled *congenital* junctional ectopic tachycardia (JET), the issue is definitional because its congenital nature has been presumed based on presentation with incessant junctional tachycardia before 6 months of age and familial tendencies.[120,121] Patients with other incessant tachycardias, including EAT and the permanent form of junctional reciprocating tachycardia (PJRT), may present as children because they are unlikely to reach maturity with their arrhythmia owing to a tendency to develop ventricular dysfunction and congestive heart failure secondary to the tachycardia.[122,123] Finally, the cardiac substrate for arrhythmia is clearly age dependent, in terms of both myocardial cellular development[124] and the presence of structural congenital heart disease.

Incessant Ectopic Atrial Tachycardia in the Child

EAT is an uncommon rhythm disorder that accounts for 5% to 20% of SVTs in children (Table 35-1) but fewer than 2% of SVTs in adult series.[119,125] It involves abnormally rapid impulse generation from a single atrial focus outside the sinus node. Because the tachycardia is frequently incessant, the presentation is accompanied by a functional left ventricular myopathy in 50% to 75% of cases.[122,123,126] Although EAT may resolve spontaneously in some patients, particularly those younger than 6 months,[52,127,128] in many cases neither conventional antiarrhythmic drug therapy[21,119,126,129] nor arrhythmia surgery has been highly successful[21,110,130,131] (Table 35-5). The fact that ventricular function usually returns to normal if the arrhythmia can be controlled[122,123] has led to an aggressive search for other therapies, most notably catheter ablation.

Mechanism

Although a precise cellular mechanism of EAT has not been determined, a variety of clinical and electrophysiologic data, as well as intracellular recordings from a single operative specimen, strongly suggest a disorder of automaticity.[129,132] EAT is a nearly incessant tachycardia with wide fluctuations in atrial rate that often parallel the autonomic state and respond to isoproterenol in a similar way to sinus rhythm (Fig. 35-11A,B).[126] Typically, the ectopic focus rate changes gradually with a "warm-up" at initiation, and a "cool-down," sometimes associated with exit block, at termination. Programmed atrial stimulation is usually of little value in initiation of EAT, and neither atrial stimulation nor direct current (DC) cardioversion is useful for terminating it. Finally, the reset response of the EAT focus to single premature atrial stimuli can be almost identical to that of the normal sinus node (Fig. 35-11C).[126] These characteristics virtually rule out reentry as the underlying mechanism, but they do not absolutely exclude triggered activity. However, microelectrode recordings from left atrial appendage tissue obtained at the time of surgical excision of an EAT focus revealed a high resting membrane potential and spontaneous phase 4 automaticity.[126,132] Therefore, although it remains possible that the clinical condition of EAT may include cases caused by a triggered mechanism, at least some characteristic ones are the result of automaticity. Alternatively, the characteristics of many EATs in adults are distinctly different, with features favoring a triggered mechanism in many patients.[133,134]

The underlying cause of EAT in the pediatric patient has not been elucidated. Most cases are not associated with specific pathologic abnormalities of either noninvolved cardiac or skeletal muscle,[126,132] nor with resected atrial tissue near the focus.[21] Pathologic findings have been either normal or limited to nonspecific fibrosis, cellular hypertrophy, and patchy fatty infiltrates, all of which may be secondary to the tachycardia-induced myopathy.[135] Other clues to the etiology of EAT may come from the use of RF catheter therapy. First, it has been observed that EAT almost always involves a small area of tissue or a single cell because it is eliminated within a few seconds after application of RF energy.[93,112] Second, just before successful elimination of the foci, the ectopic rate often accelerates, consistent with enhanced automaticity observed in response to RF energy in other tissue (Fig. 35-12).[137] Finally, the foci seem to cluster in a few specific areas of the right and left atrial appendages, and near or within the pulmonary venous ostia (Fig. 35-13). Of note, one of the primary differences between EAT in adult versus pediatric patients is a propensity for right-sided foci in adults,[133,134] whereas both left- and right-sided ones are seen in children (Table 35-5).[21,119] These findings all suggest that EAT involves subtle electrical changes in otherwise normal tissue from trabeculated atria or connections between the primitive atria and the systemic veins.

Therapy

Virtually every class of antiarrhythmic agent has been used as pharmacologic therapy for EAT. Although no single class or agent appears to be universally effective, the best results have been observed with class IC and class III agents,[21,27,138,139] with amiodarone perhaps the most effective. Occasional successes have also been reported with phenytoin and β-blockers; however, in a large series of 54 young patients, a fully effective drug was found for only 50% of cases.[21] Ventricular, but rarely atrial, rate control may occa-

TABLE 35-5

SINGLE FOCUS ECTOPIC ATRIAL TACHYCARDIA

Study	Patients				RA*	LA*	Mean age at Pres (yr)	Positive Initial Drug Response†	Mean Follow-Up (yr)	Spontaneous Resolution (No. of Patients)‡	
	Total	Age <6 mo at Pres	CHD	Incessant (vs Repetitive)						Total	Age <6 mo at Pres
Koike et al, 1988[118]	9	1	—	≥4	7	1	6.6§	6	2.0	3	0
Mehta et al, 1988[103]	10	5	1	10	8	2	0.5§	9	1.7§	4	3
Garson et al, 1990[16]	54	—	4	48	40	14	7.2	35	4.2	≤12	—
von Bernuth et al, 1992[119]	21	8	0	14	14	7	2.0§	18	2.5§	5	3
Dhala et al, 1994[105]	10	≤4	≤4	—	—	—	2.5§	≤4	—	0	0
Naheed et al, 1995[101]	6	3	0	—	5	1	2.5§	6	3.1	5	—
Walsh et al, 1994[116]	26	2	1	16	8	12	12.0	11	2.0§	0	0
Bauersfeld et al, 1995[102]	19	19	7	—	—	—	<0.5	18	1.6	17	17
Totals	155	42/101 (42%)	17/146 (12%)	92/120 (77%)	82/119 (69%)	37/119 (31%)	—	107/155 (69%)	—	46/155 (30%)	23/32 (72%)

* Ectopic focus location by either electrocardiogram or electrophysiology study for patients reported.
† Full or partial response considered clinically successful by authors.
‡ No tachycardia seen on 24-hour Holter monitoring without drug therapy.
§ Median.
CHD, congenital heart disease; LA, left atrium; Pres, presentation; RA, right atrium.

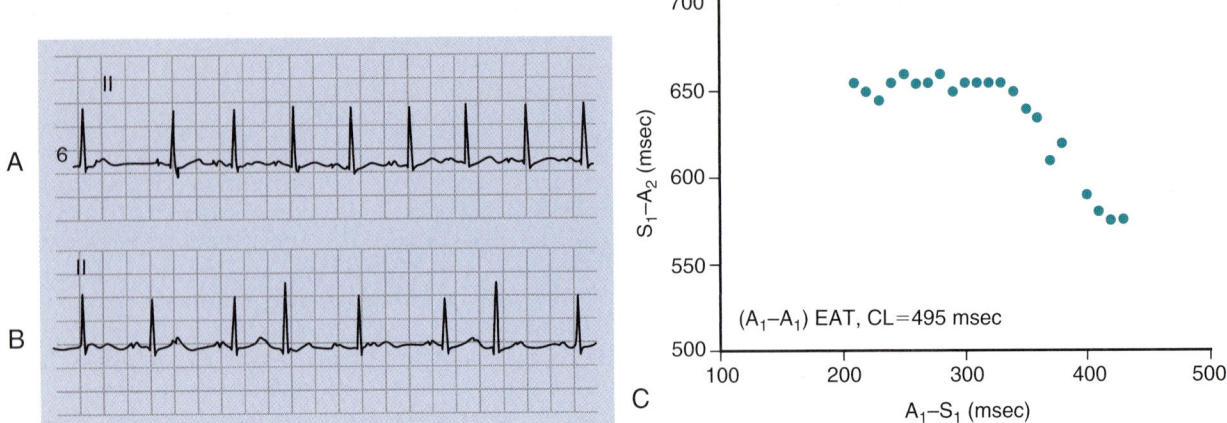

FIGURE 35-11. Surface electrocardiogram in patient with ectopic atrial tachycardia (EAT) at rest (**A**) and after mild exertion (**B**). **C,** The effect of single atrial premature stimuli (A_1-S_1) on the timing of ectopic atrial tachycardia focus discharge (S_1-A_2). The curve is similar to data generated for measurement of sinoatrial conduction time and demonstrates a clear reset zone. CL, cycle length. *(From Walsh EP. Ablation of ectopic atrial tachycardia in children. In Huang SK [ed]:* Radiofrequency Catheter Ablation of Cardiac Arrhythmias: Basic Concepts and Clinical Applications. *Mt. Kisko, NY: Futura; 1994:421–443. With permission)*

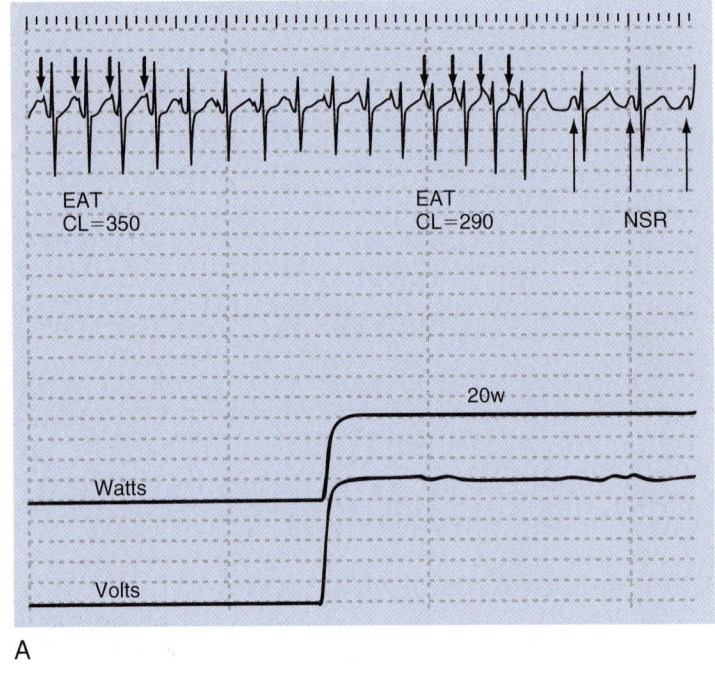

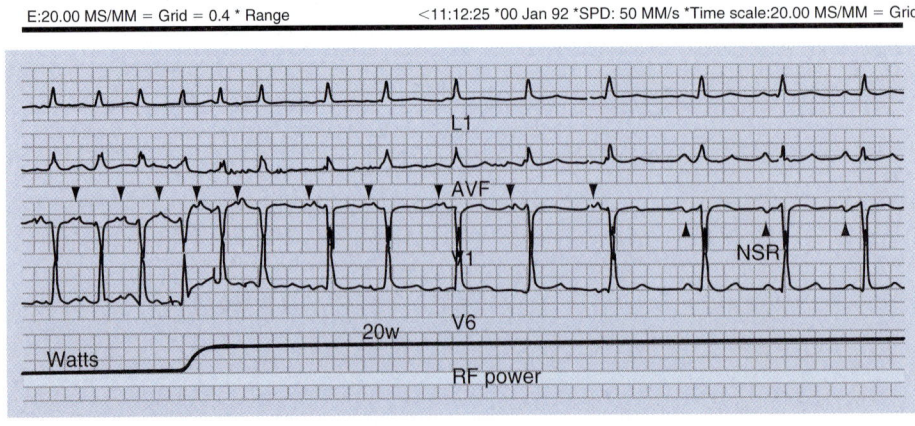

FIGURE 35-12. Ectopic atrial tachycardia (EAT) ablation. **A,** Note how ectopic P waves (*arrows*) terminate after a brief period of acceleration. **B,** EAT slows briefly, then terminates. In both cases, the changes occur soon after radiofrequency (RF) application. In other cases, the ectopic focus may stop immediately at the onset of application of RF energy. CL, cycle length; NSR, normal sinus rhythm.

EAT Focus Location

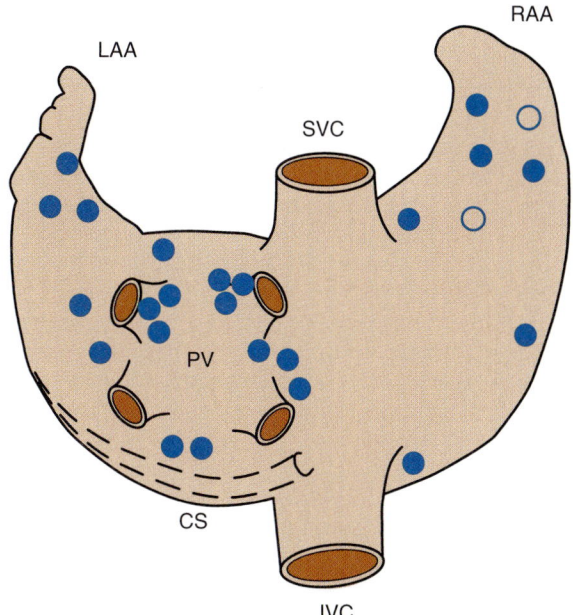

FIGURE 35-13. Location of ectopic atrial tachycardia (EAT) foci in the first 25 patients ablated at Children's Hospital in whom detailed mapping was possible. *Closed circles* (*n* = 23) indicate sites of successful ablation, and *open circles* (*n* = 2) indicate foci that could not be eliminated, in one case because of a broad area of fibrous dysplasia that was resected at surgery, and another patient because of multiple atrial foci, of which this was only one. IVC, inferior vena cava; LAA, left atrial appendage; PV, pulmonary vein; RAA, right atrial appendage; SVC, superior vena cava. *(From Walsh EP. Ablation of ectopic atrial tachycardia in children. In Huang SK [ed]:* Radiofrequency Catheter Ablation of Cardiac Arrhythmias: Basic Concepts and Clinical Applications. *Mt. Kisko, NY: Futura; 1994:421–443. With premission)*

sionally be achieved with either digoxin or verapamil. Also, adenosine may be useful diagnostically by inducing transient AV block, and it may cause transient EAT slowing and termination. Spontaneous resolution of EAT has also been reported after successful pharmacologic control, with rates ranging from 90% in a group of infants younger than 6 months of age[125,128] to 0% in a group of mostly older patients[140] and an average resolution rate from eight contemporary studies of 30% (Table 35-5).[21,127,128,130,140-143] The wide variation in these rates appears to be due to a combination of factors but is probably most influenced by age at presentation, with 72% of the spontaneous resolutions occurring in patients who presented before 6 months of age. Low spontaneous resolution rates were not associated with shorter follow-up duration among the eight studies (Table 35-5). In fact, our initial experience at the Children's Hospital, Boston[140] included no spontaneous resolutions, with a median follow-up before catheter ablation therapy of longer than 24 months, and longer than 4 years in eight patients.

In contrast to pharmacologic therapy, RF catheter ablation for EAT arising from a single focus has been acutely successful in 90% to 100% of cases without significant complications.[24,119,134,136] Because of the high success rates of RF catheter ablation and the morbidity of drug therapy, the question of drug therapy has generally been reduced to one of whether it should be attempted at all in patients with

severe ventricular dysfunction—and, if so, for how long—while waiting for spontaneous reversion to sinus rhythm.

Mapping

Most incessant EATs can be successfully mapped using a bipolar signal from the distal electrode pair of a single mapping and ablation catheter referenced to a single fixed intra-atrial signal. Comparison with the beginning of the surface P wave, when it can be identified, is very useful to identify timing in relation to some known measure of early atrial activation. Map signals that precede the surface P wave by more than 20 milliseconds are most likely to indicate a successful location.[126] Although virtually all early ablation series were done with such basic mapping techniques, there are many situations in which more sophisticated mapping is useful or even necessary. Multipoint mapping can be performed with a variety of technologies and levels of sophistication.

A simple decapolar catheter, which provides four or more nearby timing points to the distal bipole, yields a great deal of directional information. Early distal timing with sequentially later timing of the proximal pairs suggests that the tip is indeed near the ectopic focus. However, even very early timing of the distal bipole when proximal timing is equivalent indicates that activation is approaching the catheter from a different location. This situation often arises when an anterior right upper pulmonary vein focus is being mapped from within the high posterior right atrium. Timing may be early all along the catheter in the right atrium, but it will be early and sequential when the tip is in the right upper pulmonary vein. In such a case, ablation will be successful only when it is applied on the left atrial and pulmonary vein side of the atrial wall.

This example also highlights the value of three-dimensional (3D) multipoint mapping. There are a few considerations when choosing the best 3D technology for EAT mapping, including the following: (1) some foci are intermittently active, particularly under sedation or anesthesia, making sequential activation mapping frustrating or impossible; (2) the location of right pulmonary vein and near-septal foci may not be discernible from either the surface ECG or preliminary mapping, necessitating mapping in both the left and the right atrium; (3) some patients have multiple foci; and (4) some pediatric patients are too small for certain mapping technologies, particularly if remote areas of the left atrium must be accessed (such as ESI balloon mapping [St. Jude Medical, St. Paul, MN], basket mapping, or even a 7F, relatively stiff Biosense Navistar mapping catheter [Biosense Webster, Diamond Bar, CA]). Given these considerations, we have found that for clearly incessant EATs, sequential mapping technologies that allow simultaneous display and comparison of both the atria work well and provide the most flexibility. The Carto (Biosense Webster) and NavX (St. Jude Medical) systems both have all these characteristics. However, for intermittent or potentially multiple foci, sequential mapping technologies may be frustrating, particularly if the focus activity is sensitive to catheter-tip pressure. In such cases, a technology that allows for simultaneous single-beat mapping, such as the ESI balloon, works best. However, the ESI system does not allow for simultaneous display of more than one cardiac chamber and does not lend itself to easily changing the mapping chamber. Consequently, no existing system deals with all four of the considerations noted previously. Regardless of the technology employed, if foci are intermittently active and either multilead P-wave morphologies or multipolar intra-atrial activations have been recorded during EAT, pace mapping may also be a useful adjunct to identify the focus site.

Ablation

In general, failure to eliminate EAT through catheter ablation is less dependent on the ablation technology than on obtaining a good map with early activation and the number of foci present. Because the normal atria are rarely more than 3- to 4-mm thick, most ablation technologies can easily create transmural lesions using standard settings. Therefore, techniques for creating larger lesions, such as active and passive tip cooling and high-powered generators, should rarely, if ever, be necessary. In fact, because most pediatric EAT foci are in the left atrium and often near the ostium of a pulmonary vein, less destructive ablation technologies (using lower temperature, power, and duration) or cryotherapy may be most appropriate in the child. To that end, we have now used cryoablation to successfully ablate a left atrial EAT focus in a 10-year-old boy and a low right atrial EAT focus in a 15-month-old boy.

Initial procedure failure and late recurrence tend to be associated with the presence of multiple foci or intermittent EAT during the procedure. Multiple foci portend poorly for long-term success,[21] both because of the increased difficulty in differentiating the foci during mapping and because more than one foci appears to be predictive of the emergence of other foci after the ablation procedure. Fortunately, in the pediatric population, most cases of EAT are caused by a single nonsinus focus.

Complications

Beyond the usual complications of any ablation procedure, there are a few unique complications to EAT ablation. Both these topics are a covered elsewhere in this text. Although, as noted earlier, some EAT foci in children are near or within a pulmonary vein (Fig. 35-13), eliciting concerns about stenosis, clinically significant stenosis has not been reported for a pediatric case. The potential for damage to the sinus node or to the right phrenic nerve for foci that occur along the crista terminalis should be considered. Most other EAT foci are not near vital structures, such as the AV node or a coronary artery.

Junctional Ectopic Tachycardia

In children, unlike in adults, JET is seen in two relatively distinct settings: postoperative and congenital (Fig. 35-14).[121,144] The electrophysiologic characteristics of both varieties are similar to those of EAT,[121] suggesting that they are also caused by abnormal automaticity, in this case arising from either low in the AV node or high in the His-Purkinje system. However, direct intracellular recordings have not been obtained.

The postoperative and congenital forms of JET differ primarily in their duration and response to therapy.[141,145-147] Postoperative JET (1) is strongly associated with ventricular septal defect repair, either alone or at the time of repair of more complex anomalies (Table 35-6)[148]; (2) is usually transient, lasting between 1 and 4 days; and (3) responds well to cooling and intravenous amiodarone or propafenone.[141,145-147] These observations strongly suggest that the tachycardia is a response to trauma and inflammation induced at the time of the repair. In contrast, congenital JET (1) is typically not associated with structural congenital heart disease; (2) is incessant (Fig. 35-4D); (3) has a positive family history in as many as 50% of cases; (4) anecdotally does not respond to cooling; (5) is associated with the maternal lupus anti-SSA and anti-SSB antibodies in some cases[149]; and (6) may spontaneously resolve, but over a period of months to years.[150] Both JET types may result in severe hemodynamic compromise and appear to be exacerbated by both endogenous and exogenous adrenergic stimulation,[121,147] and both arrhythmias appear to respond well to intravenous amiodarone.[151]

The etiology of the congenital type, other than being "familial," is unclear. An extensive histologic evaluation was performed by Bharati and associates[147] in two patients who presented at or before 6 months of age. In one case, there were acute inflammatory changes at the summit of the ventricular septum and more chronic changes throughout the heart, including fibroelastosis, suggesting myocarditis. In the other, there were a variety of abnormal anatomic findings in the area of the AV node, including leftward displacement of the node and an abnormal central fibrous body. Multiple Purkinje-like tumor cells were found by Rossi and colleagues[152] in a third patient who did not present until 13 months of age, differentiating him slightly from the congenital group. Together, these findings remain somewhat unsatisfying because they fail to provide a unifying etiology consistent with the familial tendencies, and most patients do not present with findings of myocarditis. Dubin and coworkers[149] described a patient with both congenital AV block and JET, suggesting a link between the two diagnoses. The mother had Sjögren syndrome and was strongly positive for anti-SSA and anti-SSB antibodies. Although two other families with congenital JET and positive antibodies were identified,[149] this exciting finding has not turned out to be a unifying etiology for other cases. Thus, for most cases, JET remains an idiopathic diagnosis.

Therapy

The propensity for JET to eventually resolve spontaneously and the high theoretical risk of AV block from either catheter[153] or surgical[121] ablation of the JET focus in the AV junction suggest that JET may initially be best treated medically by minimizing adrenergic stimulation and beginning either intravenous or oral amiodarone,[9,121,154] particularly in infants. However, there are now a number of case reports[155-160] and a single multicenter series in 44 patients, which demonstrate that with both RF and cryoablation it is possible to eliminate the JET in about 85% of patients while preserving AV conduction. Importantly, despite similar success rates in the multicenter series, AV block did occur in 3 of 17 patients (18%) undergoing RF ablation and 0 of 27 undergoing cryoablation.[161] Therefore, if the JET is resistant to medical therapy, persistent after a prolonged period of control, or producing intractable hemodynamic compromise, *cryoablation* should be attempted.

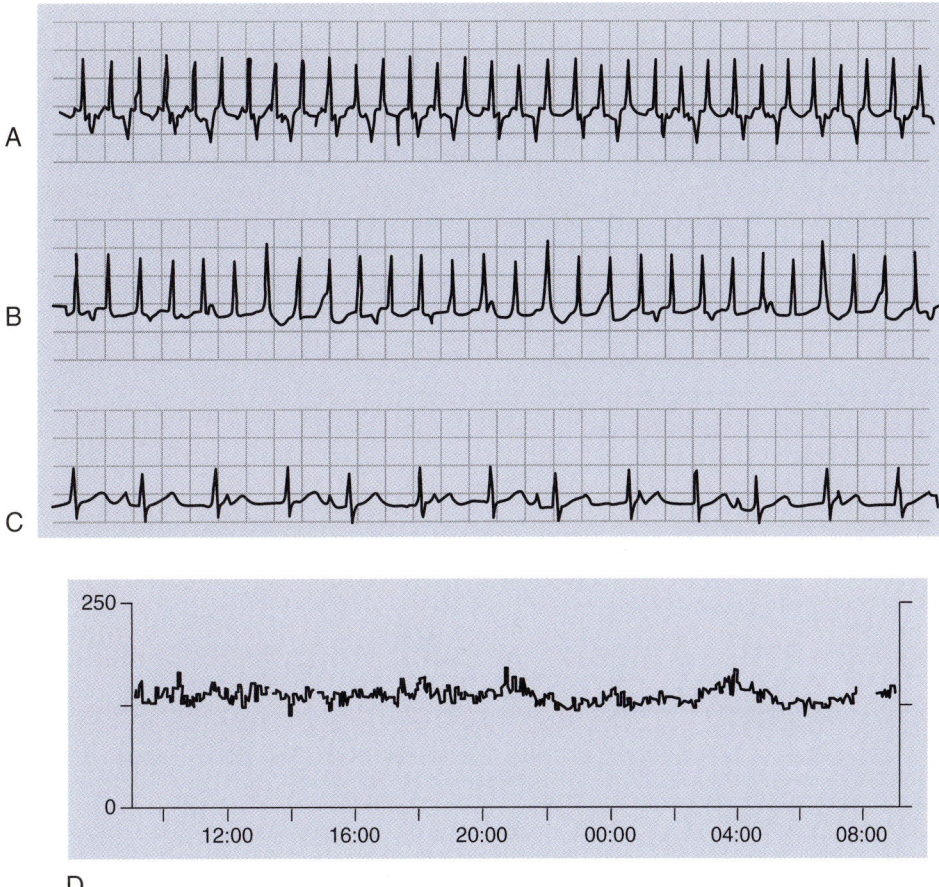

FIGURE 35-14. Junctional ectopic tachycardia in a 6-week-old infant at presentation (**A**), 24 hours after intravenous amiodarone was begun (**B**), and when controlled on oral amiodarone (**C**). Note the ventricular rate of more than 300 beats/min with ventriculoatrial (VA) Wenckebach before amiodarone (**A**). After 24 hours of intravenous amiodarone, the ventricular rate decreased to about 260 beats/min, and there was occasional VA block (**B**). After control on amiodarone, the ventricular rate was normal at about 120 to 130 beats/min (**C**). Over 24 hours (**D**), there was "normal" rate variability, but there was still junctional rhythm with occasional sinus capture throughout, as shown in **C**. *(From Saul JP, Walsh EP, Triedman JK. Mechanisms and therapy of complex arrhythmias in pediatric patients.* J Cardiovasc Electrophysiol. *1995;6:1129-1148. With permission.)*

Because of anecdotal reports of sudden death and one case of AV block with JET, some investigators have recommended ventricular demand pacing in all patients with congenital JET,[161] but the multicenter study of Collins coworkers[46] also included 50 JET patients who did not undergo ablation and demonstrated that this recommendation is no longer appropriate.

Mapping and Ablation

The multicenter series of 44 patients undergoing ablation[161] did provide evidence that cryoablation is equally successful to and much safer than RF ablation for JET; however, it did not provide specifics on exactly how the ablations were performed. The specific details in the small number of reported cases of successful JET ablation provide few overarching recommendations to use when approaching these patients. Although in most cases the region of interest has ended up in the anterior septum near the bundle of His, successful ablation in at least one case was reported in the posteroseptal region below the coronary sinus ostium, with the site identified by the use of retrograde atrial activation as a guide.[156] This region corresponds to the site used for slow pathway modification and should be associated with a low incidence of permanent AV block. However, the data

presented may be most consistent with frequent paroxysms of AVNRT triggered by junctional escape beats, and other reports have not found mapping of earliest retrograde activation to be useful.[158–160] Nonetheless, because this area is generally "safe," initial attempts at ablation may be applied in the posterior septal region. If they are unsuccessful, mapping should focus on identifying the site of the earliest His potential during JET. Before ablation, the catheter should be moved very slightly posterior to that site, attempting to increase the atrial electrogram size and minimize the His activation from the distal ablation tip, similar to the methodology used in the past for fast pathway ablation. Most prior reports of successful elimination of JET without subsequent AV block have used this technique with brief, lower-power applications of RF energy. However, there is clearly a risk for AV block in children with this technique. We have had the opportunity to use cryotherapy in two patients for ablation of JET. In one 10-year-old child with intermittently incessant tachycardia, earliest His activation during tachycardia was found with retrograde mapping just under the aortic valve (Fig. 35-15). The high degree of safety of this methodology around the AV conduction system makes it ideal for both cryomapping and cryoablation, with successful elimination of the JET and preserva-

TABLE 35-6

ASSOCIATION OF POSTOPERATIVE JUNCTIONAL ECTOPIC TACHYCARDIA AND CONGENITAL HEART LESIONS

Lesion	No. of Patients	No. of Patients with JET	Prevalence (%)	P Value
TOF	378	28	7.4	.00005
VSD	285	9	3.2	.004
TGA/VSD	57	9	15.8	.23
Fontan	266	6	2.3	.997
Truncus	33	4	1.2	.824
CCAVC	177	4	2.3	.999
PAB	111	2	1.8	.999
HLHS	94	1	1.1	.999
MVR	50	1	2.0	.999
TGA/IVS	261	—	—	.02
Coarct/Arch	375	—	—	.0001
ASD	273	—	—	.001
PDA	201	—	—	.009
Systemic-PA shunt	192	—	—	.015
Total	2753	64	2.3	—

ASD, atrial septal defect; CCAVC, complete common atrioventricular canal; coarct, coarctation; HLHS, hypoplastic left heart syndrome; IVS, intact ventricular septum; JET, junctional ectopic tachycardia; MVR, mitral valve replacement; PA, pulmonary artery; PAB, pulmonary artery band; PDA, patent ductus arteriosus; TGA, transposition of the great arteries; TOF, tetralogy of Fallot; VSD, ventricular septal defect.
Data from Children's Hospital, Boston, for years 1989-1994.

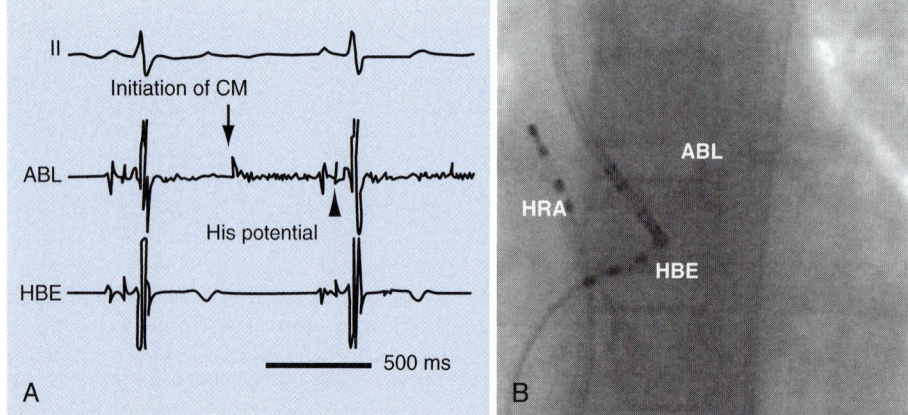

FIGURE 35-15. Successful cryoablation at location with His potential in a patient with JET. **A,** Identical His potentials are clearly seen from the ablation catheter (retrograde approach through the aortic valve) and from the His catheter (in a usual position) just before initiation of cryomapping (CM). **B,** Fluoroscopic images in the anteroposterior view shows the cryoablation catheter overlapping the image of the His position catheter. ABL, ablation; HBE, His bundle electrogram; HRA, high right atrium.

tion of the AV node, despite a catheter signal and location suggesting very close proximity to the His bundle. Our cases and the literature clearly indicate that cryotherapy is the treatment of first choice for ablation of JET.

Permanent Form of Junctional Reciprocating Tachycardia

Like EAT and JET, PJRT is an often incessant tachycardia that typically is recognized in infancy or childhood, either by detection of a rapid heart rate on a routine examina-

tion or because of the accompanying myopathy observed in many patients. First described by Coumel and coworkers,[162] the tachycardia is characterized by a narrow QRS rhythm with variable rates, a retrograde P-wave axis, and an RP interval that is longer than the PR interval. PJRT represents about 4% of the SVTs seen in infants,[125] and it accounts for up to 10% of pediatric patients referred for catheter ablation.[23] As is now clear from the results of electrophysiology studies, surgical[163,164] and catheter ablation results,[48,165-167] and anatomic data,[168,169] PJRT is caused by an orthodromic reciprocating tachycardia involving a slowly conducting concealed AP, making the name a misnomer. It is the slow and decremental retrograde conduction in the AP that leads to both the ECG characteristics and the incessant nature of the rhythm.

Therapy

As with other tachycardias caused by APs,[2] PJRT may resolve spontaneously in some patients.[169] However, in many patients, PJRT is notoriously difficult to control medically. Before the era of RF catheter ablation, both surgical ablation[110,163,164] and DC catheter ablation[170-172] techniques had been used to treat PJRT, but these techniques resulted in a significant risk for AV block as well as other complications. In addition, a false belief that the anatomic location of these APs was always posteroseptal led to a maximal success rate of only about 75%. Catheter ablation has now proved to be a highly effective technique for eliminating these fibers with minimal risk for AV block.[48,165-167,173] Also, the precise AP localization provided by current mapping techniques and the demonstrated points of successful ablation have elucidated the fact that these APs are not always posteroseptal but can occur in almost any location along the AV groove (Fig. 35-16).

Mapping and Ablation

As with any other AP, the methodology for ablation of PJRT pathways depends on their location. Because many of the pathways are posteroseptal, ablation within the mouth or veins of the coronary sinus is often necessary. Mapping should virtually always be performed during tachycardia. Electrogram characteristics, electrophysiologic techniques, and mapping techniques are somewhat different for PJRT

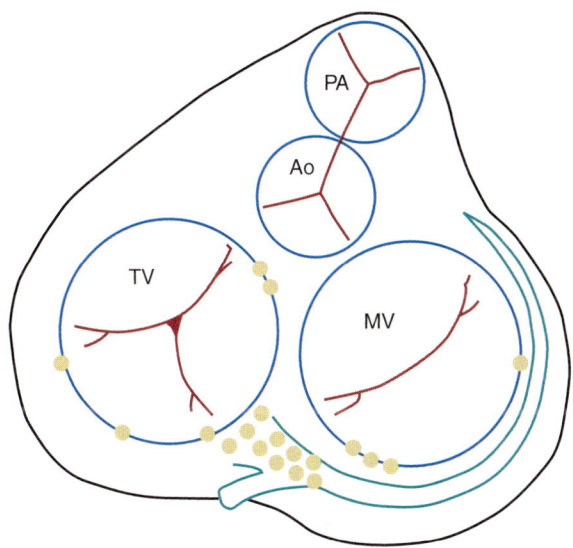

FIGURE 35-16. Schematic diagram of accessory pathway locations in patients with permanent junctional reciprocating tachycardia as identified by radiofrequency ablation. Circles represent accessory pathways causing the tachycardia. Eleven pathways were in the typical location either within or just outside the mouth of the coronary sinus, four were elsewhere along the tricuspid annulus, and four were along the mitral annulus. Ao, aorta; MV, mitral valve; PA, pulmonary artery; TV, tricuspid valve. *(From Ticho BS, Walsh EP, Saul JP. Ablation of permanent junctional reciprocating tachycardia. In Huang SK [ed]:* Radiofrequency Catheter Ablation of Cardiac Arrhythmias: Basic Concepts and Clinical Applications. *Mt. Kisko, NY: Futura; 1994:397-409. With permission.)*

pathways than for typical nondecremental APs. First, it is often impossible to confirm an AP as the retrograde conduction pathway using the standard technique of atrial preexcitation by a ventricular premature beat while the His is refractory because the retrograde conduction decrements after premature ventricular stimulation. Further, the VA interval is usually long, with a long isoelectric segment between the ventricular and atrial signals, and an AP potential may be present in as many as 75% of cases (Fig. 35-17).[174] Finally, the pathways must usually be mapped and ablated in tachycardia (Fig. 35-18) because it is often not possible to achieve reliable exclusive AP conduction during ventricular pacing, owing to either AV node conduction or retrograde block at any cycle length longer than that of the tachycardia. Given these constraints, more than 95% of pathways are still ablatable, but recurrence rates are higher than for typical APs, and some patients may require more than one procedure for initial success.[23,165-167,170,174]

Complications and Recommendations

Despite the proximity to the AV node, AV block has not been reported in the larger series of patients who have undergone RF ablation.[165-167,174] However, it is now clear from both animal[50,175] and patient data that if RF energy is used to ablate posteroseptal pathways inside the coronary sinus, there is a significant risk for coronary damage, particularly if ablation is performed near a terminating branch of the right coronary or left circumflex artery.[13] This issue and the possibility that subclinical coronary damage occurs much more often than has been previously recognized were discussed earlier in the section on AVNRT and are probably most applicable in the setting of posteroseptal PJRT pathways. In fact, Dr. Warren Jackman has often presented the unpublished case of a 15-year-old boy who was referred to him after a failed attempted ablation of a posteroseptal pathway within the mouth of the coronary sinus. A coronary angiogram performed demonstrated complete occlusion of the terminal portion of a nondominant left circumflex artery, despite the absence of any clinical or ECG changes during the first ablation attempt. Figure 35-19 is from a case of ours in a 10-year-old girl with a posteroseptal AP in which a preablation coronary angiogram demonstrated a nearby small posterior descending coronary from the left circumflex that was thought to be 2 to 3 mm from the intended ablation site. However, despite the lack of any ST changes during ablation, postablation angiography demonstrated 90% stenosis of the nearby coronary. Two months after the procedure, the coronary was still stenotic, but collateralization had taken place around it in the same region. Given the numerous anecdotes now available indicating high risk when RF energy is applied in close proximity to small coronary arteries,[13-15,17] we recommend the following for all pediatric patients undergoing posteroseptal ablation of an AP: (1) coronary angiography should be performed before application of RF energy along the posterior AV groove, particularly near the septum, or within the coronary sinus; (2) if a small coronary artery is within 2 to 3 mm of an ablation site, cryotherapy is the preferred initial ablation choice; (3) if cryotherapy is either unavailable or ineffective, RF energy application should be minimized by reducing either catheter size, the temperature set point, or maximal power or duration; and (4) high-energy RF applica-

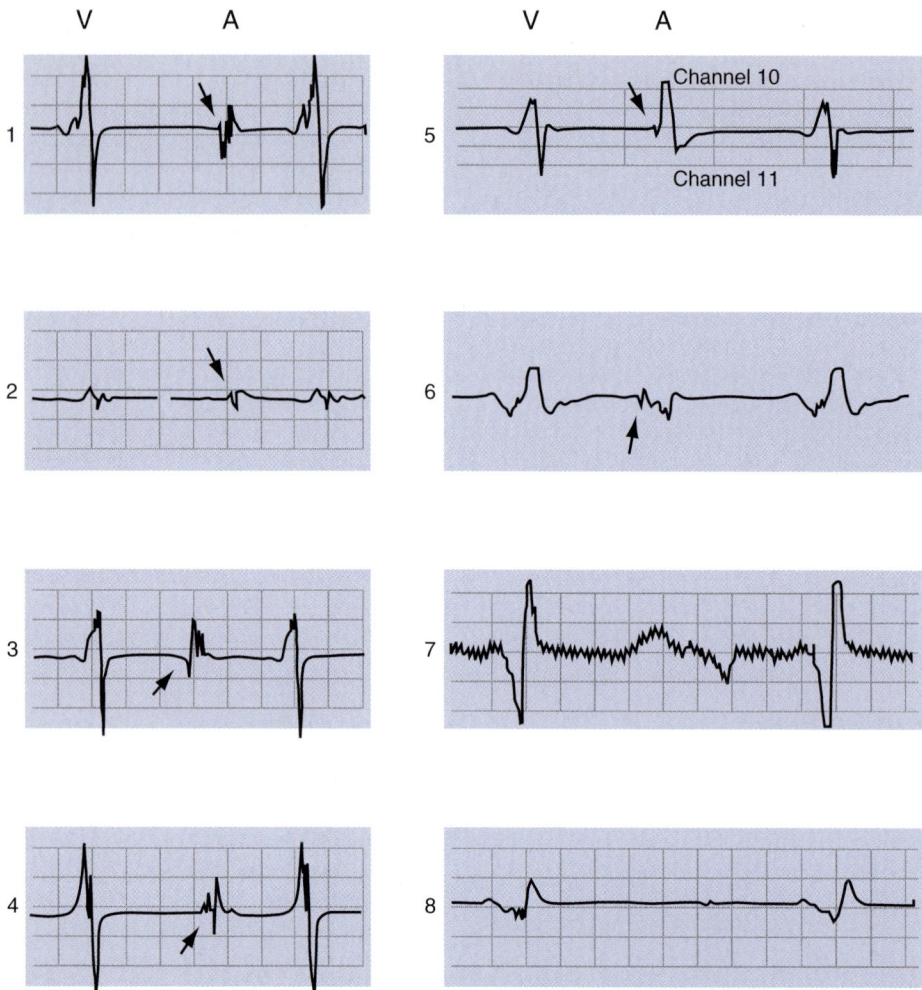

FIGURE 35-17. Electrophysiologic recordings of a single cycle of tachycardia in eight patients with permanent junctional reciprocating tachycardia. Probable accessory pathway (AP) potentials (*arrows*) are present in strips 1 through 6 and are identified as a rapid deflection that immediately precedes the atrial deflection. Strips 7 and 8 do not show such a potential. All recordings were made from the ablation catheter just before and at the location of successful ablation. After ablation, the AP potential was not present, and the ventricular signal did not change. Electrogram 7 was recorded with a catheter on the ventricular side of the tricuspid valve. *A* indicates atrial activation, and *V* ventricular activation. *(From Ticho BS, Saul JP, Hulse JE, et al. Variable location of accessory pathways associated with the permanent form of junctional reciprocating tachycardia and confirmation with radiofrequency ablation. Am J Cardiol. 1992;70:1559-1564. With permission.)*

tion with active or passive cooled-tip technology should be entirely avoided or used with extreme caution.

Despite these safety concerns, the high efficacy and relative safety of ablation for PJRT, combined with the fact that pharmacologic therapy is often ineffective, suggest that catheter ablation is reasonably appropriate as a first-line therapy for this syndrome, particularly if ventricular dysfunction is present.

General Consideration of Risk in Children

Complications

A distinct risk for vascular injury, secondary to thrombus or embolus formation, exists with any catheterization in smaller children but is particularly present with any interventional or prolonged diagnostic catheterization.[176] Therefore, it is not surprising that vascular complications, including microembolism to the foot[173] and arterial occlusion,[177] have been reported with catheter ablation. Of note,

however, the incidence of these problems appears to be quite low, even in the smallest patients, probably because of meticulous heparinization, a tendency not to use the retrograde arterial approach in most pediatric centers, and the current availability of smaller diagnostic and ablation catheters. Production of new[178] or increased[11] valvar regurgitation has been reported in pediatric patients after use of the retrograde arterial approach, providing an additional reason to avoid this approach in smaller patients. The risk for acute coronary damage has been addressed extensively, but it should also be noted that only limited data in humans are available, and no data on late coronary function have been reported in animals, children, or adults.

Sedation and Anesthesia

The pain and discomfort of an RF ablation procedure do not appear to be very much higher than for a typical diagnostic catheterization, even accounting for the pain that some patients feel during the actual RF application. Therefore, general anesthesia is by no means necessary. However, we

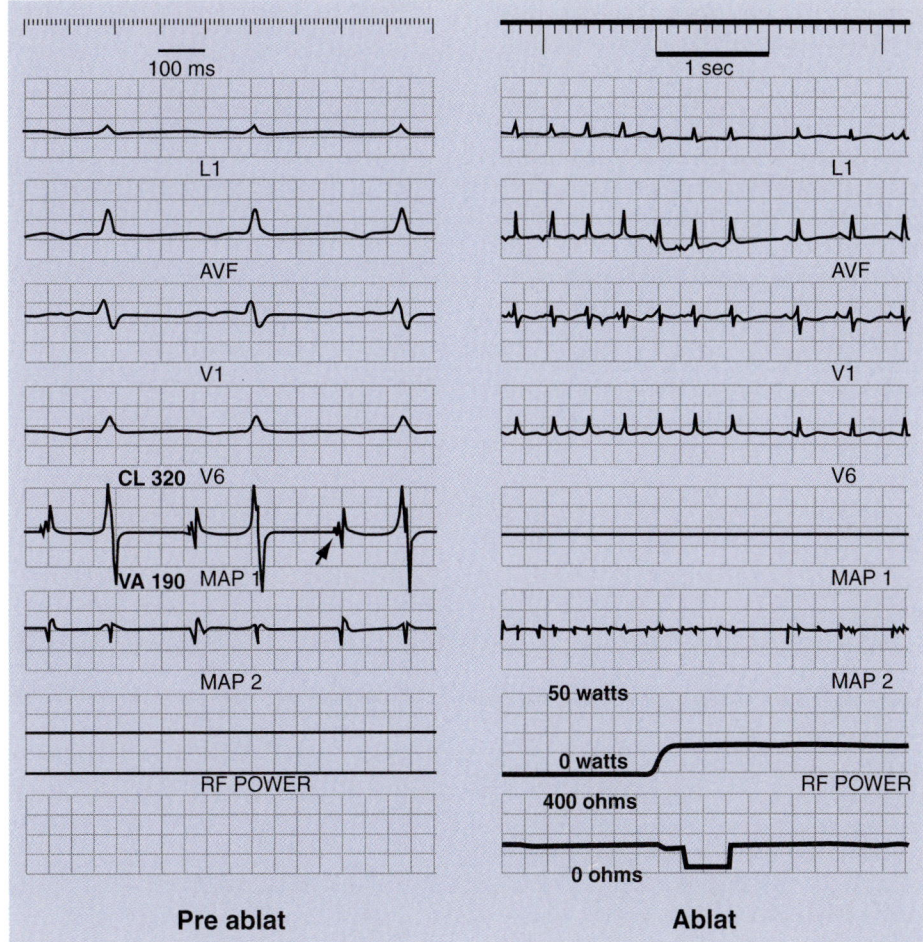

FIGURE 35-18. Electrophysiologic recordings before and during transcatheter radiofrequency (RF) ablation of permanent junctional reciprocating tachycardia. The recording on the *left* was made during tachycardia and shows a probable accessory pathway potential (*arrow*). The recording on the *right* shows conversion to sinus rhythm within 2 seconds of RF energy application. Ablat, RF ablation; CL, cycle length in msec; MAP, mapping catheter; VA, ventriculoatrial interval in msec. *(From Ticho BS, Saul JP, Hulse JE, et al. Variable location of accessory pathways associated with the permanent form of junctional reciprocating tachycardia and confirmation with radiofrequency ablation. Am J Cardiol. 1992;70:1559-1564. With permission.)*

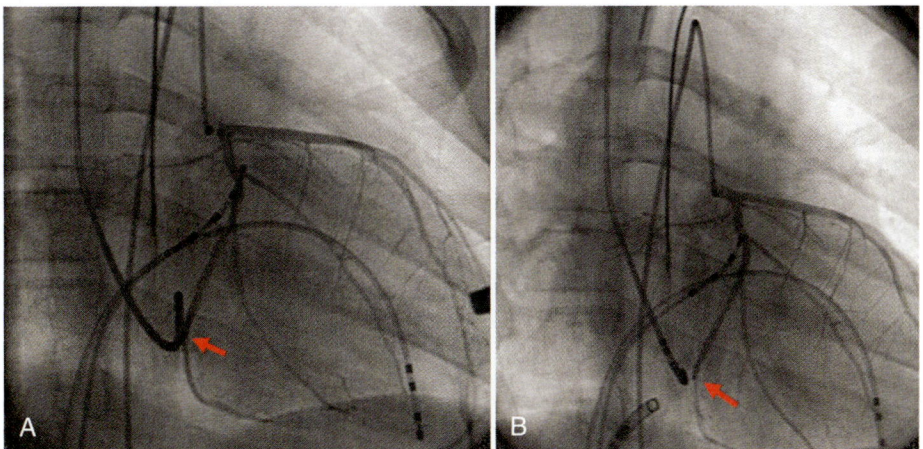

FIGURE 35-19. A, Left coronary angiogram in a 10-year-old patient with a posteroseptal accessory pathway. Earliest activation was mapped to within the mouth of the coronary sinus at the location of the *red arrow*. Despite the lack of ST changes during ablation, after radiofrequency ablation with a 7-mm-tip catheter, repeat angiography (**B**) revealed 90% stenosis of the nearby posterior descending coronary artery.

began using general or near-general anesthesia for most patients early in our experience, for two reasons. First and foremost, uncontrolled patient movement that dislodges the catheter may inadvertently occur at a critical point in the procedure, particularly if the RF application produces pain. In fact, our only case of complete heart block occurred in part as the result of untimely movement of an uncooperative patient during ablation of a mid-septal AP, leading us to replace heavy, often disorienting sedation with general anesthesia for most younger patients. Second, after beginning the use of general anesthesia, we found that even older, cooperative children and young adults find the procedure much more tolerable and are more willing to return for follow-up procedures, if needed. For similar reasons, virtually all pediatric programs use general anesthesia for ablation cases and most nonelectrophysiologic catheter interventions.

Conclusion

Children are usually smaller than adults, but in general, ablation techniques used in adults should not simply be miniaturized to fit the size of the pediatric patient. Multiple factors, including the distribution of arrhythmia mechanisms, ongoing myocardial development, and potentially increased risk for vascular injury and AV node damage, as well as the effects of smaller cardiac size, should all influence the ablation technique. An overriding theme in the child should be that safety takes precedence over efficacy. Therefore, variations of technique should be applied to the decision to ablate, the energy source and its delivery, the catheter approach to the heart and the AV ring, and the follow-up. For instance, because of its strong safety profile, despite lower efficacy, the use of cryotherapy is probably better suited to ablation in children than in adults, and has been recommended as a first choice for many of the scenarios in this chapter. Attention to these factors is probably most important in infants, a group who differ both quantitatively and qualitatively from adults. In addition, the pediatric patient is obviously more likely than an adult to have the simultaneous presence of structural congenital heart disease, which in itself has a variety of implications for the decision to ablate and the procedure technique. On the other hand, there are numerous similarities between adult and pediatric patients. Specifically, regardless of age, it seems clear that a variety of techniques and approaches are necessary to successfully ablate substrates in all locations of the heart, including the AV groove.

References

1. Garson A Jr, Dick M 2nd, Fournier A, et al. The long QT syndrome in children: an international study of 287 patients [see comments]. *Circulation.* 1993;87:1866–1872.
2. Deal BJ, Keane JF, Gillette PC, Garson A Jr. Wolff-Parkinson-White syndrome and supraventricular tachycardia during infancy: management and follow-up. *J Am Coll Cardiol.* 1985;5:130–135.
3. Kugler JD, Danford DA, Houston K, Felix G. Radiofrequency catheter ablation for paroxysmal supraventricular tachycardia in children and adolescents without structural heart disease. Pediatric EP Society, Radiofrequency Catheter Ablation Registry. *Am J Cardiol.* 1997;80:1438–1443.
4. Campbell RM, Strieper MJ, Frias PA, et al. Survey of current practice of pediatric electrophysiologists for asymptomatic Wolff-Parkinson-White syndrome. *Pediatrics.* 2003 March;111(3):e245–e247.
5. Van Hare GF, Javitz H, Carmelli D, et al. Prospective assessment after pediatric cardiac ablation: recurrence at 1 year after initially successful ablation of supraventricular tachycardia. *Heart Rhythm.* 2004;1:188–196.

6. Van Hare GF, Javitz H, Carmelli D, et al. Prospective assessment after pediatric cardiac ablation: demographics, medical profiles, and initial outcomes. *J Cardiovasc Electrophysiol.* 2004;15:759–770.
7. Van Hare GF, Carmelli D, Smith WM, et al. Prospective assessment after pediatric cardiac ablation: design and implementation of the multicenter study. *Pacing Clin Electrophysiol..* 2002;25:332–341.
8. Musto B, D'Onofrio A, Cavallaro C, Musto A. Electrophysiological effects and clinical efficacy of propafenone in children with recurrent paroxysmal supraventricular tachycardia. *Circulation.* 1988;78:863–869.
9. Perry JC, Fenrich AL, Hulse JE, et al. Pediatric use of intravenous amiodarone: efficacy and safety in critically ill patients from a multicenter protocol. *J Am Coll Cardiol.* 1996;27:1246–1250.
10. Ko JK, Deal BJ, Strasburger JF, Benson Jr DW. Supraventricular tachycardia mechanisms and their age distribution in pediatric patients. *Am J Cardiol.* 1992;69:1028–1032.
11. Saul JP, Hulse JE, De W, et al. Catheter ablation of accessory atrioventricular pathways in young patients: use of long vascular sheaths, the transseptal approach and a retrograde left posterior parallel approach. *J Am Coll Cardiol.* 1993;21:571–583.
12. Saul JP, Hulse JE, Papagiannis J, et al. Late enlargement of radiofrequency lesions in infant lambs: Implications for ablation procedures in small children. *Circulation.* 1994;90:492–499.
13. Blaufox AD, Saul JP. Acute coronary artery stenosis during slow pathway ablation for atrioventricular nodal reentrant tachycardia in a child. *J Cardiovasc Electrophysiol.* 2004;15:97–100.
14. Paul T, Kakavand B, Blaufox AD, Saul JP. Complete occlusion of the left circumflex coronary artery after radiofrequency catheter ablation in an infant. *J Cardiovasc Electrophysiol.* 2003;14:1004–1006.
15. Bertram H, Bokenkamp R, Peuster M, et al. Coronary artery stenosis after radiofrequency catheter ablation of accessory atrioventricular pathways in children with Ebstein's malformation. *Circulation.* 2001;103:538–543.
16. Hope EJ, Haigney MC, Calkins H, Resar JR. Left main coronary thrombosis after radiofrequency ablation: Successful treatment with percutaneous transluminal angioplasty. *Am Heart J.* 1995;129:1217–1219.
17. Nakagawa H, Chandrasekaren K, Pitha J, Yamanashi W. Early detection of coronary artery injury produced by radiofrequency ablation within the coronary sinus using intravascular ultrasound imaging. *Circulation.* 1995;92:I–610.
18. Rodriguez LM, de Chillou C, Schlapfer J, et al. Age of onset and gender of patients with different types of supraventricular tachycardias. *Am J Cardiol.* 1992;70:1213–1215.
19. Josephson ME, Wellens HJJ. Differential diagnosis of supraventricular tachycardia. *Cardiol Clin.* 1990;8:441–442.
20. Wellens HJJ, Brugada P. Mechanisms of supraventricular tachycardia. *Am J Cardiol.* 1988;62:10D–15D.
21. Garson A Jr, Smith RT, Moak JP, et al. Atrial automatic ectopic tachycardia in children. In: Touboul P, Waldo AL, eds. *Atrial Arrhythmias: Current Concepts and Management.* St. Louis: Mosby Year Book; 1990:282–287.
22. Silka MJ, Gillette PC, Garson A Jr, Zinner A. Transvenous catheter ablation of a right atrial automatic ectopic tachycardia. *J Am Coll Cardiol.* 1985;5:999–1001.
23. Tanel RE, Walsh EP, Triedman JK, et al. Five-year experience with radiofrequency catheter ablation: implications for management of arrhythmias in pediatric and young adult patients. *J Pediatr.* 1997;131:878–887.
24. Kugler JD, Danford DA, Deal BJ, et al. Radiofrequency catheter ablation for tachyarrhythmias in children and adolescents. The Pediatric Electrophysiology Society. *N Engl J Med.* 1994;330:1481–1487.
25. Levine JC, Walsh EP, Saul JP. Radiofrequency ablation of accessory pathways associated with congenital heart disease including heterotaxy syndrome. *Am J Cardiol.* 1993;72:689–693.
26. Saul JP, Walsh EP, Triedman JK. Mechanisms and therapy of complex arrhythmias in pediatric patients. *J Cardiovasc Electrophysiol.* 1995;6:1129–1148.
27. Schiebler GL, Adams P Jr, Anderson RC. The Wolff-Parkinson-White syndrome in infants and children: a review and a report of 28 cases. *Pediatrics.* 1959;24:585–603.
28. Dick M 2nd, Behrendt DM, Byrum CJ, et al. Tricuspid atresia and the Wolff-Parkinson-White syndrome: evaluation methodology and successful surgical treatment of the combined disorders. *Am Heart J.* 1981;101:496–500.
29. Benson DW, Smith WM, Dunnigan A. Mechanisms of regular wide QRS tachycardia in infants and children. *Am J Cardiol.* 1982;49:1776–1788.
30. Morady F, Kadish AH, DiCarlo L, et al. Long-term results of catheter ablation of idiopathic right ventricular tachycardia. *Circulation.* 1990;82:2093–2099.
31. Klein LS, Shih HT, Hackett K, et al. Radiofrequency catheter ablation of ventricular tachycardia in patients without structural heart disease. *Circulation.* 1992;85:1666–1674.
32. Laohakunakorn P, Paul T, Knick B, et al. Ventricular tachycardia in nonpostoperative pediatric patients: role of radiofrequency catheter ablation. *Pediatr Cardiol.* 2003;24:154–160.
33. Weindling SN, Walsh EP, Saul JP. Management of supraventricular tachycardia in infants. *J Am Coll Cardiol.* 2000;21:294a.
34. Benson DW Jr, Dunnigan A, Benditt DG, et al. Transesophageal study of infant supraventricular tachycardia: electrophysiologic characteristics. *Am J Cardiol.* 1983;52:1002–1006.
35. Friedman RA, Walsh EP, Silka MJ, et al. NASPE Expert Consensus Conference. Radiofrequency catheter ablation in children with and without congenital heart disease: report of the writing committee. North American

Society of Pacing and Electrophysiology [review, 127 refs]. *Pacing Clin Electrophysiol.* 2002;25:1000–1017.

36. Blaufox AD, Denslow S, Felix GL, Saul JP, Participating Members of the Pediatric Electrophysiology Society. Radiofrequency catheter ablation in Registry infants: when is it done and how do they fare? *Circulation.* 2000;102:II-698.

37. Blaufox AD, Paul T, Saul JP. Radiofrequency catheter ablation in small children: relationship of complications to application dose. *Pacing Clin Electrophysiol.* 2004;27:224–229.

38. Blaufox AD, Felix GL, Saul JP. Radiofrequency catheter ablation in infants ≤18 months old: when is it done and how do they fare? Short-term data from the pediatric ablation registry. *Circulation.* 2001;104:2803–2808.

39. Paul T, Bokenkamp R, Mahnert B, Trappe HJ. Coronary artery involvement early and late after radiofrequency current application in young pigs. *Am Heart J.* 1997;133:436–440.

40. Benson DW Jr, Dunnigan A, Benditt DG. Follow-up evaluation of infant paroxysmal atrial tachycardia: transesophageal study. *Circulation.* 1987;75:542–549.

41. Perry JC, Garson A Jr. Supraventricular tachycardia due to Wolff-Parkinson-White syndrome in children: early disappearance and late recurrence [see comments]. *J Am Coll Cardiol.* 1990;16:1215–1220.

42. Klein GJ, Yee R, Sharma AD. Longitudinal electrophysiologic assessment of asymptomatic patients with the Wolff-Parkinson-White electrocardiographic pattern [see comment]. *N Engl J Med.* 1989;320:1229–1233.

43. Zardini M, Yee R, Thakur RK, Klein GJ. Risk of sudden arrhythmic death in the Wolff-Parkinson-White syndrome: current perspectives. *Pacing Clin Electrophysiol.* 1994;17:966–975.

44. Bromberg BI, Lindsay BD, Cain ME, Cox JL. Impact of clinical history and electrophysiologic characterization of accessory pathways on management strategies to reduce sudden death among children with Wolff-Parkinson-White syndrome. *J Am Coll Cardiol.* 1996;27:690–695.

45. Maron BJ, Thompson PD, Ackerman MJ, et al. Recommendations and considerations related to preparticipation screening for cardiovascular abnormalities in competitive athletes: 2007 update: a scientific statement from the American Heart Association Council on Nutrition, Physical Activity, and Metabolism: endorsed by the American College of Cardiology Foundation. *Circulation.* 2007;115:1643–1655.

46. Zipes DP, Ackerman MJ, Estes 3rd NA, et al. Task Force 7: arrhythmias. *J Am Coll Cardiol.* 2005;45:1354–1363.

47. Gaita F, Haissaguerre M, Giustetto C, et al. Safety and efficacy of cryoablation of accessory pathways adjacent to the normal conduction system. *J Cardiovasc Electrophysiol.* 2003;14:825–829.

48. Gaita F, Antonio M, Riccardi R, et al. Cryoenergy catheter ablation: a new technique for treatment of permanent junctional reciprocating tachycardia in children. *J Cardiovasc Electrophysiol.* 2004;15:263–268.

49. Lowe MD, Meara M, Mason J, Grace AA, et al. Catheter cryoablation of supraventricular arrhythmias: a painless alternative to radiofrequency energy. *Pacing Clin Electrophysiol.* 2003;26:500–503.

50. Skanes AC, Yee R, Krahn AD, Klein GJ. Cryoablation of atrial arrhythmias. [Review] [26 refs]. *Card Electrophysiol Rev.* 2002;6:383–388.

51. Chan NY, Mok NS, Lau CL, et al. Treatment of atrioventricular nodal re-entrant tachycardia by cryoablation with a 6 mm-tip catheter vs. radiofrequency ablation. *Europace.* 2009;11:1065–1070.

52. Mehta AV, Sanchez GR, Sacks EJ, et al. Ectopic automatic atrial tachycardia in children: clinical characteristics, management and follow-up. *J Am Coll Cardiol.* 1988;11:379–385.

53. Skanes AC, Dubuc M, Klein GJ, et al. Cryothermal ablation of the slow pathway for the elimination of atrioventricular nodal reentrant tachycardia. *Circulation.* 2000;102:2856–2860.

54. Avari JN, Jay KS, Rhee EK. Experience and results during transition from radiofrequency ablation to cryoablation for treatment of pediatric atrioventricular nodal reentrant tachycardia. *Pacing Clin Electrophysiol.* 2008;31:454–460.

55. Miyazaki A, Blaufox AD, Fairbrother DL, Saul JP. Prolongation of the fast pathway effective refractory period during cryoablation in children: a marker of slow pathway modification. *Heart Rhythm.* 2005;2:1179–1185.

56. Miyazaki A, Blaufox AD, Fairbrother DL, Saul JP. Cryoablation for septal tachycardia substrates in pediatric patients: mid-term results. *J Am Coll Cardiol.* 2005;15(45):581–588.

57. Dubuc M, Roy D, Thibault B, et al. Transvenous catheter ice mapping and cryoablation of the atrioventricular node in dogs. *Pacing Clin Electrophysiol.* 1999;22:1488–1498.

58. Lustgarten DL, Bell S, Hardin N, et al. Safety and efficacy of epicardial cryoablation in a canine model. *Heart Rhythm.* 2005;2:82–90.

59. Rodriguez LM, Leunissen J, Hoekstra A, et al. Transvenous cold mapping and cryoablation of the AV node in dogs: observations of chronic lesions and comparison to those obtained using radiofrequency ablation. *J Cardiovasc Electrophysiol.* 1998;9:1055–1061.

60. Skanes AC, Jones DL, Teefy P, et al. Safety and feasibility of cryothermal ablation within the mid- and distal coronary sinus. *J Cardiovasc Electrophysiol.* 2004;15:1319–1323.

61. Khairy P, Chauvet P, Lehmann J, et al. Lower incidence of thrombus formation with cryoenergy versus radiofrequency catheter ablation. *Circulation.* 2003;107:2045–2050.

62. Schaffer MS, Silka MJ, Ross BA, Kugler JD.. Inadvertent atrioventricular block during radiofrequency catheter ablation. Results of the Pediatric Radiofrequency Ablation Registry. Pediatric Electrophysiology Society. *Circulation.* 1996;94:3214–3220.

63. Bokenkamp R, Wibbelt G, Sturm M, et al. Effects of intracardiac radiofrequency current application on coronary artery vessels in young pigs. *J Cardiovasc Electrophysiol.* 2000;11:565–571.

64. Agnoletti G, Borghi A, Vignati G, Crupi GC. Fontan conversion to total cavopulmonary connection and arrhythmia ablation: clinical and functional results. *Heart.* 2003;89(2):193–198.

65. Gist KM, Bockoven JR, Lane J, et al. Acute success of cryoablation of left-sided accessory pathways: a single institution study. *J Cardiovasc Electrophysiol.* 2009;20:637–642.

66. Gross GJ, Epstein MR, Walsh EP, Saul JP. Characteristics, management and mid-term outcome in infants with atrioventricular nodal reentry tachycardia. *Am J Cardiol.* 1998;82:956–960.

67. Silka MJ, Kron J, Halperin BD, McAnulty JH. Mechanisms of AV node reentrant tachycardia in young patients with and without dual AV node physiology. *Pacing Clin Electrophysiol.* 1994;17:2129–2133.

68. Van Hare GF, Chiesa NA, Campbell RM, et al, Pediatric Electrophysiology Society. Atrioventricular nodal reentrant tachycardia in children: effect of slow pathway ablation on fast pathway function [comment]. *J Cardiovasc Electrophysiol.* 2002;13:203–209.

69. Blaufox AD, Rhodes JF, Fishberger SB. Age related changes in dual AV nodal physiology. *Pacing Clin Electrophysiol.* 2000;477-80(2000):23.

70. Rosen KM, Bauernfeind RA, Swiryn S, et al. Dual AV nodal pathways and AV nodal reentrant paroxysmal tachycardia. *Am Heart J.* 1981;101:691–695.

71. Denes P, Wu D, Dhingra R, et al. Dual atrioventricular nodal pathways: a common electrophysiological response. *Br Heart J.* 1975;37:1069–1076.

72. Blaufox AD, Saul JP. Influences on fast and slow pathway conduction in children: Does the definition of dual atrioventricular node physiology need to be changed? [comment]. *J Cardiovasc Electrophysiol.* 2002;13:210–211.

73. Haines DE. The biophysics of radiofrequency catheter ablation in the heart: the importance of temperature monitoring. *Pacing Clin Electrophysiol.* 1993;16:586–591.

74. Haines DE, Watson DD, Verow AF. Electrode radius predicts lesion radius during radiofrequency energy heating: validation of a proposed thermodynamic model. *Circ Res.* 1990;67:124–129.

75. Dick M 2nd, O'Connor KB, Serwer GA, et al. Use of radiofrequency current to ablate accessory connections in children. *Circulation.* 1991;84:2318–2324.

76. Lesh MD, Van Hare GF, Schamp DJ, et al. Curative percutaneous catheter ablation using radiofrequency energy for accessory pathways in all locations: results in 100 consecutive patients. *J Am Coll Cardiol.* 1992;19:1303–1309.

77. Calkins H, Langberg J, Sousa J, et al. Radiofrequency catheter ablation of accessory atrioventricular connections in 250 patients: abbreviated therapeutic approach to Wolff-Parkinson-White syndrome. *Circulation.* 1992;85:1337–1346.

78. Jackman WM, Wang XZ, Friday KJ, et al. Catheter ablation of accessory atrioventricular pathways (Wolff-Parkinson-White syndrome) by radio-frequency current [see comments]. *N Engl J Med.* 1991;324:1605–1611.

79. Benito F, Sanchez C. Radiofrequency catheter ablation of accessory pathways in infants. *Heart.* 1997;78:160–162.

80. Solomon AJ, Tracy CM, Swartz JF, et al. Effect on coronary artery anatomy of radiofrequency catheter ablation of atrial insertion sites of accessory pathways. *J Am Coll Cardiol.* 1993;21:1440–1444.

81. Khanal S, Ribeiro PA, Platt M, Kuhn MA. Right coronary artery occlusion as a complication of accessory pathway ablation in a 12-year-old treated with stenting. *Cathet Cardiovasc Interv.* 1999;46:59–61.

82. Chatelain P, Zimmermann M, Weber R, et al. Acute coronary occlusion secondary to radiofrequency catheter ablation of a left lateral accessory pathway. *Eur Heart J.* 1995;16:859–861.

83. Riccardi R, Gaita F, Caponi D, et al. Percutaneous catheter cryothermal ablation of atrioventricular nodal reentrant tachycardia: efficacy and safety of a new ablation technique. *Ital Heart J.* 2003;4:35–43.

84. Okishige K, Harada T, Kawabata M, et al. Transvenous catheter cryoablation of the atrioventricular node and visual assessment of freezing of cardiac tissue using intracardiac echocardiography. *Jpn Heart J.* 2004;45:513–520.

85. Chan NY, Mok NS, Lau CL, et al. Treatment of atrioventricular nodal re-entrant tachycardia by cryoablation with a 6 mm-tip catheter vs. radiofrequency ablation. *Europace.* 2009;11:1065–1070.

86. Mantakas ME, McCue CM, Miller WW. Natural history of Wolff-Parkinson-White syndrome in infants and children: a review and a report of 28 cases. *Am J Cardiol.* 1978;41:1097–1103.

87. Erickson CC, Walsh EP, Triedman JK, Saul JP. Efficacy and safety of radiofrequency ablation in infants and young children <18 months of age. *Am J Cardiol.* 1994;74:944–947.

88. Kugler JD. Radiofrequency catheter ablation for supraventricular tachycardia: should it be used in infants and small children? [editorial; comment]. *Circulation.* 1994;90:639–641.

89. Case CL, Gillette PC, Oslizlok PC, et al. Radiofrequency catheter ablation of incessant, medically resistant supraventricular tachycardia in infants and small children. *J Am Coll Cardiol.* 1992;20:1405–1410.

90. Case CL, Gillette PC. Indications for catheter ablation in infants and small children with reentrant supraventricular tachycardia [letter]. *J Am Coll Cardiol.* 1996;27:1551–1552.

91. Zak R. Development and proliferative capacity of cardiac muscle cells. *Circ Res.* 1974;35(suppl II):17–26.

92. Denfield SW, Kearney DL, Michael L, et al. Developmental differences in canine cardiac surgical scars. *Am Heart J.* 1993;126:382–389.

93. Erickson CC, Carr D, Greer GS, et al. Emergent radiofrequency ablation of the AV node in a neonate with unstable, refractory supraventricular tachycardia. *Pacing Clin Electrophysiol.* 1995;18:1959–1962.

94. Finelli A, Rewcastle JC, Jewett MA. Cryotherapy and radiofrequency ablation: pathophysiologic basis and laboratory studies [review, 48 refs]. *Curr Opin Urol.* 2003;13:187–191.

95. Haines DE, Watson DD, Verow AF. Electrode radius predicts lesion radius during radiofrequency energy heating. Validation of a proposed thermodynamic model. *Circ Res.* 1990;67:124–129.

96. Cote JM, Epstein MR, Triedman JK, et al. Low-temperature mapping predicts site of successful ablation while minimizing myocardial damage. *Circulation.* 1996;94:253–257.

97. Chu E, Fitzpatrick AP, Chin MC, et al. Radiofrequency catheter ablation guided by intracardiac echocardiography. *Circulation.* 1994;89:1301–1305.

98. Schiebler GL, Adams P Jr, Anderson RC, et al. Clinical study of twenty-three cases of Ebstein's anomaly of the tricuspid valve. *Circulation.* 1959;19:187.

99. Anderson RH, Becker AE, Arnold R, Wilkinson JL. The conducting tissues in congenitally corrected transposition. *Circulation.* 1974;50:911–923.

100. Symons JC, Shinebourne EA, Joseph MC, et al. Criss-cross heart with congenitally corrected transposition: Report of a case with d-transposed aorta and ventricular preexcitation. *Eur J Cardiol.* 1977;5:493.

101. Van Mierop LHS, Kutsche LM, Victoria BF. Ebstein's anomaly. In: Adams FH, Emmanouilides GC, Riemenschneider TA, eds. *Heart Disease in Infants, Children and Adolescents.* Baltimore: Williams & Wilkins; 1989:361–363.

102. Lev M, Gibson S, Miller RA. Ebstein's disease with Wolff-Parkinson-White syndrome: report of a case with a histopathologic study of possible conduction pathways. *Am J Cardiol.* 1955;49:724–741.

103. Van Hare GF, Lesh MD, Stanger P. Radiofrequency catheter ablation of supraventricular arrhythmias in patients with congenital heart disease: results and technical considerations. *J Am Coll Cardiol.* 1993;22:883–890.

104. Kuck KH, Schluter M, Geiger M, et al. Radiofrequency current catheter ablation of accessory atrioventricular pathways. *Lancet.* 1991;337:1557–1561.

105. Smith WM, Gallagher JJ, Kerr CR, et al. The electrophysiologic basis and management of symptomatic recurrent tachycardia in patients with Ebstein's anomaly of the tricuspid valve. *Am J Cardiol.* 1982;49:1223–1234.

106. Twidale N, Wang X, Beckman KJ, et al. Factors associated with recurrence of accessory pathway conduction after radiofrequency catheter ablation. *Pacing Clin Electrophysiol.* 1991;14:2042–2048.

107. Gallagher JJ, Pritchett ELC, Sealy WC, et al. The preexcitation syndromes. *Prog Cardiovasc Dis.* 1978;20:285–327.

108. Cox JL, Gallagher JJ, Cain ME. Experience with 118 consecutive patients undergoing operation for the Wolff-Parkinson-White syndrome. *J Thorac Cardiovasc Surg.* 1985;90:490–501.

109. Gillette PC, Garson A Jr, Kugler JD, et al. Surgical treatment of supraventricular tachycardia in infants and children. *Am J Cardiol.* 1980;46:281–284.

110. Ott DA, Gillette PC, Garson A Jr. Surgical management of refractory supraventricular tachycardia in infants and children. *J Am Coll Cardiol.* 1985;5:124–129.

111. Weston LT, Hull RW, Laird JR. A prototype coronary electrode catheter for intracoronary electrogram recording. *Am J Cardiol.* 1992;70:1492–1493.

112. Ho SY, Anderson RH. Embryology and anatomy of the normal and abnormal conduction system. In: Gillette PC, Garson A Jr, eds. *Pediatric Arrhythmias: Electrophysiology and Pacing.* Philadelphia: Saunders; 1990:2–27.

113. Van Praagh R. Segmental approach to diagnosis. In: Fyler DC, ed. *Nadas' Pediatric Cardiology.* Philadelphia: Hanley & Belfus; 1992:27–35.

114. Walsh EP, Saul JP, Triedman JK, et al. Ablation of the "second conducting system": Mahaim fibers and "double AV nodes" in congenital heart disease. *Circulation.* 1994;90:I–100.

115. Epstein MR, Saul JP, Weindling SN, et al. Atrioventricular reciprocating tachycardia involving twin atrioventricular nodes in patients with complex congenital heart disease. *J Cardiovasc Electrophysiol.* 2001;12:671–679.

116. Langberg JJ, Calkins H, Kim YN, et al. Recurrence of conduction in accessory atrioventricular connections after initially successful radiofrequency catheter ablation. *J Am Coll Cardiol.* 1992;19:1588–1592.

117. Dunnigan A, Benson DW, Benditt DG. Atrial flutter in infancy: diagnosis, clinical features, and treatment. *Pediatrics.* 1985;75:725–729.

118. Nanthakumar K, Lau YR, Plumb VJ, et al. Electrophysiological findings in adolescents with atrial fibrillation who have structurally normal hearts. *Circulation.* 2004;110:117–123.

119. Walsh EP, Saul JP, Hulse JE, et al. Transcatheter ablation of ectopic atrial tachycardia in young patients using radiofrequency current [see comments]. *Circulation.* 1992;86:1138–1146.

120. Garson A Jr, Gillette PC. Junctional ectopic tachycardia in children: electrocardiography, electrophysiology and pharmacologic response. *Am J Cardiol.* 1979;44:298–302.

121. Villain E, Vetter VL, Garcia JM, et al. Evolving concepts in the management of congenital junctional ectopic tachycardia: a multicenter study [see comments] [review]. *Circulation.* 1990;81:1544–1549.

122. Fishberger SB, Colan SD, Saul JP, et al. Myocardial mechanics before and after ablation of chronic tachycardia. *Pacing Clin Electrophysiol.* 1996;19:42–49.

123. Gillette PC, Smith RT, Garson A Jr, et al. Chronic supraventricular tachycardia: a curable cause of congestive cardiomyopathy. *JAMA.* 1985;253:391–392.

124. Rakusan K. Cardiac growth, maturation and aging. In: Zak R, ed. *Growth of the Heart in Health and Disease.* New York: Raven Press; 1984:131–164.

125. Weindling SN, Saul JP, Walsh EP. Efficacy and risks of medical therapy for supraventricular tachycardia in neonates and infants. *Am Heart J.* 1996;131:66–72.

126. Walsh EP. Ablation of ectopic atrial tachycardia in children. In: Huang SK, ed. *Radiofrequency Catheter Ablation of Cardiac Arrhythmias: Basic Concepts and Clinical Applications.* Mt. Kisko, NY: Futura; 1994:421–443.

127. Naheed ZJ, Strasburger JF, Benson DW Jr, Deal BJ. Natural history and management strategies of automatic atrial tachycardia in children. *Am J Cardiol.* 1995;75:405–407.

128. Bauersfeld U, Gow RM, Hamilton RM, Izukawa T. Treatment of atrial ectopic tachycardia in infants <6 months old. *Am Heart J.* 1995;129:1145–1148.

129. Kunze KP, Kuck KH, Schluter M, Bleifeld W. Effect of encainide and flecainide on chronic ectopic atrial tachycardia. *J Am Coll Cardiol.* 1986;7:1121–1126.

130. Dhala AA, Case CL, Gillette PC. Evolving treatment strategies for managing atrial ectopic tachycardia in children. *Am J Cardiol.* 1994;74:283–286.

131. Garson A Jr, Gillette PC, Titus JL, et al. Surgical treatment of ventricular tachycardia in infants. *N Engl J Med.* 1984;310:1443–1445.

132. de Bakker JM, Hauer RN, Bakker PF, et al. Abnormal automaticity as mechanism of atrial tachycardia in the human heart—electrophysiologic and histologic correlation: a case report. *J Cardiovasc Electrophysiol.* 1994;5:335–344.

133. Kay GN, Chong F, Epstein AE, et al. Radiofrequency ablation for treatment of primary atrial tachycardias [see comments]. *J Am Coll Cardiol.* 1993;21:901–909.

134. Tracy CM, Swartz JF, Fletcher RD, et al. Radiofrequency catheter ablation of ectopic atrial tachycardia using paced activation sequence mapping [see comments]. *J Am Coll Cardiol.* 1993;21:910–917.

135. Spinale FG, Fulbright BM, Mukherjee R, et al. Relation between ventricular and myocyte function with tachycardia-induced cardiomyopathy. *Circ Res.* 1992;71:174–187.

136. Lesh MD, Van Hare GF, Epstein LM, et al. Radiofrequency catheter ablation of atrial arrhythmias: results and mechanisms. *Circulation.* 1994;89:1074–1089.

137. Nath S, Lynch C 3rd, Whayne JG, Haines DE. Cellular electrophysiological effects of hyperthermia on isolated guinea pig papillary muscle: implications for catheter ablation. *Circulation.* 1993;88(Pt 1):1826–1831.

138. Evans VL, Garson A Jr, Smith RT, et al. Ethmozine (moricizine HCl): a promising drug for "automatic" atrial ectopic tachycardia. *Am J Cardiol.* 1987;60:83F–86F.

139. Tanel RE, Walsh EP, Lulu JA, Saul JP. Sotalol for refractory arrhythmias in pediatric and young adult patients: initial efficacy and long-term outcome. *Am Heart J.* 1995;130:791–797.

140. Walsh EP, Saul JP, Triedman JK, et al. Natural and unnatural history of ectopic atrial tachycardia: One institution's experience. *Pacing Clin Electrophysiol.* 1994;17:746.

141. Balaji S, Sullivan I, Deanfield J, James I. Moderate hypothermia in the management of resistant automatic tachycardias in children. *Br Heart J.* 1991;66:221–224.

142. Koike K, Hesslein PS, Finlay CD, et al. Atrial automatic tachycardia in children. *Am J Cardiol.* 1988;61:1127–1130.

143. von Bernuth G, Engelhardt W, Kramer HH, et al. Atrial automatic tachycardia in infancy and childhood. *Eur Heart J.* 1992;13:1410–1415.

144. Gillette PC, Crawford FA, Fyfe DA, et al. Advances in the treatment of supraventricular tachycardia. *J S C Med Assoc.* 1989;85:275–278.

145. Sholler GF, Walsh EP, Saul JP, et al. Evaluation of a staged treatment protocol for postoperative rapid junctional ectopic tachycardia. *Circulation.* 1988;78:II–597.

146. Bash SE, Shah JJ, Albers WH. Hypothermia for the treatment of postsurgically accelerated junctional ectopic tachycardia. *J Am Coll Cardiol.* 1987;10:1095–1099.

147. Till JA, Rowland E. Atrial pacing as an adjunct to the management of postsurgical His bundle tachycardia. *Br Heart J.* 1991;66:225–229.

148. Walsh EP, Saul JP, Sholler GF, et al. Evaluation of a staged treatment protocol for rapid automatic junctional tachycardia after operation for congenital heart disease. *J Am Coll Cardiol.* 1997;29:1046–1053.

149. Dubin AM, Cuneo B, Strasburger J, et al. Congenital junctional tachycardia and congenital complete AV block: a shared etiology? *Heart Rhythm.* 2005;2:313–315.

150. Bharati S, Moskowitz WB, Scheinman M, et al. Junctional tachycardias: anatomic substrate and its significance in ablative procedures. *J Am Coll Cardiol.* 1991;18:179–186.

151. Saul JP, Scott WA, Brown S, et al. Intravenous amiodarone for incessant tachyarrhythmias in children: a randomized, double-blind, antiarrhythmic drug trial. *Circulation.* 2005;112:3470–3477.

152. Rossi L, Piffer R, Turolla E, et al. Multifocal Purkinje-like tumor of the heart: occurrence with other anatomic abnormalities in the atrioventricular junction of an infant with junctional tachycardia, Lown-Ganong-Levine syndrome, and sudden death. *Chest.* 1985;87:340–345.

153. Gillette PC, Garson A Jr, Porter CJ, et al. Junctional automatic ectopic tachycardia: New proposed treatment by transcatheter His bundle ablation. *Am Heart J.* 1983;106:619–623.

154. Figa FH, Gow RM, Hamilton RM, Freedom RM. Clinical efficacy and safety of intravenous amiodarone in infants and children. *Am J Cardiol.* 1994;74:573–577.

155. Balaji S, Gillette PC, Case CL. Successful radiofrequency ablation of permanent junctional reciprocating tachycardia in an 18-month-old child. *Am Heart J.* 1994;127:1420–1421.

156. Ehlert FA, Goldberger JJ, Deal BJ, et al. Successful radiofrequency energy ablation of automatic junctional tachycardia preserving normal atrioventricular nodal conduction. *Pacing Clin Electrophysiol*. 1993;16:54–61.

157. Rychik J, Marchlinski FE, Sweeten TL, et al. Transcatheter radiofrequency ablation for congenital junctional ectopic tachycardia in infancy. *Pediatr Cardiol*. 1997;18:447–450.

158. Van Hare GF, Velvis H, Langberg JJ. Successful transcatheter ablation of congenital junctional ectopic tachycardia in a ten-month-old infant using radiofrequency energy. *Pacing Clin Electrophysiol*. 1990;13:730–735.

159. Young ML, Mehta MB, Martinez RM, et al. Combined alpha-adrenergic blockade and radiofrequency ablation to treat junctional ectopic tachycardia successfully without atrioventricular block. *Am J Cardiol*. 1993;71:883–885.

160. Fishberger SB, Rossi AF, Messina JJ, Saul JP. Successful radiofrequency catheter ablation of congenital junctional ectopic tachycardia with preservation of atrioventricular conduction in a 9-month-old infant. *Pacing Clin Electrophysiol*. 1998;21:2132–2135.

161. Collins KK, Van Hare GF, Kertesz NJ, et al. Pediatric nonpost-operative junctional ectopic tachycardia medical management and interventional therapies. *J Am Coll Cardiol*. 2009;53:690–697.

162. Coumel P, Cabrol C, Fabiato A, et al. Tachycardie permanente par rythme reciproque. *Arch Mal Coeur*. 1967;60:1830–1864.

163. O'Neill BJ, Klein GJ, Guiraudon GM, et al. Results of operative therapy in the permanent form of junctional reciprocating tachycardia. *Am J Cardiol*. 1989;63:1074–1079.

164. Gallagher JJ, Sealy WC. The permanent form of junctional reciprocating tachycardia: further elucidation of the underlying mechanism. *Eur J Cardiol*. 1978;8:413–430.

165. Ticho BS, Saul JP, Hulse JE, et al. Variable location of accessory pathways associated with the permanent form of junctional reciprocating tachycardia and confirmation with radiofrequency ablation. *Am J Cardiol*. 1992;70: 1559–1564.

166. Ticho BS, Walsh EP, Saul JP. Ablation of permanent junctional reciprocating tachycardia. In: Huang SK, ed. *Radiofrequency Catheter Ablation of Cardiac Arrhythmias: Basic Concepts and Clinical Applications*. Mt. Kisko, NY: Futura; 1994:397–409.

167. Gaita F, Haïssaguerre M, Giustetto C, et al. Catheter ablation of permanent junctional reciprocating tachycardia with radiofrequency current. *J Am Coll Cardiol*. 1995;25:648–654.

168. Critelli G, Gallagher JJ, Monda V, et al. Anatomic and electrophysiologic substrate of the permanent form of junctional reciprocating tachycardia. *J Am Coll Cardiol*. 1984;4:601–610.

169. Guarnieri T, German LD, Gallagher JJ. The long R-P' tachycardias [review]. *Pacing Clin Electrophysiol*. 1987;10:103–117.

170. Morady F, Scheinman MM, Kou WH, et al. Long-term results of catheter ablation of a posteroseptal accessory atrioventricular connection in 48 patients. *Circulation*. 1989;79:1160–1170.

171. Chien WW, Cohen TJ, Lee MA, et al. Electrophysiological findings and long-term follow-up of patients with the permanent form of junctional reciprocating tachycardia treated by catheter ablation. *Circulation*. 1992;85:1329–1336.

172. Smith RT Jr, Gillette PC, Massumi A, et al. Transcatheter ablative techniques for treatment of the permanent form of junctional reciprocating tachycardia in young patients. *J Am Coll Cardiol*. 1986;8:385–390.

173. Van Hare GF, Lesh MD, Scheinman M, Langberg JJ. Percutaneous radiofrequency catheter ablation for supraventricular arrhythmias in children. *J Am Coll Cardiol*. 1991;17:1613–1620.

174. Haïssaguerre M, Montserrat P, Warin JF, et al. Catheter ablation of left posteroseptal accessory pathways and of long RP' tachycardias with a right endocardial approach. *Eur Heart J*. 1991;12:845–859.

175. Aoyama H, Nakagawa H, Pitha JV, et al. Comparison of cryothermia and radiofrequency current in safety and efficacy of catheter ablation within the canine coronary sinus close to the left circumflex coronary artery. *J Cardiovasc Electrophysiol*. 2005;16:1218–1226.

176. Fellows KE, Radtke WAK, Keane JF, Lock JE. Acute complications of catheter therapy for congenital heart disease. *Am J Cardiol*. 1987;60:679–683.

177. Schluter M, Kuck KH. Radiofrequency current for catheter ablation of accessory atrioventricular connections in children and adolescents: emphasis on the single-catheter technique. *Pediatrics*. 1992;89:930–935.

178. Minich LL, Snider AR, McDonald D. Doppler detection of valvular regurgitation after radiofrequency ablation of accessory connections. *Am J Cardiol*. 1992;70:116–117.

Index

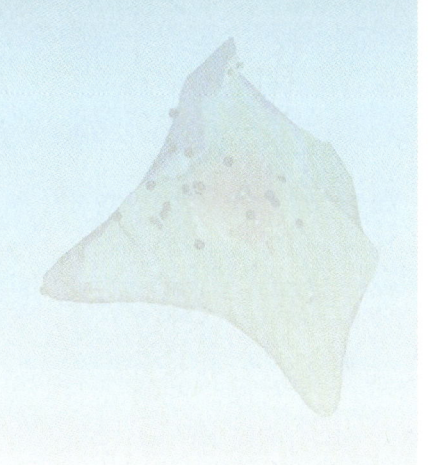